Contents

EXERCISE PHYSIOLOGY

Theory and Application to Fitness and Performance

TENTH EDITION

Scott K. Powers
University of Florida

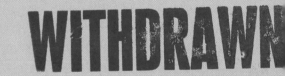

Edward T. Howley
University of Tennessee, Knoxville

EXERCISE PHYSIOLOGY

Published by McGraw-Hill Education, 2 Penn Plaza, New York, NY 10121. Copyright © 2018 by McGraw-Hill Education. All rights reserved. Printed in the United States of America. No part of this publication may be reproduced or distributed in any form or by any means, or stored in a database or retrieval system, without the prior written consent of McGraw-Hill Education, including, but not limited to, in any network or other electronic storage or transmission, or broadcast for distance learning.

Some ancillaries, including electronic and print components, may not be available to customers outside the United States.

This book is printed on acid-free paper.

1 2 3 4 5 6 7 8 9 LWI 21 20 19 18 17

ISBN 978-1-259-92205-3
MHID 1-259-92205-7

The Internet addresses listed in the text were accurate at the time of publication. The inclusion of a website does not indicate an endorsement by the authors or McGraw-Hill Education, and McGraw-Hill Education does not guarantee the accuracy of the information presented at these sites.

mheducation.com/highered

Dedicated to Lou and Ann
for their love, patience, and support.

Brief Contents

Appendices can be found in the Instructor's Resources within Connect

Preface

As with all previous editions, the tenth edition of *Exercise Physiology: Theory and Application to Fitness and Performance* is intended for students interested in exercise physiology, clinical exercise physiology, human performance, kinesiology/exercise science, physical therapy, and physical education. The overall objective of this text is to provide the student with an up-to-date understanding of the physiology of exercise. Moreover, the book contains numerous clinical applications including exercise tests to evaluate cardiorespiratory fitness and information on exercise training for improvements in health-related physical fitness and sports performance.

This book is intended for a one-semester, upper-level undergraduate or beginning graduate exercise physiology course. Clearly, the text contains more material than can be covered in a single 15-week semester. This is by design. The book was written to be comprehensive and afford instructors the freedom to select the material that they consider to be the most important for the composition of their class. Furthermore, if desired, the book could be used in a two-semester sequence of exercise physiology courses (e.g., Exercise Physiology I and II) to cover the entire 25 chapters contained in the text.

NEW TO THIS EDITION

The tenth edition of our book has undergone *major* revisions and highlights the latest research in exercise physiology. Indeed, every chapter contains new and expanded discussions, new text boxes, new figures, updated references, and contemporary suggested readings.

New Topics and Updated Content

The content of this new edition has been markedly updated. Specifically, each chapter has been revised and updated to include new and amended box features, new illustrations, new research findings, and the inclusion of up-to-date references and suggested readings. The following list describes some of the significant changes that have made the tenth edition more complete and up-to-date:

- **Chapter 0:** Two new "A Look Back" features were added to highlight the careers of Elsworth Buskirk and Frances Hellebrandt.
- **Chapter 1:** New suggested readings and updated references were added.
- **Chapter 2:** Updated discussion on the role that heat shock proteins play in the cellular adaptation to stress.
- **Chapter 3:** New illustration and box feature added to highlight the structure and function of the two subpopulations of mitochondria found in skeletal muscle.
- **Chapter 4:** Several figures were upgraded along with the addition of a new section on measurement of $\dot{V}O_2$ max.
- **Chapter 5:** Numerous new and improved figures were added along with a new table highlighting hormonal changes during exercise. New information added on the impact of both growth hormone and anabolic steroids on skeletal muscle size and function.
- **Chapter 6:** Update on the latest research findings on the impact of exercise on the immune system added.
- **Chapter 7:** Expanded discussion on muscle sense organs (i.e., Golgi tendon organ and muscle spindles). New information added about the exceptions to the size principle. Further, a new section was added discussing how central pattern generators control movement during exercise. Additionally, Clinical Applications 7.2 was expanded

to discuss the risk of chronic traumatic encephalopathy (CTE) in contact sports.

- **Chapter 8:** Updated information on the role that satellite cells play in exercise-induced skeletal muscle hypertrophy was added. Further, new information on how exercise training alters the structure and function of the neuromuscular junction was included in this chapter. Lastly, new research on the cause of exercise-related skeletal muscle cramps was added along with a new box feature discussing new pharmacological approaches to prevent muscle cramps.

- **Chapter 9:** Updated information on the prediction of maximal heart rates in older individuals. Expanded discussion highlighting new research on the regulation of muscle blood flow during exercise. Added a new A Closer Look 9.3 to discuss the impact of body position on stroke volume during exercise.

- **Chapter 10:** Updated with the newest research findings on control of breathing during exercise. Also, new research on sex differences in breathing during exercise was also added.

- **Chapter 11:** Several new and improved illustrations were added along with an expanded discussion on intracellular acid-base buffer systems. New section added about how buffering capacity differs between muscle fiber types and how exercise training impacts muscle buffer systems. Further, the chapter was improved by the addition of the latest information on nutritional supplements used to improve acid-base balance during exercise.

- **Chapter 12:** Several new illustrations were added along with a discussion on the impact of a hot environment on exercise performance. Further, a box feature was added to discuss the influence of precooling on exercise performance. Lastly, the discussion of exercise in a cold environment was expanded to discuss the latest research findings.

- **Chapter 13:** Numerous new illustrations were included in this greatly revised chapter along with the addition of two new box features that discuss (1) the impact of genetics on $\dot{V}O_2$ max and (2) the influence of endurance exercise training on skeletal muscle mitochondrial volume and turnover. Moreover, a new section was also added to discuss muscle adaptations to anaerobic exercise. Finally, new and expanded information on the signaling events that lead to resistance training-induced muscle growth was included.

- **Chapter 14:** Major revision to this chapter provides more focus on the importance of physical activity in the prevention of chronic diseases. Section on metabolic syndrome was extensively revised to include an expanded discussion of how physical activity and diet impacts the inflammation that is linked to chronic disease.

- **Chapter 15:** Wide revision of the screening process for individuals entering a physical activity program along with new figures. Latest information regarding the new national standards for $\dot{V}O_2$ max.

- **Chapter 16:** Updated references and suggested readings.

- **Chapter 17:** New information on ACSM's physical activity recommendations for all special populations. New figure added on effect of age on $\dot{V}O_2$ max along with a new Clinical Application box discussing physical activity and risk of cancer.

- **Chapter 18:** Extensive revision to include new information on vitamins and minerals along with the new dietary guidelines for Americans. Widespread revision of the discussion on how to determine body composition along with a focused analysis of the causes and treatment for obesity.

- **Chapter 19:** New "A Look Back" on Brenda Bigland-Ritchie along with an expanded discussion on the linkages between central and peripheral fatigue. Update on the role that free radicals play in exercise-induced muscle fatigue and new information on why Kenyan runners are often successful in long distance races.

- **Chapter 20:** Chapter updated with latest research findings plus the addition of new suggested readings.

- **Chapter 21:** Three new box features added to address the following: (1) What are the physiological limits to the enhancement of endurance performance?; (2) Do compression garments benefit athletes during competition and recovery from training?; and (3) Treatment of delayed onset muscle soreness.

- **Chapter 22:** New illustration was added along with the latest research findings on the female athlete triad coupled with a discussion of the recent proposal to replace the term *female athlete triad* with new terminology.

- **Chapter 23:** Updated information from the 2016 ACSM position stand on nutrition and performance along with an expanded discussion of the benefits and problems associated for athletes training with low levels of muscle glycogen. Expanded discussion of protein requirements for athletes along with a new discussion of the importance of consuming carbohydrates during long distance endurance events.

- **Chapter 24:** Updated discussion on the "Live High Train Low" training strategy. New recommendations for prevention and treatment of heat illnesses coupled with new information on how the WBGT Index fits into planning workouts in hot/humid environments.

- **Chapter 25:** Latest data on the prevalence and use of ergogenic aids. New information of dietary supplements for improving endurance performance along with additional information on the impact of stretching on performance.

connect

The tenth edition of *Exercise Physiology: Theory and Application to Fitness and Performance* is now available online with Connect, McGraw-Hill Education's integrated assignment and assessment platform. Connect also offers SmartBook™ for the new edition, which is the first adaptive reading experience proven to improve grades and help students study more effectively. All of the title's website and ancillary content is also available through Connect, including:

- A test bank of quizzes covering material from each chapter of the book.

- A full Test Bank of multiple choice questions that test students on central concepts and ideas in each chapter. Also, new to this edition is the classification of test question difficulty using Bloom's taxonomy.

- Lecture Slides for instructor use in class.

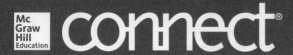

McGraw-Hill Connect®
Learn Without Limits

Connect is a teaching and learning platform that is proven to deliver better results for students and instructors.

Connect empowers students by continually adapting to deliver precisely what they need, when they need it, and how they need it, so your class time is more engaging and effective.

73% of instructors who use **Connect** require it; instructor satisfaction **increases** by 28% when **Connect** is required.

Connect's Impact on Retention Rates, Pass Rates, and Average Exam Scores

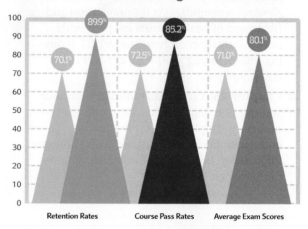

Using **Connect** improves retention rates by **19.8%**, passing rates by **12.7%**, and exam scores by **9.1%**.

Analytics

Connect Insight®

Connect Insight is Connect's new one-of-a-kind visual analytics dashboard—now available for both instructors and students—that provides at-a-glance information regarding student performance, which is immediately actionable. By presenting assignment, assessment, and topical performance results together with a time metric that is easily visible for aggregate or individual results, Connect Insight gives the user the ability to take a just-in-time approach to teaching and learning, which was never before available. Connect Insight presents data that empowers students and helps instructors improve class performance in a way that is efficient and effective.

Impact on Final Course Grade Distribution

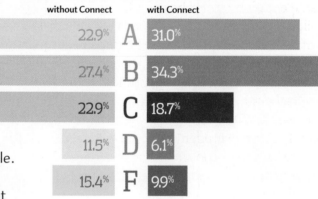

without Connect		with Connect
22.9%	A	31.0%
27.4%	B	34.3%
22.9%	C	18.7%
11.5%	D	6.1%
15.4%	F	9.9%

Students can view their results for any **Connect** course.

Mobile

Connect's new, intuitive mobile interface gives students and instructors flexible and convenient, anytime–anywhere access to all components of the Connect platform.

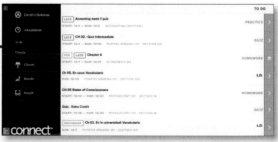

Adaptive

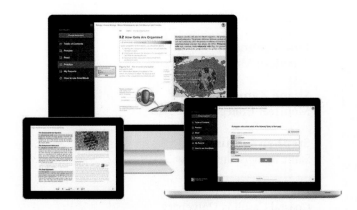

THE **ADAPTIVE** **READING EXPERIENCE** DESIGNED TO TRANSFORM THE WAY STUDENTS READ

More students earn **A's** and **B's** when they use McGraw-Hill Education **Adaptive** products.

SmartBook®

Proven to help students improve grades and study more efficiently, SmartBook contains the same content within the print book, but actively tailors that content to the needs of the individual. SmartBook's adaptive technology provides precise, personalized instruction on what the student should do next, guiding the student to master and remember key concepts, targeting gaps in knowledge and offering customized feedback, and driving the student toward comprehension and retention of the subject matter. Available on Smartphones and tablets, SmartBook puts learning at the student's fingertips—anywhere, anytime.

Over **8 billion questions** have been answered, making McGraw-Hill Education products more intelligent, reliable, and precise.

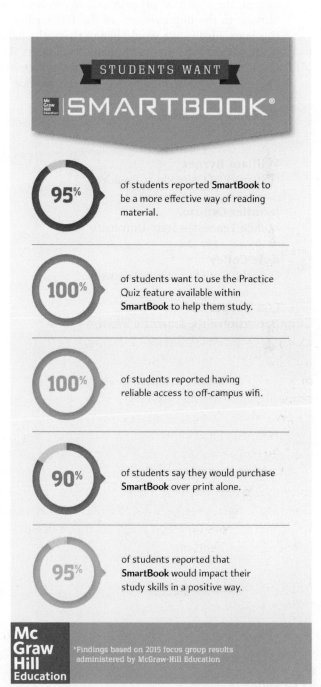

STUDENTS WANT

SMARTBOOK®

95% of students reported **SmartBook** to be a more effective way of reading material.

100% of students want to use the Practice Quiz feature available within **SmartBook** to help them study.

100% of students reported having reliable access to off-campus wifi.

90% of students say they would purchase **SmartBook** over print alone.

95% of students reported that **SmartBook** would impact their study skills in a positive way.

Mc Graw Hill Education

*Findings based on 2015 focus group results administered by McGraw-Hill Education

www.mheducation.com

ACKNOWLEDGEMENTS

This text *Exercise Physiology: Theory and Application to Fitness and Performance* is not the effort of only two authors but represents the contributions of hundreds of scientists from around the world. Although it is not possible to acknowledge every contributor to this work, we would like to recognize the following scientists who have greatly influenced our thinking, careers, and lives in general: Drs. Bruno Balke, Ronald Byrd, Jerome Dempsey, Stephen Dodd, H. V. Forster, B. D. Franks, Steven Horvath, Henry Montoye, Francis Nagle, and Hugh G. Welch.

Moreover, we would like to thank Matt Hinkley, Aaron Morton, and Brian Parr for their assistance in providing suggestions for revisions to this book. Indeed, these individuals provided numerous contributions to the improvement of the tenth edition of this book. Finally, we would like to thank the following reviewers who provided helpful comments about the ninth and tenth editions of *Exercise Physiology: Theory and Application to Fitness and Performance*:

Alexandra Auslander
Fullerton College

William Byrnes
University of Colorado at Boulder

Jennifer Caputo,
Middle Tennessee State University

Kyle Coffey
University of Massachusetts Lowell

Lisa Cooper Colvin
University of the Incarnate Word

David J. Granniss
Gardner-Webb University

Kathy Howe
Oregon State University

Jenny Johnson
American Military University

Shane Kamer
Montreat College

Stephen LoRusso
Saint Francis University

Gregory Martel
Coastal Carolina University

Erica Morley
Arizona State University

Allen C. Parcell
Brigham Young University

John Quindry
Auburn University

Brady Redus
University of Central Oklahoma

Mark Snow
Midland University

Ann M. Swartz
University of Wisconsin-Milwaukee

Eric Vlahov
The University of Tampa

Engaging Presentation of Key Concepts Supported by the Latest Research

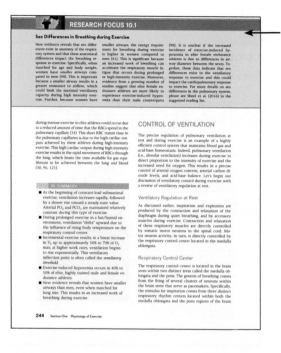

Research Focus

No matter what their career direction, students must learn how to read and think about the latest research. Research Focus presents new research and explains why it's relevant.

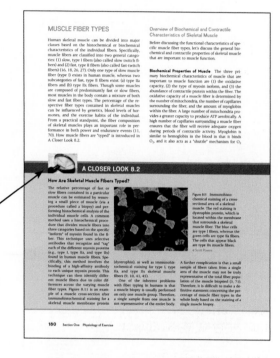

A Closer Look

A Closer Look offers an in-depth view of topics that are of special interest to students. This feature encourages students to dig deeper into key concepts.

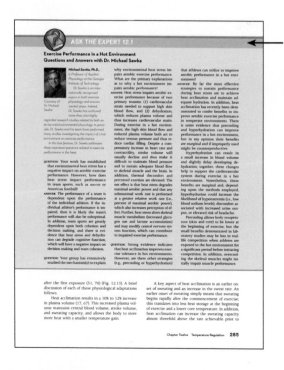

Ask the Expert

This question-and-answer feature lets you find out what leading scientists have to say about topics such as the effect of space flight on skeletal muscle and the effect of exercise on bone health.

Practical Applications of Exercise Physiology

Clinical Applications

Learn how exercise physiology is used in the clinical setting.

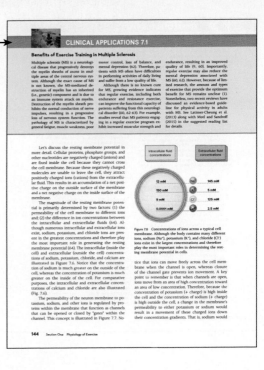

The Winning Edge

How do athletes find the "extra edge" that can make the difference between victory and defeat? These features explain the science behind a winning performance.

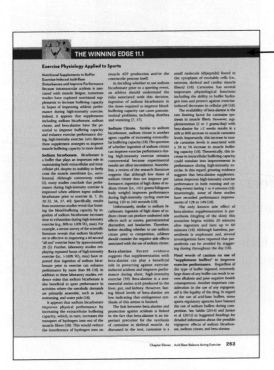

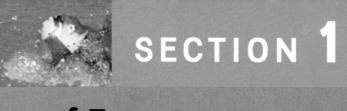

SECTION 1

Physiology of Exercise

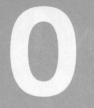
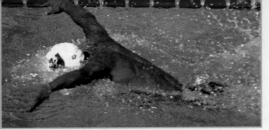

© Action Plus Sports Images/Alamy Stock Photo

Introduction to Exercise Physiology

■ Objectives

By studying this chapter, you should be able to do the following:

1. Describe the scope of exercise physiology as a branch of physiology.

2. Describe the influence of European scientists on the development of exercise physiology.

3. Name the three Nobel Prize winners whose research work involved muscle or muscular exercise.

4. Describe the role of the Harvard Fatigue Laboratory in the history of exercise physiology in the United States.

5. Describe factors influencing physical fitness in the United States over the past century.

6. List career options for students majoring in exercise science or kinesiology.

■ Outline

Does one need to have a "genetic gift" of speed to be a world-class runner, or is it all due to training? What happens to your heart rate when you take an exercise test that increases in intensity each minute? What changes occur in your muscles as a result of an endurance-training program that allows you to run at faster speeds over longer distances? What fuel—carbohydrate or fat—is most important when running a marathon? Research in exercise physiology provides answers to these and similar questions.

Physiology is the study of the function of tissues (e.g., muscle, nerve), organs (e.g., heart, lungs), and systems (e.g., cardiovascular). Exercise physiology extends this to evaluate the effect of a single bout of exercise (acute exercise) and repeated bouts of exercise (i.e., training programs) on these tissues, organs, and systems. In addition, the responses to acute exercise and training may be studied at high altitude or in extremes of heat and humidity to determine the impact of these environmental factors on our ability to respond and adapt to exercise. Finally, studies are conducted on young and old individuals, both healthy and those with disease, to understand the role of exercise in the prevention of or rehabilitation from various chronic diseases.

Consistent with this perspective, we go beyond simple statements of fact to show how information about the physiology of exercise is applied to the prevention of and rehabilitation from coronary heart disease, the performances of elite athletes, and the ability of a person to work in adverse environments such as high altitudes. The acceptance of terms such as *sports physiology, sports nutrition,* and *sports medicine* is evidence of the growth of interest in the application of physiology of exercise to real-world problems. Careers in athletic training, personal-fitness training, cardiac rehabilitation, and strength and conditioning, as well as the traditional fields of physical therapy and medicine, are of interest to students studying exercise physiology. We will expand on career opportunities later in the chapter.

In this chapter, we provide a brief history of exercise physiology to help you understand where we have been and where we are going. In addition, throughout the text a variety of scientists and clinicians are highlighted in a historical context as subject matter is presented (i.e., muscle, cardiovascular responses, altitude). We hope that by linking a person to a major accomplishment within the context of a chapter, history will come alive and be of interest to you.

BRIEF HISTORY OF EXERCISE PHYSIOLOGY

The history of exercise physiology represents a global perspective involving scientists from many different countries. In this section, we begin with the impact European scientists have had on the development of exercise physiology. We then describe the role of the Harvard Fatigue Laboratory in the growth of exercise physiology in this country.

European Heritage

A good starting place to discuss the history of exercise physiology in the United States is in Europe. Three scientists, A. V. Hill of Britain, August Krogh of Denmark, and Otto Meyerhof of Germany, received Nobel Prizes for research on muscle or muscular exercise (13). Hill and Meyerhof shared the Nobel Prize in Physiology or Medicine in 1922. Hill was recognized for his precise measurements of heat production during muscle contraction and recovery, and Meyerhof for his discovery of the relationship between the consumption of oxygen and the measurement of lactic acid in muscle. Hill was trained as a mathematician before becoming interested in physiology. In addition to his work cited for the Nobel Prize, his studies on humans led to the development of a framework around which we understand the physiological factors related to distance-running performance (6) (see Chap. 19).

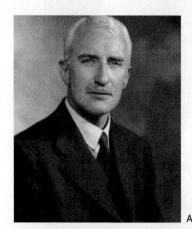 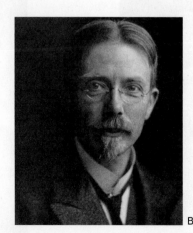 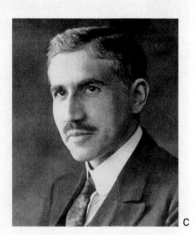

A. Archibald V. Hill, B. August Krogh, C. Otto F. Meyerhof

Although Krogh received the Nobel Prize for his research on the function of capillary circulation, he had a major impact on numerous areas of investigation. Furthermore, like many productive investigators, his influence was due not only to his own work but to that of his students and colleagues as well. Krogh's collaboration with Johannes Lindhard resulted in classic studies dealing with carbohydrate and fat metabolism during exercise, and how the cardiovascular and respiratory systems' responses are controlled during exercise (4). Three students in Krogh's lab, Erling Asmussen, Erik Hohwü-Christensen, and Marius Nielsen (called "the three musketeers" by Krogh), had a major impact on exercise physiology research throughout the middle of the twentieth century. These investigators, in turn, trained a number of outstanding physiologists, several of whom you will meet throughout this text. The August Krogh Institute in Denmark contains some of the most prominent exercise physiology laboratories in the world. Marie Krogh, his wife, was a noted scientist in her own right and was recognized for her innovative work on measuring the diffusing capacity of the lung. We recommend the biography of the Kroghs written by their daughter, Bodil Schmidt-Nielsen (see Suggested Readings), for those interested in the history of exercise physiology.

Several other European scientists must also be mentioned, not only because of their contributions to the exercise physiology but also because their names are commonly used in a discussion of exercise physiology. J. S. Haldane did some of the original work on the role of CO_2 in the control of breathing. Haldane also developed the respiratory gas analyzer that bears his name (16). C. G. Douglas did pioneering work with Haldane in the role of O_2 and lactic acid in the control of breathing during exercise, including some work conducted at various altitudes. The canvas-and-rubber gas collection bag used for many years in exercise physiology laboratories around the world carries Douglas's name. A contemporary of Douglas, Christian Bohr of Denmark, did the classic work on how O_2 binds to hemoglobin. The "shift" in the oxygen-hemoglobin dissociation curve due to the addition of CO_2 bears his name (see Chap. 10). Interestingly, it was Krogh who did the actual experiments that enabled Bohr to describe his famous "shift" (4, 16).

IN SUMMARY

- A. V. Hill, August Krogh, and Otto Meyerhof received the Nobel Prize for work related to muscle or muscular exercise.
- Numerous European scientists have had a major impact on the field of exercise physiology.

Harvard Fatigue Laboratory

A focal point in the history of exercise physiology in the United States is the Harvard Fatigue Laboratory. Professor L. J. Henderson organized the laboratory within the Business School to conduct physiological research on industrial hazards. Dr. David Bruce Dill was the research director from the time the laboratory opened in 1927 until it closed in 1947 (19). Table 0.1 shows that the scientists conducted research in numerous areas, in the laboratory and in the field, and the results of those early studies have been supported over the years. Dill's classic text, *Life, Heat, and Altitude* (15), is a recommended reading for any student of exercise and environmental physiology. Much of the careful and precise work of the laboratory was conducted using the now-classic Haldane analyzer for respiratory gas analysis and the van Slyke apparatus for blood-gas analysis. The advent of computer-controlled equipment in the 1980s has

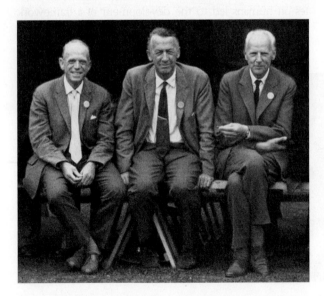

The "three musketeers": From left to right: Erling Asmussen, Erik Hohwü-Christensen, and Marius Nielsen

Courtesy of The Physiological Society

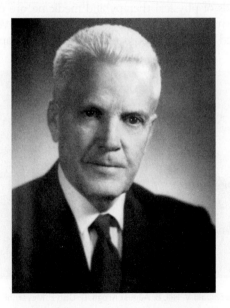

David Bruce Dill

Courtesy of American College of Sports Medicine

TABLE 0.1	Active Research Areas in the Harvard Fatigue Laboratory

Metabolism
   Maximal oxygen uptake
   Oxygen debt
   Carbohydrate and fat metabolism during
     long-term work
Environmental physiology
   Altitude
   Dry and moist heat
   Cold
Clinical physiology
   Gout
   Schizophrenia
   Diabetes
Aging
   Basal metabolic rate
   Maximal oxygen uptake
   Maximal heart rate
Blood
   Acid–base balance
   O_2 saturation: role of PO_2, PCO_2, and carbon
     monoxide
   Nutrition assessment techniques
   Vitamins
   Foods
Physical fitness
   Harvard Step Test

made data collection easier but has not improved on the accuracy of measurement (see Fig. 0.1).

The Harvard Fatigue Laboratory attracted doctoral students as well as scientists from other countries. Many of the alumni from the laboratory are recognized in their own right for excellence in research in the physiology of exercise. Two doctoral students, Steven Horvath and Sid Robinson, went on to distinguished careers at the Institute of Environmental Stress in Santa Barbara and Indiana University, respectively.

Foreign "Fellows" included the "three musketeers" mentioned in the previous section (E. Asmussen, E. Hohwü-Christensen, and M. Nielsen) and the Nobel Prize winner August Krogh. These scientists brought new ideas and technology to the lab, participated in laboratory and field studies with other staff members, and published some of the most important work in the exercise physiology between 1930 and 1980. Rudolfo Margaria, from Italy, went on to extend his classic work on oxygen debt and described the energetics of locomotion. Peter F. Scholander, from Norway, gave us his chemical gas analyzer that is a primary method of calibrating tank gas used to standardize electronic gas analyzers (19).

In summary, under the leadership of Dr. D. B. Dill, the Harvard Fatigue Laboratory became a model for research investigations into exercise and environmental physiology, especially as it relates to humans. When the laboratory closed and the staff dispersed, the ideas, techniques, and approaches to scientific inquiry were distributed throughout the world, and with them, Dill's influence in the area of environmental and exercise physiology. Dr. Dill continued his research outside Boulder City, Nevada, into the 1980s. He died in 1986 at the age of 93.

Progress toward understanding any issue in exercise physiology transcends time, national origin, and scientific training. Solutions to difficult questions require the interaction of scientists from diverse disciplines and professions such as physiology, biochemistry, molecular biology, and medicine. We recommend *Exercise Physiology–People and Ideas* (see the Suggested Readings) to further your understanding of important historical connections. In this book, internationally known scientists provide a historical treatment of a number of important issues in exercise

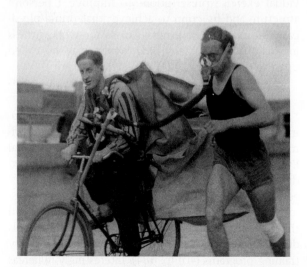
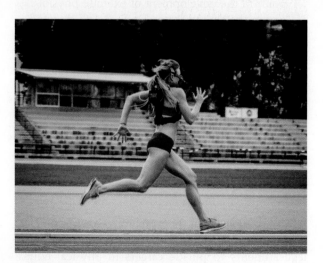

Figure 0.1 Comparison of old and new technology used to measure oxygen consumption and carbon dioxide production during exercise. (*Right:* COSMED.)

(LEFT) © Ullstein Bild/Getty Images; (RIGHT) Photo courtesy of www.cosmed.com

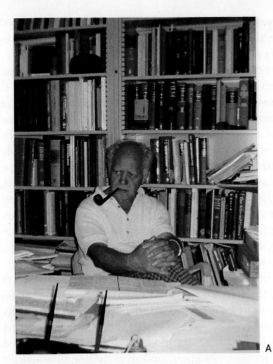

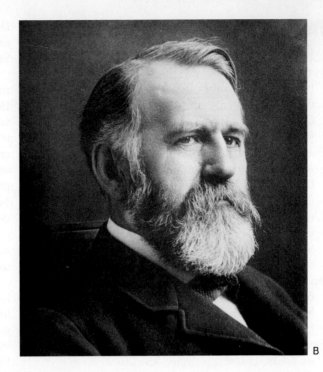

A. Steven Horvath, B. Dudley Sargent

(A) Courtesy of Steven Horvath; (B) Library of Congress [LC-B2- 1121-5]

physiology, with an emphasis on the cross-continent flow of energy and ideas. We highlight several scientists and clinicians with our "Ask the Expert" boxes throughout the text, both to introduce them to you and for them to share their current ideas. In addition, A Look Back–Important People in Science is used to recognize well-known scientists who have influenced our understanding of exercise physiology. In this context, you will get to know those who have gone before and those who are currently leading the charge.

IN SUMMARY

- The Harvard Fatigue Laboratory was a focal point in the development of exercise physiology in the United States. Dr. D. B. Dill directed the laboratory from its opening in 1927 until its closing in 1947. The body of research in exercise and environmental physiology produced by the scientists in that laboratory formed the foundation for new ideas and experimental methods that still influence us today.

PHYSIOLOGY, PHYSICAL FITNESS, AND HEALTH

Physical fitness is a popular topic today, and its popularity has been a major factor in motivating college students to pursue careers in physical education, exercise physiology, health education, nutrition,

physical therapy, and medicine. In 1980, the Public Health Service listed "physical fitness and exercise" as one of 15 areas of concern related to improving the country's overall health (32). This was far from a new idea. Similar interests and concerns about physical fitness existed in this country more than 100 years ago. Between the Civil War and the First World War (WWI), physical education was primarily concerned with the development and maintenance of fitness, and many of the leaders in physical education were trained in medicine (14) (p. 5). For example, Dr. Dudley Sargent, hired by Harvard University in 1879, set up a physical training program with individual exercise prescriptions to improve a person's structure and function to achieve "that prime physical condition called fitness–fitness for work, fitness for play, fitness for anything a man may be called upon to do" (35) (p. 297).

Sargent, D., *Physical Education*. Boston, MA: Ginn and Company, 1906.

Dr. Sargent was clearly ahead of his time in promoting health-related fitness. Later, war became a primary force driving this country's interest in physical fitness. Concerns about health and fitness were raised during WWI and WWII when large numbers of draftees failed the induction exams due to mental and physical defects (18) (p. 407). These concerns influenced the type of physical education programs in the schools during these years, making them resemble premilitary training programs (40) (p. 484). Interestingly, whereas stunted growth and being underweight were major reasons for rejecting military recruits in WWII, obesity is the major cause for rejecting recruits today (see "Still Too Fat to Fight" at **http://www.missionreadiness. org/2012/still-too-fat-to-fight/**).

The present interest in physical activity and health was stimulated in the early 1950s by two major findings: (1) autopsies of young soldiers killed during the Korean War showed that significant coronary artery disease had already developed and (2) Hans Kraus showed that American children performed poorly on a minimal muscular fitness test compared to European children (40) (p. 516). Due to the latter finding, President Eisenhower initiated a conference in 1955 that resulted in the formation of the President's Council on Youth Fitness. The American Association for Health, Physical Education, and Recreation (AAHPER) supported these activities and in 1957 developed the AAHPER Youth Fitness Test with national norms to be used in physical education programs throughout the country. Before he was inaugurated, President Kennedy expressed his concerns about the nation's fitness in an article published in *Sports Illustrated*, called "The Soft American" (24):

> For the physical vigor of our citizens is one of America's most precious resources. If we waste and neglect this resource, if we allow it to dwindle and grow soft, then we will destroy much of our ability to meet the great and vital challenges which confront our people. We will be unable to realize our full potential as a nation.
>
> Kennedy, J., "The Soft American," *Sports Illustrated*, 13, pp. 14-17, 1960.

During Kennedy's term, the council's name was changed to the "President's Council on Physical Fitness" to highlight the concern for fitness. The name was changed again in the Nixon administration to the "President's Council on Physical Fitness and Sports," which supported fitness not only in schools but also in business, industry, and for the general public. The name was most recently changed by President Obama to the "President's Council on Fitness, Sports, & Nutrition" to focus more attention on the obesity epidemic (see **www.fitness.gov**). Items in the Youth Fitness Test were changed over the years, and in 1980, the American Alliance for Health, Physical Education, Recreation, and Dance (AAHPERD) published a separate *Health-Related Physical Fitness Test Manual* (1) to distinguish between "performance testing" (e.g., 50-yard dash) and "fitness testing" (e.g., skinfold thickness). This health-related test battery is consistent with the direction of lifetime fitness programs, being concerned with obesity, cardiorespiratory fitness, and low-back function. A parallel fitness test, Fitnessgram, was developed by The Cooper Institute in 1982, including software to support the scoring and printing

of reports (see **https://www.cooperinstitute.org/ youth/fitnessgram**). The President's Council now recommends that the Fitnessgram be used to evaluate fitness in children. For readers interested in the history of fitness testing in schools, we recommend Morrow et al.'s review in the Suggested Readings.

Paralleling this interest in the physical fitness of youth was the rising concern about the death rate from coronary heart disease in the middle-aged American male population. Epidemiological studies of the health status of the population underscored the fact that degenerative diseases related to poor health habits (e.g., high-fat diet, smoking, inactivity) were responsible for more deaths than the classic infectious and contagious diseases. In 1966, a major symposium highlighted the need for more research in the area of physical activity and health (33). In the 1970s, there was an increase in the use of exercise tests to diagnose heart disease and to aid in the prescription of exercise programs to improve cardiovascular health. Large corporations developed "executive" fitness programs to improve the health status of that high-risk group. While most Americans are now familiar with such programs and some students of exercise physiology seek careers in "corporate fitness," such programs are not new. In fact, as early as 1923, *textbooks such as McKenzie's Exercise in Education and Medicine* (27) showed businessmen participating in a dance exercise class. In short, the idea that regular physical activity is an important part of a healthy lifestyle was "rediscovered." If any questions remained about the importance of physical activity to health, the publication of the Surgeon General's Report in 1996 and the appearance of the first U.S. Physical Activity Guidelines in 2008 put them to rest (see "A Closer Look 0.1").

IN SUMMARY

- Fitness has been an issue in this country from the latter part of the nineteenth century until the present. War, or the threat of war, exerted a strong influence on fitness programs in the public schools. In WWII, being underweight and small of stature were major reasons for rejecting military recruits; today, obesity is a major cause for rejection.
- Recent interest in fitness is related to the growing concern over the high death rates from disease processes that are attributable to preventable factors, such as poor diet, lack of exercise, and smoking. Government and professional organizations have responded to this need by educating the public about these problems.
- Schools use health-related fitness tests, such as the Fitnessgram, to evaluate a child's physical fitness.

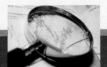
By the early to mid-1980s, it had become clear that physical inactivity was a major public health concern (32). In 1992, the American Heart Association made physical inactivity a major risk factor for cardiovascular diseases, just like smoking, high blood pressure, and high serum cholesterol (3). In 1995, the Centers for Disease Control and Prevention (CDC) and the American College of Sports Medicine published a public health physical activity recommendation that "Every U.S. adult should accumulate 30 minutes or more of moderate-intensity physical activity on most, preferably all, days of the week" (30). A year later, the *Surgeon General's Report on Physical Activity and Health* was published (39).

This report highlighted the fact that physical inactivity was killing U.S. adults, and the problem was a big one—60% of U.S. adults did not engage in the recommended amount of physical activity, and 25% were not active at all. This report was based on the large body of evidence available from epidemiological studies, small-group training studies, and clinical investigations showing the positive effects of an active lifestyle. For example, physical activity was shown to

- Lower the risk of dying prematurely and from heart disease
- Reduce the risk of developing diabetes and high blood pressure
- Help maintain weight and healthy bones, muscles, and joints
- Help lower blood pressure in those with high blood pressure and promote psychological well-being

In 2008, the first edition of the *U.S. Physical Activity Guidelines* was published (**http://www.health.gov /paguidelines/guidelines/default. aspx**). This document was developed on the basis of an Advisory Committee's comprehensive review of the research since the publication of the Surgeon General's Report in 1996 (for the Advisory Committee Report, see **http://health.gov/paguidelines /report/**). Recently, a Midcourse Report focusing on strategies to increase physical activity among youth was published (**http://www.health .gov/paguidelines/midcourse/**). The *U.S. Physical Activity Guidelines*, along with the *Dietary Guidelines for Americans 2015* (**http://health .gov/dietaryguidelines/2015 /guidelines/**), provides important information on how to address our problems of inactivity and obesity. (We discuss this in more detail in Chaps. 16, 17, and 18.)

PHYSICAL EDUCATION TO EXERCISE SCIENCE AND KINESIOLOGY

Undergraduate academic preparation in physical education has changed over the past five decades to reflect the explosion in the knowledge base related to the physiology of exercise, biomechanics, and exercise prescription. This occurred at a time of a *perceived* reduced need for school-based physical education teachers and an increased need for exercise professionals in the preventive and clinical settings. These factors, as well as others, led some college and university departments to change their names from Physical Education to Exercise Science or Kinesiology. This trend is likely to continue as programs move further away from traditional roots in education and become integrated within colleges of arts and sciences or allied health professions (38). There has been an increase in the number of programs requiring undergraduates to take one year of calculus, chemistry, and physics, and courses in organic chemistry, biochemistry, anatomy, physiology, and nutrition. In many colleges and universities, little difference now exists between the first two years of requirements in a pre-physical therapy or pre-medical track and the track associated with physical education/ kinesiology professions. The differences among these tracks lie in the "application" courses that follow. Biomechanics, physiology of exercise, fitness assessment, exercise prescription, strength and conditioning, and so on belong to the physical education/kinesiology track. However, it must again be pointed out that this new trend is but another example of a rediscovery of old roots rather than a revolutionary change. Kroll describes two 4-year professional physical education programs in the 1890s, one at Stanford and the other at Harvard, that were the forerunners of today's programs (25) (pp. 51-64). They included the detailed scientific work and application courses with clear prerequisites cited. Finally, considerable time was allotted for laboratory work. No doubt, Lagrange's 1890 text, *Physiology of Bodily Exercise* (26), served as an important reference source for these students. The expectations and goals of those programs were almost identical to those specified for current kinesiology undergraduate tracks. In fact, one of the aims of the Harvard program was to allow a student to pursue the study of medicine after completing two years of study (25) (p. 61).

GRADUATE STUDY AND RESEARCH IN THE PHYSIOLOGY OF EXERCISE

While the Harvard Fatigue Laboratory was closing in 1947, the country was on the verge of a tremendous expansion in the number of universities offering graduate study and research opportunities in exercise physiology. A 1950 survey showed that only 16 colleges or universities had research laboratories in departments of physical education (21). By 1966, 151 institutions had research facilities, 58 of them in exercise physiology (40) (p. 526). This expansion was due to the availability of more scientists trained in the research methodology of exercise physiology, the increased number of students attending college due to the GI Bill and student loans, and the increase in federal dollars to improve the research capabilities of universities (12, 38).

"The scholar's work will be multiplied many fold through the contribution of his students." This quote, taken from Montoye and Washburn (28, 29), expresses a view that has helped attract researchers and scholars to universities. Evidence to support this quote was presented in the form of genealogical charts of contributors to the *Research Quarterly* (29). These charts showed the tremendous influence a few people had through their students in the expansion of research in physical education. Probably the best example of this is Thomas K. Cureton, Jr., of the University of Illinois, a central figure in the training of productive researchers in exercise physiology and fitness. The proceedings from a symposium honoring Dr. Cureton in 1969 listed 68 Ph.D. students who completed their work under his direction (17). Although Dr. Cureton's scholarly record includes hundreds of research articles and dozens of books dealing with physical fitness, the publications of his students in the areas of epidemiology, fitness, cardiac rehabilitation, and exercise physiology represent the "multiplying effect" that students have on a scholar's productivity. For those who would like to read more about Dr. Cureton, see Berryman's article (7).

> Montoye, H., and Washburn, R., "Genealogy of Scholarship Among Academy Members," *The Academy Papers*, 13: 94-101, 1980.

An example of a major university program that can trace its lineage to the Harvard Fatigue Laboratory is found at the Laboratory for Human Performance Research (Noll Laboratory) at Pennsylvania State University (see "A Look Back–Important People in Science"). However, it is clear that excellent research in exercise and environmental physiology is conducted in laboratories other than those that have a tie to the Harvard Fatigue Laboratory. Laboratories are found in physical education/kinesiology departments, physiology departments in medical schools, clinical medicine programs at hospitals, and in independent facilities such as the Cooper Institute for Aerobics Research. The proliferation and specialization of research involving exercise is discussed in the next section.

It should be no surprise that the major issues studied by researchers in exercise physiology have changed over the years. Table 0.2, from Tipton's look at the 50 years following the closing of the Harvard Fatigue Laboratory, shows the subject matter areas that were studied in considerable detail between 1954 and 1994 (38). A great number of these topics fit into the broad area of systemic physiology or were truly applied physiology issues. Although research continues to take place in most of these areas, Tipton believes that many of the most important questions to be addressed in the future will be answered by those with special training in molecular biology. Baldwin (5) supported Tipton's viewpoint and provided a summary of important questions dealing with exercise and chronic disease whose answers are linked to functional genomics and proteomics, important new tools for the molecular biologist. However, he also noted the need for increased research to address physical activity and chronic diseases at the lifestyle and behavioral levels. This "integrated" approach, crossing disciplines and technologies, should be reflected in the academic programs educating the next generation of kinesiology students. We recommend the chapters by Tipton (38) and Buskirk and Tipton (12) for those interested in a detailed look at the development of exercise physiology in the United States.

IN SUMMARY

- The increase in research in exercise physiology was a catalyst that propelled the transformation of physical education departments into exercise science and kinesiology departments. The number of exercise physiology laboratories increased dramatically between the 1950s and 1970s, with many dealing with problems in systemic and applied physiology and the biochemistry of exercise.
- In the future, the emphasis will be on molecular biology and its developing technologies as the essential ingredients needed to solve basic science issues related to physical activity and health.
- However, there is no question about the need for additional research to better understand how to permanently change the physical activity and eating behaviors of individuals in order to realize health-related goals.

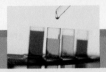

A LOOK BACK—IMPORTANT PEOPLE IN SCIENCE

Dr. Elsworth Buskirk, Noll Laboratory at Pennsylvania State University

We can trace the scientific lineage of Dr. Elsworth R. Buskirk to both the Nobel Prize winner August Krogh and to the Harvard Fatigue Laboratory. Dr. Buskirk completed his Ph.D. under the direction of Henry L. Taylor in 1954 at the Laboratory of Physiological Hygiene at the University of Minnesota.

- The director of that lab was Dr. Ancel Keys. Dr. Keys did a multiyear post-doctoral fellowship with August Krogh in Copenhagen, Denmark, in the early 1930s, where the focus of his research was on fish physiology.
- In the mid 1930s, Dr. Keys accepted a position at Harvard University to teach biochemistry and to work in the Harvard Fatigue Laboratory. Part of his research involved studying the effect of high-altitude (over 20,000 feet in the mountains of Chile) on a variety of physiological variables.
- In the late 1930s, after Dr. Keys created the Laboratory for Physiological Hygiene, he brought Henry L. Taylor, who had been a student at the Harvard Fatigue Laboratory, to complete a Ph.D. in his lab.
- Dr. Buskirk was accepted into the Ph.D. program in the early 1950s and was involved in a wide variety of studies with Dr. Taylor. One study on the measurement of maximal oxygen uptake (VO$_2$ max), which you will see later in this textbook, remains a classic.

After Dr. Buskirk received his Ph.D. in 1954, he accepted a position as physiologist at the U.S. Army Quartermaster Research and Development Lab in Natick, Massachusetts. He and his colleagues investigated the effects of nutrition, training, and acclimatization on physiological responses during exposure to exercise and environmental challenges on subjects who differed in race, fitness, fatness, and hydration level. The goals were very pragmatic–to help prepare soldiers for battle in whatever theater of war they found themselves–high altitude, extreme heat, and humidity, etc.

Three years later, in 1957, Dr. Buskirk accepted a position as physiologist at the National Institutes of Health's Institute of Arthritis and Metabolic Diseases. He was responsible for developing and directing the Metabolic Chamber Facility and Program, something that put him on the cutting edge of measuring metabolism, including when the subject was asleep! His laboratory studied the impact of exercise, cold, heat, drugs, and hormones on numerous physiological and metabolic variables in populations that differed in body composition, sex, and fitness.

In 1963, Dr. Buskirk left the National Institutes of Health and accepted a position at Penn State University as Director of the Laboratory for Human Performance Research. This laboratory grew from a small cinder block building to the current multistory Noll Laboratory of Human Performance that has two environmental chambers, a hypobaric and a hyperbaric chamber, and a Clinical Research Center. Under his direction, the laboratory did research on high altitude physiology, physical activity and heart disease, obesity, and thermal regulation. Dr. Buskirk was the major professor for 28 graduate students, and he worked with 27 post-doctoral fellows or visiting professors. He published more than 250 research articles, chapters, and scientific reviews, was on the editorial board of eight journals, and served as President of the American College of Sports Medicine (ACSM). His scientific accomplishments were recognized with the Honor Award from ACSM, and his outstanding commitment to service was recognized with the American Physiological Society's Daggs Award. He passed away in 2010, but his impact on environmental and exercise physiology lives on (10, 11, 37).

Buskirk, E., *From Harvard to Minnesota: Keys to Our History.* Baltimore, MD: Williams & Wilkins, 1992, pp. 1–26; Buskirk, E., Personal communication based on "Our Extended Family: Graduates from the Noll Lab for Human Performance Research," Noll Laboratory, Pennsylvania State University. University Park, PA, 1987.

TABLE O.2 Significant Exercise Physiology Subject Matter Areas That Were Investigated Between 1954 and 1994

A. Basic Exercise Physiology

Exercise Specificity
Exercise Prescription
Central and Peripheral Responses and Adaptations
Responses of Diseased Populations
Action of Transmitters
Regulation of Receptors
Cardiovascular and Metabolic Feed Forward and Feedback Mechanisms
Substrate Utilization Profiles
Matching Mechanisms for Oxygen Delivery and Demand
Mechanisms of Signal Transduction
Intracellular Lactate Mechanisms

Plasticity of Muscle Fibers
Motor Functions of the Spinal Cord
Hormonal Responses
The Hypoxemia of Severe Exercise
Cellular and Molecular Adaptive Responses

B. Applied Exercise Physiology

Performance of Elite Athletes
Performance and Heat Stress
Exercise at Altitude
Nutritional Aspects of Exercise
Fluid Balance During Exercise
Performance and Ergogenic Aids
Training for Physical Fitness

From Tipton, C.M., "Contemporary Exercise Physiology: Fifty years after the closure of Harvard Fatigue Laboratory," *Exercise and Sport Sciences Reviews*, vol. 26, pp. 315–339, 1998. Edited by J.O. Holloszy. Baltimore: Williams & Wilkins.

PROFESSIONAL AND SCIENTIFIC SOCIETIES AND RESEARCH JOURNALS

The expansion of interest in exercise physiology and its application to fitness and rehabilitation resulted in an increase in the number of professional societies in which scientists and clinicians could present their work. Prior to 1950, the two major societies concerned with exercise physiology and its application were the American Physiological Society (APS) and the American Association of Health, Physical Education, and Recreation (AAHPER). The need to bring together physicians, physical educators, and physiologists interested in physical activity and health into one professional society resulted in the founding of the American College of Sports Medicine (ACSM) in 1954 (see Berryman's history of the ACSM in the Suggested Readings). The ACSM now has more than 20,000 members, with 12 regional chapters throughout the country, each holding its own annual meeting to present research, sponsor symposiums, and promote sports medicine. ACSM's impact also has been enhanced by its regular publication of *Guidelines for Exercise Testing and Prescription* (2), which reaches a very diverse audience.

The explosion in exercise physiology research over the past 60 years has been accompanied by a dramatic increase in the number of professional and scientific societies and research journals communicating research findings. Table 0.3 provides a brief summary of research journals that publish research in exercise physiology.

TABLE 0.3	Sample of Research Journals for Exercise Physiology Research

Acta Physiologica (Scandinavica)
Adapted Physical Activity Quarterly
American Journal of Physiology
Aviation, Space and Environmental Medicine
Canadian Journal of Physiology and Pharmacology
European Journal of Occupational and Applied Physiology
International Journal of Sports Medicine
International Journal of Sport Nutrition
Journal of Aging and Physical Activity
Journal of Applied Physiology
Journal of Cardiopulmonary Rehabilitation
Journal of Clinical Investigation
Journal of Nutrition
Journal of Physical Activity and Health
Journal of Physiology
Journal of Sport Science
Journal of Strength and Conditioning Research
Medicine and Science in Sports and Exercise
Pediatric Exercise Physiology
Research Quarterly for Exercise and Sport

Training in Research

One of the clear consequences of this increase in research activity is the degree to which scientists must specialize to compete for research grants and to manage the research literature. Laboratories may focus on neuromuscular physiology, cardiac rehabilitation, or the influence of exercise on bone structure. Graduate students need to specialize earlier in their careers as researchers, and undergraduates must investigate graduate programs very carefully to make sure they meet their career goals (23).

This specialization in research has generated comments about the need to emphasize "basic" research examining the mechanisms underlying a physiological issue rather than "applied" research, which might describe responses of persons to exercise, environmental factors, or nutritional factors. It would appear that both types of research are needed and, to some extent, such a separation is arbitrary. For example, one scientist might study the interaction of exercise intensity and diet on muscle hypertrophy, another may characterize the changes in muscle cell size and contractile protein, a third might study changes in the energetics of muscle contraction relative to cellular enzyme activities, and a fourth might study the gene expression needed to synthesize that contractile protein. Where does "applied" research begin and "basic" research end? In the introduction to his text *Human Circulation* (34), Loring Rowell provided a quote from T. H. Huxley that bears on this issue:

> I often wish that this phrase "applied science," had never been invented. For it suggests that there is a sort of scientific knowledge of direct practical use, which can be studied apart from another sort of scientific knowledge, which is of no practical utility, and which is termed "pure science." But there is no more complete fallacy than this. What people call applied science is nothing but the application of pure science to particular classes of problems. It consists of deductions from those principles, established by reasoning and observation, which constitute pure science. No one can safely make these deductions until he has a firm grasp of the principles; and he can obtain that grasp only by personal experience of the operations of observation and of reasoning on which they are found (22).

Huxley, T., Selection from *Essays.* New York, NY: Appleton-Century-Crofts, 1948.

Solutions to chronic disease problems related to physical inactivity (e.g., type 2 diabetes, obesity) will come from a range of scientific disciplines–from epidemiologists on the one hand (39) to cell biologists on the other (8). We hope that all forms of inquiry are supported by fellow scientists so that present theories related to exercise physiology are continually questioned and modified. Last, we completely agree with the sentiments expressed in a statement ascribed to Arthur B. Otis: "Physiology is a good way to make a living and still have fun" (36).

IN SUMMARY

- The growth and development of exercise physiology over the past 60 years has resulted in dramatic increases in the number of organizations and research journals. These journals and professional meetings provide additional opportunities for research findings to be disseminated.
- A greater need exists for graduate students to identify and specialize in a particular area of research earlier in their careers in order to find the best mentor and university program to realize career goals.

CAREERS IN EXERCISE SCIENCE AND KINESIOLOGY

Over the past 30 years, there has been a sustained growth in career opportunities for those with academic training in exercise science and kinesiology. These include

- Personal fitness training in private, commercial, worksite, and hospital settings
- Strength and conditioning in commercial, rehabilitative, and sport-related environments
- Cardiac rehabilitation
- Athletic training
- Massage therapy
- Traditional allied health professions (e.g., physical or occupational therapy)
- Medicine (e.g., physician assistant, physician)

For those interested in careers in fitness and cardiac rehabilitation, coursework is not enough—students must develop the requisite skills needed to perform the job. That means that students should be completing practicum and internship experiences under the direction of a professional who can pass along what cannot be taught in a classroom or laboratory. Students should make contact with their advisors early in the program to maximize what can be gained from these experiences. Interested students should read the article by Pierce and Nagle on the internship experience (31). However, more may be needed to realize your career goal.

Those interested in cardiac rehabilitation and athletic training usually pursue graduate study (though there are exceptions) to realize their goals. If that is the case for you, apply early because there are limited spaces in most graduate programs. It is important to note that passing an appropriate certification exam is a normal part of the process to being welcomed into the community of professionals. This is simple within athletic training because there is only one official exam (offered by the National Athletic Training Association's Board of Certification). In the fitness area, it is much more complicated given the number of certification exams available. If a certification exam requires a one-day workshop with little or no formal coursework and results in a high pass rate, the certification is worthless from a professional's point of view. It is important to pass the most rigorous and respected certification exams that have, at a minimum, a formal education requirement in an appropriate field. Check out the American College of Sports Medicine (www.acsm.org) and the National Strength and Conditioning Association (https://www.nsca.com/certification/) websites for additional information for certifications that are recognized as being of high quality. If you are interested in a career in physical therapy, as many of our students are, be prepared for stiff competition for the limited number of available seats in these programs. Some undergraduate students even delay applying until they work for a year or do graduate study in an area related to physical therapy. See A Look Back–Important People in Science for someone who was a pioneer in physical therapy and whose journey began in physical education.

Over the past few years, a special initiative, Exercise Is Medicine (http://exerciseismedicine.org), was developed by the American College of Sports Medicine and the American Medical Association to encourage those working in the medical and the allied health professions to routinely promote physical activity to their patients. In addition to that goal, these health professionals need to know where to refer patients when they need more formal support for their physical activity program. For example, physical therapists need to know where to direct their patients after the mandated maximum number of rehabilitation sessions have been completed. Extensive resources for healthcare providers, fitness professionals, the public, and so on are available at the aforementioned website.

Last, but not least, if you are interested in pursuing a career in research so that you can teach and do

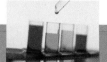
Frances A. Hellebrandt, M.D.

Frances A. Hellebrandt, M.D., made significant contributions to the fields of exercise physiology, physical education, physical therapy, and physical medicine. Her interest in muscle physiology and physical activity led her to enroll as a physical education major at the University of Wisconsin (UW), Madison, where she served as an undergraduate assistant in the Anatomy Department from 1924 to 1927, and graduated with a B.S. degree in 1928. She then entered the UW Medical School and completed her M.D. Dr. Hellebrandt then completed a general internship at Wisconsin General Hospital and did her post-graduate medical training at several major universities, focusing on Physical Medicine and Rehabilitation (PM&R). She was then hired as a faculty member at the UW Medical School and also as the director of the Exercise Physiology Lab.

Her research and training in PM&R and in exercise physiology made her a perfect candidate to lead efforts to rehabilitate soldiers returning injured from World War II (WWII). In 1944, after retirement from the UW, she accepted the position of professor of Physical Medicine and director of the Baruch Center of PM&R at the Medical College of Virginia. She established research and education programs for various modalities

(e.g., hydrotherapy) and created a new residency program in PM&R, making it only the second one in the South. The program's focus was on the rehabilitation of injured soldiers and she felt the war taught physical therapy (PT) two major lessons: the urgent need for the early use of PT to avoid contracture and disuse atrophy, and the evils of bed rest (note: she was well ahead of her time in this regard). She also emphasized the need to treat the whole person and promoted general physical fitness as part of the rehabilitation process–a view we take for granted today.

In 1951, the University of Illinois hired her as professor and head of the Department of Physical Medicine and chief of PM&R. Six years later, Dr. Hellebrandt returned to the UW where she established the Motor Learning Research Laboratory in which cross-disciplinary research was the means by which important questions were answered. She is probably best known for her theory of muscle overload and pacing, which was an extension of research by DeLorme, who developed progressive resistance training during WWII.

Over her career, Dr. Hellebrandt published over 150 papers on topics related to PM&R, exercise physiology, physical education, and physical therapy. She developed several

unique research instruments, was extremely active in professional organizations, and has had a lasting impact on the training of those who seek careers in physical therapy. She retired a second time from the UW in 1964. Her contributions were recognized with the Anderson Award from the American Association of Health, Physical Education, and Recreation, and by the American Physiological Society, which established an award in her honor (i.e., Caroline tum Suden/Frances A. Hellebrandt Professional Opportunity Award). She was both professionally and physically active throughout her long life, passing away in 1992 at the age of 90 (9, 20).

Brown, J.M., M.A. Brennan, and G. Shambes, "On the Death of Professor Emerita Frances A. Hellebrandt, M.D.," Madison Faculty Documents, University of Wisconsin. https://www.secfac.wisc.edu/senate/2002/1007/1656(mem_res).pdf. Hudak, A.M., M.E. Sandel, G. Goldberg, and A.M. Wrynn, "Dr. Frances A. Hellebrandt: Pioneering Physiologist, Physiatrist, and Physical Medicine and Rehabilitation Visionary," *Physical Medicine & Rehabilitation*, 5: 639-646, 2013; Brown, J.M., M.A. Brennan, and G. Shambes, "On the Death of Professor Emerita Frances A. Hellebrandt, M.D.," Madison Faculty Documents, University of Wisconsin. https://www.secfac.wisc.edu/senate/2002/1007/1656(mem_res).pdf.

research at a college or university, you should become involved in research while you are an undergraduate. You might volunteer as a subject for another student's research project, take course credit to assist your professor in his or her research, or use a summer break to work in a researcher's lab at another institution. If a particular area of research interests you, do a PubMed search to see who is currently active in the area; this will help you narrow down potential graduate programs. Finally, you also need to get online and determine what the requirements are for admission to the graduate programs you are interested in; this will give you time to take appropriate coursework to meet those requirements.

IN SUMMARY

- A variety of career paths exist for undergraduates majoring in exercise science and kinesiology. Get some practical experience while you are an undergraduate to help you make a decision about your future and facilitate entry to a profession or graduate school.
- Organizations such as the American College of Sports Medicine and the National Strength and Conditioning Association have developed certification programs to establish a standard of knowledge and skill to be achieved by those who lead exercise programs.

STUDY ACTIVITIES

1. If you are interested in finding new research articles about a topic, for example, "resistance training in women athletes," don't use Google. Instead, go to PubMed **(www.ncbi.nlm.nih.gov/pubmed)** and click PubMed Quick Start Guide to get the basics. Now, insert the phrase in the search box and click Search.

   Finally, select three references that might be of interest to you and send them to your e-mail address using the Send To pull-down menu.

2. Now that you know how to look up research articles on a particular topic, find out where the scientists who did that research are employed. Go to those university (departmental) websites and see what the graduate program requires for admission. If you are interested in pursuing that line of research, contact the professor and see if research or teaching assistantships are available.

3. Go to the Bureau of Labor Statistics Occupational Outlook Handbook **(http://www.bls.gov/ooh/)** and search on your career interest(s) to obtain estimates of salary, projected needs, degrees required, and so forth. Then, locate the office at your college or university that provides advising support for your interest.

4. Identify the primary scientific meeting your professors attend. Find out if the organization that sponsors that meeting has a membership category for students, how much it costs, and what you would receive (e.g., journals) if you joined.

SUGGESTED READINGS

Berryman, J.W. 1995. *Out of Many, One: A History of the American College of Sports Medicine.* Champaign, IL: Human Kinetics.

Morrow, J.R., Jr., W. Zhu, B.D. Franks, M.D. Meredith, and C. Spain. 1958-2008: 50 years of youth fitness tests in the United States. *Research Quarterly for Exercise and Sport.* 80: 1-11, 2009.

Schmidt-Nielsen, B. 1995. *August & Marie Krogh–Lives in Science.* New York, NY: Oxford University Press.

Tipton, C.M. 2003. *Exercise Physiology–People and Ideas.* New York, NY: Oxford University Press.

REFERENCES

1. **American Alliance for Health, Physical Education, Recreation, and Dance.** *Lifetime Health Related Physical Fitness: Test Manual.* Reston, VA, 1980.

2. **American College of Sports Medicine.** *ACSM's Guidelines for Exercise Testing and Prescription.* Baltimore, MD: Lippincott, Williams & Wilkins, 2014.

3. **American Heart Association.** Statement on exercise. *Circulation* 86: 340-344, 1992.

4. **Åstrand P-O.** Influence of Scandinavian scientists in exercise physiology. *Scandinavian Journal of Medicine & Science in Sports* 1: 3-9, 1991.

5. **Baldwin K.** Research in the exercise sciences: where do we go from here? *Journal of Applied Physiology* 88: 332-336, 2000.

6. **Bassett D, Jr. and Howley E.** Maximal oxygen uptake: "classical" versus "contemporary" viewpoints. *Medicine & Science in Sports & Exercise* 29: 591-603, 1997.

7. **Berryman J.** Thomas K. Cureton, Jr.: pioneer researcher, proselytizer, and proponent for physical fitness. *Research Quarterly for Exercise and Sport* 67: 1-12, 1996.

8. **Booth F, Chakravarthy M, Gordon S, and Spangenburg E.** Waging war on physical inactivity: using modern molecular ammunition against an ancient enemy. *Journal of Applied Physiology* 93: 3-30, 2002.

9. **Brown JM, Brennan MA, and Shambes G.** On the death of professor emerita Frances A. Hellebrandt, M.D. University of Wisconsin, Madison Faculty Documents. https://www.secfac.wisc.edu /senate/2002/1007/1656(mem_res).pdf

10. **Buskirk E.** *From Harvard to Minnesota: Keys to Our History.* Baltimore, MD: Williams & Wilkins, 1992, pp. 1-26.

11. **Buskirk E.** Personal communication based on "Our extended family: graduates from the Noll Lab for Human Performance Research." Noll Laboratory, Pennsylvania State University. University Park, PA, 1987.

12. **Buskirk E and Tipton C.** *Exercise Physiology.* Champaign, IL: Human Kinetics, 1977, pp. 367-438.

13. **Chapman C and Mitchell J.** The physiology of exercise. *Scientific American* 212: 88-96, 1965.

14. **Clarke H and Clark D.** *Developmental and Adapted Physical Education.* Englewood Cliffs, NJ: Prentice-Hall, 1978.

15. **Dill D.** *Life, Heat, and Altitude.* Cambridge, MA: Harvard University Press, 1938.

16. **Fenn W and Rahn H.** *Handbook of Physiology: Respiration.* Washington, D.C.: American Physiological Society, 1964.

17. **Franks B.** *Exercise and Fitness.* Chicago, IL: The Athletic Institute, 1969.

18. **Hackensmith C.** *History of Physical Education.* New York, NY: Harper & Row, 1966.

19. **Horvath S and Horvath E.** *The Harvard Fatigue Laboratory: Its History and Contributions.* Englewood Cliffs, NJ: Prentice-Hall, 1973.

20. **Hudak AM, Sandel ME, Goldberg G, and Wrynn AM.** Dr. Frances A. Hellebrandt: pioneering physiologist, physiatrist, and physical medicine and rehabilitation visionary. *Physical Medicine & Rehabilitation* 5: 639-646, 2013.

21. **Hunsicker P.** A survey of laboratory facilities in college physical education departments. *Research Quarterly for Exercise and Sport* 21: 420-423, 1950.

22. **Huxley T.** *Selection from Essays.* New York, NY: Appleton-Century-Crofts, 1948.

23. **Ianuzzo D and Hutton R.** A prospectus for graduate students in muscle physiology and biochemistry. *Sports Medicine Bulletin* 22: 17-18, 1987.

24. **Kennedy J.** The soft American. *Sports Illustrated* 13: 14-17, 1960.
25. **Kroll W.** *Perspectives in Physical Education.* New York, NY: Academic Press, 1971.
26. **Lagrange F.** *Physiology of Bodily Exercise.* New York, NY: D. Appleton and Company, 1890.
27. **McKenzie R.** *Exercise in Education and Medicine.* Philadelphia, PA: W. B. Saunders, 1923.
28. **Montoye H and Washburn R.** Genealogy of scholarship among academy members. *The Academy Papers* 13: 94-101, 1980.
29. **Montoye H and Washburn R.** Research quarterly contributors: an academic genealogy. *Research Quarterly for Exercise and Sport* 51: 261-266, 1980.
30. **Pate R, Pratt M, Blair S, Haskell W, Macera C, Bouchard C, et al.** Physical activity and public health. A recommendation from the Centers for Disease Control and Prevention and the American College of Sports Medicine. *Journal of the American Medical Association* 273: 402-407, 1995.
31. **Pierce P and Nagle E.** Uncommon sense for the apprentice! Important steps for interns. *ACSM's Health & Fitness Journal* 9: 18-23, 2005.
32. **Powell K and Paffenbarger R.** Workshop on epidimiologic and public health aspects of physical activity and exercise: a summary. *Public Health Reports* 100: 118-126, 1985.
33. **Shephard RJ.** Proceedings of the International Symposium on Physical Activity and Cardiovascular Health. *Canadian Medical Association Journal* 96: 695-915, 1967.
34. **Rowell L.** *Human Circulation: Regulation During Physical Stress.* New York, NY: Oxford University Press, 1986.
35. **Sargent D.** *Physical Education.* Boston, MA: Ginn and Company, 1906.
36. **Stainsby W.** Part two: "For what is a man profited?" *Sports Medicine Bulletin* 22: 15, 1987.
37. **Tipton CM.** Living history: Elsworth R. Buskirk. *Advances in Physiology Education* 33: 243-252, 2009.
38. **Tipton C.** Contemporary exercise physiology: fifty years after the closure of Harvard Fatigue Laboratory. *Exercise and Sport Sciences Review* 26: 315-339, 1998.
39. **US Department of Health and Human Services.** *Physical Activity and Health: A Report of the Surgeon General.* Atlanta, GA: U.S. Department of Health and Human Services, 1996.
40. **Van Dalen D and Bennett B.** *A World History of Physical Education: Cultural, Philosophical, Comparative.* Englewood Cliffs, NJ: Prentice-Hall, 1971.

1

Common Measurements in Exercise Physiology

■ Objectives

By studying this chapter, you should be able to do the following:

1. Express work, power, and energy in standardized (SI) units and convert those units to others commonly used in exercise physiology.

2. Give a brief explanation of the procedure used to calculate work performed during step, cycle ergometer, and treadmill exercise.

3. Describe the concept behind the measurement of energy expenditure using (a) direct calorimetry and (b) indirect calorimetry.

4. Calculate the following expressions of energy expenditure when given the oxygen uptake in liters per minute: $kcal \cdot min^{-1}$, $ml \cdot kg^{-1} \cdot min^{-1}$, METs, and $kcal \cdot kg^{-1} \cdot hr^{-1}$.

5. Estimate energy expenditure during horizontal treadmill walking and running, and cycle ergometry.

6. Describe the procedure used to calculate net efficiency during steady-state exercise; distinguish efficiency from economy.

■ Outline

■ Key Terms

cycle ergometer
direct calorimetry
ergometer
ergometry
indirect calorimetry
kilocalorie (kcal)
MET (metabolic equivalent)
net efficiency
open-circuit spirometry
percent grade
power
relative $\dot{V}O_2$
System International (SI) units
work

How much energy do you expend when you run a mile? How fast can you run 100 m? How high can you jump? These questions deal with energy, speed, and explosive power—and so will you as you study exercise physiology. Throughout this text, we will discuss such terms as *aerobic and anaerobic power*, *efficiency*, *work capacity*, and *energy expenditure*. The purpose of this chapter is to introduce you to some of the most common pieces of equipment and measurements linked to these terms. It is very important to understand this information at the outset, as it is used throughout the text. However, the details associated with specific exercise tests for fitness and performance are covered in detail in Chaps. 15 and 20. Let's begin with the most basic units of measurement.

UNITS OF MEASURE

Metric System

In the United States, the English system of measurement remains in common use. In contrast, the metric system, which is used in most countries, is the standard system of measurement for scientists and is used by almost all scientific journals. In the metric system, the basic units of length, volume, and mass are the meter, the liter, and the gram, respectively. The main advantage of the metric system is that subdivisions or multiples of its basic units are expressed in factors of 10 using prefixes attached to the basic unit. Students not familiar with the metric system should refer to Table 1.1 for a list of the basic prefixes used in metric measurements.

SI Units

An ongoing problem in exercise science is the failure of scientists to standardize units of measurement employed in presenting research data. In an effort to eliminate this problem, a uniform system of reporting scientific measurement has been developed through international cooperation. This system, known as **System International units**, or SI units, has been endorsed by almost all exercise and sports medicine

TABLE 1.1	Common Metric Prefixes
mega: one million (1,000,000)	
kilo: one thousand (1000)	
centi: one-hundredth (0.01)	
milli: one-thousandth (0.001)	
micro: one-millionth (0.000001)	
nano: one-billionth (0.000000001)	
pico: one-trillionth (0.000000000001)	

TABLE 1.2	SI Units of Importance in the Measurement of Human Exercise Performance
Units for Quantifying Human Exercise	SI Unit
Mass	kilogram (kg)
Distance	meter (m)
Time	second (s)
Force	newton (N)
Work	joule (J)
Energy	joule (J)
Power	watt (W)
Velocity	meters per second ($m \cdot s^{-1}$)
Torque	newton-meter ($N \cdot m$)

journals for the publication of research data (24, 25). The SI system ensures standardization in the reporting of scientific data and makes comparison of published values easy. Table 1.2 contains SI units of importance in the measurement of exercise performance.

IN SUMMARY

- The metric system is the system of measurement used by scientists to express mass, length, and volume.
- In an effort to standardize terms for the measurement of energy, force, work, and power, scientists have developed a common system of terminology called System International (SI) units.

WORK AND POWER DEFINED

Work

Work is defined as the product of force and the distance through which that force acts:

$$\text{Work} = \text{Force} \times \text{Distance}$$

The SI unit for force is newtons (N), whereas the SI unit for distance is meters (m). The following example shows how to calculate work when a 10-kg weight is lifted upward a distance of 2 m. At the earth's surface, a mass of 1 kg exerts a force of 9.81 N due to the force of gravity. Therefore,

Convert kg to N, where 1 kg = 9.81 N,
so 10 kg = 98.1 N

Work = 98.1 N × 2 m
= 196.2 newton-meters (N · m) or
196.2 joules (J)

TABLE 1.3	Common Units Used to Express the Amount of Work Performed or Energy Expended
Term	Conversion
Kilopond-meter (kpm)*	1 kpm = 9.81 joules (J)
Kilocalorie (kcal)	1 kcal = 4186 J or 4.186 kJ
	1 kcal = 426.8 kpm
joule (J)†	1 J = 1 newton-meter (N · m)
	1 J = 2.39 × 10⁻⁴ kcal
	1 J = 0.102 kpm

*The kilopond is a unit of force describing the effect of gravity on a mass of 1 kg.

†The joule is the basic unit adopted by the System International (called SI unit) for expression of energy expenditure or work.

The work performed was computed by multiplying the force (expressed in N) times the distance traveled (expressed in m), with the resulting work being expressed in joules, which is the SI unit for work (where 1 joule = 1 N · m; Table 1.3).

Although the SI units are the preferred units for quantifying exercise performance and energy expenditure, you will encounter situations in which a number of traditional units are used to express both work and energy. For example, body weight (a force) is commonly given in kilograms, the unit for mass. To avoid confusion in the calculation of work, the term *kilopond* (kp) is used as the force unit, representing the effect of gravity on a mass of 1 kilogram. Using the preceding example, work may be expressed in kilopond-meters (kpm). In the preceding example, the 10-kg weight is considered 10-kg force (or 10 kiloponds), which when moved through 2 m, results in work of 20 kpm. Since 1 kpm is equal to 9.81 J (see Table 1.3), the work performed is 196.2 J (20 kpm × 9.81 J/kpm). Table 1.3 contains a list of terms that are in common use today to express work and energy–remember that the SI unit for both work and energy is the joule. For example, the energy content of commercial food products is often listed on the label in kilocalories. However, the SI unit for energy content and expenditure is joules, where 1 kilocalorie is equal to 4186 joules (J) or 4.186 kilojoules (kJ).

Power

Power is the term used to describe how much work is accomplished per unit of time. The SI unit for power is the watt (W) and is defined as 1 joule per second (Table 1.4). Power can be calculated as:

$$\text{Power} = \text{Work} \div \text{Time}$$

The concept of power is important because it describes the rate at which work is being performed (work rate). It is the work rate, or power output, that

TABLE 1.4	Common Terms and Units Used to Express Power
Term	Conversion
Watt (W)*	1 W = 1 J · s⁻¹
	1 W = 6.12 kpm · min⁻¹
Horsepower (hp)	1 hp = 745.7 W or J · s⁻¹
	1 hp = 10.69 kcal · min⁻¹
Kilopond-meter · min⁻¹ (kpm · min⁻¹)	1 kpm · min⁻¹ = 0.163 W

*The watt is the basic unit adopted by the System International (called SI unit) for expression of power.

describes the intensity of exercise. Given enough time, any healthy adult could perform a total work output of 20,000 J. However, only a few highly trained athletes could perform this amount of work in 60 seconds (s). The power output of these athletes can be calculated as follows:

$$\text{Power} = 20,000 \text{ joules}/60 \text{ seconds}$$
$$= 333.3 \text{ watts (W)}$$

Note that the SI unit for power is the watt. Table 1.4 contains a list of both the SI and more traditional terms and units used to express power. The ability to convert from one expression of work, energy, or power to another is important, as we will see later in the chapter when we calculate mechanical efficiency.

MEASUREMENT OF WORK AND POWER

The term **ergometry** refers to the measurement of work output. The word **ergometer** refers to the apparatus or device used to measure a specific type of work. It is important to point out that the determination of work and power requires that a force is moved against some resistance. This could be a person's body weight (a force) moving up a step against gravity (a resistance) or pedaling a stationary bike when a resistance has been applied to the wheel. Many types of ergometers are in use today in exercise physiology laboratories (Fig. 1.1). A brief introduction to commonly used ergometers follows.

Bench Step

One of the earliest ergometers used to measure work capacity in humans was the bench step. This ergometer is still in use today and simply involves the subject stepping up and down on a bench at a specified rate. Calculation of the work performed during bench stepping is very easy. Suppose a 70-kg man steps up

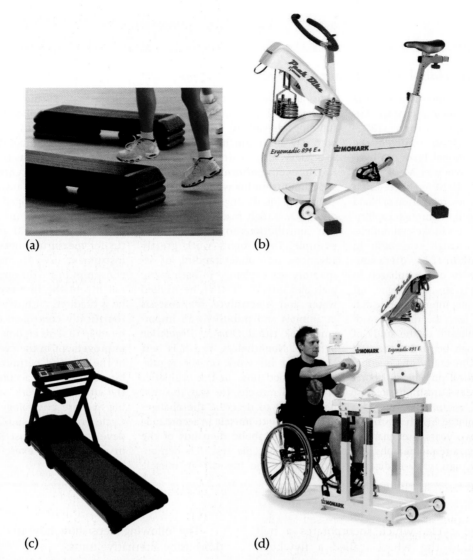

Figure 1.1 Illustrations of four different ergometers used in the measurement of human work output and power. (a) A bench step. (b) Friction-braked cycle ergometer. (c) Motor-driven treadmill. Both the treadmill elevation and the horizontal speed can be adjusted by electronic controls. (d) Arm crank ergometer. Arm crank ergometry can be used to measure work output with the arms and is based on the same principle as cycle ergometry.

and down on a 30-centimeter (0.3-meter) bench for 10 minutes (min) at a rate of 30 steps per minute. The amount of work performed during this 10-minute task can be computed as follows:

$$\text{Force} = 686.7 \text{ N (i.e., 70 kg} \times 9.81 \text{ N/kg)}$$

$$\text{Distance} = 0.3 \text{ m} \cdot \text{step}^{-1} \times 30 \text{ steps} \cdot \text{min}^{-1} \times 10 \text{ min}$$
$$= 90 \text{ m}$$

Therefore, the total work performed is:

$$686.7 \text{ N} \times 90 \text{ m} = 61,803 \text{ joules or } 61.8 \text{ kilojoules (kJ)}$$
$$\text{(rounded to nearest 0.1)}$$

The power output during this 10 minutes (600 seconds) of exercise can be calculated as:

$$\text{Power} = 61,803 \text{ J/600 seconds}$$
$$= 103 \text{ J} \cdot \text{s}^{-1} \text{ or 103 watts (W)}$$

Using a more traditional unit of work, the kilopond-meter (kpm), power can be calculated as follows:

$$\text{Work} = 70 \text{ kp} \times 0.3 \text{ m} \times 30 \text{ steps} \cdot \text{min}^{-1} \times 10 \text{ min}$$
$$= 6300 \text{ kpm}$$

$$\text{Power} = 6300 \text{ kpm} \div 10 \text{ min} = 630 \text{ kpm} \cdot \text{min}^{-1} \text{ or}$$
$$103 \text{ watts (See Table 1.4 for conversions)}$$

Cycle Ergometer

The **cycle ergometer** was developed more than 100 years ago and remains a popular ergometer in exercise physiology laboratories today (see "A Look Back–Important People in Science"). This type of ergometer is a stationary exercise cycle that permits accurate measurement of the work performed. A common type of cycle ergometer is the Monark

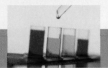
August Krogh: Nobel Prize Winner and Inventor

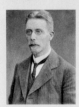

© Library of Congress/Science Source

As mentioned in the previous chapter, **August Krogh** (1872–1949) received the Nobel Prize in Physiology or Medicine in 1920 for his research on regulation of blood flow through capillaries in skeletal muscle. Krogh was born in Grenaa, Denmark in 1874. After entering the University of Copenhagen in 1893, he began to study medicine, but developed a strong interest in research and decided to leave his medical studies to devote himself to the study of physiology. Krogh began his research career at the University of Copenhagen in the medical physiology laboratory of the famous Danish physiologist Christian Bohr.

Krogh completed his Ph.D. studies in 1903 and two years later married Marie Jørgensen, a renowned physiologist. August Krogh was a dedicated physiologist with extreme curiosity. He devoted his entire life to understanding physiology, and he worked both day and night in his laboratory to achieve his research goals. In fact, Krogh even performed physiology experiments on his wedding day!

During his distinguished research career, Dr. Krogh made many important contributions to physiology. For example, Dr. Krogh's work greatly advanced our understanding of respiratory gas exchange in both mammals and insects. Further, he studied water and electrolyte homeostasis in animals and published an important book titled *Osmotic Regulation* in 1939. Nonetheless, Krogh is best known for his work on the regulation of blood flow in the capillaries of skeletal muscle. He was the first physiologist to describe the changes in blood flow to muscle in accordance with the metabolic demands of the tissue. Indeed, his research demonstrated that the increase in muscle blood flow during contractions was achieved by the opening of arterioles and capillaries. This is the work that earned him the Nobel Prize.

In addition to physiology research, August Krogh invented many important scientific instruments. For instance, he developed both the spirometer (a device used to measure pulmonary volumes) and an apparatus for measuring metabolic rate (an instrument used to measure oxygen consumption). Although Krogh did not invent the first cycle ergometer, he is credited with developing an automatically controlled cycle ergometer in 1913. This ergometer was a large improvement in the cycle ergometers of the day and permitted Krogh and his colleagues to accurately measure the amount of work performed during exercise physiology experiments. Cycle ergometers similar to the one developed by August Krogh are still in use today in exercise physiology laboratories.

---

friction-braked cycle, which incorporates a belt wrapped around the wheel (called a flywheel) (Fig. 1.1(*b*)). The belt can be loosened or tightened to provide a change in resistance. The distance the wheel travels can be determined by computing the distance covered per revolution of the pedals (6 meters per revolution on a standard Monark cycle) times the number of pedal revolutions. Consider the following example for the computation of work and power using the cycle ergometer. Calculate work given:

> Duration of exercise = 10 min
> Resistance against flywheel = 1.5 kp or 14.7 N
> Distance traveled per pedal revolution = 6 m
> Pedaling speed = 60 rev · min^{-1}
> Therefore, the total revolutions in 10 min
> = 10 min × 60 rev · min^{-1} = 600 rev

Hence, total work = 14.7 N × (6 m · rev^{-1} × 600 rev)
= 52,920 J or 52.9 kJ

The power output in this example is computed by dividing the total work performed by time:

> Power = 52,920 joules ÷ 600 seconds
> = 88.2 watts

The following steps show how to do the calculations using alternative units:

Work = 1.5 kp × 6 m · rev^{-1} × 60 rev · min^{-1} × 10 min
= 5400 kpm

Power = 5400 kpm ÷ 10 min = 540 kpm · min^{-1}
= 88.2 watts (See Table 1.4 for conversions)

Treadmill

When a person walks or runs on a treadmill at 0% grade, the center of mass (imagine a point at the hip) of that person rises and falls with each stride, more for running than walking since there is a period of flight during each running stride. However, it is very difficult to measure that small vertical displacement of the center of mass, and consequently "work" cannot be easily determined when walking or running on a horizontal treadmill. In contrast, it is very easy to measure work when a person is walking or running up a slope (grade). The incline of the treadmill is expressed in units called "percent grade." **Percent grade** is defined as the amount of vertical rise per 100 units of belt travel. For instance, a subject walking on a treadmill at a 10% grade travels 10 meters

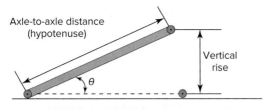

Axle-to-axle distance
(hypotenuse)

Vertical
rise

θ

Fixed rear-axle treadmill
Grade = Sine θ = Rise ÷ Hypotenuse

Figure 1.2   Determination of the "percent grade" on an inclined treadmill. Theta (θ) represents the angle of inclination. Percent grade is computed as the sine of angle $\theta \times 100$.

vertically for every 100 meters of the belt travel. Percent grade is calculated by multiplying the sine of the treadmill angle by 100. In practice, the treadmill angle (expressed in degrees) can be determined by simple trigonometric computations (Fig. 1.2) or by using a measurement device called an inclinometer (9).

To calculate the work output during treadmill exercise, you must know both the subject's body weight and the distance traveled vertically. Vertical travel can be computed by multiplying the distance the belt travels by the percent grade. This can be written as:

Vertical displacement = % Grade × Distance

where percent grade is expressed as a fraction and the total distance traveled is calculated by multiplying the treadmill speed (m · min⁻¹) by the total minutes of exercise. Consider the following sample calculation of work output during treadmill exercise:

Body weight = 60 kg (force = 60 kp or 588.6 N)
Treadmill speed = 200 m · min⁻¹
Treadmill angle = 7.5% grade (7.5 ÷ 100 = 0.075 as
       fractional grade)
Exercise time = 10 min
Total vertical distance traveled
       = 200 m · min⁻¹ × 0.075 × 10 min = 150 m
Therefore, total work performed = 588.6 N × 150 m
       = 88,290 J or 88.3 kJ

Using more traditional units, the following calculations can be made:

Work = 60 kp × 0.075 × 200 m · min⁻¹ × 10 min
     = 9000 kpm or 88,290 J (88.3 kJ)

IN SUMMARY

- An understanding of the terms *work* and *power* is necessary to compute human work output and the associated exercise efficiency.
- Work is defined as the product of force times distance:

   Work = Force × Distance

- Power is defined as work divided by time:

   Power = Work ÷ Time

MEASUREMENT OF ENERGY EXPENDITURE

Measurement of an individual's energy expenditure at rest or during a particular activity has many practical applications. One direct application applies to exercise-assisted weight-loss programs. Clearly, knowledge of the energy cost of walking, running, or swimming at various speeds is useful to individuals who use these modes of exercise as an aid in weight loss. Furthermore, an industrial engineer might measure the energy cost of various tasks around a job site and use this information in making the appropriate job assignments to workers (17, 35). In this regard, the engineer might recommend that the supervisor assign those jobs that demand large energy requirements to workers who are physically fit and possess high work capacities. In general, two techniques are employed in the measurement of human energy expenditure: (1) direct calorimetry and (2) indirect calorimetry.

Direct Calorimetry

When the body uses energy to do work, heat is liberated. This production of heat by cells occurs via both cellular respiration (bioenergetics) and cell work. The general process can be drawn schematically as (5, 36, 37):

$$\text{Nutrients} + O_2 \rightarrow \text{ATP} + \text{Heat}$$
$$\downarrow$$
$$\text{Cell work} + \text{Heat}$$

The process of cellular respiration is discussed in detail in Chap. 3. Note that the rate of heat production in an individual is directly proportional to the metabolic rate. Therefore, measuring heat production (calorimetry) of a person gives a direct measurement of metabolic rate.

The SI unit to measure heat energy is the joule (the same as for work). However, a common unit employed to measure heat energy is the calorie (see Table 1.3). A calorie is defined as the amount of heat required to raise the temperature of one gram of water by one degree Celsius. Because the calorie is very small, the term **kilocalorie (kcal)** is commonly used to express energy expenditure and the energy value of foods. One kcal is equal to 1000 calories. In converting kcals to SI units, 1 kcal is equal to 4186 joules or 4.186 kilojoules (kJ) (see Table 1.3 for conversions). The process of measuring a person's metabolic rate via the measurement of heat production is called **direct calorimetry**, and it has been used by scientists since the eighteenth century. This technique involves placing the person in a closed chamber (called a calorimeter), which is insulated from the environment (usually by a jacket of water surrounding the chamber), and allowance is made for the free exchange of

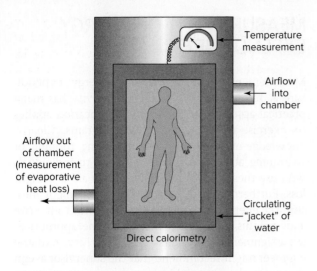

Figure 1.3 Diagram of a simple calorimeter used to measure metabolic rate by measuring the production of body heat. This method of determining metabolic rate is called direct calorimetry.

O_2 and CO_2 from the chamber (Fig. 1.3). The person's body heat raises the temperature of the water circulating around the chamber. Therefore, by measuring the temperature change per unit of time, the amount of heat production can be computed. In addition, heat is lost from the person by evaporation of water from the skin and respiratory passages. This heat loss is measured and is added to the total heat picked up by the water to yield an estimate of the rate of energy expenditure by the person (5, 9).

Indirect Calorimetry

Although direct calorimetry is considered to be a precise technique for the measurement of metabolic rate, construction of a chamber that is large enough for doing exercise physiology research on humans is expensive. Also, the use of direct calorimetry to measure metabolic rate during exercise is complicated because the ergometer itself may produce heat. Fortunately, another procedure can be used to calculate metabolic rate. This technique is termed **indirect calorimetry** because it does not involve the direct measurement of heat production. The principle of indirect calorimetry can be explained by the following relationship:

$$\text{Nutrients} + O_2 \rightarrow \text{Heat} + CO_2 + H_2O$$
(Indirect calorimetry)　　(Direct calorimetry)

Because a direct relationship exists between O_2 consumed and the amount of heat produced in the body, measuring O_2 consumption provides an estimate of metabolic rate (3, 5, 15). To convert the amount of O_2 consumed into heat equivalents, it is necessary to know the type of nutrient (i.e., carbohydrate, fat, or protein) that was metabolized. The

energy liberated when fat is the only nutrient metabolized is 4.7 kcal (or 19.7 kJ) $\cdot$ L O_2^{-1}, whereas the energy released when only carbohydrates are used is 5.05 kcal (or 21.13 kJ) $\cdot$ L O_2^{-1}. Although it is not exact, the caloric expenditure of exercise is often estimated to be approximately 5 kcal (or 21 kJ) per liter of O_2 consumed (19). Therefore, a person exercising at an oxygen consumption of 2.0 L $\cdot$ min^{-1} would expend approximately 10 kcal (or 42 kJ) of energy per minute.

The most common technique used to measure oxygen consumption today is termed **open-circuit spirometry**. In the classic technique, the subject wore a nose clip to prevent nasal breathing and a respiratory valve that allowed room air to be breathed in while the exhaled gas was directed to a collection bag (Douglas bag) that was later analyzed for gas volume and percent of O_2 and CO_2. Gas volume was measured in a gasometer, and the O_2 and CO_2 were either analyzed chemically or with the aid of calibrated gas analyzers. The steps provided in Appendix A were followed to calculate O_2 consumption and CO_2 production. (All appendices can be accessed through the Instructor Resources within Connect.) Modern-day, open-circuit spirometry (see Fig. 1.4) employs

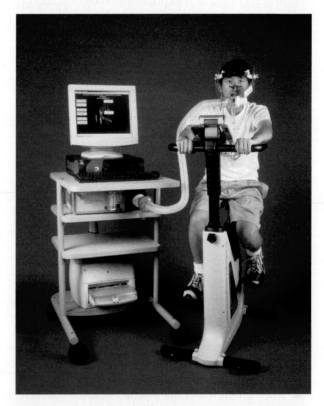

Figure 1.4 The TrueOne metabolic measurement system utilizes electronic flow sensors, gas analyzers, and computer technology. These devices are used to measure oxygen uptake and carbon dioxide production at rest and during exercise.

© ParvoMedics

computer technology that measures the volume of the exhaled gas on a breath-by-breath basis, which is then directed to a mixing chamber where samples are taken for continuous gas analysis. The calculations of O_2 consumption and CO_2 production are done automatically. Although the computer-based system certainly makes the process of measuring oxygen consumption easier, the traditional method is used as the "gold standard" to make sure the automated system is working correctly (4).

IN SUMMARY

- Measurement of energy expenditure at rest or during exercise is possible using either direct or indirect calorimetry.
- Direct calorimetry uses the measurement of heat production as an indication of metabolic rate.
- Indirect calorimetry estimates metabolic rate via the measurement of oxygen consumption.

COMMON EXPRESSIONS OF ENERGY EXPENDITURE

The oxygen consumption can be used to express energy expenditure in different ways (21).

$\dot{V}O_2$ ($L \cdot min^{-1}$) By following the steps outlined in Appendix A, oxygen consumption ($\dot{V}O_2$) can be calculated in liters of oxygen used per minute (L/min). (All appendices can be accessed through the Instructor Resources within Connect.) For example, the following data were collected on a 60-kg trained woman during a submaximal run on a treadmill:

$$\text{Ventilation (STPD)} = 60\ L \cdot min^{-1}$$
$$= \text{inspired } O_2\ 20.93\%$$
$$= \text{expired } O_2\ 16.93\%$$
$$\dot{V}O_2\ (L \cdot min^{-1}) = 60\ L \cdot min^{-1} \times (20.93\%\ O_2$$
$$-\ 16.93\%\ O_2) = 2.4\ L \cdot min^{-1}$$

kcal $\cdot$ min^{-1} Oxygen uptake can also be expressed in kilocalories used per minute. The caloric equivalent of 1 L of O_2 varies from 4.7 kcal $\cdot$ L^{-1} for fats to 5.05 kcal $\cdot$ L^{-1} for carbohydrates. However, for practical reasons, and with little error, 5 kcal $\cdot$ L^{-1} of O_2 is used to convert the $\dot{V}O_2$ to kilocalories per minute. Total energy expenditure is calculated by multiplying the kilocalories expended per minute (kcal $\cdot$ min^{-1}) by the duration of the activity in minutes. For example, if the 60-kg woman mentioned previously runs on the treadmill for 30 minutes at a $\dot{V}O_2$ = 2.4 L $\cdot$ min^{-1}, the total energy expenditure can be calculated as follows:

$$2.4\ L \cdot min^{-1} \times 5\ kcal \cdot L^{-1}\ O_2 = 12\ kcal \cdot min^{-1}$$
$$12\ kcal \cdot min^{-1} \times 30\ min = 360\ kcal$$

$\dot{V}O_2$ ($ml \cdot kg^{-1} \cdot min^{-1}$) When the measured oxygen uptake, expressed in liters per minute, is multiplied by 1000 to yield milliliters per minute and then divided by the subject's body weight in kilograms, the value is expressed in milliliters of O_2 per kilogram of body weight per minute, or ml $\cdot$ $kg^{-1} \cdot min^{-1}$. This allows comparisons among people of different body sizes. For example, for the 60-kg woman with a $\dot{V}O_2$ = 2.4 L $\cdot$ min^{-1}:

$$2.4\ L \cdot min^{-1} \times 1000\ ml \cdot L^{-1} \div 60\ kg$$
$$= 40\ ml \cdot kg^{-1} \cdot min^{-1}$$

METs The resting metabolic rate is usually measured with an individual at quiet supine rest, after a period of fasting and not participating in exercise. The resting metabolic rate varies with age and gender, being less in females than males, and decreases with age (23). The **MET (metabolic equivalent)** is a term used to represent resting metabolism and is taken, by convention, to be 3.5 ml $\cdot$ $kg^{-1} \cdot min^{-1}$. This is called 1 MET. In essence, the energy cost of activities can be expressed in terms of multiples of the MET unit. METs are useful for comparing the relative intensity of various activities. Using the preceding information:

$$40\ ml \cdot kg^{-1} \cdot min^{-1} \div 3.5\ ml \cdot kg^{-1} \cdot min^{-1} = 11.4\ \text{METs}$$

kcal $\cdot$ $kg^{-1} \cdot hr^{-1}$ The MET expression can also be used to express the number of calories the subject uses per kilogram of body weight per hour. In the example mentioned previously, the subject is working at 11.4 METs, or 40 ml $\cdot$ $kg^{-1}\ min^{-1}$. When this value is multiplied by 60 min $\cdot$ hr^{-1}, it equals 2400 ml $\cdot$ $kg^{-1} \cdot hr^{-1}$, or 2.4 L $\cdot$ $kg^{-1} \cdot hr^{-1}$. If the person is using a mixture of carbohydrates and fats as the fuel, the $\dot{V}O_2$ is multiplied by 4.85 kcal $\cdot$ L^{-1} of O_2 (average between 4.7 and 5.05 kcal/L O_2) to give 11.6 kcal $\cdot$ $kg^{-1} \cdot hr^{-1}$. The following steps show the detail.

$$11.4\ \text{METs} \times 3.5\ ml \cdot kg^{-1} \cdot min^{-1} = 40\ ml \cdot kg^{-1} \cdot min^{-1}$$
$$40\ ml \cdot kg^{-1} \cdot min^{-1} \times 60\ min \cdot hr^{-1}$$
$$= 2400\ ml \cdot kg^{-1} \cdot hr^{-1} = 2.4\ L \cdot kg^{-1} \cdot hr^{-1}$$
$$2.4\ L \cdot kg^{-1} \cdot hr^{-1} \times 4.85\ kcal \cdot L^{-1}\ O_2$$
$$= 11.6\ kcal \cdot kg^{-1} \cdot hr^{-1}$$

IN SUMMARY

- Energy expenditure can be expressed in terms of oxygen consumption ($\dot{V}O_2$) in units of L $\cdot$ min^{-1} and ml $\cdot$ $kg^{-1} \cdot min^{-1}$.
- Based on $\dot{V}O_2$, energy expenditure can also be expressed as METs, where 1 MET = 3.5 ml $\cdot$ $kg^{-1} \cdot min^{-1}$.
- Energy expenditure can also be expressed in terms of kcal $\cdot$ min^{-1} and kcal $\cdot$ $kg^{-1} \cdot min^{-1}$.

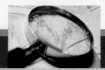

A CLOSER LOOK 1.1

Estimation of the O_2 Requirement of Treadmill Walking

The O_2 requirement of horizontal treadmill walking can be estimated with reasonable accuracy for speeds between 50 and 100 m · min⁻¹ using the following formula:

$\dot{V}O_2$ (ml · kg⁻¹ · min⁻¹) = 0.1 ml · kg⁻¹ · min⁻¹/(m · min⁻¹) × speed (m · min⁻¹) + 3.5 ml · kg⁻¹ · min⁻¹ (resting $\dot{V}O_2$)

For example, the O_2 cost of walking at 80 m · min⁻¹ is

$\dot{V}O_2$ (ml kg⁻¹ min⁻¹) = 0.1 ml · kg⁻¹ · min⁻¹ × 80 m · min⁻¹ + 3.5 ml · kg⁻¹ · min⁻¹
= 11.5 ml · kg⁻¹ · min⁻¹ or 3.3 METs (11.5 ÷ 3.5)

Estimation of the O_2 Requirement of Treadmill Running

The O_2 requirements of horizontal treadmill running for speeds greater than 134 m · min⁻¹ can be estimated in a manner similar to the procedure used to estimate the O_2 requirement for treadmill walking. The O_2 cost of the horizontal component is calculated using the following formula:

$\dot{V}O_2$ (ml · kg⁻¹ · min⁻¹) = 0.2 ml · kg⁻¹ · min⁻¹/m · min⁻¹ × speed (m · min⁻¹) + 3.5 ml · kg⁻¹· min⁻¹ (resting $\dot{V}O_2$)

What is the oxygen cost of a person running at 6 mph (161 m/min or 9.7 km/hr)?

$\dot{V}O_2$ (ml · kg⁻¹ · min⁻¹) = 0.2 ml · kg⁻¹· min⁻¹/m · min⁻¹ × 161 m · min⁻¹ + 3.5 ml · kg⁻¹ · min⁻¹
= 35.7 ml · kg⁻¹ · min⁻¹ or 10.2 METs (35.7 ÷ 3.5)

Formulas are taken from reference (2).

ESTIMATION OF ENERGY EXPENDITURE

Researchers studying the oxygen cost (O_2 cost = $\dot{V}O_2$ at steady state) of exercise have demonstrated that it is possible to estimate the energy expended during certain types of physical activity with reasonable precision (8, 10, 11, 19, 31). Walking, running, and cycling are activities that have been studied in detail. The O_2 requirements of walking and running graphed as a function of speed are presented in Figure 1.5. Expressing $\dot{V}O_2$ as a function of the body weight is referred to as **relative $\dot{V}O_2$**, and it is appropriate when describing the O_2 cost of weight-bearing activities such as walking, running, and climbing steps. Note that the relationships between the relative O_2 requirement (ml · kg⁻¹ · min⁻¹) and walking/running speed are straight lines (2, 19). A similar relationship exists for cycling, up to a power output of about 200 W (see Fig. 1.6). The fact that this relationship is linear over a wide range of speeds and power outputs makes the calculation of the O_2 cost (or energy cost) very easy (see A Closer Look 1.1 and 1.2 for examples). Estimation of the energy expenditure of other types of activities is more complex. For example, estimation of energy expenditure during tennis is dependent on whether the match is singles or doubles and is also influenced by the participants'

skill level. That said, modern portable oxygen uptake devices allow direct measurement of $\dot{V}O_2$ outside the laboratory to estimate energy expenditure of almost any activity. See the Compendium of Physical Activities **(http://sites.google.com/site/compendiumofphysicalactivities/)** for a detailed list of the oxygen cost (MET values) of numerous physical activities (1).

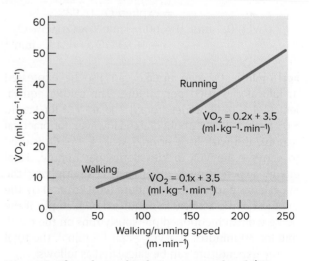

Figure 1.5 The relationship between speed and $\dot{V}O_2$ cost is linear for both walking and running. Note that x equals the walking/running speed in m · min⁻¹.

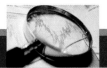

A CLOSER LOOK 1.2

Estimation of the O₂ Requirement of Cycling

Similar to the energy cost of walking and running, the oxygen requirement of cycling is also linear (straight line) over a range of work rates up to about 200 W (Fig. 1.6). Because of this linear relationship, the O_2 requirement of cycling can be easily estimated for power outputs between 50 and 200 watts (i.e., ~300 and 1200 kpm · min⁻¹). The total O_2 cost of cycling on a cycle ergometer is composed of three components. These include the resting O_2 consumption, the O_2 demand associated with unloaded cycling (i.e., energy cost of moving the legs), and the O_2 requirement that is directly proportional to the external load on the cycle. An explanation of how the O_2 cost of these components is computed follows.

First, the resting O_2 consumption is estimated at 3.5 ml · kg⁻¹ · min⁻¹. Second, at a cranking speed of 50 to 60 rpm, the oxygen cost of unloaded cycling is also approximately 3.5 ml · kg⁻¹ · min⁻¹. Finally, the relative O_2 cost of cycling against an external load is 1.8 ml · kpm⁻¹ × work rate × body mass⁻¹. Putting these three components together, the collective formula to compute the O_2 of cycling is:

$$\dot{V}O_2 \text{ (ml · kg}^{-1} \text{· min}^{-1}) = \\ 1.8 \text{ ml · kpm}^{-1} \text{ (work rate)} \times M^{-1} \\ + 7 \text{ ml · kg}^{-1} \text{· min}^{-1}$$

where:

- work rate on the cycle ergometer is expressed in kpm · min⁻¹
- M is body mass in kilograms
- 7 ml · kg⁻¹ · min⁻¹ is the sum of resting O_2 consumption (3.5) and the O_2 cost of unloaded cycling (3.5)

For example, the O_2 cost of cycling at 600 kpm/min (~100 W) for a 70-kg man is:

$$1.8 \text{ ml · kpm}^{-1} \text{ (600 kpm · min}^{-1}) \times \\ 70 \text{ kg}^{-1} + 7 \text{ ml · kg}^{-1} \text{· min}^{-1} = 22.4 \\ \text{ml · kg}^{-1} \text{· min}^{-1}$$

Formulas are from reference (2).

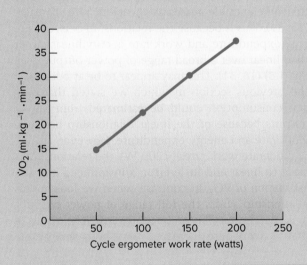

Figure 1.6 The relationship between work rate and $\dot{V}O_2$ cost is linear for cycling over a wide range of workloads. This figure illustrates the relative oxygen cost (i.e., $\dot{V}O_2$ per kilogram of body mass) of cycling for a 70-kg individual.

IN SUMMARY

- The energy cost of horizontal treadmill walking or running and cycling can be estimated with reasonable accuracy because the O_2 requirements increase as a linear function of speed and power, respectively.

CALCULATION OF EXERCISE EFFICIENCY

Efficiency describes the capacity to convert energy expenditure into work; it is expressed as the ratio of the work done to the energy put in to do the work. A more efficient individual uses less energy to do the same amount of work. Exercise physiologists have long searched for ways to mathematically describe the efficiency of human movement. Although measurements of gross, net, delta, and instantaneous efficiency have been used to describe exercise efficiency, one of the most common and simple expressions is **net efficiency** (6, 7, 10, 13, 16, 30, 31, 38, 39). Net efficiency is defined as the mathematical ratio of work output divided by the energy expended above rest:

$$\% \text{ Net Efficiency} = \frac{\text{Work Output}}{\text{Energy Expenditure}} \times 100$$

No machine is 100% efficient, because some energy is lost due to friction of the moving parts.

Likewise, the human machine is not 100% efficient because energy is lost as heat. It is estimated that the gasoline automobile engine operates with an efficiency of approximately 20% to 25%. Similarly, net efficiency for humans exercising on a cycle ergometer ranges from 15% to 27%, depending on work rate (13, 16, 31, 34, 39).

The calculation of net efficiency during cycle ergometer or treadmill exercise requires measurement of work output and the subject's energy expenditure during the exercise and at rest. It should be emphasized that $\dot{V}O_2$ measurements must be made during steady-state conditions. The work rate on the cycle ergometer or treadmill is calculated as discussed earlier and is generally expressed in kpm · min^{-1}. The energy expenditure during these types of exercise is usually estimated by first measuring $\dot{V}O_2$ (L · min^{-1}) using open-circuit spirometry and then converting it to either kcal or kJ using the exact conversion based on the specific nutrients being used as fuel (see Chap. 4 for details). In the following example, we will use 5 kcal · L^{-1} O_2 to show how to do this calculation. To do the computation using the net efficiency formula, both numerator and denominator must be expressed in similar terms. Because the numerator (work rate) is expressed in kpm · min^{-1} and energy expenditure is expressed in kcal · min^{-1}, we have to convert one unit to match the other. Consider the following sample calculation of net efficiency during submaximal, steady-state cycle ergometer exercise. Given:

Resistance against the cycle flywheel = 2 kp (19.6 N)
Cranking speed = 50 rpm
Resting $\dot{V}O_2$ = 0.25 L · min^{-1}
Steady-state exercise $\dot{V}O_2$ = 1.5 L · min^{-1}
Distance traveled per revolution = 6 m · rev^{-1}
Therefore:
Work rate = [2 kp × (50 m · rev^{-1} × 6 m · rev^{-1})]
    = 600 kpm · min^{-1}
Net energy expenditure = [1.5 L · min^{-1} − 0.25 L · min^{-1}]
    × 5 kcal · L^{-1} = 6.25 kcal · min^{-1}

To convert kpm to kcal: 600 kpm · min^{-1} ÷ 426.8 kpm · kcal^{-1} = 1.41 kcal · min^{-1}

$$\text{Hence, net efficiency} = \frac{1.41 \text{ kcal} \cdot \text{min}^{-1}}{6.25 \text{ kcal} \cdot \text{min}^{-1}} \times 100\%$$
$$= -22.6\%$$

Factors That Influence Exercise Efficiency

The efficiency of exercise is influenced by several factors: (1) the exercise work rate, (2) the speed of movement, and (3) the fiber composition of the muscles performing the exercise. A brief discussion of each of these factors follows.

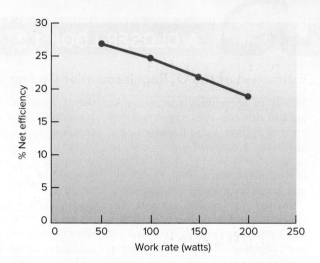

Figure 1.7 Changes in net efficiency during arm crank ergometry as a function of work rate.

Work Rate and Exercise Efficiency Figure 1.7 depicts the changes in net efficiency during cycle ergometry exercise as a function of work rate. Note that efficiency decreases as the work rate increases (13, 31). This is because the relationship between energy expenditure and work rate is curvilinear rather than linear over a broad range of power outputs (see Fig. 1.8) (16, 31). This may appear to be at odds with the previous section in which we stated that oxygen consumption could be estimated from power outputs because of the linear relationship between work rate and energy expenditure. However, at low-to-moderate work rates (<200 W), the relationship is close to linear and little error is introduced into the estimation of $\dot{V}O_2$. In contrast, when we look at this relationship across the full range of power outputs, it is clearly curvilinear (see Fig. 1.8). The result is that as work rate increases, total body energy ex-

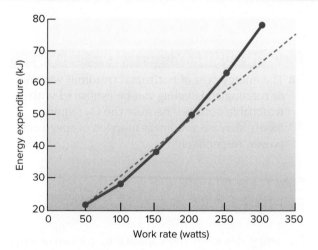

Figure 1.8 Relationship between energy expenditure and work rate. Note that energy expenditure increases as a curvilinear function of work rate.

penditure increases out of proportion to the work rate; this is indicative of a lower efficiency at higher power outputs.

Movement Speed and Efficiency Research has shown that there is an "optimum" speed of movement for any given work rate. Evidence suggests that the optimum speed of movement increases as the power output increases (8). In other words, at higher power outputs, a greater speed of movement is required to obtain optimum efficiency. At low-to-moderate work rates, a pedaling speed of 40 to 60 rpm is generally considered optimum during arm or cycle ergometry (12, 14, 16, 28, 31, 33). Note that any change in the speed of movement away from the optimum results in a decrease in efficiency (Fig. 1.9). This decline in efficiency at low speeds of movement is probably due to inertia (31). That is, there may be an increased energy cost of performing work when movements are slow and the limbs involved must repeatedly stop and start. The decline in efficiency associated with high-speed movement (at low-to-moderate work rates) may be because increasing speeds might augment muscular friction and thus increase internal work (6, 31).

Fiber Type and Efficiency People differ in their net efficiency during cycle ergometer exercise. Why? Recent evidence suggests that subjects with a high percentage of slow muscle fibers display a higher exercise efficiency compared to subjects with a high percentage of fast muscle fibers (see Chap. 8 for a discussion of muscle fiber types) (20, 22, 26, 32). The physiological explanation for this observation is that slow muscle fibers are more efficient than fast fibers. That is, slow fibers require less ATP per unit of work performed compared to fast fibers. It is clear that a higher efficiency is associated with better performance (20).

IN SUMMARY

- Net efficiency is defined as the mathematical ratio of work performed divided by the energy expenditure above rest and is expressed as a percentage:

$$\% \text{ Net Efficiency} = \frac{\text{Work Output}}{\text{Energy Expenditure}} \times 100$$

- The efficiency of exercise decreases as the exercise work rate increases. This occurs because the relationship between work rate and energy expenditure is curvilinear.
- To achieve maximal efficiency at any work rate, there is an optimal speed of movement.
- Exercise efficiency is greater in subjects who possess a high percentage of slow muscle fibers compared to subjects with a high percentage of fast fibers. This occurs because slow muscle fibers are more efficient than fast fibers.

RUNNING ECONOMY

As discussed previously, the computation of work is not generally possible during horizontal treadmill running, and thus a calculation of exercise efficiency cannot be performed. However, the measurement of the steady-state $\dot{V}O_2$ requirement (O_2 cost) of running at various speeds offers a means of comparing running economy (not efficiency) between two runners or groups of runners (10, 18, 19, 27, 29). Although these terms appear similar, the distinction is that efficiency refers to the ratio of work output to energy expenditure, and if "work" cannot be measured, efficiency cannot be calculated. In contrast, it is very easy to measure an individual's energy expenditure (oxygen uptake) at a specific running speed to determine running economy. Figure 1.10 compares the O_2

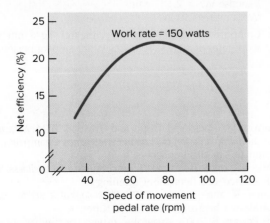

Figure 1.9   Effects of speed of movement (pedal rate) on exercise efficiency at 150 W. Note the optimum pedal rate for maximum efficiency at this work rate.

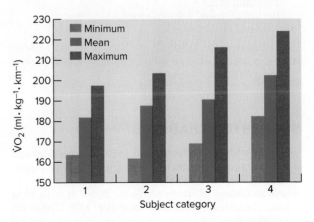

Figure 1.10   Minimum, mean, and maximum values for the oxygen cost of running, expressed in $ml \cdot kg^{-1} \cdot km^{-1}$, for elite runners (Category 1), sub-elite runners (Category 2), good runners (Category 3), and untrained individuals (Category 4).

cost of running among groups differing in running ability, from elite runners to untrained individuals (29). The economy of running is expressed (on the y-axis) in milliliters of oxygen used per kilogram of weight per kilometer ($ml \cdot kg^{-1} \cdot km^{-1}$). Not surprisingly, the average (mean) oxygen cost of running was lowest in elite runners and increased as ability level decreased. However, the average difference between the elite runners and the untrained individuals was only 10%, suggesting that systematic training has a limited effect on running economy. In contrast, one of the most interesting aspects of this study was the incredible variability in running economy within each group. There was about a 20% difference between the least and most economical runner in each group, independent of running ability. This amplifies the point that factors other than systematic training influence running economy.

That being said, there is no question that a better running economy is associated with a better performance in distance running events. This is addressed in more detail in Chaps. 19 and 20.

IN SUMMARY

- Although it is not easy to compute efficiency during horizontal running, the measurement of the O_2 cost of running ($ml \cdot kg^{-1} \cdot min^{-1}$) at any given speed offers a measure of running economy.
- Running economy is better, on average, in elite runners compared to those with less ability or untrained individuals. However, there is considerable variation in running economy between individuals, independent of running ability.

STUDY QUESTIONS

1. Define the following terms:
   a. work
   b. power
   c. percent grade
   d. relative $\dot{V}O_2$
   e. net efficiency
   f. metric system
   g. SI units

2. Calculate the total amount of work performed in 5 minutes of exercise on the cycle ergometer, given the following:

   Resistance on the flywheel = 25 N
   Cranking speed = 60 rpm
   Distance traveled per revolution = 6 meters

3. Compute total work and power output per minute for 10 minutes of treadmill exercise, given the following:

   Treadmill grade = 15%
   Horizontal speed = 90 $m \cdot min^{-1}$
   Subject's weight = 70 kg

4. Briefly describe the procedure used to estimate energy expenditure using (a) direct calorimetry and (b) indirect calorimetry.

5. Compute the estimated energy expenditure ($ml \cdot kg^{-1} \cdot min^{-1}$) during horizontal treadmill walking for the following examples:
   a. Treadmill speed = 50 $m \cdot min^{-1}$
      Subject's weight = 62 kg
   b. Treadmill speed = 80 $m \cdot min^{-1}$
      Subject's weight = 75 kg

6. Calculate the estimated O_2 cost of horizontal treadmill running ($ml \cdot kg^{-1} \cdot min^{-1}$) for a 70-kg subject at 150, 200, and 235 $m \cdot min^{-1}$.

7. Calculate the power output ($kpm \cdot min^{-1}$ and watts) during cycle ergometer exercise, given the following:

   Resistance on the flywheel = 3.0 kp
   Cranking speed = 50 rpm
   Distance traveled per revolution = 6 meters

8. Calculate net efficiency, given the following:

   Resting $\dot{V}O_2$ = 0.3 $L \cdot min^{-1}$
   Exercise $\dot{V}O_2$ = 2.1 $L \cdot min^{-1}$
   Work rate = 150 W

9. Compute the oxygen cost of cycling ($ml \cdot kg^{-1} \cdot min^{-1}$) at work rates of 50, 75, 100, 125 W for a 60-kg person.

SUGGESTED READINGS

American College of Sports Medicine. 2014. *Guidelines for Exercise Testing and Prescription.* Baltimore, MD: Lippincott, Williams & Wilkins.

American College of Sports Medicine. 2006. *ACSM's Metabolic Calculations Handbook.* Baltimore, MD: Lippincott, Williams & Wilkins.

Bentley, D., J. Newell, and D. Bishop. 2007. Incremental exercise test design and analysis: implications for performance diagnostics in endurance athletes. *Sports Medicine.* 37: 575–586.

Kenney, W.L., J. Wilmore, and D. Costill. 2015. *Physiology of Sport and Exercise.* Champaign, IL: Human Kinetics.

Morrow, J., A. Jackson, J. Disch, and D. Mood. 2016. *Measurement and Evaluation in Human Performance.* Champaign, IL: Human Kinetics Publishers.

Powers, S. and S. Dodd. 2017. *Total Fitness and Wellness.* San Francisco, CA: Benjamin Cummings.

Tanner, R. and C. Gore. 2013. *Physiological Tests for Elite Athletes.* Champaign, IL: Human Kinetics.

Van Praagh, E. 2007. Anaerobic fitness tests: what are we measuring? *Medicine and Sport Science.* 50: 26–45.

REFERENCES

1. **Ainsworth BE, Haskell WL, Herrmann SD, Meckes N, Bassett DR, Jr., Tudor-Locke C, et al**. Compendium of physical activities: a second update of codes and MET values. *Medicine & Science in Sports & Exercise* 43: 1575-1581, 2011.

2. **American College of Sports Medicine**. *Guidelines for Exercise Testing and Prescription*. Baltimore, MD: Lippincott, Williams & Wilkins, 2014.

3. **Åstrand P**. *Textbook of Work Physiology*. Champaign, IL: Human Kinetics, 2003.

4. **Bassett DRJ, Howley ET, Thompson DL, King GA, Strath SJ, McLaughlin JE, et al**. Validity of inspiratory and expiratory methods of measuring gas exchange with a computerized system. *Journal of Applied Physiology* 91: 218-224, 2001.

5. **Brooks G, Fahey T, and Baldwin K**. *Exercise Physiology: Human Bioenergetics and Its Applications*. New York, NY: McGraw-Hill, 2005.

6. **Cavanagh PR and Kram R**. Mechanical and muscular factors affecting the efficiency of human movement. *Medicine & Science in Sports & Exercise* 17: 326-331, 1985.

7. **Cavanagh PR and Kram R**. The efficiency of human movement—a statement of the problem. *Medicine & Science in Sports & Exercise* 17: 304-308, 1985.

8. **Coast JR and Welch HG**. Linear increase in optimal pedal rate with increased power output in cycle ergometry. *European Journal of Applied Physiology and Occupational Physiology* 53: 339-342, 1985.

9. **Consolazio C, Johnson R, and Pecora L**. *Physiological Measurements of Metabolic Function in Man*. New York, NY: McGraw-Hill, 1963.

10. **Daniels J and Daniels N**. Running economy of elite male and elite female runners. *Medicine & Science in Sports & Exercise* 24: 483-489, 1992.

11. **Daniels JT**. A physiologist's view of running economy. *Medicine & Science in Sports & Exercise* 17: 332-338, 1985.

12. **Deschenes MR, Kraemer WJ, McCoy RW, Volek JS, Turner BM, and Weinlein JC**. Muscle recruitment patterns regulate physiological responses during exercise of the same intensity. *American Journal of Physiology - Regulatory, Integrative and Comparative Physiology* 279: R2229-R2236, 2000.

13. **Donovan CM and Brooks GA**. Muscular efficiency during steady-rate exercise. II. Effects of walking speed and work rate. *Journal of Applied Physiology* 43: 431-439, 1977.

14. **Ferguson RA, Ball D, Krustrup P, Aagaard P, Kjaer M, Sargeant AJ, et al**. Muscle oxygen uptake and energy turnover during dynamic exercise at different contraction frequencies in humans. *Journal of Physiology* 536: 261-271, 2001.

15. **Fox E, Foss M, and Keteyian S**. *Fox's Physiological Basis for Exercise and Sport*. New York, NY: McGraw-Hill, 1998.

16. **Gaesser GA and Brooks GA**. Muscular efficiency during steady-rate exercise: effects of speed and work rate. *Journal of Applied Physiology* 38: 1132-1139, 1975.

17. **Grandjean E**. *Fitting the Task to the Man: An Ergonomic Approach*. New York, NY: International Publications Service, 1982.

18. **Hagan RD, Strathman T, Strathman L, and Gettman LR**. Oxygen uptake and energy expenditure during horizontal treadmill running. *Journal of Applied Physiology* 49: 571-575, 1980.

19. **Hopkins P and Powers SK**. Oxygen uptake during submaximal running in highly trained men and women. *American Corrective Therapy Journal* 36: 130-132, 1982.

20. **Horowitz JF, Sidossis LS, and Coyle EF**. High efficiency of type I muscle fibers improves performance. *International Journal of Sports Medicine* 15: 152-157, 1994.

21. **Howley ET and Thompson, DL**. *Health Fitness Instructor's Handbook*. Champaign, IL: Human Kinetics, 2017.

22. **Hunter GR, Newcomer BR, Larson-Meyer DE, Bamman MM, and Weinsier RL**. Muscle metabolic economy is inversely related to exercise intensity and type II myofiber distribution. *Muscle Nerve* 24: 654-661, 2001.

23. **Knoebel LK**. Energy metabolism. In: *Physiology*, edited by E. Selkurt Boston, MA: Little Brown & Co., 1984, pp. 635-650.

24. **Knuttgen H and Komi P**. Basic definitions for exercise. In: *Strength and Power in Sport*, edited by P. Komi Oxford, UK: Blackwell Scientific, 1992.

25. **Knuttgen HG**. Force, work, power, and exercise. *Medicine & Science in Sports* 10: 227-228, 1978.

26. **Lucia A, Rivero JL, Perez M, Serrano AL, Calbet JA, Santalla A, et al**. Determinants of $\dot{V}O_2$ kinetics at high power outputs during a ramp exercise protocol. *Medicine & Science in Sports & Exercise* 34: 326-331, 2002.

27. **Margaria R, Cerretelli P, Aghemo P, and Sassi G**. Energy cost of running. *Journal of Applied Physiology* 18: 367-370, 1963.

28. **Michielli DW and Stricevic M**. Various pedaling frequencies at equivalent power outputs. Effect on heart-rate response. *New York State Journal of Medicine* 77: 744-746, 1977.

29. **Morgan DW, Bransford DR, Costill DL, Daniels JT, Howley ET, and Krahenbuhl GS**. Variation in the aerobic demand of running among trained and untrained subjects. *Medicine & Science in Sports & Exercise* 27: 404-409, 1995.

30. **Moseley L and Jeukendrup AE**. The reliability of cycling efficiency. *Medicine & Science in Sports & Exercise* 33: 621-627, 2001.

31. **Powers SK, Beadle RE, and Mangum M**. Exercise efficiency during arm ergometry: effects of speed and work rate. *Journal of Applied Physiology* 56: 495-499, 1984.

32. **Scheuermann BW, Tripse McConnell JH, and Barstow TJ**. EMG and oxygen uptake responses during slow and fast ramp exercise in humans. *Experimental Physiology* 87: 91-100, 2002.

33. **Seabury JJ, Adams WC, and Ramey MR**. Influence of pedalling rate and power output on energy expenditure during bicycle ergometry. *Ergonomics* 20: 491-498, 1977.

34. **Shephard R**. *Physiology and Biochemistry of Exercise*. New York, NY: Praeger, 1982.

35. **Singleton W**. *The Body at Work*. London: Cambridge University Press, 1982.

36. **Spence A and Mason E**. *Human Anatomy and Physiology*. Menlo Park, CA: Benjamin-Cummings, 1992.

37. **Stegeman J**. *Exercise Physiology: Physiological Bases of Work and Sport*. Chicago, IL: Year Book Publishers, 1981.

38. **Stuart MK, Howley ET, Gladden LB, and Cox RH**. Efficiency of trained subjects differing in maximal oxygen uptake and type of training. *Journal of Applied Physiology* 50: 444-449, 1981.

39. **Whipp BJ and Wasserman K**. Efficiency of muscular work. *Journal of Applied Physiology* 26: 644-648, 1969.

2

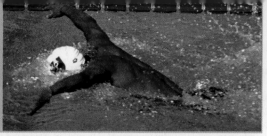

© Action Plus Sports Images/Alamy Stock Photo

Control of the Internal Environment

■ Objectives

By studying this chapter, you should be able to do the following:

1. Define the terms *homeostasis* and *steady state*.

2. Diagram and discuss a biological control system.

3. Give an example of a biological control system.

4. Explain the term *negative feedback*.

5. Define what is meant by the gain of a control system.

■ Outline

■ Key Terms

acclimation
adaptation
autocrine signaling
biological control system
cell signaling
control center
effectors
endocrine signaling
endocrine system
gain
heat shock proteins
homeostasis
intracrine signaling
juxtacrine signaling
negative feedback
paracrine signaling
sensor
steady state
stress proteins

More than 100 years ago, the French physiologist Claude Bernard observed that the "milieu interior" (internal environment) of the body remained remarkably constant despite a changing external environment (see A Look Back–Important People in Science). The fact that the body maintains a relatively constant internal environment in spite of stressors (e.g., heat, cold, exercise) is not an accident but is the result of many control systems (15). Control mechanisms that are responsible for maintaining a stable internal environment constitute a major chapter in exercise physiology, and it is helpful to examine their function in light of simple control theory. Therefore, this chapter introduces the concept of "control systems" and discusses how the body maintains a relatively constant internal environment during periods of stress. However, before you begin to read this chapter, take time to review Research Focus 2.1. This box provides an overview of how to interpret graphs and gain useful information from these important tools of science.

HOMEOSTASIS: DYNAMIC CONSTANCY

The term **homeostasis** is defined as the maintenance of a relatively constant internal environment. A similar term, **steady state,** is often used to denote a steady and unchanging level of some physiological variable (e.g., heart rate). Although the terms *homeostasis* and *steady state* are similar, they differ in the following way. The term *homeostasis* is commonly used to denote a relatively constant and normal internal environment during resting conditions (8, 16). In contrast, a steady state does not mean that a physiological variable is at resting values but that the physiological variable is constant and unchanging.

An example that is useful in distinguishing between these two terms is the case of body temperature during exercise. Figure 2.2 illustrates the changes in body core temperature during 60 minutes of constant-load submaximal exercise in a thermoneutral environment (i.e., low

RESEARCH FOCUS 2.1

How to Understand Graphs: A Picture Is Worth a Thousand Words

Throughout this book, we use line graphs to illustrate important concepts in exercise physiology. Although these same concepts can be explained in words, graphs are useful visual tools that can illustrate complicated relationships in a way that is easy to understand. Let's briefly review the basic concepts behind the construction of a line graph.

A line graph is used to illustrate relationships between two variables, that is, how one thing is affected by another. You may recall from one of your math courses that a variable is the generic term for any characteristic that changes. For example, in exercise physiology, heart rate is a variable that changes as a function of exercise intensity. Figure 2.1 is a line graph illustrating the relationship between heart rate and exercise intensity. In this illustration, exercise intensity (independent variable) is placed on the x-axis (horizontal) and heart rate (dependent variable) is

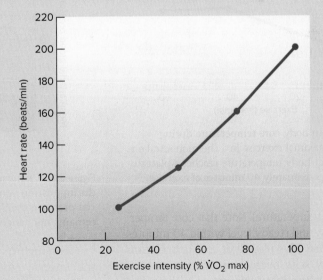

Figure 2.1
The relationship between heart rate and exercise intensity (expressed as a percent of $\dot{V}O_2$ max).

located on the *y*-axis (vertical). Heart rate is considered the dependent variable because it changes as a function of exercise intensity. Because exercise intensity is independent of heart rate, it is the independent variable. Note in Figure 2.1 that heart rate increases as a linear (straight-line) function of the exercise intensity. This type of line graph makes it easy to see what happens to heart rate when exercise intensity is increased.

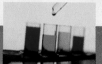

Claude Bernard—A Founding Father of Physiology

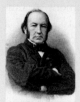

© Boyer/Roger Viollet/Getty Image

Claude Bernard (1813-1878) was a French physician and physiologist who is considered one of the founding "fathers of physiology." Indeed, Dr. Bernard's research and writings greatly improved our understanding of physiology during the nineteenth century, and he is credited with recognizing the importance of a constant internal environment. A brief overview of Dr. Bernard's life and contributions to physiology follows.

Claude Bernard was born in the French village of Saint-Julien and received his early education at the local Jesuit school. He attended Lyon College briefly, but left college to devote his efforts toward becoming a successful writer. At the age of 21, Dr. Bernard went to Paris to formally launch his writing career. However, following discussions with literature critics, Dr. Bernard abandoned writing and decided to study medicine as a career. As a medical intern at a Paris hospital, Dr. Bernard began to work with a senior French physician/physiologist, Francois Magendie, who was involved in research and teaching medical students. Dr. Bernard quickly became Magendie's deputy professor and later succeeded him as a professor.

During his research and medical career, Claude Bernard made many important contributions to physiology and medicine. One of his first important studies was aimed at understanding the role of the pancreas in digestion. He also discovered that the liver was capable of synthesizing glucose from products (e.g., lactate) removed from the blood. Additionally, Dr. Bernard discovered the vasomotor system, and this important discovery led to our understanding that the nervous system can act to both dilate and constrict blood vessels. Finally, although Dr. Bernard proposed the idea that maintaining a stable internal environment is a requirement for the body to remain healthy, he is not responsible for the concept of homeostasis. Indeed, the maintenance of a stable internal environment was termed "homeostasis" by Walter Cannon in 1932. The word *homeostasis* comes from the Greek words *homoios* (meaning the same) and *stasis* (meaning to stay or stand). For more details on the work of Walter Cannon, see A Look Back—Important People in Science in Chap. 5.

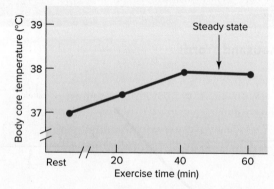

Figure 2.2 Changes in body core temperature during 60 minutes of submaximal exercise in a thermoneutral environment. Note that body temperature reaches a plateau (steady state) by approximately 40 minutes of exercise.

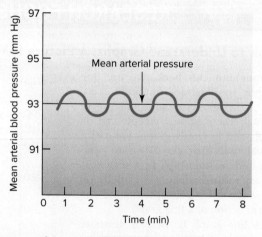

Figure 2.3 Changes in arterial blood pressure across time during resting conditions. Notice that although the arterial pressure oscillates across time, the mean pressure remains unchanged.

humidity and low temperature). Note that core temperature reaches a new and steady level within 40 minutes after start of exercise. This plateau of core temperature represents a steady state because temperature is constant; however, this constant temperature is above the normal resting body temperature and thus does not represent a true homeostatic condition. Therefore, the term *homeostasis* is generally reserved for describing normal resting conditions, and the term *steady state* is often applied to exercise wherein the physiological variable in question (i.e., body temperature) is constant but may not equal the "homeostatic" resting value.

Although the concept of homeostasis means that the internal environment is unchanging, this does not mean that the internal environment remains absolutely constant. In fact, most physiological variables vary around some "set" value, and thus homeostasis represents a rather dynamic constancy. An example of this dynamic constancy is the arterial blood pressure. Figure 2.3 shows the mean (average) arterial blood pressure during eight minutes of rest. Note the oscillatory change in arterial pressure, but the mean (average) arterial pressure remains around 93 mm Hg. The reason such an oscillation occurs in physiological variables is related to the "feedback" nature of biological control systems (16). This is discussed later in the chapter in the "Negative Feedback" section.

IN SUMMARY

- Homeostasis is defined as the maintenance of a constant or unchanging "normal" internal environment during unstressed conditions.
- The term *steady state* is also defined as a constant internal environment, but this does not necessarily mean that the internal environment is normal. When the body is in a steady state, a physiological variable (e.g., heart rate) is relatively constant.

CONTROL SYSTEMS OF THE BODY

The body has literally hundreds of different control systems, and the overall goal of most is to regulate some physiological variable at or near a constant value (16). The most intricate of these control systems reside inside the cell itself. These cellular control systems regulate cell activities such as protein breakdown and synthesis, energy production, and maintenance of the appropriate amounts of stored nutrients. Almost all organ systems of the body work to help maintain homeostasis (14). For example, the lungs (pulmonary system) and heart (circulatory system) work together to replenish oxygen and to remove carbon dioxide from the extracellular fluid. The fact that the cardiopulmonary system is usually able to maintain normal levels of oxygen and carbon dioxide even during periods of strenuous exercise is not an accident but the end result of a good control system.

NATURE OF THE CONTROL SYSTEMS

To develop a better understanding of how the body maintains a stable internal environment, let's begin with the analogy of a simple, nonbiological control system, such as a thermostat-regulated heating and cooling system in a home. Suppose the thermostat is set at 20°C. Any change in room temperature away from the 20°C "set point" results in the appropriate response by the temperature "control center" to return the room temperature to 20°C. If the room temperature rises above the set point, the thermostat signals the control center to turn off the furnace, which gradually returns the room temperature to 20°C. In contrast, a decrease in temperature below the set point results in the thermostat signaling the furnace to begin operation. In both cases, the response

by the control center was to correct the condition–low or high temperature–that initially turned it on.

Similar to the example of a mechanical control system, a **biological control system** is a series of interconnected components that maintain a chemical or physical parameter of the body near a constant value (16). Biological control systems are composed of three elements: (1) a sensor (or receptor); (2) a control center (i.e., center to integrate response); and (3) effectors (i.e., organs that produce the desired effect) (Fig. 2.4). The signal to begin the operation of a control system is the stimulus that represents a change in the internal environment (i.e., too much or too little of a regulated variable). The stimulus excites a **sensor** that is a receptor in the body capable of detecting change in the variable in question. The excited sensor then sends a message to the control center. The **control center** integrates the strength of the incoming signal from the sensor and sends a message to the **effectors** to bring about the appropriate response to correct the disturbance (i.e., desired effect). The return of the internal environment to normal (i.e., homeostasis) results in a decrease in the original stimulus that triggered the control system into action. This type of feedback loop is termed *negative feedback* and is the primary method responsible for maintaining homeostasis in the body (16) (Fig. 2.4). A more detailed discussion of negative feedback follows.

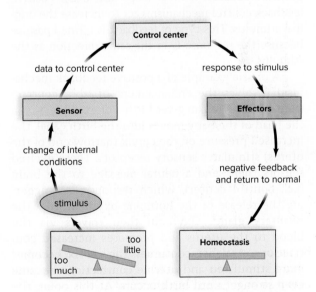

Figure 2.4 This schematic illustrates the components of a biological control system. The process begins with a change in the internal environment (i.e., stimulus), which excites a sensor to send information about the change to a control center. The control center makes an assessment of the amount of response that is needed to correct the problem and sends the appropriate message to the appropriate organs to bring about the desired effect. This effect is responsible for correcting the disturbance, and thus the stimulus is removed.

Negative Feedback

Most control systems of the body operate via **negative feedback** (16). Negative feedback is an important class of biological control systems in the body that serves to restore normal values of a variable to maintain homeostasis. An example of negative feedback is the respiratory system's regulation of the CO_2 concentration in extracellular fluid. In this case, an increase in extracellular CO_2 above normal levels triggers a receptor, which sends information to the respiratory control center to increase breathing and bring more air into the lungs. The effectors in this example are the respiratory muscles, which act to increase breathing. This increase in breathing will reduce extracellular CO_2 concentrations back to normal, thus reestablishing homeostasis. This type of feedback is termed *negative* because the response of the control system is negative (opposite) to the stimulus. In other words, this type of feedback is negative because the high concentration of carbon dioxide causes physiological events that decrease the concentration back to normal, which is negative to the initiating stimulus.

Positive Feedback

Although negative feedback is the primary type of feedback used to maintain homeostasis in the body, positive feedback control loops also exist. Positive feedback control mechanisms act to increase the original stimulus. This type of feedback is termed *positive* because the response is in the same direction as the stimulus.

A classic example of a positive feedback mechanism involves the enhancement of labor contractions when a woman gives birth. For example, when the head of the baby moves into the birth canal, the increased pressure on the cervix (narrow end of the uterus) stimulates sensory receptors. These excited sensors then send a neural message to the brain (i.e., control center), which responds by triggering the release of the hormone oxytocin from the pituitary gland. Oxytocin then travels via the blood to the uterus and promotes increased contractions. As labor continues, the cervix becomes more stimulated and uterine contractions become even stronger until birth occurs. At this point, the stimulus (i.e., the pressure) for oxytocin release stops and thus shuts off the positive feedback mechanism.

Gain of a Control System

The precision with which a control system maintains homeostasis is called the **gain** of the system. Gain can be thought of as the "capability" of the control system.

This means that a control system with a large gain is more capable of correcting a disturbance in homeostasis than a control system with a low gain. As you might predict, the most important control systems of the body have large gains. For example, control systems that regulate body temperature, breathing (i.e., pulmonary system), and delivery of blood (i.e., cardiovascular system) all have large gains. The fact that these systems have large gains is not surprising, given that these control systems all deal with life-and-death issues.

IN SUMMARY

- A biological control system is composed of a receptor, a control center, and an effector.
- Most control systems act by way of negative feedback.
- The degree to which a control system maintains homeostasis is termed the *gain* of the system. A control system with a large gain is more capable of maintaining homeostasis than a system with a low gain.

EXAMPLES OF HOMEOSTATIC CONTROL

To better understand biological control systems, let's consider a few examples of homeostatic control.

Regulation of Body Temperature

An excellent example of a homeostatic control system that uses negative feedback is the regulation of body temperature (15). The sensors in this system are thermal receptors located in several body locations. The control center for temperature regulation is located in the brain, and when body temperature increases above normal, temperature sensors send a neural message to the control center that temperature is above normal (top portion of Fig. 2.5). The control center responds to this stimulus by directing a response to promote heat loss (i.e., skin blood vessels dilate and sweating occurs). When body temperature returns to normal, the control center is inactivated.

When body temperature falls below normal, temperature sensors send these data to the control center in the brain, which responds by preventing the loss of body heat (e.g., blood vessels in the skin constrict); this action serves to conserve heat (bottom portion of Fig. 2.5). Again, when body temperature returns to normal, the control center becomes inactive. Complete details about how the body regulates temperature during exercise are presented in Chap. 12.

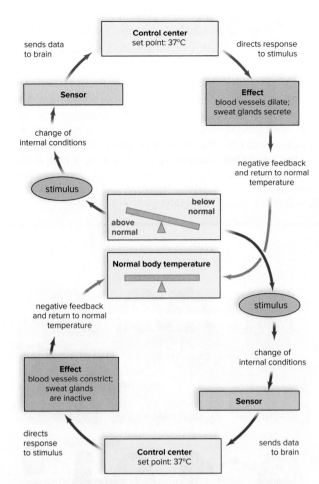

Figure 2.5 Illustration of the negative feedback that is used to regulate body temperature. See text for details of how this system operates.

Regulation of Blood Glucose

Maintaining homeostasis is an important function of the **endocrine system** (see Chap. 5). The body contains eight major endocrine glands, which synthesize and secrete blood-borne chemical substances called *hormones*. Hormones are transported via the circulatory system throughout the body as an aid to regulate circulatory and metabolic functions (4, 16). An example of the endocrine system's role in the maintenance of homeostasis is the control of blood glucose levels. Indeed, in health, the blood glucose concentration is carefully regulated by the endocrine system. For example, the hormone insulin regulates cellular uptake and the metabolism of glucose and is therefore important in the regulation of the blood glucose concentration. After consuming a large carbohydrate meal, blood glucose levels increase above normal. This rise in blood glucose signals the pancreas to release insulin, which then lowers blood glucose by increasing cellular uptake. Failure of the blood glucose control system results in disease (diabetes) and is discussed in Clinical Applications 2.1.

EXERCISE: A TEST OF HOMEOSTATIC CONTROL

Muscular exercise presents a dramatic test of the body's homeostatic control systems because exercise has the potential to disrupt many homeostatic variables. For example, during heavy exercise, skeletal muscle produces large amounts of heat, which pose a challenge for the body to prevent overheating. Additionally, heavy exercise results in large increases in muscle O_2 requirements, and large amounts of CO_2 are produced. These changes must be countered by increases in breathing (pulmonary ventilation) and blood flow to increase O_2 delivery to the exercising muscle and remove metabolically produced CO_2. The body's control systems must respond rapidly to prevent drastic alterations in the internal environment.

In a strict sense, the body rarely maintains true homeostasis while performing intense exercise or during prolonged exercise in a hot or humid environment. Heavy exercise or prolonged work results in disturbances in the internal environment that are generally too great for even the highest gain control systems to overcome, and thus a steady state is not possible. Severe disturbances in homeostasis result in fatigue and, ultimately, cessation of exercise (3, 7, 13). Understanding how various body control systems minimize exercise-induced disturbances in homeostasis is extremely important to the exercise physiology student and is thus a major theme of this textbook. Specific details about individual control systems (e.g., circulatory, respiratory) that affect the internal environment during exercise are discussed in Chaps. 4 through 12. Furthermore, improved exercise performance following exercise training is largely due to training adaptations that result in a better maintenance of homeostasis; this is discussed in Chap. 13. In the next segment, we highlight the processes that promote exercise-induced improvements in the body's homeostatic control mechanisms.

EXERCISE IMPROVES HOMEOSTATIC CONTROL VIA CELLULAR ADAPTATION

The term **adaptation** refers to a change in the structure and function of a cell or an organ system that results in an improved ability to maintain homeostasis during stressful conditions. Indeed, a cell's ability to respond to a challenge is not fixed and can be improved by prolonged exposure to a specific stress (e.g., regular bouts of exercise). Also, cells can adapt to environmental stresses, such as heat stress due to a hot environment. This type of environmental

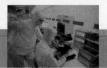
Failure of a Biological Control System Results in Disease

Failure of any component of a biological control system results in a disturbance in homeostasis. A classic illustration of the failure of a biological control system is the disease diabetes. Although there are two forms of diabetes (type 1 and type 2), both types are characterized by abnormally high blood glucose levels (called hyperglycemia). In type 1 diabetes, the beta cells in the pancreas do not function properly (beta cells produce insulin). Hence, insulin is no longer produced and released into the blood to promote the transport of glucose into tissues. Therefore, this malfunction of pancreatic beta cells represents a failure of the "effector" component of this control system. If insulin cannot be released in response to an increase in blood glucose following a high-carbohydrate meal, glucose transport into cells is impaired and the end result is hyperglycemia and diabetes.

---

adaptation–the improved function of an existing homeostatic system–is known as **acclimation** (16).

It is well known that regular bouts of exercise promote cellular changes that result in an improved ability to preserve homeostasis during the "stress" of exercise (11, 12). This improved ability of cells and organ systems to maintain homeostasis occurs via a variety of cell signaling mechanisms. The term **cell signaling** refers to a system of communication between cells that coordinates cellular activities. The ability of cells to detect changes in their internal environment and correctly respond to this change is essential in the maintenance of homeostasis. It should be no surprise that a variety of cell signaling mechanisms coordinate all the different functions of the body. As you read this text, you will encounter five different cell signaling mechanisms. These signaling mechanisms are illustrated in Figure 2.6 and are briefly defined next.

■ **Intracrine signaling.** Intracrine signaling occurs when a chemical messenger is produced inside a cell that triggers a signaling pathway within the same cell that leads to a specific response. Examples of intracrine signaling are provided in Chap. 13, where we discuss the cell signaling mechanisms responsible for skeletal muscle adaptation to exercise training.

■ **Juxtacrine signaling.** Some cells communicate by cell-to-cell contact, in which the cytoplasm of one cell is in contact with the cytoplasm of another through small junctions that connect the two cell membranes. This type of cell signaling is called juxtacrine signaling. You will see this in Chap. 9 as the method by which one heart cell signals to an adjacent cell to contract; this signaling mechanism ensures that the heart contracts in a smooth and effective manner.

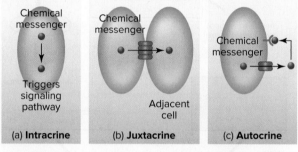

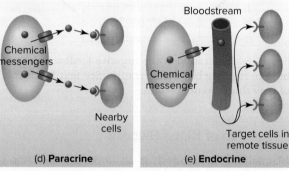

Figure 2.6 Illustration of the five major cell signaling mechanisms that participate in the control of homeostasis and cellular adaptation. (*a*) Intracrine signaling occurs when a chemical messenger is produced inside a cell and triggers an intracellular signaling pathway that leads to a specific cellular response. (*b*) Juxtacrine signaling occurs when the cytoplasm of one cell is in contact with the cytoplasm of another cell through small junctions that bridge the two cell membranes. This permits a chemical messenger from one cell to move into the neighboring cell. (*c*) Autocrine signaling occurs when a cell produces and releases a chemical messenger into the extracellular fluid that acts upon the cell producing the signal. (*d*) Paracrine signaling occurs when one cell produces and releases a chemical messenger that acts on nearby cells to bring about a coordinated response. (*e*) Endocrine signaling occurs when a cell releases a chemical messenger (hormone) into the blood and this hormone is then carried by the blood stream throughout the body to target cells.

- **Autocrine signaling.** Autocrine signaling occurs when a cell produces and releases a chemical messenger into the extracellular fluid that acts upon the cell producing the signal. For example, during resistance training, autocrine signaling within the muscle cell triggers the DNA in the nucleus to produce more contractile protein, which in turn increases the size of that muscle cell. This type of cell signaling is discussed in Chap. 13. A Closer Look 2.1 presents an overview of how cell signaling can promote protein synthesis in cells.

- **Paracrine signaling.** Some cells produce signals that act locally on nearby cells (paracrine signals) to bring about a coordinated response. For example, we will see in Chap. 6 how immune cells communicate with each other to generate a coordinated attack to protect the body from infection and injury. Synaptic signaling is another type of paracrine signaling that occurs in the nervous system (Chap. 7).

- **Endocrine signaling.** Finally, some cells release chemical signals (hormones) into the blood, and these hormones are then carried throughout the body. However, the cells that respond to the hormone are only cells with a receptor specific to this hormone. This is called endocrine signaling and is covered in Chap. 5.

STRESS PROTEINS ASSIST IN THE REGULATION OF CELLULAR HOMEOSTASIS

A disturbance in cellular homeostasis occurs when a cell is faced with a "stress" that surpasses its ability to defend against this particular type of disturbance. A classic illustration of how cells use control systems to combat stress (i.e., disturbances in homeostasis) is termed the *cellular stress response*. The cellular stress response is a biological control system in cells that battles homeostatic disturbances by manufacturing proteins designed to defend against stress. A brief overview of the cellular stress response system and how it protects cells against homeostatic disturbances follows.

At the cellular level, proteins are important in maintaining homeostasis. For example, proteins play critical roles in normal cell function by serving as intracellular transporters or as enzymes that catalyze chemical reactions. Damage to cellular proteins by stress (e.g., low pH or free radicals) can result in cell damage and a disturbance in homeostasis. To combat this type of disruption in homeostasis, cells respond by rapidly manufacturing protective proteins called **stress proteins**

(5, 9, 10). The term *stress protein* refers to a family of proteins that are manufactured in cells in response to a variety of stresses (e.g., high temperature). One of the most important families of stress proteins are called **heat shock proteins.** It is well known that exercise training results in significant increases in the production of numerous heat shock proteins within the heart and the trained skeletal muscle (10, 12).

Heat shock proteins were discovered by an Italian scientist following the observation that exposure of flies to heat stress resulted in the synthesis of select proteins in the cells of the flies. Note that production of heat shock proteins can also be triggered by other types of stress such as free radical production, low pH, and inflammation. As a consequence, heat shock proteins are also referred to as stress proteins.

The process of synthesizing heat shock proteins begins with a stressor that promotes protein damage (e.g., heat or free radicals). After synthesis, heat shock proteins go to work to protect the cell by repairing damaged proteins and restoring homeostasis. Many families of heat shock proteins exist and each family plays a specific role in protecting cells and maintaining homeostasis. For a detailed discussion of heat shock proteins and their effect on protecting skeletal muscle fibers against damage see Kim (2015) in the suggested readings.

IN SUMMARY

- Exercise presents a challenge to the body's control systems to maintain homeostasis. In general, the body's many control systems are capable of maintaining a steady state during most types of submaximal exercise in a cool environment. However, intense exercise or prolonged work in a hot environment (i.e., high temperature/ humidity) may exceed the ability of a control system to maintain a steady state, and severe disturbances in homeostasis often occur.

- Acclimation is the change that occurs in response to repeated environmental stresses and results in the improved function of an existing homeostatic system.

- Cell signaling is defined as a system of communication that governs cellular activities and coordinates cell actions.

- A variety of cell signaling mechanisms participate in the regulation of homeostasis and are required to regulate cellular adaptation. The major cell signaling mechanisms include (1) intracrine signaling, (2) juxtacrine signaling, (3) autocrine signaling, (4) paracrine signaling, and (5) endocrine signaling.

- Exercise-induced protein synthesis occurs via cell signaling events that lead to the activation of genes, which leads to protein synthesis and to an improved ability to maintain homeostasis during the "stress" of exercise (Closer Look 2.1).

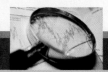

An Overview of Cellular Protein Synthesis

Often, the exercise-induced improved ability of cells to maintain homeostasis results from increased synthesis of the specific proteins that participate in maintaining cellular balance. Exercise-induced protein synthesis occurs via cell signaling events that ultimately lead to the activation of genes and, subsequently, protein synthesis (1, 2). A brief overview of how cell signaling results in protein synthesis follows.

Human cells contain between 20,000 and 25,000 genes, and each gene is responsible for the synthesis of a specific protein (6). Cellular signals regulate protein synthesis by "turning on" or "turning off" specific genes. Figure 2.7 illustrates the process of exercise-induced protein synthesis in a muscle fiber. The process begins with the "stress" of exercise stimulating a specific cell signaling pathway that results in the activation of a molecule called a transcriptional activator. Transcriptional activators are responsible for "turning

on" specific genes to synthesize new proteins. Once activated in the sarcoplasm, the transcriptional activator moves into the nucleus and binds to the promoter region of the gene. Activation of the gene's promoter provides the stimulus for transcription. Transcription results in the formation of a message called messenger RNA (mRNA), which contains the genetic information for a specific protein's amino acid sequence. The message (i.e., mRNA) leaves the nucleus and travels through the sarcoplasm to the ribosome, which is the site of protein synthesis. At the ribosome, the mRNA is translated into a specific protein. Individual proteins differ in structure and function; this is important because the types of proteins contained in a muscle fiber determine the fiber characteristic and its ability to perform specific types of exercise. Therefore, understanding the cellular signaling pathways that promote or inhibit gene activation in skeletal muscle is of major

importance to exercise physiologists. Details of how exercise promotes skeletal muscle adaptation by altering gene expression are discussed in Chap. 13.

Note that dissimilar modes of exercise promote the expression of different genes in the active muscle fibers. For example, resistance exercise and endurance exercise promote the activation of different cell signaling pathways; therefore, different genes are activated, resulting in the expression of diverse proteins. However, you will also learn that resistance exercise and endurance exercise activate several common genes, such as the genes that express stress proteins. Numerous stress proteins exist in cells and play an important role in maintaining cellular homeostasis. A brief introduction to stress proteins and their role in the control of cellular homeostasis is discussed in the section titled "Stress Proteins Assist in the Regulation of Cellular Homeostasis."

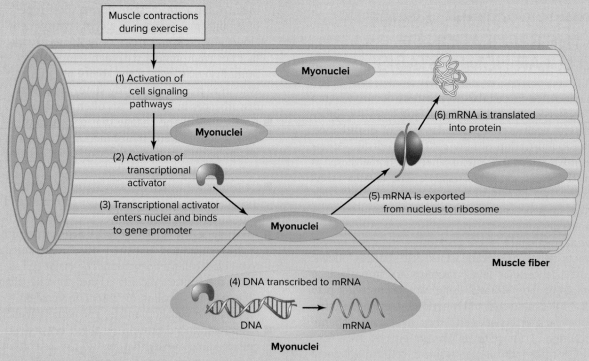

Figure 2.7 Illustration of how exercise promotes the activation of cell signaling pathways in muscle fibers that lead to increased gene expression and the synthesis of new proteins.

STUDY QUESTIONS

1. Define the term *homeostasis*. How does it differ from the term *steady state*?
2. Cite an example of a biological homeostatic control system.
3. Draw a simple diagram that demonstrates the relationships between the components of a biological control system.
4. Briefly explain the role of the receptor, the integrating center, and the effector organ in a biological control system.
5. Explain the term *negative feedback*. Give a biological example of negative feedback.
6. Discuss the concept of gain associated with a biological control system.
7. Define cell signaling and outline the five types of cell signaling mechanisms that participate in the regulation of homeostasis and cellular adaptation.
8. List the steps that lead to exercise-induced increases in protein synthesis in skeletal muscles.

SUGGESTED READINGS

Fox, S. 2015. *Human Physiology*. New York, NY: McGraw-Hill.

Kim, K. 2015. Interaction between HSP70 and iNOS in skeletal muscle injury and repair. *Journal of Exercise Rehabilitation*. 11: 240-243.

Widmaier, E., H. Raff, and K. Strang. 2015. *Vander's Human Physiology*. New York, NY: McGraw-Hill.

REFERENCES

1. **Alberts B, Johnson A, and Raff J.** *Molecular Biology of the Cell*. New York, NY: Garland Science, 2014.
2. **Berk H, Kaiser C, and Krieger M.** *Molecular Cell Biology*. New York, NY: W. H. Freeman, 2012.
3. **Fitts RH.** The cross-bridge cycle and skeletal muscle fatigue. *Journal of Applied Physiology* 104: 551-558, 2008.
4. **Fox S.** *Human Physiology*. New York, NY: McGraw-Hill, 2015.
5. **Harkins MS.** Exercise regulates heat shock proteins and nitric oxide. *Exercise and Sport Sciences Reviews* 37: 73-77, 2009.
6. **Karp G, Iwasa J, and Marshall W.** *Karp's Cell and Molecular Biology*. Hoboken, NJ: Wiley, 2016.
7. **Lamb GD.** Mechanisms of excitation-contraction uncoupling relevant to activity-induced muscle fatigue. *Applied Physiology, Nutrition, and Metabolism (Physiologie appliquee, nutrition et metabolisme)* 34: 368-372, 2009.
8. **Marieb E and Hoehn K.** *Human Anatomy and Physiology*. Menlo Park, CA: Benjamin-Cummings, 2015.
9. **Morton JP, Kayani AC, McArdle A, and Drust B.** The exercise-induced stress response of skeletal muscle, with specific emphasis on humans. *Sports Medicine* 39: 643-662, 2009.
10. **Noble EG, Milne KJ, and Melling CW.** Heat shock proteins and exercise: a primer. *Applied Physiology, Nutrition, and Metabolism (Physiologie appliquee, nutrition et metabolisme)* 33: 1050-1065, 2008.
11. **Powers S, Nelson W, and Hudson M.** *Free Radical Biology and Medicine* 51: 942-950, 2011.
12. **Powers S, Smuder A, Kavazis A, and Quindry A.** Mechanisms of exercise-induced cardioprotection. *Physiology* 29: 27-38, 2014.
13. **Reid MB.** Free radicals and muscle fatigue: of ROS, canaries, and the IOC. *Free Radical Biology & Medicine* 44: 169-179, 2008.
14. **Saladin K.** *Anatomy and Physiology*. Boston, MA: McGraw-Hill, 2014.
15. **Schlader ZJ, Stannard SR, and Mundel T.** Human thermoregulatory behavior during rest and exercise—a prospective review. *Physiology & Behavior* 99: 269-275, 2010.
16. **Widmaier E, Raff H, and Strang K.** *Vander's Human Physiology*. Boston, MA: McGraw-Hill, 2015.

3

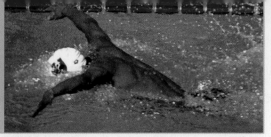

© Action Plus Sports Images/Alamy Stock Photo

Bioenergetics

■ Objectives

By studying this chapter, you should be able to do the following:

1. Discuss the function of the cell membrane, nucleus, and mitochondria.

2. Define the following terms: (1) *endergonic reactions*, (2) *exergonic reactions*, (3) *coupled reactions*, and (4) *bioenergetics*.

3. Describe the role of enzymes as catalysts in cellular chemical reactions.

4. List and discuss the nutrients that are used as fuels during exercise.

5. Describe the structure and function of ATP in the cell.

6. Discuss the biochemical pathways involved in anaerobic ATP production.

7. Describe the aerobic production of ATP.

8. Describe how the metabolic pathways involved in bioenergetics are regulated.

9. Discuss the interaction between aerobic and anaerobic ATP production during exercise.

10. Identify the enzymes that are considered rate limiting in glycolysis and the citric acid cycle.

■ Outline

■ Key Terms

acetyl-CoA
activation energy
adenosine diphosphate (ADP)
adenosine triphosphate (ATP)
aerobic
anaerobic
ATPase
ATP-PC system
beta oxidation
bioenergetics
cell membrane
chemiosmotic hypothesis
citric acid cycle (also called the Krebs cycle)
coupled reactions
cytoplasm
electron transport chain
endergonic reactions
enzymes
exergonic reactions
flavin adenine dinucleotide (FAD)
glucose
glycogen
glycogenolysis
glycolysis
inorganic
inorganic phosphate (P_i)
isocitrate dehydrogenase
Krebs cycle (also called citric acid cycle)
lactate
metabolism
mitochondrion
molecular biology
nicotinamide adenine dinucleotide (NAD^+)
nucleus
organic
oxidation
oxidative phosphorylation
phosphocreatine (PC)
phosphofructokinase (PFK)
reduction

Thousands of chemical reactions occur throughout the body during each minute of the day. Collectively, these reactions are called **metabolism**. Metabolism is broadly defined as the total of all cellular reactions and includes chemical pathways that result in the synthesis of molecules (anabolic reactions), as well as the breakdown of molecules (catabolic reactions).

Because energy is required by all cells, it is not surprising that cells possess chemical pathways that are capable of converting foodstuffs (i.e., fats, proteins, carbohydrates) into a biologically usable form of energy. This metabolic process is termed **bioenergetics**. For you to run, jump, or swim, skeletal muscle cells must be able to continuously extract energy from food nutrients. Indeed, in order to continue to contract, muscle cells must have a continuous source of energy. Given the importance of cellular energy production during exercise, it is essential that students of exercise physiology develop a thorough understanding of bioenergetics. Therefore, this chapter will introduce both general and specific concepts associated with bioenergetics.

CELL STRUCTURE

Cells were discovered in the seventeenth century by the English scientist Robert Hooke. Advancements in the microscope over the past 300 years have led to improvements in our understanding of cell structure and function. To understand bioenergetics, it is important to have some appreciation of cell structure and function. Four elements (an element is a basic chemical substance) compose over 95% of the human body. These include oxygen (65%), carbon (18%), hydrogen (10%), and nitrogen (3%) (10). Additional elements found in rather small amounts in the body include sodium, iron, zinc, potassium, magnesium, chloride, and calcium. These various elements are linked by chemical bonds to form molecules or compounds. Compounds that contain carbon are called **organic** compounds, whereas those that do not contain carbon are termed **inorganic**. For example, water (H_2O) lacks carbon and is thus inorganic. In contrast, proteins, fats, and carbohydrates contain carbon and are organic compounds.

As the basic functional unit of the body, the cell is a highly organized factory capable of synthesizing the large number of compounds necessary for normal cellular function. Figure 3.1 illustrates the structure of a muscle cell (muscle cells are also called muscle fibers). Note that not all cells are alike, nor do they all perform the same functions. Nonetheless, in general, cell structure can be divided into three major parts:

1. **Cell membrane** The cell membrane (also called the *sarcolemma* in skeletal muscle fibers) is a semipermeable barrier that separates the cell from the extracellular environment. Two important functions of the cell membrane are to enclose the components of the cell and to regulate the passage of various types of substances in and out of the cell (1, 10, 21).

2. **Nucleus** The nucleus is a large, round body within the cell that contains the cellular genetic components (genes). Genes are composed of double strands of deoxyribonucleic acids (DNA), which serve as the basis for the genetic code. Genes regulate protein synthesis, which determines cell composition and controls cellular activity. The field of **molecular biology** is concerned with understanding the regulation of genes and is introduced in A Closer Look 3.1. Note that although most cells have only one nucleus, skeletal muscle fibers are unique in that they have many nuclei along the entire length of the muscle fiber.

3. **Cytoplasm** (called *sarcoplasm* in muscle cells) This is the fluid portion of the cell between the nucleus and the cell membrane. Contained within the cytoplasm are various organelles (tiny structures) that are concerned with specific cellular functions. One such organelle, the **mitochondrion,** is called the powerhouse of the cell and is involved in the oxidative conversion of foodstuffs into usable cellular energy. The important role that mitochondria plays in skeletal muscle bioenergetics will be discussed later in this chapter. See Research Focus 3.1 for details about the structure and cellular locations of mitochondria contained in skeletal muscle fibers. Also contained in the cytoplasm are the enzymes that regulate the breakdown of glucose (i.e., glycolysis). Further, in muscle cells, the contractile proteins (also called myofibrillar proteins) occupy a large portion of the cytoplasm.

BIOLOGICAL ENERGY TRANSFORMATION

All energy on earth comes from the sun. Plants use light energy from the sun to drive chemical reactions to form carbohydrates, fats, and proteins. Animals (including humans) then eat plants and other animals to obtain the energy required to maintain cellular activities.

Energy exists in several forms (e.g., electrical, mechanical, chemical), and all forms of energy are interchangeable (21). For example, muscle fibers convert chemical energy obtained from carbohydrates, fats, or proteins into mechanical energy to perform movement. The bioenergetic process of converting chemical energy to mechanical energy requires a series of tightly controlled chemical reactions. Before discussing the specific reactions involved, we provide a review of cellular chemical reactions.

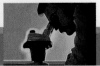
Skeletal Muscle Fibers Contain Two Distinct Subpopulations of Mitochondria

As discussed in the text, in order to perform physical activity (e.g., running), skeletal muscle must have a continuous supply of energy. Much of this cellular energy comes from aerobic metabolism in the mitochondrion, which harnesses the energy from food and converts this chemical energy into usable energy for muscle contraction (details of this process are provided later in this chapter). To supply the muscle with a constant supply of usable energy, skeletal muscle fibers contain two subpopulations of mitochondria that differ in cellular location: (1) subsarcolemmal mitochondria that are located directly beneath the cell membrane (sarcolemma) and (2) intermyofibrillar mitochondria that are found near the myofibrillar (i.e., contractile) proteins (Fig. 3.1) (14). The different cellular locations for these two subpopulations are by design. The subsarcolemma mitochondria produce the cellular energy needed to maintain active transport of ions (e.g., sodium) across the sarcolemma. In contrast, the primary job of the intermyofibrillar mitochondria is to provide the energy needed to sustain muscle contraction (Chap. 8). Together, these mitochondria form a network to provide all regions of the muscle fiber with a constant supply of energy.

Mitochondria are usually pictured as small bean-shaped structures (Fig. 3.1). However, in muscle cells, mitochondria are dynamic and are constantly changing to form a mitochondrial network (called a reticulum) (14). Moreover, muscle fibers are constantly producing new mitochondria (i.e., mitochondrial biogenesis), and damaged mitochondria are continuously degraded and eliminated from the fiber. Regular bouts of endurance exercise (e.g., running) promote a significant increase in mitochondrial biogenesis and will be discussed in detail in Chap. 13.

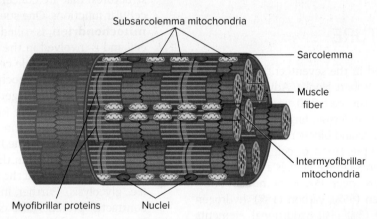

Figure 3.1 A muscle cell (fiber) and some of its key components including the nucleus, contractile proteins (myofibrillar proteins), and the two subpopulations of mitochondria (i.e., subsarcolemmal mitochondria and myofibrillar mitochondria). See text for details.

Cellular Chemical Reactions

Energy transfer in the body occurs via the release of energy trapped within chemical bonds of various molecules. Chemical bonds that contain relatively large amounts of potential energy are termed *high-energy bonds*. As mentioned previously, bioenergetics is concerned with the transfer of energy from foodstuffs into a biologically usable form. This energy transfer in the cell occurs as a result of a series of chemical reactions. Many of these reactions require that energy be added to the reactants **(endergonic reactions)** before the reaction will "proceed." However, when energy is added to the reaction, the products contain more free energy than the original reactants.

Reactions that give off energy as a result of chemical processes are known as **exergonic reactions.** Note that the words *endergonic* and *endothermic* can be used interchangeably. The same applies for the words *exergonic* and *exothermic*. Figure 3.3 illustrates that the amount of total energy released via exergonic reactions is the same whether the energy is released in one single reaction (combustion) or many small, controlled steps (i.e., cellular oxidation) that usually occur in cells.

Coupled Reactions Many of the chemical reactions that occur within the cell are called **coupled reactions**. Coupled reactions are reactions that are linked, with the liberation of free energy in one reaction being used to "drive" a second reaction.

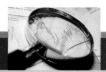

A CLOSER LOOK 3.1

Molecular Biology and Exercise Physiology

Molecular biology is the branch of biology that deals with the molecular basis of cellular function. More specifically, molecular biology is concerned with how cells regulate gene activity and the synthesis of proteins that determine the characteristics of cells. The field of molecular biology overlaps with other areas of biology, including physiology, biochemistry, and genetics (Fig. 3.2).

Recall from Chap. 2 that each gene is responsible for the synthesis of a specific cellular protein. Cellular signals regulate protein synthesis by "turning on" or "turning off" specific genes. Therefore, understanding the signals that promote or inhibit protein synthesis is of importance to exercise physiologists.

The technical revolution in the field of molecular biology offers another opportunity to make use of scientific information for the improvement of human health and athletic performance. For example, exercise training results in modifications in the amounts and types of proteins synthesized in the exercised muscles (see Chap. 13 for details). Indeed, it is well known that regular strength training results in an increase in muscle size due to an increase in contractile proteins. The techniques of molecular biology provide the exercise physiologist with the "tools" to understand how exercise controls gene function and the synthesis of new proteins. Ultimately, understanding how exercise promotes the synthesis of specific proteins in muscles will allow the exercise scientist to design the most effective training program to achieve the desired training effects.

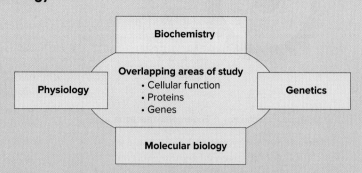

Figure 3.2 The different fields of biology have overlapping areas of study.

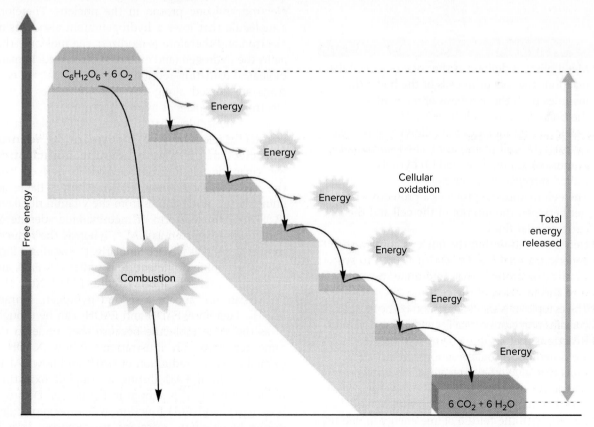

Figure 3.3 The breakdown of glucose into carbon dioxide and water via cellular oxidation results in a release of energy. Reactions that result in the release of free energy are termed *exergonic*.

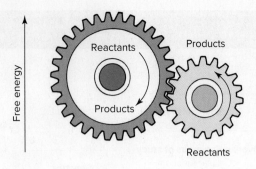

Free energy

Reactants
Products
Products
Reactants

Exergonic reactions   Endergonic reactions

Figure 3.4 Illustration of exergonic and endergonic reactions. Note that the energy given off by the exergonic reaction (larger, left gear) powers the endergonic reactions (smaller, right gear).

Figure 3.4 illustrates this point. In this example, energy released by an exergonic reaction is used to drive an energy-requiring reaction (endergonic reaction) in the cell. This is like two meshed gears in which the turning of one (energy-releasing, exergonic gear) causes the movement of the second (endergonic gear). In other words, energy-liberating reactions are "coupled" to energy-requiring reactions. Oxidation-reduction reactions are an important type of coupled reaction and are discussed in the next section.

IN SUMMARY

- Metabolism is defined as the total of all cellular reactions that occur in cells of the body; this includes both the synthesis of molecules and the breakdown of molecules.
- Cell structure includes the following three major parts: (1) cell membrane (called *sarcolemma* in muscle), (2) nucleus, and (3) cytoplasm (called *sarcoplasm* in muscle).
- The cell membrane provides a protective barrier between the interior of the cell and the extra cellular fluid.
- Genes located within the nucleus contain the genetic material (i.e., DNA) that is used to synthesize the proteins that determine the structure and function of the cell.
- The cytoplasm is the fluid portion of the cell and contains numerous organelles and cellular proteins.
- Reactions that require energy to be added are called endergonic reactions, whereas reactions that give off energy are called exergonic reactions.
- Coupled reactions are reactions that are connected, with the release of free energy in one reaction being used to drive the second reaction.

Oxidation–Reduction Reactions

The process of removing an electron from an atom or molecule is called **oxidation**. The addition of an electron to an atom or molecule is referred to as **reduction**. Oxidation and reduction are always coupled reactions because a molecule cannot be oxidized unless it donates electrons to another atom. The molecule that donates the electron is known as the *reducing agent*, whereas the one that accepts the electrons is called an *oxidizing agent*. Note that some molecules can act as both an oxidizing agent and a reducing agent. For example, when molecules play both roles, they can gain electrons in one reaction and then pass these electrons to another molecule to produce an oxidation-reduction reaction. Hence, coupled oxidation-reduction reactions are analogous to a bucket brigade, with electrons being passed along in the buckets.

Note that the term *oxidation* does not mean that oxygen participates in the reaction. This term is derived from the fact that oxygen tends to accept electrons and therefore acts as an oxidizing agent. This important property of oxygen is used by cells to produce a usable form of energy and is discussed in detail in the section "Electron Transport Chain."

Keep in mind that oxidation-reduction reactions in cells often involve the transfer of hydrogen atoms (with their electrons) rather than free electrons alone. This occurs because a hydrogen atom contains one electron and one proton in the nucleus. Therefore, a molecule that loses a hydrogen atom also loses an electron and therefore is oxidized; the molecule that gains the hydrogen (and electron) is reduced. In many biological oxidation-reduction reactions, pairs of electrons are passed along between molecules as free electrons or as pairs of hydrogen atoms.

Two molecules that play important roles in the transfer of electrons are **nicotinamide adenine dinucleotide** and **flavin adenine dinucleotide**. Nicotinamide adenine dinucleotide is derived from the vitamin niacin (vitamin B_3), whereas flavin adenine dinucleotide comes from the vitamin riboflavin (B_2). The oxidized form of nicotinamide adenine dinucleotide is written as NAD^+, whereas the reduced form is written as NADH. Similarly, the oxidized form of flavin adenine dinucleotide is written as FAD, and the reduced form is abbreviated as FADH. Note that FADH can also accept a second hydrogen, forming $FADH_2$. Therefore, FADH and $FADH_2$ can be thought of as the same molecule because they undergo the same reactions. An illustration of how NADH is formed from the reduction of NAD^+ and how $FADH_2$ is formed from FAD during a coupled oxidation-reduction reaction is shown in Figure 3.5. Details of how NAD^+ and FAD function as "carrier molecules" during bioenergetic reactions are discussed later in this chapter in the section "Electron Transport Chain."

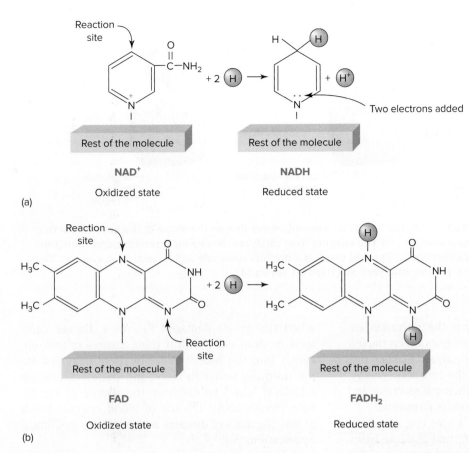

(a)

NAD⁺
Oxidized state

NADH
Reduced state

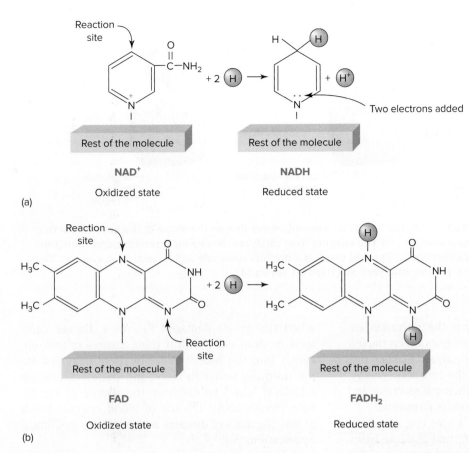

(b)

FAD
Oxidized state

FADH₂
Reduced state

Figure 3.5 Structural formulas for NAD⁺, NADH, FAD, and FADH₂. (*a*) When NAD⁺ reacts with two hydrogen atoms, it binds to one of them and accepts the electron from the other. This is shown by two dots above the nitrogen (N̈) in the formula for NADH. (*b*) When FAD reacts with two hydrogen atoms to form FADH₂, it binds each of them to a nitrogen atom at the reaction sites.

Enzymes

The speed of cellular chemical reactions is regulated by catalysts called **enzymes**. Enzymes are proteins that play a major role in the regulation of metabolic pathways in the cell. Enzymes do not cause a reaction to occur but simply regulate the rate or speed at which the reaction takes place. Furthermore, the enzyme does not change the nature of the reaction nor its final result.

Chemical reactions occur when the reactants have sufficient energy to proceed. The energy required to initiate chemical reactions is called the **activation energy** (8, 31). Enzymes work as catalysts by lowering the activation energy. The end result is to increase the rate at which these reactions take place. Figure 3.6

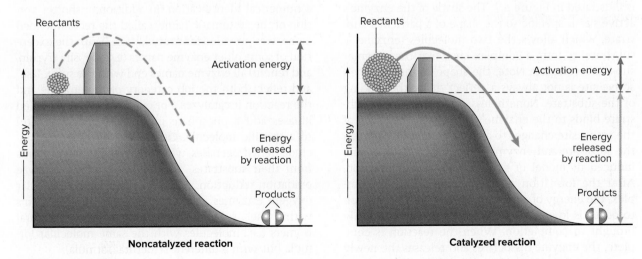

Noncatalyzed reaction

Catalyzed reaction

Figure 3.6 Enzymes catalyze reactions by lowering the energy of activation. That is, the energy required to achieve the reaction is reduced, which increases the probability that the reaction will occur. This point is illustrated in the two graphs. Notice in the left picture that in a noncatalyzed reaction (i.e., no enzyme present), the energy of activation is high; this high barrier reduces the possibility that the reaction will occur. However, note in the picture on the right that when an enzyme is present, the energy of activation is lowered (i.e., barrier lowered), the reaction occurs, and the reaction products are produced.

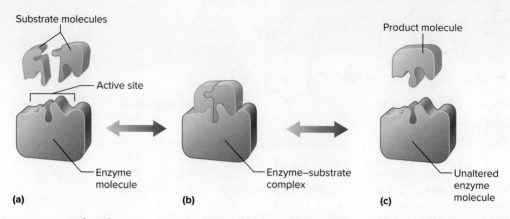

Figure 3.7 An enzyme-catalyzed reaction. On the far left (*a*), two substrates fit into the shape of the enzyme's active site; this forms the enzyme–substrate complex. (*b*) The enzyme then catalyzes the chemical reaction that results in the formation of the new product molecule. (*c*) The end result is a product molecule and an unaltered enzyme. The "double arrows" indicate that many enzyme-catalyzed reactions are reversible.

Shier et al, *Hole's Human Anatomy & Physiology.* New York, NY: McGraw-Hill Education, 2016, P 124. Copyright © 2016 by McGraw-Hill Education.

illustrates this concept. Note that the activation energy is greater in the noncatalyzed reaction on the left when compared to the enzyme-catalyzed reaction pictured on the right. By reducing the activation energy, enzymes increase the speed of chemical reactions and therefore increase the rate of product formation.

The ability of enzymes to lower the activation energy results from unique structural characteristics. In general, enzymes are large protein molecules with a unique shape. Each type of enzyme has characteristic ridges and grooves. The pockets that are formed from the ridges or grooves located on the enzyme are called active sites. These active sites are important because it is the unique shape of the active site that causes a specific enzyme to adhere to a particular reactant molecule (called a *substrate*). The concept of how enzymes fit with a particular substrate molecule is illustrated in Figure 3.7. The shape of the enzyme's active site is specific to the shape of a particular substrate, which allows the two molecules (enzyme + substrate) to form a complex known as the enzyme–substrate complex. Note, the shape of the enzyme's active site is not always a perfect fit for the binding of the substrate. Nonetheless, once the correct substrate binds to the enzyme's active site, the shape of the active site changes to allow a perfect fit between the substrate and enzyme; this process is called the induced fit model of enzyme–substrate interaction. After the formation of the enzyme-substrate complex, the energy of activation needed for the reaction to occur is lowered, and the reaction is more easily brought to completion. When the reaction is complete, the enzyme dissociates and releases the newly formed product. Note that the ability of an enzyme to work as a catalyst is not constant and can be modified by several factors; this will be discussed shortly.

Note that cellular enzymes can often play a key role in diagnosing specific illnesses. For example, when tissues are damaged due to a disease, damaged or dead cells within these tissues release enzymes into the blood. Many of these enzymes are not normally found in blood and therefore provide a clinical "clue" to diagnose the source of the illness. Details about the use of blood enzyme levels in the diagnosis of diseases are contained in Clinical Applications 3.1.

Classification of Enzymes In the early days of biochemistry, enzymes were named by the scientist who discovered them. Often, these names did not provide a clue as to the function of the enzyme. Therefore, to reduce confusion, an international committee developed a system that names the enzyme according to the type of chemical reaction it catalyzes. In this scheme, enzymes are provided a systematic name and a numerical identification. In addition, a shorter version of the systematic name, called the recommended name, was provided for everyday use. With the exception of some older enzyme names (e.g., pepsin, trypsin, and rennin) all enzyme names end with the suffix "ase" and reflect both the job category of the enzyme and the reaction it catalyzes. For example, enzymes called kinases add a phosphate group (i.e., phosphorylate) to a specific molecule. Other enzyme categories include dehydrogenases, which remove hydrogen atoms from their substrates, and oxidases, which catalyze oxidation–reduction reactions involving molecular oxygen. Enzymes called isomerases rearrange atoms within their substrate molecules to form structural isomers (i.e., molecules with the same molecular formula but with a different structural formula).

Factors That Alter Enzyme Activity The activity of an enzyme, as measured by the rate at which its substrates are converted into products, is influenced by several factors. Two of the more important factors

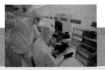

CLINICAL APPLICATIONS 3.1

Diagnostic Value of Measuring Enzyme Activity in the Blood

When tissues become diseased, damaged dead cells often release their enzymes into the blood. Because many of these intracellular enzymes are not normally found in blood, the presence of a specific enzyme in blood provides important diagnostic information regarding the source of the medical problem. In practice, the diagnostic test proceeds as follows. A doctor obtains a blood sample from the patient and forwards the sample to a clinical laboratory for analysis. The laboratory then determines the activity of a specific enzyme in a test tube. The results of this test can often assist in making a diagnosis. For example, the finding that the blood sample contains high levels of the enzyme lactate dehydrogenase (cardiac-specific isoform) suggests that the patient experienced a myocardial infarction (i.e., heart attack). Similarly, elevated blood levels of the enzyme creatine kinase would also indicate cardiac injury and would provide additional evidence that the patient suffered a heart attack. See Table 3.1 for additional examples of the diagnostic usage for specific enzymes found in blood.

TABLE 3.1	Examples of the Diagnostic Value of Enzymes Found in Blood
Enzyme	**Diseases Associated with High Blood Levels of Enzyme**
Lactate dehydrogenase (cardiac-specific isoform)	Myocardial infarction
Creatine kinase	Myocardial infarction, muscular dystrophy
Alkaline phosphatase	Carcinoma of bone, Paget's disease, obstructive jaundice
Amylase	Pancreatitis, perforated peptic ulcer
Aldolase	Muscular dystrophy

include temperature and pH (pH is a measure of acidity or alkalinity) of the solution.

Individual enzymes have an optimum temperature at which they are most active. In general, a small rise in body temperature above normal (i.e., 37°C) increases the activity of most enzymes. This is useful during exercise because muscular work results in an increase in body temperature. The resulting elevation in enzyme activity would enhance bioenergetics (ATP production) by speeding up the rate of reactions involved in the production of biologically useful energy. This point is illustrated in Figure 3.8. Notice that enzyme activity is less than maximum at normal body temperature (37°C). Also, note that an exercise-induced increase in body temperature (e.g., 40°C) results in a temperature-induced increase in enzyme activity.

The pH of body fluids also has a large effect on enzyme activity. The relationship between pH and enzyme activity is similar to the temperature/enzyme activity relationship; that is, individual enzymes have a pH optimum. If the pH is altered from the optimum, the enzyme activity is reduced (Fig. 3.9). This has important implications during exercise. For example, during intense exercise, skeletal muscles can produce large amounts of hydrogen ions (34). Accumulation of large quantities of hydrogen ions results in a decrease in the pH (i.e., increased acidity) of body fluids below the optimum pH of important bioenergetic enzymes. The end result is a decreased ability to provide the energy (i.e., ATP) required for muscular contraction. In fact, extreme acidity is an important limiting factor in various types of intense exercise. This will be discussed again in Chaps. 10, 11, and 19.

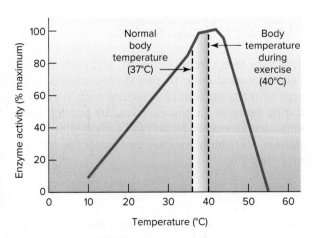

Figure 3.8 The effect of body temperature on enzyme activity. Notice that an optimal range of temperatures exist for enzyme activity. An increase or decrease in temperature away from the optimal temperature range results in diminished enzyme activity.

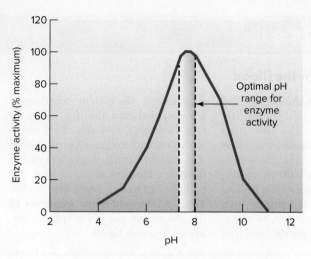

Figure 3.9 The effect of pH on enzyme activity. Note that every enzyme has a narrow range of optimal pH. An increase or decrease of pH away from this optimum range results in a decrease in enzyme activity.

IN SUMMARY

- Oxidation is the process of removing an electron from an atom or molecule.
- Reduction is the addition of an electron to an atom or molecule.
- Oxidation–reduction reactions are always coupled because a molecule cannot be oxidized unless it donates an electron to another atom.
- Enzymes serve as catalysts for cellular reactions and regulate the speed of chemical reactions.
- Enzymes are classified into categories based upon the type of reaction that the enzyme performs.
- Two important factors that regulate enzyme activity are temperature and pH. Individual enzymes have an optimum temperature and pH at which they are most active.

FUELS FOR EXERCISE

The body uses carbohydrate, fat, and protein nutrients consumed daily to provide the necessary energy to maintain cellular activities both at rest and during exercise. During exercise, the primary nutrients used for energy are fats and carbohydrates, with protein contributing a small amount of the total energy used (3).

Carbohydrates

Carbohydrates are composed of carbon, hydrogen, and oxygen atoms. Stored carbohydrates provide the body with a rapidly available form of energy, with 1 gram of carbohydrate yielding approximately 4 kcal of energy (36). As mentioned earlier, plants synthesize carbohydrates from the interaction of

CO_2, water, and solar energy in a process called photosynthesis. Carbohydrates exist in three forms (36): (1) monosaccharides, (2) disaccharides, and (3) polysaccharides. Monosaccharides are simple sugars such as glucose and fructose. **Glucose** is familiar to most of us and is often referred to as "blood sugar." It can be found in foods or can be formed in the digestive tract as a result of cleavage of more complex carbohydrates. Fructose is contained in fruits or honey and is considered to be the sweetest of the simple carbohydrates (33).

Disaccharides are formed by combining two monosaccharides. For example, table sugar is called sucrose and is composed of glucose and fructose. Maltose, also a disaccharide, is composed of two glucose molecules. Sucrose is considered to be the most common dietary disaccharide in the United States (28). It occurs naturally in many carbohydrates, such as cane sugar, beets, honey, and maple syrup.

Polysaccharides are complex carbohydrates that contain three or more monosaccharides. Polysaccharides can exist as small molecules (i.e., three monosaccharides) or relatively large molecules containing hundreds of monosaccharides. The two most common forms of polysaccharides are cellulose and starch. Humans lack the enzymes necessary to digest cellulose, and thus cellulose is discarded as waste in the fecal material. On the other hand, starch–found in corn, grains, beans, potatoes, and peas–is easily digested by humans and is an important source of carbohydrate in the diet (28). After ingestion, starch is broken down to form monosaccharides and can be used as energy immediately by cells or stored in another form within cells for future energy needs.

Glycogen is a polysaccharide stored in animal tissue. It is synthesized within cells by linking glucose molecules using the action of the enzyme *glycogen synthase*. Glycogen molecules are generally large and consist of hundreds to thousands of glucose molecules. Cells store glycogen as a means of supplying carbohydrates as an energy source. For example, during exercise, individual muscle cells break down glycogen into glucose (this process is called **glycogenolysis**) and use the glucose as a source of energy for contraction. Note that glycogenolysis also occurs in the liver, with the free glucose being released into the bloodstream and transported to tissues throughout the body.

Important to exercise metabolism is that glycogen is stored in both muscle fibers and the liver. However, total glycogen stores in the body are relatively small and can be depleted within a few hours as a result of prolonged exercise. Therefore, glycogen synthesis is an ongoing process within cells. Diets low in carbohydrates tend to hamper glycogen synthesis, whereas high-carbohydrate diets enhance glycogen synthesis (see Chap. 23).

Fats

Although fats contain the same chemical elements as carbohydrates, the ratio of carbon to oxygen in fats is much greater than that found in carbohydrates. Stored body fat is an ideal fuel for prolonged exercise because fat molecules contain large quantities of energy per unit of weight. One gram of fat contains about 9 kcal of energy, which is more than twice the energy content of either carbohydrates or protein (33). Fats are insoluble in water and can be found in both plants and animals. In general, fats can be classified into four groups: (1) fatty acids, (2) triglycerides, (3) phospholipids, and (4) steroids. Fatty acids consist of chains of carbon atoms linked to a carboxyl group at one end (a carboxyl group contains a carbon, oxygen, and hydrogen group). Importantly, fatty acids are the primary type of fat used by muscle cells for energy.

Fatty acids are stored in the body as triglycerides. Triglycerides are composed of three molecules of fatty acids and one molecule of glycerol (not a fat but a type of alcohol). Although the largest storage site for triglycerides is fat cells, these molecules are also stored in many cell types, including skeletal muscle. In times of need, fats are broken down into their component parts, with fatty acids being used as energy substrates by muscle and other tissues. The process of breaking down triglycerides into fatty acids and glycerol is termed *lipolysis* and is regulated by a family of enzymes called *lipases*. The glycerol released by lipolysis is not a direct energy source for muscle, but can be used by the liver to synthesize glucose. Therefore, the entire triglyceride molecule is a useful source of energy for the body.

Phospholipids are not used as an energy source by skeletal muscle during exercise (17). Phospholipids are lipids combined with phosphoric acid and are synthesized in virtually every cell in the body. The biological roles of phospholipids vary from providing the structural integrity of cell membranes to providing an insulating sheath around nerve fibers (10).

The final classification of fats is the steroids. Again, these fats are not used as an energy source during exercise but will be mentioned briefly to provide a clearer understanding of the nature of biological fats. The most common steroid is cholesterol. Cholesterol is a component of all cell membranes. It can be synthesized in every cell in the body and, of course, can be consumed in foods. In addition to its role in membrane structure, cholesterol is needed for the synthesis of the sex hormones estrogen, progesterone, and testosterone (10). Although cholesterol has many useful biological functions, high blood cholesterol levels have been implicated in the development of coronary artery disease (38) (this issue will be addressed in a later chapter).

Proteins

Proteins are composed of many tiny subunits called amino acids. At least 20 types of amino acids are needed by the body to form various tissues, enzymes, blood proteins, and so on. Nine amino acids, called essential amino acids, cannot be synthesized by the body and therefore must be consumed in foods. Proteins are formed by linking amino acids by chemical bonds called peptide bonds. As a potential fuel source, proteins contain approximately 4 kcal per gram (8). For proteins to be used as substrates for the formation of high-energy compounds, they must be broken down into their constituent amino acids. Proteins can contribute energy for exercise in two ways. First, the amino acid alanine can be converted in the liver to glucose, which can then be used to synthesize glycogen. Liver glycogen can be degraded into glucose and transported to working skeletal muscle via the circulation. Second, many amino acids (e.g., isoleucine, alanine, leucine, valine) can be converted into metabolic intermediates (i.e., compounds that may directly participate in bioenergetics) in muscle cells and directly contribute as fuel in the bioenergetic pathways (12).

IN SUMMARY

- The body uses carbohydrate, fat, and protein nutrients consumed daily to provide the necessary energy to maintain cellular activities both at rest and during exercise.
- During exercise, the primary nutrients used for energy are fats and carbohydrates, with protein contributing a relatively small amount of the total energy used.
- Glucose is stored in animal cells as a polysaccharide called glycogen.
- Fatty acids are the primary form of fat used as an energy source in cells. Fatty acids are stored as triglycerides in muscle and fat cells.
- Proteins are composed of amino acids, and 20 different amino acids are required to form the various proteins contained in cells. The use of protein as an energy source requires that cellular proteins be broken down into amino acids.

HIGH-ENERGY PHOSPHATES

The immediate source of energy for muscular contraction is the high-energy phosphate compound **adenosine triphosphate (ATP)** (33). Although ATP is not the only energy-carrying molecule in the cell, it is the most important one, and without sufficient amounts of ATP, most cells die quickly.

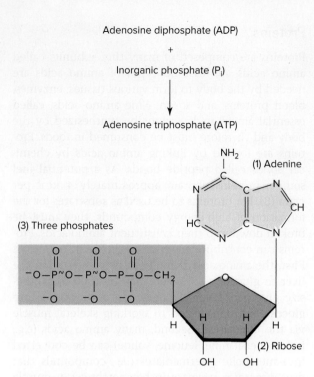

Adenosine diphosphate (ADP)

+

Inorganic phosphate (Pᵢ)

↓

Adenosine triphosphate (ATP)

Figure 3.10 The structural formation of adenosine triphosphate (ATP).

The structure of ATP consists of three main parts: (1) an adenine portion, (2) a ribose portion, and (3) three linked phosphates (Fig. 3.10). The formation of ATP occurs by combining **adenosine diphosphate (ADP)** and **inorganic phosphate (Pᵢ)** and requires energy. Some of this energy is stored in the chemical bond joining ADP and P_i. Accordingly, this bond is called a high-energy bond. When the enzyme **ATPase** breaks this bond, energy is released, and this energy can be used to do work (e.g., muscular contraction):

$$ATP \xrightarrow{\text{ATPase}} ADP + P_i + Energy$$

ATP is often called the universal energy donor. It couples the energy released from the breakdown of foodstuffs into a usable form of energy required by all cells. For example, Figure 3.11 presents a model depicting ATP as the universal energy donor in the cell. The cell uses exergonic reactions (breakdown of foodstuffs) to form ATP via endergonic reactions. This newly formed ATP can then be used to drive the energy-requiring processes in the cell. Therefore, energy-liberating reactions are linked to energy-requiring reactions like two meshed gears.

BIOENERGETICS

Muscle cells store limited amounts of ATP. Therefore, because muscular exercise requires a constant supply of ATP to provide the energy needed for contraction, metabolic pathways must exist in the cell with the capability to produce ATP rapidly. Indeed, muscle cells produce ATP using a combination of three metabolic pathways that are activated at the beginning of muscle contractions: (1) formation of ATP by **phosphocreatine (PC)** breakdown, (2) formation of ATP via the degradation of glucose or glycogen (called glycolysis), and (3) oxidative formation of ATP. Formation of ATP via the PC pathway and glycolysis does not involve the use of oxygen (O_2); these pathways are

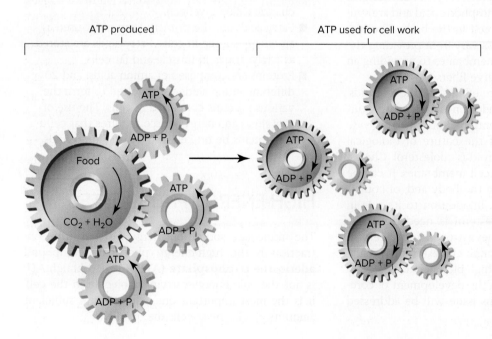

Figure 3.11 A model of ATP as the universal energy carrier of the cell. Exergonic reactions are shown as blue gears with arrows going down. Endergonic reactions are shown as green gears with arrows going up.

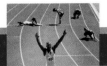
Exercise Physiology Applied to Sports

Does Creatine Supplementation Improve Exercise Performance?

The depletion of phosphocreatine (PC) may limit exercise performance during short-term, high-intensity exercise (e.g., 100- to 200-meter dash) because the depletion of PC results in a reduction in the rate of ATP production by the ATP-PC system. Studies have shown that ingestion of large amounts of creatine monohydrate (20 grams/day) over a five-day period results in increased stores of muscle PC (2, 6, 19, 26, 39). Although some controversy exists, creatine supplementation has been shown to improve performance in laboratory settings during short-duration (e.g., 30 seconds), high-intensity exercise (2, 19, 26, 39).

Interestingly, studies also suggest that creatine supplementation in conjunction with resistance exercise training results in an enhanced physiologic adaptation to weight training (2, 5, 15, 23, 32, 39). Specifically, these studies indicate that creatine supplementation combined with resistance training promotes an increase in both dynamic muscular strength and fat-free mass.

Does oral creatine supplementation result in adverse physiological side effects and pose health risks? Unfortunately, a definitive answer to this question is not available. Although anecdotal reports indicate that creatine supplementation can be associated with negative side effects, such as nausea, neurological dysfunction, minor gastrointestinal distress, and muscle cramping, these reports are not well documented (2, 7, 14, 20, 39). At present, due to limited data, a firm conclusion about the long-term health risks of creatine supplementation cannot be reached. However, current evidence suggests that creatine supplementation for up to eight weeks does not appear to produce major health risks, but the safety of more prolonged creatine supplementation has not been established.

An important issue related to the use of creatine and other dietary supplements is the possibility of contamination within the product; that is, the supplement product may contain other chemical compounds in addition to creatine (27). Indeed, this is an important safety issue in the "over-the-counter supplement" industry because a large study has reported a high level of variability in the purity of over-the-counter products (27). For more information on creatine and exercise performance, see Devries and Phillips (2014), Lanhers et al. (2015), and Sahlin (2014) in the Suggested Readings.

---

called **anaerobic** (without O_2) pathways. Oxidative formation of ATP by the use of O_2 is termed **aerobic** metabolism. A detailed discussion of the operation of the three metabolic pathways involved in the formation of ATP during exercise follows.

Anaerobic ATP Production

The simplest and, consequently, the most rapid method of producing ATP involves the donation of a phosphate group and its bond energy from PC to ADP to form ATP (33, 36, 37):

$$PC + ADP \xrightarrow{\text{Creatine kinase}} ATP + C$$

The reaction is catalyzed by the enzyme creatine kinase. As rapidly as ATP is broken down to ADP + P_i at the onset of exercise, ATP is resynthesized via the PC reaction. However, muscle cells store only small amounts of PC, and thus the total amount of ATP that can be formed via this reaction is limited. The combination of stored ATP and PC is called the **ATP-PC system,** or the "phosphagen system." It provides energy for muscular contraction at the onset of exercise and during short-term, high-intensity exercise (i.e., lasting fewer than five seconds). PC reformation requires ATP and occurs only during recovery from exercise (11).

The importance of the ATP-PC system in athletics can be appreciated by considering short-term, intense exercise such as sprinting 50 meters, high jumping, performing a rapid weight-lifting move, or a football player racing 10 yards downfield. All these activities require only a few seconds to complete and thus need a rapid supply of ATP. The ATP-PC system provides a simple one-enzyme reaction to produce ATP for these types of activities. The fact that depletion of PC is likely to limit short-term, high-intensity exercise has led to the suggestion that ingesting large amounts of creatine can improve exercise performance (see The Winning Edge 3.1).

A second metabolic pathway capable of producing ATP rapidly without the involvement of O_2 is termed **glycolysis**. Glycolysis involves the breakdown of glucose or glycogen to form two molecules of pyruvate (also called pyruvic acid) or **lactate** (Fig. 3.13). Simply stated, glycolysis is an anaerobic pathway used to transfer bond energy from glucose to rejoin P_i to ADP. This process involves a series of enzymatically catalyzed, coupled reactions. Glycolysis occurs in the sarcoplasm of the muscle cell and produces a net gain of two molecules of ATP and two molecules of pyruvate or lactate per glucose molecule (see A Closer Look 3.2).

Let's consider glycolysis in more detail. First, the reactions between glucose and pyruvate can be considered as two distinct phases: (1) an energy investment phase and (2) an energy generation phase (Fig. 3.13). The first reactions make up the "energy investment phase" where stored ATP must be used

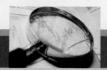

A CLOSER LOOK 3.2

Lactic Acid or Lactate?

In many textbooks, the terms *lactic acid* and *lactate* are used interchangeably. This is often confusing to students, who ask, "Are lactic acid and lactate the same molecule?" The answer is that lactic acid and lactate are related but are technically different molecules. Here's the explanation:

The term *lactate* refers to the base of lactic acid (Fig. 3.12) (4). You may recall from another science course that when acids dissociate and release hydrogen ions, the remaining molecule is called the *conjugate base* of the acid. It follows that lactate is the conjugate base of lactic acid. Because of the close relationship between lactic acid and lactate, many authors use these terms interchangeably (3). Remembering the relationship between lactic acid and lactate will reduce confusion when you read about these molecules in future chapters within this text.

Figure 3.12   The ionization of lactic acid forms the conjugate base called lactate. At normal body pH, lactic acid will rapidly dissociate to form lactate.

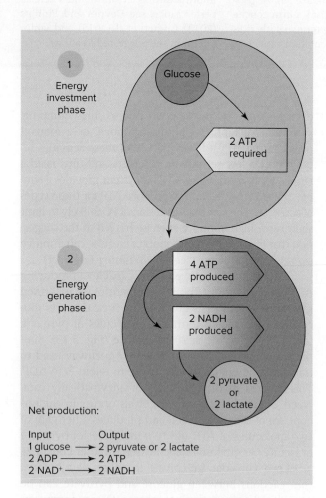

Net production:

Input		Output
1 glucose	→	2 pyruvate or 2 lactate
2 ADP	→	2 ATP
2 NAD⁺	→	2 NADH

Figure 3.13   Illustration of the two phases of glycolysis and the products of glycolysis.

Mathews and van Holde, *Biochemistry*. The Benjamin/Cummings Publishing Company, 1990.

to form sugar phosphates. Although the end result of glycolysis is the release of energy, glycolysis must be "primed" by the addition of ATP at two points at the beginning of the pathway (Figs. 3.14 and 3.15). The purpose of the ATP priming is to add phosphate groups (called phosphorylation) to glucose and to fructose 6-phosphate. Note that if glycolysis begins with glycogen as the substrate, the addition of only one ATP is required. That is, glycogen does not require phosphorylation by ATP but is phosphorylated

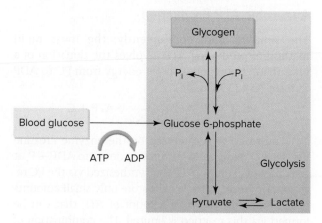

Figure 3.14   Illustration of the interaction between blood glucose and muscle glycogen for the provision of glucose for glycolysis. Regardless of the source of glucose for glycolysis, glucose must be phosphorylated to form glucose 6-phosphate as the first step in glycolysis. Note, however, that phosphorylation of glucose obtained from the blood requires 1 ATP, whereas the phosphorylation of glucose obtained from glycogen is achieved by using inorganic phosphate (P_i) located in the cell.

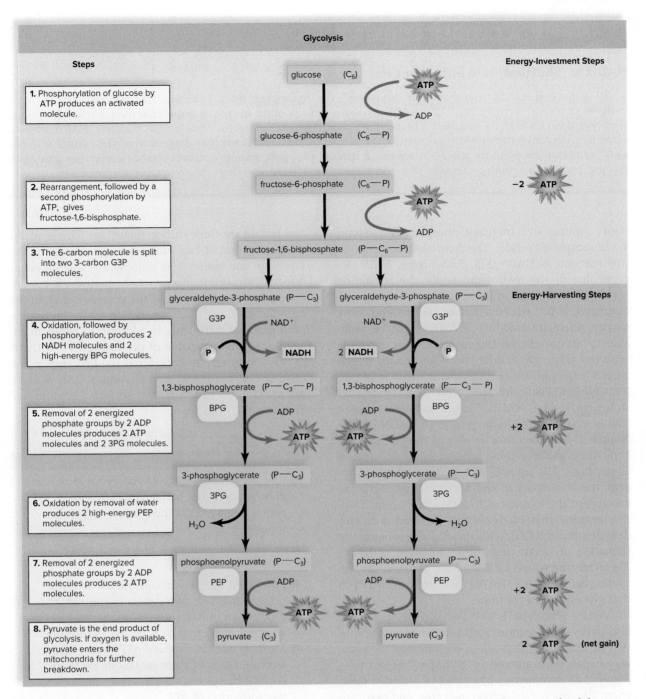

Figure 3.15 Summary of the anaerobic metabolism of glucose that is called glycolysis. Note that the net result of the anaerobic breakdown of one molecule of glucose is the production of two molecules of ATP and two molecules of pyruvate.

by inorganic phosphate instead (Fig. 3.14). The last steps of glycolysis represent the "energy generation phase." Figure 3.15 points out that two molecules of ATP are produced at each of two separate reactions near the end of the glycolytic pathway; thus, the net gain of glycolysis is two ATP if glucose is the substrate and three ATP if glycogen is the substrate.

Hydrogens are frequently removed from nutrient substrates in bioenergetic pathways and are transported by "carrier molecules." Two biologically important carrier molecules are nicotinamide adenine dinucleotide (NAD^+) and flavin adenine dinucleotide (FAD). Both NAD^+ and FAD transport hydrogens and their associated electrons to be used for later generation of ATP in the mitochondrion via aerobic processes. For the chemical reactions in glycolysis to proceed, two hydrogens must be removed from glyceraldehyde 3-phosphate, which

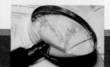
NADH Is "Shuttled" into Mitochondria

NADH generated during glycolysis must be converted back to NAD$^+$ if glycolysis is to continue. As discussed in the text, the conversion of NADH to NAD$^+$ can occur by pyruvate accepting the hydrogens (forming lactate) or "shuttling" the hydrogens from NADH across the mitochondrial membrane. The "shuttling" of hydrogens across the mitochondrial membrane requires a specific transport system. Figure 4.9 (see Chap. 4) illustrates this process. This transport system is located within the mitochondrial membrane and transfers NADH-released hydrogens from the cytosol into the mitochondria, where they can enter the electron transport chain.

then combines with inorganic phosphate (P$_i$) to form 1,3-biphosphoglycerate. The hydrogen acceptor in this reaction is NAD$^+$ (Fig. 3.15). Here, NAD$^+$ accepts one of the hydrogens, while the remaining hydrogen is free in solution. Upon accepting the hydrogen, NAD$^+$ is converted to its reduced form, NADH. Adequate amounts of NAD$^+$ must be available to accept the hydrogen atoms that must be removed from glyceraldehyde 3-phosphate if glycolysis is to continue (3, 31). How is NAD$^+$ reformed from NADH? There are two ways that the cell restores NAD$^+$ from NADH. First, if sufficient oxygen (O$_2$) is available, the hydrogens from NADH can be "shuttled" into the mitochondria of the cell and can contribute to the aerobic production of ATP (see A Closer Look 3.3). Second, if O$_2$ is not available to accept the hydrogens in the mitochondria, pyruvate can accept the hydrogens to form lactate (Fig. 3.16). The enzyme that catalyzes this reaction is lactate dehydrogenase (LDH), with the end result being the formation of lactate and the reformation of NAD$^+$. Therefore, the reason for lactate formation is the "recycling" of NAD$^+$ (i.e., NADH converted to NAD$^+$) so that glycolysis can continue.

Again, glycolysis is the breakdown of glucose into pyruvate or lactate, with the net production of two or three ATP, depending on whether the pathway began with glucose or glycogen, respectively. Figure 3.15 summarizes glycolysis in a simple flowchart. Glucose is a six-carbon molecule, and pyruvate and lactate are three-carbon molecules. This explains the production of two molecules of pyruvate or lactate from one molecule of glucose. Because O$_2$ is not directly involved in glycolysis, the pathway is considered anaerobic. However, in the presence of O$_2$ in the mitochondria, pyruvate can participate in the aerobic production of ATP. Thus, in addition to being an anaerobic pathway capable of producing ATP without O$_2$, glycolysis can be considered the first step in the aerobic degradation of carbohydrates. This will be discussed in detail in the next section, "Aerobic ATP Production."

IN SUMMARY

- The immediate source of energy for muscular contraction is the high-energy phosphate ATP. ATP is degraded via the enzyme ATPase as follows:

$$ATP \xrightarrow[\text{ATPase}]{} ADP + P_i + Energy$$

- Formation of ATP without the use of O$_2$ is termed *anaerobic metabolism*. In contrast, the production of ATP using O$_2$ as the final electron acceptor is referred to as *aerobic metabolism*.
- Muscle cells can produce ATP by any one or a combination of three metabolic pathways: (1) ATP-PC system, (2) glycolysis, and (3) oxidative formation of ATP.
- The ATP-PC system and glycolysis are two anaerobic metabolic pathways that are capable of producing ATP without O$_2$.

Aerobic ATP Production

Aerobic production of ATP occurs inside the mitochondria and involves the interaction of two cooperating metabolic pathways: (1) the **citric acid cycle** and (2) the **electron transport chain**. The primary function of the citric acid cycle (also called the Krebs cycle or tricarboxylic acid cycle) is to complete the oxidation (hydrogen removal)

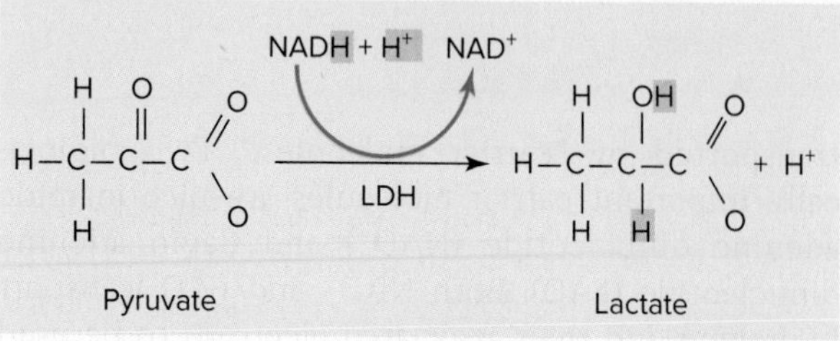

Figure 3.16 The addition of hydrogen atoms to pyruvate forms lactate and NAD$^+$, which can be used again in glycolysis. The reaction is catalyzed by the enzyme lactate dehydrogenase (LDH).

of carbohydrates, fats, or proteins using NAD$^+$ and FAD as hydrogen (energy) carriers. The importance of hydrogen removal is that hydrogens (by virtue of the electrons that they possess) contain the potential energy in the food molecules. This energy can be used in the electron transport chain to combine ADP + P$_i$ to reform ATP. Oxygen does not participate in the reactions of the citric acid cycle, but is the final hydrogen acceptor at the end of the electron transport chain (i.e., water is formed, H$_2$ + O → H$_2$O). The process of aerobic production of ATP is termed **oxidative phosphorylation**. To understand the processes involved in aerobic ATP generation, it is convenient to think of aerobic ATP production as a multi-stage process (Fig. 3.17). This process begins with the formation of two molecules of acetyl-CoA. Acetyl-CoA can be formed from pyruvate produced by glycolysis or from the oxidation of fatty acids or amino acids. Acetyl-CoA then enters the citric acid cycle and undergoes oxidation resulting in the release of electrons into the electron transport chain. The transport of electrons down the electron transport chain results in the aerobic formation of ATP, which is commonly called as oxidative phosphorylation. A detailed look at the citric acid cycle and electron transport chain follows.

Glycolysis

(1) The 6-carbon sugar glucose is broken down in the cytosol into two 3-carbon pyruvic acid molecules with a net gain of 2 ATP and the release of high-energy electrons.

Citric Acid Cycle

(2) The 3-carbon pyruvic acids generated by glycolysis enter the mitochondria separately. Each loses a carbon (generating CO$_2$) and is combined with a coenzyme to form a 2-carbon acetyl coenzyme A (acetyl CoA). More high-energy electrons are released.

(3) Each acetyl CoA combines with a 4-carbon oxaloacetic acid to form the 6-carbon citric acid, for which the cycle is named. For each citric acid, a series of reactions removes 2 carbons (generating 2 CO$_2$'s), synthesizes 1 ATP, and releases more high-energy electrons. The figure shows 2 ATP resulting directly from 2 turns of the cycle per glucose molecule that enters glycolysis.

Electron Transport Chain

(4) The high-energy electrons still contain most of the chemical energy of the original glucose molecule. Special carrier molecules bring the high-energy electrons to a series of enzymes that transfer much of the remaining energy to more ATP molecules. The electrons eventually combine with hydrogen ions and an oxygen atom to form water. The function of oxygen as the final electron acceptor in this last step is why the overall process is called aerobic respiration.

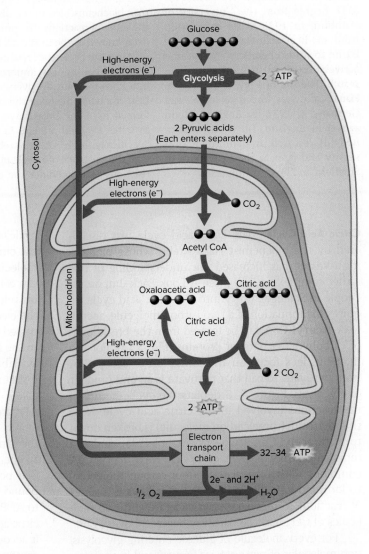

Figure 3.17 The steps lead to oxidative phosphorylation. Glycolysis takes place in the cytosol and does not require oxygen. Oxidative phosphorylation (also called aerobic metabolism) takes place in the mitochondria and requires oxygen. The process of aerobic metabolism begins with glycolysis producing two molecules of pyruvic acid (also called pyruvate), which enters the mitochondria to form two molecules of acetyl-CoA. Acetyl-CoA then undergoes oxidation in the citric acid cycle within the matrix (i.e., center) of the mitochondria. The end products of aerobic metabolism include ATP, heat, carbon dioxide (CO$_2$), and water (H$_2$O). Note that the size of mitochondria relative to size of the cytosol is exaggerated to emphasize the metabolic pathways. See Figure 3.1 for a more realistic ratio of the mitochondrial size relative to the cytosol.

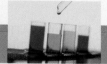

A LOOK BACK—IMPORTANT PEOPLE IN SCIENCE

Hans Krebs and the Discovery of the Citric Acid Cycle

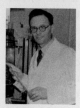

© Keystone/
Getty Images

Hans Krebs (1900–1981) received the Nobel Prize in Physiology or Medicine in 1953 for his research on a series of important chemical reactions in cells that became known as the "Krebs cycle." Krebs was born in Germany and earned his M.D. degree from the University of Hamburg in 1925. After graduation from medical school, he moved to Berlin to study chemistry and became actively involved in biochemical research. The son of a Jewish physician, Hans Krebs was forced to leave Nazi Germany in 1933 for England. Upon arrival in England, Dr. Krebs continued his research at Cambridge University and later at the University of Sheffield and Oxford University.

During his distinguished research career, Hans Krebs made many important contributions to physiology and biochemistry. One of his first significant areas of research was how protein is metabolized in cells. An important outcome of this early work was the finding that the liver produces a nitrogenous waste product of protein metabolism called urea. Further work by Dr. Krebs and his colleague Kurt Henseleit (another German biochemist) led to the discovery of the series of reactions that produce urea (later known as the urea cycle).

Although Dr. Krebs's research on protein metabolism was important, he is best known for his discovery of the cellular reactions involving the substances formed from the breakdown of carbohydrates, fats, and proteins in the body. Specifically, in 1937, Dr. Krebs discovered the existence of a cycle of chemical reactions that combines the end prod-uct of carbohydrate breakdown (this product was later named acetyl-CoA) with oxaloacetic acid to form citric acid. Dr. Krebs's work showed that this cycle regenerates oxaloacetic acid through a series of intermediate compounds while liberating carbon dioxide and electrons. This cycle is known by three different names, including the citric acid cycle, Krebs cycle, and the tricarboxylic acid cycle. However, this chemical cycle is commonly referred to as either the citric acid cycle or the Krebs cycle. Therefore, the Krebs cycle and the citric acid cycle are different names for the same chemical pathway. The discovery of the citric acid cycle and how chemical foodstuffs are converted into usable energy was of vital importance to our basic understanding of cellular energy metabolism and paved the way for exercise physiologists to further investigate skeletal muscle bioenergetics during exercise.

Citric Acid Cycle The citric acid cycle was discovered by the biochemist Hans Krebs, whose pioneering research has increased our understanding of this rather complex pathway (see A Look Back–Important People in Science). Entry into the citric acid cycle requires the formation of a two-carbon molecule, acetyl-CoA. **Acetyl-CoA** can be formed from the breakdown of carbohydrates, fats, or proteins (Fig. 3.17). For the moment, let's focus on the formation of acetyl-CoA from pyruvate. Recall that pyruvate is an end product of glycolysis. Figure 3.18 depicts the cyclic nature of the reactions involved in the citric acid cycle. Note that pyruvate (three-carbon molecule) is broken down to form acetyl-CoA (two-carbon molecule), and the remaining carbon is given off as CO_2. Next, acetyl-CoA combines with oxaloacetate (four-carbon molecule) to form citrate (six carbons). What follows is a series of reactions to regenerate oxaloacetate and two molecules of CO_2, and the pathway begins all over again.

For every molecule of glucose entering glycolysis, two molecules of pyruvate are formed, and in the presence of O_2, they are converted to two molecules of acetyl-CoA. This means that each molecule of glucose results in two turns of the citric acid cycle. With this in mind, let's examine the citric acid cycle in more detail. The primary function of the citric acid cycle is to remove hydrogens and the energy associated with those hydrogens from various substrates involved in the cycle. Figure 3.18 illustrates that during each turn of the citric acid cycle, three molecules of NADH and one molecule of FADH are formed. Both NADH and FADH can return to their oxidized form (i.e., NAD and FAD) by releasing electrons to the electron carriers within the electron transport chain. For every pair of electrons passed through the electron transport chain from NADH to the final electron acceptor oxygen, enough energy is available to form 2.5 molecules of ATP (10). For every FADH molecule that is formed, enough energy is available to produce 1.5 molecules of ATP. Thus, in terms of ATP production, FADH is not as energy rich as NADH.

In addition to the production of NADH and FADH, the citric acid cycle results in the direct formation of an energy-rich compound guanosine triphosphate (GTP) (see bottom of Fig. 3.18). GTP is a high-energy compound that can transfer its terminal phosphate group to ADP to form ATP. The direct formation of GTP in the citric acid cycle is called substrate-level phosphorylation. It accounts for only a small amount of the total energy conversion in the citric acid cycle because most of the citric acid cycle energy yield (i.e., NADH and FADH) is coupled with the electron transport chain to form ATP.

Up to this point, we have focused on the role that carbohydrates play in producing acetyl-CoA to enter the citric acid cycle. How do fats and proteins undergo aerobic metabolism? The answer can be found in Figure 3.19. Note that fats (triglycerides) are

---

56 Section One Physiology of Exercise

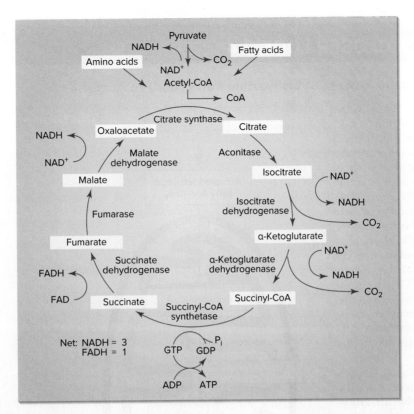

Figure 3.18 Compounds and reactions involved in the citric acid cycle. Note that each turn of the citric acid produces two ATP molecules directly and two CO_2 molecules. Eight hydrogens with high-energy electrons are also released. Each glucose molecule metabolized in glycolysis results in the production of two molecules of acetyl-CoA and two turns of the citric acid cycle. Also, please note that the size of mitochondria relative to size of the cytosol is exaggerated to emphasize the metabolic pathways. See Figure 3.1 for a more realistic ratio of the mitochondrial size relative to the cytosol.

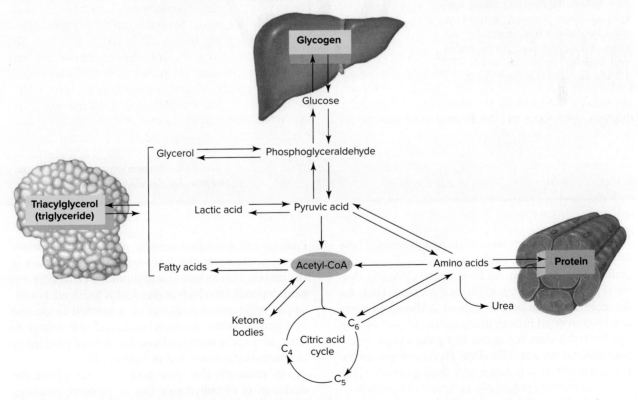

Figure 3.19 The relationships among the metabolism of proteins, carbohydrates, and fats. The overall interaction between the metabolic breakdown of these three foodstuffs is often referred to as the metabolic pool.

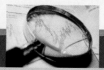
Beta Oxidation Is the Process of Converting Fatty Acids to Acetyl-CoA

Fats are stored in the body in the form of triglycerides within fat cells and within the muscle fiber itself. Release of fat from these storage depots occurs by the breakdown of triglycerides, which results in the liberation of fatty acids (see Chap. 4). However, for fatty acids to be used as a fuel during aerobic metabolism, they must first be converted to acetyl-CoA. **Beta oxidation** is the process of oxidizing fatty acids to form acetyl-CoA. This occurs in the mitochondria and involves a series of enzymatically catalyzed steps, starting with an "activated fatty acid" and ending with the production of acetyl-CoA.

A simple illustration of this process is presented in Figure 3.20. This process begins with the "activation" of the fatty acid; the activated fatty acid is then transported into the mitochondria, where the process of beta oxidation begins. In short, beta oxidation is a sequence of four reactions that "chops" fatty acids into two carbon fragments forming acetyl-CoA. Once formed, acetyl-CoA then becomes a fuel source for the citric acid cycle (i.e., Krebs cycle) and leads to the production of ATP via the electron transport chain.

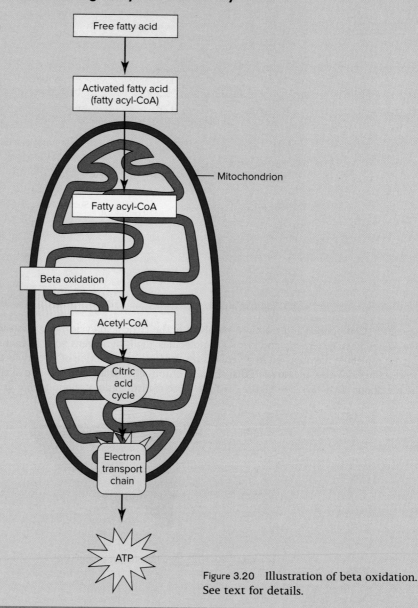

Figure 3.20 Illustration of beta oxidation. See text for details.

broken down to form fatty acids and glycerol. These fatty acids can then undergo a series of reactions (called beta oxidation) to form acetyl-CoA and thus enter the citric acid cycle (8) (see A Closer Look 3.4 for more details on beta oxidation). Although glycerol can be converted into an intermediate of glycolysis in the liver, this does not occur to a great extent in human skeletal muscle. Therefore, glycerol is not an important direct muscle fuel source during exercise (16).

As mentioned previously, protein is not considered a major fuel source during exercise because it contributes only 2% to 15% of the fuel during exercise (9, 25).

Proteins can enter bioenergetic pathways in a variety of places. However, the first step is the breakdown of the protein into its amino acid subunits. What happens next depends on which amino acid is involved. For example, some amino acids can be converted to glucose or pyruvate, some to acetyl-CoA, and still others to citric acid cycle intermediates. The role of proteins in bioenergetics is illustrated in Figure 3.19.

In summary, the citric acid cycle completes the oxidation of carbohydrates, fats, or proteins; produces CO_2; and supplies electrons to be passed through the electron transport chain to provide the energy for the aerobic production of ATP. Enzymes catalyzing citric acid cycle reactions are located inside the mitochondria.

Electron Transport Chain   The aerobic production of ATP (called oxidative phosphorylation) occurs in the mitochondria. The pathway responsible for this process is called the electron transport chain (also called the respiratory chain or cytochrome chain). Aerobic production of ATP is possible due to a mechanism that uses the potential energy available in reduced hydrogen carriers such as NADH and FADH to rephosphorylate ADP to ATP. Note that NADH and FADH do not directly react with oxygen. Instead, electrons removed from the hydrogen atoms transported by NADH and FADH are passed down a series of electron carriers known as cytochromes. During this passage of electrons down the cytochrome chain, enough energy is released to rephosphorylate ADP to form ATP (8) (Fig. 3.21). Interestingly, as electrons pass down the electron transport chain, highly reactive molecules called *free radicals* are also formed. However, during muscular exercise, the increased rates of electron flow through the electron transport chain do not increase the rate of radical production in the mitochondrion (see Research Focus 3.2).

The hydrogen carriers that bring the electrons to the electron transport chain come from a variety of sources. Recall that two NADH are formed per glucose molecule that is degraded via glycolysis (Fig. 3.15). These NADH are outside the mitochondria, and their hydrogens must be transported across the mitochondrial membrane by special "shuttle" mechanisms. However, the bulk of the electrons that enter the electron transport chain come from those NADH and FADH molecules formed as a result of citric acid cycle oxidation.

Figure 3.21 outlines the pathway for electrons entering the electron transport chain. Pairs of electrons from NADH or FADH are passed down a series of compounds that undergo oxidation and reduction, with enough energy being released to synthesize ATP.

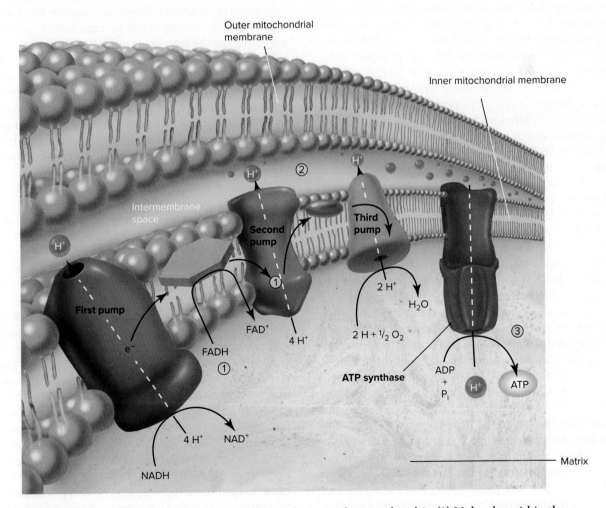

Figure 3.21   The steps leading to oxidative phosphorylation in the mitochondria. (1) Molecules within the electron transport chain function to pump H⁺ from the mitochondrial matrix into the intermembrane space. (2) This results in an increased concentration of H⁺ ions in the intermembrane space and therefore a large H⁺ gradient between the intermembrane space and the matrix of the mitochondria. (3) The movement of H⁺ through the ATP synthase provides the energy required to produce ATP.

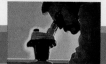
Free Radicals Are Formed in the Mitochondria

Although the passage of electrons down the electron transport chain performs an essential role in the process of aerobic ATP production, this pathway also produces free radicals (30). Free radicals are molecules that have an unpaired electron in their outer orbital, which makes them highly reactive. That is, free radicals quickly react with other molecules in the cell, and this combination results in damage to the molecule combining with the radical.

Historically, it was believed that increased aerobic metabolism during exercise promotes increased production of free radicals in the mitochondria of the working muscles (30). However, new research indicates that this is not the case. Indeed, although exercise results in increased production of free radicals in the active skeletal muscles, this increase in muscle free radical production is not due to oxidative phosphorylation in the mitochondrion (22). For additional information on the sources of free radical production during exercise, see Sakellariou et al. (2013) in the Suggested Readings.

Notice that FADH enters the cytochrome pathway at a point just below the entry level for NADH (Fig. 3.21). This is important because the level of FADH entry bypasses one of the sites of ATP formation, and thus each molecule of FADH that enters the electron transport chain has enough energy to form only 1.5 ATP. In contrast, NADH entry into the electron transport chain results in the formation of 2.5 ATP (details will be mentioned later). At the end of the electron transport chain, oxygen accepts the electrons that are passed along and combines with hydrogen to form water. If O_2 is not available to accept those electrons, oxidative phosphorylation is not possible, and ATP formation in the cell must occur via anaerobic metabolism.

How does this ATP formation occur? The mechanism to explain the aerobic formation of ATP is known as the **chemiosmotic hypothesis.** As electrons are transferred along the cytochrome chain, the energy released is used to "pump" hydrogens (protons; H^+) released from NADH and FADH from the inside (i.e., matrix) of the mitochondria across the inner mitochondrial membrane (Fig. 3.21). This results in an accumulation of hydrogen ions within the space between the inner and outer mitochondrial membranes. The accumulation of H^+ is a source of potential energy that can be captured and used to recombine P_i with ADP to form ATP (17). For example, this collection of H^+ is similar to the potential energy of water at the top of a dam; when the water accumulates and runs over the top of the dam, falling water becomes kinetic energy, which can be used to do work (17).

Three pumps move H^+ (i.e., protons) from mitochondrial matrix to the intermembrane space (Fig. 3.21). The first pump (using NADH) moves four H^+ into the intermembrane space for every two electrons that move along the electron transport chain. The second pump also transports four H^+ into the intermembrane space, while the third pump moves only two H^+ into the intermembrane space. As a result, there is a higher concentration of H^+ within the intermembrane space compared to that in the matrix; this gradient creates a strong drive for these H^+ to diffuse back into the matrix. However, because the inner mitochondrial membrane is not permeable to H^+, these ions can cross the membrane only through specialized H^+ channels (called *respiratory assemblies*). This idea is illustrated in Figure 3.21. Notice that as H^+ cross the inner mitochondrial membrane through these channels, ATP is formed from the addition of phosphate to ADP (called *phosphorylation*). This occurs because the movement of H^+ across the inner mitochondrial membrane activates the enzyme ATP synthase, which is responsible for catalyzing the reaction:

$$ADP + P_i \rightarrow ATP$$

So, why is oxygen essential for the aerobic production of ATP? Remember that the purpose of the electron transport chain is to move electrons down a series of cytochromes to provide energy to drive ATP production in the mitochondria. This process, illustrated in Figure 3.21, requires each element in the electron transport chain to undergo a series of oxidation–reduction reactions. If the last cytochrome (i.e., cytochrome a_3) remains in a reduced state, it would be unable to accept more electrons, and the electron transport chain would stop. However, when oxygen is present, the last cytochrome in the chain can be oxidized by oxygen. That is, oxygen, derived from the air we breathe, allows electron transport to continue by functioning as the final electron acceptor of the electron transport chain. Oxygen is the ultimate electron acceptor in the electron transport chain because oxygen has a high capacity to accept electrons; this property is called electronegativity. Indeed, the ability of oxygen to accept electrons is an essential step in the electron transport chain that allows electron transport and oxidative phosphorylation to continue. Therefore, at the last step in the electron transport

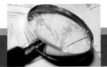
A New Look at the ATP Balance Sheet

Historically, it was believed that aerobic metabolism of one molecule of glucose resulted in the production of 38 ATP. However, recent research suggests that this number overestimates the total ATP production and that only 32 molecules of ATP actually reach the cytoplasm. The explanation for this conclusion is that new evidence indicates that the energy provided by NADH and FADH is required not only for ATP production but also to transport ATP across the mitochondrial membrane. This added energy cost of ATP metabolism reduces the estimates of the total ATP yield from glucose. Specific details of this process follow.

For many years, it was believed that for every three H+ pumped into the intermembrane space, one molecule of ATP was produced and could be used for cellular energy. Although it is true that approximately three H+ must pass through the H+ channels (i.e., respiratory assemblies) to produce one ATP, it is now known that another H+ is required to move the ATP molecule across the mitochondrial membrane into the cytoplasm. The ATP and H+ are transported into the cytoplasm in exchange for ADP and P_i, which are transported into the mitochondria to resynthesize ATP. Therefore, while the theoretical yield of ATP from glucose is 38 molecules, the actual ATP yield, allowing for the energy cost of transport, is only 32 molecules of ATP per glucose. For details of how these numbers are obtained, see the section "Aerobic ATP Tally."

chain, oxygen accepts two electrons that were passed along the electron transport chain from either NADH or FADH. This reduced oxygen molecule now binds with two protons (H+) to form water (Fig. 3.21).

As mentioned earlier, NADH and FADH differ in the amount of ATP that can be formed from each of these molecules. Each NADH formed in the mitochondria donates two electrons to the electron transport system at the first proton pump (Fig. 3.21). These electrons are then passed to the second and third proton pumps until they are finally passed along to oxygen. The first and second electron pumps transport four protons each, whereas the third electron pump transports two protons, for a total of ten. Because four protons are required to produce and transport one ATP from the mitochondria to the cytoplasm, the total ATP production from one NADH molecule is 2.5 ATP (10 protons 4 protons per ATP = 2.5 ATP). Note that ATP molecules do not exist in halves and that the decimal fraction of ATP indicates an average number of ATP molecules that are produced per NADH.

Compared to NADH, each FADH molecule produces less ATP because the electrons from FADH are donated later in the electron transport chain than those by NADH (Fig. 3.21). Therefore, the electrons from FADH activate only the second and third proton pumps. Because the first proton pump is bypassed, the electrons from FADH result in the pumping of six protons (four by the second pump and two by the third pump). Because four protons are required to produce and transport one ATP from the mitochondria to the cytoplasm, the total ATP production from one FAD molecule is 1.5 ATP (6 protons 4 protons per ATP = 1.5 ATP). See A Closer Look 3.5 for more details on the quantity of ATP produced in cells.

IN SUMMARY

■ Oxidative phosphorylation or aerobic ATP production occurs in the mitochondria as a result of a complex interaction between the citric acid cycle and the electron transport chain. The primary role of the citric acid cycle is to complete the oxidation of substrates and form NADH and FADH to enter the electron transport chain. The end result of the electron transport chain is the formation of ATP and water. Water is formed by oxygen accepting electrons; hence, the reason we breathe oxygen is to use it as the final acceptor of electrons in aerobic metabolism.

AEROBIC ATP TALLY

It is now possible to compute the overall ATP production as a result of the aerobic breakdown of glucose or glycogen. Let's begin by counting the total energy yield of glycolysis. Recall that the net ATP production of glycolysis was two ATP per glucose molecule. Furthermore, when O_2 is present in the mitochondria, two NADH produced by glycolysis can then be shuttled into the mitochondria, with the energy used to synthesize an additional five ATP (Table 3.2). Thus, glycolysis can produce two ATP directly via substrate-level phosphorylation and an additional five ATP by the energy contained in the two molecules of NADH.

How many ATP are produced as a result of the oxidation–reduction activities of the citric acid cycle? Table 3.2 shows that two NADH are formed when pyruvate is converted to acetyl-CoA, which results in

Metabolic Process	High-Energy Products	ATP from Oxidative Phosphorylation	ATP Subtotal
Glycolysis	2 ATP	–	2 (total if anaerobic)
	2 NADH*	5	7 (if aerobic)
Pyruvate to acetyl-CoA	2 NADH	5	12
Citric acid cycle	2 GTP	–	14
	6 NADH	15	29
	2 FADH'	3	32
			Grand total: 32 ATP

*2.5 ATP per NADH.

†1.5 ATP per FADH.

the formation of five ATP. Note that two GTP (similar to ATP) are produced via substrate-level phosphorylation. A total of six NADH and two FADH are produced in the citric acid cycle from one glucose molecule. Hence, the six NADH formed via the citric acid cycle results in the production of a total of 15 ATP (6 NADH × 2.5 ATP per NADH = 15 ATP), with 3 ATP being produced from the 2 FADH. Therefore, the total ATP yield for the aerobic degradation of glucose is 32 ATP. The aerobic ATP yield for glycogen breakdown is 33 ATP, because the net glycolytic production of ATP by glycogen is one ATP more than that of glucose.

EFFICIENCY OF OXIDATIVE PHOSPHORYLATION

How efficient is oxidative phosphorylation as a system of converting energy from foodstuffs into biologically usable energy? This can be calculated by computing the ratio of the energy contained in the ATP molecules produced via aerobic respiration divided by the total potential energy contained in the glucose molecule. For example, a mole (a mole is 1 gram molecular weight) of ATP, when broken down, has an energy yield of 7.3 kcal. The potential energy released from the oxidation of a mole of glucose is 686 kcal. Thus, an efficiency figure for aerobic respiration can be computed as follows (18):

$$\text{Efficiency of respiration} = \frac{32 \text{ moles ATP/mole glucose} \times 7.3 \text{ kcal/mole ATP}}{686 \text{ kcal/mole glucose}}$$

Therefore, the efficiency of aerobic respiration is approximately 34%, with the remaining 66% of the free energy of glucose oxidation being released as heat.

IN SUMMARY

- The aerobic metabolism of one molecule of glucose results in the production of 32 ATP molecules, whereas the aerobic ATP yield for glycogen breakdown is 33 ATP.
- The overall efficiency of aerobic respiration is approximately 34%, with the remaining 66% of the energy being released as heat.

CONTROL OF BIOENERGETICS

The biochemical pathways that result in the production of ATP are regulated by very precise control systems. Each of these pathways contains a number of reactions that are catalyzed by specific enzymes. In general, if ample substrate is available, an increase in the number of enzymes present results in an increased rate of chemical reactions. Therefore, the regulation of one or more enzymes in a biochemical pathway would provide a means of controlling the rate of that particular pathway. Indeed, metabolism is regulated by the control of enzymatic activity. Most metabolic pathways have one enzyme that is considered "rate limiting." This rate-limiting enzyme determines the speed of the particular metabolic pathway involved.

How does a rate-limiting enzyme control the speed of reactions? First, as a rule, rate-limiting enzymes are found early in a metabolic pathway. This position is important because products of the pathway might accumulate if the rate-limiting enzymes were located near the end of a pathway. Second, the activity of rate-limiting enzymes is regulated by modulators. Modulators are substances that increase or decrease enzyme activity. Enzymes that are regulated by modulators are called *allosteric enzymes*. In the con-

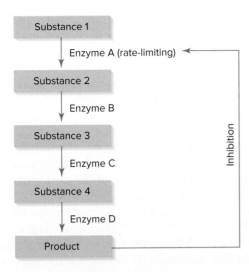

Figure 3.22 An example of a "rate-limiting" enzyme in a simple metabolic pathway. Here, a buildup of the product serves to inhibit the rate-limiting enzyme, which in turn slows down the reactions involved in the pathway.

trol of energy metabolism, ATP is the classic example of an inhibitor, whereas ADP and P_i are examples of substances that stimulate enzymatic activity (31). The fact that large amounts of cellular ATP would inhibit the metabolic production of ATP is logical because large amounts of ATP would indicate that ATP usage in the cell is low. An example of this type of negative feedback is illustrated in Figure 3.22. In contrast, an increase in cell levels of ADP and P_i (low ATP) would indicate that ATP utilization is high. Therefore, it makes sense that ADP and P_i stimulate the production of ATP to meet the increased energy need.

Control of ATP-PC System

Phosphocreatine breakdown is regulated by creatine kinase activity. Creatine kinase is activated when sarcoplasmic concentrations of ADP increase and is inhibited by high levels of ATP. At the onset of exercise, ATP is split into ADP + P_i to provide energy for muscular contraction. This immediate increase in ADP concentrations stimulates creatine kinase to trigger the breakdown of PC to resynthesize ATP. If

exercise is continued, glycolysis and finally aerobic metabolism begin to produce adequate ATP to meet the muscles' energy needs. The increase in ATP concentration, coupled with a reduction in ADP concentration, inhibits creatine kinase activity (Table 3.3). Regulation of the ATP-PC system is an example of a "negative feedback" control system, which was introduced in Chap. 2.

Control of Glycolysis

Although several factors control glycolysis, the most important rate-limiting enzyme in glycolysis is **phosphofructokinase (PFK)** (1). Note that PFK is located near the beginning of glycolysis. Table 3.3 lists known regulators of PFK. When exercise begins, ADP + P_i levels rise and enhance PFK activity, which serves to increase the rate of glycolysis. In contrast, at rest, when cellular ATP levels are high, PFK activity is inhibited and glycolytic activity is slowed. Further, high cellular levels of hydrogen ions (i.e., decreased pH) or citrate (produced via citric acid cycle) also inhibit PFK activity (35). Similar to the control of the ATP-PC system, regulation of PFK activity operates via negative feedback.

Another important regulatory enzyme in carbohydrate metabolism is phosphorylase, which is responsible for degrading glycogen to glucose. Although this enzyme is not technically considered a glycolytic enzyme, the reaction catalyzed by phosphorylase plays an important role in providing the glycolytic pathway with the necessary glucose at the origin of the pathway. With each muscle contraction, calcium (Ca^{++}) is released from the sarcoplasmic reticulum in muscle. This rise in sarcoplasmic Ca^{++} concentration indirectly activates phosphorylase, which immediately begins to break down glycogen to glucose for entry into glycolysis. In addition, phosphorylase activity may be stimulated by high levels of the hormone epinephrine. Epinephrine is released at a faster rate during heavy exercise and results in the formation of the compound cyclic AMP (see Chap. 5). It is cyclic AMP, not epinephrine, that directly activates phosphorylase. Thus, the influence of epinephrine on phosphorylase is indirect.

TABLE 3.3	Factors Known to Affect the Activity of Rate-Limiting Enzymes of Metabolic Pathways Involved in Bioenergetics		
Pathway	**Rate-Limiting Enzyme**	**Stimulators**	**Inhibitors**
ATP-PC system	Creatine kinase	ADP	ATP
Glycolysis	Phosphofructokinase	AMP, ADP, P_i, pH↑	ATP, CP, citrate, pH↓
Citric acid cycle	Isocitrate dehydrogenase	ADP, Ca^{++}, NAD^+	ATP, NADH
Electron transport chain	Cytochrome oxidase	ADP, P_i	ATP

Control of Citric Acid Cycle and Electron Transport Chain

The citric acid cycle, like glycolysis, is subject to enzymatic regulation. Although several citric acid cycle enzymes are regulated, the rate-limiting enzyme is **isocitrate dehydrogenase**. Isocitrate dehydrogenase, like PFK, is inhibited by ATP and stimulated by increasing levels of ADP + P_i (31). Further, growing evidence suggests that increased levels of calcium (Ca^{++}) in the mitochondria also stimulates isocitrate dehydrogenase activity (13, 29). This is a logical signal to turn on energy metabolism in muscle cells because an increase in free calcium in muscle is the signal to begin muscular contraction (see Chap. 8).

The electron transport chain is also regulated by the amount of ATP and ADP + P_i present (31). The rate-limiting enzyme in the electron transport chain is cytochrome oxidase. When exercise begins, ATP levels decline, ADP + P_i levels increase, and cytochrome oxidase is stimulated to begin aerobic production of ATP. When exercise stops, cellular levels of ATP increase and ADP + P_i concentrations decline, and thus the electron transport activity is reduced when normal levels of ATP, ADP, and P_i are reached.

IN SUMMARY

- Metabolism is regulated by enzymatic activity. An enzyme that controls the rate of a metabolic pathway is termed the *rate-limiting enzyme*.
- The rate-limiting enzyme for glycolysis is phosphofructokinase, and the rate-limiting enzymes for the citric acid cycle and electron transport chain are isocitrate dehydrogenase and cytochrome oxidase, respectively.
- In general, cellular levels of ATP and ADP + P_i regulate the rate of metabolic pathways involved in the production of ATP. High levels of ATP inhibit further ATP production, whereas low levels of ATP and high levels of ADP + P_i stimulate ATP production. Evidence also exists that calcium may stimulate aerobic energy metabolism.

INTERACTION BETWEEN AEROBIC/ANAEROBIC ATP PRODUCTION

It is important to emphasize the interaction of anaerobic and aerobic metabolic pathways in the production of ATP during exercise. Although it is common to hear someone speak of aerobic versus anaerobic exercise, in reality, the energy to perform most types of exercise comes from a combination of anaerobic and aerobic sources (11). Indeed, ATP production by the ATP-PC system, glycolysis, and oxidative phosphorylation occurs simultaneously in contracting skeletal muscles. However, during very short bouts of exercise (i.e., one to three seconds), the total contribution of aerobically produced ATP to this movement is small because of the time required to achieve the many reactions involved in the citric acid cycle and the electron transport chain. This point is illustrated in The Winning Edge 3.2. Notice that the contribution of anaerobic ATP production is greater in short-term, high-intensity activities, whereas aerobic metabolism predominates in longer activities. For example, approximately 90% of the energy required to perform a 100-meter dash would come from anaerobic sources, with most of the energy coming via the ATP-PC system. Similarly, energy to run 400 meters (i.e., 55 seconds) would be largely anaerobic (70% to 75%). However, ATP and PC stores are limited, and thus glycolysis must supply much of the ATP during this type of event (11).

On the other end of the energy spectrum, events like the marathon (i.e., 26.2-mile race) rely on aerobic production of ATP for the bulk of the needed energy. Where does the energy come from in events of moderate length (i.e., 2 to 30 minutes)? The Winning Edge 3.2 provides an estimation of the percentage of anaerobic/aerobic yield in events over a wide range of durations. Although these estimates are based on laboratory measurements of running or exercising on a cycle ergometer, they can be related to other athletic events that require intense effort by comparing the length of time spent in the activity. In review, the shorter the duration of all-out activity, the greater the contribution of anaerobic energy production; conversely, the longer the duration, the greater the contribution of aerobic energy production. A more detailed discussion of the metabolic responses to various types of exercise is presented in Chap. 4.

IN SUMMARY

- Energy to perform exercise comes from an interaction of anaerobic and aerobic pathways.
- In general, the shorter the activity (high intensity), the greater the contribution of anaerobic energy production. In contrast, long-term activities (low to moderate intensity) utilize ATP produced from aerobic sources.

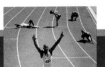

THE WINNING EDGE 3.2

Exercise Physiology Applied to Sports

Contributions of Anaerobic/ Aerobic Energy Production During Various Sporting Events

Because sports differ widely in both the intensity and the duration of physical effort, it is not surprising that the source of energy production differs widely among sporting events. Figure 3.23 provides an illustration of the anaerobic versus aerobic energy production during selected sports. Knowledge of the interaction between the anaerobic and aerobic energy production in exercise is useful to coaches and trainers in planning conditioning programs for athletes. See Chap. 21 for more details.

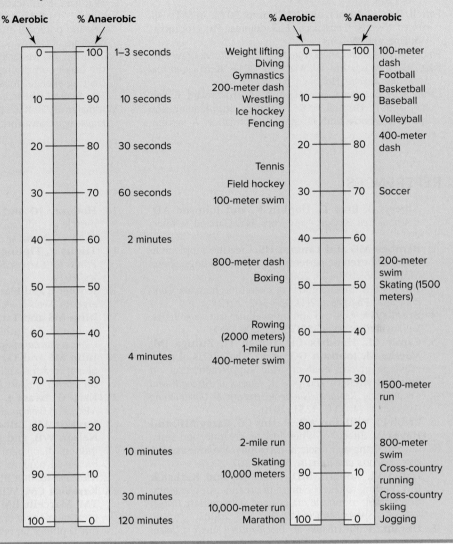

Figure 3.23 Contribution of anaerobically and aerobically produced ATP for use during sports.

STUDY ACTIVITIES

1. List and briefly discuss the function of the three major components of cell structure.
2. Briefly explain the concept of coupled reactions.
3. Define the following terms: (1) *bioenergetics*, (2) *endergonic reactions*, and (3) *exergonic reactions*.
4. Discuss the role of enzymes as catalysts. What is meant by the expression "energy of activation"?
5. Where do glycolysis, the citric acid cycle, and oxidative phosphorylation take place in the cell?
6. Define the terms *glycogen*, *glycogenolysis*, and *glycolysis*.
7. What are high-energy phosphates? Explain the statement that "ATP is the universal energy donor."
8. Define the terms *aerobic* and *anaerobic*.
9. Briefly discuss the function of glycolysis in bioenergetics. What role does NAD$^+$ play in glycolysis?
10. Discuss the operation of the citric acid cycle and the electron transport chain in the aerobic production of ATP. What is the function of NAD$^+$ and FAD in these pathways?
11. What is the efficiency of the aerobic degradation of glucose?
12. What is the role of oxygen in aerobic metabolism?
13. What are the rate-limiting enzymes for the following metabolic pathways: ATP-PC system, glycolysis, citric acid cycle, and electron transport chain?
14. Briefly discuss the interaction of anaerobic versus aerobic ATP production during exercise.
15. Discuss the chemiosmotic theory of ATP production.
16. Briefly discuss the impact of changes in both temperature and pH on enzyme activity.
17. Discuss the relationship between lactic acid and lactate.

SUGGESTED READINGS

Devries, M.C. and S. Phillips. 2014. Creatine supplementation during resistance training in older adults-a meta-analysis. *Medicine and Science in Sports and Exercise.* 46: 1194-1203.

Farrell, P.A., M. Joyner, and V. Caiozzo. 2012. ACSM's *Advanced Exercise Physiology.* Philadelphia, PA: Lippincott Williams and Wilkins.

Fox, S. 2016. *Human Physiology.* New York, NY: McGraw-Hill.

Karp, G., J. Iwasa, and W. Marshall. 2016. *Karp's Cell and Molecular Biology.* Hoboken, NJ: Wiley.

Lanhers, C., B. Pereira, G. Naughton, M. Trousselard, F. Lesage, and F. Dutheil. 2015. Creatine supplementation and lower body limb strength performance: A system-atic review and metabolic analysis. *Sports Medicine.* 45: 1285-1294.

Nicholls, D.G. and S. Ferguson. 2013. *Bioenergetics 4.* Waltham, MA: Academic Press.

Sahlin, K. 2014. Muscle energetics during explosive activities and potential effects of nutrition and training. *Sports Medicine.* 44: S167-S173.

Sakellariou, G., M. Jackson, and A. Vasilaki. 2014. Refining the major contributors to superoxide production in contracting skeletal muscle. The role of NAD(P)H oxidases. *Free Radical Research.* Epub. 48:12-29.

Widmaier, E., H. Raff, and K. Strang. 2014. *Vander's Human Physiology.* New York, NY: McGraw-Hill.

REFERENCES

1. **Alberts B, Bray D, Hopkin K, and Johnson AD.** *Essential Cell Biology.* New York, NY: Garland Science, 2014.

2. **Bemben MG and Lamont HS.** Creatine supplementation and exercise performance: recent findings. *Sports Medicine* 35: 107-125, 2005.

3. **Brooks GA.** Bioenergetics of exercising humans. *Comprehensive Physiology* 2(1): 537-562, 2012.

4. **Brooks GA.** Cell-cell and intracellular lactate shuttles. *Journal of Physiology* 587: 5591-5600, 2009.

5. **Camic CL, Hendrix CR, Housh TJ, Zuniga JM, Mielke M, Johnson GO, et al.** The effects of poly-ethylene glycosylated creatine supplementation on muscular strength and power. *Journal of Strength and Conditioning Research/National Strength & Conditioning Association* 24: 3343-3351, 2010.

6. **Cribb PJ, Williams AD, Stathis CG, Carey MF, and Hayes A.** Effects of whey isolate, creatine, and resistance training on muscle hypertrophy. *Medicine and Science in Sports and Exercise* 39: 298-307, 2007.

7. **Dalbo VJ, Roberts MD, Stout JR, and Kerksick CM.** Putting to rest the myth of creatine supplementation leading to muscle cramps and dehydration. *British Journal of Sports Medicine* 42: 567-573, 2008.

8. **Devlin T.** *Textbook of Biochemistry with Clinical Correlations.* Hoboken, NJ: Wiley, 2010.

9. **Dolny DG and Lemon PW.** Effect of ambient temperature on protein breakdown during prolonged exercise. *Journal of Applied Physiology* 64: 550-555, 1988.

10. **Fox S.** *Human Physiology.* New York, NY: McGraw-Hill, 2015.

11. **Gastin PB.** Energy system interaction and relative contribution during maximal exercise. *Sports Medicine* 31: 725-741, 2001.

12. **Gibala MJ.** Protein metabolism and endurance exercise. *Sports Medicine* 37: 337-340, 2007.

13. **Glancy B, Willis WT, Chess DJ, and Balaban RS.** Effect of calcium on the oxidative phosphorylation cascade in skeletal muscle mitochondria. *Biochemistry* 52: 2793-2809, 2013.

14. **Glancy B, Hartnell L, Malide D, Yu Z, Combs C, Connelly P, et al.** Mitochondrial reticulum for cellular energy distribution in muscle. *Nature* 523: 617-620, 2015.

15. **Hespel P and Derave W.** Ergogenic effects of creatine in sports and rehabilitation. *Sub-cellular Biochemistry* 46: 245-259, 2007.

16. **Holloszy JO and Coyle EF.** Adaptations of skeletal muscle to endurance exercise and their metabolic consequences. *Journal of Applied Physiology* 56: 831-838, 1984.

17. **Tiidus P, Tipling R, and Houston M.** *Biochemistry Primer for Exercise Science.* Champaign, IL: Human Kinetics, 2012.

18. **Jequier E and Flatt J.** Recent advances in human bioenergetics. *News in Physiological Sciences* 1: 112-114, 1986.

19. **Juhn MS and Tarnopolsky M.** Oral creatine supplementation and athletic performance: a critical review. *Clinical Journal of Sport Medicine* 8: 286-297, 1998.

20. **Juhn MS and Tarnopolsky M.** Potential side effects of oral creatine supplementation: a critical review. *Clinical Journal of Sport Medicine* 8: 298-304, 1998.

21. **Karp G, Iwasa J, and Marshall W.** *Karp's Cell and Molecular Biology* Hoboken, NJ: Wiley, 2016.

22. **Kavazis AN, Talbert EE, Smuder AJ, Hudson MB, Nelson WB, and Powers SK.** Mechanical ventilation induces diaphragmatic mitochondrial dysfunction and increased oxidant production. *Free Radical Biology & Medicine* 46: 842-850, 2009.

23. **Kerksick CM, Wilborn CD, Campbell WI, Harvey TM, Marcello BM, Roberts MD, et al.** The effects of creatine monohydrate supplementation with and without D-pinitol on resistance training adaptations. *Journal of Strength and Conditioning Research/National Strength & Conditioning Association* 23: 2673-2682, 2009.

24. **Law YL, Ong WS, GillianYap TL, Lim SC, and Von Chia E.** Effects of two and five days of creatine loading on muscular strength and anaerobic power in trained athletes. *Journal of Strength and Conditioning Research/National Strength & Conditioning Association* 23: 906-914, 2009.

25. **Lemon PW and Mullin JP.** Effect of initial muscle glycogen levels on protein catabolism during exercise. *Journal of Applied Physiology* 48: 624-629, 1980.

26. **Maughan RJ.** Creatine supplementation and exercise performance. *International Journal of Sport Nutrition* 5: 94-101, 1995.

27. **Maughan RJ, King DS, and Lea T.** Dietary supplements. *Journal of Sports Sciences* 22: 95-113, 2004.

28. **McArdle W, Katch F, and Katch V.** *Exercise Physiology: Energy, Nutrition, and Human Performance.* Baltimore, MD: Lippincott Williams & Wilkins, 2006.

29. **McCormack J and Denton R.** Signal transduction by intramitochondrial calcium in mammalian energy metabolism. *News in Physiological Sciences* 9: 71-76, 1994.

30. **Powers S, Nelson W, and Hudson M.** Exercise-induced oxidative stress in humans: cause and consequences. *Free Radical Biology and Medicine* 51: 942-950, 2011.

31. **Pratt CW and Cornely K.** *Essential Biochemistry.* Hoboken, NJ: Wiley, 2013.

32. **Rawson ES and Volek JS.** Effects of creatine supplementation and resistance training on muscle strength and weightlifting performance. *Journal of Strength and Conditioning Research/National Strength & Conditioning Association* 17: 822-831, 2003.

33. **Reed S.** *Essential Physiological Biochemistry: An Organ-Based Approach.* Hoboken, NJ: Wiley, 2010.

34. **Sahlin K.** Muscle energetics during explosive activities and potential effects of nutrition and training. *Sports Medicine* 44: S167-S173, 2014.

35. **Spriet LL.** Phosphofructokinase activity and acidosis during short-term tetanic contractions. *Canadian Journal of Physiology and Pharmacology* 69: 298-304, 1991.

36. **Tymoczko J, Berg J, and Stryer L.** *Biochemistry: A Short Course.* London, UK: Macmillan Higher Education, 2016.

37. **Voet D, Voet J, and Pratt C.** *Fundamentals of biochemistry: Life at the molecular level.* Hoboken, NJ: Wiley, 2015.

38. **Tandon O.** *Best and Taylor's Physiological Basis of Medical Practice.* Baltimore, MD: Lippincott Williams & Wilkins, 2011.

39. **Williams MH and Branch JD.** Creatine supplementation and exercise performance: an update. *Journal of the American College of Nutrition* 17: 216-234, 1998.

4

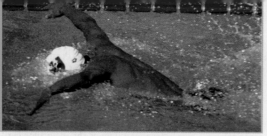

© Action Plus Sports Images/Alamy Stock Photo

Exercise Metabolism

■ Objectives

By studying this chapter, you should be able to do the following:

1. Discuss the relationship between exercise intensity/duration and the bioenergetic pathways that are most responsible for the production of ATP during various types of exercise.

2. Describe graphically the change in oxygen uptake during the transition from rest to steady-state exercise and then recovery from exercise. Identify the oxygen deficit, oxygen requirement, and oxygen debt (excess post-exercise oxygen uptake).

3. Describe graphically the changes in oxygen uptake during an incremental (graded) exercise test and identify the maximal oxygen uptake ($\dot{V}O_2$ max).

4. Describe the various criteria for having achieved ($\dot{V}O_2$ max).

5. Describe graphically the changes in the blood lactate concentration during an incremental

(graded) exercise test and identify the lactate threshold.

6. Discuss several possible explanations for the sudden rise in blood-lactate concentration during incremental exercise.

7. List the factors that regulate fuel selection during exercise.

8. Describe the changes in the respiratory exchange ratio (R) with increasing intensities of exercise and during prolonged exercise of moderate intensity.

9. Describe the types of carbohydrates and fats used during increasing intensities of exercise and during prolonged exercise of moderate intensity.

10. Describe the lactate shuttle, with examples of how it is used during exercise.

■ Outline

■ Key Terms

anaerobic threshold
Cori cycle
excess post-exercise oxygen consumption (EPOC)
free fatty acids (FFAs)
gluconeogenesis
graded (or incremental) exercise test
incremental exercise test
lactate threshold
lipase
lipolysis
maximal oxygen uptake ($\dot{V}O_2$ max)
oxygen debt
oxygen deficit
respiratory exchange ratio (R)

Exercise poses a serious challenge to the bioenergetic pathways in the working muscle. For example, during heavy exercise, the body's total energy expenditure may increase 15 to 25 times above expenditure at rest. Most of this increase in energy production is used to provide ATP for contracting skeletal muscles, which may increase their energy utilization 200 times over utilization at rest (1). Clearly, skeletal muscles have a great capacity to produce and use large quantities of ATP during exercise. This chapter describes (a) the metabolic responses at the beginning of exercise and during recovery from exercise; (b) the metabolic responses to high-intensity, incremental, and prolonged exercise; (c) the selection of fuels used to produce ATP; and (d) how exercise metabolism is regulated.

We begin with an overview of the energy requirements of the body at rest, followed by a discussion of which bioenergetic pathways are activated at the onset of exercise.

ENERGY REQUIREMENTS AT REST

Recall that homeostasis is defined as a steady and an unchanging internal environment (see Chap. 2). During resting conditions, the healthy human body is in homeostasis, and therefore the body's energy requirement is also constant. At rest, almost 100% of the energy (i.e., ATP) required to sustain bodily functions is produced by aerobic metabolism. It follows that resting blood lactate levels are also steady and low (e.g., 1.0 millimole per liter).

Because the measurement of oxygen (O_2) consumption (oxygen consumed by the body) is an index of aerobic ATP production, measurement of O_2 consumption during rest provides an estimate of the body's "baseline" energy requirement. At rest, the total energy requirement of an individual is relatively low. For example, a 70-kilogram young adult would consume approximately 0.25 liter of oxygen each minute; this translates to a relative O_2 consumption of 3.5 ml of O_2 per kilogram (body weight) per minute. As mentioned earlier, muscular exercise can greatly increase the body's need for energy. Let's begin our discussion of exercise metabolism by considering which bioenergetic pathways are active during the transition from rest to exercise.

REST-TO-EXERCISE TRANSITIONS

Assume you are standing alongside a treadmill with its belt moving at 7 mph, and you jump onto the belt and start running. Within one step, you go from zero to 7 mph, and in that one step your muscles increase their rate of ATP production from that required for standing to that required for running at 7 mph (see Fig. 4.1(a) and (b)). If ATP production did not increase instantaneously, you would have fallen off the back of the treadmill! What metabolic changes must occur in skeletal muscle at the beginning of exercise to provide

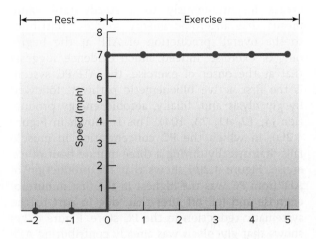

(b)

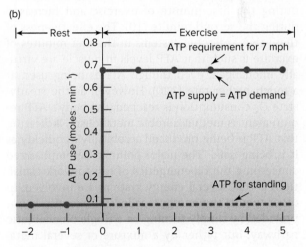

(c)

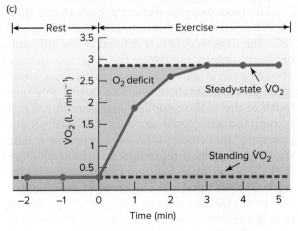

Figure 4.1 The time course of speed (a), rate of ATP use (b), and oxygen uptake ($\dot{V}O_2$) (c) in the transition from rest to submaximal exercise.

the necessary energy to continue movement? Similar to the measurement of O_2 consumption during rest, the measurement of O_2 consumption during exercise can provide information about aerobic metabolism during exercise. For example, in the transition from rest to light or moderate exercise, O_2 consumption increases rapidly and reaches a steady state within one to four minutes (12, 22, 99) (Fig. 4.1(c)).

The fact that O_2 consumption does not increase instantaneously to a steady-state value means that anaerobic energy sources contribute to the overall production of ATP at the beginning of exercise. Indeed, much evidence suggests that at the onset of exercise, the ATP-PC system is the first active bioenergetic pathway, followed by glycolysis and, finally, aerobic energy production (4, 17, 41, 73, 104). This is shown in Figure 4.2(a), in which the PC concentration in muscle falls dramatically during a three-minute bout of exercise. Figure 4.2(b) shows that the production of ATP from PC was the highest in the first minute of exercise and fell off after that, due in part to the systematic reduction in the PC store. Figure 4.2(c) shows that glycolysis was already contributing ATP during the first minute of exercise and increased during the second minute (10). The effectiveness of these two anaerobic systems in the first minutes of exercise is such that ATP levels in muscle are virtually unchanged, even though ATP is being used at a much higher rate (120). However, as the steady-state O_2 consumption is reached, the body's ATP requirement is met via aerobic metabolism, indicating that ATP is being produced aerobically as quickly as it is being used. The major point to be emphasized concerning the bioenergetics of rest-to-work transitions is that several energy systems are involved. In other words, the energy needed for exercise is not provided by simply turning on a single bioenergetic pathway, but rather by a mixture of several metabolic systems operating with considerable overlap.

The term **oxygen deficit** applies to the lag in oxygen uptake at the beginning of exercise. Specifically, the oxygen deficit is defined as the difference between oxygen uptake in the first few minutes of exercise and an equal time period after steady state has been obtained (90, 97). During this time, much of the ATP is supplied anaerobically (ATP-PC system and glycolysis) since aerobic ATP production is insufficient until the oxygen uptake reaches steady state. This is represented as the shaded area in the left portion of Figure 4.1(c). What causes this lag in oxygen uptake at the onset of exercise? Is it due to inadequate oxygen delivery to the muscle, or is it a failure of oxidative phosphorylation to increase immediately when exercise begins (82)? Dr. Bruce Gladden answers those questions in Ask the Expert 4.1.

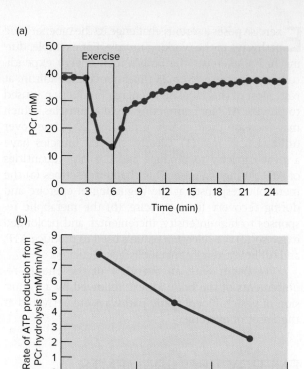

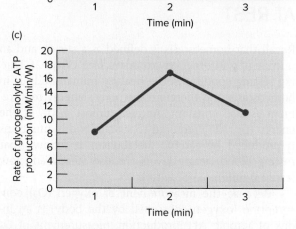

Figure 4.2 Figure (a) shows the rapid change of phosphocreatine (PC) concentration in muscle during a three-minute bout of exercise. Figures (b) and (c) show the rate of ATP production during this three-minute bout from PC and glycolysis, respectively.

Trained adults (64, 99) and adolescents (88) reach the steady-state $\dot{V}O_2$ faster than untrained subjects, resulting in a smaller oxygen deficit. What is the explanation for this difference? It seems likely that the trained subjects have a better developed aerobic bioenergetic capacity, resulting from either cardiovascular or muscular adaptations induced by endurance training (33, 64, 97, 99). Practically speaking, this means that aerobic ATP production is active earlier at the beginning of exercise and results in less production of lactate and H^+ in the trained individual when compared to the untrained individual. Chapter 13 provides a detailed analysis of this adaptation to training.

Oxygen Uptake Kinetics at the Onset of Constant Work-Rate Exercise: Questions and Answers with Dr. Bruce Gladden

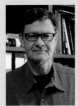

Courtesy of Bruce Gladden

Bruce Gladden, Ph.D., a professor in the School of Kinesiology at Auburn University, is an internationally known expert in muscle metabolism during exercise. Dr. Gladden's research has addressed important questions relative to those factors that regulate oxygen consumption in skeletal muscle during exercise. Examples of Dr. Gladden's work can be found in prestigious international physiology journals. In this feature, Dr. Gladden answers questions about the time course of oxygen consumption at the onset of submaximal exercise.

QUESTION: What is so important about the oxygen consumption response at the onset of submaximal, constant work-rate exercise?

ANSWER: First, it is critical to realize that O_2 consumption is a reliable indicator of the energy supplied by oxidative phosphorylation (i.e., the oxidative or aerobic energy system). The fact that there is a "lag" or delay before oxygen consumption rises to a steady-state level tells us that aerobic metabolism (i.e., oxidative phosphorylation in the mitochondria) is not fully activated at the onset of exercise. The importance of this response is that it can provide information about the control or regulation of oxidative phosphorylation. Further, this delayed response tells us that the anaerobic energy systems must also be activated to supply the needed energy at the beginning of exercise; that is, there is an oxygen deficit.

QUESTION: Why is oxidative phosphorylation not fully activated instantaneously at the onset of exercise?

ANSWER: Historically, two alternative hypotheses have been offered. First, it has been suggested that there is an inadequate oxygen supply to the contracting muscles at the onset of exercise. What this means is that in at least some mitochondria, at least some of the time, there may not be molecules of oxygen available to accept electrons at the end of the electron transport chains. Clearly, if this is correct, the oxidative phosphorylation rate, and therefore the whole-body oxygen consumption, would be restricted. The second hypothesis holds that there is a delay because the stimuli for oxidative phosphorylation require some time to reach their final levels and to have their full effects for a given exercise intensity. As discussed in Chap. 3, the electron transport chain is stimulated by ADP and P_i (e.g., Table 3.3). Shortly after the onset of exercise, the concentrations of ADP and P_i are barely above resting levels because the ATP concentration is being maintained by the creatine kinase reaction ($PC + ADP \rightarrow ATP + C$) and accelerated glycolysis (with lactate accumulation). However, the concentrations of ADP and P_i will continue to rise as PC is broken down, gradually providing additional stimulation to "turn on" oxidative phosphorylation until this aerobic pathway is providing essentially 100% of the energy requirement of the exercise. The key point is that these stimulators of oxidative phosphorylation rate do not instantaneously rise from resting concentrations to the steady-state concentration levels. This has sometimes been referred to as the "inertia of metabolism."

QUESTION: Which of the two hypotheses is correct?

ANSWER: This is a difficult question because the two hypotheses are not mutually exclusive. My research with numerous colleagues (especially Drs. Bruno Grassi, Mike Hogan, and Harry Rossiter) provides support for the second hypothesis (i.e., "slowness" in the stimuli required to fully activate oxidative phosphorylation). In particular, there is evidence for a significant role of the creatine kinase reaction in "buffering" some of the most important signals (e.g., ADP concentration) for activating oxidative phosphorylation. Nevertheless, oxygen supply limitation can also play a role, a role that likely becomes more important at higher exercise intensities. None of the possible regulators or controllers of oxidative phosphorylation should be considered separately. All of them interact with each other to provide the overall stimulus to oxidative phosphorylation under any given exercise condition.

IN SUMMARY

- In the transition from rest to light or moderate exercise, oxygen uptake increases rapidly, generally reaching a steady state within one to four minutes.
- The term *oxygen deficit* applies to the lag in oxygen uptake at the beginning of exercise.
- The failure of oxygen uptake to increase instantly at the beginning of exercise means that anaerobic pathways contribute to the overall production of ATP early in exercise. After a steady state is reached, the body's ATP requirement is met via aerobic metabolism.

RECOVERY FROM EXERCISE: METABOLIC RESPONSES

If a subject is running on the treadmill at a speed that can be maintained comfortably for 20 or 30 minutes, and then jumps off to the side, the metabolic rate ($\dot{V}O_2$) does not fall instantaneously from the steady-state value measured during the exercise to the resting $\dot{V}O_2$ value associated with standing by the treadmill. The metabolic rate remains elevated for several minutes immediately following exercise. This is shown in Figure 4.3(*a*), with a steady-state $\dot{V}O_2$ being achieved

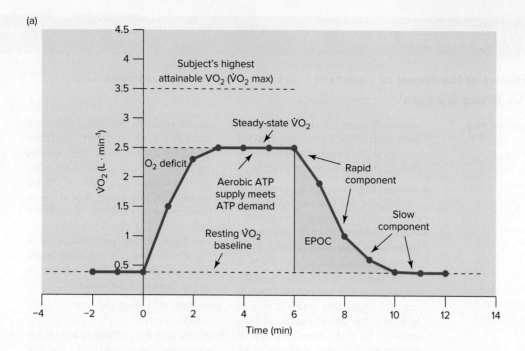

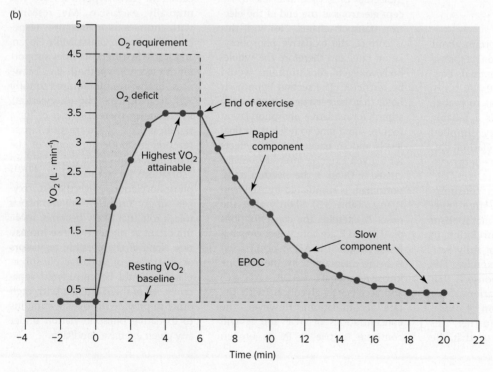

Figure 4.3 Oxygen deficit and the excess post-exercise O_2 consumption (EPOC) during moderate exercise (*a*) and during heavy, exhausting exercise (*b*).

by minute 3 of submaximal exercise, and the oxygen uptake returning to resting levels by five minutes after exercise. This means that, for several minutes after exercise, the oxygen uptake is above the level needed to meet the demands of standing on the treadmill. In contrast, Figure 4.3(*b*) shows the subject doing nonsteady-state exercise that can be maintained for only six minutes before exhaustion occurs. This test is set at an intensity that exceeds the highest $\dot{V}O_2$ the subject can attain ($\dot{V}O_2$ max). In this case, the subject could not meet the oxygen requirement for the task as shown by the much larger oxygen deficit, and the subject's $\dot{V}O_2$

is still not back to the resting level by 14 minutes after exercise. Clearly, the magnitude and duration of this elevated post-exercise metabolic rate are influenced by the intensity of the exercise (6, 53, 97). The reason(s) for this observation will be discussed shortly.

Historically, the term **oxygen debt** has been applied to the elevated oxygen uptake (above resting levels) following exercise. The prominent British physiologist A. V. Hill (65) first used the term O_2 debt and reasoned that the excess oxygen consumed (above rest) following exercise was repayment for the O_2 deficit incurred at the onset of exercise

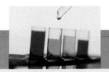

A.V. Hill Was a Pioneer in Exercise Physiology

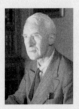

© AP Images

Archibald Vivian (A.V.) Hill (1886-1977) received the Nobel Prize in Physiology or Medicine in 1922 for his research on heat production in skeletal muscle. This work precisely described the magnitude of heat production in isolated skeletal muscle during both contraction and relaxation. Professor Hill was born in Bristol, England, and his family had little money to support his education. Nonetheless, he was both motivated and resourceful as he earned scholarships to support his studies in mathematics and natural sciences (chemistry, physics, and physiology) at Trinity College, Cambridge.

After graduation, Hill was encouraged to focus on physiology by one of his teachers, Dr. Walter Fletcher. Hill initiated his physiology research career at Cambridge in 1909 and began to investigate the nature of muscular contraction using frog muscle as a model. Hill later held faculty positions at Manchester University (1920-1923) and at University College, London (1923-1951).

In addition to his Nobel Prize winning research on heat production in skeletal muscle, A.V. Hill made many other contributions to our understanding of exercise physiology. For example, he was the first physiologist to demonstrate that contracting skeletal muscle can produce energy anaerobically. This work was important because the general view at the time was that all energy for muscular performance was derived from aerobic metabolism. A.V. Hill also introduced the concept of the oxygen debt (i.e., oxygen consumption following exercise), and he was the first scientist to clearly describe the concept of maximal oxygen consumption in exercising humans. Other important scientific contributions of Hill include his discovery of heat production in nerves and the force-velocity equation in skeletal muscle.

For more information on A.V. Hill and his scientific contributions to exercise physiology, see the paper by Bassett in the Suggested Readings.

(see A Look Back–Important People in Science). Evidence collected in the 1920s and 1930s by Hill and other researchers in Europe and the United States suggested that the oxygen debt could be divided into two portions: the rapid portion immediately following exercise (i.e., approximately two to three minutes post-exercise) and the slow portion, which persisted for greater than 30 minutes after some types of exercise. The rapid portion is represented by the steep decline in oxygen uptake following exercise, and the slow portion is represented by the slow decline in O_2 across time following exercise (Fig. 4.3(a) and (b)). The rationale for the two divisions of the O_2 debt was based on the belief that the rapid portion of the O_2 debt represented the oxygen that was required to resynthesize stored ATP and PC and replace tissue stores of O_2 (~20% of the O_2 debt), while the slow portion of the debt was due to the oxidative conversion of lactate to glucose in the liver (~80% of the O_2 debt).

Contradicting previous beliefs, current evidence shows that only about 20% of the oxygen debt is used to convert the lactate produced during exercise to glucose (the process of glucose synthesis from noncarbohydrate sources is called **gluconeogenesis**) (14, 17). Several investigators have argued that the term *oxygen debt* be eliminated from the literature because the elevated oxygen consumption following exercise does not appear to be entirely due to the "borrowing" of oxygen from the body's oxygen stores (14, 15, 17, 46). In recent years, several replacement terms have been suggested. One such term is **EPOC,** which stands for "**excess post-exercise oxygen consumption**" (15, 46).

If the EPOC is not exclusively used to convert lactate to glucose, why does oxygen consumption remain elevated post-exercise? Several possibilities exist. First, at least part of the O_2 consumed immediately following exercise is used to restore PC in muscle and O_2 stores in blood and tissues (12, 46).

Restoration of both PC and oxygen stores in muscle is completed within two to three minutes of recovery (59). This is consistent with the classic view of the rapid portion of the oxygen debt. Further, heart rate and breathing remain elevated above resting levels for several minutes following exercise; therefore, both of these activities require additional O_2 above resting levels. Other factors that may result in the EPOC are an elevated body temperature and specific circulating hormones. Increases in body temperature result in an increased metabolic rate (called the Q_{10} effect) (19, 57, 101). Further, it has been argued that high levels of epinephrine or norepinephrine result in increased oxygen consumption after exercise (48). However, both of these hormones are rapidly removed from the blood following exercise and therefore may not exist long enough to have a significant impact on the EPOC.

Compared to moderate-intensity exercise, the EPOC is greater during high-intensity exercise because (53)

- Heat production and body temperature are higher
- PC is depleted to a greater extent and more O_2 is required for its resynthesis

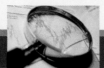

A CLOSER LOOK 4.1

Removal of Lactate Following Exercise

What happens to the lactate that is formed during exercise? Classical theory proposed that the majority of the post-exercise lactate was converted into glucose in the liver and resulted in an elevated post-exercise oxygen uptake (i.e., O_2 debt). However, recent evidence suggests that this is not the case and that lactate is mainly oxidized after exercise (14, 17). That is, lactate is converted to pyruvate and used as a substrate by the heart and skeletal muscle. It is estimated that approximately 70% of the lactate produced during exercise is oxidized, while 20% is converted to glucose and the remaining 10% is converted to amino acids.

Figure 4.4 demonstrates the time course of lactate removal from the blood following strenuous exercise. Note that lactate removal is more rapid if continuous light exercise is performed as compared to a resting recovery. The explanation for these findings is linked to the fact that light exercise enhances the oxidation of lactate by the working muscle (34, 47, 63). It is estimated that the optimum intensity of recovery exercise to promote blood lactate removal is around 30% to 40% of $\dot{V}O_2$ max (34). Higher

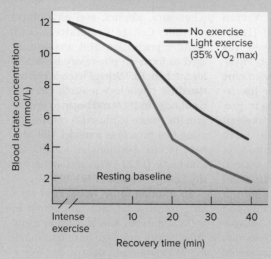

Figure 4.4 Blood lactate removal following strenuous exercise. Note that lactate can be removed more rapidly from the blood during recovery if the subject engages in continuous light exercise.

exercise intensities would likely result in an increased muscle production of lactate and therefore hinder removal.

In one study, the intensity of the active recovery was set at a percentage of the lactate threshold (LT), rather than a percentage of $\dot{V}O_2$ max. They found that when subjects did their active recovery at intensities just below the LT (the point at which lactate accumulation occurs), blood lactate was removed faster than at lower intensities (e.g., 40% to 60% of the LT) (92).

Due to the increase in muscle oxidative capacity observed with endurance training, some authors have speculated that trained subjects might have a greater capacity to remove lactate during recovery from intense exercise (7, 9). However, two well-designed investigations have reported no differences in blood lactate disappearance between trained and untrained subjects during resting recovery from a maximal exercise bout (7, 42).

- Higher blood lactate levels mean more O_2 is required for lactate conversion to glucose in gluconeogenesis
- Epinephrine and norepinephrine levels are much higher.

All these factors may contribute to the EPOC being greater following high-intensity exercise than following moderate-intensity exercise. This observation has been used to make claims that high intensity exercise is better for weight loss because of the prolonged "after-burn." However, it isn't as important for weight loss as people might hope. It has been shown that when subjects are tested at the same absolute work rate following an endurance training program, the majority of these factors are reduced in magnitude, and with it, the EPOC (110). Figure 4.5 contains a summary of factors thought to contribute to the excess post-exercise

oxygen consumption. Further, see A Closer Look 4.1 for more details on removal of lactate following exercise.

IN SUMMARY

- The oxygen debt (also called excess post-exercise oxygen consumption [EPOC]) is the O_2 consumption above rest following exercise.
- Several factors contribute to the EPOC. First, some of the O_2 consumed early in the recovery period is used to resynthesize stored PC in the muscle and replace O_2 stores in both muscle and blood. Other factors that contribute to the "slow" portion of the EPOC include an elevated body temperature, O_2 required to convert lactate to glucose (gluconeogenesis), and elevated blood levels of epinephrine and norepinephrine.

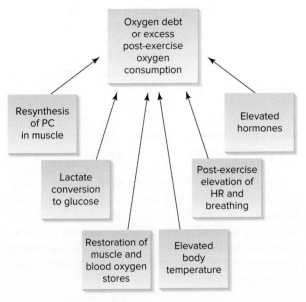

Factors Contributing to Excess Post-Exercise Oxygen Consumption

Figure 4.5 A summary of factors that might contribute to excess post-exercise oxygen consumption (EPOC). See text for details.

METABOLIC RESPONSES TO EXERCISE: INFLUENCE OF DURATION AND INTENSITY

The point was made in Chap. 3 that short-term, high-intensity exercise lasting less than ten seconds utilizes primarily anaerobic metabolic pathways to produce ATP. In contrast, an event like the marathon makes primary use of aerobic ATP production to provide the needed ATP for work. However, events lasting longer than 10 to 20 seconds and less than 10 minutes generally produce the needed ATP for muscular contraction via a combination of both anaerobic and aerobic pathways. In fact, most sports use a combination of anaerobic and aerobic pathways to produce the ATP needed for muscular contraction. The next three sections consider which bioenergetic pathways are involved in energy production in specific types of exercise.

Short-Term, Intense Exercise

The energy to perform short-term exercise of high intensity comes primarily from anaerobic metabolic pathways. Whether the ATP production is dominated by the ATP-PC system or glycolysis depends primarily on the length of the activity (1, 4, 73, 80). For example, the energy to run a 50-meter dash or to complete a single play in a football game comes principally from the ATP-PC system. In contrast, the energy to complete the 400-meter dash (i.e., 55 seconds) comes from a combination of the ATP-PC system, glycolysis, and aerobic

metabolism, with glycolysis producing most of the ATP. In general, the ATP-PC system can supply almost all the needed ATP for work for events lasting one to five seconds; intense exercise lasting longer than five seconds begins to utilize the ATP-producing capability of glycolysis. It should be emphasized that the transition from the ATP-PC system to an increased dependence upon glycolysis during exercise is not an abrupt change but rather a gradual shift from one pathway to another.

Events lasting longer than 45 seconds use a combination of all three energy systems (i.e., ATP-PC, glycolysis, and aerobic systems). This point was emphasized in Figure 3.23 in Chap. 3. In general, intense exercise lasting approximately 60 seconds utilizes 70%/30% (anaerobic/aerobic) energy production, whereas competitive events lasting 2 to 3 minutes utilize anaerobic and aerobic bioenergetic pathways almost equally to supply the needed ATP (see Fig. 3.23). Clearly, the contribution of aerobic energy production to the total energy requirement increases with the duration of the competition.

IN SUMMARY

- During high-intensity, short-term exercise (i.e., 2 to 20 seconds), the muscle's ATP production is dominated by the ATP-PC system.
- Intense exercise lasting more than 20 seconds relies more on anaerobic glycolysis to produce much of the needed ATP.
- Finally, high-intensity events lasting longer than 45 seconds use a combination of the ATP-PC system, glycolysis, and the aerobic system to produce the needed ATP for muscular contraction, with a 50%/50% (anaerobic/aerobic) contribution needed for exercise lasting between two and three minutes.

Prolonged Exercise

The energy to perform long-term exercise (i.e., more than ten minutes) comes primarily from aerobic metabolism. A steady-state oxygen uptake can generally be maintained during submaximal, moderate-intensity exercise. However, two exceptions to this rule exist. First, prolonged exercise in a hot/humid environment results in a "drift" upward of oxygen uptake; therefore, a steady state is not maintained in this type of exercise even though the work rate is constant (101) (see Fig. 4.6(a)). Second, continuous exercise at a high relative work rate (i.e., >75% $\dot{V}O_2$ max) results in a slow rise in oxygen uptake across time (57) (Fig. 4.6(b)). In each of these two types of exercise, the drift upward in $\dot{V}O_2$ is due principally to the effects of increasing body temperature and to rising blood levels of the hormones epinephrine and norepinephrine (19, 46, 48, 57, 78). Both of these variables tend to increase the

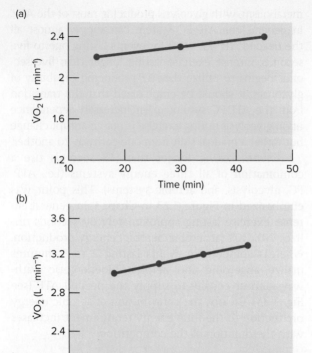

(a)

(b)

Figure 4.6 Comparison of oxygen uptake ($\dot{V}O_2$) across time during prolonged exercise in a hot and humid environment (*a*) and during prolonged exercise at a high relative work rate (>75% $\dot{V}O_2$ max) (*b*). Note that in both conditions there is a steady "drift" upward in $\dot{V}O_2$. See text for details.

metabolic rate, resulting in increased oxygen uptake across time. Use of a drug that blocks the receptors that epinephrine and norepinephrine bind to (to block their effects) results in an elimination of the drift in $\dot{V}O_2$, confirming the link between the two (78). In contrast, even though an eight-week endurance training program was shown to reduce the drift in $\dot{V}O_2$ during heavy exercise, it was not linked to a lower body temperature (21). Could lower epinephrine and norepinephrine levels be the cause, as was shown for the lower EPOC following endurance training (110)? Clearly, additional research is needed to explain the causes of this drift in $\dot{V}O_2$ in heavy exercise.

IN SUMMARY

- The energy to perform prolonged exercise (i.e., more than 10 minutes) comes primarily from aerobic metabolism.
- A steady-state oxygen uptake can generally be maintained during prolonged, moderate-intensity exercise. However, exercise in a hot/humid environment or exercise at a high relative work rate results in an upward "drift" in oxygen consumption over time; therefore, a steady state is not obtained in these types of exercise.

Incremental Exercise

Incremental exercise tests (also called **graded exercise tests**) are often employed by physicians to examine patients for possible heart disease and by exercise scientists to determine a subject's cardiovascular fitness. These tests are usually conducted on a treadmill or a cycle ergometer. However, an arm crank ergometer can be employed for testing individuals who have lost use of their legs or athletes whose sport involves arm work (e.g., swimmers). The test generally begins with the subject performing a brief warm-up, followed by an increase in the work rate every one to three minutes until the subject cannot maintain the desired power output. This increase in work rate can be achieved on the treadmill by increasing either the speed of the treadmill or the incline. On the cycle or arm ergometer, the increase in power output is obtained by increasing the resistance against the flywheel.

Maximal Oxygen Uptake The maximal capacity to transport and utilize oxygen during exercise (**maximal oxygen uptake, or $\dot{V}O_2$ max**) is considered by many exercise scientists to be the most valid measurement of cardiovascular fitness.

Figure 4.7 illustrates the change in oxygen uptake during a typical incremental exercise test on a cycle ergometer. Oxygen uptake increases systematically with work rate until $\dot{V}O_2$ max is reached. When $\dot{V}O_2$ max is reached, an increase in power output does not result in an increase in oxygen uptake; thus, $\dot{V}O_2$ max represents a "physiological ceiling" for the ability of the oxygen transport system to deliver O_2 to contracting muscles. In the classic presentation of this test, the $\dot{V}O_2$ levels off or exhibits a "plateau" when the subject completes one stage further in the test (66, 117); Figure 4.7 shows this as a dashed line. The reason for using a dashed line is that many subjects

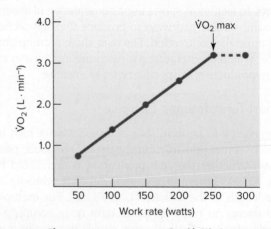

Figure 4.7 Changes in oxygen uptake ($\dot{V}O_2$) during an incremental exercise test. The dashed line indicates a plateau in $\dot{V}O_2$ at a higher work rate; however, this is not observed in many cases.

do not demonstrate this plateau at the end of an incremental test; they simply cannot do one more stage beyond the one at which the highest $\dot{V}O_2$ was achieved. However, there are ways to demonstrate that the highest value reached is $\dot{V}O_2$ max (3, 32, 71, 72, 76, 106) (see A Closer Look 4.2 for more on this). The physiological factors that influence $\dot{V}O_2$ max include the following: (a) the maximum ability of the cardiorespiratory system to deliver oxygen to the contracting muscle and (b) the muscle's ability to take up the oxygen and produce ATP aerobically. Both genetics and exercise training are known to influence $\dot{V}O_2$ max; this will be discussed in Chap. 13. Chapter 15 describes tests to measure or estimate $\dot{V}O_2$ max.

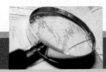

A CLOSER LOOK 4.2

$\dot{V}O_2$ max and Its Verification

The concept of $\dot{V}O_2$ max and its dependence on cardiac output was described by Hill and Lupton in 1923 (66). Over the following decades, investigators had to deal with a central issue in the measurement of $\dot{V}O_2$ max: How can one be certain that a true $\dot{V}O_2$ max had actually been obtained? The concept of a plateau in oxygen uptake with increasing intensities of exercise (the "primary" criterion) was central to Hill and Lupton's description of $\dot{V}O_2$ max. Taylor et al. (117) operationally defined the plateau for their test procedures (7 mph, 2.5% grade change per stage) as a $\dot{V}O_2$ increase of <2.1 ml · kg^{-1} · min^{-1} between stages of the test. However, no matter what criterion was used, in practice, great variation existed in the percentage of subjects who achieved a plateau at the end of a continuous incremental exercise test (72). This led investigators to use a variety of "secondary" criteria to provide objective evidence that the highest $\dot{V}O_2$ was, in fact, $\dot{V}O_2$ max. For example, measuring a very high level of lactate in the blood (≥8 times resting levels) after the test or measuring a very high respiratory exchange ratio of ≥1.15 (see later discussion in this chapter) was evidence that the subject was probably working maximally at the time the highest $\dot{V}O_2$ was measured (3, 76). However, there was still considerable variation in how subjects responded, limiting the use of these secondary criteria (see Chap. 15 for more on this).

There is now a renewed interest in obtaining a confirmation of the $\dot{V}O_2$ max value on the same test day by having the subject do a single-stage follow-up test at a work rate higher than the last one just completed on a maximal incremental exercise test. In this sense, a verification of the $\dot{V}O_2$ max value would indicate that a "plateau" had been achieved. The following studies provide some insights into current approaches to this issue. In a study by Foster et al. (44), the treadmill grade was set at 3% for female runners and at 4% for male runners, with the initial speed set at 134 m · min^{-1} (5 mph). The speed was increased by 27 m · min^{-1} (1 mph) at 3-min intervals until exhaustion. Following a 3-min recovery while walking at 53 m · min^{-1} (2 mph) and 0% grade, the subjects ran at a speed 13.4 m · min^{-1} (0.5 mph) or 26.8 m · min^{-1} (1 mph) faster than the last stage of the previous test. The same $\dot{V}O_2$ max was measured. These results were similar to a study on highly trained runners by Hawkins et al. (60) in which the follow-up test was done on a separate day and at a work rate equal to 130% of the final stage of the exercise test. Both studies clearly supported the underlying proposition of Hill and Lupton—that there really is an upper limit to oxygen uptake. In 2009, Midgley and Carroll (93) did a review of studies, including the two just mentioned, that used follow-up tests to verify that a true $\dot{V}O_2$ max had been achieved in the incremental exercise test. In general, across all of the studies, there was no difference between the average $\dot{V}O_2$ max value measured on the follow-up test and the average value measured at the end of the incremental exercise test. However, the authors expressed appropriate concern that without looking at individual data, that is, how much of a difference existed between the first and follow-up test for each person, the average values could disguise inherent within-subject variability. In effect, they are asking, what is the largest difference in $\dot{V}O_2$ max between the tests that you would accept as signifying no difference in response? This is similar to the issue Taylor et al. (117) dealt with in establishing their criterion $\dot{V}O_2$ difference of 2.1 ml · kg^{-1} · min^{-1} for one additional stage of their exercise test protocol. In addition, the authors indicate that to firm up procedures for the verification protocol, there is a need to:

- use only a work rate higher than the one achieved in the incremental exercise test for the follow-up test;

- establish the minimum duration of the follow-up test consistent with allowing the subject time to achieve $\dot{V}O_2$ max;

- identify a consistent rest interval and warm-up prior to the verification test; and

- establish the minimum gas sampling interval (e.g., 20s, 30s) to minimize error in estimating a one-minute $\dot{V}O_2$ value.

We are sure to hear more about these follow-up tests to verify that the $\dot{V}O_2$ max achieved on an incremental exercise test is, in fact, the true $\dot{V}O_2$ max.

Lactate Threshold During light and moderate intensity exercise, most of the ATP production used to provide energy for muscular contraction comes from aerobic sources (86, 98, 111). However, as the exercise intensity increases during an incremental exercise test, blood levels of lactate begin to rise in an exponential fashion (Fig. 4.8). This appears in untrained subjects around 50% to 60% of $\dot{V}O_2$ max, whereas it occurs at higher work rates in trained subjects (i.e., 65% to 80% $\dot{V}O_2$ max) (51). Early on, a common term used to describe the point of a systematic rise in blood lactate during incremental exercise was the **anaerobic threshold** (16, 31, 40, 67, 77, 100, 123, 125, 129) because of the obvious link between anaerobic metabolism and the appearance of lactate. However, because of arguments over terminology (discussed next), a more neutral term, the **lactate threshold,** has been widely adopted (30, 34, 116).

Another commonly used term that is related to the systematic rise in the blood lactate concentration is the *onset of blood lactate accumulation* (abbreviated as OBLA). This term, OBLA, differs from the lactate threshold in one important way. Rather than describing the blood lactate inflection point, the OBLA is defined as the exercise intensity (or oxygen consumption) at which a specific blood lactate concentration is reached (e.g., 4 millimoles per liter) (15, 61, 116). To avoid confusion, we will refer to the sudden rise in blood lactate levels during incremental exercise as the lactate threshold.

Some investigators believed that this sudden rise in the blood lactate concentration during incremental exercise represented a point of increasing reliance on anaerobic metabolism (i.e., glycolysis) (29, 121-125). Consequently, the term *anaerobic threshold* was adopted. The basic argument against the term *anaerobic threshold* centers

around the question of whether the rise in blood lactate during incremental exercise is due to a lack of oxygen (hypoxia) in the working muscle or occurs for other reasons. Historically, rising blood lactate levels were considered an indication of increased anaerobic metabolism within the contracting muscle because of low levels of O_2 in the individual muscle cells (123, 125). However, whether the end product of glycolysis is pyruvate or lactate depends on a variety of factors. First, if the rate of glycolysis is rapid, NADH production may exceed the transport capacity of the shuttle mechanisms that move hydrogens from the sarcoplasm into the mitochondria (113, 115, 128). Indeed, blood levels of epinephrine begin to rise at 50% to 65% of $\dot{V}O_2$ max during incremental exercise and have been shown to stimulate the glycolytic rate; this increase in glycolysis increases the rate of NADH production (115). Failure of the shuttle system to keep up with the rate of NADH production by glycolysis would result in pyruvate accepting some "unshuttled" hydrogens, and the formation of lactate could occur independent of whether the muscle cell had sufficient oxygen for aerobic ATP production (Fig. 4.9).

A second explanation for the formation of lactate in exercising muscle is related to the enzyme that catalyzes the conversion of pyruvate to lactate. The enzyme responsible for this reaction is lactate dehydrogenase (LDH), and it exists in several forms (different forms of the same enzyme are called isozymes). Recall that the reaction is as follows:

$$\underset{\text{Pyruvate}}{\overset{\displaystyle CH_3}{\underset{\displaystyle COO^-}{\mid}} \atop C=O} + NADH + H^+ \overset{LDH}{\longleftrightarrow} \underset{\text{Lactate}}{\overset{\displaystyle CH_3}{\underset{\displaystyle COO^-}{\mid}} \atop H-C-OH} + NAD$$

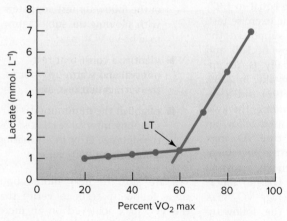

Figure 4.8 Changes in blood lactate concentration during incremental exercise. The sudden rise in lactate is known as the lactate threshold (LT).

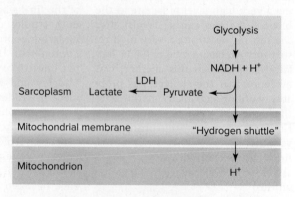

Figure 4.9 Failure of the mitochondrial "hydrogen shuttle" system to keep pace with the rate of glycolytic production of NADH + H$^+$ results in the conversion of pyruvate to lactate.

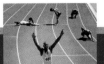

Exercise Physiology Applied to Sports

Does Lactate Cause Muscle Soreness?
A belief among some athletes and coaches is that lactate production during exercise is a primary cause of delayed-onset muscle soreness (i.e., soreness occurring 24 to 48 hours after exercise). Nonetheless, physiological evidence indicates that lactate is not a primary cause of this type of muscle soreness. Several lines of "physiological reasoning" can be used to support this position. First, although lactate production occurs in active skeletal muscle during high-intensity exercise, lactate removal from the muscle and blood is rapid following an exercise session. In fact, blood levels of lactate return to resting levels within 60 minutes after exercise (see A Closer Look 4.1). Therefore, it seems unlikely that lactate production during a single exercise bout would result in muscle soreness one or two days later.

A second argument against lactate causing delayed-onset muscle soreness is that if lactate production caused muscle soreness, power athletes would experience soreness after each workout. Clearly, this is not the case. Indeed, well-conditioned power athletes (e.g., track sprinters) rarely experience muscle soreness after a routine training session.

If lactate is not the cause of delayed-onset muscle soreness, what is the cause? Growing evidence indicates that this type of muscle soreness originates from microscopic injury to muscle fibers. This kind of injury results in a slow cascade of biochemical events leading to inflammation and edema within the injured muscles. Because these events are slow to develop, the resulting pain generally doesn't appear until 24 to 48 hours after exercise. Details of the events leading to delayed-onset muscle soreness are discussed in Chap. 21.

This reaction is reversible in that lactate can be converted back to pyruvate under the appropriate conditions. Human skeletal muscle can be classified into three fiber types (see Chap. 8). One of these is a "slow" fiber (sometimes called slow-twitch), whereas the remaining two are called "fast" fibers (sometimes called fast-twitch). As the names imply, fast fibers are recruited during intense, rapid exercise, whereas slow fibers are used primarily during low-intensity activity. The LDH isozyme found in fast fibers has a greater affinity for attaching to pyruvate, promoting the formation of lactate (69, 111). In contrast, slow fibers contain an LDH form that promotes the conversion of lactate to pyruvate. Therefore, lactate formation might occur in fast fibers during exercise simply because of the type of LDH present. Thus, lactate production would again be independent of oxygen availability in the muscle cell. Early in an incremental exercise test, it is likely that slow fibers are the first called into action. However, as the exercise intensity increases, the amount of muscular force produced must be increased. This increased muscular force is supplied by recruiting more and more fast fibers. Therefore, the involvement of more fast fibers may result in increased lactate production and thus may be responsible for the lactate threshold.

A final explanation for the lactate threshold may be related to the rate of removal of lactate from the blood during incremental exercise. When a researcher obtains a blood sample from a subject during an exercise test, the concentration of lactate in that sample is the difference between the rate at which lactate enters the blood and the rate at which lactate is removed from the blood. At any given time during exercise, some muscles are producing lactate and releasing it into the blood, and some tissues (e.g., liver, skeletal muscles, heart) are removing lactate. Therefore, the concentration of lactate in the blood at any given time can be expressed mathematically in the following way:

$$\text{Blood lactate concentration} = \text{Lactate entry into the blood} - \text{Blood lactate removal}$$

Thus, a rise in the blood lactate concentration can occur due to either an increase in lactate production or a decrease in lactate removal. Recent evidence suggests that the rise in blood lactate levels in animals during incremental exercise may be the result of both an increase in lactate production and a decrease in the rate of lactate removal (17, 37). See Chap. 13 for a discussion of how endurance training affects lactate production. Also, see The Winning Edge 4.1.

To summarize, controversy exists over both the terminology and the mechanism to explain the sudden rise in blood lactate concentration during incremental exercise. It is possible that any one or a combination of the explanations (including lack of O_2) might explain the lactate threshold. Figure 4.10 contains a summary of possible mechanisms to explain the lactate threshold. The search for definitive evidence to explain the mechanism(s) altering the blood lactate concentration during incremental exercise will continue for years to come.

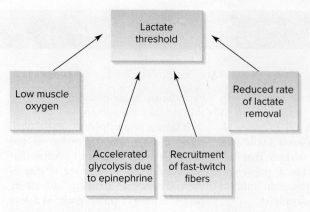

Figure 4.10 Possible mechanisms to explain the lactate threshold during incremental exercise. See text for details.

Practical Use of the Lactate Threshold Regardless of the physiological mechanism to explain the lactate threshold, it has important implications for predicting sports performance and perhaps in planning training programs for endurance athletes. For example, several studies have demonstrated that the lactate threshold, used in combination with other physiological measurements (e.g., $\dot{V}O_2$ max), is a useful predictor of success in distance running (43, 87). If $\dot{V}O_2$ max is the "physiological ceiling" for aerobic ATP production during exercise, then the LT sets the upper limit for sustainable exercise intensity (e.g., $\%\dot{V}O_2$ max or running speed). Consequently, the lactate threshold might serve as a guideline for coaches and athletes in planning the level of exercise intensity needed to optimize training results (e.g., choose a training heart rate based on the LT). This is discussed in more detail in Chaps. 16 and 21.

IN SUMMARY

- Oxygen uptake increases in a linear fashion during incremental exercise until $\dot{V}O_2$ max is reached.
- The point at which there is a sudden increase in the blood lactate concentration during an incremental (graded) exercise test is termed the *lactate threshold.*
- Controversy exists over the mechanism to explain the sudden rise in blood lactate concentration during incremental exercise. It is possible that any one or a combination of the following factors might provide an explanation for the lactate threshold: (1) low muscle oxygen, (2) accelerated glycolysis due to epinephrine, (3) recruitment of fast muscle fibers, and (4) a reduced rate of lactate removal.
- The lactate threshold has practical uses, such as predicting endurance performance and as a marker of training intensity.

ESTIMATION OF FUEL UTILIZATION DURING EXERCISE

A noninvasive technique that is commonly used to estimate the percent contribution of carbohydrate or fat to energy metabolism during exercise is the ratio of the volume of carbon dioxide produced ($\dot{V}CO_2$) to the volume of oxygen consumed ($\dot{V}O_2$) (45, 127). This $\dot{V}CO_2/\dot{V}O_2$ ratio is called the **respiratory exchange ratio (R)**. During steady-state conditions, the $\dot{V}CO_2/\dot{V}O_2$ ratio is often termed the *respiratory quotient* (RQ), as it is thought to reflect CO_2 production and O_2 consumption by the mitochondria of the active muscles. For simplicity, we will refer to the $\dot{V}CO_2/\dot{V}O_2$ ratio as the respiratory exchange ratio (R). How can the R be used to estimate whether fat or carbohydrate is being used as a fuel? The answer is related to the fact that fat and carbohydrate differ in the amount of O_2 used and CO_2 produced during oxidation. When using R as a predictor of fuel utilization during exercise, the role that protein contributes to ATP production during exercise is ignored. This is reasonable because protein generally plays a small role as a substrate during physical activity. Therefore, the R during exercise is often termed a *nonprotein R.*

Let's consider the R for fat first. When fat is oxidized, O_2 combines with carbon to form CO_2 and joins with hydrogen to form water. The chemical relationship is as follows:

Fat (palmitic acid) $C_{16}H_{32}O_2$
Oxidation: $C_{16}H_{32}O_2 + 23\ O_2 \rightarrow 16\ CO_2 + 16\ H_2O$
Therefore, the R $= \dot{V}CO_2 \div \dot{V}O_2 = 16\ CO_2 \div 23\ O_2$
$= 0.70$

For R to be used as an estimate of substrate utilization during exercise, the subject must have reached a steady state. This is important because only during steady-state exercise are the $\dot{V}CO_2$ and $\dot{V}O_2$ reflective of O_2 uptake and CO_2 production in the tissues. For example, if a person is hyperventilating due to the buildup of hydrogen ions in heavy work, excessive CO_2 loss from the body's CO_2 stores (see Chaps. 10 and 11) could bias the ratio of $\dot{V}CO_2$ to $\dot{V}O_2$ and invalidate the use of R to estimate which fuel is being consumed. That said, the elevated R measured at the end of a maximal incremental exercise test has been used as a secondary criterion for having achieved $\dot{V}O_2$ max (see previous section on $\dot{V}O_2$ max).

Carbohydrate oxidation also results in a predictable ratio of the volume of CO_2 produced to the volume of O_2 consumed. The oxidation of carbohydrate results in an R of 1.0:

Glucose $= C_6H_{12}O_6$
Oxidation: $C_6H_{12}O_6 + 6\ O_2 \rightarrow 6\ CO_2 + 6\ H_2O$
R $= \dot{V}CO_2 \div \dot{V}O_2 = 6\ CO_2 \div 6\ O_2 = 1.0$

TABLE 4.1	Percentage of Fat and Carbohydrate Metabolized as Determined by a Nonprotein Respiratory Exchange Ratio (R) and the Caloric Equivalent for Oxygen (kcal·L^{-1} O$_2$)		
R	% Fat	% Carbohydrate	kcal · L^{-1} O$_2$
0.70	100	0	4.69
0.75	83	17	4.74
0.80	67	33	4.80
0.85	50	50	4.86
0.90	33	67	4.92
0.95	17	83	4.99
1.00	0	100	5.05

Knoebel, K.L., "Energy Metabolism," *Physiology*, edited by E. Selkurt. Boston, MA: Little Brown & Company, 1984, pp. 635–650.

Fat oxidation requires more O$_2$ than carbohydrate oxidation because carbohydrate contains more O$_2$ than fat (116). The amount of energy released when one liter of oxygen is used (the caloric equivalent) is approximately 4.70 kcal when fats alone are used, and approximately 5.0 kcal when carbohydrates alone are used. Consequently, about 6% more energy (ATP) per liter of oxygen is obtained when using carbohydrate, compared to fat, as the sole fuel for exercise.

It is unlikely that either fat or carbohydrate would be the only substrate used during most types of submaximal exercise. Therefore, the R would likely be somewhere between 1.0 and 0.70. Table 4.1 lists a range of R values and the percentage of fat or carbohydrate metabolism they represent. Note that a nonprotein R of 0.85 represents a condition wherein fat and carbohydrate contribute equally as energy substrates. Further, notice that the higher the R, the greater the role of carbohydrate as an energy source, and the lower the R, the greater the contribution of fat. Table 4.1 shows how the caloric equivalent of oxygen changes with the mixture of fuel used (79).

IN SUMMARY

- The respiratory exchange ratio (R) is the ratio of carbon dioxide produced to the oxygen consumed ($\dot{V}CO_2 / \dot{V}O_2$).
- For R to be used as an estimate of substrate utilization during exercise, the subject must have reached steady state. This is important because only during steady-state exercise are the $\dot{V}CO_2$ and $\dot{V}O_2$ reflective of metabolic exchange of gases in tissues.
- The caloric equivalent for oxygen is approximately 4.7 kcal/L when fat alone is used and 5.0 kcal/L when carbohydrate alone is used, about a 6% difference.

FACTORS GOVERNING FUEL SELECTION

Proteins contribute less than 2% of the substrate used during exercise of less than one hour's duration. However, the role of proteins as a fuel source may increase slightly during prolonged exercise (i.e., three to five hours' duration). During this type of exercise, the total contribution of protein to the fuel supply may reach 5% to 10% during the final minutes of work (11, 15, 70, 83, 84, 103, 126). Therefore, proteins play only a minor role as a substrate during most types of exercise, with fat and carbohydrate serving as the major sources of energy in healthy individuals consuming a balanced diet. Whether fat or carbohydrate is the primary substrate during work is determined by several factors, including (a) diet, (b) the intensity and duration of exercise, and (c) whether the subject is endurance trained. For example, consuming a high-fat/low-carbohydrate diet promotes a high rate of fat metabolism. In regard to exercise intensity, low-intensity exercise relies primarily on fat as fuel, whereas carbohydrate is the primary energy source during high-intensity exercise. Fuel selection is also influenced by the duration of exercise. During low-intensity, prolonged exercise, there is a progressive increase in the amount of fat oxidized by the working muscles. Endurance-trained subjects use more fat and less carbohydrate than less-fit subjects during prolonged exercise at the same intensity. In the next two sections, we discuss in detail the influence of exercise intensity and duration on fuel selection. The role of endurance training is discussed in detail in Chap. 13, and diet and performance is covered in Chap. 23.

Exercise Intensity and Fuel Selection

Again, fats are a primary fuel source for muscle during low-intensity exercise (i.e., 30% $\dot{V}O_2$ max), whereas carbohydrate is the dominant substrate during high-intensity exercise (i.e., 70% $\dot{V}O_2$ max) (20, 25, 94, 109). Consequently, the R increases as exercise intensity increases. The influence of exercise intensity on muscle fuel selection is illustrated in Figure 4.11. Note that as the exercise intensity increases, there is a progressive increase in carbohydrate metabolism and a decrease in fat metabolism. Also notice that as the exercise intensity increases, there is an exercise intensity at which the energy derived from carbohydrate exceeds that of fat; this work rate has been labeled the *crossover point* (20). That is, as the exercise intensity increases above the crossover point, a progressive shift occurs from fat to carbohydrate metabolism.

McArdle's Syndrome: A Genetic Error in Muscle Glycogen Metabolism

McArdle's syndrome is a genetic disease in which the person is born with a gene mutation and cannot synthesize the enzyme phosphorylase. This metabolic disorder prevents the individual from breaking down muscle glycogen as a fuel source during exercise. This inability to use glycogen during exercise also prevents the muscle from producing lactate, as indicated by the observation that blood lactate levels do not increase in McArdle's patients during high-intensity exercise. It should be no surprise then that during submaximal exercise, McArdle's patients use more fat as a fuel compared to control subjects (96). However, despite rising levels of fatty acids in the blood of McArdle's patients, they are not able to oxidize more fat. This indicates that carbohydrate availability limits fat oxidation even during steady-state exercise in these patients. See the section "Interaction of Fat/Carbohydrate Metabolism" for more on this.

An unfortunate side effect of this genetic disorder is that McArdle's patients often complain of exercise intolerance and muscle pain during exertion. This clinical observation provides a practical illustration of the importance of muscle glycogen as an energy source during exercise. McArdle's syndrome is but one of many genetic disorders of metabolism. See van Adel and Tarnopolsky's review on these metabolic myopathies in Suggested Readings.

What causes this shift from fat to carbohydrate metabolism as the exercise intensity increases? Two primary factors are involved: (1) recruitment of fast fibers and (2) increasing blood levels of epinephrine. As the exercise intensity increases, more and more fast muscle fibers are recruited (50). These fibers have an abundance of glycolytic enzymes but few mitochondrial and lipolytic enzymes (enzymes responsible for fat breakdown). In short, this means that fast fibers are better equipped to metabolize carbohydrates than fats. Therefore, the increased recruitment of fast fibers results in greater carbohydrate metabolism and less fat metabolism (20).

A second factor that regulates carbohydrate metabolism during exercise is epinephrine. As exercise intensity increases, there is a progressive rise in blood levels of epinephrine. High levels of epinephrine increase phosphorylase activity, which causes an increase in muscle glycogen breakdown; this results in an increased rate of glycolysis and lactate production (20). Interestingly, there are some individuals who lack phosphorylase and cannot produce lactate (see Clinical Applications 4.1). This increased production of lactate inhibits fat metabolism by reducing the availability of fat as a substrate (119). The lack of fat as a substrate for working muscles under these conditions dictates that carbohydrate will be the primary fuel (see Chap. 5 for more details on how this occurs).

Many individuals use exercise as a means of keeping body weight and body fat in check, and you are probably familiar with pieces of exercise equipment having a selection for a "fat burning" workout. In such a workout, the emphasis is on low intensity and long duration. But is that really the best way to burn fat? See A Closer Look 4.3 for the answer.

Exercise Duration and Fuel Selection

During prolonged (i.e., greater than 30 minutes), moderate-intensity (40% to 59% $\dot{V}O_2$ max) exercise the R decreases over time, indicating a gradual shift from carbohydrate metabolism toward an increasing reliance on fat as a substrate (5, 49, 68, 81, 94, 102). Figure 4.12 demonstrates this point.

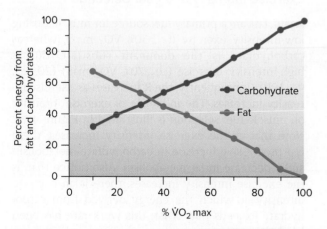

Figure 4.11 Illustration of the "crossover" concept. Note that as the exercise intensity increases, there is a progressive increase in the contribution of carbohydrate as a fuel source.

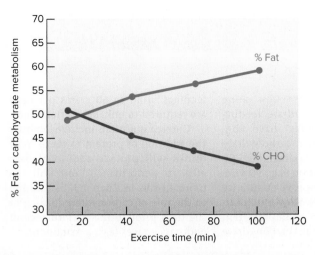

Figure 4.12 Shift from carbohydrate metabolism toward fat metabolism during prolonged exercise.

What factors control the rate of fat metabolism during prolonged exercise? Fat metabolism is regulated by those variables that control the rate of fat breakdown (a process called lipolysis). Triglycerides are broken down into **free fatty acids (FFAs)** and glycerol by enzymes called **lipases**. These lipases are generally inactive until stimulated by the hormones epinephrine, norepinephrine, and glucagon (68). For example, during low-intensity, prolonged exercise, blood levels of epinephrine rise, which increases lipase activity and thus promotes lipolysis. This increase in lipolysis results in an increase in blood and muscle levels of FFA and promotes fat metabolism. In general, **lipolysis** is a slow process, and an increase in fat metabolism occurs only after several minutes of exercise. This point is illustrated in Figure 4.12 by the slow increase in fat metabolism across time during prolonged submaximal exercise.

The mobilization of FFA into the blood is inhibited by the hormone insulin and high blood levels of lactate. Insulin inhibits lipolysis by the direct inhibition of lipase activity. Normally, blood insulin levels decline during prolonged exercise (see Chap. 5). However, if a high-carbohydrate meal or drink is

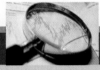

A CLOSER LOOK 4.3

Exercise and Fat Metabolism: Is Low-Intensity Exercise Best for Burning Fat?

What intensity of exercise is optimal for burning fat? At first glance, it would appear that low-intensity exercise would be best because a high percentage of the energy expenditure is derived from fat oxidation (see Fig. 4.11). However, one must keep in mind that because overall energy expenditure is also very low at these low exercise intensities, only a small amount of fat is oxidized. For example, let's assume an individual is working at 20% $\dot{V}O_2$ max and the metabolic rate is 3 kcal $\cdot$ min^{-1}. If the R is 0.80, two-thirds of the energy (2 kcal $\cdot$ min^{-1}) is coming from fat and one-third (1 kcal $\cdot$ min^{-1}) from carbohydrate (see Table 4.1). If the individual is now working at 60% $\dot{V}O_2$ max, the metabolic rate is 9 kcal $\cdot$ min^{-1}. If the R is 0.90, only one-third of the energy is coming from fat. However, because the metabolic rate is three times higher, 3 kcal $\cdot$ min^{-1} are derived from fat–50% more fat oxidation than at 20% $\dot{V}O_2$ max. Figure 4.13 shows changes in R and in fat oxidation over a range of exercise intensities. Fat oxidation increased until about 60% $\dot{V}O_2$

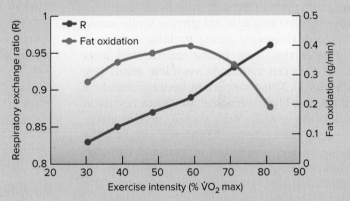

Figure 4.13 Changes in the respiratory exchange ratio (R) and in fat oxidation with increasing exercise intensity in active men and women. Fat oxidation increased from light exercise and reached a peak around 60% $\dot{V}O_2$ max.

max and then decreases thereafter. This is a fairly typical pattern of fat oxidation.

The highest rate of fat oxidation is sometimes termed FAT_{max}, and there is support for a connection between the LT and FAT_{max}. In effect, the acceleration of glycolysis that is related to the rising lactate concentration in the blood signifies an overall increase in carbohydrate oxidation. Consistent with that, the FAT_{max} appears to be reached just before the LT (107). In addition, fat oxidation appears to be higher at the same relative work load (%$\dot{V}O_2$ max) during running compared to cycling in both adults (24) and children (130). Any discussion of which exercise or exercise intensity is best for fat oxidation must keep in mind that the total energy expenditure is key in any weight maintenance or weight loss program. See Chap. 16 for details on prescribing exercise.

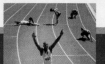
Exercise Physiology Applied to Sports

Carbohydrate Feeding via Sports Drinks Improves Endurance Performance

The depletion of muscle and blood carbohydrate stores can contribute to muscular fatigue during prolonged exercise. Therefore, can the ingestion of carbohydrates during prolonged exercise improve endurance performance? The clear answer to this question is yes! Studies investigating the effects of carbohydrate feeding through "sports drinks" have convincingly shown that carbohydrate feedings during submaximal (i.e., 70% $\dot{V}O_2$ max), long-duration (e.g., 90 minutes) exercise can improve endurance performance (28, 89). How much carbohydrate is required to improve performance? In general, carbohydrate feedings of 30 to 60 grams per hour are required to enhance performance.

Current questions include whether the addition of protein to these sport drinks will provide additional benefits to performance. You will see more on this in Chap. 23, in addition to the role of carbohydrate loading in the days prior to the performance of endurance races (e.g., a marathon).

---

consumed 30 to 60 minutes prior to exercise, blood glucose levels rise and more insulin is released from the pancreas. This elevation in blood insulin may result in diminished lipolysis and a reduction in fat metabolism, leading to a greater use of carbohydrate as a fuel (see Chap. 23 for more on this).

Interaction of Fat/Carbohydrate Metabolism

During short-term exercise, it is unlikely that muscle stores of glycogen or blood glucose levels would be depleted. However, during prolonged exercise (e.g., greater than two hours) muscle and liver stores of glycogen can reach very low levels (15, 26, 50, 55, 62). This is important because depletion of muscle and blood carbohydrate stores results in muscular fatigue (55). Why do low muscle glycogen levels produce fatigue? Evidence suggests the following answer. Depletion of available carbohydrate reduces the rate of glycolysis, and therefore the concentration of pyruvate in the muscle is also reduced (55). This lowers the rate of aerobic production of ATP by reducing the number of Krebs-cycle compounds (intermediates). In human muscle with adequate glycogen stores, submaximal exercise (i.e., 70% $\dot{V}O_2$ max) results in a ninefold increase (above resting values) in the number of Krebs-cycle intermediates (108). This elevated pool of Krebs-cycle intermediates is required for the Krebs cycle to "speed up" in an effort to meet the high ATP demands during exercise. Pyruvate (produced via glycolysis) is important in providing this increase in Krebs-cycle intermediates. For example, pyruvate is a precursor of several Krebs-cycle intermediates (e.g., oxaloacetate, malate). When the rate of glycolysis is reduced due to the unavailability of glucose or glycogen, pyruvate levels in the sarcoplasm decline, and the levels of Krebs-cycle intermediates decrease as well. This decline in Krebs-cycle intermediates slows the rate of Krebs-cycle activity, with the end result being a reduction in the rate of aerobic ATP production. This reduced rate of muscle ATP production limits muscular performance and may result in fatigue.

It is important to appreciate that a reduction in Krebs-cycle intermediates (due to glycogen depletion) results in a diminished rate of ATP production from fat metabolism because fat can be metabolized only via Krebs-cycle oxidation. Hence, when carbohydrate stores are depleted in the body, the rate at which fat is metabolized is also reduced (108). Therefore, "fats burn in the flame of carbohydrates" (115). The role that depletion of body carbohydrate stores may play in limiting performance during prolonged exercise is introduced in The Winning Edge 4.2 and is further discussed in both Chaps. 19 and 23.

Body Fuel Sources

In this section, we outline the storage sites in the body for carbohydrates, fats, and proteins. Further, we define the role that each of these fuel storage sites plays in providing energy during exercise. Finally, we discuss the use of lactate as a fuel source during work.

Sources of Carbohydrate During Exercise Carbohydrate is stored as glycogen in both the muscle and the liver (see Table 4.2). Muscle glycogen stores provide a direct source of carbohydrate for muscle energy metabolism, whereas liver glycogen stores serve as a means of replacing blood glucose. For example, when blood glucose levels decline during prolonged exercise, liver glycogenolysis is stimulated and

Note that dietary intake of carbohydrate influences the amount of glycogen stored in both the liver and muscle. Mass units for storage are grams (g) and kilograms (kg). Energy units are kilocalories (kcal) and kilojoules (kJ). Data are from references 31, 33, and 69.

| | | CARBOHYDRATE (CHO) | |
Storage Site	Mixed Diet	High-CHO Diet	Low-CHO Diet
Liver glycogen	60 g (240 kcal or 1005 kJ)	90 g (360 kcal or 1507 kJ)	<30 g (120 kcal or 502 kJ)
Glucose in blood and extracellular fluid	10 g (40 kcal or 167 kJ)	10 g (40 kcal or 167 kJ)	10 g (40 kcal or 167 kJ)
Muscle glycogen	350 g (1400 kcal or 5860 kJ)	600 g (2400 kcal or 10,046 kJ)	300 g (1200 kcal or 5023 kJ)

| | FAT | | |
Storage Site	Mixed Diet		
Adipocytes	14 kg (107,800 kcal or 451,251 kJ)		
Muscle	0.5 kg (3850 kcal or 16,116 kJ)		

glucose is released into the blood. This glucose can then be transported to the contracting muscle and used as fuel.

Carbohydrate used as a substrate during exercise comes from both glycogen stores in muscle and from blood glucose (23, 27, 50, 74, 114). The relative contribution of muscle glycogen and blood glucose to energy metabolism during exercise varies as a function of the exercise intensity and duration. Blood glucose plays the greater role during low-intensity exercise, whereas muscle glycogen is the primary source of carbohydrate during high-intensity exercise (see Fig. 4.14). As mentioned earlier, the increased glycogen usage during high-intensity exercise can be explained by the increased rate of glycogenolysis that occurs due to recruitment of fast-twitch fibers and elevated blood epinephrine levels.

During the first hour of submaximal (i.e., 65% to 75% V̇O$_2$ max) prolonged exercise, much of the carbohydrate metabolized by muscle comes from muscle glycogen. However, as muscle glycogen levels decline across time, blood glucose becomes an increasingly important source of fuel (see Fig. 4.15).

Sources of Fat During Exercise When an individual consumes more energy (i.e., food) than he or she expends, this additional energy is stored in the form of fat. A gain of 3500 kcal of energy results in the storage of 1 pound of fat. Most fat is stored in the form of triglycerides in adipocytes (fat cells), but some is stored in muscle cells as well (see Table 4.2). As mentioned earlier, the major factor

that determines the role of fat as a substrate during exercise is its availability to the muscle cell. To be metabolized, triglycerides must be degraded to FFA (three molecules) and glycerol (one molecule). The FFA can be converted into acetyl-CoA and enter the Krebs cycle.

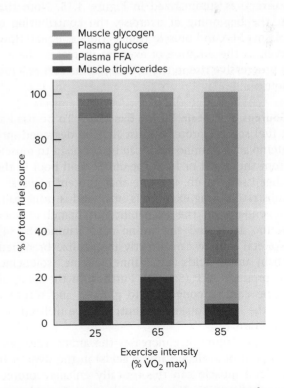

Figure 4.14 Influence of exercise intensity on muscle fuel source. Data are from highly trained endurance athletes.

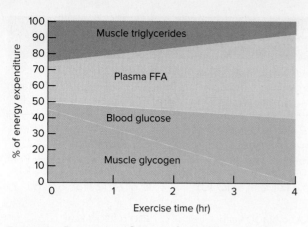

Figure 4.15 Percentage of energy derived from the four major sources of fuel during submaximal exercise (i.e., 65% to 75% $\dot{V}O_2$ max). Data are from trained endurance athletes.

Which fat stores are used as a fuel source varies as a function of the exercise intensity and duration. For example, plasma FFAs (i.e., FFA from adipocytes) are the primary source of fat during low-intensity exercise. At higher work rates, metabolism of muscle triglycerides increases (see Fig. 4.14). At exercise intensities between 65% and 85% $\dot{V}O_2$ max, the contribution of fat as a muscle fuel source is approximately equal between plasma FFA and muscle triglycerides (25, 58, 105).

The contribution of plasma FFA and muscle triglycerides to exercise metabolism during prolonged exercise is summarized in Figure 4.15. Note that at the beginning of exercise, the contribution of plasma FFA and muscle triglycerides is equal. However, as the duration of exercise increases, there is a progressive rise in the role of plasma FFA as a fuel source.

Sources of Protein During Exercise To be used as a fuel source, proteins must first be degraded into amino acids. Amino acids can be supplied to muscle from the blood or from the amino acid pool in the fiber itself. Again, the role that protein plays as a substrate during exercise is small and is principally dependent on the availability of branch-chained amino acids and the amino acid alanine (8, 54). Skeletal muscle can directly metabolize branched-chain amino acids (e.g., valine, leucine, isoleucine) to produce ATP (52, 70). Further, in the liver, alanine can be converted to glucose and returned via the blood to skeletal muscle to be utilized as a substrate.

Any factor that increases the amino acid pool (amount of available amino acids) in the liver or in skeletal muscle can theoretically enhance protein metabolism (70, 85). One such factor is prolonged exercise (i.e., more than two hours). Numerous investigators have demonstrated that enzymes ca-

pable of degrading muscle proteins (proteases) are activated during long-term exercise (2, 35, 36, 95). The mechanism responsible for activation of these proteases during prolonged exercise appears to be exercise-induced increases in calcium levels within muscle fibers (2, 91). Indeed, several families of proteases are activated by increases in cellular levels of calcium (2, 91). As a result of this activation, amino acids are liberated from their parent proteins and increase the use of amino acids as fuel during exercise (94). The use of protein as a fuel during exercise is also related to carbohydrate availability (see Chap. 23).

Lactate as a Fuel Source During Exercise For many years, lactate was considered to be a waste product of glycolysis with limited metabolic use. However, evidence has shown that lactate plays a beneficial role during exercise by serving as both a substrate for the liver to synthesize glucose (see A Closer Look 4.4) and as a direct fuel source for skeletal muscle and the heart (13, 17, 58). That is, in slow skeletal muscle fibers and the heart, lactate removed from the blood can be converted to pyruvate, which can then be transformed to acetyl-CoA. This acetyl-CoA can then enter the Krebs cycle and contribute to oxidative metabolism. The concept that lactate can be produced in one tissue and then transported to another to be used as an energy source has been termed the *lactate shuttle* (13, 14, 16–18). This has implications well beyond lactate being used as a fuel or participating in gluconeogenesis. Lactate shuttles have been implicated in the growth of cancer cells (38, 75, 112).

IN SUMMARY

- The regulation of fuel selection during exercise is under complex control and is dependent upon several factors, including diet and the intensity and duration of exercise.
- In general, carbohydrates are used as the major fuel source during high-intensity exercise.
- During prolonged exercise, there is a gradual shift from carbohydrate metabolism toward fat metabolism.
- Proteins contribute less than 2% of the fuel used during exercise of less than one hour's duration. During prolonged exercise (i.e., three to five hours' duration), the total contribution of protein to the fuel supply may reach 5% to 10% during the final minutes of prolonged work.

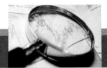

A CLOSER LOOK 4.4

The Cori Cycle: Lactate as a Fuel Source

During exercise, some of the lactate that is produced by skeletal muscles is transported to the liver via the blood (56, 118). Upon entry into the liver, lactate can be converted to glucose via gluconeogenesis. This "new" glucose can be released into the blood and transported back to skeletal muscles to be used as an energy source during exercise. The cycle of lactate glucose between the muscle and liver is called the **Cori cycle** and is illustrated in Figure 4.16. Recent evidence indicates that gluconeogenesis plays an essential role in maintaining total glucose production during exercise in fasted subjects, independent of training state (39).

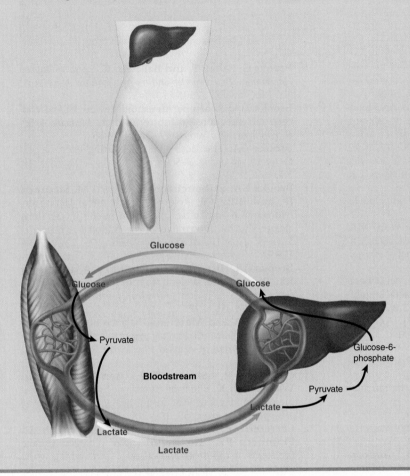

Glucose

Glucose

Glucose

Pyruvate

Bloodstream

Glucose-6-phosphate

Pyruvate

Lactate

Lactate

Lactate

Figure 4.16 The Cori cycle. During intense exercise, lactate is formed in muscle fibers. The lactate formed in muscle can then be transported via the blood to the liver and converted to glucose by gluconeogenesis.

STUDY ACTIVITIES

1. Identify the predominant energy systems used to produce ATP during the following types of exercise:
   a. Short-term, intense exercise (i.e., less than ten seconds' duration)
   b. 400-meter dash
   c. 20-kilometer race (i.e., 12.4 miles)
2. Graph the change in oxygen uptake during the transition from rest to steady-state, submaximal exercise. Label the oxygen deficit. Where does the ATP come from during the transition period from rest to steady state?
3. Graph the change in oxygen uptake during recovery from exercise. Label the excess post-exercise oxygen consumption (EPOC) (i.e., oxygen debt).
4. Graph the change in oxygen uptake and blood lactate concentration during incremental exercise. Label the point on the graph that might be considered the lactate threshold.
5. Discuss several possible reasons why blood lactate begins to rise rapidly during incremental exercise.
6. Briefly explain how the respiratory exchange ratio is used to estimate which substrate is being utilized during exercise. What is meant by the term nonprotein R?
7. List the factors that play a role in the regulation of carbohydrate metabolism during exercise.
8. Discuss the influence of exercise intensity on muscle fuel selection.
9. How does the duration of exercise influence muscle fuel selection?
10. List those variables that regulate fat metabolism during exercise.
11. What is the "lactate shuttle"?

SUGGESTED READINGS

Bassett, D.R. 2002. Scientific contributions of A. V. Hill: Exercise physiology pioneer. *Journal of Applied Physiology.* 93: 1567-1582.

Brooks, G., T. Fahey, and K. Baldwin. 2005. *Exercise Physiology: Human Bioenergetics and Its Applications*, 4th ed. New York, NY: McGraw-Hill.

Fox, S. 2016. *Human Physiology*. New York, NY: McGraw-Hill.

Gladden, L.B. 2004. Lactate metabolism: A new paradigm for the third millennium. *Journal of Physiology.* 558: 5-30.

Svedahl, K. and B. MacIntosh. 2003. Anaerobic threshold: the concept and methods of measurement. *Canadian Journal of Applied Physiology.* 28: 299-323.

Van Adel, B.A. and M.A. Tarnopolsky. 2009. Metabolic myopathies: Update 2009. *Journal of Clinical Neuromuscular Disease.* 10: 97-121.

Widmaier, E., H. Raff, and K. Strang. 2014. *Vander's Human Physiology*, 13th ed. New York, NY: McGraw-Hill.

REFERENCES

1. **Armstrong R.** Biochemistry: energy liberation and use. In *Sports Medicine and Physiology*, edited by R. Strauss Philadelphia, PA: W. B. Saunders, 1979.

2. **Arthur GD, Booker TS, and Belcastro AN.** Exercise promotes a subcellular redistribution of calcium-stimulated protease activity in striated muscle. *Canadian Journal of Physiology and Pharmacology* 77: 42-47, 1999.

3. **Åstrand PO.** *Experimental Studies of Physical Working Capacity in Relation to Sex and Age*. Copenhagen, DK: Manksgaard, 1952.

4. **Åstrand P.** *Textbook of Work Physiology*. Champaign, IL: Human Kinetics, 2003.

5. **Ball-Burnett M, Green HJ, and Houston ME.** Energy metabolism in human slow and fast twitch fibres during prolonged cycle exercise. *Journal of Physiology* 437: 257-267, 1991.

6. **Barnard RJ and Foss ML.** Oxygen debt: effect of beta-adrenergic blockade on the lactacid and alactacid components. *Journal of Applied Physiology* 27: 813-816, 1969.

7. **Bassett DR, Jr., Merrill PW, Nagle FJ, Agre JC, and Sampedro R.** Rate of decline in blood lactate after cycling exercise in endurance-trained and untrained subjects. *Journal of Applied Physiology* 70: 1816-1820, 1991.

8. **Bates P.** Exercise and protein turnover in the rat. *Journal of Physiology (Lond).* 303: 41P, 1980.

9. **Belcastro AN and Bonen A.** Lactic acid removal rates during controlled and uncontrolled recovery exercise. *Journal of Applied Physiology* 39: 932-936, 1975.

10. **Bendahan D, Mattei JP, Ghattas B, Confort-Gouny S, LeGuern ME, and Cozzone PJ.** Citrulline/malate promotes aerobic energy production in human exercising muscle. *British Journal of Sports Medicine* 36: 282-289, 2002.

11. **Berg A and Keul J.** Serum alanine during long-lasting exercise. *International Journal of Sports Medicine* 1: 199-202, 1980.

12. **Boutellier U, Giezendanner D, Cerretelli P, and di Prampero PE.** After effects of chronic hypoxia on $\dot{V}O_2$ kinetics and on O_2 deficit and debt. *European Journal of Applied Physiology and Occupational Physiology* 53: 87-91, 1984.

13. **Brooks G.** Lactate production under fully aerobic conditions: the lactate shuttle during rest and exercise. *Federation Proceedings* 45: 2924-2929, 1986.

14. **Brooks G.** Lactate: glycolytic end product and oxidative substrate during sustained exercise in mammals—the lactate shuttle. In: *Comparative Physiology and Biochemistry: Current Topics and Trends, Volume A, Respiration-Metabolism-Circulation*, edited by R. Gilles. Berlin: Springer-Verlag, 1985, pp. 208-218.

15. **Brooks G, Fahey T, and Baldwin K.** *Exercise Physiology: Human Bioenergetics and Its Applications*. New York, NY: McGraw-Hill, 2005.

16. **Brooks GA.** Anaerobic threshold: review of the concept and directions for future research. *Medicine & Science in Sports & Exercise* 17: 22-34, 1985.

17. **Brooks GA.** The lactate shuttle during exercise and recovery. *Medicine & Science in Sports & Exercise* 18: 360-368, 1986.

18. **Brooks GA, Dubouchaud H, Brown M, Sicurello JP, and Butz CE.** Role of mitochondrial lactate dehydrogenase and lactate oxidation in the intracellular lactate shuttle. *Proceedings of the National Academy of Sciences of the United States of America* 96: 1129-1134, 1999.

19. **Brooks GA, Hittelman KJ, Faulkner JA, and Beyer RE.** Temperature, skeletal muscle mitochondrial functions, and oxygen debt. *American Journal of Physiology* 220: 1053-1059, 1971.

20. **Brooks GA and Mercier J.** Balance of carbohydrate and lipid utilization during exercise: the "crossover" concept. *Journal of Applied Physiology* 76: 2253-2261, 1994.

21. **Casaburi R, Storer TW, Ben-Dov I, and Wasserman K.** Effect of endurance training on possible determinants of $\dot{V}O_2$ during heavy exercise. *Journal of Applied Physiology* 62: 199-207, 1987.

22. **Cerretelli P, Shindell D, Pendergast DP, Di Prampero PE, and Rennie DW.** Oxygen uptake transients at the onset and offset of arm and leg work. *Respiration Physiology* 30: 81-97, 1977.

23. **Coggin A.** Plasma glucose metabolism during exercise in humans. *Sports Medicine* 11: 102-124, 1991.

24. **Capostagno B and Bosch A.** Higher fat oxidation in running than cycling at the same exercise intensities. *International Journal of Sport Nutrition and Exercise Metabolism* 20: 44-55, 2010.

25. **Coyle EF.** Substrate utilization during exercise in active people. *American Journal of Clinical Nutrition* 61: 968S-979S, 1995.

26. **Coyle EF, Coggan AR, Hemmert MK, and Ivy JL.** Muscle glycogen utilization during prolonged strenuous exercise when fed carbohydrate. *Journal of Applied Physiology* 61: 165-172, 1986.

27. **Coyle EF, Hamilton MT, Alonso JG, Montain SJ, and Ivy JL.** Carbohydrate metabolism during intense exercise when hyperglycemic. *Journal of Applied Physiology* 70: 834-840, 1991.

28. **Coyle EF and Montain SJ.** Carbohydrate and fluid ingestion during exercise: are there trade-offs? *Medicine & Science in Sports & Exercise* 24: 671-678, 1992.

29. **Davis JA.** Anaerobic threshold: review of the concept and directions for future research. *Medicine & Science in Sports & Exercise* 17: 6-21, 1985.

30. **Davis JA, Rozenek R, DeCicco DM, Carizzi MT, and Pham PH.** Comparison of three methods for detection of the lactate threshold. *Clinical Physiology and Functional Imaging* 27: 381-384, 2007.

31. **Davis JA, Vodak P, Wilmore JH, Vodak J, and Kurtz P.** Anaerobic threshold and maximal aerobic power for three modes of exercise. *Journal of Applied Physiology* 41: 544-550, 1976.

32. **Day JR, Rossiter HB, Coats EM, Skasick A, and Whipp BJ.** The maximally attainable $\dot{V}O_2$ during exercise in humans: the peak vs. maximal issue. *Journal of Applied Physiology* 95: 1910-1907, 2003.

33. **Dodd S, Powers S, O'Malley N, Brooks E, and Sommers H.** Effects of beta-adrenergic blockade on ventilation and gas exchange during incremental exercise. *Aviation, Space, and Environmental Medicine* 59: 718-722, 1988.

34. **Dodd S, Powers SK, Callender T, and Brooks E.** Blood lactate disappearance at various intensities of recovery exercise. *Journal of Applied Physiology* 57: 1462-1465, 1984.

35. **Dohm GL, Beecher GR, Warren RQ, and Williams RT.** Influence of exercise on free amino acid concentrations in rat tissues. *Journal of Applied Physiology* 50: 41-44, 1981.

36. **Dohm GL, Puente FR, Smith CP, and Edge A.** Changes in tissue protein levels as a result of endurance exercise. *Life Science* 23: 845-849, 1978.

37. **Donovan CM and Brooks GA.** Endurance training affects lactate clearance, not lactate production. *American Journal of Physiology* 244: E83-E92, 1983.

38. **Draoui N and Feron O.** Lactate shuttles at a glance: from physiological paradigms to anti-cancer treatment. *Disease Models & Mechanisms* 4: 727-732, 2011.

39. **Emhoff CW, Messonnier LA, Horning MA, Fattor JA, Carlson TJ, and Brooks GA.** Gluconeogenesis and hepatic glycogenolysis during exercise at the lactate threshold. *Journal of Applied Physiology* 114: 297-306, 2013.

40. **England P.** The effect of acute thermal dehydration on blood lactate accumulation during incremental exercise. *Journal of Sports Sciences* 2: 105-111, 1985.

41. **Essen B and Kaijser L.** Regulation of glycolysis in intermittent exercise in man. *Journal of Physiology* 281: 499-511, 1978.

42. **Evans BW and Cureton KJ.** Effect of physical conditioning on blood lactate disappearance after supramaximal exercise. *British Journal of Sports Medicine* 17: 40-45, 1983.

43. **Farrell PA, Wilmore JH, Coyle EF, Billing JE, and Costill DL.** Plasma lactate accumulation and distance running performance. *Medicine and Science in Sports* 11: 338-344, 1979.

44. **Foster C, Kuffel E, Bradley N, Battista RA, Wright G, Porcari JP, et al.** $\dot{V}O_2$ max during successive maximal efforts. *European Journal of Applied Physiology* 102: 67-72, 2007.

45. **Fox S.** *Human Physiology.* New York, NY: McGraw-Hill, 2016.

46. **Gaesser GA and Brooks GA.** Metabolic bases of excess post-exercise oxygen consumption: a review. *Medicine & Science in Sports & Exercise* 16: 29-43, 1984.

47. **Gladden LB.** Net lactate uptake during progressive steady-level contractions in canine skeletal muscle. *Journal of Applied Physiology* 71: 514-520, 1991.

48. **Gladden LB, Stainsby WN, and MacIntosh BR.** Norepinephrine increases canine skeletal muscle $\dot{V}O_2$ during recovery. *Medicine & Science in Sports & Exercise* 14: 471-476, 1982.

49. **Gollnick P and Saltin B.** Fuel for muscular exercise: role of fat. In *Exercise, Nutrition, and Energy Metabolism,* edited by E. Horton and R. Terjung. New York, NY: Macmillan, 1988.

50. **Gollnick PD.** Metabolism of substrates: energy substrate metabolism during exercise and as modified by training. *Federation Proceedings* 44: 353-357, 1985.

51. **Gollnick PD, Bayly WM, and Hodgson DR.** Exercise intensity, training, diet, and lactate concentration in muscle and blood. *Medicine & Science in Sports & Exercise* 18: 334-340, 1986.

52. **Goodman M.** Amino acid and protein metabolism. In *Exercise, Nutrition, and Energy Metabolism,* edited by E. Horton and R. Terjung. New York, NY: Macmillan, 1988.

53. **Gore CJ and Withers RT.** Effect of exercise intensity and duration on postexercise metabolism. *Journal of Applied Physiology* 68: 2362-2368, 1990.

54. **Graham T.** Skeletal muscle amino acid metabolism and ammonia production during exercise. In *Exercise Metabolism.* Champaign, IL: Human Kinetics, 1995.

55. **Green H.** How important is endogenous muscle glycogen to fatigue during prolonged exercise? *Canadian Journal of Physiology and Pharmacology* 69: 290-297, 1991.

56. **Green H, Halestrap A, Mockett C, O'Toole D, Grant S, and Ouyang J.** Increases in muscle MCT are associated with reductions in muscle lactate after a single exercise session in humans. *American Journal of Physiology. Endocrinology and Metabolism* 282: E154-E160, 2002.

57. **Hagberg JM, Mullin JP, and Nagle FJ.** Oxygen consumption during constant-load exercise. *Journal of Applied Physiology* 45: 381-384, 1978.

58. **Hargreaves M.** Skeletal muscle carbohydrate metabolism during exercise. In *Exercise Metabolism.* Champaign, IL: Human Kinetics, 1995.

59. **Harris RC, Edwards RH, Hultman E, Nordesjo LO, Nylind B, and Sahlin K.** The time course of phosphorylcreatine resynthesis during recovery of the quadriceps muscle in man. *Pflügers Archiv - European Journal of Physiology* 367: 137-142, 1976.

60. **Hawkins MN, Raven PB, Snell PG, Stray-Gundersen J, and Levine BD.** Maximal oxygen uptake as a parametric measure of cardiorespiratory capacity. *Medicine & Science in Sports & Exercise* 39: 103-107, 2007.

61. **Heck H, Mader A, Hess G, Mucke S, Muller R, and Hollmann W.** Justification of the 4-mmol/l lactate threshold. *International Journal of Sports Medicine* 6: 117-130, 1985.

62. **Helge JW, Rehrer NJ, Pilegaard H, Manning P, Lucas SJ, Gerrard DF, et al.** Increased fat oxidation and regulation of metabolic genes with ultraendurance exercise. *Acta Physiologica (Oxford)* 191: 77-86, 2007.

63. **Hermansen L and Stensvold I.** Production and removal of lactate during exercise in man. *Acta Physiologica Scandinavica* 86: 191-201, 1972.

64. **Hickson RC, Bomze HA, and Hollozy JO.** Faster adjustment of O_2 uptake to the energy requirement of exercise in the trained state. *Journal of Applied Physiology* 44: 877-881, 1978.

65. **Hill A.** The oxidative removal of lactic acid. *Journal of Physiology (London)* 48: x-xi, 1914.

66. **Hill A and Lupton H.** Muscular exercise, lactic acid, and the supply and utilization of oxygen. *Quarterly Journal of Medicine* 16: 135-171, 1923.

67. **Hollmann W.** Historical remarks on the development of the aerobic-anaerobic threshold up to 1966. *International Journal of Sports Medicine* 6: 109-116, 1985.

68. **Holloszy J.** Utilization of fatty acids during exercise. In *Biochemistry of Exercise VII*, edited by A. Taylor Champaign, IL: Human Kinetics, 1990, pp. 319-328.

69. **Holloszy JO.** Muscle metabolism during exercise. *Archives of Physical Medicine and Rehabilitation* 63: 231-234, 1982.

70. **Hood DA and Terjung RL.** Amino acid metabolism during exercise and following endurance training. *Sports Medicine* 9: 23-35, 1990.

71. **Howley ET.** $\dot{V}O_2$ max and the plateau—needed or not? *Medicine & Science in Sports & Exercise* 39: 101-102, 2007.

72. **Howley ET, Bassett DR, and Welch HG.** Criteria for maximal oxygen uptake: review and commentary. *Medicine & Science in Sports & Exercise* 27: 1292-1301, 1995.

73. **Hultman E.** Energy metabolism in human muscle. *J Physiol* 231: 56P, 1973.

74. **Hultman E and Sjoholm H.** Substrate availability. In *Biochemistry of Exercise*, edited by H. Knuttgen, J. Vogel and J. Poortmans. Champaign, IL: Human Kinetics, 1983.

75. **Hussien R and Brooks GA.** Mitochondrial and plasma membrane lactate transporter and lactate dehydrogenase isoform expression in breast cancer cell lines. *Physiological Genomics* doi:10.1152:PG-00177-02010, 2010.

76. **Issekutz B, Birkhead NC, and Rodahl K.** The use of respiratory quotients in assessment of aerobic power capacity. *Journal of Applied Physiology* 17: 47-50, 1962.

77. **Jones NL and Ehrsam RE.** The anaerobic threshold. *Exercise and Sport Sciences Reviews* 10: 49-83, 1982.

78. **Kalis JK, Freund BJ, Joyner MJ, Jilka SM, Nittolo J, and Wilmore JH.** Effect of ß-blockade on the drift in O_2 consumption during prolonged exercise. *Journal of Applied Physiology* 64: 753-758, 1988.

79. **Knoebel KL.** Energy metabolism. In: *Physiology*, edited by E. Selkurt. Boston, MA: Little Brown & Co., 1984, pp. 635-650.

80. **Knuttgen HG, and Saltin B.** Muscle metabolites and oxygen uptake in short-term submaximal exercise in man. *Journal of Applied Physiology* 32: 690-694, 1972.

81. **Ladu MJ, Kapsas H, and Palmer WK.** Regulation of lipoprotein lipase in muscle and adipose tissue during exercise. *Journal of Applied Physiology* 71: 404-409, 1991.

82. **Lai N, Gladden LB, Carlier PG, and Cabrera ME.** Models of muscle contraction and energetics. *Drug Discovery Today: Disease Models, Kinetic Models* 5: 273-288, 2009.

83. **Lemon PW and Mullin JP.** Effect of initial muscle glycogen levels on protein catabolism during exercise. *Journal of Applied Physiology* 48: 624-629, 1980.

84. **Lemon PW and Nagle FJ.** Effects of exercise on protein and amino acid metabolism. *Medicine & Science in Sports & Exercise* 13: 141-149, 1981.

85. **MacLean DA, Spriet LL, Hultman E, and Graham TE.** Plasma and muscle amino acid and ammonia responses during prolonged exercise in humans. *J Appl Physiol* 70: 2095-2103, 1991.

86. **Mader A and Heck H.** A theory of the metabolic origin of "anaerobic threshold." *International Journal of Sports Medicine* 7 Suppl 1: 45-65, 1986.

87. **Marti B, Abelin T, and Howald H.** A modified fixed blood lactate threshold for estimating running speed for joggers in 16-km races. *Scandinavian Journal of Sports Sciences* 9: 41-45, 1987.

88. **Marwood S, Roche D, Rowland T, Garrard M, and Unnithan VB.** Faster pulmonary oxygen uptake kinetics in trained versus untrained male adolescents. *Medicine & Science in Sports & Exercise* 42: 127-134, 2010.

89. **Maughan R.** Carbohydrate-electrolyte solutions during prolonged exercise. Perspectives in exercise science and sports medicine. In *Ergogenics: Enhancements of Performance in Exercise and Sport*, edited by D. Lamb and M.H. Williams. New York, NY: McGraw-Hill, 1991.

90. **Medbo JI, Mohn AC, Tabata I, Bahr R, Vaage O, and Sejersted OM.** Anaerobic capacity determined by maximal accumulated O_2 deficit. *Journal of Applied Physiology* 64: 50-60, 1988.

91. **Menconi MJ, Wei W, Yang H, Wray CJ, and Hasselgren PO.** Treatment of cultured myotubes with the calcium ionophore A23187 increases proteasome activity via a CaMK II-caspase-calpain-dependent mechanism. *Surgery* 136: 135-142, 2004.

92. **Menzies P, Menzies C, McIntyre L, Paterson P, Wilson J, and Kemi OJ.** Blood lactate clearance during active recovery after an intense running bout depends on the intensity of the active recovery. *Journal of Sports Sciences* 28: 975-982, 2010.

93. **Midgley AW and Carroll S.** Emergence of the verification phase procedure for confirming "true" $\dot{V}O_2$ max. *Scandinavian Journal of Medicine and Science in Sports* 19: 313-322, 2009.

94. **Mooren F and Volker K.** *Molecular and Cellular Exercise Physiology.* Champaign, IL: Human Kinetics, 2011.

95. **Ordway GA, Neufer PD, Chin ER, and DeMartino GN.** Chronic contractile activity upregulates the proteasome system in rabbit skeletal muscle. *Journal of Applied Physiology* 88: 1134-1141, 2000.

96. **Ørngreen MC, Jeppesen TD, Andersen ST, Taivassalo T, Hauerslev S, Preisler N, et al.** Fat metabolism during exercise in patients with McArdle disease. *Neurology* 72: 718-724, 2009.

97. **Powers S.** Oxygen deficit-debt relationships in ponies during submaximal treadmill exercise. *Respiratory Physiology* 70: 251-263, 1987.

98. **Powers SK, Byrd RJ, Tulley R, and Callender T.** Effects of caffeine ingestion on metabolism and performance during graded exercise. *European Journal of Applied Physiology and Occupational Physiology* 50: 301-307, 1983.

99. **Powers SK, Dodd S, and Beadle RE.** Oxygen uptake kinetics in trained athletes differing in $\dot{V}O_2$ max. *European Journal of Applied Physiology and Occupational Physiology* 54: 306-308, 1985.

100. **Powers SK, Dodd S, and Garner R.** Precision of ventilatory and gas exchange alterations as a predictor of the anaerobic threshold. *European Journal of Applied Physiology and Occupational Physiology* 52: 173-177, 1984.

101. **Powers SK, Howley ET, and Cox R.** Ventilatory and metabolic reactions to heat stress during prolonged exercise. *Journal of Sports Medicine and Physical Fitness* 22: 32-36, 1982.

102. **Powers SK, Riley W, and Howley ET.** Comparison of fat metabolism between trained men and women during prolonged aerobic work. *Research Quarterly for Exercise and Sport* 51: 427-431, 1980.

103. **Refsum HE, Gjessing LR, and Stromme SB.** Changes in plasma amino acid distribution and urine amino acids excretion during prolonged heavy exercise. *Scandinavian Journal of Clinical and Laboratory Investigation* 39: 407-413, 1979.

104. **Riley WW, Jr., Powers SK, and Welch HG.** The effect of two levels of muscular work on urinary creatinine excretion. *Research Quarterly for Exercise and Sport* 52: 339-347, 1981.

105. **Romijn JA, Coyle EF, Sidossis LS, Gastaldelli A, Horowitz JF, Endert E, et al.** Regulation of endogenous fat and carbohydrate metabolism in relation to exercise intensity and duration. *American Journal of Physiology* 265: E380-E391, 1993.

106. **Rossiter HB, Kowalchuk JM, and Whipp BJ.** A test to establish maximum O_2 uptake despite no plateau in the O_2 uptake response to ramp incremental exercise. *Journal of Applied Physiology* 100: 764-770, 2006.

107. **Rynders CA, Angadi SS, Weltman NY, Gaesser GA, and Weltman A.** Oxygen uptake and ratings of perceived exertion at the lactate threshold and maximal fat oxidation rate in untrained adults. *European Journal of Applied Physiology* 111: 2063-2068, 2011.

108. **Sahlin K, Katz A, and Broberg S.** Tricarboxylic acid cycle intermediates in human muscle during prolonged exercise. *American Journal of Physiology* 259: C834-C841, 1990.

109. **Saltin B and Gollnick P.** Fuel for muscular exercise: Role of carbohydrate. In: *Exercise, Nutrition, and Energy Metabolism*, edited by E. Horton and R. Terjung. New York, NY: Macmillan, 1988, pp. 45-71.

110. **Sedlock, DA, Lee MG, Flynn, MG, Park KS, and Kamimori, GH.** Excess postexercise oxygen consumption after aerobic exercise training. *International Journal of Sport Nutrition and Exercise Metabolism* 20: 336-349, 2010.

111. **Skinner JS and McLellan TH.** The transition from aerobic to anaerobic metabolism. *Research Quarterly for Exercise and Sport* 51: 234-248, 1980.

112. **Sonveaux P, Végran F, Schroeder T, Wergin MC, Verrax J, Rabbani ZN, et al.** Targeting lactate-fueled respiration selectively kills hypoxic tumor cells in mice. *Journal of Clinical Investigation* 118: 3930-3942, 2008.

113. **Stainsby WN.** Biochemical and physiological bases for lactate production. *Medicine & Science in Sports & Exercise* 18: 341-343, 1986.

114. **Stanley WC and Connett RJ.** Regulation of muscle carbohydrate metabolism during exercise. *FASEB Journal* 5: 2155-2159, 1991.

115. **Stryer L.** *Biochemistry.* New York, NY: W. H. Freeman, 2002.

116. **Svedahl K and MacIntosh BR.** Anaerobic threshold: the concept and methods of measurement. *Canadian Journal of Applied Physiology* 28: 299-323, 2003.

117. **Taylor HL, Buskirk E, and Henschel A.** Maximal oxygen intake as an objective measure of cardiorespiratory performance. *Journal of Applied Physiology* 8: 73-80, 1955.

118. **Tonouchi M, Hatta H, and Bonen A.** Muscle contraction increases lactate transport while reducing sarcolemmal MCT4, but not MCT1. *American Journal of Physiology. Endocrinology and Metabolism* 282: E1062-E1069, 2002.

119. **Turcotte L.** Lipid metabolism during exercise. In *Exercise Metabolism.* Champaign, IL: Human Kinetics, 1995, pp. 99-130.

120. **van Hall G.** Lactate kinetics in human tissues at rest and during exercise. *Acta Physiologica* 199: 499-508, 2010.

121. **Wasserman K.** Anaerobiosis, lactate, and gas exchange during exercise: the issues. *Federation Proceedings* 45: 2904-2909, 1986.

122. **Wasserman K, Beaver WL, and Whipp BJ.** Mechanisms and patterns of blood lactate increase during exercise in man. *Medicine & Science in Sports & Exercise* 18: 344-352, 1986.

123. **Wasserman K and McIlroy MB.** Detecting the threshold of anaerobic metabolism in cardiac patients during exercise. *American Journal of Cardiology* 14: 844-852, 1964.

124. **Wasserman K, Whipp BJ, and Davis JA.** Respiratory physiology of exercise: metabolism, gas exchange, and ventilatory control. *International Review of Physiology* 23: 149-211, 1981.

125. **Wasserman K, Whipp BJ, Koyl SN, and Beaver WL.** Anaerobic threshold and respiratory gas exchange during exercise. *Journal of Applied Physiology* 35: 236-243, 1973.

126. **White TP and Brooks GA.** [U-14C]glucose, -alanine, and -leucine oxidation in rats at rest and two intensities of running. *American Journal of Physiology* 240: E155-E165, 1981.

127. **Widmaier E, Raff H, and Strang K.** *Vander's Human Physiology.* New York, NY: McGraw-Hill, 2006.

128. **Wilson DF, Erecinska M, Drown C, and Silver IA.** Effect of oxygen tension on cellular energetics. *American Journal of Physiology* 233: C135-C140, 1977.

129. **Yoshida T.** Effect of dietary modifications on the anaerobic threshold. *Sports Medicine* 3: 4-9, 1986.

130. **Zakrezewski JK and Tolfrey K.** Comparison of fat metabolism over a range of intensities during treadmill and cycling exercise in children. *European Journal of Applied Physiology* 112: 163-171, 2012.

5

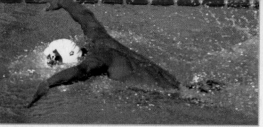

© Action Plus Sports Images/Alamy Stock Photo

Cell Signaling and the Hormonal Responses to Exercise

■ Objectives

By studying this chapter, you should be able to do the following:

1. Describe the concept of hormone–receptor interaction.

2. Identify the factors influencing the concentration of a hormone in the blood.

3. Describe the mechanisms by which hormones act on cells.

4. Describe the role of the hypothalamus in the control of hormone secretion from the anterior and posterior pituitary glands.

5. Identify the site of release, stimulus for release, and the predominant action of the following hormones: epinephrine, norepinephrine, glucagon, insulin, cortisol, aldosterone, thyroxine, growth hormone, estrogen, and testosterone.

6. Discuss the use of testosterone (and its synthetic analogs) and growth hormone on muscle growth and their potential side effects.

7. Contrast the role of plasma catecholamines with intracellular factors in the mobilization of muscle glycogen during exercise.

8. Discuss the four mechanisms by which blood glucose homeostasis is maintained.

9. Graphically describe the changes in the following hormones during graded and prolonged exercise: insulin, glucagon, cortisol, growth hormone, epinephrine, and norepinephrine.

10. Describe the effect of changing hormone and substrate levels in the blood on the mobilization of free fatty acids from adipose tissue.

■ Outline

acromegaly
adenylate cyclase
adiponectin
adrenal cortex
adrenocorticotrophic hormone
  (ACTH)
aldosterone
alpha receptors
anabolic steroids
androgenic steroid
androgens
angiotensin I and II
anterior pituitary
antidiuretic hormone (ADH)
beta receptors
calcitonin
calmodulin
catecholamines
cortisol
cyclic AMP
diabetes mellitus
diacylglycerol

endocrine glands
epinephrine (E)
estrogens
follicle-stimulating hormone
  (FSH)
G protein
glucagon
glucocorticoids
growth hormone (GH)
hormones
hypothalamic somatostatin
hypothalamus
incretins
inositol triphosphate (IP_3)
insulin
insulin-like growth factors (IGFs)
leptin
luteinizing hormone (LH)
melanocyte-stimulating hormone
  (MSH)
mineralocorticoids
neuroendocrinology

norepinephrine (NE)
pancreas
phosphodiesterase
phospholipase C
pituitary gland
posterior pituitary gland
prolactin
protein kinase C
receptors
releasing hormones
renin
second messengers
sex steroids
somatostatin
steroids
testosterone
thyroid gland
thyroid-stimulating hormone
  (TSH)
thyroxine (T_4)
triiodothyronine (T_3)

As presented in Chap. 4, the fuels for muscular exercise include muscle glycogen and fat, plasma glucose and free fatty acids (FFAs), and, to a lesser extent, amino acids. These fuels must be provided at an optimal rate for activities as diverse as the 400-meter run and the 26-mile, 385-yard marathon, or performance will suffer. What controls the mixture of fuel used by the muscles? What stimulates the adipose tissue to release more FFA? How is the liver made aware of the need to replace the glucose that is being removed from the blood by exercising muscles? If glucose is not replaced, a hypoglycemic (low blood glucose) condition will occur. Hypoglycemia is a topic of crucial importance in discussing exercise as a challenge to homeostasis. Blood glucose is the primary fuel for the central nervous system (CNS), and without optimal CNS function during exercise, the chance of fatigue and the risk of serious injury increase. Although blood glucose was used as an example, it should be noted that sodium, calcium, potassium, and water concentrations, as well as blood pressure and pH, are also maintained within narrow limits during exercise. It should be no surprise then that there are a variety of automatic control systems maintaining these variables within these limits.

Chapter 2 presented an overview of automatic control systems that maintain homeostasis. In that context, you also were introduced to cell signaling—the fact that a wide variety of signals, some acting locally and others reaching all tissues, are needed for our adaptation to a single bout of exercise, or to repeated bouts of exercise (training) that lead to changes in muscle structure and function. Although this chapter focuses primarily on endocrine signals,

the other types of signals (i.e., autocrine, paracrine, and synaptic) are crucial—not only for muscular adaptations but also for the health-related benefits such as reduced risks of type 2 diabetes and coronary heart disease. This chapter provides additional information on cell signaling, with an emphasis on **neuroendocrinology,** a branch of physiology dedicated to the systematic study of control systems. The first part of the chapter presents a brief introduction to each hormone, indicates the factors controlling its secretion, and discusses its role in homeostasis. Following that, we discuss how **hormones** control the delivery of carbohydrates and fats during exercise.

NEUROENDOCRINOLOGY

Two of the major homeostatic systems involved in the control and regulation of various functions (cardiovascular, renal, metabolic, etc.) are the nervous and endocrine systems. Both are structured to sense information, organize an appropriate response, and then deliver the message to the proper organ or tissue. Often, the two systems work together to maintain homeostasis; the term *neuroendocrine response* is reflective of that interdependence. The two systems differ in the way the message is delivered: The endocrine system releases hormones (endocrine signals) into the blood to circulate to tissues, whereas nerves use neurotransmitters (synaptic signals) to relay messages from one nerve to the other, or from a nerve to a tissue.

Endocrine glands release hormones (chemical messengers) directly into the blood, which carries the

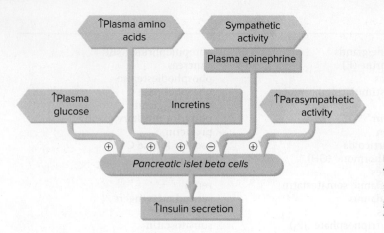

Figure 5.1   Major controls of insulin secretion. The ⊕ and ⊖ symbols represent stimulatory and inhibitory actions, respectively. Incretions are gastrointestinal hormones that act as feedforward signals to the pancreas.

hormone to a tissue to exert an effect. It is the binding of the hormone to a specific protein receptor that allows the hormone to exert its effect. In that way, the hormone can circulate to all tissues while affecting only a few–those with the specific receptor.

Hormones can be divided into several classes based on chemical makeup: amino acid derivatives, peptides, proteins, and **steroids.** The chemical structure influences the way in which the hormone is transported in the blood and the manner in which it exerts its effect on the tissue. For example, while steroid hormones' lipid-like structure requires that they be transported bound to plasma protein (to "dissolve" in the plasma), that same lipid-like structure allows them to diffuse through cell membranes to exert their effects (96).

Blood Hormone Concentration

The effect a hormone exerts on a tissue is directly related to the concentration of the hormone in the plasma and the number of active receptors to which it can bind. The hormone concentration in the plasma is dependent upon the following factors:

■ The rate of secretion of the hormone from the endocrine gland

■ The rate of metabolism or excretion of the hormone

■ The quantity of transport protein (for some hormones)

■ Changes in the plasma volume

Control of Hormone Secretion   The rate at which a hormone is secreted from an endocrine gland is dependent on the magnitude of the input and whether it is stimulatory or inhibitory in nature. The input in every case is a chemical one, be it an ion (e.g., Ca⁺⁺) or a substrate (e.g., glucose) in the plasma, a neurotransmitter such as acetylcholine or norepinephrine, or another hormone. Most endocrine glands are under the direct influence of more than one type of input, which may either reinforce or interfere with each other's effect. An example of this interaction is found in the control of **insulin** release from the pancreas. Figure 5.1 shows that the **pancreas,** which produces insulin, responds to changes in plasma glucose and amino acids, to norepinephrine released from sympathetic neurons as well as circulating epinephrine, to parasympathetic neurons, which release acetylcholine, and to a variety of hormones, including **incretins.** Elevations of plasma glucose and amino acids increase insulin secretion (+), whereas an increase in sympathetic nervous system activity (epinephrine and norepinephrine) decreases (−) insulin secretion. The incretins are a group of hormones secreted by endocrine cells in the GI tract when food is being ingested; these hormones anticipate and augment the insulin response due to the rising blood glucose or amino acid levels (151). This magnitude of inhibitory versus excitatory input determines whether there will be an increase or a decrease in the secretion of insulin.

Metabolism and Excretion of Hormones   The concentration of a hormone in the plasma is also influenced by the rate at which it is metabolized (inactivated) and/or excreted. Inactivation can take place at or near the receptor or in the liver, the major site for hormone metabolism. In addition, the kidneys can metabolize a variety of hormones or excrete them in their free (active) form. In fact, the rate of excretion of a hormone in the urine has been used as an indicator of its rate of secretion during exercise (8, 35, 63, 64). Because blood flow to the kidneys and liver decreases during exercise, the rate at which hormones are inactivated or excreted decreases. This results in an elevation of the plasma level of the hormone over and above that due to higher rates of secretion.

Transport Protein   The concentration of some hormones is influenced by the quantity of transport protein in the plasma. Steroid hormones and thyroxine are transported bound to plasma proteins. For a hormone to exert its effect on a cell, it must be "free" to interact with the receptor and not "bound" to the transport protein. The amount of free hormone is dependent on the quantity of transport protein and the capacity and affinity of the protein to bind the hormone molecules. *Capacity* refers to the maximal quantity of hormone that can be bound to the transport protein, and *affinity* refers to the tendency of the transport protein to bind to the hormone. An increase in the quantity, capacity, or affinity of transport protein would reduce the amount of free hormone and its effect on tissue (38, 76). For example, high levels of estrogen during pregnancy increase the quantity of thyroxine's transport protein, causing a reduction in free thyroxine. The **thyroid gland** produces more thyroxine to counteract this effect.

Plasma Volume Changes in plasma volume will change the hormone concentration independent of changes in the rate of secretion or inactivation of the hormone. During exercise, plasma volume decreases due to the movement of water out of the cardiovascular system. This causes a small increase in the concentration of hormones in the plasma. By measuring changes in plasma volume, it is possible to "correct" the concentration of the hormone to obtain a more accurate assessment of endocrine gland activity (76).

IN SUMMARY

- Endocrine glands release hormones directly into the blood to alter the activity of tissues possessing receptors to which the hormone can bind.
- The free plasma hormone concentration determines the magnitude of the effect at the tissue level.
- The free hormone concentration can be changed by altering the rate of secretion or inactivation of the hormone, the quantity of transport protein, and the plasma volume.

Hormone–Receptor Interaction

Hormones are carried by the circulation to all tissues, but they affect only certain tissues. Tissues responsive to specific hormones have specific protein receptors capable of binding to those hormones. These protein receptors should not be viewed as static fixtures associated with cells, but like any cellular structure, they are subject to change. The number of receptors varies from 500 to 100,000 per cell, depending on the receptor. Receptor number may decrease when exposed to a chronically elevated level of a hormone (down-regulation), resulting in a diminished response for the same hormone concentration. The opposite case, chronic exposure to a low concentration of a hormone, may lead to an increase in receptor number (up-regulation), with the tissue becoming very responsive to the available hormone. Because there are a finite number of receptors on or in a cell, a situation can arise in which the concentration of a hormone is so high that all receptors are bound to the hormone; this is called saturation. Any additional increase in the plasma hormone concentration will have no additional effect (38). Further, because the receptors are specific to a hormone, any chemical similar in "shape" will compete for the limited receptor sites. A major way in which endocrine function is studied is to use chemicals (drugs) to block receptors and observe the consequences. For example, patients with heart disease may receive a drug that blocks the receptors to which epinephrine (adrenaline) binds; this prevents the heart rate from getting too high during exercise. After the hormone binds to a receptor, cellular activity is altered by a variety of mechanisms.

Mechanisms of Hormone Action Mechanisms by which hormones modify cellular activity include:

- Altering activity of DNA in the nucleus to initiate or suppress the synthesis of a specific protein
- Activation of special proteins in the cells by "second messengers"
- Alteration of membrane transport mechanisms

Altering Activity of DNA in the Nucleus Due to their lipid-like nature, steroid hormones diffuse easily through cell membranes, where they become bound to a protein receptor in the cytoplasm of the cell. Figure 5.2 shows that the steroid-receptor complex enters the nucleus and binds to hormone-responsive elements on DNA, which contains the instruction codes for protein synthesis. This activates (or, in a few cases, suppresses) genes that lead to the synthesis of a specific messenger RNA (mRNA) that carries the codes from the nucleus to the cytoplasm where the specific protein is synthesized. Although thyroid hormones are not steroid hormones, they act in a similar manner. These processes—the activation of DNA and the synthesis of specific protein—take time to turn on (making the hormones involved "slow-acting" hormones), but their effects are longer lasting than those generated by "second messengers" (38).

Second Messengers Many hormones, because of their size or highly charged structure, cannot easily cross cell membranes. These hormones exert their effects by binding to a receptor on the membrane surface and activating a **G protein** located in the membrane of the cell. The G protein is the link between the hormone–receptor interaction on the surface of the membrane and the subsequent events inside the cell. The G protein may open an ion channel to allow Ca^{++} to enter the cell, or it may activate an enzyme in the membrane. If the G protein activates

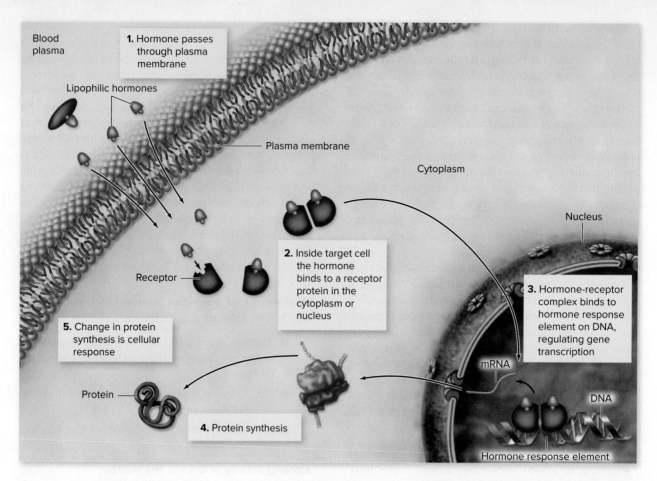

Figure 5.2   The mechanism by which steroid hormones act on target cells. A lipophilic hormone (e.g., steroid hormone) diffuses through the plasma membrane (1) and binds to a cytoplasmic receptor (2). This hormone–receptor complex translocates to the nucleus, where it binds to hormone-response elements on DNA that regulate the production of mRNA (3). The outcome may either increase or decrease protein synthesis (4), which alters cellular activity (5).

adenylate cyclase, then **cyclic AMP** (cyclic 3′,5′-adenosine mono-phosphate) is formed from ATP (see Fig. 5.3). The cyclic AMP concentration increases in the cell and activates protein kinase A that, in turn, activates response proteins to alter cellular activity. For example, this mechanism is used to break down glycogen to glucose (by activating phosphorylase) and break down triglyceride molecules to free fatty acids (by activating hormone-sensitive lipase [HSL]). The cyclic AMP is inactivated by **phosphodiesterase,** an enzyme that converts cyclic AMP to 5′AMP. Factors that interfere with phosphodiesterase activity, such as caffeine, would increase the effect of the hormone by allowing cyclic AMP to exert its effect for a longer period. For example, caffeine may exert this effect on adipose tissue, causing free fatty acids to be mobilized at a faster rate (see Chap. 25).

A G protein may activate a membrane-bound enzyme **phospholipase C.** When this occurs, a phospholipid in the membrane, phosphatidylinositol (PIP₂), is hydrolyzed into two intracellular molecules, **inositol triphosphate (IP₃),** which causes Ca++ release from

intracellular stores, and **diacylglycerol** (DAG). The calcium binds to and activates a protein called calmodulin, which alters cellular activity in much the same way as cyclic AMP does. The diacylglycerol activates **protein kinase C** (PKC) that, in turn, activates proteins in the cell (see Fig. 5.4). Cyclic AMP, Ca++, inositol triphosphate, and diacylglycerol are viewed as **second messengers** in the events following the hormone's binding to a receptor on the cell membrane. These second messengers should not be viewed as being independent of one another because changes in one can affect the action of the others (112, 143).

Membrane Transport   After binding to a receptor on a membrane, the major effect of some hormones is to activate carrier molecules in or near the membrane to increase the movement of substrates or ions from outside to inside the cell. For example, insulin binds to receptors on the surface of the cell and mobilizes glucose transporters to the membrane of the cell. The transporters link up with glucose on the outside of the cell membrane where the concentration of glucose is

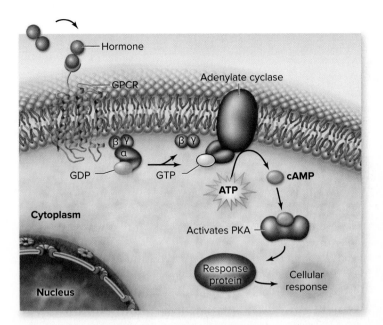

Figure 5.3 The cyclic AMP "second messenger" mechanism by which hormones act on target cells. A hormone binds to a G protein coupled receptor (GPCR) on the plasma membrane, which activates a G protein. The G protein activates adenylate cyclase, which causes ATP to be converted to cyclic AMP. The cyclic AMP activates protein kinase A (PKA) that, in turn, activates response proteins to alter cellular activity.

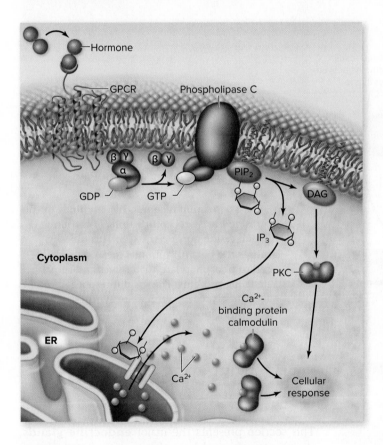

Figure 5.4 The phospholipase C second messenger mechanism by which hormones act on target cells. A hormone binds to a G protein coupled receptor (GPCR) on the plasma membrane and activates a G protein. The G protein activates the effector protein phospholipase C, which causes phosphotidylinositol (PIP_2) to be broken down into inositol triphosphate (IP_3) and diacylglycerol (DAG). The IP_3 causes release of calcium from intracellular organelles that activates the calcium-binding protein calmodulin, and the DAG activates protein kinase C to bring about additional cellular responses.

high, and the glucose diffuses to the inside of the membrane for use in the cell (71). If an individual does not have adequate insulin, as exists in uncontrolled diabetes, glucose accumulates in the plasma because the glucose transporters are not activated. Insulin does not use second messenger mechanisms to bring about its effects on the cell. Instead, insulin binds to a tyrosine kinase receptor's alpha (α) subunits, which reside outside the cell (see Fig. 5.5). This binding causes the beta (β) subunits located inside the cell to phosphorylate themselves. The activated tyrosine kinase phosphorylates insulin-response proteins that lead to the movement of glucose transporters (called GLUT4) from the cytoplasm to the membrane so glucose can enter the cell. The insulin-response protein also activates the enzyme glycogen synthase to form glycogen from the glucose molecules brought into the cell, as shown in Figure 5.5 (112).

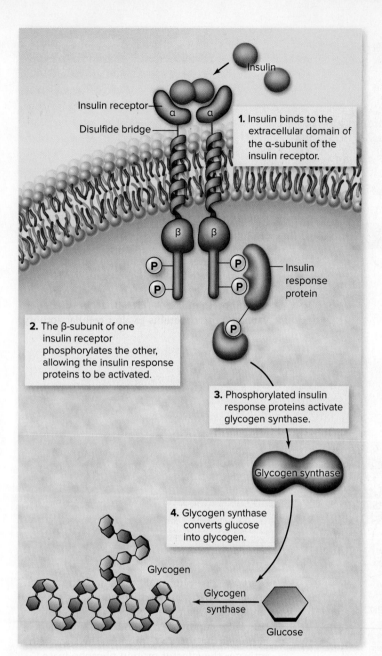

1. Insulin binds to the extracellular domain of the α-subunit of the insulin receptor.

2. The β-subunit of one insulin receptor phosphorylates the other, allowing the insulin response proteins to be activated.

3. Phosphorylated insulin response proteins activate glycogen synthase.

4. Glycogen synthase converts glucose into glycogen.

Figure 5.5 Insulin receptor. Insulin binds to the tyrosine kinase receptor's alpha (α) subunits, which reside outside the cell. This binding causes the beta (β) subunits located inside the cell to phosphorylate themselves and activate signaling proteins. The insulin-response proteins activate glycogen synthase to synthesize glycogen from glucose.

IN SUMMARY

- The hormone–receptor interaction triggers events at the cell, and changing the concentration of the hormone, the number of receptors on the cell or the affinity of the receptor for the hormone will all influence the magnitude of the effect.
- Hormones bring about their effects by activating/suppressing genes to alter protein synthesis, activating second messengers (e.g., cyclic AMP, Ca^{++}, inositol triphosphate, and diacylglycerol), and modifying membrane transport (e.g., tyrosine kinase).

HORMONES: REGULATION AND ACTION

This section presents the major **endocrine glands,** their hormones and how they are regulated, the effects the hormones have on tissues, and how some of the hormones respond to exercise. This information is essential to discuss the role of the neuroendocrine system in the mobilization of fuel for exercise.

Hypothalamus and the Pituitary Gland

The **pituitary gland** is located at the base of the brain, attached to the hypothalamus. The gland has two lobes–the anterior lobe (adenohypophysis), which is a true endocrine gland, and the posterior lobe (neurohypophysis), which is neural tissue extending from the hypothalamus. Both lobes are under the direct control of the hypothalamus. In the case of the **anterior pituitary,** hormone release is controlled principally by chemicals (**releasing hormones** or factors) that originate in neurons located in the hypothalamus. These releasing hormones stimulate or inhibit the release of specific hormones from the anterior pituitary. The **posterior pituitary gland** receives its hormones from special neurons originating in the hypothalamus. The hormones move down the axon to blood vessels in the posterior hypothalamus where they are discharged into the general circulation (38, 77).

Anterior Pituitary Gland   The anterior pituitary hormones include **adrenocorticotrophic hormone (ACTH), follicle-stimulating hormone (FSH), luteinizing hormone (LH), melanocyte-stimulating hormone (MSH), thyroid-stimulating hormone (TSH), growth hormone (GH),** and **prolactin.** While prolactin directly stimulates the breast to produce milk, the majority of the hormones secreted from the anterior pituitary control the release of other hormones. TSH controls the rate of thyroid hormone formation and secretion from the thyroid gland; ACTH stimulates the production and secretion of **cortisol** in the adrenal cortex; LH stimulates the production of testosterone in the testes and estrogen in the ovaries; and GH stimulates the release of **insulin-like growth factors (IGFs)** from the liver and other tissues. However, IGFs can be produced by a variety of other means. In fact, the IGF-1 produced in muscle due to muscle contraction acts locally via autocrine and paracrine mechanisms and is a principal driver of muscle hypertrophy (51, 80, 127). However, as we will see, growth hormone exerts important effects on protein, fat, and carbohydrate metabolism.

Growth Hormone   Growth hormone is secreted from the anterior pituitary gland and exerts profound effects on the growth of all tissues through the action of IGFs. Growth hormone secretion is controlled by releasing hormones secreted from the **hypothalamus.** Growth hormone-releasing hormone (GHRH) stimulates GH release from the anterior pituitary, whereas another factor, **hypothalamic somatostatin,** inhibits it. The GH and IGF levels in blood exert a negative feedback effect on the continued secretion of GH. As shown in Figure 5.6, additional input to the hypothalamus that can influence the secretion of GH includes exercise, stress (broadly defined), a low plasma-glucose concentration, and sleep (151). However, exercise is the most potent stimulus (149). GH

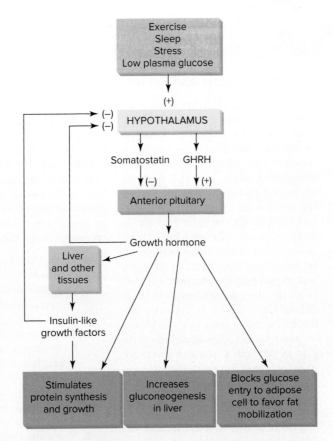

Figure 5.6   Summary of the positive and negative input to the hypothalamus, influencing growth hormone secretion.

"Summary of the Positive and Negative Input to the Hypothalamus, Influencing Growth Hormone Secretion," from Vander, A. J., et al., *Human Physiology: The Mechanisms of Body Function,* 4th ed. New York: McGraw-Hill, Inc., 1985.

and IGFs stimulate tissue uptake of amino acids, the synthesis of new protein, and long-bone growth. In addition, GH spares plasma glucose by

- Opposing the action of insulin ("anti-insulin effect") to reduce the use of plasma glucose
- Increasing the synthesis of new glucose in the liver (gluconeogenesis) from amino acids, glycerol, and lactate
- Increasing the mobilization of fatty acids from adipose tissue to increase the use of fat as a fuel

Given these characteristics, it should be no surprise that GH increases with exercise to help maintain the plasma glucose concentration (this will be covered in detail in a later section, "Permissive and Slow-Acting Hormones"). However, it is important to keep in mind that GH is also important after exercise to stimulate protein synthesis. Consistent with this view, a recent study showed that prolonged aerobic exercise was associated with large increases in the pulsatile release of GH and in total GH secretion (100). Because of GH's

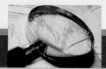
Growth Hormone and Performance

An excess of growth hormone (GH) during childhood is tied to gigantism, whereas an inadequate secretion causes dwarfism. The latter condition requires the administration of GH (along with other growth-promoting hormones) during the growing years if the child is to regain his or her normal position on the growth chart. In addition, in GH-deficient adults, therapeutic doses of GH cause increases in fat oxidation, $\dot{V}O_2$ max and strength, and improve body composition (149). However, the gain in strength in these GH-deficient adults is typically observed in longer-term (>1 year) studies; short-term studies show little or no gain in strength (150). GH was originally obtained by extracting it from the pituitary glands of cadavers—an expensive and time-consuming proposition. Due to the success of genetic engineering, recombinant human GH (rhGH) is now available.

If an excess of GH occurs during adulthood, a condition called **acromegaly** occurs. The additional GH during adulthood does not affect growth in height because the epiphyseal growth plates at the ends of the long bones have closed. Unfortunately, the excess GH causes permanent deformities, as seen in a thickening of the bones in the face, hands, and feet. Until recently, the usual cause of acromegaly was a tumor in the anterior pituitary gland that resulted in excess secretion of GH. This is no longer the case. In a drive to take advantage of the anabolic effects of GH, young adults with normal GH levels are injecting the now readily available human GH, along with other hormones (see A Closer Look 5.3). Does GH work on these individuals? Based on three systematic reviews, there appears to be consensus on the following (60, 84, 149):

- Normal adults show an increase in lean body mass, but this is due more to an increase in water retention than an increase in cell mass.
- There are minimal gains in lean body mass, muscle mass, and strength in normal, healthy men when GH is used with resistance training, compared to the use of resistance training alone.
- There are a variety of adverse events when GH is used, and these events are dose dependent. Adverse events include suppression of the GH/IGF axis, water retention and edema, joint and muscle aches, and an increased risk of injection-related diseases (e.g., HIV/AIDS).

But it is not only the athletes who are interested in the use of GH. A great deal of attention has been focused on the role that GH might have on older adults (≥65 years) relative to slowing or stopping the loss of bone and muscle mass that occurs with age. In general, older adults experience an increase in lean mass and a decrease in body fatness with GH therapy, but muscle strength does not change. In addition, because a wide variety of adverse effects are associated with this therapy, some recommend that GH not be used as an anti-aging therapy (85). That said, Giannoulis and colleagues (44) suggest that the reason for poor outcomes in these studies may be related to the following:

- Study was not long enough, and a multi-year study is needed
- GH should be used in combination with testosterone, a potent anabolic hormone (see A Close Look 5.3)
- Doses of both hormones should be lowered to achieve physiological levels in order to reduce adverse effects
- Exercise should be used in conjunction with the hormone replacement therapy

It is important to remember that while the focus of this discussion has been on GH and protein synthesis, it is clear that it is the IGFs produced by contracting skeletal muscle, as well as those secreted by the liver, that are responsible for bringing about muscular adaptations (127, 128).

---

role in protein synthesis, it is being used by some athletes to enhance muscle mass and by older adults to slow down the aging process. However, there are problems with this approach (see A Closer Look 5.1).

IN SUMMARY

- The hypothalamus controls the activity of both the anterior pituitary and posterior pituitary glands.
- GH is released from the anterior pituitary gland and is essential for normal growth.
- GH increases during exercise to mobilize fatty acids from adipose tissue and to aid in the maintenance of blood glucose.

Posterior Pituitary Gland The posterior pituitary gland provides a storage site for two hormones, oxytocin and antidiuretic hormone (ADH, also called arginine vasopressin), which are produced in the hypothalamus to which the posterior pituitary is attached. Oxytocin is a powerful stimulator of smooth muscle, especially at the time of childbirth, and is also involved in the milk "let down" response needed for the release of milk from the breast.

Antidiuretic Hormone Antidiuretic hormone (**ADH**) does what its name implies: It reduces water loss from the body. ADH favors the reabsorption of water from the kidney tubules back into the

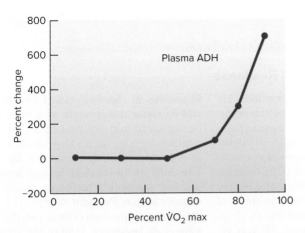

Figure 5.7 **Percent change in the plasma antidiuretic hormone (ADH) concentration with increasing exercise intensity.**

capillaries to maintain body fluid. Two major stimuli cause an increased secretion of ADH:

- High plasma osmolality (a low water concentration) that can be caused by excessive sweating without water replacement
- A low plasma volume, which can be due either to the loss of blood or to inadequate fluid replacement

There are osmoreceptors in the hypothalamus that sense the water concentration in the interstitial fluid. When the plasma has a high concentration of particles (low water concentration), the osmoreceptors shrink, and a neural reflex to the hypothalamus stimulates ADH release, which causes a reduction in water loss at the kidney. If the osmolality of the plasma is normal but the volume of plasma is low, stretch receptors in the left atrium initiate a reflex leading to ADH release to attempt to maintain body fluid. During exercise, plasma volume decreases and osmolality increases, and for exercise intensities in excess of 60% of $\dot{V}O_2$ max, ADH secretion is increased, as shown in Figure 5.7 (23). This favors the conservation of water to maintain plasma volume (145). Recently, it has been hypothesized that nonosmotic signals associated with exercise may override the usual controls and lead to excessive water retention and dilution of the body's sodium concentration, which may result in hyponatremia (low blood sodium concentration). This has potentially deadly consequences (see Chap. 23 for more on this) (55).

Thyroid Gland

The thyroid gland is stimulated by TSH to synthesize two iodine-containing hormones: **triiodothyronine (T_3)** and **thyroxine (T_4).** T_3 contains three iodine atoms and T_4 contains four. TSH is also the primary stimulus for the release of T_3 and T_4 into the circulation, where they are bound to plasma proteins. Remember, it is the "free" hormone concentration (that which is not bound to plasma proteins) that is important in bringing about an effect on tissue.

Thyroid Hormones Thyroid hormones are central in establishing the overall metabolic rate (i.e., a hypothyroid [low T_3] individual would be characterized as being lethargic and hypokinetic). It is this effect of the hormone that has been linked to weight-control problems, but only a small percentage of obese individuals are hypothyroid. T_3 and T_4 act as permissive hormones in that they permit other hormones to exert their full effect. There is a relatively long latent period between the time T_3 and T_4 are elevated and the time when their effects are observed. The latent period is 6 to 12 hours for T_3 and 2 to 3 days for T_4. However, once initiated, their effects are long lasting (38). The control of T_3 and T_4 secretion is another example of the negative feedback mechanism introduced in Chap. 2. At rest, as the plasma concentrations of T_3 and T_4 increase, they inhibit the release of TSH-releasing hormone from the hypothalamus as well as TSH itself. This self-regulating system ensures the necessary level of T_3 and T_4 for the maintenance of a normal metabolic rate. During exercise, the "free" hormone concentration increases due to changes in the binding characteristic of the transport protein, and the hormones are taken up at a faster rate by tissues. To counter the higher rate of removal of T_3 and T_4, TSH secretion increases and causes an increased secretion of these hormones from the thyroid gland (139). There is some evidence to suggest that the exercise-induced increases in prolactin and cortisol (see later) also influence TSH release (50). Finally, evidence suggests that resistance training has little effect on the pituitary (TSH)-thyroid (T_3, T_4) function (2).

IN SUMMARY

- Thyroid hormones T_3 and T_4 are important for maintaining the metabolic rate and allowing other hormones to bring about their full effect.

Calcitonin The thyroid gland also secretes **calcitonin,** which is involved in a minor way in the regulation of plasma calcium (Ca^{++}), a crucial ion for normal muscle and nerve function. The secretion of this hormone is controlled by another negative feedback mechanism. As the plasma Ca^{++} concentration increases, calcitonin release is increased. Calcitonin blocks the release of Ca^{++} from bone and stimulates Ca^{++} excretion at the kidneys to lower the plasma Ca^{++} concentration. As the Ca^{++} concentration is decreased, the rate of calcitonin secretion is reduced.

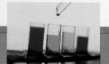

Walter B. Cannon (1871–1945) and the Fight or Flight Response

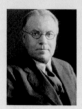

© BettmannGetty Images

Walter B. Cannon was born and raised in Wisconsin and attended Harvard College from 1892-1896. He then entered Harvard University to study medicine. During his first year, he worked in Dr. Henry Bowditch's lab and began to use the new technique of X-rays to study gastrointestinal motility. He completed his medical degree in 1900 and stayed on as an instructor in the Department of Physiology, of which Bowditch was chairman. Bowditch was a well-known physiologist who was one of the five founders of the American Physiological Society. Two years later, Dr. Cannon was promoted to assistant professor, and in 1906, he succeeded Dr. Bowditch as chairman of the department–a post he held until his retirement in 1942.

Dr. Cannon's research included work on gastrointestinal motility and the physiology of the emotions. He developed the concept of the emergency function of the sympathetic nervous system–the "fight or flight" response–the importance of epinephrine and norepinephrine in mobilizing the resources to the body to stay and fight or to take flight in times of extreme stress. In addition to these important contributions, he was responsible for the development of the concept of homeostasis–the idea that a dynamic constancy exists in the internal environment that is maintained by complex regulatory systems, of which the neuroendocrine system, described in this chapter, is a major part. Homeostasis is one of the most fundamental theories in biology, and a theme that we use through this textbook.

Dr. Cannon provided outstanding leadership, not only to the Physiology Department at Harvard but also to the broader field of physiology. He was the sixth president of the American Physiological Society (1914-1916), and he spoke out strongly on a number of social and political issues, including fighting anti-vivisectionists, as did his mentor, Dr. Bowditch, before him. He published several important textbooks, including *Bodily Changes in Pain, Fear, and Rage* (1915), *The Wisdom of the Body* (1932), and *The Way of an Investigator* (1945), the latter being an autobiography that describes his personal experiences as a scientist. It provides keen insights for those interested in pursuing the life of a scientist. Dr. Cannon is regarded as the greatest American physiologist of the first half of the twentieth century.

For those interested in more detail about this man's life, see *Walter B. Cannon, The Life and Times of a Young Scientist* and *Walter B. Cannon, Science and Society*, both published by Harvard University Press.

American Physiological Society (http://www.the-aps.org/fm/presidents/introwbc.html)

Calcitonin is not increased as a result of exercise, an appropriate response given its function (88).

Parathyroid Gland

Parathyroid hormone is the primary hormone involved in plasma Ca^{++} regulation. The parathyroid gland releases parathyroid hormone in response to a low plasma Ca^{++} concentration. The hormone stimulates bone to release Ca^{++} into the plasma and simultaneously increases the renal absorption of Ca^{++}; both raise the plasma Ca^{++} level. Parathyroid hormone also stimulates the kidney to convert a form of vitamin D (vitamin D_3) into a hormone that increases the absorption of Ca^{++} from the gastrointestinal tract. Parathyroid hormone increases during both intense and prolonged exercise (10, 90). The increase is related to a lower Ca^{++} concentration and the exercise-induced increases in plasma H^+ and catecholamine concentrations (88).

Adrenal Gland

The adrenal gland is really two different glands–the adrenal medulla, which secretes the **catecholamines,** **epinephrine (E),** and **norepinephrine (NE),** and the **adrenal cortex,** which secretes steroid hormones.

Adrenal Medulla The adrenal medulla is part of the sympathetic nervous system. Eighty percent of the gland's hormonal secretion is epinephrine, which affects receptors in the cardiovascular and respiratory systems, gastrointestinal (GI) tract, liver, other endocrine glands, muscle, and adipose tissue. E and NE are involved in the maintenance of blood pressure and the plasma glucose concentration. Their role in the cardiovascular system is discussed in Chap. 9, and their involvement in the mobilization of substrate for exercise is discussed later in this chapter in the section "Fast-Acting Hormones." E and NE also respond to strong emotional stimuli, and they form the basis for Cannon's "fight or flight" hypothesis of how the body responds to challenges from the environment (14). Cannon's view was that the activation of the sympathetic nervous system prepared you either to confront a danger or to flee from it. Statements by sportscasters, such as "The adrenalin must really be pumping now," are a rough translation of this hypothesis. See A Look Back–Important People in Science for more on Dr. Walter B. Cannon.

Receptor Type	Effect of E/NE	Membrane-Bound Enzyme	Intracellular Mediator	Effects on Various Tissues
β_1	E = NE	Adenylate cyclase	↑cyclic AMP	↑Heart rate ↑Glycogenolysis ↑Lipolysis
β_2	E ≫ NE	Adenylate cyclase	↑cyclic AMP	↑Bronchodilation ↑Vasodilation
β_3	NE > E	Adenylate cyclase	↑cyclic AMP	↑Lipolysis
α_1	E ≥ E	Phospholipase C	↑Ca^{++}	↑Phosphodiesterase ↑Vasoconstriction
α_2	E ≥ NE	Adenylate cyclase	↓cyclic AMP	Opposes action of β_1 and β_2 receptors ↓Insulin secretion

Tepperman, J., and H. M. Tepperman, *Metabolic and Endocrine Physiology*. Chicago, IL: Year Book Medical Publishers, 1987; Brunton, L., J. S. Lazo, and K. L. Parker, eds., *Goodman & Gilman's The Pharmacological Basis of Therapeutics*. New York, NY: McGraw-Hill, 2005; Zouhal, H., C. Jacob, P. Delamarche, and A. Gratas-Delamarche, "Catecholamines and the Effects of Exercise, Training, and Gender," *Sports Medicine* 38: 401–423, 2008.

E and NE bind to adrenergic (from adrenaline, the European name for epinephrine) receptors on target tissues. The **receptors** are divided into two major classes: **alpha** (α) and **beta** (β), with subgroups (α_1 and α_2; β_1, β_2, and β_3). E and NE bring about their effects via the second messenger mechanisms mentioned earlier. The response generated in the target tissue, both size and direction (inhibitory or excitatory), is dependent on the receptor type and whether E or NE is involved. This is an example of how important the receptors are in determining the cell's response to a hormone. Table 5.1 summarizes the effects of E and NE relative to the type of adrenergic receptor involved (132). The different receptors cause changes in the cell's activity by increasing or decreasing the cyclic AMP or Ca^{++} concentrations. From this table, it can be seen that if a cell experienced a loss of β_1 receptors and a gain in α_2 receptors, the same epinephrine concentration would bring about very different effects in the cell.

IN SUMMARY

- The adrenal medulla secretes the catecholamines epinephrine (E) and norepinephrine (NE). E is the adrenal medulla's primary secretion (80%), and NE is primarily secreted from the adrenergic neurons of the sympathetic nervous system.
- Epinephrine and norepinephrine bind to α- and β-adrenergic receptors and bring about changes in cellular activity (e.g., increased heart rate, mobilization of fatty acids from adipose tissue) via second messengers.

Adrenal Cortex The adrenal cortex secretes a variety of steroid hormones with rather distinct physiological functions. The hormones can be grouped into three categories:

- **Mineralocorticoids** (aldosterone), involved in the maintenance of the Na^+ and K^+ concentrations in plasma
- **Glucocorticoids** (cortisol), involved in plasma glucose regulation
- **Sex steroids** (androgens and estrogens), which support prepubescent growth, with androgens being associated with postpubescent sex drive in women

The chemical precursor common to all of these steroid hormones is cholesterol; although the final active hormones possess minor structural differences, their physiological functions differ greatly.

Aldosterone Aldosterone (mineralocorticoid) is an important regulator of Na^+ reabsorption and K^+ secretion at the kidney. Aldosterone is directly involved in Na^+/H_2O balance and, consequently, plasma volume and blood pressure (see Chap. 9). There are two levels of control over aldosterone secretion. The release of aldosterone from the adrenal cortex is controlled directly by the plasma K^+ concentration. An increase in K^+ concentration increases aldosterone secretion, which stimulates the kidney's active transport mechanism to secrete K^+ ions. This control system uses the negative feedback loop we have already seen. Aldosterone secretion is also controlled by another more complicated mechanism. A decrease in plasma volume, a fall in blood pressure at the kidney, or an increase in sympathetic nerve activity to the kidney stimulates special cells in the kidney to secrete an enzyme called **renin.** Renin enters the plasma and converts renin substrate (angiotensinogen) to **angiotensin I,** which is, in turn, converted to **angiotensin II** by angiotensin-converting enzyme (ACE) in the lungs. Angiotensin II is a powerful vasoconstrictor, and individuals with hypertension may be prescribed an ACE inhibitor to lower blood pressure. Angiotensin II stimulates aldosterone release, which increases Na$^+$ reabsorption. The stimuli for aldosterone and ADH secretion are also the signals that stimulate thirst, a necessary ingredient to restore body fluid volume. During light exercise, little or no change occurs in plasma renin activity or aldosterone (87). However, when a heat load is imposed during light exercise, both renin and aldosterone secretion are increased (39). When exercise intensity approaches 50% $\dot{V}O_2$ max (Fig. 5.8), renin, angiotensin, and aldosterone increase in parallel, showing the linkage within this homeostatic system (87, 139). Further, liver production of renin substrate increases to maintain the plasma concentration (93). In contrast, a sustained elevation of blood volume triggers the release of atrial natriuretic hormone (ANH) from heart muscle cells (not from an endocrine gland). ANH opposes the action of aldosterone to decrease blood volume (151).

Cortisol The primary glucocorticoid secreted by the adrenal cortex is cortisol. By a variety of mechanisms, cortisol contributes to the maintenance of plasma glucose during long-term fasting and exercise. These mechanisms

- Promote the breakdown of tissue protein (by inhibiting protein synthesis) to form amino acids, which are then used by the liver to form new glucose (gluconeogenesis)

- Stimulate the mobilization of free fatty acids from adipose tissue
- Stimulate liver enzymes involved in the metabolic pathway leading to glucose synthesis
- Block the entry of glucose into tissues, forcing those tissues to use more fatty acids as fuel (38, 151)

A summary of cortisol's actions and its regulation is presented in Figure 5.9. Cortisol secretion is controlled in the same manner as thyroxine. The hypothalamus secretes corticotrophic-releasing hormone (CRH), which causes the anterior pituitary gland to secrete more ACTH into the general circulation. ACTH binds to receptors on the adrenal cortex and increases cortisol secretion. As the cortisol level increases, CRH and ACTH are inhibited in another negative feedback system. However, the hypothalamus, like any brain center, receives neural input from other areas of the brain. This input can influence the secretion of hypothalamic-releasing hormones beyond the level seen in a negative feedback system. More than 70 years ago, Hans Selye observed that a wide variety of stressful events, such as burns,

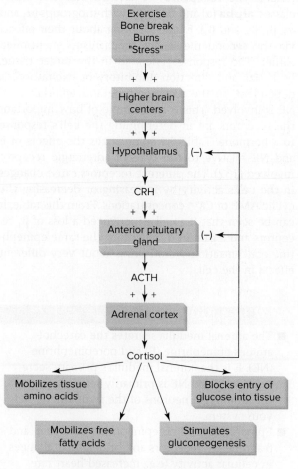

Figure 5.9 Control of cortisol secretion, showing the balance of positive and negative input to the hypothalamus, and cortisol's influence on metabolism.

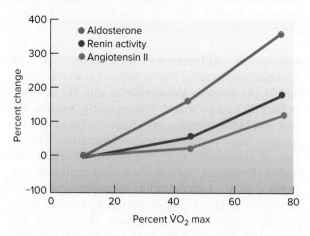

Figure 5.8 Parallel increases in renin activity, angiotensin II, and aldosterone with increasing intensities of exercise. Data are expressed as the percent change from resting values.

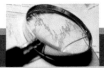

Adipose Tissue Is an Endocrine Organ

Many of you know that a connection exists between the obesity epidemic in this country and the dramatic increase in the number of people with type 2 diabetes and other chronic diseases (e.g., coronary artery disease, cancer). However, until recently, the direct link or cause between obesity and these diseases has remained a mystery. Fortunately, new evidence provides clues as to why too much adipose tissue has a negative impact on health.

Adipose tissue has been viewed, simply, as the principal storage site for fat, primarily triglycerides. When caloric intake exceeds expenditure, fat stores increase. Conversely, when caloric intake cannot meet energy demands, adipose tissue releases free fatty acids into the circulation to provide energy for the cells. Over the past 15 years, this picture of adipose tissue as a passive energy supply depot changed markedly as it became clear that adipose tissue secretes a variety of hormones and other factors that have a direct effect on metabolism and energy balance; they act through endocrine, paracrine, or autocrine mechanisms.

In the mid-1990s, the hormone **leptin** was discovered. This hormone, secreted by adipose cells (adipocytes), influences appetite through a direct effect on the "feeding centers" in the hypothalamus. In addition, leptin acts on peripheral tissues to enhance insulin sensitivity (allowing insulin to act) and promotes the oxidation of free fatty acids in muscle. **Adiponectin** is another hormone secreted by adipocytes. This hormone also increases insulin sensitivity and fatty acid oxidation in muscle (37, 47, 146), and reduces the risk

of cardiovascular disease by protecting both vascular endothelial cells and cardiac muscle cells (97).

As fat mass increases, leptin secretion also increases, but strangely, food intake is not restrained. Another molecule that blocks leptin's signal from reaching the hypothalamus is also produced, leading to what is known as leptin resistance. In contrast, adiponectin secretion decreases with an increase in fat mass, leading to a reduced sensitivity of tissues to insulin (insulin resistance) and the development of type 2 diabetes (a condition in which there is plenty of insulin, but the tissues are unresponsive to it). In addition, the risk of cardiovascular disease is increased (97).

In addition, as fat mass increases, adipocytes produce a variety of proinflammatory cytokines (e.g., tumor necrosis factor alpha [TNF-α] and interleukin-6 [IL-6]), and obesity is now recognized as contributing to a state of low-grade systemic inflammation (101, 122). See Chap. 6 for more on inflammation and see Chap. 14 for the connection between inflammation and chronic disease. Adiponectin has the ability to suppress this systemic inflammation, but because its secretion is reduced in obesity, it cannot carry out that role. These proinflammatory cytokines (also called adipokines in adipose tissue) can lead to both insulin resistance and atherosclerosis (37, 47, 146). What causes these changes in the adipocyte? One potential trigger is hypoxia (a relative lack of oxygen). As the mass of adipose tissue increases in obesity, some adipocytes will be farther away from existing capillaries, and O_2 will not be as available. It has been shown that when

normal adipocytes are made hypoxic, anaerobic metabolism is increased, lactate and hydrogen ion levels increase, and the cells respond with a decrease in adiponectin secretion and an increase in leptin and IL-6 secretion (141).

Given the importance of adiponectin in insulin sensitivity, one might expect that exercise, which is known to improve insulin sensitivity (see Chap. 17), would increase its concentration. Interestingly, neither an acute bout of exercise nor exercise training has any effect on the adiponectin concentration in blood. In contrast, the adiponectin level increases when there is a decrease in fat mass, whether it is brought about by exercise, diet, or a combined intervention. This suggests that the positive effects of exercise and weight loss on insulin sensitivity are independent and occur by different pathways. The same appears to be true for leptin; it is more responsive to changes in body weight than any exercise intervention (6, 9, 81, 136).

Recently, it has been shown that adipose tissue releases other factors (e.g., resistin, visfatin) that also influence health and disease (19). Clearly, adipose tissue is not a simple passive depot for energy storage but is directly involved in appetite, energy expenditure, and the development of inflammation-related diseases, including cardiovascular disease and type 2 diabetes. It is clear that being physically active and maintaining a normal body weight are reasonable goals to minimize the risks of developing chronic diseases. See A Closer Look 5.4 for more on how muscle counters adipose tissue's tendency to promote inflammation.

---

bone breaks, and heavy exercise, led to predictable increases in ACTH and cortisol; he called this response the General Adaptation Syndrome (GAS). A key point in this response was the release of ACTH and cortisol to aid in the adaptation. His GAS had three stages: (1) the alarm reaction, involving cortisol secretion, (2) the stage of resistance, where repairs are made, and (3) the stage of exhaustion, in which repairs are not adequate, and sickness or death results (130). The usefulness of the GAS is seen in times of

"stress" caused by tissue damage. Cortisol stimulates the breakdown of tissue protein to form amino acids, which can then be used at the site of the tissue damage for repair. While it is clear that muscle tissue is a primary source of amino acids, the functional overload of muscle with resistance or endurance training can prevent the muscle atrophy the glucocorticoids can cause (3, 56, 57). Throughout this section, we summarize the role of hormones secreted from various endocrine glands. A Closer Look 5.2

provides a new addition to this list that will have profound implications in our understanding of obesity and its disease-related consequences.

IN SUMMARY

- The adrenal cortex secretes aldosterone (mineralocorticoid), cortisol (glucocorticoid), and estrogens and androgens (sex steroids).
- Aldosterone regulates Na^+ and K^+ balance. Aldosterone secretion increases with strenuous exercise, driven by the renin-angiotensin system.
- Cortisol responds to a variety of stressors, including exercise, to ensure that fuel (glucose and free fatty acids) is available and to make amino acids available for tissue repair.

Pancreas

The pancreas is both an exocrine and an endocrine gland. The exocrine secretions include digestive enzymes and bicarbonate, which are secreted into ducts leading to the small intestine. The hormones, released from groups of cells in the endocrine portion of the pancreas called the islets of Langerhans, include insulin, **glucagon,** and **somatostatin.**

Insulin   Insulin is secreted from beta (β) cells of the islets of Langerhans. Insulin is the most important hormone during the absorptive state, when nutrients are entering the blood from the small intestine. Insulin stimulates tissues to take up nutrient molecules such as glucose and amino acids and store them as glycogen, proteins, and fats. Insulin's best-known role is in the facilitated diffusion of glucose across cell membranes. A lack of insulin causes an accumulation of glucose in the plasma because the tissues cannot take it up. The plasma glucose concentration can become so high that reabsorption mechanisms in the kidney are overwhelmed and glucose is lost to the urine, taking large volumes of water with it. This condition is called **diabetes mellitus.**

As mentioned earlier in this chapter, insulin secretion is influenced by a variety of factors: plasma glucose concentration, plasma amino acid concentration, sympathetic and parasympathetic nerve stimulation, and various hormones. The rate of secretion of insulin is dependent on the level of excitatory and inhibitory input to the beta cells of the pancreas (see Fig. 5.1). The blood glucose concentration is a major source of input that is part of a simple negative feedback loop; as the plasma glucose concentration increases (following a meal), the beta cells directly monitor this increase and secrete additional insulin to enhance tissue uptake of glucose. This increased uptake lowers the plasma glucose concentration, and insulin secretion is reduced (38, 96).

Glucagon   Glucagon, secreted from the alpha (α) cells in the islets of Langerhans, exerts effects opposite those of insulin. Glucagon secretion increases in response to a low plasma glucose concentration, which is monitored by the alpha cells. Glucagon stimulates both the mobilization of glucose from liver stores (glycogenolysis) and free fatty acids from adipose tissue (to spare blood glucose as a fuel), using the adenylate cyclase second messenger mechanism mentioned earlier. Last, along with cortisol, glucagon stimulates gluconeogenesis in the liver. Glucagon secretion is also influenced by factors other than the glucose concentration, notably the sympathetic nervous system (138). A complete description of the role of insulin and glucagon in the maintenance of blood glucose during exercise is presented later in this chapter in "Fast-Acting Hormones."

IN SUMMARY

- Insulin is secreted by the β cells of the islets of Langerhans in the pancreas and promotes the storage of glucose, amino acids, and fats.
- Glucagon is secreted by the α cells of the islets of Langerhans in the pancreas and promotes the mobilization of glucose and fatty acids.

Somatostatin   Pancreatic somatostatin is secreted by the delta cells of the islets of Langerhans. Pancreatic somatostatin secretion is increased during the absorptive state, and it modifies the activity of the GI tract to control the rate of entry of nutrient molecules into the circulation. It may also be involved in the regulation of insulin secretion (138).

Testes and Ovaries

Testosterone and **estrogen** are the primary sex steroids secreted by the testes and ovaries, respectively. These hormones are not only important in establishing and maintaining reproductive function but they also determine the secondary sex characteristics associated with masculinity and femininity.

Testosterone   Testosterone is secreted by the interstitial cells of the testes and is controlled by interstitial cell stimulating hormone (ICSH–also known as LH), which is produced in the anterior pituitary. LH is, in turn, controlled by a releasing hormone secreted by the hypothalamus. Sperm production from the seminiferous tubules of the testes requires follicle-stimulating hormone (FSH) from the anterior pituitary and testosterone. Figure 5.10 shows testosterone secretion to be controlled by a negative feedback loop involving the anterior pituitary gland and the hypothalamus. Sperm production is controlled, in

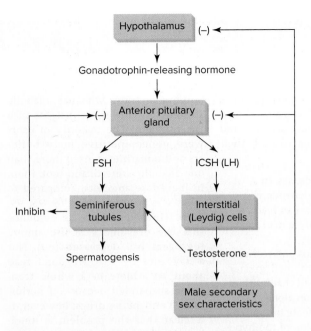

Figure 5.10 Control of testosterone secretion and sperm production by hypothalamus and anterior pituitary.

part, by another negative feedback loop involving the hormone inhibin (96, 151).

Testosterone is both an anabolic (tissue building) and androgenic (promoter of masculine characteristics) steroid because it stimulates protein synthesis and is responsible for the characteristic changes in boys at adolescence that lead to the high muscle-mass to fat-mass ratio. The plasma testosterone concentration is increased 10% to 37% during prolonged submaximal work (144), during exercise taken to maximum levels (26), and during endurance or strength training workouts (73). Some feel that these small changes are due to a reduction in plasma volume or to a decrease in the rate of inactivation and removal of testosterone (139). However, others have concluded on the basis of a parallel increase in the LH concentration that the increase in plasma testosterone is due to an increased rate of production (26). The exercise-induced increase in testosterone has been viewed as a primary stimulus of muscle protein synthesis and hypertrophy, but new information suggests that testosterone alone accounts for ~10% of the variation in hypertrophy observed as a result of resistance training (128). That said, there is considerable individual variation in hypertrophy as a result of resistance training, and part of that variation is believed to be due to differences in the testosterone response to exercise. With such a developing story, we are sure to hear more on this (128). Most readers probably recognize testosterone or one of its synthetic analogs as one of the most abused drugs in the drive to increase muscle mass and performance. Such use is not without its problems (see A Closer Look 5.3).

Estrogen and Progesterone Estrogen is a group of hormones that exerts similar physiological effects. These hormones include estradiol, estrone, and estriol, with estradiol being the primary estrogen. Estrogen stimulates breast development, female fat deposition, and other secondary sex characteristics (see Fig. 5.11). During the early part of the menstrual cycle called the follicular phase, LH stimulates the production of **androgens** in the follicle, which are subsequently converted to estrogens under the influence of FSH. Following ovulation, the luteal phase of the menstrual cycle begins, and both estrogens and progesterone are produced by the corpus luteum, a secretory structure occupying the space where the ovum was located (151). How does exercise affect these hormones, and vice versa? In one study (74), the plasma levels of LH, FSH, estradiol, and progesterone were measured at rest and at three different work rates during both the follicular and luteal phases of the menstrual cycle. The patterns of response of these hormones during graded exercise were very similar in the two phases of the menstrual cycle (74). Figure 5.12 shows only small changes in progesterone and estradiol with increasing intensities of work. Given that LH and FSH changed little or not at all during the luteal phase, the small increases in progesterone and estradiol were believed to be due to changes in plasma volume and to a decreased rate of removal rather than an increased rate of secretion (13, 139).

The effect of the phase of the menstrual cycle on exercise metabolism is not clear cut. This is due, in part, to variations in the research design, methods of measurement, and intensity of exercise used in the

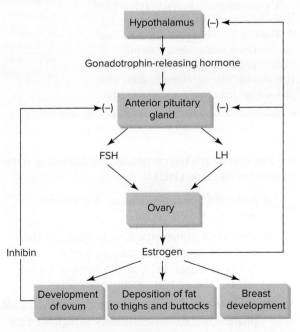

Figure 5.11 Control of estrogen production in the early and middle follicular phases.

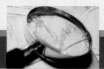

A CLOSER LOOK 5.3

Anabolic Steroids and Performance

Testosterone, as both an anabolic and an **androgenic steroid,** causes size changes as well as male secondary sexual characteristics, respectively. Due to these combined effects, scientists developed steroids to maximize the anabolic effects and minimize the androgenic effects. However, these effects can never be completely separated. These synthetic steroids were originally developed to promote tissue growth in patients who had experienced atrophy as a result of prolonged bed rest. Before long, the thought occurred that these **anabolic steroids** might be helpful in developing muscle mass and strength in athletes.

The use of anabolic steroids to enhance athletic performance has an interesting history. Results from early studies were inconsistent due to variations in the dose and type of steroid used, the training status of the subjects, length of the study, etc. (4, 99, 154, 155, 158). However, before long there was clear evidence that these steroids worked. This led to mandatory testing of athletes in international competitions and in both college and professional sports. The problem escalated when athletes started to take pure testosterone rather than the anabolic steroid. Part of the reason for the switch was to reduce the chance of detection when drug testing was conducted, and part was related to the availability of testosterone. The following information, taken from two major position stands, provides a good summary of what we know about the use of these steroids and what should be done to curb their abuse (60, 99):

- Androgen use causes, in a concentration-dependent manner, increases in lean body mass, muscle mass, and strength in men.
- When androgens and resistance training are combined, greater gains are realized than with either intervention alone.
- The adverse effects in men include suppression of the hypothalamic–pituitary–gonadal axis, mood and behavior disorders, increased risk of cardiovascular disease, liver dysfunction (with oral androgens), insulin resistance, glucose intolerance, acne, and gynecomastia (breast development). A recent study's findings of cognitive deficits in long-term anabolic steroid users supports these concerns (75).
- The adverse effects in women are similar to that of men, but in addition, the androgens may have virilizing effects, such as enlargement of the clitoris, deepening of the voice, hirsutism, and change in body build. These changes may not be reversible when androgen use is stopped.

Surveys of those who use anabolic steroids provide some insights into the problem: The majority of users were noncompetitive body builders and nonathletes, used more than one anabolic steroid, and took them in megadose amounts, compared to what was recommended (5, 95, 99, 108). However, there is evidence that the prevalence of use among teenagers has decreased (60). Not a day goes by that we don't read about an athlete or a whole team being suspended because of performance-enhancing drugs; however, it is clear that the problem is much broader than realized by the general public. The same position stands mentioned earlier emphasize the need for continued efforts to educate the athletes, coaches, parents, physicians, athletic trainers, and the general public about androgen use and abuse (60, 99). For more information on a list of prohibited substances, go to the World Anti-Doping Agency's website (**www.wada-ama.org).** One last comment: as the number of older adults ($\geq$65 years) increases, considerable attention is being directed at the use of testosterone as a way to slow down or stop the loss of muscle mass and strength that occurs with age. This is not new, and as discussed in A Closer Look 5.1, testosterone is not the only hormone being used to achieve that goal (44).

studies. Based on a recent review, the following statements can be made (102):

- Anaerobic performances are not affected by menstrual cycle phase.
- The effect of menstrual cycle phase on time-trial endurance performances is mixed, and it has been suggested that the focus of future research be on ultra-endurance events.
- Glucose mobilization is lower during the luteal phase when exercise intensity is high enough to create an energy demand for carbohydrate. However, when exercise takes place soon after a meal or when glucose is provided during the exercise, the impact of menstrual cycle phase is reduced or eliminated.
- Although animal studies show that estrogen increases lipolysis and plasma FFA, human studies do not support these findings.
- There is an increase in protein catabolism at rest and during exercise in the luteal phase. This appears to be due to the effect of progesterone, since estrogen has the opposite effect.

Consistent with this, there is strong evidence that the response of the glucose-regulatory hormones

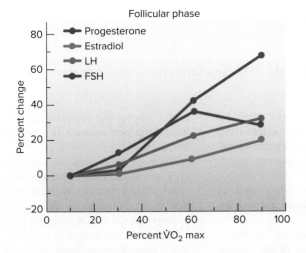

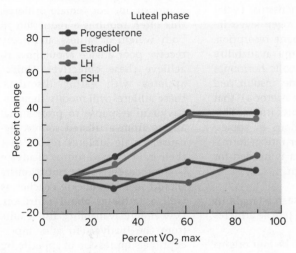

Figure 5.12 Percent change (from resting values) in the plasma FSH, LH, progesterone, and estradiol concentrations during graded exercise in the follicular and luteal phases of the menstrual cycle.

to prolonged exercise is unaffected by menstrual cycle phase (82). In addition, there is a general agreement that there are no menstrual cycle phase effects on $\dot{V}O_2$ max and the lactate, plasma volume, heart rate, and ventilation responses to exercise (156). Finally, there does not appear to be an increased risk of heat illness during the luteal phase of the menstrual cycle, even though body temperature is higher (89).

There is an ongoing debate about whether estrogen influences indices of muscle damage, inflammation, and tissue repair. Animal studies provide consistent evidence that estrogen offers protective benefits; however, studies on humans fail to confirm these results (33). For those interested in having a ringside seat in this debate, read the Point: Counterpoint on this topic in which Tiidus and Enns debate Huber and Clarkson (140).

Because female athletes have a four- to six-fold greater risk of anterior cruciate injury compared to male athletes, there is interest as to whether the phase of the menstrual cycle might influence the risk.

A review by Zazulak et al. (160) suggests that greater knee laxity occurs at 10 to 14 days into the cycle, compared to days 15 to 28, and the latter was greater than that measured during days 1 to 9. However, biomechanical analysis of the forces and the magnitude of knee flexion experienced when doing jumping tasks showed no differences between phases of the menstrual cycle or between genders (17).

Although the changes in estrogen and progesterone during an acute exercise bout are small, concern is being raised about the effect of chronic heavy exercise on the menstrual cycle of athletes. The two principal menstrual disorders are primary amenorrhea (absence of menstrual cycles in a girl who has not menstruated by 15 years of age) and secondary amenorrhea (onset of amenorrhea sometime after menarche). The incidence of menstrual disorders in athletes varies greatly but is higher in aesthetic, endurance, and weight-class sports and, at younger ages, higher training volumes, and lower body weights. Typically, the prevalence of amenorrhea in college-age women is about 2% to 5%. In contrast, in collegiate runners, the incidence ranged from about 3% to 60% as training volume increased from <10 miles (16 km) to >68 miles (113 km) per week, and body weight decreased from >60 kg to <50 kg. In addition, the incidence is much higher in younger (69%) than older (9%) runners (113). There is evidence that amenorrheic athletes demonstrate blunted hormonal responses to both aerobic (126) and resistance (98) exercise. Special attention is now being directed at the issue of secondary amenorrhea because the chronically low estradiol levels can have a deleterious effect on bone mineral content. Osteoporosis, usually associated with the elderly (see Chap. 17), is common in athletes with amenorrhea (58). Interested readers are referred to Redman and Loucks's review of the possible causes of exercise-induced menstrual cycle irregularities (113). What is most interesting is that exercise itself may not suppress reproductive function, but rather the impact of the energy cost of the exercise on energy availability. For some first-hand insights into this issue, see Ask the Expert 5.1.

IN SUMMARY

- Testosterone and estrogen establish and maintain reproductive function and determine secondary sex characteristics.
- Chronic exercise (training) can decrease testosterone levels in males and estrogen levels in females. The latter adaptation has potentially negative consequences related to osteoporosis.

The endocrine system is set up to automatically respond when homeostasis is threatened; this is especially true for plasma glucose, the principal fuel for

Reproductive Disorders and Low Bone Mass in Female Athletes Questions and Answers with Dr. Anne B. Loucks

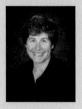

Courtesy of
Anne B. Loucks

Dr. Loucks is Professor of Biological Sciences at Ohio University. She is a productive researcher in the area of reproductive and skeletal disorders in female athletes, the author of numerous research articles and reviews on this topic, and is recognized internationally as an expert in the field. Dr. Loucks was involved in the development and revision of the American College of Sports Medicine's position stand on the Female Athlete Triad. Her many accomplishments in research and scholarship were recognized by the American College of Sports Medicine in 2008 when she received that organization's prestigious Citation Award.

QUESTION: Are reproductive disorders in female athletes caused by low body fatness?

ANSWER: No. Few studies have found any difference in body composition between amenorrheic and eumenorrheic athletes. Physiological systems, including the reproductive system, depend on energy availability, which is the amount of dietary energy remaining after exercise for all other physiological functions. Resting energy expenditure is about 30 kcal/kgFFM/day. When energy availability is less than 30 kcal/kgFFM/day, the brain activates mechanisms that reduce energy expenditure. In the reproductive system, the pulsatile secretion of gonadotropin-releasing hormone by the hypothamus slows down and this suppresses ovarian function. Reproductive disorders have been induced, prevented, and reversed experimentally by changing energy availability without any change in body composition. Because menstrual disorders are

also symptoms of many diseases, however, a medical examination and endocrine measurements are needed to properly diagnose them.

QUESTION: Is the low bone mass in some female athletes caused by amenorrhea?

ANSWER: In part, but not entirely. Bone mass declines in proportion to the number of menstrual cycles missed, and low estrogen levels increase the rate of bone resorption. However, low energy availability also suppresses anabolic hormones (e.g. thyroid hormone, insulin, and insulin-like growth factor-1) that stimulate bone formation. This is especially hazardous in adolescence, when a faster rate of formation than resorption is needed for skeletal development.

QUESTION: What has research taught us about why so many female athletes do not eat enough?

ANSWER: There seem to be four origins of low energy availability. Two originate outside of sport. Some athletes undereat obsessively as part of an eating disorder. Because eating disorders have one of the highest rates of premature death of all mental illnesses, sports programs should institute procedures for identifying cases of eating disorders, referring them for psychiatric care, and excluding them from participation until they receive medical clearance. Other athletes undereat in intentional efforts to improve appearance for social reasons. Worldwide, at all deciles of BMI, about twice as many young women as young men perceive themselves to be overweight, and the multiple of young women more than young men who are actively trying to lose weight increases to 5 to 9 times as BMI declines! Indeed, more athletes

report improving appearance than improving performance as a reason for dieting.

Two other origins of low energy availability are found inside sport. Many female athletes undereat in intentional efforts to improve performance, because performance is optimized by acquiring a sport-specific body size and composition. For female athletes, this often requires a reduction in body weight or fatness, and many receive poor advice about how to achieve these objectives. Unlike athletes with eating disorders, these athletes will modify their behavior in response to professional advice from a trusted source. Because female athletes report that their most trusted source of advice is their coach, sports nutritionists should seek to educate coaches as well as athletes about nutrition. Low energy availability also results from the inadvertent and imperceptible suppression of appetite by prolonged exercise and the high carbohydrate diet recommended to endurance athletes. Together, these two factors can suppress *ad libitum* energy intake enough to reduce energy availability below 30 kcal/kgFFM/day. So, athletes in endurance sports need to eat by discipline (i.e., specific amounts of particular foods at planned times) instead of appetite.

QUESTION: What are the most important issues remaining to be solved?

ANSWER: We think we know how much athletes need to eat to compensate for the energy they expend in exercise, but we need applied research to develop practical techniques for monitoring and managing energy availability to achieve sports objectives without compromising health.

Hormone	Gland	Exercise Response	Action	Effect on Fuel Utilization
Epinephrine Norepinephrine	Adrenal medulla	↑	↑ Muscle and liver glycogenolysis ↑ FFA mobilization	Mobilizes both fat and carbohydrate fuels
Cortisol	Adrenal cortex	↑	↑ FFA mobilization ↑ Gluconeogenesis ↓ Glucose uptake	Mobilizes fat fuels Preserves blood glucose
Growth hormone	Anterior pituitary	↑	↑ FFA mobilization ↑ Gluconeogenesis ↓ Glucose uptake	Mobilizes fat fuels Preserves blood glucose
Glucagon	Pancreas (α-cells)	↑	↑ FFA mobilization ↑ Glycogenolysis ↓ Glucose uptake	Mobilizes fat fuels Preserves blood glucose
Insulin	Pancreas (β-cells)	↓	↑ Glucose, amino acid, and FFA uptake into tissues	Stores fuels Lowers blood glucose

the brain. The four mechanisms, presented earlier in the chapter, by which the plasma glucose concentration is protected, include the following:

- Mobilize existing glucose from liver glycogen stores
- Mobilize FFA from adipose tissue to increase the use of fat as a fuel, and thus spare plasma glucose
- Synthesize new glucose from amino acids, glycerol, and lactate (gluconeogenesis)
- Block glucose entry into cells (an "anti-insulin" effect), forcing the cells to use fat as a fuel, and thus spare plasma glucose

Table 5.2 contains a summary of the most important hormones responsible for protecting the plasma glucose concentration when glucose is being used rapidly (i.e., exercise) or when the dietary intake of carbohydrate is inadequate (i.e., starvation). Each of these will be discussed in detail in the next section of the chapter. However, before we leave this section, we need to introduce you to a new member of the endocrine family–muscle itself (see A Closer Look 5.4).

HORMONAL CONTROL OF SUBSTRATE MOBILIZATION DURING EXERCISE

The type of substrate and the rate at which it is utilized during exercise depend to a large extent on the intensity and duration of the exercise. During strenuous exercise, there is an obligatory demand for carbohydrate oxidation that must be met; fatty acid oxidation cannot substitute. In contrast, there is an increase in fat oxidation during prolonged, moderate exercise as carbohydrate fuels are depleted (61). Although diet and the training state of the person are important (see Chaps. 13, 21, and 23), the factors of intensity and duration of exercise ordinarily have prominence. Because of this, our discussion of the hormonal control of substrate mobilization during exercise will be divided into two parts. The first will deal with the control of muscle glycogen utilization, and the second with the control of glucose mobilization from the liver and FFA from adipose tissue.

Muscle-Glycogen Utilization

At the onset of the most types of exercise, and for the entire duration of very strenuous exercise, muscle glycogen is the primary carbohydrate fuel for muscular work (124). The intensity of exercise, which is inversely related to exercise duration, determines the rate at which muscle glycogen is used as fuel. Figure 5.13 shows a series of lines describing the rates of glycogen breakdown for various exercise intensities expressed as a percent of $\dot{V}O_2$ max (124). The heavier the exercise, the faster glycogen is broken down. This process of glycogen breakdown (glycogenolysis) is initiated by second messengers, which activate protein kinases in the muscle cell (described in Fig. 5.3). Plasma epinephrine, a powerful stimulator of cyclic AMP formation when bound to β-adrenergic receptors on a cell, was believed

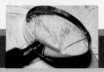
Muscle as an Endocrine Gland

Three of the major causes of death are cardiovascular disease, diabetes, and cancer. These diseases are linked to the presence of a low-grade chronic inflammation as shown by elevated blood levels of proinflammatory cytokines such as tumor necrosis factor alpha (TNF-α). What is important to know is that doing moderate-to-vigorous physical activity on a regular basis (e.g., 3 to 5 d/wk) is associated with positive health outcomes, including a reduction in the risk of type 2 diabetes, heart disease, and certain cancers. What is the connection between exercise and the reduced risk of these diseases? Until recently, little was known about the connection, but now it appears that it is muscle itself that brings about these favorable changes (11, 31, 90, 106, 111). Over the past ten years, it has become clear that muscle is an endocrine organ–that is, it produces small signaling molecules called myokines (muscle cytokines) when it contracts. The number and types of these myokines continue to grow (111), indicating that muscle contraction

plays a much larger role than simply getting us down the road. Some of these myokines act locally as autocrine agents to stimulate glucose uptake and increase fatty acid oxidation, and as paracrine agents to promote blood vessel growth in muscle. However, other myokines are released into the blood so that they can act as hormones and affect a variety of tissues and organs. For example, some myokines can increase liver production of glucose and stimulate triglyceride breakdown in adipose tissue to provide free fatty acids for fuel (11, 90, 106).

Interleukin 6 (IL-6) is the principal myokine produced by muscle during exercise. IL-6 can act as both a proinflammatory cytokine and an antiinflammatory cytokine–that is, it can both promote inflammation and reduce it. IL-6 is the first myokine to appear in the muscle and blood during exercise, and plasma IL-6 levels can be elevated 100-fold compared to resting conditions, though smaller changes are more typical (107). It is important that other proinflammatory cytokines

associated with chronic inflammation (e.g., TNF-α) are suppressed with exercise, suggesting that the IL-6 released during exercise promotes an antiinflammatory environment (31). Consistent with that, IL-6 has been shown to inhibit the production of TNF-α and stimulate the production of other anti-inflammatory cytokines (106).

In effect, the relatively large and short-lived hormonal (e.g., epinephrine, cortisol) and myokine (e.g., IL-6) responses to exercise are adaptive, that is, they help maintain homeostasis. In contrast, the sustained chronic elevation of IL-6, as seen in obesity, leads to chronic disease (31, 111). There is a growing body of evidence that skeletal muscle, via its myokines, engages in "cross talk" with the pancreas, liver, and adipose tissue to facilitate our adaptation to exercise and enhance our overall health (31, 148). Consequently, maintaining a healthy amount of body fat and a regular exercise program goes a long way in preventing chronic diseases (see Chap. 14 for more on this).

---

to be primarily responsible for glycogenolysis. Figure 5.14 also shows a family of lines, the slopes of which describe how fast plasma E changes with increasing intensities of exercise (78). Clearly, the data presented in Figures 5.13 and 5.14 are consistent

with the view that a linkage exists between changes in plasma E during exercise and the increased rate of glycogen degradation. However, there is more to this story.

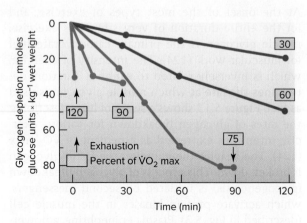

Figure 5.13 Glycogen depletion in the quadriceps muscle during bicycle exercise of increasing intensities.

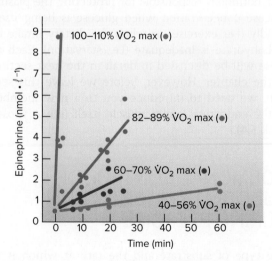

Figure 5.14 Changes in the plasma epinephrine concentration during exercises of different intensities and durations.

To test the hypothesis that glycogenolysis in muscle is controlled by circulating E during exercise, investigators had subjects take propranolol, a drug that blocks both β_1- and β_2-adrenergic receptors on the cell membrane. This procedure should block glycogenolysis because cyclic AMP formation would be affected. In the control experiment, subjects worked for two minutes at an intensity of exercise that caused the muscle glycogen to be depleted to half its initial value and the muscle lactate concentration to be elevated 10-fold. Surprisingly, as shown in Figure 5.15, when the subjects took the propranolol and repeated the test on another day, there was no difference in glycogen depletion or lactate formation (52). Other experiments have also shown that β-adrenergic blocking drugs have little effect on slowing the rate of glycogen breakdown during exercise (142). How can this be?

As mentioned in Chap. 3, enzymatic reactions in a cell are under the control of both intracellular and extracellular factors. In the aforementioned example with propranolol, plasma E may not have been able to activate adenylate cyclase to form the cyclic AMP needed to activate the protein kinases to initiate glycogen breakdown. However, when a muscle cell is stimulated to contract, Ca^{++}, which is stored in the sarcoplasmic reticulum, floods the cell. Some Ca^{++} ions are used to initiate contractile events (see Chap. 8), but other Ca^{++} ions bind to **calmodulin,** which, in turn, activates the protein kinases needed for glycogenolysis (see Fig. 5.4). In this case, the increased intracellular Ca^{++} (rather than cAMP) is the initial event stimulating muscle glycogen breakdown.

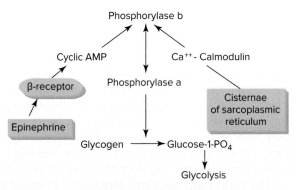

Figure 5.16 The breakdown of muscle glycogen, glycogenolysis, can be initiated by either the Ca^{++}-calmodulin mechanism or the cyclic AMP mechanism. When a drug blocks the β-receptor, glycogenolysis can still occur.

Figure 5.16 summarizes these events. Experiments in which the increased secretion of catecholamines was blocked during exercise confirmed the propranolol experiments, showing that an intact sympathoadrenal system was not necessary to initiate glycogenolysis in skeletal muscle (16).

Observations of glycogen-depletion patterns support this view. Individuals who do heavy exercise with one leg will cause elevations in plasma E, which circulates to all muscle cells. The muscle glycogen, however, is depleted only from the exercised leg (66), suggesting that intracellular factors (e.g., Ca^{++}) are more responsible for these events. Further, in experiments in which individuals engaged in intermittent, intense exercise interspersed with a rest period (interval work), the glycogen was depleted faster from fast-twitch fibers (32, 34, 45). The plasma E concentration should be the same outside both fast- and slow-twitch muscle fibers, but the glycogen was depleted at a faster rate from the fibers used in the activity. This is reasonable because a "resting" muscle fiber should not be using glycogen (or any other fuel) at a high rate. The rate of glycogenolysis would be expected to parallel the rate at which ATP is used by the muscle, and this has been shown to be the case, independent of E (113). This discussion does not mean that E cannot or does not cause glycogenolysis (18, 157). There is ample evidence to show that a surge of E will, in fact, cause this to occur (72, 132–134).

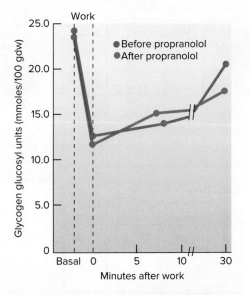

Figure 5.15 Changes in muscle glycogen due to two minutes of work at 1200 kpm/min, before and after propranolol administration. Blocking the beta-adrenergic receptors had no effect on glycogen breakdown.

IN SUMMARY

- Glycogen breakdown to glucose in muscle is under the dual control of epinephrine-cyclic AMP and Ca^{++}-calmodulin. The latter's role is enhanced during exercise due to the increase in Ca^{++} from the sarcoplasmic reticulum. In this way the delivery of fuel (glucose) parallels the activation of contraction.

Blood Glucose Homeostasis During Exercise

As mentioned in the introduction, a focal point of hormonal control systems is the maintenance of the plasma glucose concentration during times of inadequate carbohydrate intake (fasting/starvation) and accelerated glucose removal from the circulation (exercise). In both cases, body energy stores are used to meet the challenge, and the hormonal response to these two different situations, exercise and starvation, is quite similar.

The plasma glucose concentration is maintained through four processes that

- Mobilize existing glucose from liver glycogen stores to maintain the plasma glucose level
- Mobilize plasma FFA from adipose tissue to increase the use of fat as a fuel and spare plasma glucose
- Synthesize new glucose in the liver (gluconeogenesis) from amino acids, lactate, and glycerol to have it available as needed
- Block glucose entry into cells (an "anti-insulin effect") to force the cell to use fat as a fuel, and thus spare plasma glucose

The overall aim of these four processes is to provide fuel for work while maintaining the plasma glucose concentration. This is a major task when you consider that the liver may have only 80 grams of glucose before exercise begins, and the rate of blood glucose oxidation approaches 1 g/min in heavy exercise or in prolonged (≥3 hours) moderate exercise (21, 25).

Although the hormones will be presented separately, keep in mind that each of the four processes is controlled by more than one hormone, and all four processes are involved in the adaptation to exercise. Some hormones act in a "permissive" way, or are "slow acting," while others are "fast-acting" controllers of substrate mobilization. For this reason, this discussion of the hormonal control of plasma glucose will be divided into two sections—one dealing with permissive and slow-acting hormones and the other dealing with fast-acting hormones.

Permissive and Slow-Acting Hormones Thyroxine, cortisol, and growth hormone are involved in the regulation of carbohydrate, fat, and protein metabolism. These hormones are discussed in this section because they either facilitate the actions of other hormones or respond to stimuli in a slow manner. Remember that to act in a permissive manner, the hormone concentration doesn't have to change. However, as you will see, in certain stressful situations, permissive hormones can achieve such elevated plasma concentrations that they act directly to influence carbohydrate and fat metabolism rather than to simply facilitate the actions of other hormones.

Thyroid Hormones The discussion of substrate mobilization during exercise must include the thyroid hormones T_3 and T_4, whose free concentrations do not change dramatically from resting to the exercising state. As mentioned earlier, T_3 and T_4 are important in establishing the overall metabolic rate and in allowing other hormones to exert their full effect (permissive hormone). They accomplish this latter function by influencing either the number of receptors on the surface of a cell (for other hormones to interact with) or the affinity of the receptor for the hormone. For example, without T_3, epinephrine has little effect on the mobilization of free fatty acids from adipose tissue. During exercise, there is an increase in "free" T_3 due to changes in the binding characteristics of the transport protein (139). T_3 and T_4 are removed from the plasma by tissues during exercise at a greater rate than at rest. In turn, TSH secretion from the anterior pituitary is increased to stimulate the secretion of T_3 and T_4 from the thyroid gland to maintain the plasma level (43). Low levels of T_3 and T_4 (hypothyroid state) would interfere with the ability of other hormones to mobilize fuel for exercise (105, 139).

Cortisol The primary glucocorticoid in humans is cortisol. As Figure 5.17 shows, cortisol (38)

- Stimulates FFA mobilization from adipose tissue
- Mobilizes tissue protein to yield amino acids for glucose synthesis in the liver (gluconeogenesis)
- Decreases the rate of glucose utilization by cells

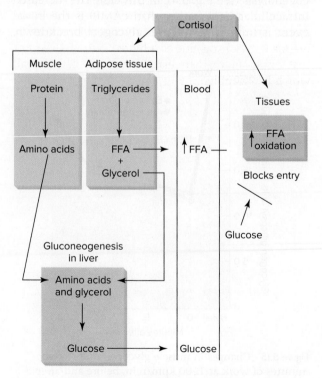

Figure 5.17 Role of cortisol in the maintenance of plasma glucose.

There are problems, however, when attempting to describe the cortisol response to exercise. Given the GAS of Selye, events other than exercise can influence the cortisol response. Imagine how a naive subject might view a treadmill test on first exposure. The wires, noise, nose clip, mouthpiece, and blood sampling could all influence the level of arousal of the subject and result in a cortisol response that is not related to a need to mobilize additional substrate.

As exercise intensity increases, one might expect the cortisol secretion to increase. This is true, but only within certain limits. For example, Bonen (8) showed that the urinary excretion of cortisol was not changed by exercise at 76% $\dot{V}O_2$ max for 10 minutes but was increased about two-fold when the duration was extended to 30 minutes. Davies and Few (27) extended our understanding of the cortisol response to exercise when they studied subjects who completed several one-hour exercise bouts. Each test was set at a constant intensity between 40% and 80% $\dot{V}O_2$ max. Exercise at 40% $\dot{V}O_2$ max resulted in a decrease in plasma cortisol over time, while the response was considerably elevated for exercise at 80% $\dot{V}O_2$ max. Figure 5.18 shows the plasma cortisol concentration measured at 60 minutes into each of the exercise tests plotted against % $\dot{V}O_2$ max. When the exercise intensity exceeded 60% $\dot{V}O_2$ max, the cortisol concentration increased; below that, the cortisol concentration decreased. What caused these changes? Using radioactive cortisol as a tracer, the researchers found that during light exercise, cortisol was removed faster than the adrenal cortex secreted it, and during intense exercise, the increase in plasma cortisol was due to a higher rate of secretion that could more than match the rate of removal, which had doubled.

What is interesting is that for low-intensity, long-duration exercise where the effects of cortisol would go a long way in maintaining the plasma glucose concentration, the concentration of cortisol does not change very much. Even if it did, the effects on metabolism would not be immediately noticeable. The direct effect of cortisol is mediated through the stimulation of DNA and the resulting mRNA formation, which leads to protein synthesis, a slow process. In essence, cortisol, like thyroxine, exerts a permissive effect on substrate mobilization during acute exercise, allowing other fast-acting hormones such as epinephrine and glucagon to deal with glucose and FFA mobilization. Support for this was provided in a study in which a drug was used to lower plasma cortisol before and during submaximal exercise; the overall metabolic response was not affected compared to a normal cortisol condition (29). Given that athletic competitions (triathlon, ultra marathon, most team sports) can result in tissue damage, the reason for changes in the plasma cortisol concentration might not be for the mobilization of fuel for exercising muscles. In these situations, cortisol's role in dealing with tissue repair might come to the forefront.

Growth Hormone Growth hormone plays a major role in the synthesis of tissue protein, acting either directly or through the enhanced secretion of IGFs from the liver. However, GH can also influence fat and carbohydrate metabolism. Figure 5.19 shows that growth hormone supports the action of cortisol; it

- Decreases glucose uptake by tissue
- Increases FFA mobilization
- Enhances gluconeogenesis in the liver

The net effect is to preserve the plasma glucose concentration.

Describing the plasma GH response to exercise is as difficult as describing cortisol's response to exercise because GH can also be altered by a variety of physical, chemical, and psychological stresses (24, 48, 137). Given that, the earlier comments about

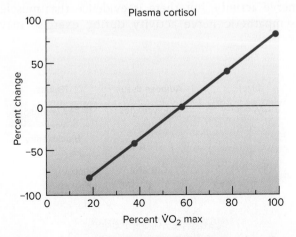

Figure 5.18 Percent change (from resting values) in the plasma cortisol concentration with increasing exercise intensity.

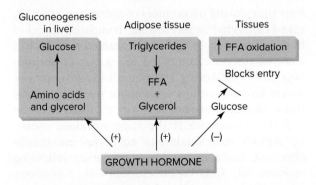

Figure 5.19 Role of plasma growth hormone in the maintenance of plasma glucose.

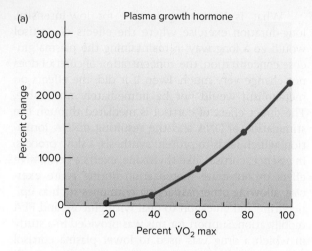

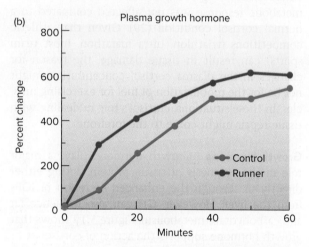

Figure 5.20 (*a*) Percent change (from resting values) in the plasma growth hormone concentration with increasing exercise intensity. (*b*) Percent change (from resting values) in the plasma growth hormone concentration during exercise at 60% V̇O₂ max for runners and nonrunners (controls).

cortisol should be kept in mind. Figure 5.20(*a*) shows plasma GH to increase with increasing intensities of exercise, achieving, at maximal work, values 25 times those at rest (137). Figure 5.20(*b*) shows the plasma GH concentration to increase over time during 60 minutes of exercise at 60% V̇O₂ max (13). What is interesting, compared to other hormonal responses, is that the trained runners had a higher response compared to a group of nonrunners (see "Fast-Acting Hormones"). By 60 minutes, values for both groups were about five to six times those measured at rest. It must be added that the higher GH response at the same workload shown by trained individuals has not been universally observed. Some report lower responses following training (91, 135). In conclusion, GH, a hormone primarily concerned with protein synthesis, can achieve plasma concentrations during exercise that

can exert a direct but "slow-acting" effect on carbohydrate and fat metabolism.

IN SUMMARY

- The hormones thyroxine, cortisol, and growth hormone act in a permissive manner to support the actions of other hormones during exercise.
- Growth hormone and cortisol also provide a "slow-acting" effect on carbohydrate and fat metabolism during exercise.

Fast-Acting Hormones In contrast to the aforementioned "permissive" and slow-acting hormones, there are very fast-responding hormones whose actions quickly return the plasma glucose to normal. Again, although each will be presented separately, they behave collectively and in a predictable way during exercise to maintain the plasma glucose concentration (20).

Epinephrine and Norepinephrine Epinephrine and norepinephrine have already been discussed relative to muscle glycogen mobilization. However, as Figure 5.21 shows, they are also involved in the following (22, 119):

- The mobilization of glucose from the liver
- The mobilization of FFA from adipose tissue
- Interference with the uptake of glucose by tissues

Although plasma NE can increase 10- to 20-fold during exercise and can achieve a plasma concentration that can exert a physiological effect (131), the primary means by which NE acts is when released from sympathetic neurons onto the surface of the tissue under consideration. The plasma level of NE is usually taken as an index of overall sympathetic nerve activity, but there is evidence that muscle sympathetic nerve activity during exercise may

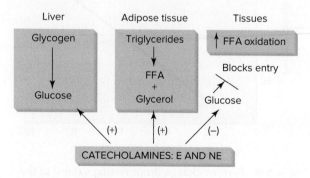

Figure 5.21 Role of catecholamines in substrate mobilization.

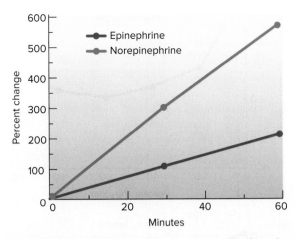

Figure 5.22 Percent change (from resting values) in the plasma epinephrine and norepinephrine concentrations during exercise at ~60% V̇O₂ max.

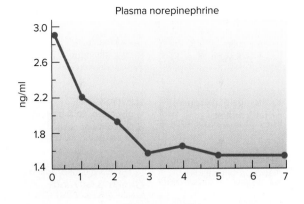

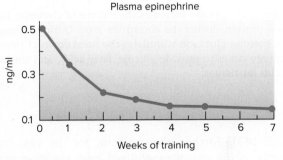

Figure 5.23 Changes in plasma epinephrine and norepinephrine responses to a fixed workload over seven weeks of endurance training.

be a better indicator than that of plasma NE (129). Epinephrine, released from the adrenal medulla, is viewed as the primary catecholamine in the mobilization of glucose from the liver and FFA from adipose tissue (28, 40).

Figure 5.22 shows plasma E and NE to increase linearly with duration of exercise (65, 109, 161). These changes are related to cardiovascular adjustments to exercise–the increased heart rate and blood pressure–as well as to the mobilization of fuel. These responses favor the mobilization of glucose and FFA to maintain the plasma glucose concentration. While it is sometimes difficult to separate the effect of E from NE, E seems to be more responsive to changes in the plasma glucose concentration. A low plasma glucose concentration stimulates a receptor in the hypothalamus to increase E secretion while having only a modest effect on plasma NE. In contrast, when the blood pressure is challenged, as during an increased heat load, the primary catecholamine involved is norepinephrine (109). Epinephrine binds to β-adrenergic receptors on the liver and stimulates the breakdown of liver glycogen to form glucose for release into the plasma. For example, when arm exercise is added to existing leg exercise, the adrenal medulla secretes a large amount of E. This causes the liver to release more glucose than muscles are using, and the blood glucose concentration actually increases (79). What happens if we block the effects of E and NE? If β-adrenergic receptors are blocked with propranolol (a β-adrenergic receptor blocking drug), the plasma glucose concentration is more difficult to maintain during exercise, especially if the subject has fasted (142). In addition, since the propranolol blocks β-adrenergic receptors on adipose tissue cells, fewer FFAs are released, and the muscles have to rely more on their limited glycogen supply for fuel (42).

Figure 5.23 shows that endurance training causes a very rapid decrease in the plasma E and NE responses to a fixed exercise bout. Within three weeks, the concentration of both catecholamines is greatly reduced (152). Paralleling this rapid decrease in E and NE with endurance exercise training is a reduction in glucose mobilization (92). In spite of this, the plasma glucose concentration is maintained because there is also a reduction in glucose uptake by muscle at the same fixed workload following endurance training (118, 153). Interestingly, during a very stressful event, a trained individual has a greater capacity to secrete E than an untrained individual does. In addition, when exercise is performed at the same relative workload (% V̇O₂ max) after training (in contrast to the same fixed workload as in Fig. 5.23), the plasma NE concentration is higher. This suggests that physical training, which stimulates the sympathetic nervous system on a regular basis, increases its capacity to respond to extreme challenges (161).

Insulin and Glucagon These two hormones will be discussed together because they respond to the same stimuli but exert opposite actions relative to the mobilization of liver glucose and adipose tissue FFA. In fact, the ratio of glucagon to insulin provides control over the mobilization of these fuels

Absorption of a Meal   During Fasting and Exercise

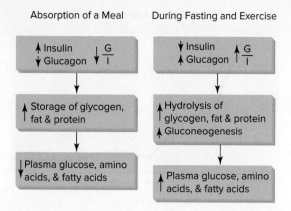

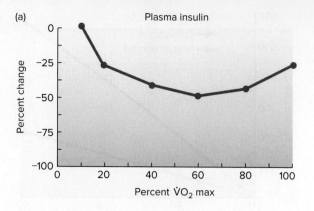

Figure 5.24 Insulin increases the storage of glycogen, fat and protein, during the absorptive state. During fasting or exercise glucagon stimulates the breakdown of these energy stores to provide glucose, fatty acids, and amino acids for tissues.

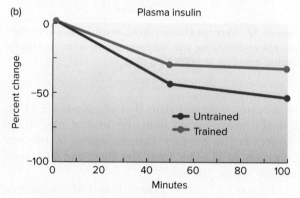

Figure 5.25 (*a*) Percent change (from resting values) in the plasma insulin concentration with increasing intensities of exercise. (*b*) Percent change (from resting values) in the plasma insulin concentration during prolonged exercise at 60% V̇O$_2$ max showing the effect of endurance training on that response.

(20, 143). Further, they account for the vast majority of the glucose mobilized from the liver during moderate to vigorous exercise (22). Figure 5.24 shows that when a meal is being absorbed, the elevated insulin (and the resulting low glucagon-to-insulin ratio) drives the uptake and storage of glucose, amino acids, and fatty acids to lower their levels in the plasma. In contrast, during fasting or exercise, the elevated glucagon (and the high glucagon-to-insulin ratio) stimulates the hydrolysis (breakdown) of glycogen, fat and protein, and increases gluconeogenesis; the result is an increase in the availability of fuel in the plasma.

Given that insulin is directly involved in the uptake of glucose into tissue, and that glucose uptake by muscle can increase 7- to 20-fold during exercise (36), what should happen to the insulin concentration during exercise? Figure 5.25(*a*) shows that the insulin concentration decreases during exercise of increasing intensity (41, 53, 110); this, of course, is an appropriate response. If exercise were associated with an increase in insulin, the plasma glucose would be taken up into all tissues (including adipose tissue) at a faster rate, leading to an immediate hypoglycemia. The lower insulin concentration during exercise favors the mobilization of glucose from the liver and FFA from adipose tissue, both of which are necessary to maintain the plasma glucose concentration. Figure 5.25(*b*) shows that the plasma insulin concentration decreases during moderate-intensity, long-term exercise (49).

With plasma insulin decreasing with long-term exercise, it should be no surprise that the plasma glucagon concentration increases (49). This increase in plasma glucagon (shown in Fig. 5.26) favors the mobilization of FFA from adipose tissue and glucose

from the liver, as well as an increase in gluconeogenesis. Overall, the reciprocal responses of insulin and glucagon favor the maintenance of the plasma glucose concentration at a time when the muscle is using plasma glucose at a high rate. Figure 5.26 also shows that following an endurance training program, the glucagon response to a fixed exercise task is diminished to the point that there is no increase during exercise. In effect, endurance training allows the plasma glucose concentration to be maintained with little or no change in insulin and glucagon. This is related in part to an increase in glucagon sensitivity in the liver (30, 83), a decrease in glucose uptake by muscle (118), and an increase in the muscle's use of fat as a fuel.

These findings raise several questions. If the plasma glucose concentration is relatively constant during exercise and the plasma glucose concentration is a primary stimulus for insulin and glucagon secretion, what causes the insulin secretion to decrease and glucagon secretion to increase? The answer lies in the multiple levels of control over hormonal secretion mentioned earlier in the

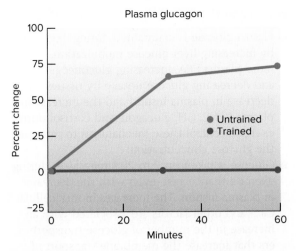

Figure 5.26 Percent change (from resting values) in the plasma glucagon concentration during prolonged exercise at 60% $\dot{V}O_2$ max showing the effect of endurance training on that response.

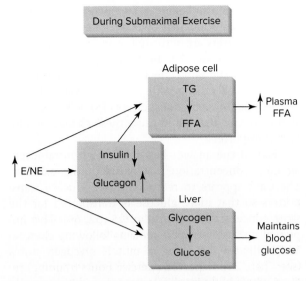

During Submaximal Exercise

Figure 5.28 Effect of increased sympathetic nervous system activity on free fatty acid and glucose mobilization during submaximal exercise.

chapter (see Fig. 5.1). There is no question that changes in the plasma glucose concentration provide an important level of control over the secretion of glucagon and insulin (42). However, when the plasma glucose concentration is relatively constant, the sympathetic nervous system can modify the secretion of insulin and glucagon. Figure 5.27 shows that E and NE stimulate α-adrenergic receptors on the beta cells of the pancreas to decrease insulin secretion during exercise when the plasma glucose concentration is normal. Figure 5.27 also shows that E and NE stimulate β-adrenergic receptors on the alpha cells of the pancreas to increase glucagon secretion when the plasma glucose concentration is normal (22). These effects have

been confirmed through the use of adrenergic receptor blocking drugs. When phentolamine, an α-adrenergic receptor blocker, is given, insulin secretion increases with exercise. When propranolol, a β-adrenergic receptor blocker, is given, the glucagon concentration remains the same or decreases with exercise (86). Figure 5.28 summarizes the effect the sympathetic nervous system has on the mobilization of fuel for muscular work. Endurance training decreases the sympathetic nervous system response to a fixed exercise bout, resulting in less stimulation of adrenergic receptors on the pancreas and less change in insulin and glucagon (see Figs. 5.25(b) and 5.26).

The observation that plasma insulin decreases with prolonged, submaximal exercise raises another question. How can exercising muscle take up glucose 7 to 20 times faster than at rest if the insulin concentration is decreasing? Part of the answer lies in the large (10- to 20-fold) increase in blood flow to muscle during exercise. Glucose delivery is the product of muscle blood flow and the blood glucose concentration. Therefore, during exercise, more glucose and insulin are delivered to muscle than at rest, and because the muscle is using glucose at a higher rate, a gradient for its facilitated diffusion is created (69, 118, 153). Another part of the answer relates to exercise-induced changes in the number of glucose transporters in the membrane. It has been known for some time that acute (a single bout) and chronic (training program) exercise increase a muscle's sensitivity to insulin so that less insulin is needed to have the same effect on glucose uptake into tissue (7, 54, 70). The

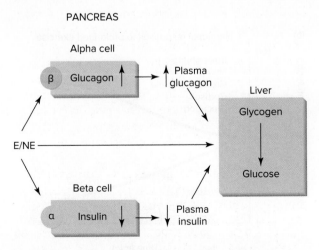

Figure 5.27 Effect of epinephrine and norepinephrine on insulin and glucagon secretion from the pancreas during exercise.

effects of insulin and exercise on glucose transport are additive, suggesting that two separate pools of glucose transporters are activated or translocated in the membrane (46, 68, 70, 147). Interestingly, hypoxia brings about the same effect as exercise, but it is not an additive effect, suggesting that hypoxia and exercise recruit the same transporters (15). What is there about exercise that could cause these changes in glucose transporters?

Part of the answer lies in the high intramuscular Ca^{++} concentration that exists during exercise. The Ca^{++} appears to recruit inactive glucose transporters so that more glucose is transported for the same concentration of insulin (15, 62, 69). This improved glucose transport remains following exercise and facilitates the filling of muscle glycogen stores (see Chap. 23). Repeated exercise bouts (training) reduce whole-body insulin resistance, making exercise an important part of therapy for those with diabetes (69, 95, 159). Consistent with this, bed rest (94) and limb immobilization (117) increase insulin resistance. However, it is clear that glucose transporters in contracting muscle are regulated by more than changes in the calcium concentration. Factors such as protein kinase C, nitric oxide, AMP-activated protein kinase, and others play a role (116, 121, 123).

In summary, Figure 5.29(*a*) and (*b*) shows the changes in epinephrine, norepinephrine, growth hormone, cortisol, glucagon, and insulin to exercise of varying intensity and duration. The decrease in insulin and the increase in all the other hormones favor the mobilization of glucose from the liver, FFA from adipose tissue, and gluconeogenesis in the liver, while inhibiting the uptake of glucose. These combined actions maintain homeostasis relative to the plasma glucose concentration so that the central nervous system and the muscles can have the fuel they need.

IN SUMMARY

- Plasma glucose is maintained during exercise by increasing liver glucose mobilization, using more plasma FFA, increasing gluconeogenesis, and decreasing glucose uptake by tissues. The decrease in plasma insulin and the increase in plasma E, NE, GH, glucagon, and cortisol during exercise control these mechanisms to maintain the glucose concentration.
- Glucose is taken up 7 to 20 times faster during exercise than at rest—even with the decrease in plasma insulin. The increases in intracellular Ca^{++} and other factors are associated with an increase in the number of glucose transporters that increase the membrane transport of glucose.
- Training causes a reduction in E, NE, glucagon, and insulin responses to exercise.

Hormone–Substrate Interaction

In the examples mentioned previously, insulin and glucagon responded as they did during exercise with a normal plasma glucose concentration due to the influence of the sympathetic nervous system. It must be mentioned that if there were a sudden change in the plasma glucose concentration during exercise, these hormones would respond to that change. For example, if the ingestion of glucose before exercise caused an elevation of plasma glucose, the plasma concentration of insulin would increase. This hormonal change would reduce FFA mobilization and force the muscle to use additional muscle glycogen (1).

During intense exercise, plasma glucagon, GH, cortisol, E, and NE are elevated and insulin is decreased. These hormonal changes favor the mobilization of FFA from adipose tissue that would spare

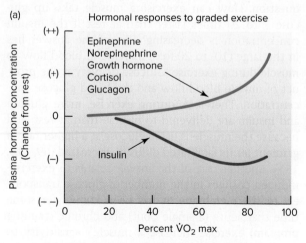

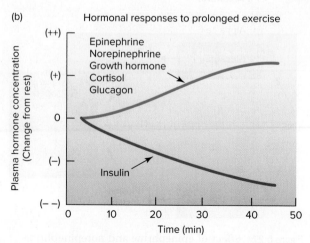

Figure 5.29 (*a*) Summary of the hormonal responses to exercise of increasing intensity. (*b*) Summary of the hormonal responses to moderate exercise of long duration.

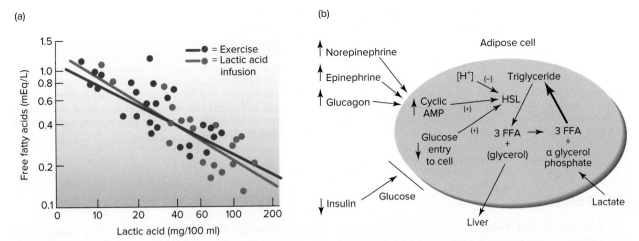

Figure 5.30 (*a*) Changes in plasma free fatty acids due to increases in lactic acid. (*b*) Effect of lactate and H⁺ on the mobilization of free fatty acids from the adipose cell.

carbohydrate and help maintain the plasma glucose concentration. If this is the case, why does plasma FFA use decrease with increasing intensities of exercise (120)? Part of the answer seems to be that there is an upper limit in the adipose cell's ability to deliver FFA to the circulation during exercise. For example, in trained subjects, the rate of release of FFA from adipose tissue was the highest at 25% $\dot{V}O_2$ max, and decreased at 65% and 85% $\dot{V}O_2$ max (120). Given that the hormone sensitive lipase (HSL) involved in triglyceride breakdown to FFA and glycerol is under stronger hormonal stimulation at the higher work rates, the FFA actually appears to be "trapped" in the adipose cell (59, 120). This may be due to a variety of factors, one of which is lactate. Figure 5.30(*a*) shows that as the blood lactate concentration increases, the plasma FFA concentration decreases (67). The elevated lactate has been linked to an increase in alpha glycerol phosphate, the activated form of glycerol needed to make triglycerides. In effect, as fast as the FFA becomes available from the breakdown of triglycerides, the alpha glycerol phosphate recycles the FFA to generate a new triglyceride molecule (see Fig. 5.30(*b*)). In addition, the elevated H⁺ concentration (associated with the high lactate level) can inhibit HSL. The result is that the FFAs are not released from the adipose cell (104). Other explanations of the reduced availability of adipose tissue FFA during heavy exercise include a reduced blood supply to adipose tissue, resulting in less FFA to transport to muscle (40, 120), and an inadequate amount of albumin, the plasma protein needed to transport the FFA in the plasma (59). The result is that FFAs are not released from the adipose cell, the plasma FFA level falls, and the muscle must use more carbohydrate as fuel. One of the effects of endurance training is to decrease the lactate concentration at any fixed work rate, which reduces this inhibition to FFA mobilization from adipose tissue. When this is combined with the training-induced increase in mitochondria, the trained person can use more fat as a fuel, spare the limited carbohydrate stores, and improve performance.

IN SUMMARY

- The plasma FFA concentration decreases during heavy exercise even though the adipose cell is stimulated by a variety of hormones to increase triglyceride breakdown to FFA and glycerol. This may be due to (1) the higher H⁺ concentration, which may inhibit HSL, (2) the high levels of lactate during heavy exercise that promote the resynthesis of triglycerides, (3) an inadequate blood flow to adipose tissue, or (4) insufficient albumin needed to transport the FFA in the plasma.

STUDY ACTIVITIES

1. Draw and label a diagram of a negative feedback mechanism for hormonal control using cortisol as an example.
2. List the factors that can influence the blood concentration of a hormone.
3. Discuss the use of testosterone and growth hormone as aids to increase muscle size and strength, and discuss the potential long-term consequences of such use.
4. List each endocrine gland, the hormone(s) secreted from that gland, and its (their) action(s).

5. Describe the two mechanisms by which muscle glycogen is broken down to glucose (glycogenolysis) for use in glycolysis. Which one is activated at the same time as muscle contraction?
6. Identify the four mechanisms involved in maintaining the blood glucose concentration.
7. Draw a summary graph of the changes in the following hormones with exercise of increasing intensity or duration: epinephrine, norepinephrine, cortisol, growth hormone, insulin, and glucagon.

8. What is the effect of training on the responses of epinephrine, norepinephrine, and glucagon to the same exercise task?
9. Briefly explain how glucose can be taken into the muscle at a high rate during exercise when plasma insulin is reduced. Include the role of glucose transporters.
10. Explain how free fatty acid mobilization from the adipose cell decreases during maximal work in spite of the cell being stimulated by all the hormones to break down triglycerides.

REFERENCES

1. **Ahlborg G and Felig P.** Influence of glucose ingestion on fuel-hormone response during prolonged exercise. *Journal of Applied Physiology: Respiratory, Environmental and Exercise Physiology* 41: 683–688, 1976.
2. **Alen M, Pakarinen A, and Hakkinen K.** Effects of prolonged training on serum thyrotropin and thyroid hormones in elite strength athletes. *Journal of Sports Sciences* 11: 493–497, 1993.
3. **Almon RR and Dubois DC.** Fiber-type discrimination in disuse and glucocorticoid-induced atrophy. *Medicine and Science in Sports and Exercise* 22: 304–311, 1990.
4. **American College of Sports Medicine.** The use of anabolic-androgenic steroids in sports. In *Position Stands and Opinion Statements.* Indianapolis: The American College of Sports Medicine, 1984.
5. **Angell P, Chester N, Green D, Somauroo J, Whyte G, and George K.** Anabolic steroids and cardiovascular risk. *Sports Medicine* 42: 119–134, 2012.
6. **Berggren JR, Hulver MW, and Houmard JA.** Fat as an endocrine organ: influence of exercise. *Journal of Applied Physiology: Respiratory, Environmental and Exercise Physiology* 99: 757–764, 2005.
7. **Berggren JR, Tanner CJ, Koves TR, Muoio DM, and Houmard JA.** Glucose uptake in muscle cell cultures from endurance-trained men. *Medicine and Science in Sports and Exercise* 37: 579–584, 2005.
8. **Bonen A.** Effects of exercise on excretion rates of urinary free cortisol. *Journal of Applied Physiology: Respiratory, Environmental and Exercise Physiology* 40: 155–158, 1976.
9. **Bouassida A, Chamari K, Zaouali M, Feki Y, Zbidi A, and Tabka Z.** Review on leptin and adiponectin responses and adaptations to acute and chronic exercise. *British Journal of Sports Medicine* 44: 620–630, 2010.
10. **Bouassida A, Latiri I, Bouassida S, Zalleg D, Zaouali M, Feki Y, et al.** Parathyroid hormone and physical exercise: a brief review. *J Sport Science and Medicine* 5: 367–374, 2006.
11. **Brandt C and Pedersen BK.** The role of exercise-induced myokines in muscle homeostasis and the defense against chronic disease. *Journal of Biomedicine and Biotechnology:* Article ID: 520258, 2010.
12. **Brunton L, Lazo JS, and Parker KL.** *Goodman & Gilman's The Pharmacological Basis of Therapeutics.* New York, NY: McGraw-Hill, 2005.
13. **Bunt JC, Boileau RA, Bahr JM, and Nelson RA.** Sex and training differences in human growth hormone levels during prolonged exercise. *Journal of Applied Physiology: Respiratory, Environmental and Exercise Physiology* 61: 1796–1801, 1986.

14. **Cannon W.** *Bodily Changes in Pain, Hunger, Fear and Rage.* Boston, MA: Charles T. Branford Company, 1983.
15. **Cartee GD, Douen AG, Ramlal T, Klip A, and Holloszy JO.** Stimulation of glucose transport in skeletal muscle by hypoxia. *Journal of Applied Physiology: Respiratory, Environmental and Exercise Physiology* 70: 1593–1600, 1991.
16. **Cartier LJ and Gollnick PD.** Sympathoadrenal system and activation of glycogenolysis during muscular activity. *Journal of Applied Physiology: Respiratory, Environmental and Exercise Physiology* 58: 1122–1127, 1985.
17. **Chaudhari AM, Lindenfeld TN, Andriacchi TP, Hewett TE, Riccobene J, Myer GD, et al.** Knee and hip loading patterns at different phases in the menstrual cycle: implications for the gender difference in anterior cruciate ligament injury rates. *The American Journal of Sports Medicine* 35: 793–800, 2007.
18. **Christensen NJ and Galbo H.** Sympathetic nervous activity during exercise. *Annual Review of Physiology* 45: 139–153, 1983.
19. **Coelho M, Oliveira T, and Fernandes R.** Biochemistry of adipose tissue: an endocrine organ. *Archives of Medical Science* 2: 191–200, 2013.
20. **Coggan AR.** Plasma glucose metabolism during exercise in humans. *Sports Medicine* 11: 102–124, 1991.
21. **Coggan AR and Coyle EF.** Carbohydrate ingestion during prolonged exercise: effects on metabolism and performance. *Exercise and Sport Sciences Reviews* 19: 1–40, 1991.
22. **Coker RH and Kjaer M.** Glucoregulation during exercise: the role of the neuroendocrine system. *Sports Medicine* 35: 575–583, 2005.
23. **Convertino VA, Keil LC, and Greenleaf JE.** Plasma volume, renin, and vasopressin responses to graded exercise after training. *Journal of Applied Physiology: Respiratory, Environmental and Exercise Physiology* 54: 508–514, 1983.
24. **Copinschi G, Hartog M, Earll JM, and Havel RJ.** Effect of various blood sampling procedures on serum levels of immunoreactive human growth hormone. *Metabolism: Clinical and Experimental* 16: 402–409, 1967.
25. **Coyle EF.** Substrate utilization during exercise in active people. *American Journal of Clinical Nutrition* 61: 968S–979S, 1995.
26. **Cumming DC, Brunsting LA, 3rd, Strich G, Ries AL, and Rebar RW.** Reproductive hormone increases in response to acute exercise in men. *Medicine and Science in Sports and Exercise* 18: 369–373, 1986.
27. **Davies CT and Few JD.** Effects of exercise on adrenocortical function. *Journal of Applied Physiology:*

Respiratory, Environmental and Exercise Physiology 35: 887-891, 1973.

28. **De Glisezinski I, Larrouy D, Bajzova M, Koppo K, Polak J, Berlan M, et al.** Adrenaline but not noradrenaline is a determinant of exercise-induced lipid mobilization in human subcutaneous adipose tissue. *Journal of Physiology* 13: 3393-3404, 2009.

29. **Del Corral P, Howley ET, Hartsell M, Ashraf M, and Younger MS.** Metabolic effects of low cortisol during exercise in humans. *Journal of Applied Physiology: Respiratory, Environmental and Exercise Physiology* 84: 939-947, 1998.

30. **Drouin R, Lavoie C, Bourque J, Ducros F, Poisson D, and Chiasson JL.** Increased hepatic glucose production response to glucagon in trained subjects. *American Journal of Physiology* 274: E23-E28, 1998.

31. **Eckardt K, Görgens S, Raschke S, and Eckel J.** Myokines in insulin resistance and type 2 diabetes. *Diabetologia* 57: 1087-1099, 2014.

32. **Edgerton VR.** *Glycogen Depletion in Specific Types of Human Skeletal Muscle Fibers in Intermittent and Continuous Exercise.* Verlag Basel: Birkhauser, 1975, pp. 402-415.

33. **Enns DL and Tiidus PM.** The influence of estrogen on skeletal muscle-sex matters. *Sports Medicine* 40: 41-58, 2010.

34. **Essen B.** Glycogen depletion of different fibre types in human skeletal muscle during intermittent and continuous exercise. *Acta Physiologica Scandinavica* 103: 446-455, 1978.

35. **Euler U.** *Sympatho-Adrenal Activity and Physical Exercise.* New York, NY: Karger, Basal, 1969, pp. 170-181.

36. **Felig P and Wahren J.** Fuel homeostasis in exercise. *New England Journal of Medicine* 293: 1078-1084, 1975.

37. **Fischer-Posovszky P, Wabitsch M, and Hochberg Z.** Endocrinology of adipose tissue–an update. *Hormone and Metabolic Research (Hormon- und Stoffwechselforschung = Hormones et metabolisme)* 39: 314-321, 2007.

38. **Fox SI.** *Human Physiology,* 12th ed. New York, NY: McGraw-Hill, 2011.

39. **Francesconi RP, Sawka MN, and Pandolf KB.** Hypohydration and heat acclimation: plasma renin and aldosterone during exercise. *Journal of Applied Physiology: Respiratory, Environmental and Exercise Physiology* 55: 1790-1794, 1983.

40. **Frayn KN.** Fat as a fuel: emerging understanding of the adipose tissue-skeletal muscle axis. *Acta Physiologica Scandinavica* 199: 509-518, 2010.

41. **Galbo H, Holst JJ, and Christensen NJ.** Glucagon and plasma catecholamine responses to graded and prolonged exercise in man. *Journal of Applied Physiology: Respiratory, Environmental and Exercise Physiology* 38: 70-76, 1975.

42. **Galbo H, Holst JJ, Christensen NJ, and Hilsted J.** Glucagon and plasma catecholamines during beta-receptor blockade in exercising man. *Journal of Applied Physiology: Respiratory, Environmental and Exercise Physiology* 40: 855-863, 1976.

43. **Galbo H, Hummer L, Peterson IB, Christensen NJ, and Bie N.** Thyroid and testicular hormone responses to graded and prolonged exercise in man. *European Journal of Applied Physiology and Occupational Physiology* 36: 101-106, 1977.

44. **Giannoulis M, Martin F, Nair S, Umpleby A, and Sonksen P.** Hormone replacement therapy and physical function in healthy older men. Time to talk hormones? *Endocrine Reviews* 33: 314-377, 2012.

45. **Gollnick PD.** *Glycogen Depletion Patterns in Human Skeletal Muscle Fibers after Varying Types and Intensities of Exercise.* Verlag Basel: Birkhauser, 1975.

46. **Goodyear LJ and Kahn BB.** Exercise, glucose transport, and insulin sensitivity. *Annual Review of Medicine* 49: 235-261, 1998.

47. **Greenberg AS and Obin MS.** Obesity and the role of adipose tissue in inflammation and metabolism. *American Journal of Clinical Nutrition* 83: 461S-465S, 2006.

48. **Greenwood FC and Landon J.** Growth hormone secretion in response to stress in man. *Nature* 210: 540-541, 1966.

49. **Gyntelberg F, Rennie MJ, Hickson RC, and Holloszy JO.** Effect of training on the response of plasma glucagon to exercise. *Journal of Applied Physiology: Respiratory, Environmental and Exercise Physiology* 43: 302-305, 1977.

50. **Hackney AC and Dobridge JD.** Thyroid hormones and the relationship of cortisol and prolactin: influence of prolonged, exhaustive exercise. *Polish Journal of Endocrinology* 60: 252-257, 2009.

51. **Hameed M, Harridge SD, and Goldspink G.** Sarcopenia and hypertrophy: a role for insulin-like growth factor-1 in aged muscle? *Exercise and Sport Sciences Reviews* 30: 15-19, 2002.

52. **Harris RC, Bergström J, and Hultman E.** *The Effect of Propranolol on Glycogen Metabolism during Exercise.* New York, NY: Plenum Press, 1971, pp. 301-305.

53. **Hartley LH, Mason JW, Hogan RP, Jones LG, Kotchen TA, Mougey EH, et al.** Multiple hormonal responses to prolonged exercise in relation to physical training. *Journal of Applied Physiology: Respiratory, Environmental and Exercise Physiology* 33: 607-610, 1972.

54. **Heath GW, Gavin JR, 3rd, Hinderliter JM, Hagberg JM, Bloomfield SA, and Holloszy JO.** Effects of exercise and lack of exercise on glucose tolerance and insulin sensitivity. *Journal of Applied Physiology: Respiratory, Environmental and Exercise Physiology* 55: 512-517, 1983.

55. **Hew-Butler T.** Arginine vasopressin, fluid balance and exercise. *Sports Medicine* 40: 459-479, 2010.

56. **Hickson RC, Czerwinski SM, Falduto MT, and Young AP.** Glucocorticoid antagonism by exercise and androgenic-anabolic steroids. *Medicine and Science in Sports and Exercise* 22: 331-340, 1990.

57. **Hickson RC and Marone JR.** Exercise and inhibition of glucocorticoid-induced muscle atrophy. *Exercise and Sport Sciences Reviews* 21: 135-167, 1993.

58. **Highet R.** Athletic amenorrhoea. An update on aetiology, complications and management. *Sports Medicine* 7: 82-108, 1989.

59. **Hodgetts V, Coppack S, Frayn K, and Hockaday T.** Factors controlling fat mobilization from human subcutaneous adipose tissue during exercise. *Journal of Applied Physiology* 71: 445-451, 1991.

60. **Hoffman JR, Kraemer WJ, Bhasin S, Storer T, Ratamess NA, Haff GG, et al.** Position stand on androgen and human growth hormone use. *J Strength and Conditioning Research* 23 (Suppl 5): S1-S59, 2009.

61. **Holloszy JO, Kohrt WM, and Hansen PA.** The regulation of carbohydrate and fat metabolism during and after exercise. *Frontiers in Bioscience* 3: D1011-D1027, 1998.

62. **Holloszy JO and Narahara HT.** Enhanced permeability to sugar associated with muscle contraction. Studies of the role of Ca^{++}. *Journal of General Physiology* 50: 551-562, 1967.

63. **Howley ET.** The effect of different intensities of exercise on the excretion of epinephrine and norepinephrine. *Medicine and Science in Sports* 8: 219-222, 1976.

64. **Howley ET.** *The Excretion of Catecholamines as an Index of Exercise Stress.* Springfield, MA: Charles C. Thomas, 1980, pp. 171-183.

65. **Howley ET, Cox RH, Welch HG, and Adams RP.** Effect of hyperoxia on metabolic and catecholamine responses to prolonged exercise. *Journal of Applied Physiology: Respiratory, Environmental and Exercise Physiology* 54: 59-63, 1983.

66. **Hultman E.** *Physiological Role of Muscle Glycogen in Man with Special Reference to Exercise.* New York, NY: The American Heart Association, 1967, pp. 1-114.

67. **Issekutz B and Miller H.** Plasma free fatty acids during exercise and the effect of lactic acid. *Proceedings of the Society of Experimental Biology and Medicine* 110: 237-239, 1962.

68. **Ivy JL.** Role of exercise training in the prevention and treatment of insulin resistance and non-insulin-dependent diabetes mellitus. *Sports Medicine* 24: 321-336, 1997.

69. **Ivy JL.** The insulin-like effect of muscle contraction. *Exercise and Sport Sciences Reviews* 15: 29-51, 1987.

70. **Ivy JL, Young JC, McLane JA, Fell RD, and Holloszy JO.** Exercise training and glucose uptake by skeletal muscle in rats. *Journal of Applied Physiology: Respiratory, Environmental and Exercise Physiology* 55: 1393-1396, 1983.

71. **James DE.** The mammalian facilitative glucose transporter family. *News in Physiological Sciences* 10, 67-71, 1995.

72. **Jansson E, Hjemdahl P, and Kaijser L.** Epinephrine-induced changes in muscle carbohydrate metabolism during exercise in male subjects. *Journal of Applied Physiology: Respiratory, Environmental and Exercise Physiology* 60: 1466-1470, 1986.

73. **Jensen J, Oftebro H, Breigan B, Johnsson A, Ohlin K, Meen HD, et al.** Comparison of changes in testosterone concentrations after strength and endurance exercise in well trained men. *European Journal of Applied Physiology and Occupational Physiology* 63: 467-471, 1991.

74. **Jurkowski JE, Jones NL, Walker C, Younglai EV, and Sutton JR.** Ovarian hormonal responses to exercise. *Journal of Applied Physiology: Respiratory, Environmental and Exercise Physiology* 44: 109-114, 1978.

75. **Kanayama G, Kean J, Hudson JI, and Pope Jr. HG.** Cognitive deficits in long-term anabolic-androgenic steroid users. *Drug and Alcohol Dependence* 130: 208-214, 2013.

76. **Kargotich S, Goodman C, Keast D, Fry RW, Garcia-Webb P, Crawford PM, et al.** Influence of exercise-induced plasma volume changes on the interpretation of biochemical data following high-intensity exercise. *Clinical Journal of Sport Medicine* 7: 185-191, 1997.

77. **Keizer HA and Rogol AD.** Physical exercise and menstrual cycle alterations. What are the mechanisms? *Sports Medicine* 10: 218-235, 1990.

78. **Kjaer M.** Epinephrine and some other hormonal responses to exercise in man: with special reference to physical training. *International Journal of Sports Medicine* 10: 2-15, 1989.

79. **Kjaer M, Kiens B, Hargreaves M, and Richter EA.** Influence of active muscle mass on glucose homeostasis during exercise in humans. *Journal of Applied Physiology: Respiratory, Environmental and Exercise Physiology* 71: 552-557, 1991.

80. **Kostek MC, Delmonico MJ, Reichel JB, Roth SM, Douglass L, Ferrell RE, et al.** Muscle strength response to strength training is influenced by insulin-like growth factor 1 genotype in older adults. *Journal of Applied Physiology: Respiratory, Environmental and Exercise Physiology* 98: 2147-2154, 2005.

81. **Kraemer RR and Castracane VD.** Exercise and humoral mediators of peripheral energy balance: ghrelin and adiponectin. *Experimental Biology and Medicine* 232: 184-194, 2007.

82. **Kraemer RR, Francois M, Webb ND, Worley JR, Rogers SN, Norman RL, et al.** No effect of menstrual cycle phase on glucose and glucoregulatory endocrine responses to prolonged exercise. *European Journal of Applied Physiology* 113: 2401-2408, 2013.

83. **Lavoie C.** Glucagon receptors: effect of exercise and fasting. *Canadian Journal of Applied Physiology (Revue canadienne de physiologie appliquee)* 30: 313-327, 2005.

84. **Liu H, Bravata DM, Olkin I, Friedlander AL, Liu V, Roberts B, et al.** Systematic review: the effects of growth hormone on athletic performance. *Annals of Internal Medicine* 148: 2008.

85. **Liu H, Bravata DM, Olkin I, Nayak S, Roberts B, Garber AM, et al.** Systematic review: the safety and efficacy of growth hormone in the healthy elderly. *Annals of Internal Medicine* 146: 104-115, 2007.

86. **Luyckx AS and Lefebvre PJ.** Mechanisms involved in the exercise-induced increase in glucagon secretion in rats. *Diabetes* 23: 81-93, 1974.

87. **Maher JT, Jones LG, Hartley LH, Williams GH, and Rose LI.** Aldosterone dynamics during graded exercise at sea level and high altitude. *Journal of Applied Physiology: Respiratory, Environmental and Exercise Physiology* 39: 18-22, 1975.

88. **Maïmoun L and Sultan C.** Effect of physical activity on calcium homeostasis and calciotrophic hormones: a review. *Calcified Tissue International* 85: 277-286, 2009.

89. **Marsh SA and Jenkins DG.** Physiological responses to the menstrual cycle: implications for the development of heat illness in female athletes. *Sports Medicine* 32: 601-614, 2002.

90. **Mathur N and Pedersen BK.** Exercise as a means to control low-grade systemic inflammation. *Mediators of Inflammation* 2008: 1-6, 2008.

91. **McMurray RG and Hackney AC.** Interactions of metabolic hormones, adipose tissue and exercise. *Sports Medicine* 35: 393-412, 2005.

92. **Mendenhall LA, Swanson SC, Habash DL, and Coggan AR.** Ten days of exercise training reduces glucose production and utilization during moderate-intensity exercise. *American Journal of Physiology* 266: E136-E143, 1994.

93. **Metsarinne K.** Effect of exercise on plasma renin substrate. *International Journal of Sports Medicine* 9: 267-269, 1988.

94. **Mikines KJ, Richter EA, Dela F, and Galbo H.** Seven days of bed rest decrease insulin action on glucose uptake in leg and whole body. *Journal of Applied Physiology: Respiratory, Environmental and Exercise Physiology* 70: 1245-1254, 1991.

95. **Mikines KJ, Sonne B, Tronier B, and Galbo H.** Effects of acute exercise and detraining on insulin action in trained men. *Journal of Applied Physiology: Respiratory, Environmental and Exercise Physiology* 66: 704-711, 1989.

96. **Molina PE.** *Endocrine Physiology.* New York, NY: McGraw-Hill. 2013.

97. **Nakamura K, Fuster J, and Walsh K.** Adipokines: a link between obesity and cardiovascular disease. *Journal of Cardiology* 63: 250-259, 2014.

98. **Nakamura Y, Aizawa K, Imai T, Kono I, and Mesaki N.** Hormonal responses to resistance exercise during different menstrual cycle phases. *Medicine and Science in Sports and Exercise* 43: 967-973, 2011.

99. **National Athletic Trainers' Association.** Position statement: anabolic-androgenic steroids. *Journal of Athletic Training* 47: 567-588, 2012.

100. **Nindl B, Pierce J, Rarick K, Tuckow A, Alemany J, Sharp M, et al.** Twenty-hour growth hormone secretory profiles after aerobic and resistance exercise. *Medicine and Science in Sport and Exercise* 46: 1917-1927, 2014.

101. **Ogawa W and Kasuga M.** Fat stress and liver resistance. *Science* 322: 1483-1484, 2008.

102. **Oosthuyse T and Bosch AN.** The effect of the menstrual cycle on exercise metabolism. *Sports Medicine* 40: 207-227, 2010.

103. **Parkinson AB and Evans NA.** Anabolic androgenic steroids: a survey of 500 users. *Medicine and Science in Sports and Exercise* 38: 644-651, 2006.

104. **Paul P.** FFA metabolism of normal dogs during steady-state exercise at different work loads. *Journal of Applied Physiology: Respiratory, Environmental and Exercise Physiology* 28: 127-132, 1970.

105. **Paul P.** Uptake and Oxidation of Substrates in the Intact Animal during Exercise. In *Muscle Metabolism During Exercise*, edited by B. Pernow and B. Saltin. New York, NY: Plenum Press, 1971, pp. 225-248.

106. **Pedersen BK.** Edward F. Adolph Distinguished Lecture: Muscle as an endocrine organ: IL-6 and other myokines. *Journal of Applied Physiology: Respiratory, Environmental and Exercise Physiology* 107: 1006-1014, 2009.

107. **Pedersen BK and Febbraio MA.** Muscles, exercise and obesity: skeletal muscle as a secretory organ. *Nature Reviews–Endocrinology* 8: 457-465, 2012.

108. **Perry PJ, Lund BC, Deninger MJ, Kutscher EC, and Schneider J.** Anabolic steroid use in weightlifters and bodybuilders: an internet survey of drug utilization. *Clinical Journal of Sport Medicine* 15: 326-330, 2005.

109. **Powers SK, Howley ET, and Cox R.** A differential catecholamine response during prolonged exercise and passive heating. *Medicine and Science in Sports and Exercise* 14: 435-439, 1982.

110. **Pruett ED.** Glucose and insulin during prolonged work stress in men living on different diets. *Journal of Applied Physiology: Respiratory, Environmental and Exercise Physiology* 28: 199-208, 1970.

111. **Raschke S and Eckel J.** Adipo-Myokines: two sides of the same coin: mediators of inflammation and mediators of exercise. *Mediators of Inflammation* DOI: 10.1155/2013/320724, 2013.

112. **Raven PH, Johnson GB, Losos JB, Mason KA, and Singer SR.** *Biology.* New York, NY: McGraw-Hill, 2008.

113. **Redman LM and Loucks AB.** Menstrual disorders in athletes. *Sports Medicine* 35: 747-755, 2005.

114. **Ren JM and Hultman E.** Regulation of glycogenolysis in human skeletal muscle. *Journal of Applied Physiology: Respiratory, Environmental and Exercise Physiology* 67: 2243-2248, 1989.

115. **Rennie MJ.** Claims for the anabolic effects of growth hormone: a case of the emperor's new clothes? *British Journal of Sports Medicine* 37: 100-105, 2003.

116. **Richter EA, Derave W, and Wojtaszewski JF.** Glucose, exercise and insulin: emerging concepts. *Journal of Physiology* 535: 313-322, 2001.

117. **Richter EA, Kiens B, Mizuno M, and Strange S.** Insulin action in human thighs after one-legged immobilization. *Journal of Applied Physiology: Respiratory, Environmental and Exercise Physiology* 67: 19-23, 1989.

118. **Richter EA, Kristiansen S, Wojtaszewski J, Daugaard JR, Asp S, Hespel P, et al.** Training effects on muscle glucose transport during exercise. *Advances in Experimental Medicine and Biology* 441: 107-116, 1998.

119. **Rizza R, Haymond M, Cryer P, and Gerich J.** Differential effects of epinephrine on glucose production and disposal in man. *American Journal of Physiology* 237: E356-E362, 1979.

120. **Romijn JA, Coyle EF, Sidossis LS, Gastaldelli A, Horowitz JF, Endert E, et al.** Regulation of endogenous fat and carbohydrate metabolism in relation to exercise intensity and duration. *American Journal of Physiology* 265: E380-E391, 1993.

121. **Ryder JW, Chibalin AV, and Zierath JR.** Intracellular mechanisms underlying increases in glucose uptake in response to insulin or exercise in skeletal muscle. *Acta Physiologica Scandinavica* 171: 249-257, 2001.

122. **Sabio G, Das M, Mora A, Zhang Z, Jun JY, Ko HJ, et al.** A stress signaling pathway in adipose tissue regulates hepatic insulin resistance. *Science* 322: 1539-1543, 2008.

123. **Sakamoto K and Goodyear LJ.** Invited review: intracellular signaling in contracting skeletal muscle. *Journal of Applied Physiology: Respiratory, Environmental and Exercise Physiology* 93: 369-383, 2002.

124. **Saltin B and Karlsson J.** *Muscle Glycogen Utilization during Work of Different Intensities.* New York, NY: Plenum Press, 1971.

125. **Saugy M, Robinson N, Saudan C, Baume N, Avois L, and Mangin P.** Human growth hormone doping in sport. *British Journal of Sports Medicine* 40 Suppl 1: i35-i39, 2006.

126. **Schaal K, Van Loan MD, and Casazza GA.** Reduced catecholamine response to exercise in amenorrheic athletes. *Medicine and Science in Sports and Exercise* 43: 34-43, 2011.

127. **Schoenfeld BJ.** Potential mechanisms for a role of metabolic stress in hypertrophic adaptations to resistance training. *Sports Medicine* 43: 179-194, 2013a.

128. **Schoenfeld BJ.** Postexercise hypertrophic adaptations: a reexamination of the hormone hypothesis and its applicability to resistance training program design. *Journal of Strength and Conditioning Research* 27: 1720-1730, 2013b.

129. **Seals DR, Victor RG, and Mark AL.** Plasma norepinephrine and muscle sympathetic discharge during rhythmic exercise in humans. *Journal of Applied Physiology: Respiratory, Environmental and Exercise Physiology* 65: 940-944, 1988.

130. **Selye H.** *The Stress of Life.* New York, NY: McGraw-Hill, 1976.

131. **Silverberg AB, Shah SD, Haymond MW, and Cryer PE.** Norepinephrine: hormone and neurotransmitter in man. *American Journal of Physiology* 234: E252-E256, 1978.

132. **Spriet LL, Ren JM, and Hultman E.** Epinephrine infusion enhances muscle glycogenolysis during prolonged electrical stimulation. *Journal of Applied Physiology: Respiratory, Environmental and Exercise Physiology* 64: 1439-1444, 1988.

133. **Stainsby WN, Sumners C, and Andrew GM.** Plasma catecholamines and their effect on blood lactate and muscle lactate output. *Journal of Applied*

Physiology: Respiratory, Environmental and Exercise Physiology 57: 321-325, 1984.

134. **Stainsby WN, Sumners C, and Eitzman PD.** Effects of catecholamines on lactic acid output during progressive working contractions. *Journal of Applied Physiology: Respiratory, Environmental and Exercise Physiology* 59: 1809-1814, 1985.

135. **Stokes K.** Growth hormone responses to sub-maximal and sprint exercise. *Growth Hormone & IGF Research* 13: 225-238, 2003.

136. **Sun Y, Xun K, Wang C, Zhao H, Bi H, Chen X, et al.** Adiponectin, an unlocking adipocytokine. *Cardiovascular Therapeutics* 27: 59-75, 2009.

137. **Sutton J and Lazarus L.** Growth hormone in exercise: comparison of physiological and pharmacological stimuli. *Journal of Applied Physiology: Respiratory, Environmental and Exercise Physiology* 41: 523-527, 1976.

138. **Tepperman J and Tepperman HM.** *Metabolic and Endocrine Physiology.* Chicago, IL: Year Book Medical Publishers, 1987.

139. **Terjung R.** *Endocrine Response to Exercise.* New York, NY: Macmillan, 1979.

140. **Tiidus PM, Enns DL, Hubal MJ, and Clarkson PM.** Point: counterpoint: estrogen and sex do/do not influence post-exercise indexes of muscle damage, inflammation, and repair. *Journal of Applied Physiology: Respiratory, Environmental and Exercise Physiology* 106: 1010-1015, 2009.

141. **Trayhurn P.** Hypoxia and adipose tissue function and dysfunction in obesity. *Physiological Reviews* 93: 1-21, 2013.

142. **Van Baak MA.** ß-Adrenoceptor blockade and exercise: an update. *Sports Medicine* 5: 209-225, 1988.

143. **Voet D and Voet JG.** *Biochemistry* New York, NY: John Wiley & Sons, 1995.

144. **Vogel RB, Books CA, Ketchum C, Zauner CW, and Murray FT.** Increase of free and total testosterone during submaximal exercise in normal males. *Medicine and Science in Sports and Exercise* 17: 119-123, 1985.

145. **Wade CE.** Response, regulation, and actions of vasopressin during exercise: a review. *Medicine and Science in Sports and Exercise* 16: 506-511, 1984.

146. **Waki H and Tontonoz P.** Endocrine functions of adipose tissue. *Annual Review of Pathology* 2: 31-56, 2007.

147. **Wallberg-Henriksson H, Constable SH, Young DA, and Holloszy JO.** Glucose transport into rat skeletal muscle: interaction between exercise and insulin. *Journal of Applied Physiology: Respiratory, Environmental and Exercise Physiology* 65: 909-913, 1988.

148. **Welc SS and Clanton TL.** The regulation of interleukin-6 implicates skeletal muscle as an integrative stress sensor and endocrine organ. *Experimental Physiology* 98: 359-371, 2013.

149. **Widdowson WM, Healy M-L, Sönksen PH, and Gibney J.** The physiology of growth hormone and sport. *Growth Hormone & IGF Research* 19: 308-319, 2009.

150. **Widdowson WM and Gibney J.** The effect of growth hormone (GH) replacement on muscle strength in patients with GH-deficiency: a meta-analysis. *Clinical Endocrinology* 72: 787-792, 2010.

151. **Widmaier EP, Raff H, and Strang KT.** *Vander's Human Physiology.* New York, NY: McGraw-Hill, 2014.

152. **Winder WW, Hagberg JM, Hickson RC, Ehsani AA, and McLane JA.** Time course of sympathoadrenal adaptation to endurance exercise training in man. *Journal of Applied Physiology: Respiratory, Environmental and Exercise Physiology* 45: 370-374, 1978.

153. **Wojtaszewski JF and Richter EA.** Glucose utilization during exercise: influence of endurance training. *Acta Physiologica Scandinavica* 162: 351-358, 1998.

154. **Wright JE.** *Anabolic Steroids and Athletics.* New York, NY: Macmillan, 1980.

155. **Wright JE.** *Anabolic Steroids and Sports.* New York, NY: Sports Science Consultants, 1982.

156. **Xanne A and Janse de Jonge X.** Effects of the menstrual cycle on exercise performance. *Sports Medicine* 33: 833-851, 2003.

157. **Yakovlev NN and Viru AA.** Adrenergic regulation of adaptation to muscular activity. *International Journal of Sports Medicine* 6: 255-265, 1985.

158. **Yesalis CE and Bahrke MS.** Anabolic-androgenic steroids. Current issues. *Sports Medicine* 19: 326-340, 1995.

159. **Young JC, Enslin J, and Kuca B.** Exercise intensity and glucose tolerance in trained and nontrained subjects. *Journal of Applied Physiology: Respiratory, Environmental and Exercise Physiology* 67: 39-43, 1989.

160. **Zazulak BT, Paterno M, Myer GD, Romani WA, and Hewett TE.** The effects of the menstrual cycle on anterior knee laxity: a systematic review. *Sports Medicine* 36: 847-862, 2006.

161. **Zouhal H, Jacob C, Delamarche P, and Gratas-Delamarche A.** Catecholamines and the effects of exercise, training, and gender. *Sports Medicine* 38: 401-423, 2008.

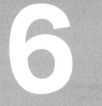

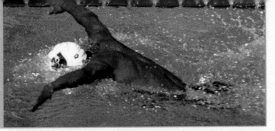

© Action Plus Sports Images/Alamy Stock Photo

Exercise and the Immune System

■ Objectives

By studying this chapter, you should be able to do the following:

1. Describe how the innate and acquired immune systems work together to protect against infection.

2. Discuss the key components that make up the innate immune system, and describe how the major elements of the innate immune system protect the body against infection.

3. Outline the primary components that compose the acquired immune system and explain how they protect against infection.

4. Explain the differences between acute and chronic inflammation.

5. Discuss the effects of moderate exercise training on the immune system and the risk of infection.

6. Explain how an acute bout of intense and prolonged (>90 minutes) exercise impacts immune function and the risk of infection.

7. Discuss how exercise in environmental extremes (heat, cold, and high altitude) influence immune function.

8. Explain the guidelines for exercise when you have a cold.

■ Outline

■ Key Terms

B-cells
complement system
cytokines
exercise immunology
immunity
inflammation
leukocytes
macrophages
natural killer cell
neutrophils
phagocytes
T-cells

The concept of homeostasis and the control systems that regulate the internal environment were introduced in Chap. 2. The immune system is a critical homeostatic system that recognizes and destroys foreign agents in the body. Obviously, this is important because the body is constantly under attack from foreign agents (e.g., bacteria, viruses, and fungi) that promote infection. By protecting the body against infection, the immune system plays an important role in maintaining homeostasis in the body.

Everyone has suffered from the unpleasant symptoms (i.e., runny nose and fever) of an upper respiratory tract infection (URTI). These URTIs are commonly referred to as colds and are caused by more than 200 different viruses (16). Currently, URTIs are the most common types of infections worldwide, and the average adult suffers from two to five colds a year (10, 25). Although colds are not usually life threatening in healthy individuals, colds have many negative consequences because of increased healthcare costs and lost days from work, school, and exercise training (12). Because of the high occurrence of colds, these illnesses present a real concern to the health of athletes and the general population. Since exercise and other stresses (e.g., emotional stress, loss of sleep, etc.) are known to influence the immune system, it is important to understand the relationship between physical activity and the immune system. Therefore, this chapter will introduce the primary components of the immune system and to discuss how exercise training affects this important homeostatic system. We begin with a brief overview of how the immune system works to prevent infection.

OVERVIEW OF THE IMMUNE SYSTEM

The term **immunity** refers to all of the mechanisms used in the body to protect against foreign agents. The origin of this term is from the Latin *immunitas* (meaning "freedom from") (4). Immunity results from a well-coordinated immune system that consists of complex cellular and chemical components that provide overlapping protection against infectious agents. This overlapping of immune system components is designed to ensure that these redundant systems are efficient in protecting the body against infection from pathogens (disease-causing agents) such as bacteria, viruses, and fungi. The redundancy of the immune system is achieved by the teamwork of two arms of the immune system referred to as the innate and acquired immune system (also called the adaptive or specific immune system). A short introduction to these two immune systems follows.

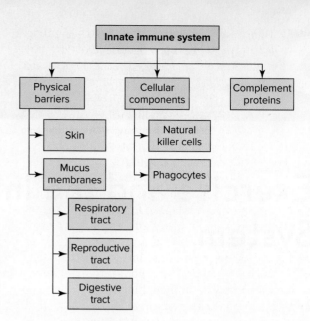

Figure 6.1 **Major components of innate immunity. See text for complete details.**

Innate Immune System

Humans and other animals are born with an innate, nonspecific immune system that is made up of a diverse collection of both cellular and protein elements. This system provides both physical barriers and internal defenses against foreign invaders (Fig. 6.1). Physical barriers are the first line of innate defense and are composed of barriers such as the skin and the mucus membranes (i.e., mucosa) that line our respiratory, digestive (gut), and genitourinary tracts. So, in order to cause trouble, bacteria and other foreign agents must cross these barriers. An invader that crosses the physical barrier of skin or mucosa is greeted by a second line of innate defense. This internal defense is composed of both specialized cells (e.g., phagocytes and natural killer cells) designed to destroy the invader, and a group of proteins called the complement system, which is located in the blood and tissues. The complement system is composed of more than 20 different proteins that work together to destroy foreign invaders; this system also signals other components of the immune system that the body has been attacked. Let's discuss each of these components of innate immunity in more detail.

Physical Barriers Again, the first line of defense against invaders is the physical barrier of the skin and the mucosa. Although we tend to think about the skin as being the primary barrier against foreign agents, the area covered by the skin is only about 2 square meters (29). In contrast, the area covered by the mucosa (i.e., respiratory, digestive, and genitourinary tracts) measures about 400 square meters (an area about the size of two tennis courts) (29). The key point here is that there is a larger perimeter that must be defended to keep unwanted foreign agents from entering the body.

Cellular Components Numerous types of immune cells exist to protect the body against infection, but a complete discussion of all these cells is beyond the scope of this chapter. Therefore, we will focus the discussion on a few types of cells that play a major role in the immune system. Specifically, we will direct our attention toward select members of the leukocyte family of immune cells that work together with another key immune cell, macrophages, to protect the body against infection. **Leukocytes** (also called white blood cells) are an important class of immune cells designed to recognize and remove foreign invaders (e.g., bacteria) in the body. Similarly, **macrophages** are another type of immune cell that is capable of engulfing bacteria and protecting against infection. Let's begin with a discussion of how the body produces these key cellular players in immune function.

Where do leukocytes come from? All blood cells (red and white) are made in the bone marrow, where they are produced from common "self-renewing" stem cells. These cells are self-renewing because when stem cells divide into two daughter cells, one of the daughter cells remains a stem cell (unspecialized cell), whereas the second daughter cell becomes a mature blood cell. This strategy of renewal ensures that there will always be stem cells available to produce mature blood cells.

When stem cells divide, the maturing daughter cell must make a choice as to what type of blood cell it will become when it matures. These choices are not random but are highly regulated by complicated control systems. Figure 6.2 illustrates the process of stem cells forming a bipotential stem cell that then can form a variety of different leukocytes. Table 6.1 provides a brief description of the function of each

of these leukocytes. Also, notice that macrophages are derived from a specific type of leukocyte called a monocyte (Fig. 6.2). In the next segments, we discuss the role that both leukocytes and monocytes play in innate immunity by protecting against both bacterial and viral infections.

Immune cells that consume (i.e., engulf) bacteria are classified as phagocytes. Specifically, **phagocytes** are cells that engulf foreign agents in a process called phagocytosis. To remove unwanted bacteria, the body produces several different types of phagocytes that participate in the innate immune system. Two key phagocytes are macrophages and neutrophils. Together, these important phagocytes form an important line of defense against infection.

As illustrated in Figure 6.2, macrophages are derived from monocytes. Macrophages are located in tissues throughout the body and are often called "professional" phagocytes because they make their living by destroying bacteria (29). When bacteria enter the body, macrophages recognize these invading cells and attach to the bacteria. This results in the bacteria being engulfed into a pouch (vesicle) that is moved inside the macrophage. When the bacterium is engulfed by the macrophage, the bacterium is killed by powerful chemicals and enzymes contained within the macrophage (4).

Macrophages can also contribute to innate immunity in two other important ways. First, when macrophages are destroying bacteria, they give off chemicals to increase the amount of blood flow to the infected site. This increased blood flow brings additional leukocytes to the area to assist in the battle of removing the invading bacteria.

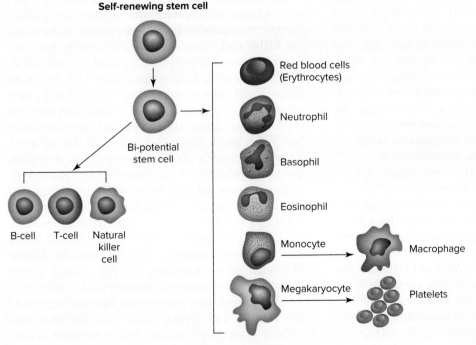

Figure 6.2 The formation of immune cells from stem cells within the bone marrow. See text for details.

TABLE 6.1 A Brief Overview of Leukocytes (White Blood Cells) and Their Function in Protecting against Foreign Invaders

Leukocyte (White Blood Cell)	Site Produced	Innate or Acquired Immunity	Functions
Neutrophils	Bone marrow	Innate	1. Phagocytosis 2. Release chemicals involved in inflammation (vasodilators, chemotaxins, etc.)
Basophils	Bone marrow	Innate	Release chemicals (e.g., histamine) involved in inflammation
Eosinophils	Bone marrow	Innate	1. Destroy multicellular parasites 2. Involved in hypersensitivity reactions
Monocytes	Bone marrow	Innate	Precursors of macrophages—Macrophages are important phagocytes involved in innate immunity.
Megakaryocytes	Bone marrow	Not involved in immune function	Precursors of platelets—platelets play an important role in blood clotting
B-cell (also called B-lymphocyte)	Bone marrow	Acquired	1. Initiate antibody-mediated reactions 2. Precursors of plasma cells—mature plasma cells secrete antibodies
T-cell (also called T-lymphocyte)	Bone marrow-activated in thymus	Acquired	Several different types of T-cells exist collectively; these cells participate in cell-mediated responses of the acquired immune system
Natural killer cells	Bone marrow	Innate	1. Bind directly to virus-infected cells and cancer cells to kill them 2. Function as killer cells in antibody-dependent immune response

Further, during the battle with bacteria, macrophages also produce proteins called cytokines. **Cytokines** are cell signals that regulate the immune system by facilitating communication between cells within the immune system (4). For example, some cytokines alert immune cells that the battle is on and cause these cells to exit the blood to help fight the rapidly multiplying bacteria (29). In this case, cytokines serve as a chemoattractant. Chemoattractants are chemicals that recruit other immune system "soldiers" to the battle site to assist in protecting the body from infection. Other cytokines promote fever, stimulate production of other components of the immune response, and promote inflammation (8).

Macrophages are not the only phagocytes involved in innate immunity. Indeed, neutrophils may be the most important phagocyte in innate immunity (29). **Neutrophils** are leukocytes that also participate as phagocytes during a bacterial invasion. Neutrophils have been called professional killers that are "on call" in the blood (29). After neutrophils have been summoned to the infected area, these important phagocytes exit the blood and become activated to begin destroying the foreign invaders. Similar to macrophages, neutrophils also produce cytokines that can alert other immune cells. Further, activated neutrophils also release chemicals that promote increased blood flow to the infected area.

In addition to the professional phagocytes (i.e., macrophages and neutrophils), another key cellular component of the innate immune system is the **natural killer cell**. These cells are produced in the bone marrow from stem cells (Fig. 6.2) and are "on call" to fight an infection. Most natural killer cells are found in the blood, liver, or spleen and when called to fight an infection, these cells exit the blood and move to the battle ground to take part in the fight. When they reach the battle site (i.e., location of the bacteria), natural killer cells play two key roles in defending us against infections. First, natural killer cells can destroy virus-infected cells, bacteria, parasites, fungi, and cancer cells. Second, natural killer cells also give off cytokines that help with immune defense. So, natural killer cells are an important part of the innate immune system because they are versatile "killers" of foreign agents, including bacteria, viruses, cancer cells, and other unwanted invaders of the body.

To summarize, phagocytes (macrophages and neutrophils) and natural killer cells are important cellular components of the innate immune system

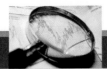

A CLOSER LOOK 6.1

Inflammation Is a Normal Part of the Immune Response

The word *inflammation* comes from the Latin word *inflammare*, which means "to set on fire." **Inflammation** is a normal part of the biological response to harmful stimuli, such as bacteria entering the body. In short, the goal of inflammation is to restore homeostasis by helping the injured tissue return to its normal state. Inflammation can be classified as either acute or chronic. A brief explanation of the differences between acute and chronic inflammation follows.

Acute Inflammation The following example illustrates an acute inflammatory response. At some time in your life, you have probably experienced a small cut on your finger or hand. In this case, the break in your skin allows bacteria to enter through the wound and results in an acute (i.e., brief) and localized inflammatory response. The clinical signs of localized inflammation are redness, swelling, heat, and pain. This occurs because of a cascade of events triggered by the innate immune system. The redness, swelling, and heat around the injured tissue result from the increased blood flow to the damaged area. This increased blood flow is triggered by the release of chemicals from phagocytes that are summoned to the infected area. Indeed, both macrophages and neutrophils release chemicals (e.g., bradykinin) that promote vasodilation (i.e., widening of the diameter of blood vessels). This vasodilation increases blood flow and fluid collection (i.e., edema) around the injured tissue. The pain associated with this type of local inflammatory response comes from chemicals (e.g., kinins) that stimulate pain receptors in the inflamed area.

Chronic Inflammation Typically, a small cut on your finger results in acute inflammation that is resolved within a few days when the immune system removes the invading bacteria, a scab forms, and the tissue returns to normal. However, chronic (i.e., unending) systemic inflammation occurs in situations of persistent infection (e.g., tuberculosis) or constant activation of the immune response as seen in diseases such as cancer, heart failure, rheumatoid arthritis, or chronic obstructive lung disease. Interestingly, both obesity and aging are also associated with chronic inflammation (1, 2). Regardless of the cause, chronic inflam-mation is associated with increased circulating cytokines and the so-called "acute-phase proteins" such as c-reactive protein. This is significant because chronically elevated blood levels of both cytokines and c-reactive proteins are thought to contribute to the risk of many diseases, including heart disease (1).

It is also important to appreciate that chronic systemic inflammation is not "all or none," but can exist in differing levels that are often described as "high grade" or "low grade" inflammation. A severe "high grade" level of inflammation might occur in patients suffering from certain types of cancers or rheumatoid arthritis. In contrast, even in the absence of diagnosed diseases, low grade inflammation can exist in both older and obese individuals (2). The health significance of "low grade" systemic inflammation is a hot topic in medicine because low grade inflammation has been linked to increased risks of cancer, Alzheimer disease, diabetes, and heart disease (1, 2). However, whether chronic inflammation actually causes all of these diseases or merely accompanies them is currently unknown.

and form the second line of defense against infection. Collectively, these cells remove dangerous invading agents and protect the body against infection whenever the physical barriers of defense are compromised (e.g., skin wound). When these cellular components of the innate immune system are activated following an infection, a physiologic response known as inflammation occurs. The hallmark signs of inflammation are redness, swelling, heat, and pain. More details about inflammation can be found in A Closer Look 6.1.

Complement System The **complement system** plays an important role in innate immunity and consists of numerous proteins that circulate in the blood in inactive forms. Like phagocytes and natural killer cells, the complement system is another component of the innate defense against infection. The more than 20 proteins that make up the complement system are produced primarily by the liver and are present in high concentrations in the blood and tissues (29). When the body is exposed to a foreign agent (e.g., bacterium), the complement system is activated to attack the invader. These activated complement proteins recognize the surface of the bacterium as a foreign agent and attach to the surface of the foreign cell. This triggers a rapid series of events resulting in the binding of more and more complement proteins on the surface of the bacteria. The addition of multiple complement proteins to the surface of the bacterium forms a "hole" (i.e., channel) in the surface of the bacterium. And once a bacterium has a hole in its membrane, the bacterium dies.

In addition to forming membrane attack complexes, the complement system performs two other jobs in innate immunity. The second function is to "tag" the cell surface of invading bacteria so that other cellular components (e.g., phagocytes) of the innate immune system can recognize and kill the invader. The third and final role of complement proteins is to serve as chemoattractants. As mentioned earlier, a chemoattractant recruits other immune players to the battle site to assist in protecting the body from infection.

To summarize, the complement system performs three important jobs when the body is invaded by

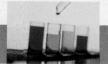
Edward Jenner Was the Pioneer of the Smallpox Vaccine

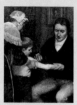

© Popperfoto/
Getty Images

Edward Jenner (1749–1823) was an English physician who played a major role in developing the smallpox vaccine. Because of this accomplishment, he is sometimes referred to as the "father of immunology." Here is the story behind Jenner's discovery of the smallpox vaccine.

After discovering that the immune system was adaptive, Jenner began vaccinating the English against smallpox in 1796. During the life of Jenner, smallpox was a huge health problem, and approximately 30 percent of the people infected with smallpox died. In fact, hundreds of thousands of people died from the disease, and many others were horribly disfigured (29). Two

observations led Edward Jenner to develop a vaccination procedure against smallpox. First, Jenner observed that milkmaids often contracted a disease called cowpox, which caused them to develop lesions that were similar to the sores associated with smallpox. Second, Jenner observed that the milkmaids that contracted cowpox almost never got smallpox, which, as it turns out, is a close relative of the cowpox virus (29). Based upon these observations, Jenner reasoned that exposure to a small amount of cowpox virus can promote immunity against smallpox.

To test this hypothesis, Jenner decided to perform a bold experiment. He collected pus from the sores of milkmaids infected with cowpox. He then injected this fluid into the arm of a young boy named James Phipps. This inoculation produced a

fever, but no great illness resulted. A few weeks following this treatment, Jenner then injected Phipps with pus collected from sores of a patient infected with smallpox. This daring experiment was a huge success because, remarkably, the young boy did not contract smallpox. However, Phipps was still able to contract other childhood diseases (e.g., measles). This illustrates one of the hallmarks of the adaptive immune system. That is, the acquired immune system adapts to defend against specific invaders.

Obviously, Jenner's experiments on this boy would not be performed today because of ethical concerns. Nonetheless, we can be thankful that Jenner's experiments were a success because it paved the way for future vaccines that have saved the lives of countless numbers of people around the world.

---

foreign agents. First, this system can destroy invaders by punching a hole in the surface of the invading bacterium. Second, it can enhance the function of other cells (e.g., phagocytes) within the immune system by tagging the invading agent for destruction. Third, it can alert other cells in the immune system that the body is being attacked. Importantly, all these functions of the complement system can respond rapidly to protect the body during invasion.

Acquired Immune System

Over 95 percent of all animals get along fine with only the innate immune system to protect them (29). However, for humans and other vertebrates, Mother Nature developed another layer of protection against disease, the acquired immune system. This system of immunity adapts to protect us against almost any type of invader. The primary purpose of the acquired immune system is to protect us against viruses because the innate immune system cannot eliminate many viruses (29). The first evidence that the acquired immune system existed was provided by Dr. Edward Jenner in the 1790s (see A Look Back—Important People in Science).

The acquired immune system is composed of highly specialized cells and processes that prevent or eliminate invading pathogens. This adaptive immune response provides us with the ability to recognize and remember specific pathogens (i.e., to generate

immunity) and to mount stronger attacks each time a repeating pathogen is encountered. Therefore, this system is sometimes called the *adaptive immune system* because it prepares itself for future pathogen challenges.

The major cells involved in the acquired immune system are B-cells (also called B-lymphocytes) and T-cells (also called T-lymphocytes). Both B- and T-cells are members of the leukocyte family of blood cells that have their origin from stem cells located within bone marrow (Fig. 6.2). A brief overview of how B- and T-cells function in acquired immunity follows.

B-Cells These cells are produced in the bone marrow and play a key role in specific immunity and combat both bacterial and viral infections by secreting antibodies into the blood. **B-cells** function as antibody factories and can produce more than 100 million different types of antibodies that are required to protect us against a wide variety of invading antigens. Antibodies (also called immunoglobulins) are proteins manufactured by B-cells to help fight against foreign substances called *antigens*. Antigens are any substance that stimulates the immune system to produce antibodies. For example, bacteria, viruses, or fungi are all antigens. Further, antigens that promote an allergic response are commonly called allergens. Common allergens include pollen, animal dander, dust, and the contents of certain foods. When the body is confronted by these antigens, B-cells respond by producing antibodies to protect against this invasion.

Although the body can produce more than 100 million different antibodies, there are five general classes of antibodies, and each has a different function. The five classes of antibodies are IgG, IgA, IgM, IgD, and IgE. The abbreviation Ig stands for immunoglobulin (i.e., antibody). A detailed discussion of the specific function of each of these classes of antibodies exceeds the goals of this chapter. However, an example of how two classes of antibodies function is useful in understanding the role of antibodies in protecting against disease.

When B-cells are activated by an invading antigen, IgM is one of the first classes of antibodies produced. Producing this antibody early during an infection is a good strategy because IgM antibodies can protect against invaders in two important ways. First, IgM antibodies can activate the complement cascade to assist in removing the unwanted invader. In fact, the term *complement* was coined by immunologists when they discovered that antibodies were much more effective in dealing with invaders if they are complemented by other proteins—the complement system (29). Second, IgM antibodies are good at neutralizing viruses by binding to them and preventing the virus from infecting cells. Hence, because of these combined properties, the IgM is the perfect "first" antibody to protect against viral or bacterial invasions (29).

IgG antibodies are another important class of antibodies. These antibodies circulate in the blood and other body fluids and defend against invading bacteria and viruses (33). The binding of IgG antibodies to bacterial or viral antigens activates other immune cells (e.g., macrophages, neutrophils, and natural killer cells) that destroy these invaders and protect us against disease.

T-Cells **T-cells** are a family of immune cells produced in the bone marrow. T-cells and B-cells differ in several ways. First, while B-cells mature in the bone marrow, T-cells mature in a specialized immune organ called the thymus; this is why they are called T-cells. Further, T-cells do not produce antibodies but specialize in recognizing protein antigens in the body. There are three main types of T-cells: (1) killer T-cells (also called cytotoxic T-cells); (2) helper T-cells; and (3) regulatory T-cells. Killer T-cells are a potent weapon against viruses because they can recognize and kill virus-infected cells (6). Helper T-cells secrete cytokines that have a dramatic effect on other immune system cells. In this way, helper T-cells serve as the quarterback of the immune system by directing the action of other immune cells. Finally, as the name implies, the regulatory T-cells are involved in regulation of immune function. Specifically, these cells play a role in inhibiting responses to both self-antigens (i.e., preventing the immune system from attacking

normal body cells) and foreign antigens. In this way, regulatory T-cells help to regulate self-tolerance and prevent autoimmune diseases (4).

IN SUMMARY

- The human immune system is a complex and redundant system designed to protect us against invading pathogens.
- A healthy immune system requires the teamwork of two layers of immune protection: (1) innate immune system and (2) acquired immune system.
- The innate system protects against foreign invaders and is composed of three major components: (1) physical barriers such as the skin and the mucous membranes that line our respiratory, digestive, and genitourinary tracts; (2) specialized cells (e.g., phagocytes and natural killer cells) designed to destroy invaders; and (3) a group of proteins called the complement system, which are located throughout the body to protect against invaders.
- The acquired immune system adapts to protect against almost any type of invading pathogen. The primary purpose of the acquired immune system is to provide protection against viruses that the innate immune system cannot provide. B- and T-cells are the major cells involved in the acquired immune system. B-cells produce antibodies, whereas T-cells specialize in recognizing and removing antigens in the body.

EXERCISE AND THE IMMUNE SYSTEM

The field of **exercise immunology** is defined as the study of exercise, psychological, and environmental influences on immune function. Compared to other areas of exercise physiology research, exercise immunology is relatively new. However, interest in the field of exercise immunology has grown rapidly during the past two decades. In the following sections, we will discuss several important topics related to the effects of exercise on resistance to infection.

Exercise and Resistance to Infection

The concept that exercise can have both a positive and a negative effect on the risk of infection is almost two decades old. This idea was introduced by Dr. David Nieman when he described the risk of a URTI as a J-shaped curve that changed as a function of the intensity and amount of exercise being performed (Fig. 6.3). Note in Figure 6.3 that people engaging

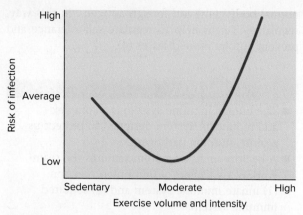

Figure 6.3 "J" shaped model of the relationship between varying amounts of exercise and the risk of URTI. This model suggests that moderate aerobic exercise reduces the risk of infection, whereas high-intensity/long-duration exercise may increase the risk of infection (19).

in regular bouts of moderate exercise are at a lower risk of a URTI compared to sedentary individuals and people who engage in intense and/or long-duration exercise sessions. For example, marathon runners represent those at the high end of the exercise intensity and duration scale. Indeed, running a marathon increases the risk of a URTI in the days following the run (24). In the next two segments, we discuss the reasons why moderate- and high-intensity exercise have different effects on the risk of infection.

Moderate Aerobic Exercise Protects against Infection Although controversy exists, several studies support the concept that people who engage in regular bouts of moderate aerobic exercise catch fewer colds (i.e., URTIs) than both sedentary individuals and people who engage in high-intensity/long-duration exercise (22, 23). For example, both epidemiological and randomized studies consistently report that regular exercise results in an 18% to 67% reduction in the

risk of URTI (9). Interestingly, this exercise-induced protection against infection can be achieved with many types of aerobic activity (e.g., walking, jogging, cycling, swimming, sports play, and aerobic dance). In general, it appears that 20 to 40 minutes of moderate-intensity exercise (i.e., 40% to 60% of $\dot{V}O_2$ max) per day is adequate to promote a beneficial effect on the immune system. Importantly, this exercise-induced reduction in the risk of URTI occurs in both young adult and middle age men and women (22). Further, regular aerobic exercise appears to benefit the immune system in older individuals as well (28). See Clinical Applications 6.1 for more details on the impact of exercise on the aging immune system.

The explanation as to why moderate-intensity exercise protects against URTI remains a topic of debate. Nonetheless, there are several possible reasons to explain this. First, each bout of moderate aerobic exercise causes an increase in blood levels of natural killer cells, neutrophils, and antibodies (9). Therefore, an acute bout of exercise provides a positive boost to both the innate immune system (natural killer cells and neutrophils) and the acquired immune system (antibodies). Note that this exercise-induced boost in immune function is transient and that the immune system returns to pre-exercise levels within three hours. Nonetheless, it seems that each bout of exercise improves immune function against pathogens over a short period, which results in a reduced risk of infection (22). Other factors might also contribute to the positive impact of routine exercise on the reduced risk of infection. For example, people who engage in regular exercise may also benefit from an improved psychological well-being (i.e., less emotional stress), good nutritional status, and a healthy lifestyle (e.g., adequate sleep). Each of these factors has been linked to a reduced risk of infection and, therefore, may also contribute to the connection between regular exercise and lowered risk for URTI.

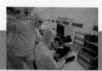

CLINICAL APPLICATIONS 6.1

Is Regular Exercise a Friend or Foe of the Aging Immune System?

Aging is associated with a decline in the normal function of the immune system, which is referred to as "immunosenescence." For example, older individuals (e.g., >70 years old) often have poor vaccine responses and an increased risk of infection and cancer (28). Although the possibility exists that high-intensity exercise may suppress the immune

system in older individuals, most research suggests that regular bouts of moderate-intensity aerobic exercise can improve immune function in older individuals (28, 32). The positive effects of exercise on the immune system in older persons is evidenced by enhanced vaccination responses, increased numbers of T-cells, lower circulating levels

of inflammatory cytokines, and increased neutrophil phagocytic activity (28). Nonetheless, whether exercise can completely reverse or prevent immunosenescence remains a debated topic, and more research is required to reveal the optimal volume and intensity of exercise to improve immune function in older individuals.

Although it appears that aerobic exercise provides protection against colds, it remains unknown if resistance exercise training provides the same level of protection against infection. This is because few studies have systematically investigated the impact of resistance exercise on immune function. Nonetheless, based on the available evidence, it appears that an acute bout of resistance exercise results in a transient increase in natural killer cells (15). However, this immune boost is temporary because blood levels of primary immune cells return to normal within a short period following a resistance training session (5). To summarize, it appears that regular bouts of resistance exercise might protect against infection, but additional research is required to firmly establish that resistance exercise alone is effective in providing protection against URTIs.

High-Intensity/Long-Duration Aerobic Exercise Increases the Risk of Infection

The idea that athletes engaged in intense training are more susceptible to infections originated from anecdotal reports from coaches and athletes. For instance, the marathon runner Alberto Salazar reported that he caught 12 colds in 12 months while training for the 1984 Olympic marathon (17). Because Salazar was engaged in intense exercise training, many people reasoned that the high level of exercise training was responsible for his increased number of colds. However, anecdotal reports do not prove cause and effect, and scientific studies were required to determine if intense exercise training leads to an increased risk of infection. Although controversy exists (31), several studies support the concept that athletes engaged in intense endurance training suffer a higher incidence of URTI compared to sedentary individuals or people engaged in moderate exercise (Fig. 6.3) (9, 21, 24). For example, compared to the general population, evidence indicates that sore throats and flu-like symptoms are more common in athletes involved in intense training (11, 24). Indeed, the risk of developing a URTI is two- to sixfold higher in athletes following a marathon compared to the general public (24). This increased risk of illness is a concern for athletes because even minor infections can impair exercise performance and the ability to sustain intense exercise training (27). Further, prolonged viral infections are often associated with the development of persistent fatigue, which poses another threat to the athlete (7).

There are several reasons why high-intensity and long-duration exercise promotes an increased risk of infection (9). First, prolonged (>90 minutes) and intense exercise has a temporary depressive effect on the immune system. For example, after a marathon,

the following major changes occur in immune function:

- Decreased blood levels of B-cells, T-cells, and natural killer cells
- Decrease in natural killer cell activity and T-cell function
- Decrease in nasal neutrophil phagocytosis
- Decrease in nasal and salivary IgA levels
- Increase in pro- and anti-inflammatory cytokines

Collectively, these changes result in a depression of the immune system's ability to defend against invading pathogens. It has been argued that this immune suppression following a marathon provides an "open window," during which viruses and bacteria can gain a foothold and increase the risk of infection (see Fig. 6.4).

The biological reason to explain why intense exercise promotes immune depression is probably related to the immunosuppressive effects of stress hormones such as cortisol (8). You may recall from Chap. 5 that prolonged strenuous exercise results in large increases in the circulating levels of cortisol. High cortisol levels have been reported to depress immune system function in several ways (8). For example, high levels of cortisol can inhibit the function of specific cytokines, suppress natural killer cell function, and depress both the production and function of T-cells (20).

Although strenuous exercise can depress immune function, other factors may also contribute to the increased risk of infection in athletes engaged in intense training. For example, athletes engaged in intense training may also be exposed to other potential stressors, including a lack of sleep, mental stress, increased exposure to pathogens due to large crowds, air travel, and inadequate diet to support immune health

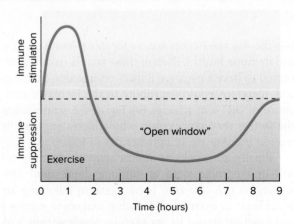

Figure 6.4 The open window theory is a potential explanation for why high-intensity exercise increases the risk of infection. In brief, prolonged exercise (e.g., marathon-type exertion) leads to immune depression that increases the likelihood for opportunistic upper respiratory tract infections (21).

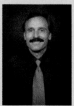

Courtesy of David C. Nieman

Dr. David Nieman, a professor in the Department of Health, Leisure, and Exercise Science at Appalachian State University, is an internationally known expert on stress and human immune function. Specifically, Dr. Nieman's research has addressed numerous important questions related to the impact of both exercise and nutrition on the risk of infection in athletes. In this feature, Dr. Nieman answers questions about the impact of diet and nutritional supplements on immune function in athletes.

QUESTION: Nutritional deficiencies have been shown to impair immune function. What nutritional advice can you provide to athletes regarding the importance of adequate energy intake and the balance of macronutrient consumption during periods of intense training?

ANSWER: Low energy intake leading to rapid weight loss and muscle wasting has a profound, negative effect on immune function. However, when energy intake matches energy expenditure, a wide range in the macronutrient and micronutrient content of the diet is compatible with healthy immune function. Low energy intake is just one of several lifestyle factors that influence immune function, and others include heavy exertion, mental stress, sleep disruption, and poor hygienic practices. All of these factors together can seriously undermine immune function, increasing the risk for certain infections, including URTI.

QUESTION: Some reports suggest that consumption of carbohydrate (30–60 g CHO/hour) during prolonged exercise can reduce the degree of exercise-induced immunosuppression. How strong is the experimental evidence to support this claim?

ANSWER: Multiple research teams have investigated this question since the mid-1990s. In general, ingesting 30 to 60 grams carbohydrate during each hour of running, cycling, or similar aerobic exercise keeps blood glucose higher when compared to no-carbohydrate conditions, lowers blood levels of stress hormones such as cortisol and epinephrine, and, as a result, takes the edge off post-exercise immune inflammatory responses. Nonetheless, consumption of carbohydrates during exercise does not protect against the transient decrease in immune function that is experienced by athletes after long exercise bouts.

QUESTION: Numerous advertisements claim that specific nutritional supplements can improve immune function and reduce the risk of infection. In your opinion, are there nutritional supplements that can provide the athlete with increased protection against the risk of URTI?

ANSWER: There is a growing realization that extra vitamins, minerals, and amino acids do not provide countermeasure immune benefits for healthy and well-fed athletes during heavy training. As a result, the focus has shifted to other types of nutritional components such as probiotics, bovine colostrum, β-glucan, flavonoids, and polyphenols such as quercetin, resveratrol, curcumin, and epigallicatechin-3-gallate (EGCG), N-3 polyunsaturated fatty acids (N-3 PUFAs or fish oil), herbal supplements, and unique plant extracts (e.g., green tea extract, black currant extract, tomato extract with lycopene, anthocyanin-rich extract from bilberry, polyphenol-rich pomegranate fruit extract). More well-designed studies with human subjects are needed before enthusiastic support is given to any of these supplements. Some exert impressive effects when cultured with specialized cells and in animal-based models, but then fail when studied under double-blinded, placebo-controlled conditions in human athletes.

(see the Ask the Expert feature for more details on diet and immune health). Each of these factors has been reported to have a negative impact on immune function and, therefore, could contribute to the increased incidence of URTIs in athletes (9). Figure 6.5 summarizes the factors that may explain why athletes engaged in intense training are at a greater risk of infection.

Finally, do weeks of intense exercise training result in a chronic state of immune depression? The answer to this question is no, because following an acute bout of exercise, circulating leukocyte number and function return to pre-exercise levels within 3 to 24 hours (8). Further, comparisons of leukocyte number and other markers of immune function between athletes and nonathletes do not differ markedly (8). Therefore, in the resting state, immune function is not different between athletes and nonathletes.

Factors affecting susceptibility to infection in athletes

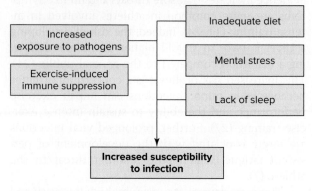

Figure 6.5 Several factors may explain why athletes engaged in intense training are at a greater risk of infection; these include increased exposure to pathogens, exercise-induced immune suppression, inadequate diet, mental stress, and lack of sleep.

- Exercise can have both a positive and a negative effect on the risk of infection. The relationship between the intensity/amount of exercise and the risk of developing a URTI is described as a J-shaped curve (Fig. 6.3). This J-shaped curve illustrates that moderate-intensity aerobic exercise decreases the risk of infection, whereas high-intensity/prolonged exercise increases the risk of infection.
- Regular aerobic exercise can reduce the risk of infection in several ways. In particular, an acute bout of moderate exercise increases blood levels of antibodies, natural killer cells, and neutrophils that provide a positive boost to the immune system.
- The fact that moderate aerobic exercise provides a transient boost to the immune system is another example of how regular exercise can enhance a control system in the body to preserve homeostasis. Indeed, by protecting the body against infection, the immune system plays an important role in maintaining homeostasis.
- High-intensity/long-duration exercise has been shown to have a temporary depressive effect on the immune system. This acute immune suppression following an intense exercise session provides an "open window" during which viruses and bacteria can grow, resulting in an infection.

EXERCISING IN ENVIRONMENTAL EXTREMES: INCREASED RISK FOR INFECTION?

Exercise in environmental extremes (e.g., heat, cold, and high altitude) can increase circulating stress hormones such as cortisol (31). Given that high levels of cortisol can depress immune function, does exercise in environmental extremes result in immune depression and increase the risk of infection? Let's review the evidence regarding the effects of exercise in hot, cold, and high-altitude environments on the immune system.

Exercising in a hot versus cool environment results in significant increases in body temperature and elevates circulating levels of stress hormones (31). In theory, this increase in circulating stress hormones could pose a threat to immune function. Nonetheless, laboratory studies indicate that exercise in a hot environment does not significantly impair the function of key cells involved in immune function (e.g., neutrophils and natural killer cells) (26, 31). Therefore, exercising in the heat does not pose a greater threat to immune function than exercise in a cool environment.

It is commonly believed that being exposed to cold weather increases the susceptibility to URTIs. Indeed, the use of the term *colds* may have come from the belief that cold exposure causes URTI (31). Several studies have investigated the impact of short- and long-term cold exposure with/without exercise on key elements of the immune system. Collectively, these investigations provide limited evidence to indicate that cold exposure increases your risk of infection. For example, both acute exposure and repeated bouts of cold exposure increase the number of circulating neutrophils, T- and B-cells, and natural killer cells in non-exercising subjects (13). Therefore, cold exposure alone does not have a negative impact on the immune system; indeed, cold exposure appears to have a positive effect on the immune system (31). Studies also demonstrate that exercise in a cold environment does not suppress immune function (31). Therefore, current evidence does not support the popular belief that short- or long-term cold exposure, with or without exercise, suppresses immune function and increases the risk of infection (31).

Endurance exercise performed at high altitudes (e.g., >6,000 feet above sea level) impairs performance and is associated with increased levels of stress hormones that could depress immune function. Nonetheless, laboratory studies indicate that acute exercise at simulated high altitude does not impair immune function. In fact, a single bout of exercise in a simulated high-altitude condition results in increased circulating levels of leukocytes (14). In contrast to these laboratory studies, field studies conducted in the mountains suggest that living and exercising at high altitude depresses immune function and increases the risk of URTI (3, 30). The increased risk of infection that occurs during prolonged exposure to high altitudes may arise from a combination of stresses, such as low arterial oxygen levels, high altitude-related sleep disorders, and acute mountain sickness. Regardless of the mechanisms involved, prolonged high-altitude exposure combined with exercise appears to impair the immune system and increase the risk of URTI (31).

- Although exercise in the heat can increase circulating levels of stress hormones, exercise in a hot environment does not pose a greater threat to immune function compared to exercise in a cool environment.
- Research does not support the popular belief that short- or long-term cold exposure, with or without exercise, suppresses immune function and increases the risk of infection.
- Prolonged high-altitude exposure (i.e., living in the mountains) combined with exercise can increase the risk of URTI.

SHOULD YOU EXERCISE WHEN YOU HAVE A COLD?

Anyone who exercises on a regular basis has been faced with the decision of whether to skip a workout or exercise during a cold. This is often a difficult decision because of the uncertainty as to whether a bout of exercise will worsen your illness or perhaps make you feel better. The next time that you are faced with a cold, here are some general guidelines to follow when you are making the decision as to whether you should exercise or take the day off. It is typically okay to exercise with a cold if your symptoms are above the neck (18). That is, if your cold symptoms are limited to a runny nose, nasal congestion, and a mild sore throat (18). Nonetheless, you should probably reduce the intensity of workout during a cold and avoid high-intensity/long-duration workouts. If your cold symptoms get worse with physical activity, stop exercise and rest. You can restart your workout routine gradually as you begin to feel better.

In contrast to this advice there are some situations when you should not exercise. For example, postpone your workout if your cold symptoms are below the neck (i.e., chest congestion, cough, or stomach pain). Further, don't exercise if you have a fever, general fatigue, or widespread muscle aches (18). You can resume training when the below-the-neck cold symptoms have passed and your fever is no longer present. For more details on when athletes can return to training and competition following a URTI, see Ahmadinejad et al. (2014) in the suggested reading list.

IN SUMMARY

- It is reasonable to exercise during a cold if your symptoms are limited to a runny nose, nasal congestion, and a mild sore throat.
- It is not wise to exercise if your cold symptoms are below the neck (i.e., chest congestion, cough, or stomach pain). Also, don't exercise if you have a fever, general fatigue, or widespread muscle aches.

STUDY ACTIVITIES

1. Describe how the innate and acquired immune systems work as a unit to protect the body against infection.
2. Define the key components that make up the innate immune system (e.g., macrophages, neutrophils, natural killer cells, and complement system), and describe how these elements protect against infection.
3. List the primary components of the acquired immune system (e.g., B-cells, antibodies, and T-cells), and explain how they protect against infection.
4. Describe the differences between acute and chronic inflammation.
5. Outline the effects of moderate exercise training on the immune system and the risk of infection.
6. Explain how an acute bout of intense and prolonged (>90 minutes) exercise affects immune function and the risk of infection.
7. Discuss the impact of exercise in hot, cold, and high-altitude environments on the immune system and the risk of infection.
8. Discuss the guidelines for deciding whether it is wise to exercise when you have a cold.

SUGGESTED READINGS

Ahmadinejad, A., N. Alijani, S. Mansori, and V. Ziaee. 2014. Common sports-related infections: a review on clinical pictures, management, and time to return to sports. *Asian Journal of Sports Medicine.* 5: 1–9.

Coico, R., and G. Sunshine. 2015. *Immunology: A Short Course.* Hoboken, NJ: Wiley-Blackwell.

Gleeson, M., and N. Walsh. 2012. The BASES expert statement on exercise, immunity, and infection. *Journal of Sports Science.* 30: 321–324.

Simpson, R. J., T. Lowder, G. Spielmann, A. Bigley, and E. LaVoy. 2012. Exercise and the aging immune system. *Ageing Research Reviews.* 11: 404–420.

Somppayrac, L. 2015. *How the Immune System Works.* Hoboken, NJ: Wiley-Blackwell.

Walsh, N., and S. Oliver. 2015. Exercise, immune function, and respiratory infection: an update on the influence of training and environmental stress. *Immunology and Cell Biology.* 5th edition. 1–8.

REFERENCES

1. **Ahmad A, Banerjee S, Wang Z, Kong D, Majumdar AP, and Sarkar FH.** Aging and inflammation: etiological culprits of cancer. *Current Aging Science* 2: 174–186, 2009.
2. **Balistreri CR, Caruso C, and Candore G.** The role of adipose tissue and adipokines in obesity-related inflammatory diseases. *Mediators of Inflammation.* doi:10.1155/2010/802078.
3. **Chouker A, Demetz F, Martignoni A, Smith L, Setzer F, Bauer A, et al.** Strenuous physical exercise inhibits granulocyte activation induced by high altitude. *Journal of Applied Physiology* 98: 640–647, 2005.
4. **Coico R and Sunshine G.** *Immunology: A Short Course.* Hoboken, NJ: Wiley-Blackwell, 2015.
5. **Flynn MG, Fahlman M, Braun WA, Lambert CP, Bouillon LE, Brolinson PG, et al.** Effects of

resistance training on selected indexes of immune function in elderly women. *Journal of Applied Physiology* 86: 1905-1913, 1999.

6. **Fox S.** *Human Physiology.* Boston, MA: McGraw-Hill, 2015.

7. **Friman G and Ilback NG.** Acute infection: metabolic responses, effects on performance, interaction with exercise, and myocarditis. *International Journal of Sports Medicine* 19 (Suppl 3): S172-182, 1998.

8. **Gleeson M.** *Immune Function in Sport and Exercise.* Philadelphia, PA: Elsevier, 2006.

9. **Gleeson M.** Immune function in sport and exercise. *Journal of Applied Physiology* 103: 693-699, 2007.

10. **Graham N.** The epidemiology of acute respiratory tract infections in children and adults: a global perspective. *Epidemiological Reviews* 12: 149-178, 1990.

11. **Heath GW, Ford ES, Craven TE, Macera CA, Jackson KL, and Pate RR.** Exercise and the incidence of upper respiratory tract infections. *Medicine & Science in Sports & Exercise* 23: 152-157, 1991.

12. **Heath GW, Macera CA, and Nieman DC.** Exercise and upper respiratory tract infections. Is there a relationship? *Sports Medicine* 14: 353-365, 1992.

13. **Jansky L, Pospisilova D, Honzova S, Ulicny B, Sramek P, Zeman V, et al.** Immune system of cold-exposed and cold-adapted humans. *European Journal of Applied Physiology and Occupational Physiology* 72: 445-450, 1996.

14. **Klokker M, Kjaer M, Secher NH, Hanel B, Worm L, Kappel M, et al.** Natural killer cell response to exercise in humans: effect of hypoxia and epidural anesthesia. *Journal of Applied Physiology* 78: 709-716, 1995.

15. **Miles MP, Kraemer WJ, Grove DS, Leach SK, Dohi K, Bush JA, et al.** Effects of resistance training on resting immune parameters in women. *European Journal of Applied Physiology* 87: 506-508, 2002.

16. **Monto A.** Epidemiology of viral infections. *American Journal of Medicine* 112: 4S-12S, 2002.

17. **Nieman DC.** Can too much exercise increase the risk of sickness? *Sports Science Exchange* 11 (Suppl): 69, 1998.

18. **Nieman DC.** Current perspective on exercise immunology. *Current Sports Medicine Reports* 2: 239-242, 2003.

19. **Nieman DC.** Exercise, upper respiratory tract infection, and the immune system. *Medicine & Science in Sports & Exercise* 26: 128-139, 1994.

20. **Nieman DC.** Immune response to heavy exertion. *Journal of Applied Physiology* 82: 1385-1394, 1997.

21. **Nieman DC.** Marathon training and immune function. *Sports Medicine* 37: 412-415, 2007.

22. **Nieman DC, Henson DA, Austin MD, and Sha W.** Upper respiratory tract infection is reduced in physically fit and active adults. *British Journal of Sports Medicine* 45: 987-992, 2011.

23. **Nieman DC, Henson DA, Gusewitch G, Warren BJ, Dotson RC, Butterworth DE, et al.** Physical activity and immune function in elderly women. *Medicine & Science in Sports & Exercise* 25: 823-831, 1993.

24. **Nieman DC, Johanssen LM, Lee JW, and Arabatzis K.** Infectious episodes in runners before and after the Los Angeles Marathon. *Journal of Sports Medicine and Physical Fitness* 30: 316-328, 1990.

25. **NIH.** The common cold. **www.niaidnihgov/topics/commoncold**, 2010.

26. **Peake J, Peiffer JJ, Abbiss CR, Nosaka K, Okutsu M, Laursen PB, et al.** Body temperature and its effect on leukocyte mobilization, cytokines and markers of neutrophil activation during and after exercise. *European Journal of Applied Physiology* 102: 391-401, 2008.

27. **Roberts JA.** Viral illnesses and sports performance. *Sports Medicine* 3: 298-303, 1986.

28. **Simpson RJ, Lowder T, Spielmann G, Bigley A, and LaVoy E.** Exercise and the aging immune system. *Ageing Research Reviews* 11: 404-420, 2012.

29. **Somppayrac, L.** *How the Immune System Works.* Hoboken, NJ: Wiley-Blackwell, 2012.

30. **Tiollier E, Schmitt L, Burnat P, Fouillot JP, Robach P, Filaire E, et al.** Living high-training low altitude training: effects on mucosal immunity. *European Journal of Applied Physiology* 94: 298-304, 2005.

31. **Walsh N and Oliver S.** Exercise, immune function, and respiratory infection: an update on the influence of training and environmental stress. *Immunology and Cell Biology.* doi: 10.1038: 1-8, 2015.

32. **Walsh N, et al.** Position statement. Part one. Immune system and exercise. *Exercise Immunology Reviews* 17: 6-63, 2011.

33. **Widmaier E, Raff H, and Strang K.** *Vander's Human Physiology.* Boston, MA: McGraw-Hill, 2015.

7

© Action Plus Sports Images/Alamy Stock Photo

The Nervous System: Structure and Control of Movement

■ Objectives

By studying this chapter, you should be able to do the following:

1. Discuss the general organization of the nervous system.
2. Describe the structure and function of a nerve.
3. Draw and label the pathways involved in a withdrawal reflex.
4. Define depolarization, action potential, and repolarization.
5. Discuss the role of position receptors in the control of movement.
6. Describe the role of the vestibular apparatus in maintaining equilibrium.
7. Discuss the areas of the brain involved in voluntary control of movement.
8. Describe the structure and function of the autonomic nervous system.

■ Outline

■ Key Terms

action potential
afferent fibers
autonomic nervous system
axon
brain stem
cell body
central nervous system (CNS)
cerebellum
cerebrum
conductivity
dendrites
efferent fibers
excitatory postsynaptic potentials (EPSPs)
Golgi tendon organs (GTOs)
homeostasis
inhibitory postsynaptic potential (IPSP)
irritability
kinesthesia
motor cortex
motor neuron
motor unit
muscle spindle
neurons
neurotransmitter
parasympathetic nervous system
peripheral nervous system (PNS)
proprioceptors
reciprocal inhibition
resting membrane potential
Schwann cells
size principle
spatial summation
sympathetic nervous system
synapses
temporal summation
vestibular apparatus

The nervous system provides the body with a rapid means of internal communication that allows us to move about, talk, and coordinate the activity of billions of cells. Thus, neural activity is critically important in the body's ability to maintain homeostasis. This chapter will provide an overview of the nervous system, with emphasis on neural control of voluntary movement. We will begin with a discussion of the general function of the nervous system.

GENERAL NERVOUS SYSTEM FUNCTIONS

The nervous system is the body's means of perceiving and responding to events in the internal and external environments. Receptors capable of sensing touch, pain, temperature changes, and chemical stimuli send information to the **central nervous system (CNS)** concerning changes in our environment (5). The CNS can respond to these stimuli in several ways. The response may be involuntary movement (e.g., rapid removal of a hand from a hot surface) or alteration in the rate of release of some hormone from the endocrine system (see Chap. 5). In addition to integrating body activities and controlling voluntary movement, the nervous system is responsible for storing experiences (memory) and establishing patterns of response based on previous experiences (learning). Let's begin our discussion of the nervous system by reviewing the general organization.

ORGANIZATION OF THE NERVOUS SYSTEM

Anatomically, the nervous system can be divided into two main parts: the CNS and the **peripheral nervous system (PNS).** The CNS is the portion of the nervous system contained in the skull (brain) and the spinal cord; the PNS consists of nerve cells (neurons) outside the CNS (see Fig. 7.1). Recall from your previous courses in physiology that the term *innervation* refers to the supply of nerves to a particular organ (e.g., skeletal muscle). In other words, the term *innervation* means that nerves are connected to a particular organ.

The PNS can be further subdivided into two sections: (1) the sensory portion and (2) the motor portion. The sensory division is responsible for transmission of neuron impulses from sense organs (receptors) to the CNS. These sensory nerve fibers, which conduct information toward the CNS, are called **afferent fibers.** The motor portion of the

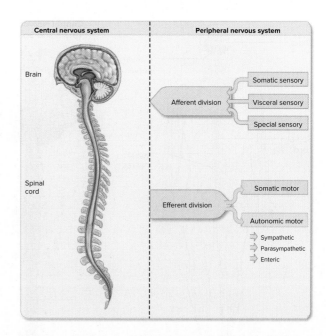

Figure 7.1 Overview of the anatomical divisions of the nervous system.

PNS can be further subdivided into the somatic motor division (which innervates skeletal muscle) and autonomic motor division (which innervates involuntary effector organs like smooth muscle surrounding blood vessels, cardiac muscle, and glands). Motor nerve fibers, which conduct impulses away from the CNS, are referred to as **efferent fibers.** The relationships between the CNS and the PNS are visualized in Figure 7.2.

IN SUMMARY

- The nervous system is the body's means of perceiving and responding to events in the internal and external environments. Receptors capable of sensing touch, pain, temperature, and chemical stimuli send information to the CNS concerning changes in our environment. The CNS responds by either voluntary movement or a change in the rate of release of specific hormones from the endocrine system, depending on which response is appropriate.
- The nervous system is divided into two major divisions: (1) the central nervous system and (2) the peripheral nervous system. The central nervous system includes the brain and the spinal cord, whereas the peripheral nervous system includes the nerves outside the central nervous system.
- The PNS is divided into afferent and efferent divisions.

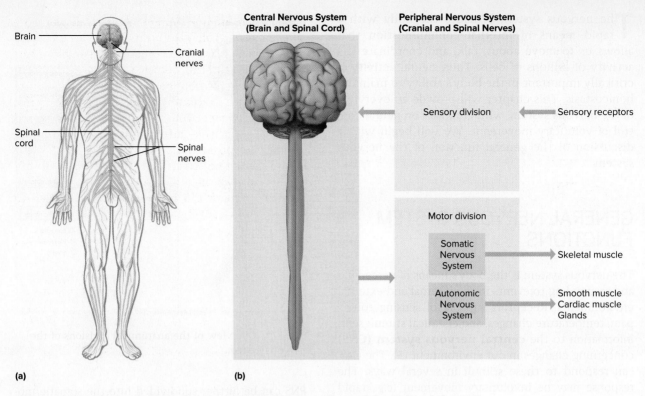

Figure 7.2 The relationship between the motor and sensory fibers of the PNS and the CNS.

Structure of the Neuron

The functional unit of the nervous system is the **neuron.** Anatomically, neurons are cells that are typically composed of three regions: (1) **cell body,** (2) dendrites, and (3) axon (see Fig. 7.3). The center of operation for the neuron is the **cell body,** which contains the nucleus. Dendrites and axons are processes (i.e., extensions) from the cell body. Dendrites are thin, branched processes that extend from the neuron cell body. **Dendrites** serve as a receptive area that can conduct electrical impulses toward the cell body. The **axon** (also called the nerve fiber) is a longer process that carries the electrical message (called action potentials) away from the cell body toward another neuron or effector organ. Axons vary in length from a few millimeters to a meter (14). Each neuron has only one axon; however, the axon can divide into several collateral branches that terminate at other neurons, muscle cells, or glands (Fig. 7.3). Contact points between an axon of one neuron and the dendrite of another neuron are called **synapses** (see Fig. 7.4).

In large nerve fibers like those innervating skeletal muscle, the axons are covered with an insulating layer of cells called **Schwann cells.** The membranes of Schwann cells contain a large amount of a lipid-protein substance called myelin, which forms a discontinuous

sheath that covers the outside of the axon. The gaps or spaces between the myelin segments along the axon are called nodes of Ranvier and play an important role in neural transmission. In general, the larger the diameter of the axon, the greater the speed of neural transmission (14). Thus, those axons with large myelin sheaths conduct impulses more rapidly than small, nonmyelinated fibers. Damage or destruction of myelin along myelinated nerve fibers results in nervous system dysfunction. Indeed, damage to myelin is the basis for the neurological disease multiple sclerosis (see Clinical Applications 7.1 for more information about multiple sclerosis).

Electrical Activity in Neurons

Neurons are considered "excitable tissue" because of their specialized properties of irritability and conductivity. **Irritability** is the ability of the dendrites and neuron cell body to respond to a stimulus and convert it to a neural impulse. **Conductivity** refers to the transmission of the impulse along the axon. In simple terms, a nerve impulse is an electrical signal carried the length of the axon. This electrical signal is initiated by a stimulus that causes a change in the electrical charge of the neuron. Let's begin our discussion of this process with a definition of the resting membrane potential.

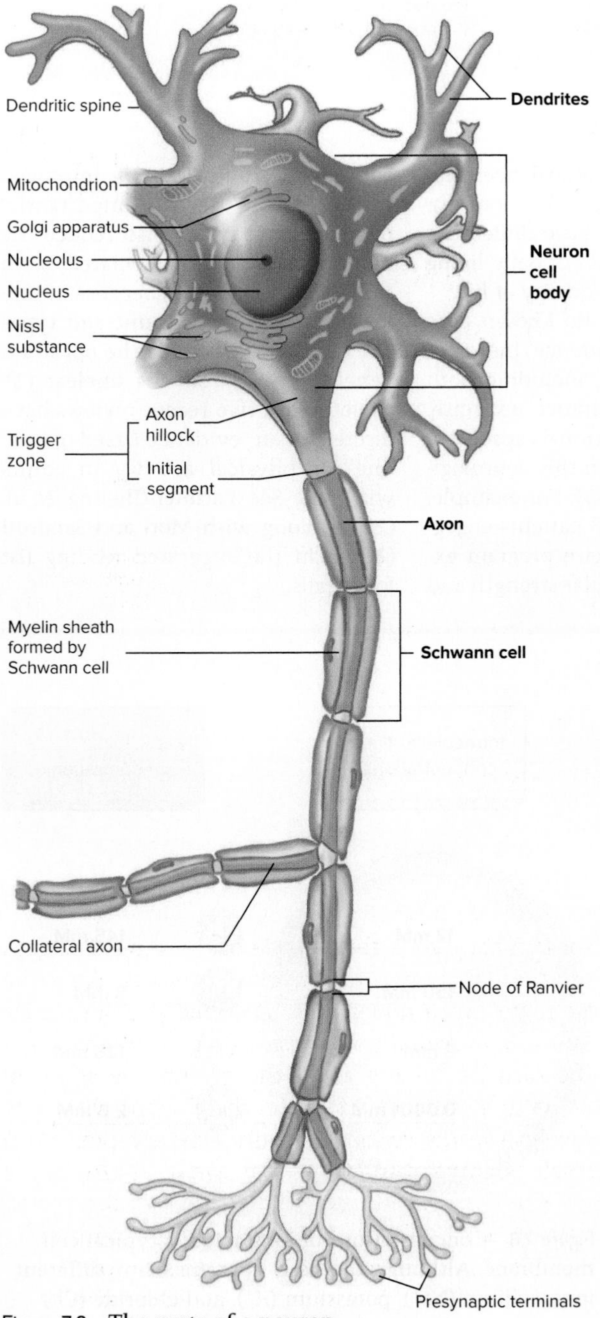

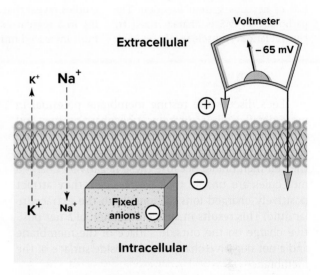

Figure 7.3   The parts of a neuron.

Labels on figure:
- Dendritic spine
- Mitochondrion
- Golgi apparatus
- Nucleolus
- Nucleus
- Nissl substance
- Trigger zone
  - Axon hillock
  - Initial segment
- Myelin sheath formed by Schwann cell
- Collateral axon
- Dendrites
- Neuron cell body
- Axon
- Schwann cell
- Node of Ranvier
- Presynaptic terminals

Resting Membrane Potential   At rest, all cells (including neurons) are negatively charged on the inside of the cell with respect to the charge that exists outside the cell. This negative charge is the result of an unequal distribution of charged ions (ions are elements with a positive or negative charge) across the cell membrane. Thus, a neuron is polarized, and this electrical charge difference is called the **resting membrane potential.** The magnitude of the resting membrane potential varies from –5 to –100 mV depending upon the cell type. The resting membrane potential of neurons is generally in the range of –40 mv to –75 mV (58) (Fig. 7.5).

Figure on right:
- Voltmeter: –65 mV
- Extracellular
- K^+, Na^+
- K^+, Na^+
- Fixed anions
- Intracellular

Figure 7.5   Illustration of the resting membrane potential in cells. Compared to the outside of the cell, more negatively charged (fixed) ions exist inside the cell; this results in a negative resting membrane potential. Also, notice that both sodium and potassium can diffuse across the plasma membrane with potassium diffusing from the inside of the cell to the extracellular fluid, whereas sodium diffuses into the cell from the extracellular fluid.

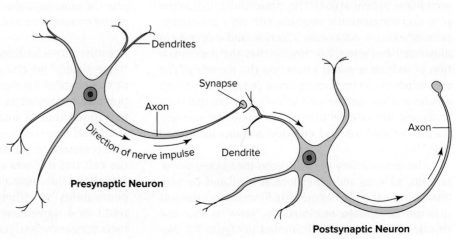

Figure 7.4   An illustration of synaptic transmission. For a nerve impulse to continue from one neuron to another, it must cross the synaptic cleft at a synapse.

Labels on figure:
- Dendrites
- Synapse
- Axon
- Direction of nerve impulse
- Dendrite
- Axon
- Presynaptic Neuron
- Postsynaptic Neuron

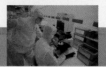

Benefits of Exercise Training in Multiple Sclerosis

Multiple sclerosis (MS) is a neurological disease that progressively destroys the myelin sheaths of axons in multiple areas of the central nervous system. Although the exact cause of MS is not known, the MS-mediated destruction of myelin has an inherited (i.e., genetic) component and is due to an immune system attack on myelin. Destruction of the myelin sheath prohibits the normal conduction of nerve impulses, resulting in a progressive loss of nervous system function. The pathology of MS is characterized by general fatigue, muscle weakness, poor motor control, loss of balance, and mental depression (62). Therefore, patients with MS often have difficulties in performing activities of daily living and suffer from a low quality of life.

Although there is no known cure for MS, growing evidence indicates that regular exercise, including both endurance and resistance exercise, can improve the functional capacity of patients suffering from this neurological disorder (60, 62-63). For example, studies reveal that MS patients engaging in a regular exercise program exhibit increased muscular strength and endurance, resulting in an improved quality of life (9, 60). Importantly, regular exercise may also reduce the mental depression associated with MS (60, 62). However, because of limited research, the amount and types of exercise that provide the optimum benefit for MS remains unclear (1). Nonetheless, two recent reviews have discussed an evidence-based guideline for physical activity in adults with MS. See Latimer-Cheung et al. (2013) along with Motl and Sandroff (2015) in the suggested reading list for details.

Let's discuss the resting membrane potential in more detail. Cellular proteins, phosphate groups, and other nucleotides are negatively charged (anions) and are fixed inside the cell because they cannot cross the cell membrane. Because these negatively charged molecules are unable to leave the cell, they attract positively charged ions (cations) from the extracellular fluid. This results in an accumulation of a net positive charge on the outside surface of the membrane and a net negative charge on the inside surface of the membrane.

The magnitude of the resting membrane potential is primarily determined by two factors: (1) the permeability of the cell membrane to different ions and; (2) the difference in ion concentrations between the intracellular and extracellular fluids (64). Although numerous intracellular and extracellular ions exist, sodium, potassium, and chloride ions are present in the greatest concentrations and therefore play the most important role in generating the resting membrane potential (64). The intracellular (inside the cell) and extracellular (outside the cell) concentrations of sodium, potassium, chloride, and calcium are illustrated in Figure 7.6. Notice that the concentration of sodium is much greater on the outside of the cell, whereas the concentration of potassium is much greater on the inside of the cell. For comparative purposes, the intracellular and extracellular concentrations of calcium and chloride are also illustrated (Fig. 7.6).

The permeability of the neuron membrane to potassium, sodium, and other ions is regulated by proteins within the membrane that function as channels that can be opened or closed by "gates" within the channel. This concept is illustrated in Figure 7.7. No-

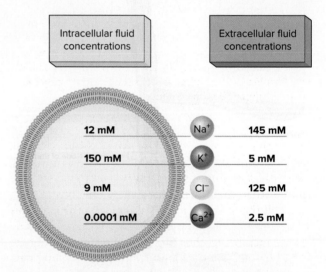

Figure 7.6 Concentrations of ions across a typical cell membrane. Although the body contains many different ions, sodium (Na^+), potassium (K^+), and chloride (Cl^-) ions exist in the largest concentrations and therefore play the most important roles in determining the resting membrane potential in cells.

tice that ions can move freely across the cell membrane when the channel is open, whereas closure of the channel gate prevents ion movement. A key point to remember is that when channels are open, ions move from an area of high concentration toward an area of low concentration. Therefore, because the concentration of potassium (+ charge) is high inside the cell and the concentration of sodium (+ charge) is high outside the cell, a change in the membrane's permeability to either potassium or sodium would result in a movement of these charged ions down their concentration gradients. That is, sodium would

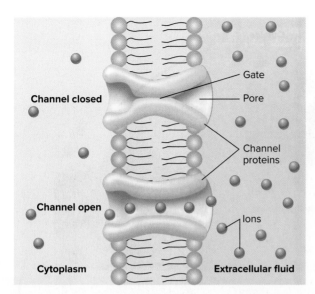

Figure 7.7 Illustration of channels that regulate ion passage across the plasma membrane. Ion channels are composed of proteins that span the entire membrane from the inside to the outer surface. Ion passage through the channels is regulated by the opening or closing of "gates" that serve as doors in the middle of the channel. For example, when channels are open (i.e., gate is open), ions are free to pass through the channel (lower portion of figure). In contrast, when the channel gate is closed, ions' movement through the channel is halted (upper portion of figure).

enter the cell, and potassium would leave the cell. At rest, almost all the sodium channels are closed, whereas a few potassium channels are open. This means that there are more potassium ions leaving the cell than sodium ions "leaking" into the cell. This results in a net loss of positive charges from the inside of the membrane, thus making the resting membrane potential negative. In short, the negative membrane potential in a resting neuron is due primarily to the diffusion of potassium out of the cell, caused by (1) the higher permeability of the membrane for potassium than sodium and (2) the concentration gradient for potassium promotes movement of potassium ions out of the cell.

As mentioned previously, a small number of ions are always moving across the cell membrane. If potassium ions continued to diffuse out of the cell and the sodium ions continued to diffuse into the cell, the concentration gradients for these ions would decrease. This would result in a loss of the negative membrane potential. What prevents this from happening? The cell membrane has a sodium/potassium pump that uses energy from ATP to maintain the intracellular/extracellular ion concentrations by pumping sodium out of the cell and potassium into the cell. Interestingly, this pump not only maintains the concentration gradients that are needed to maintain the resting

membrane potential but it also helps to generate the potential because it exchanges three sodium ions for every two potassium ions (5, 62) (Fig. 7.8).

Action Potential Research that explained how neurons transmit impulses from the periphery to the brain was completed more than 50 years ago. A neural message is generated when a stimulus of sufficient strength reaches the neuron membrane and opens sodium gates, which allows sodium ions to diffuse into the neuron, making the inside of the cell more and more positive (depolarizing the cell). When depolarization reaches a critical value called "threshold," more sodium gates open and an **action potential,** or nerve impulse, is formed (see Figs. 7.9 and 7.10(b)). After an action potential has been generated, a sequence of ionic exchanges occurs along the axon to propagate the nerve impulse. This ionic exchange along the neuron occurs in a sequential fashion at the nodes of Ranvier (Fig. 7.3).

Repolarization occurs immediately following depolarization, resulting in a return of the resting membrane potential with the nerve ready to be stimulated again (Figs. 7.9 and 7.10). How does repolarization occur? To explain, let's take a closer look at depolarization. Depolarization of the cell, with a slight time delay, causes a brief increase in membrane permeability to potassium. As a result, potassium leaves the cell rapidly, making the inside of the membrane more negative (see Fig. 7.10(c)). Further, after the depolarization stimulus is removed, the sodium gates within the cell membrane close, and sodium entry into the cell is slowed (therefore, few positive charges are entering the cell). The combined result of these activities quickly restores the resting membrane potential to the original negative charge, thus repolarizing the cell. To summarize, the events leading to neuron depolarization and repolarization are illustrated step by step in Figures 7.10(a) through 7.10(c). Specifically, the resting membrane potential is illustrated in Figure 7.10(a), whereas the events that lead to an action potential are highlighted in Figure 7.10(b). Finally, the ionic movements that lead to repolarization of the neuron are illustrated in Figure 7.10(c).

All-or-None Law The development of a nerve impulse is considered to be an "all-or-none" response and is referred to as the "all-or-none" law of action potentials. This means that if a nerve impulse is initiated, the impulse will travel the entire length of the axon without a decrease in voltage. In other words, the neural impulse is just as strong after traveling the length of the axon as it was at the initial point of stimulation.

Neurotransmitters and Synaptic Transmission As mentioned previously, neurons communicate with other neurons at junctions called synapses. A synapse

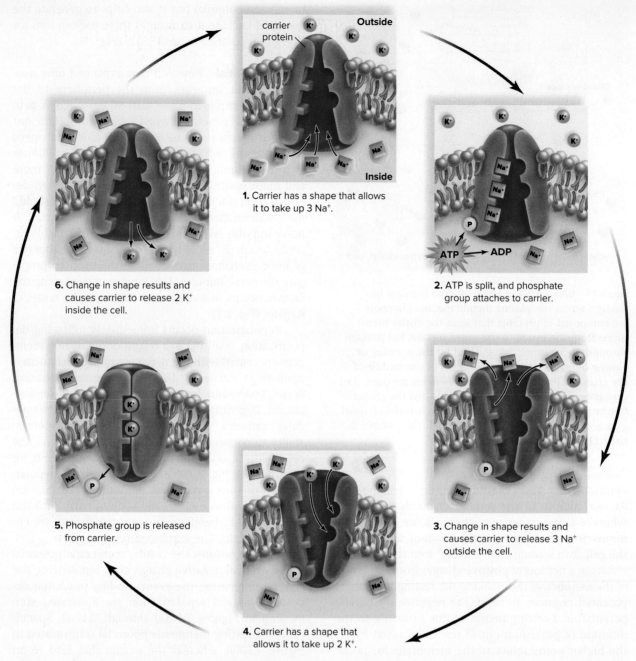

1. Carrier has a shape that allows it to take up 3 Na⁺.

2. ATP is split, and phosphate group attaches to carrier.

3. Change in shape results and causes carrier to release 3 Na⁺ outside the cell.

4. Carrier has a shape that allows it to take up 2 K⁺.

5. Phosphate group is released from carrier.

6. Change in shape results and causes carrier to release 2 K⁺ inside the cell.

carrier protein

Outside

Inside

ATP → ADP

Figure 7.8   Exchange of sodium and potassium across the plasma membrane by the sodium/potassium pump. The sodium/potassium pump requires energy (ATP) and is therefore an active transport pump that moves three molecules of sodium out of the cell and returns two molecules of potassium into the cell. The sodium/potassium pump process is summarized by steps 1 through 6.

is a small gap (20–30 nanometers) between the synaptic endfoot of the presynaptic neuron and a dendrite of a postsynaptic neuron (see Fig. 7.11).

Communication between neurons occurs via a process called synaptic transmission. Synaptic transmission occurs when sufficient amounts of a specific **neurotransmitter** (a neurotransmitter is a chemical messenger that neurons use to communicate with each other) are released from synaptic vesicles

contained in the presynaptic neuron (Fig. 7.11). The nerve impulse results in the synaptic vesicles releasing stored neurotransmitter into the synaptic cleft (space between presynaptic neuron and postsynaptic membrane; see Fig. 7.11). Neurotransmitters that cause the depolarization of membranes are termed *excitatory transmitters*. After release into the synaptic cleft, these neurotransmitters bind to "receptors" on the target membrane, which produces a series of

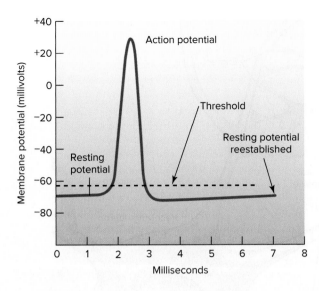

Figure 7.9 An action potential is produced by an increase in sodium conductance into the neuron. As sodium enters the neuron, the charge becomes more and more positive, and an action potential is generated.

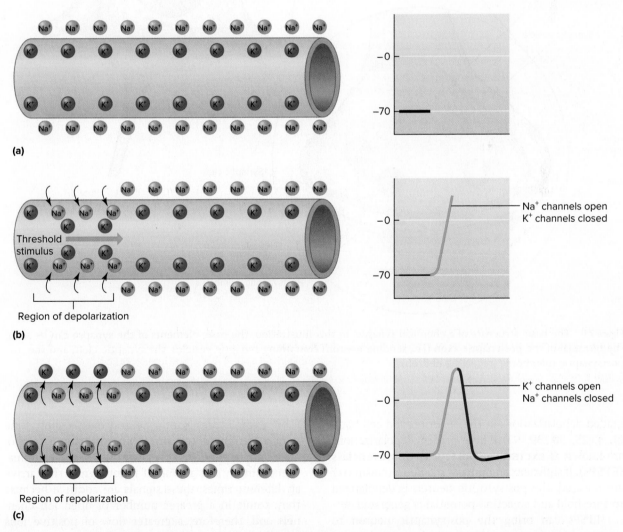

Figure 7.10 (*a*) At rest, the membrane is about −70 millivolts. (*b*) When the membrane reaches threshold, sodium channels open, some sodium ions diffuse inward, and the membrane is depolarized. (*c*) When the potassium channels open, potassium channels diffuse outward, and the membrane is repolarized.

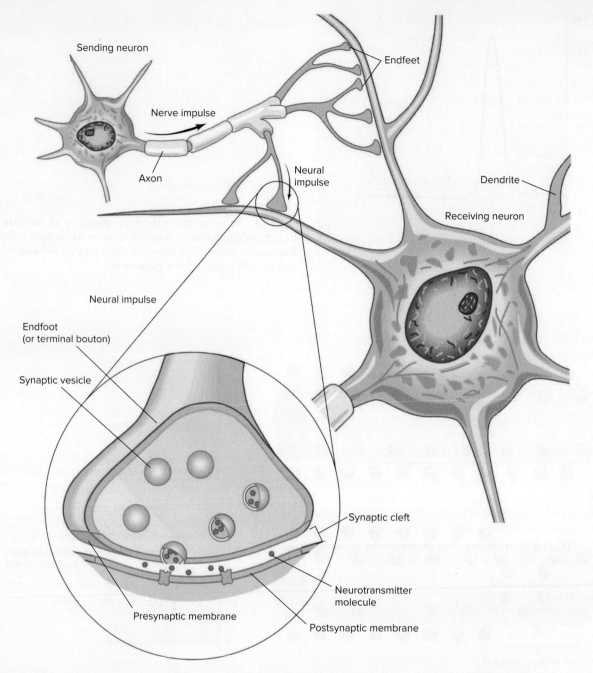

Figure 7.11 The basic structure of a chemical synapse. In this illustration, the basic elements of the synapse can be seen: the terminal of the presynaptic axon (i.e., sending neuron) containing synaptic vesicles, the synaptic cleft, and the postsynaptic membrane (receiving neuron).

Vander, A. J., et al., *Human Physiology: The Mechanisms of Body Function*, 8th ed. New York: McGraw-Hill, Inc., 2005.

graded depolarizations in the dendrites and cell body (3, 4, 25, 30, 39, 53). These graded depolarizations are known as **excitatory postsynaptic potentials (EPSPs).** If sufficient amounts of the neurotransmitter are released, the postsynaptic neuron is depolarized to threshold and an action potential is generated.

EPSPs can bring the postsynaptic neuron to threshold in two ways: (1) temporal summation and (2) spatial summation. The summing of several EPSPs from a single presynaptic neuron over a short time period is termed **temporal summation** ("temporal" refers to time). In other words, temporal summation is simply the adding of input signals that arrive at different times; these signals are additive because they result in a greater number of open ion channels and, therefore, a greater flow of positive ions into the cell. The number of EPSPs required to bring the postsynaptic neuron to threshold varies, but it is estimated that the addition of up to 50 EPSPs might be required to produce an action potential within some neurons. Regardless of how many EPSPs are required, one way by which an action potential can be generated is through rapid, repetitive excitation from a single excitatory presynaptic neuron (i.e., temporal summation).

A second means of achieving an action potential at the postsynaptic membrane is to sum EPSPs from several different presynaptic inputs (i.e., several different axons), known as spatial summation. In **spatial summation,** concurrent EPSPs come into a postsynaptic neuron from numerous different excitatory inputs. As with temporal summation, up to 50 EPSPs arriving simultaneously on the postsynaptic membrane may be required to produce an action potential (5).

A common neurotransmitter, which also happens to be the transmitter at the nerve/muscle junction, is acetylcholine. Upon release into the synaptic cleft, acetylcholine binds to receptors on the postsynaptic membrane and opens "channels" that permit sodium to enter the nerve or muscle cell. As discussed previously, when enough sodium enters the postsynaptic membrane of a neuron or muscle, depolarization results. To prevent chronic depolarization of the postsynaptic neuron, the neurotransmitter must be broken down into less active molecules via enzymes located within the synaptic cleft. In the case of acetylcholine, the degrading enzyme is called acetylcholinesterase. This enzyme breaks down acetylcholine into acetyl and choline and thus removes the stimulus for depolarization (14). Following breakdown of the neurotransmitter, the postsynaptic membrane repolarizes and is prepared to receive additional neurotransmitters and generate a new action potential. Note that not all neurotransmitters are excitatory. In fact, some neurotransmitters have just the opposite effect of excitatory transmitters (5). These inhibitory transmitters cause a hyperpolarization (increased negativity) of the postsynaptic membrane. This hyperpolarization of the membrane is called an **inhibitory postsynaptic potential (IPSP).** The end result of an IPSP is that the neuron develops a more negative resting membrane potential, is pushed further from threshold, and thus resists depolarization. In general, whether a neuron reaches threshold or not is dependent on the ratio of the number of EPSPs to the number of IPSPs. For example, a neuron that is simultaneously bombarded by an equal number of EPSPs and IPSPs will not reach threshold and generate an action potential. On the other hand, if the EPSPs outnumber the IPSPs, the neuron is moved toward threshold and an action potential may be generated.

IN SUMMARY

- Nerve cells (i.e., neurons) are divided anatomically into three parts: (1) the cell body, (2) dendrites, and (3) the axon. Axons are generally covered by Schwann cells, with gaps between these cells called nodes of Ranvier.
- Neurons are specialized cells that respond to physical or chemical changes in their environment. At rest, neurons are negatively charged in the interior with respect to the electrical charge outside the cell. This difference in electrical charge is called the resting membrane potential.
- A neuron "fires" when a stimulus changes the permeability of the membrane, allowing sodium to enter at a high rate, which depolarizes the cell. When the depolarization reaches threshold, an action potential or nerve impulse is initiated. Repolarization occurs immediately following depolarization due to an increase in membrane permeability to potassium and a decreased permeability to sodium.
- Neurons communicate with other neurons at junctions called synapses. Synaptic transmission occurs when sufficient amounts of a specific neurotransmitter are released from the presynaptic neuron. Upon release, the neurotransmitter binds to a receptor on the post-synaptic membrane and causes ion channels to open.
- Neurotransmitters can be excitatory or inhibitory. An excitatory transmitter increases neuronal permeability to sodium and results in excitatory postsynaptic potentials (EPSPs). Inhibitory neurotransmitters cause the neuron to become more negative (hyperpolarized). This hyperpolarization of the membrane is called an inhibitory postsynaptic potential (IPSP).

SENSORY INFORMATION AND REFLEXES

The CNS receives a constant bombardment of messages from receptors throughout the body about changes in both the internal and external environment. These receptors are sense organs that change forms of energy in the "real world" into the energy of nerve impulses, which are conducted to the CNS by sensory neurons. A complete discussion of sense organs is beyond the scope of this chapter, so we will limit our discussion to those receptors responsible for position sense. Receptors that provide the CNS with information about body position are called **proprioceptors,** or kinesthetic receptors, and include muscle spindles, Golgi tendon organs, and joint receptors.

Joint Proprioceptors

The term **kinesthesia** (also called kinesthetic sense) means conscious recognition of the position of body parts with respect to one another as well as recognition of the speed of limb-movement (32, 33, 42, 48, 49). This sense of body position is important in performing both everyday activities (e.g., walking down the stairs) and athletic skills. Indeed, a keen sense of body position is essential to perform complex skills such as those movements involved in gymnastics, diving, and basketball. In fact, it is predicted that individual differences in kinesthetic sense likely plays an important role in defining differences in athletic performance between athletes competing in sports (e.g., gymnastics, diving) that require a high level of kinesthetic sense to be successful. A brief discussion of the three primary sensory devices involved in proprioception follows.

There are three principal types of joint proprioceptors: (1) free nerve endings, (2) Golgi-type receptors, and (3) Pacinian corpuscles. The most abundant of these are free nerve endings, which are sensitive to touch and pressure. These receptors are stimulated strongly at the beginning of movement; they adapt (i.e., become less sensitive to stimuli) slightly at first, but then transmit a steady signal until the movement is complete (7, 17, 29, 34, 48). A second type of position receptor, Golgi-type receptors (not to be confused with Golgi tendon organs found in muscle tendons), are found in ligaments around joints. These receptors are not as abundant as free nerve endings, but they work in a similar manner. Pacinian corpuscles are found in the tissues around joints and adapt rapidly following the initiation of movement. This rapid adaptation presumably helps detect the rate of joint rotation (29). To summarize, the joint receptors work together to provide a conscious means of recognition of the orientation of body parts as well as feedback about the rates of limb movement.

Muscle Proprioceptors

Skeletal muscle contains several types of sensory receptors. These include muscle spindles and Golgi tendon organs (29, 34, 49). Collectively, these sensory receptors are often called muscle mechanoreceptors because these receptors are sensitive to mechanical (pressure/length) changes in the muscle. Importantly, these mechanoreceptors not only send information to higher brain centers about movement patterns but these receptors also send afferent neural information to both the cardiovascular and respiratory control centers; this information is used to regulate the cardiovascular and respiratory response to exercise. This topic will be discussed in more detail in Chaps. 9 and 10, respectively.

For the nervous system to properly control skeletal muscle movements, it must receive continuous sensory feedback from the contracting muscle. This sensory feedback includes (1) information concerning the tension developed by a muscle; and (2) an account of the muscle length. Golgi tendon organs provide the central nervous system with feedback concerning the tension developed by the muscle, whereas the muscle spindle provides sensory information concerning the relative length of the muscle (8, 34, 49). A discussion of each sensory organ follows.

Muscle Spindle As previously stated, the **muscle spindle** functions as a length detector. Muscle spindles are found in large numbers in most human locomotor muscles (49). Muscles that require the finest degree of control, such as the muscles of the hands, have the highest density of spindles. In contrast, muscles that are responsible for gross movements (e.g., quadriceps) contain relatively few spindles.

The muscle spindle is composed of several thin muscle cells (called intrafusal fibers) that are surrounded by a connective tissue sheath. Like normal skeletal muscle fibers (called extrafusal fibers), muscle spindles insert into connective tissue within the muscle. Therefore, muscle spindles run parallel with muscle fibers (see Fig. 7.12).

Muscle spindles contain two types of sensory nerve endings. The primary endings respond to dynamic changes in muscle length. The second type of sensory ending is called the secondary ending, and it does not respond to rapid changes in muscle length, but provides the central nervous system with continuous information concerning static muscle length.

In addition to the sensory neurons, muscle spindles are innervated by gamma motor neurons, which stimulate the intrafusal fibers to contract simultaneously along with extrafusal fibers. Gamma motor neuron stimulation causes the central region of the intrafusal fibers to shorten, which serves to tighten the spindle. The need for contraction of the intrafusal fibers can be explained as follows: When skeletal muscles are shortened by motor neuron stimulation, muscle spindles are passively shortened along with the skeletal muscle fibers. If the intrafusal fibers did not compensate accordingly, this shortening would result in "slack" in the spindle and make them less sensitive. Therefore, their function as length detectors would be compromised.

Muscle spindles are responsible for the observation that rapid stretching of skeletal muscles results in a reflex contraction. This is called the stretch reflex or myotatic reflex; it is present in all muscles but is most dramatic in the extensor muscles of the limbs.

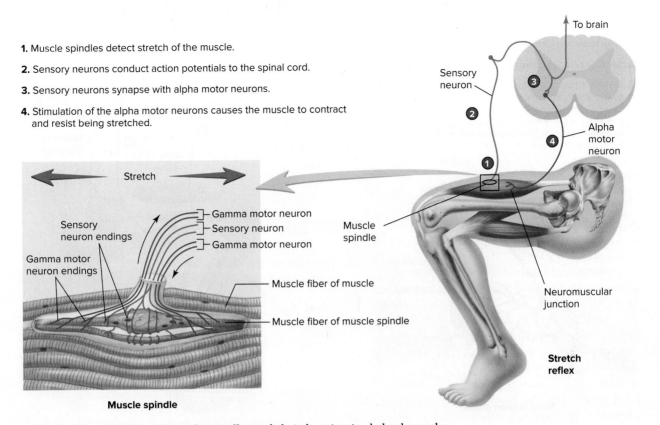

1. Muscle spindles detect stretch of the muscle.

2. Sensory neurons conduct action potentials to the spinal cord.

3. Sensory neurons synapse with alpha motor neurons.

4. Stimulation of the alpha motor neurons causes the muscle to contract and resist being stretched.

Figure 7.12 The structure of muscle spindles and their location in skeletal muscle.

The so-called knee-jerk reflex is often evaluated by the physician by tapping the patellar tendon with a rubber mallet. The blow by the mallet stretches the entire muscle and thus "excites" the primary nerve endings located in muscle spindles. The neural impulse from the muscle spindle synapses at the spinal cord level with a motor neuron, which then stimulates the extrafusal fibers of the extensor muscle, resulting in an isotonic contraction.

The function of the muscle spindle is to assist in the regulation of movement and to maintain posture. This is accomplished by the muscle spindle's ability to detect and cause the central nervous system to respond to changes in the length of skeletal muscle fibers. The following practical example shows how the muscle spindle assists in the control of movement. Suppose a person is holding a single book in front of their body with the arm extended. This type of load poses a tonic stretch on the muscle spindle, which sends information to the CNS concerning the final length of the extrafusal muscle fibers. If a second book is suddenly placed upon the first book, the muscles would be suddenly stretched (arm would drop) and a burst of impulses from the muscle spindle would alert the CNS about the change in muscle length due to the increased

load. The ensuing reflex would recruit additional motor units to raise the arm back to the original position. Generally, this type of reflex action results in an overcompensation. That is, more motor units are recruited than are needed to bring the arm back to the original position. However, immediately following the overcompensation movement, an additional adjustment rapidly occurs and the arm is quickly returned to the original position.

Golgi Tendon Organs The **Golgi tendon organs (GTOs)** continuously monitor the tension produced by muscle contraction. Golgi tendon organs are located within the tendon and thus are in series with the extrafusal fibers (Fig. 7.13). In essence, GTOs serve as "safety devices" that help prevent excessive force during muscle contraction. When activated, GTOs send information to the spinal cord via sensory neurons, which in turn excite inhibitory neurons (i.e., send IPSPs). This inhibitory reflex prevents motor neurons from firing, reduces muscle force production, and therefore protects the muscle against contraction-induced injury. This process is pictured in Figure 7.13.

It seems possible that GTOs play an important role in the performance of strength activities. For

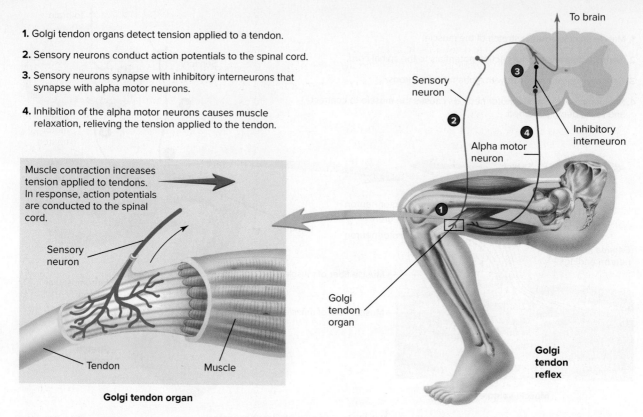

1. Golgi tendon organs detect tension applied to a tendon.

2. Sensory neurons conduct action potentials to the spinal cord.

3. Sensory neurons synapse with inhibitory interneurons that synapse with alpha motor neurons.

4. Inhibition of the alpha motor neurons causes muscle relaxation, relieving the tension applied to the tendon.

Muscle contraction increases tension applied to tendons. In response, action potentials are conducted to the spinal cord.

Sensory neuron

Tendon

Muscle

Golgi tendon organ

To brain

Sensory neuron

Inhibitory interneuron

Alpha motor neuron

Golgi tendon organ

Golgi tendon reflex

Figure 7.13 The Golgi tendon organ. The Golgi tendon organ is located in series with muscle and serves as a "tension monitor" that acts as a protective device for muscle. See text for details.

instance, the amount of force that can be produced by a muscle group may be dependent on the ability of the individual to voluntarily oppose the inhibition of the GTO. Because resistance training increases tendon stiffness, it is feasible that the inhibitory influences of the GTO on force production could be gradually reduced in response to strength training (20, 61). This would allow an individual to produce a greater amount of muscle force and, in many cases, improve sport performance.

Finally, the GTO is also responsible for a reflex known as the inverse stretch reflex (also called inverse myotatic reflex). As the name implies, the inverse stretch reflex is the opposite of the stretch reflex and results in decreased muscle tension by GTO-mediated inhibition of motor neurons in the spinal cord supplying the muscle. Here's how the inverse stretch reflex works. A vigorous contraction of a muscle group activates the GTO. The GTO responds by sending a message to the spinal cord to inhibit motor neuron firing and reduce the amount of force generated by the muscle. Interestingly, passive stretching of a muscle also activates the GTO and results in relaxation of the stretched muscle.

IN SUMMARY

- Proprioceptors are position receptors located in joint capsules, ligaments, and muscles. The three most abundant joint and ligament receptors are free nerve endings, Golgi-type receptors, and Pacinian corpuscles. These receptors provide the body with a conscious means of recognizing the orientation of body parts, as well as feedback about the rates of limb movement.
- The muscle spindle functions as a length detector in muscle.
- Golgi tendon organs continuously monitor the tension developed during muscular contraction. In essence, Golgi tendon organs serve as safety devices that help prevent excessive force during muscle contractions.
- Collectively, proprioceptors provide important information to the CNS about body position and speed of limb movement, which is essential for the successful performance of complex sports skills.

MUSCLE CHEMORECEPTORS

In addition to proprioceptors, skeletal muscles contain chemoreceptors that respond to chemical changes within the muscle (26, 28, 35). Specifically, these receptors are a type of free nerve ending and are sensitive to changes in the chemical environment surrounding the muscle. When stimulated by changes in the concentrations of hydrogen ions (i.e., pH changes), carbon dioxide, and potassium around the muscle, these receptors send information to the CNS via nerve fibers classified as group III (myelinated) and group IV (nonmyelinated) fibers. The physiological role of muscle chemoreceptors is to provide the CNS with information about the metabolic rate of muscular activity (i.e., how hard the muscle is working). This information is important in the control of the cardiovascular and pulmonary responses to exercise (6, 28, 35) and will be discussed in Chaps. 9 and 10.

IN SUMMARY

- Muscle chemoreceptors are sensitive to chemical changes around muscle fibers.
- When stimulated, muscle chemoreceptors send information back to the CNS about the metabolic rate of muscular activity, and these messages play a role in the regulation of both the cardiovascular and pulmonary response to exercise.

SOMATIC MOTOR FUNCTION AND MOTOR NEURONS

The term *somatic* refers to the outer (i.e., nonvisceral) regions of the body. The somatic motor portion of the peripheral nervous system is responsible for carrying neural messages from the spinal cord to skeletal muscle fibers. These neural messages are the signals for muscular contraction to occur. Muscular contraction will be discussed in detail in Chap. 8.

The organization of the somatic motor nervous system is illustrated in Figure 7.14. The somatic neuron that innervates skeletal muscle fibers is called a **motor neuron** (also called an alpha motor neuron). Note that the cell body of motor neurons is located within the spinal cord (Fig. 7.14). The axon of the motor neuron leaves the spinal cord as a spinal nerve and extends to the muscle that it is responsible for innervating. After the axon reaches the muscle, the axon splits into collateral branches; each collateral branch innervates a single muscle fiber. Each motor neuron and all the muscle fibers that it innervates is known as a **motor unit.**

When a single motor neuron is activated, all of the muscle fibers that it innervates are stimulated to contract. However, note that the number of muscle fibers that a motor neuron innervates is not constant and varies from muscle to muscle. The number of muscle fibers innervated by a single motor neuron

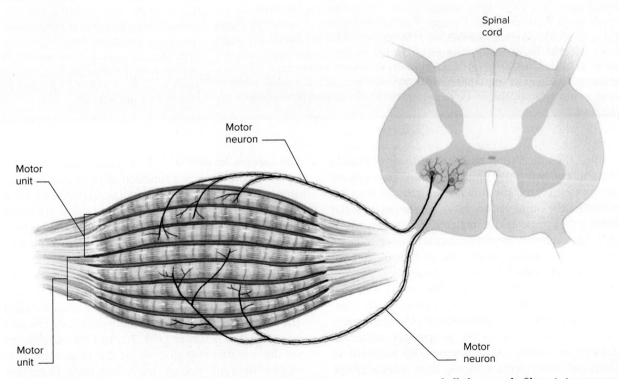

Figure 7.14   Illustration of a motor unit. A motor unit is defined as a motor neuron and all the muscle fibers it innervates.

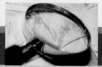
Motor Unit Recruitment and the Size Principle

As introduced in the text, motor unit recruitment is the progressive activation of more and more muscle fibers by the successive recruitment of additional motor units. Recall that a motor unit consists of one motor neuron and all of the muscle fibers that it is responsible for activating. All muscles in the body contain many motor units, and the fibers belonging to a motor unit are spread out across the entire muscle. When a single motor unit is activated, all the muscle fibers innervated by the motor neuron are stimulated to contract. The activation of a single motor unit results in a weak muscle contraction (i.e., limited force production). To increase muscle force production, more motor units must be recruited. This process of motor unit recruitment occurs in an orderly fashion, beginning with the smallest motor neurons and eventually activating larger and larger motor neurons (37). This concept was developed by Elwood Henneman and is known as the size principle.

Henneman proposed that the mechanism responsible for the size principle was that the smaller motor neurons had a smaller surface area and would produce a larger EPSP, which would reach threshold sooner, resulting in an action potential. Further, he predicted that larger motor neurons (with a larger surface area) would produce smaller EPSPs; therefore, these motor neurons would be more difficult to depolarize and achieve an action potential. Taken together, the size principle predicts that motor unit recruitment will occur in order of their increasing size, with the smallest motor neurons firing first, followed by larger and larger motor neurons.

To better understand how the size principle works, let's discuss the three main types of motor units in the body:

1. Type S (slow)–These small motor neurons innervate the slow and highly oxidative muscle fibers. These fibers are called type I muscle fibers; muscle fiber types are discussed in detail in Chap. 8.

2. Type FR (fast, fatigue resistant)–These larger motor neurons innervate the "intermediate" muscle fibers (called type IIa fibers).

3. Type FF (fast, fatigable)–These are the largest motor neurons and innervate the "fast" muscle fibers (called type IIx fibers).

An incremental exercise test is a good example to illustrate how the size principle works during exercise. Recall from Chap. 4 that an incremental exercise test consists of numerous stages lasting one to three minutes per stage. The test begins at a low work rate and with each progressive stage, the work rate increases until the subject cannot maintain the desired power output. So, during the first stage of a graded exercise test, only a low level of muscle force production is required; therefore, you would recruit only the slow, type S motor units. The recruitment of the smaller motor neurons that innervate slow (highly oxidative) muscle fibers first helps to delay fatigue when high force production is not required to perform the exercise. However, as the test progresses, you will need to produce more muscular force and therefore you will recruit more and more of the type S motor units and eventually progress to the type FR motor units. As the exercise test becomes more difficult, any further increase in muscle force production would come from recruiting the type FF motor units.

Note that exceptions to the size principle exist during the performance of high intensity and short duration exercise. For instance, in the human performance example of a high velocity and high power output activity (e.g., Olympic weight lifting, baseball pitchers, or sprinters), fast motor units are recruited first in order to allow for a faster movement. The recruitment of fast motor units first is achieved by inhibiting the activation of slow motor units; this allows the activation of the fast motor units first. The size principle and its role in muscle force production is discussed again in Chap. 8 and is illustrated in Figure 19.3 in Chap. 19.

is called the innervation ratio (i.e., number of muscle fibers/motor neuron). In muscle groups that require fine motor control, the innervation ratio is low. For example, the innervation ratio of the extraocular muscles (i.e., muscles that regulate eye movement) is 23/1. In contrast, innervation ratios of large muscles that are not involved in fine motor control (e.g., leg muscles) may range from 1000/1 to 2000/1.

One of the ways that the CNS can increase the force of muscle contraction is by increasing the number of motor units that are recruited. The term *motor unit recruitment* refers to the progressive activation of more and more motor neurons. Recruitment of additional motor units activates more muscle fibers, which increases the strength of a voluntary muscle contraction. In general, motor units are recruited in an orderly fashion as a function of their size. For example, when a muscle is initially activated to lift a light weight, the first motor units to fire are small in size; this results in a limited amount of force generation. However, when more force is required (i.e., lifting a heavy weight), there is a progressive increase in the recruitment of more large motor neurons to increase muscle force production. This orderly and sequential recruitment of larger motor units is called the **size principle** (37). For more details on the size principle, see A Closer Look 7.1, and for information on the scientist that discovered this important principle of neurophysiology, see A Look Back–Important People in Science.

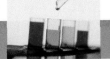

Elwood Henneman Discovered the Size Principle of Motor Neuron Recruitment

Elwood Henneman (1915-1995) was an American scientist interested in understanding how the nervous system controls the actions of skeletal muscles. Dr. Henneman completed his medical education at McGill University, and following his post-doctoral training at Johns Hopkins, he became a faculty member at Harvard.

Although Dr. Henneman's research advanced our understanding of many aspects of the nervous system, one of his most important discoveries was that the susceptibility of a motor neuron to "fire" is a function of its size. That is, the smallest motor neurons are the most easily excited, whereas large motor neurons are the least susceptible to excitation. This important discovery is referred to as the *size principle* (also called the *Henneman size principle*) and is discussed in A Closer Look 7.1.

Dr. Henneman's research interest in skeletal muscles developed from his lifelong pursuit of sports and physical activity. During his undergraduate studies, Henneman was a star on the Harvard tennis team. Dr. Henneman was also an excellent downhill skier, and he remained physically active throughout his life. In fact, his strong physique is credited with allowing him to survive a series of major operations, including installation of an artificial aortic valve, coronary bypass surgery, and an aortic aneurysm (i.e., tear in the aorta). The latter operation was described as "colorful" because the aneurysm occurred when Dr. Henneman was delivering a lecture to Harvard medical students. He diagnosed the problem himself from behind the speakers' podium and ordered a student in the front row to call the hospital and alert the surgery department that Professor Henneman would be arriving to the emergency room with an aortic aneurysm. Although this was a close call, Dr. Henneman survived the surgery and remained active in science until his death.

IN SUMMARY

- The somatic motor portion of the peripheral nervous system is responsible for carrying neural messages from the spinal cord to skeletal muscle fibers.
- A motor neuron and all the muscle fibers that it innervates are known as a motor unit.
- The number of muscle fibers innervated by a single motor neuron is called the innervation ratio (i.e., number of muscle fibers/motor neuron).
- The size principle is defined as the progressive recruitment of motor units, beginning with the smallest motor neurons and progressing to larger and larger motor neurons.
- Recruiting smaller motor neurons that innervate slow (highly oxidative) muscle fibers first helps to delay muscle fatigue when high force production is not required to perform the exercise.
- Exceptions to the size principle exist as fast motor neurons are recruited first during the performance of high velocity and high power output movements (e.g., Olympic weight lifters, sprinters, etc.).

VESTIBULAR APPARATUS AND EQUILIBRIUM

Before we begin a discussion of how the brain controls motor functions, it is important to understand how the body maintains balance (i.e., equilibrium). The **vestibular apparatus,** an organ located in the inner ear, is responsible for maintaining general equilibrium. Although a detailed discussion of the anatomy of the vestibular apparatus will not be presented here, a brief discussion of the function of the vestibular apparatus is appropriate. The receptors contained within the vestibular apparatus are sensitive to any change in head position or movement direction (5, 25, 47). Movement of the head excites these receptors, and nerve impulses are sent to the CNS regarding this change in position. Specifically, these receptors provide information about both linear and angular acceleration of the head. This mechanism allows us to have a sense of acceleration or deceleration when running or traveling by car. Further, a sense of angular acceleration helps us maintain balance when the head is turning or spinning (e.g., performing gymnastics or diving).

The neural pathways involved in the control of equilibrium are outlined in Figure 7.15. Any head movement results in the stimulation of receptors in the vestibular apparatus, which transmits neural information to the cerebellum and the vestibular nuclei located in the brain stem. Further, the vestibular nuclei relay a message to the oculomotor center (controls eye movement) and to neurons in the spinal cord that control movements of the head and limbs. Thus, the vestibular apparatus controls head and eye movement during physical activity, which serves to maintain balance and visually track the events of movement. In summary, the vestibular apparatus is sensitive to the position of the head

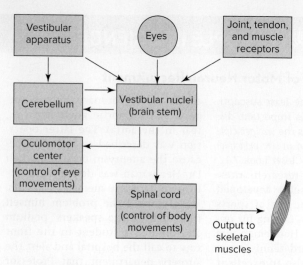

Figure 7.15 The role of the vestibular apparatus in the maintenance of equilibrium and balance.

■ The vestibular apparatus is responsible for maintaining general equilibrium and is located in the inner ear. Specifically, these receptors provide information about linear and angular acceleration.

MOTOR CONTROL FUNCTIONS OF THE BRAIN

The brain can be subdivided into three major parts: the cerebrum, cerebellum, and brain stem. Figure 7.16 demonstrates the anatomical relationship of these components. Each of these structures makes important contributions to the regulation of movement. The next several paragraphs will outline the brain's role in regulating the performance of sports skills.

Cerebrum

The **cerebrum** is the large dome of the brain that is divided into right and left cerebral hemispheres. The outermost layer of the cerebrum is called the cerebral cortex and is composed of tightly arranged neurons. Although the cortex is only about one-fourth of an inch thick, it contains over eight million neurons. The cortex performs three very important motor behavior functions (14): 1) the organization of complex

in space and to sudden changes in the direction of body movement. Its primary function is to maintain equilibrium and preserve a constant plane of head position. Failure of the vestibular apparatus to function properly would prevent the accurate performance of any athletic task that requires head movement. Since most sporting events require at least some head movement, the importance of the vestibular apparatus is obvious.

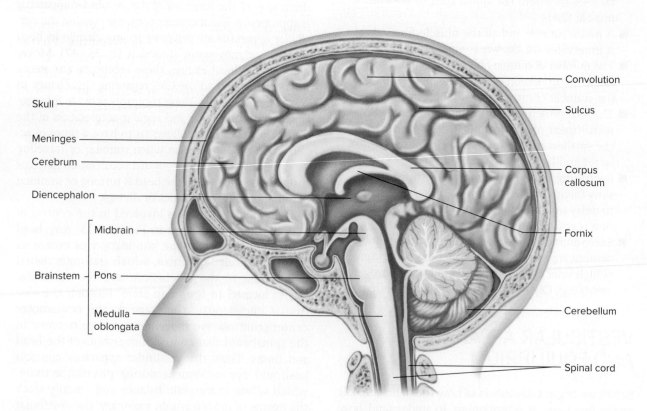

Figure 7.16 The anatomical relationship among the cerebrum, the cerebellum, and the brain stem.

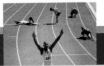

Mind Over Matter? The Central Governor Theory of Exercise-Induced Fatigue

Everyone that has engaged in long-duration or a high intensity exercise training session has experienced fatigue. In theory, exercise-induced fatigue could be due to central factors (e.g., higher brain centers and/or motor neurons) or peripheral factors (fatigue within skeletal muscle fibers). Let's discuss central fatigue and peripheral fatigue during exercise in more detail. In regard to peripheral fatigue, it is clear that prolonged or intense exercise can disturb homeostasis within the contracting muscle fibers resulting in decreased force production (45, 46). However, it is also possible that exercise-induced fatigue could result from dysfunction of the central nervous system (i.e., central fatigue) resulting in a reduced motor output to the exercising skeletal muscles (43, 52, 56). This type of central fatigue could occur during prolonged endurance exercise due to the depletion of excitatory neurotransmit-

ters in the motor cortex. This depletion of excitatory neurotransmitters would impair the activation of motor neurons and the muscle fibers that they innervate. In fact, some investigators have proposed that higher brain centers act as a "governor" to control exercise tolerance (40, 41). This "central governor" theory of fatigue proposes that exercise-induced fatigue is regulated by the action of a central (brain) control center that regulates exercise performance (40). It is proposed that this type of control system would limit muscle activation during exercise by reducing motor output from higher brain centers. A theorized advantage of the central governor theory of exercise fatigue is that this system would protect the body against catastrophic disturbances in homeostasis by promoting fatigue and the cessation of exercise before damage occurs to the working muscles.

So, is exercise-induced fatigue controlled solely by the brain, as predicted by the central governor theory? Unfortunately, the answer to this question remains unknown because this is a difficult problem to study. Nonetheless, current evidence suggests that both central and peripheral factors can contribute to exercise-induced fatigue, and that the relative contribution of central or peripheral factors may depend upon the environmental conditions and the type of exercise (e.g., intensity and duration) performed to induce fatigue. Therefore, the "central governor" theory of exercise-induced fatigue remains a theory, and future research will be required to fully support or reject this concept (57). More will be said about muscle fatigue in Chap. 8. See Shei and Mickleborough (2013) and Rauch (2013) in the suggested reading list for more details on the central governor theory of exercise-induced fatigue.

movement, 2) the storage of learned experiences, and 3) the reception of sensory information. We will limit our discussion to the role of the cortex in the organization of movement. The portion of the cerebral cortex that is most concerned with voluntary movement is the motor cortex. Although the motor cortex plays a significant role in motor control, it appears that input to the motor cortex from subcortical structures (i.e., cerebellum, etc.) is absolutely essential for coordinated movement to occur (14, 23, 55). Thus, the **motor cortex** can be described as the final relay point upon which subcortical inputs are focused. After the motor cortex sums these inputs, the final movement plan is formulated and the motor commands are sent to the spinal cord. This "movement plan" can be modified by both subcortical and spinal centers, which supervise the fine details of the movement. See the Winning Edge 7.1 for a discussion of the role that the CNS plays in exercise-induced fatigue.

Cerebellum

The **cerebellum** lies behind the pons and medulla (Fig. 7.16). Although complete knowledge about cerebellar function is not currently available, much is known about the role of this structure in movement control. It is clear that the cerebellum plays an important role in coordinating and monitoring complex movement. This

work is accomplished via connections leading from the cerebellum to the motor cortex, the brain stem, and the spinal cord. Evidence exists to suggest that the primary role of the cerebellum is to aid in the control of movement in response to feedback from proprioceptors (29, 55). Further, the cerebellum may initiate fast, ballistic movements via its connection with the motor cortex (5). Damage to the cerebellum results in poor movement control and muscular tremor that is most severe during rapid movement. Head injuries due to sport-related injuries can lead to damage and dysfunction in the cerebrum and/or cerebellum. For an overview of sport-related concussions, see Clinical Applications 7.2.

Brain Stem

The **brain stem** is located inside the base of the skull just above the spinal cord. It consists of a complicated series of nerve tracts and nuclei (clusters of neurons) and is responsible for many metabolic functions, cardiorespiratory control, and some highly complex reflexes. The major structures of the brain stem are the medulla, pons, and midbrain. In addition, there is a series of complex neurons scattered throughout the brain stem that is collectively called the reticular formation. The reticular formation receives and integrates information from all regions of the CNS and works with higher brain centers in controlling muscular activity (5).

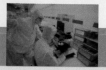

Sport-Related Traumatic Brain Injuries and Development of Chronic Traumatic Encephalopathy (CTE)

Although head injuries can occur in many activities, sports with the greatest risk of head injury include football, gymnastics, ice hockey, wrestling, and boxing. Other sporting activities that pose a significant risk for head injury include horse racing, motorcycle and automobile racing, martial arts, soccer, and rugby.

A forceful blow to the head during sports (e.g., a football collision) can result in a traumatic brain injury (TBI) that is classified by the amount of damage to brain tissue. One of the most common brain injuries in sports is the concussion, and it is estimated that approximately 3.8 million sports-related concussions occur each year in the United States (22, 51). A concussion is defined as a complex TBI resulting from a traumatic force to the head, neck, or body (36). Concussions differ in their degree of severity, but most concussions share several common features (see Table 7.1). Note that a concussion does not always result in a loss of consciousness. Indeed, only 10% of athletes who suffer a sport-related concussion are rendered unconscious (2).

Interestingly, girls appear to have a higher rate of concussion than boys in the same sport (e.g., basketball) (11, 22). The reason for this difference is unknown, but some experts suggest that gender differences exist in the ability to withstand equivalent blows to the head and neck (11, 22). It is also possible that, compared to female athletes, some male athletes may be reluctant to report their head injuries to coaches or parents for fear of being removed from athletic competition (22). Therefore, the incidence of TBI in male athletes may be underestimated (22). If this is the case, the occurrence of concussions may not differ between girls and boys.

What health risks are associated with sustaining a concussion? In general, most concussions result in a short-lived impairment of brain function that typically resolves naturally within a few days (36). Nonetheless, there are some atypical outcomes of a concussion that present serious health risks. These major health risks associated with a concussion include (51): (1) permanent brain damage or death associated with delayed brain swelling; (2) second-impact syndrome; (3) same season repeat concussion; and (4) late-life consequences of repeated concussions. A brief discussion of these concussion-related risks follows.

The risk of permanent brain damage or death in most sports is low. For example, although American football is considered a high-risk sport for head injury, it is estimated that only 1 out of every 20,500 football players develop an acute injury that results in permanent brain injury each year (51). The second-impact syndrome occurs when an athlete who has sustained an initial concussion suffers a second head injury before the first injury has healed. This second-impact syndrome promotes brain vascular congestion, which can progress to cerebral swelling and death. Also, after sustaining a concussion, the brain is in a state of vulnerability for an extended period. Therefore, an additional risk of a sports-related concussion is the increased vulnerability to a second concussion within the same season (51). This concussion-related health risk is often called the *same-season repeat concussion*. The final risk associated with repeated sports-related TBI (i.e., concussions) is the increased risk of the development of degenerative brain disorders resulting in impaired mental function later in life (i.e., dementia) (22a, 51). Indeed, compared to a nonathletic population, evidence indicates that American professional football players are at a higher risk of developing Alzheimer's disease and other forms of dementia (19). Moreover, abundant evidence exists that exposure to repeated TBI from other sports (e.g., boxing) is also associated with an increased risk of neurodegenerative disease (22a). The disease process responsible for TBI-induced dementia is called chronic traumatic encephalopathy (CTE); this is a complex disease that is associated with neuronal death, loss of axons, and chronic inflammation within the brain (22a). For more details on sports-related TBI and CTE see Hay et al. (2016) and Pfister et al. (2015) in the suggested reading list.

TABLE 7.1	Signs and Symptoms of a Concussion		
Physical	**Cognitive**	**Emotional**	**Sleep**
Headache	Difficulty remembering	Irritability	Drowsiness
Nausea	Difficulty concentrating	Sadness	Sleeping more than usual
Vomiting	Feeling mentally "foggy"	Emotional	Sleeping less than usual
Visual problems	Answers questions slowly	Nervousness	Difficulty falling asleep

In general, the neuronal circuits in the brain stem are thought to be responsible for the control of eye movement and muscle tone, equilibrium, support of the body against gravity, and many special reflexes. One of the most important roles of the brain stem in control of locomotion is that of maintaining postural tone. That is, centers in the brain stem provide the nervous activity necessary to maintain normal upright posture and therefore support the body against gravity. It is clear that the maintenance of upright posture requires that the brain stem receive information from several sensory modalities (e.g., vestibular receptors, pressure receptors of the skin, vision). Damage to any portion of the brain stem results in impaired movement control (5, 13, 25).

IN SUMMARY

- The brain can be subdivided into three parts: (1) the cerebrum, (2) the cerebellum, and (3) the brain stem.
- The motor cortex controls motor activity with the aid of input from subcortical areas.
- Sports with a high risk of traumatic brain injury (i.e., concussions) include American football, gymnastics, ice hockey, and boxing.
- Repeated sports related brain injuries are associated with a higher risk of neurodegenerative diseases (e.g., dementia) in later life.
- The disease process responsible for traumatic brain injury-induced dementia is called chronic traumatic encephalopathy (CTE).

MOTOR FUNCTIONS OF THE SPINAL CORD

Growing evidence indicates that the spinal cord contributes to the control of movement. Indeed, there is increasing evidence that normal motor function is influenced by spinal reflexes. Specifically, although signals originating in the motor cortex are required to drive spinal motor neuron activation, growing evidence reveals that the final movement pattern is influenced by spinal cord neural circuitry (5, 23, 27, 59). This occurs by intrinsic spinal networks known as central pattern generators.

The spinal cord makes a major contribution to the control of movement by preparing spinal centers to perform the desired movement. The spinal mechanism by which a voluntary movement is translated into appropriate muscle action is termed *spinal tuning*. Spinal tuning involves intrinsic spinal neuronal networks (i.e., central pattern generators) and operates in the following way (27). Higher brain centers of the motor system are concerned with only the general parameters of movement. The specific details of the movement are refined at the spinal cord level via interaction of spinal cord neurons and higher brain centers. In other words, although the general pattern of the anticipated movement is controlled by higher motor centers, additional refinement of this movement may occur by a complex interaction of spinal cord neurons and higher centers (5). Thus, spinal centers play an important role in volitional movement.

Another motor control function of the spinal cord is the withdrawal reflex, which occurs via a reflex arc.

A reflex arc is the nerve pathway from the receptor to the CNS and from the CNS along a motor pathway back to the effector organ. Reflex contraction of skeletal muscles can occur in response to sensory input and is not dependent on the activation of higher brain centers. One purpose of a reflex is to provide a rapid means of removing a limb from a source of pain. Consider the case of a person touching a sharp object. The obvious reaction to this painful stimulus is to quickly remove the hand from the source of pain. This rapid removal is accomplished via reflex action. Again, the pathways for this neural reflex are as follows (21): (1) a sensory nerve (pain receptor) sends a nerve impulse to the spinal column; (2) interneurons within the spinal cord are excited and in turn stimulate motor neurons; (3) the excited interneurons cause depolarization of specific motor neurons, which control the flexor muscles necessary to withdraw the limb from the point of injury. The antagonistic muscle group (e.g., extensors) is simultaneously inhibited via IPSPs. This simultaneous excitatory and inhibitory activity is known as **reciprocal inhibition** (see Fig. 7.17).

Another interesting feature of the withdrawal reflex is that the opposite limb is extended to support the body during the removal of the injured limb. This event is called the crossed-extensor reflex and is illustrated by the left portion of Figure 7.17. Notice that the extensors are contracting as the flexors are inhibited.

IN SUMMARY

- Evidence exists that the spinal cord plays an important role in voluntary movement, with groups of neurons controlling certain aspects of motor activity.
- The spinal mechanism by which a voluntary movement is translated into appropriate muscle action is termed *spinal tuning*.
- Reflexes provide the body with a rapid, unconscious means of reacting to a painful stimuli.

CONTROL OF MOTOR FUNCTIONS

Watching a highly skilled athlete perform a sports skill is exciting, but it really does not help us to appreciate the complex integration of the many parts of the nervous system required to perform this act. A pitcher throwing a baseball seems to the observer to be accomplishing a simple act, but in reality, this movement consists of a complex interaction of higher brain centers with spinal reflexes performed together with precise timing. How the nervous system produces a coordinated movement has been

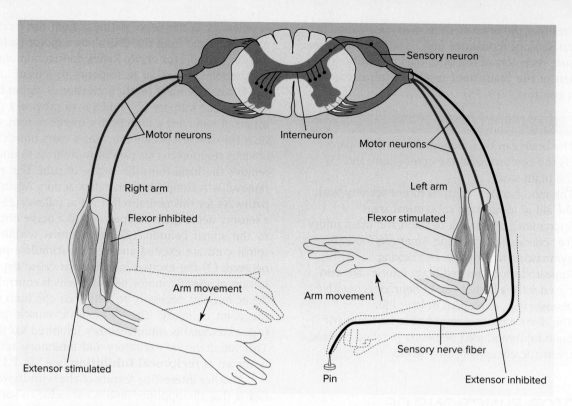

Figure 7.17 When the flexor muscle on one side of the body is stimulated to contract via a withdrawal reflex, the extensor on the opposite side also contracts.

one of the major unresolved mysteries facing neurophysiologists for many decades. Although progress has been made toward answering the basic question of "How do humans control voluntary movement?" much is still unknown about this process. Our purpose here will be to provide the reader with a simplistic overview of the brain and the control of movement.

Traditionally, it was believed that the motor cortex controlled voluntary movement with little input from subcortical areas. However, evidence suggests that this is not the case (23, 55). Although the motor cortex is the final executor of movement programs, it appears that the motor cortex does not give the initial signal to move, but rather is at the end of the chain of neurophysiological events involved in volitional movement (44). The first step in performing a voluntary movement occurs in subcortical and cortical motivational areas, which play a key role in consciousness. This conscious "prime drive" sends signals to the so-called association areas of the cortex (different from the motor cortex), which forms a "rough draft" of the planned movement from a stock of stored subroutines (12, 38). Information concerning the nature of the plan of movement is then sent to both the cerebellum and the basal nuclei (clusters of neurons located in the cerebral hemispheres)

(see Fig. 7.18). These structures cooperate to convert the "rough draft" into precise temporal and spatial excitation programs (23). The cerebellum is possibly more important for making fast movements, whereas the basal nuclei are more responsible for slow or deliberate movements. From the cerebellum and basal nuclei, the precise program is sent through the thalamus to the motor cortex, which forwards the message down to spinal neurons for "spinal tuning" and finally to skeletal muscle (16, 18). Feedback to the CNS from muscle receptors and proprioceptors allows for modification of motor programs if necessary. The ability to change movement patterns allows the individual to correct "errors" in the original movement plan.

To summarize, the control of voluntary movement is complex and requires the cooperation of many areas of the brain as well as several subcortical areas. Evidence indicates that the motor cortex does not by itself formulate the signals required to initiate voluntary movement. Instead, the motor cortex receives input from a variety of cortical and subcortical structures. Feedback to the CNS from muscle and joint receptors allows for adjustments to improve the movement pattern. Much is still unknown about the details of the control of complex movement, and this topic provides an exciting frontier for future research.

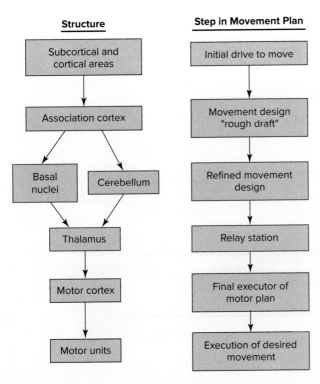

Structure	Step in Movement Plan
Subcortical and cortical areas	Initial drive to move
Association cortex	Movement design "rough draft"
Basal nuclei / Cerebellum	Refined movement design
Thalamus	Relay station
Motor cortex	Final executor of motor plan
Motor units	Execution of desired movement

Figure 7.18 Block diagram of the structures and processes leading to voluntary movement.

IN SUMMARY

- Control of voluntary movement is complex and requires the cooperation of many areas of the brain as well as several subcortical areas.
- The first step in performing a voluntary movement occurs in subcortical and cortical motivational areas, which send signals to the association cortex, which forms a "rough draft" of the planned movement.
- The movement plan is then sent to both the cerebellum and the basal nuclei. These structures cooperate to convert the "rough draft" into precise temporal and spatial excitation programs.
- The cerebellum is important for making fast movements, whereas the basal nuclei are more responsible for slow or deliberate movements.
- From the cerebellum and basal nuclei, the precise program is sent through the thalamus to the motor cortex, which forwards the message down to spinal neurons for "spinal tuning" and finally to skeletal muscle.
- Feedback to the CNS from muscle receptors and proprioceptors allows for the modification of motor programs if necessary.

AUTONOMIC NERVOUS SYSTEM

The **autonomic nervous system** plays an important role in maintaining homeostasis. In contrast to somatic motor nerves, autonomic motor nerves innervate effector organs that are not usually under voluntary control. For example, autonomic motor nerves innervate cardiac muscle, glands, and smooth muscle found in airways, the gut, and blood vessels. In general, the autonomic nervous system operates below the conscious level, although some individuals can learn to control some portions of this system by learning relaxation skills using biofeedback to gain a greater awareness of physiological functions (e.g., heart rate). Although involuntary, it appears that the function of the autonomic nervous system is closely linked to emotion. For example, all of us have experienced an increase in heart rate following extreme excitement or fear. Further, the secretions from the digestive glands and sweat glands are affected by periods of excitement. It should not be surprising that participation in intense exercise results in an increase in autonomic activity.

The autonomic nervous system can be separated both functionally and anatomically into two divisions: (1) **sympathetic nervous system** and (2) **parasympathetic nervous system** (see Fig. 7.19). Most organs receive dual innervation by both the parasympathetic and sympathetic branches of the autonomic nervous system (62). In general, the sympathetic portion of the autonomic nervous system tends to activate an organ (e.g., increases heart rate), whereas parasympathetic impulses tend to inhibit it (e.g., slows heart rate). Therefore, the activity of a particular organ can be regulated according to the ratio of sympathetic/parasympathetic impulses to the tissue. In this way, the autonomic nervous system may regulate the activities of involuntary muscles (i.e., smooth muscle) and glands in accordance with the needs of the body (see Chap. 5).

The sympathetic division of the autonomic nervous system has its cell bodies of the preganglionic neurons in the thoracic and lumbar regions of the spinal cord. These fibers leave the spinal cord and enter the sympathetic ganglion (a ganglion is a mass of neural tissue outside the CNS) (Fig. 7.19). The neurotransmitter between the preganglionic neurons and postganglionic neurons is acetylcholine. Postganglionic sympathetic fibers leave these sympathetic ganglia and innervate a wide variety of tissues. The neurotransmitter released at the effector organ is primarily norepinephrine. Recall from Chap. 5 that norepinephrine exerts its action on the effector organ by binding to either an alpha or a beta receptor on the membrane of the target organ (21).

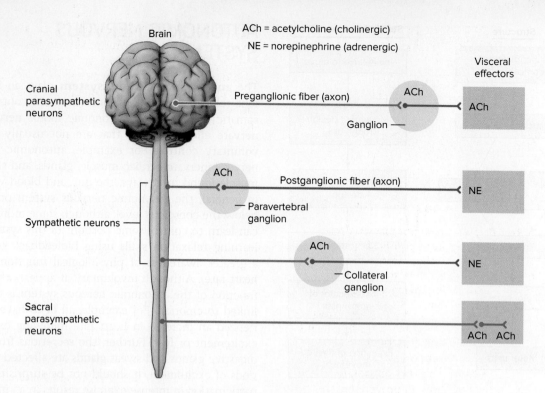

ACh = acetylcholine (cholinergic)
NE = norepinephrine (adrenergic)

Figure 7.19   A simple schematic demonstrating the neurotransmitters of the autonomic nervous system.

Following sympathetic stimulation, norepinephrine is removed in two ways: (1) reuptake into the postganglionic fiber and/or (2) broken down into nonactive by-products (21).

The parasympathetic division of the autonomic nervous system has its cell bodies located within the brain stem and the sacral portion of the spinal cord. Parasympathetic fibers leave the brain stem and the spinal cord and converge on ganglia in a wide variety of anatomical areas. Acetylcholine is the neurotransmitter in both preganglionic and postganglionic fibers. After parasympathetic nerve stimulation, acetylcholine is released and rapidly degraded by the enzyme acetyl-cholinesterase.

At rest, the activities of the sympathetic and parasympathetic divisions of the autonomic nervous system are in balance. However, during a bout of exercise, the activity of the parasympathetic nervous system decreases and activation of the sympathetic nervous system increases. A major role of the sympathetic nervous system during exercise is to regulate blood flow to the working muscles (54). This is achieved by increasing cardiac output and a redistribution of blood flow toward the contracting muscles (discussed in Chap. 9). At the cessation of exercise, sympathetic activity decreases and parasympathetic activity increases, allowing the body to return to a resting state (15).

EXERCISE ENHANCES BRAIN HEALTH

Although it is well known that regular exercise can benefit overall health, a large body of evidence also reveals that exercise can also improve brain (cognitive) function, particularly in later life. Maintaining brain health throughout life is an important goal, and both mental stimulation (e.g., reading) and exercise are interventions that can contribute to good brain health. Therefore, daily exercise is a simple and inexpensive way to help maintain the health of the CNS.

How strong is the evidence that regular exercise improves brain function and protects against age-related deterioration? In short, the evidence is extremely strong. Specifically, numerous studies reveal that exercise targets many aspects of brain function and has broad effects on overall brain health, learning, memory, and depression, particularly in older populations (8). Moreover, regular exercise can protect against several types of dementia (e.g., Alzheimer's disease) and certain types of brain injury (e.g., stroke) (8, 24, 50). Therefore, exercise increases brain health, just as it improves body health, and thus represents an important lifestyle intervention to improve brain function and resistance to neurodegenerative diseases (10, 31, 50).

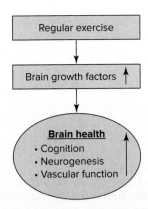

Figure 7.20 Regular exercise targets many aspects of brain function and has broad positive benefits on overall brain health. Specifically, exercise promotes an increase in several brain growth factors that lead to improved brain health by improving cognition, neurogenesis, and vascular function.

How does exercise enhance brain health? Regular aerobic exercise promotes a cascade of brain growth factor signaling that (1) enhances learning and memory; (2) stimulates neurogenesis (i.e., formation of new neurons); (3) improves brain vascular function and blood flow; and (4) attenuates the mechanisms driving depression (7). In addition to these central mechanisms, exercise reduces several peripheral risk factors for cognitive decline, including inflammation, hypertension, and insulin resistance (8). Figure 7.20 summarizes the exercise-induced cascade of events that lead to improved brain function and health.

IN SUMMARY

- The autonomic nervous system is responsible for maintaining the constancy of the body's internal environment.
- Anatomically and functionally, the autonomic nervous system can be divided into two divisions: (1) the sympathetic division and (2) the parasympathetic division.
- In general, the sympathetic portion (releasing norepinephrine) tends to excite an organ, whereas the parasympathetic portion (releasing acetylcholine) tends to inhibit the same organ.
- Research indicates that exercise can improve brain (cognitive) function, particularly in older individuals.

STUDY ACTIVITIES

1. Identify the location and functions of the central nervous system.
2. Draw a simple chart illustrating the organization of the nervous system.
3. Define *synapses*.
4. Define *membrane potential* and *action potential*.
5. Discuss an IPSP and an EPSP. How do they differ?
6. What are proprioceptors? Give some examples.
7. Describe the location and function of the vestibular apparatus.
8. What is meant by the term *spinal tuning*?
9. List the possible motor functions played by the brain stem, the motor cortex, and the cerebellum.
10. Describe the divisions and functions of the autonomic nervous system.
11. Define the terms *motor unit* and *innervation ratio*.
12. Briefly describe the positive benefits of exercise on brain function.
13. How does regular exercise maintain neuronal health?
14. Describe the withdrawal reflex.
15. Outline the functions of both muscle spindles and the Golgi tendon organ.
16. Describe the general anatomical design of a muscle spindle and discuss its physiological function.
17. Discuss the function of Golgi tendon organs in monitoring muscle tension.

SUGGESTED READINGS

Fox, S. *Human Physiology*. New York, NY: McGraw-Hill Companies, 2015.

Halstead, M.E., and K.D. Walter. American Academy of Pediatrics. Clinical report–sport-related concussion in children and adolescents. *Pediatrics* 126: 597-615, 2010.

Hay, J., V. Johnson, D. Smith, and W. Stewart. Chronic traumatic encephalopathy: the neurological legacy of traumatic brain injury. *Annual Review of Pathology and Mechanisms of Disease*. 11: 21-45, 2016.

Intlekofer, K., and C. Cotman. Exercise counteracts declining hippocampal function in aging and Alzheimer's disease. *Neurobiology of Disease*. 57: 47-55, 2013.

Latimer-Cheung, A. et al. Development of evidence-informed physical activity guidelines for adults with multiple sclerosis. *Archives of Physical Medicine and Rehabilitation*. 94: 1829-1836, 2013.

Motl, R.W., and B.M. Sandroff. Benefits of exercise training in multiple sclerosis. *Current Neurology and Neuroscience Reports*. (doi: 10.1007/s11910-015-0585-6) 15: 62, 2015.

Noakes, T. Time to move beyond a brainless exercise physiology: the evidence for complex regulation of human exercise performance. *Applied Physiology, Nutrition, and Metabolism*. 36: 23-35, 2011.

Pfister, T.K. Pfister, B. Hagel, W. Ghali, and P. Ronksley. The incidence of concussion in youth sports: a systematic review and meta-analysis. *British Journal of Sports Medicine*. Published online first. November 30, 2015. doi: 10.1136/bjsports-2015-094978.

Rauch, H., G. Schonbachler, and T. Noakes. Neural correlates of motor vigor and motor urgency during exercise. *Sports Medicine.* doi: 10.1007/s40279-013-0025-1, 2013.

Roatta, S., and Farina, D. Sympathetic actions on the skeletal muscle. *Exercise and Sport Science Reviews* 38: 31-35, 2011.

Shei, R., and T. Mickleborough. Relative contributions of central and peripheral factors in human muscle fatigue during exercise: a brief review. *Journal of Exercise Physiology Online.* 16: 1-17, 2013.

REFERENCES

1. **Asano M, Dawes DJ, Arafah A, Moriello C, and Mayo NE.** What does a structured review of the effectiveness of exercise interventions for persons with multiple sclerosis tell us about the challenges of designing trials? *Multiple Sclerosis* (Houndmills, UK) 15: 412-421, 2009.

2. **Bailes J.** Sports-related concussion: what we know in 2009–a neurosurgeon's perspective. *Journal of the International Neuropsychological Society* 15: 509-511, 2009.

3. **Barchas JD, Akil H, Elliott GR, Holman RB, and Watson SJ.** Behavioral neurochemistry: neuroregulators and behavioral states. *Science* 200: 964-973, 1978.

4. **Barde YA, Edgar D, and Thoenen H.** New neurotrophic factors. *Annu Rev Physiol* 45: 601-612, 1983.

5. **Brodal P.** *Central Nervous System.* New York, NY: Oxford University Press, 2010.

6. **Busse MW, Maassen N, and Konrad H.** Relation between plasma K+ and ventilation during incremental exercise after glycogen depletion and repletion in man. *The Journal of Physiology* 443: 469-476, 1991.

7. **Clark FJ and Burgess PR.** Slowly adapting receptors in cat knee joint: can they signal joint angle? *Journal of Neurophysiology* 38: 1448-1463, 1975.

8. **Cotman CW, Berchtold NC, and Christie LA.** Exercise builds brain health: key roles of growth factor cascades and inflammation. *Trends Neurosci* 30: 464-472, 2007.

9. **De Souza-Teixeira F, Costilla S, Ayan C, Garcia-Lopez D, Gonzalez-Gallego J, and de Paz JA.** Effects of resistance training in multiple sclerosis. *International Journal of Sports Medicine* 30: 245-250, 2009.

10. **Desai AK, Grossberg GT, and Chibnall JT.** Healthy brain aging: a road map. *Clinics in Geriatric Medicine* 26: 1-16, 2010.

11. **Dick RW.** Is there a gender difference in concussion incidence and outcomes? *British Journal of Sports Medicine* 43 (Suppl 1): i46-50, 2009.

12. **Dietz V.** Human neuronal control of automatic functional movements: interaction between central programs and afferent input. *Physiological Reviews* 72: 33-69, 1992.

13. **Eccles JC.** *The Understanding of the Brain.* New York, NY: McGraw-Hill, 1977.

14. **Fox S.** *Human Physiology.* New York, NY: McGraw-Hill, 2015.

15. **Freeman JV, Dewey FE, Hadley DM, Myers J, and Froelicher VF.** Autonomic nervous system interaction with the cardiovascular system during exercise. *Progress in Cardiovascular Diseases* 48: 342-362, 2006.

16. **Fregni F and Pascual-Leone A.** Hand motor recovery after stroke: tuning the orchestra to improve hand motor function. *Cognitive and Behavioral Neurology* 19: 21-33, 2006.

17. **Goodwin GM, McCloskey DI, and Matthews PB.** The contribution of muscle afferents to kinaesthesia shown by vibration induced illusions of movement and by the effects of paralysing joint afferents. *Brain* 95: 705-748, 1972.

18. **Grillner S.** Control of locomotion in bipeds, tetrapods, and fish. In: *Handbook of Physiology: The Nervous System Motor Control.* Washington, DC: American Physiological Society, 1981, 1179-1236.

19. **Guskiewicz KM, Marshall SW, Bailes J, McCrea M, Cantu RC, Randolph C, and Jordan BD.** Association between recurrent concussion and late-life cognitive impairment in retired professional football players. *Neurosurgery* 57: 719-726; discussion 719-726, 2005.

20. **Hakkinen K, Pakarinen A, Kyrolainen H, Cheng S, Kim DH, and Komi PV.** Neuromuscular adaptations and serum hormones in females during prolonged power training. *International Journal of Sports Medicine* 11: 91-98, 1990.

21. **Hall J.** *Guyton and Hall: Texbook of Medical Physiology.* Philadelphia, PA: Saunders, 2016.

22. **Halstead ME and Walter KD.** American Academy of Pediatrics. Clinical report–sport-related concussion in children and adolescents. *Pediatrics* 126: 597-615, 2010.

22a. **Hay J, Johnson V, Smith D, and Stewart W.** Chronic traumatic encephalopathy: the neurological legacy of traumatic brain injury. *Annual Review of Pathology and Mechanisms of Disease.* 11: 21-45, 2016.

23. **Henatsch HD and Langer HH.** Basic neurophysiology of motor skills in sport: a review. *International Journal of Sports Medicine* 6: 2-14, 1985.

24. **Intlekofer K and Cotman C.** Exercise counteracts declining hippocampal function in aging and Alzheimer's disease. *Neurobiology of Disease.* 57: 47-55, 2013.

25. **Kandel E, Schwartz J, Jessell D, Siegelbaum S, and Hudspeth A.** *Principles of Neural Science.* New York, NY: McGraw-Hill, 2012.

26. **Kaufman MP, Rybicki KJ, Waldrop TG, and Ordway GA.** Effect of ischemia on responses of group III and IV afferents to contraction. *Journal of Applied Physiology* 57: 644-650, 1984.

27. **Kiehn O.** Locomotor circuits in the mammalian spinal cord. *Annual Review of Neuroscience.* 29: 279-306, 2006.

28. **Kniffki K, Mense S, and Schmidt R.** Muscle receptors with fine afferent fibers which may evoke circulatory reflexes. *Circulation Research* 48 (Suppl): 25-31, 1981.

29. **Konczak J, Corcos DM, Horak F, Poizner H, Shapiro M, Tuite P, Volkmann J, and Maschke M.** Proprioception and motor control in Parkinson's disease. *Journal of Motor Behavior* 41: 543-552, 2009.

30. **Krieger DT and Martin JB.** Brain peptides (first of two parts). *The New England Journal of Medicine* 304: 876-885, 1981.

31. **Marks BL, Katz LM, and Smith JK.** Exercise and the aging mind: buffing the baby boomer's body and brain. *The Physician and Sportsmedicine* 37: 119-125, 2009.

32. **Matthews PB.** Muscle afferents and kinaesthesia. *British Medical Bulletin* 33: 137-142, 1977.

33. **McAuley E, Kramer AF, and Colcombe SJ.** Where does Sherrington's muscle sense originate? *Annual Review of Neuroscience* 5: 189-218, 1982.

34. **McCloskey D.** Sensing position and movements of the fingers. *News in Physiological Sciences* 2: 226-230, 1987.

35. **McCloskey DI and Mitchell JH.** Reflex cardiovascular and respiratory responses originating in exercising muscle. *The Journal of Physiology* 224: 173-186, 1972.

36. **McCrory P, Meeuwisse W, Johnston K, Dvorak J, Aubry M, Molloy M, and Cantu R.** Consensus statement on concussion in sport–the Third International Conference on Concussion in Sport held in Zurich, November 2008. *The Physician and Sportsmedicine* 37: 141-159, 2009.

37. **Mendell LM.** The size principle: a rule describing the recruitment of motoneurons. *Journal of Neurophysiology* 93: 3024-3026, 2005.

38. **Morton SM and Bastian AJ.** Cerebellar contributions to locomotor adaptations during splitbelt treadmill walking. *Journal of Neuroscience* 26: 9107-9116, 2006.

39. **Nicoll RA, Malenka RC, and Kauer JA.** Functional comparison of neurotransmitter receptor subtypes in mammalian central nervous system. *Physiological Reviews* 70: 513-565, 1990.

40. **Noakes T.** Time to move beyond a brainless exercise physiology: the evidence for complex regulation of human exercise performance. *Applied Physiology, Nutrition, and Metabolism* 36: 23-35, 2011.

41. **Noakes TD, St Clair Gibson A, and Lambert EV.** From catastrophe to complexity: a novel model of integrative central neural regulation of effort and fatigue during exercise in humans: summary and conclusions. *British Journal of Sports Medicine* 39: 120-124, 2005.

42. **O'Donovan MJ.** Developmental regulation of motor function: an uncharted sea. *Medicine & Science in Sports & Exercise* 17: 35-43, 1985.

43. **Ogoh S and Ainslie PN.** Cerebral blood flow during exercise: mechanisms of regulation. *Journal of Applied Physiology* 107: 1370-1380, 2009.

44. **Petersen TH, Rosenberg K, Petersen NC, and Nielsen JB.** Cortical involvement in anticipatory postural reactions in man. *Experimental Brain Research Experimentelle Hirnforschung* 193: 161-171, 2009.

45. **Place N, Bruton JD, and Westerblad H.** Mechanisms of fatigue induced by isometric contractions in exercising humans and in mouse isolated single muscle fibres. *Clinical and Experimental Pharmacology & Physiology* 36: 334-339, 2009.

46. **Powers S, Nelson WB, and Hudson M.** Exercise-induced oxidative stress in humans: cause and consequences. *Free Radical Biology and Medicine.* 51: 942-950, 2011.

47. **Pozzo T, Berthoz A, Lefort L, and Vitte E.** Head stabilization during various locomotor tasks in humans. II. Patients with bilateral peripheral vestibular deficits. *Experimental Brain Research Experimentelle Hirnforschung* 85: 208-217, 1991.

48. **Proske U.** Kinesthesia: the role of muscle receptors. *Muscle & Nerve* 34: 545-558, 2006.

49. **Proske U and Gandevia SC.** The kinaesthetic senses. *The Journal of Physiology* 587: 4139-4146, 2009.

50. **Radak Z, Hart N, Sarga L, Koltai E, Atalay M, Ohno H, and Boldogh I.** Exercise plays a preventive role against Alzheimer's disease. *Journal of Alzheimer's Disease* 20: 777-783, 2010.

51. **Randolph C and Kirkwood MW.** What are the real risks of sport-related concussion, and are they modifiable? *Journal of the International Neuropsychological Society* 15: 512-520, 2009.

52. **Rauch H, Schonbachler G, and Noakes T.** Neural correlates of motor vigor and motor urgency during exercise. *Sports Medicine* 43: 227-241, (doi 10.1007/s40279-013-0025-1), 2013.

53. **Redman S.** Monosynaptic transmission in the spinal cord. *News in Physiological Sciences* 1: 171-174, 1986.

54. **Roatta S and Farina D.** Sympathetic actions on the skeletal muscle. *Exercise and Sport Sciences Reviews* 38: 31-35, 2010.

55. **Sage GH.** *Motor Learning and Control: A Neuropsychological Approach.* New York, NY: McGraw-Hill, 1984.

56. **Saldanha A, Nordlund Ekblom MM, and Thorstensson A.** Central fatigue affects plantar flexor strength after prolonged running. *Scandinavian Journal of Medicine & Science in Sports* 18: 383-388, 2008.

57. **Shephard RJ.** Is it time to retire the "central governor"? *Sports Medicine* (Auckland, NZ) 39: 709-721, 2009.

58. **Shier D, Butler J, and Lewis R.** *Hole's Human Anatomy and Physiology.* New York, NY: McGraw-Hill, 2007.

59. **Soechting J and Flanders M.** Arm movements in three-dimensional space: computation, theory, and observation. In: *Exercise and Sport Science Reviews*, edited by Holloszy J. Baltimore, MD: Lippincott Williams & Wilkins, 1991, 389-418.

60. **Stroud NM and Minahan CL.** The impact of regular physical activity on fatigue, depression and quality of life in persons with multiple sclerosis. *Health and Quality of Life Outcomes* 7: 68, 2009.

61. **Waugh C, Korff T, and Blazevich A.** Effects of resistance training on tendon mechanical properties and rapid force production in prepubertal children. *Journal of Applied Physiology.* 117: 257-266, 2014.

62. **White LJ and Dressendorfer RH.** Exercise and multiple sclerosis. *Sports Medicine* (Auckland, NZ) 34: 1077-1100, 2004.

63. **White LJ, McCoy SC, Castellano V, Gutierrez G, Stevens JE, Walter GA, and Vandenborne K.** Resistance training improves strength and functional capacity in persons with multiple sclerosis. *Multiple Sclerosis* (Houndmills, UK) 10: 668-674, 2004.

64. **Widmaier E, Raff H, and Strang K.** *Vander's Human Physiology.* New York, NY: McGraw-Hill, 2015.

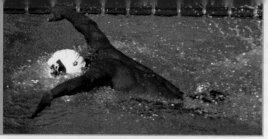

Skeletal Muscle: Structure and Function

■ Objectives

By studying this chapter, you should be able to do the following:

1. Draw and label the microstructure of a skeletal muscle fiber.

2. Define satellite cells. What role do satellite cells play in muscle repair from injury?

3. List the chain of events that occur during muscular contraction.

4. Define both dynamic and static exercise. What types of muscle action occur during each form of exercise?

5. Describe the three factors that determine the amount of force produced during muscular contraction.

6. Compare and contrast the major biochemical and mechanical properties of the three primary types of muscle fibers found in human skeletal muscle.

7. Describe how skeletal muscle fiber types influence athletic performance.

8. Graph and describe the relationship between movement velocity and the amount of force exerted during muscular contraction.

■ Outline

■ Key Terms

actin
concentric action
dynamic
eccentric action
endomysium
end-plate potential (EPP)
epimysium
extensors
fascicle
fast-twitch fibers
flexors
intermediate fibers
isometric action
lateral sac
motor neurons
motor unit
muscle action
myofibrils
myosin
neuromuscular junction (NMJ)

perimysium
postactivation potentiation (PAP)
sarcolemma
sarcomeres
sarcoplasmic reticulum
satellite cells
sliding filament model
slow-twitch fibers
summation
swinging lever-arm model
terminal cisternae
tetanus
transverse tubules
tropomyosin
troponin
twitch
type I fibers
type IIa fibers
type IIx fibers

The human body contains more than 600 skeletal muscles, which constitute 40% to 50% of the total body weight (61). Skeletal muscle performs three important functions: (1) force generation for locomotion and breathing, (2) force generation for postural support, and (3) heat production during cold stress. The most obvious function of skeletal muscle is to enable an individual to move freely and breathe. New evidence also suggests that skeletal muscles are endocrine organs and play an important role in the regulation of a variety of organ systems in the body. This concept was introduced in Chap. 5 and will be mentioned again in this chapter.

Skeletal muscles are attached to bones by tough connective tissue called tendons. One end of the muscle is attached to a bone that does not move (origin), and the opposite end is fixed to a bone (insertion) that is moved during muscular contraction. A variety of different movements are possible, depending on the type of joint and muscles involved. Muscles that decrease joint angles are called **flexors,** and muscles that increase joint angles are called **extensors.**

Given the role of skeletal muscles in determining sports performance, a thorough understanding of muscle structure and function is important to the exercise scientist, physical educator, physical therapist, and coach. Therefore, this chapter will discuss the structure and function of skeletal muscle.

STRUCTURE OF SKELETAL MUSCLE

Skeletal muscle is composed of several kinds of tissue. These include muscle cells (also called muscle fibers) themselves, nerve tissue, blood, and various types of connective tissue. Figure 8.1 displays the relationship

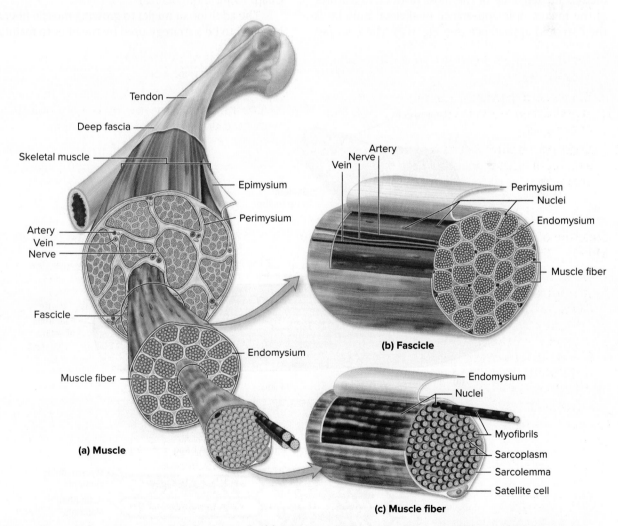

Figure 8.1 Structural organization of skeletal muscle. (*a*) An entire skeletal muscle is covered by a connective tissue layer called the epimysium. (*b*) Each fascicle (i.e., bundle of muscle fibers) is wrapped within a layer of connective tissue called the perimysium. (*c*) Each individual muscle fiber is surrounded by a delicate connective tissue layer called the endomysium.

between muscle and the various connective tissues. Individual muscles are separated from each other and held in position by connective tissue called fascia. Three separate layers of connective tissue exist in skeletal muscle. The outermost layer that surrounds the entire muscle is called the **epimysium.** As we move inward from the epimysium, connective tissue called the **perimysium** surrounds individual bundles of muscle fibers. These individual bundles of muscle fibers are called a **fascicle.** Each muscle fiber within the fasciculus is surrounded by connective tissue called the **endomysium.** Just below the endomysium and surrounding each muscle fiber is another layer of protective tissue called the basal lamina (also called the basement membrane).

Despite their unique shape, muscle fibers contain most of the same organelles that are present in other cells. That is, they contain mitochondria, lysosomes, and so on. However, unlike most other cells in the body, muscle cells are multinucleated (i.e., contain numerous nuclei). One of the most distinctive features of the microscopic appearance of skeletal muscles is their striated appearance (see Fig. 8.2). These stripes are produced by alternating light and dark bands that appear across the length of the fiber; the dark bands contain the primary muscle contractile proteins and will be discussed in detail later.

Each individual muscle fiber is a thin, elongated cylinder that generally extends the length of the muscle. The cell membrane surrounding the muscle fiber cell is called the **sarcolemma.** Located above the sarcolemma and below the basal lamina are a group of muscle precursor cells called satellite cells. **Satellite cells** are undifferentiated cells that are predicted to play a key role in muscle growth and repair (80). In response to resistance exercise training, satellite cells become activated and divide; this increases the number of nuclei (called myonuclei) in the muscle fiber. In theory, an increase in myonuclei in a muscle fiber should enhance the fibers' ability to synthesize proteins and, therefore, assist in muscle growth (80). Nonetheless, debate exists as to whether the addition of nuclei to muscle is required for muscle growth (see Chap. 13 for more details).

The addition of nuclei to growing muscle fibers is believed to be a strategy used by the fiber to maintain

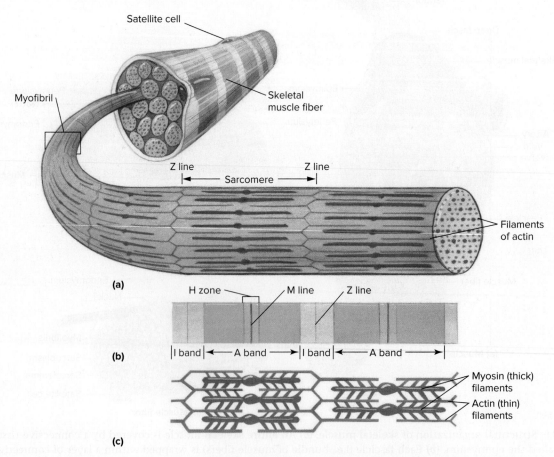

Figure 8.2 The microstructure of muscle. Note that a skeletal muscle fiber contains numerous myofibrils, each consisting of units called sarcomeres.

a constant ratio of cell volume per nucleus. The volume of cytoplasm surrounding an individual nucleus is termed the *myonuclear domain* (1). The biological significance of the myonuclear domain is that a single nucleus can sustain the necessary gene expression (i.e., production of proteins) only for a limited area of cell volume. Therefore, to maintain a constant myonuclear domain, new nuclei (obtained from satellite cells) are incorporated into skeletal muscle fibers during growth (49, 79). It follows that to maintain a stable myonuclear domain, nuclei are lost from fibers when a reduction in muscle fiber size occurs (i.e., muscle atrophy).

Beneath the sarcolemma lies the sarcoplasm (also called cytoplasm), which contains the cellular proteins, organelles, and myofibrils. **Myofibrils** are numerous threadlike structures that contain the contractile proteins (Fig. 8.2). In general, myofibrils are composed of two major types of protein filaments: (1) thick filaments composed of the protein **myosin** and (2) thin filaments composed primarily of the protein **actin.** The arrangement of these two protein filaments gives skeletal muscle its striated appearance (Fig. 8.2). Located on the actin molecule itself are two additional proteins: troponin and tropomyosin. These proteins make up only a small portion of the muscle, but they play an important role in the regulation of the contractile process.

Myofibrils can be further subdivided into individual segments called **sarcomeres.** Sarcomeres are divided from each other by a thin sheet of structural proteins called a *Z line* or *Z disk.* Myosin filaments are located primarily within the dark portion of the sarcomere, which is called the *A band*, while actin filaments occur principally in the light regions of the sarcomere called *I bands* (Fig. 8.2). In the center of the sarcomere is a portion of the myosin filament with no overlap of the actin. This is the *H zone.*

Within the sarcoplasm of muscle is a network of membranous channels that surrounds each myofibril. These channels are called the **sarcoplasmic reticulum** and are storage sites for calcium (Fig. 8.3). This is important because calcium release from the sarcoplasmic reticulum is required to trigger muscular contraction. Another set of membranous channels called the **transverse tubules** extends from the sarcolemma into the muscle fiber and passes completely through the fiber. These transverse tubules pass between two enlarged portions of the sarcoplasmic reticulum called the **terminal cisternae.** All of these parts serve a function in muscular contraction and are discussed in detail later in this chapter.

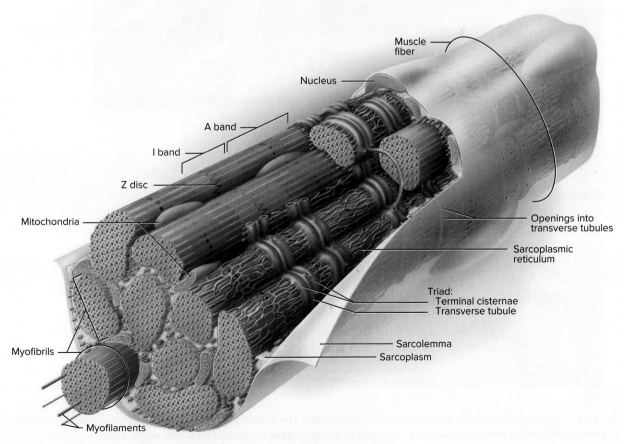

Figure 8.3 Structure of an individual skeletal muscle fiber. See text for details.

NEUROMUSCULAR JUNCTION

Recall from Chap. 7 that each skeletal muscle cell is connected to a nerve fiber branch coming from a nerve cell. These nerve cells are called **motor neurons,** and they extend outward from the spinal cord. The motor neuron and all the muscle fibers it innervates are called a **motor unit.** Stimulation from motor neurons initiates the contraction process. The site where the motor neuron and muscle cell meet is called the **neuromuscular junction (NMJ).** At this junction the sarcolemma forms a pocket that is called the synpaptic cleft (see Fig. 8.4).

The end of the motor neuron does not physically make contact with the muscle fiber, but is separated by a short gap called the synaptic cleft (also called the neuromuscular cleft). When a nerve impulse reaches the end of the motor nerve, the neurotransmitter acetylcholine is released and diffuses across the synaptic cleft to bind with receptor sites on the motor end plate. This causes an increase in the permeability of the sarcolemma to sodium, resulting in a depolarization called the **end-plate potential (EPP).** The EPP is always large enough to exceed threshold and is the signal to begin the contractile process.

From the description above, it is clear that the NMJ is a key component of both the nervous system and the muscle system. Indeed, the NMJ is the synapse that allows communication from the motor neuron to the muscle fiber it innervates. Note that the NMJ is a potential site of neuromuscular fatigue (see Chap. 19). However, both endurance exercise and resistance exercise training promote positive adaptations to the NMJ. Specifically, both forms of exercise training increase the size of the NMJ. Importantly, this increase in NMJ size is accompanied by an increased number of synaptic vesicles (containing acetylcholine) and an expanded number of acetylcholine receptors on the postsynaptic

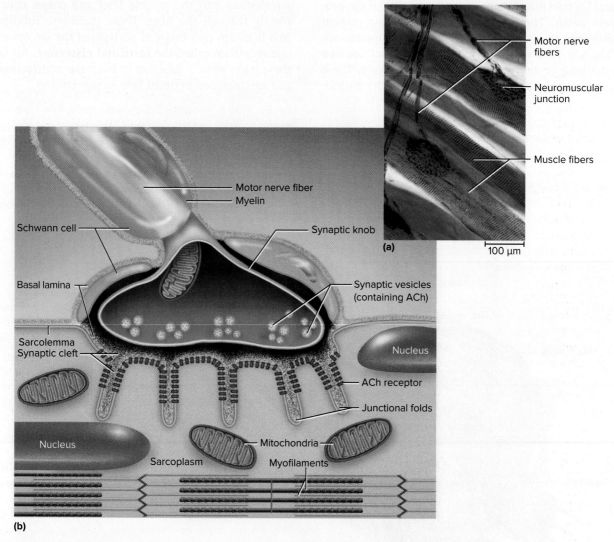

Figure 8.4   The connecting point between a motor neuron and the muscle fiber is called the neuromuscular junction. The neurotransmitter acetylcholine (ACh) is stored in synaptic vesicles at the end of the nerve fiber.
(A) © Victor B. Eichler, Ph.D.

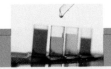

A LOOK BACK—IMPORTANT PEOPLE IN SCIENCE

Andrew F. Huxley Developed the "Sliding Filament Theory of Muscle Contraction"

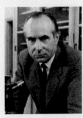

© Keystone/Getty Images

Andrew Huxley (1917-2012) received the Nobel Prize in Physiology and Medicine in 1963 for his research on nerve transmission. Huxley was born in London, England, and was educated at the University of Cambridge.

During his distinguished research career, Huxley made many important contributions to physiology. One of his first significant areas of research was the process of how neural transmission occurs. Working with Alan Hodgkin, the pair hypothesized that neural transmission (i.e., development of an action potential) occurs due to ions passing through ion channels on cell membranes. This hypothesis was confirmed years later, and Dr. Huxley

and Dr. Hodgkin shared the Nobel Prize in 1963 for this work.

Although he won the Nobel Prize for his research on neural transmission, Professor Huxley is probably best known for his work on how skeletal muscles contract. Dr. Huxley and his research colleagues developed the "sliding filament theory of muscle contraction," and many investigators have since confirmed the basic principles of this original theory.

---

membrane (53). These exercise-induced adaptations are predicted to improve the ability of the motor neuron to activate muscle contraction, which could improve performance in many sports.

IN SUMMARY

- The human body contains more than 600 voluntary skeletal muscles, which constitute 40% to 50% of the total body weight. Skeletal muscle performs three major functions: (1) force production for locomotion and breathing, (2) force production for postural support, and (3) heat production during cold stress.
- Individual muscle fibers are composed of hundreds of threadlike protein filaments called myofibrils. Myofibrils contain two major types of contractile protein: (1) actin (part of the thin filaments) and (2) myosin (major component of the thick filaments).
- The region of cytoplasm surrounding an individual nucleus is termed the *myonuclear domain*. The importance of the myonuclear domain is that a single nucleus is responsible for the gene expression for its surrounding cytoplasm.
- Motor neurons extend outward from the spinal cord and innervate individual muscle fibers. The site where the motor neuron and muscle cell meet is called the neuromuscular junction. Acetylcholine is the neurotransmitter that stimulates the muscle fiber to depolarize, which is the signal to start the contractile process.
- Both endurance training and resistance exercise training stimulate positive adaptations to the NMJ that include the following: (1) increasing the size of the NMJ, (2) expanding the number of synaptic vesicles (containing acetylcholine), and (3) increasing the number of acetylcholine receptors on the postsynaptic membrane.

MUSCULAR CONTRACTION

Muscular contraction is a complex process involving numerous cellular proteins and energy production systems. The final result is the sliding of actin over myosin, which causes the muscle to shorten and therefore develop tension. Although complete details of muscular contraction at the molecular level continue to be investigated, the basic steps that lead to muscular contraction are well defined. The process of muscular contraction is explained by the **sliding filament model** of contraction, which is also called the **swinging lever-arm model** of muscle contraction (31, 40, 69). For a historical overview of the sliding filament theory of muscle contraction, see A Look Back–Important People in Science.

Overview of the Sliding Filament/ Swinging Lever-Arm Model

The general process or "big picture" of muscular contraction is illustrated in Figure 8.5. Muscle fibers contract by a shortening of their myofibrils due to actin sliding over the myosin. This results in a reduction in the distance from Z line to Z line. Understanding the details of how muscular contraction occurs requires an appreciation of the microscopic structure of the myofibril. Note that the "heads" of the myosin cross-bridges are oriented toward the actin molecule (see Fig. 8.6). The actin and myosin filaments slide across each other during muscular contraction due to the action of the numerous cross-bridges extending out as "arms" from myosin and attaching to actin. The binding of the myosin cross-bridge to actin results in the myosin cross-bridge moving the actin molecule toward the center of the sarcomere. This "pulling" of actin over the myosin molecule results in muscle shortening and the generation of force.

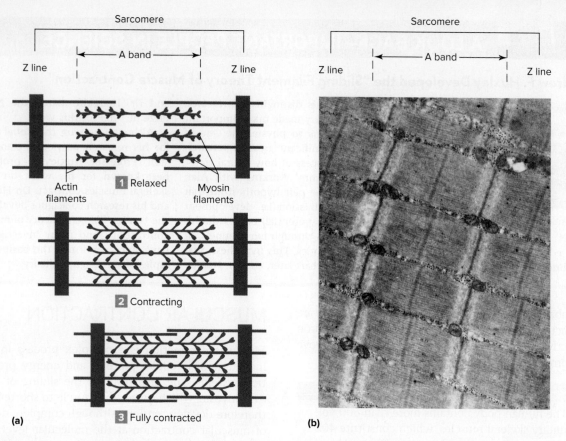

Figure 8.5 When a skeletal muscle contracts, (*a*) individual sarcomeres shorten as thick (myosin) and thin (actin) filaments slide past one another. (*b*) Photograph taken with an electron microscope that illustrates a shortened sarcomere during muscle contraction (magnification to 40,000×).

(B) © Biophoto Associates/Science Source

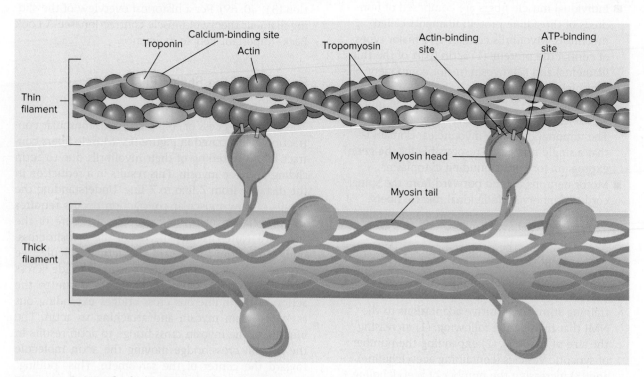

Figure 8.6 Proposed relationships among troponin, tropomyosin, myosin cross-bridges, and calcium. Note that when Ca++ binds to troponin, tropomyosin is removed from the active sites on actin and cross-bridge attachment can occur.

The term *excitation-contraction coupling* refers to the sequence of events in which a nerve impulse (action potential) reaches the muscle membrane and leads to muscle shortening by cross-bridge activity. This process will be discussed step-by-step next. Let's begin with a discussion of the energy source for contraction.

Energy for Contraction

The energy for muscular contraction comes from the breakdown of ATP by the enzyme myosin ATPase (21, 32, 36, 37, 41, 43). This enzyme is located on the "head" of the myosin cross-bridge. Recall that the bioenergetic pathways responsible for the synthesis of ATP were discussed in Chap. 3 and are resummarized in Figure 8.7. The breakdown of ATP to ADP and inorganic phosphate (Pi) and the release of energy serves to energize the myosin cross-bridges, which in turn pull the actin molecules over myosin and thus shorten the muscle (25, 37, 50, 75).

Note that a single contraction cycle or "power stroke" of all the cross-bridges in a muscle would shorten the muscle by only 1% of its resting length. Because some muscles can shorten up to 60% of their resting length, it is clear that the contraction cycle must be repeated over and over again.

Regulation of Excitation-Contraction Coupling

Again, the term *excitation-contraction coupling* refers to the sequence of events that produce depolarization of the muscle (excitation), which leads to muscle shortening and force production (contraction). In the next sections, we will provide a big-picture overview of the excitation-contraction coupling process, followed by a discussion of the events leading to muscle relaxation. Let's begin with the process of excitation.

Excitation The process of excitation begins with the nerve impulse arriving at the neuromuscular junction. The action potential from the motor neuron causes the release of acetylcholine into the synaptic cleft of the neuromuscular junction; acetylcholine binds to receptors on the motor end plate, producing an end-plate potential that leads to depolarization of the muscle cell (61). This depolarization (i.e., excitation) is conducted down the transverse tubules deep into the muscle fiber. This excitation process leads to depolarization of the muscle, which results in the release of calcium from the sarcoplasmic reticulum into the sacroplasm of the muscle. The "big picture" of how the release of free calcium results in muscular contraction is summarized in the next section.

Contraction When the action potential reaches the sarcoplasmic reticulum, calcium is released and diffuses into the muscle to bind to a protein called troponin. This is the "trigger" step in the control of muscular contraction because the regulation of contraction is controlled by two regulatory proteins, **troponin** and **tropomyosin,** which are located on the actin molecule. Troponin and tropomyosin regulate muscular contraction by controlling the interaction of actin and myosin.

To understand how the release of calcium from the sarcoplasmic reticulum interacts with troponin and tropomyosin to control muscular contraction, let's examine the anatomical relationship between actin, troponin, and tropomyosin (see Fig. 8.6). Notice that the actin filament is formed from many protein subunits arranged in a double row and twisted. Tropomyosin is a thin molecule that lies in a groove between the double rows of actin. Note that troponin is attached directly to the tropomyosin. This arrangement allows troponin and tropomyosin to work together to regulate the attachment of myosin cross-bridges to their binding site on the actin molecule. In a relaxed

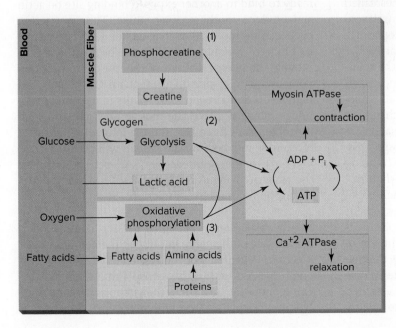

Figure 8.7 The three sources of ATP production in muscle during contraction: (1) phosphocreatine, (2) glycolysis, and (3) oxidative phosphorylation.

Vander, A. J., et al., *Human Physiology: The Mechanisms of Body Function*, 8th ed. New York: McGraw-Hill, Inc., 2005.

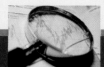
Step-by-Step Summary of Excitation-Contraction Coupling and Relaxation

In the sections below, we highlight the steps involved in muscle excitation, contraction, and relaxation. Note that each numbered step below corresponds to the numbered events illustrated in Figure 8.8.

Excitation

Excitation is illustrated in the first three steps of Figure 8.8.

1. A nerve signal arrives at the synaptic knob.

2. The synaptic vesicles release acetylcholine (ACh) that diffuses across the synaptic cleft and binds to receptors on the sarcolemma of the muscle fiber. This opens ion channels on the sarcolemma that results in the movement of sodium into the fiber.

3. The inward movement of positive sodium ions depolarizes the fiber and sends a wave of depolarization through the T-tubules.

Contraction

Muscle contraction occurs following depolarization (i.e., excitation) of the muscle fiber and is illustrated in steps 4 to 8 in Figure 8.8.

4. Depolarization of the T-tubules results in the release of calcium from the sarcoplasmic reticulum (SR) into the cytosol of the muscle fiber.

5. Calcium ions bind to troponin (located on actin molecule). Calcium binding to troponin results in a shift in the position of tropomyosin so that the myosin binding sites on actin are exposed.

6-8. Steps 6 to 8 illustrate cross-bridge cycling and development of muscle force production. Briefly, an energized myosin cross-bridge binds to the active site on actin and pulls on the actin molecule to produce movement (i.e., fiber shortens). Steps 6 to 8 occur repeatedly as long as neural stimulation to

the muscle continues. To view an illustration of the process of muscular contraction, please see Figure 8.9 that illustrates the step-by-step events involved in myosin cross-bridge cycling.

Relaxation

9. The first step in muscle relaxation occurs when the motor neuron stops to fire. Indeed, when neural stimulation of the muscle ceases, ACh is no longer released and the muscle fiber is repolarized.

10. When the motor neuron ceases to fire and muscle excitation ceases, calcium is pumped from the cytosol into the SR for storage. Without free calcium in the cytosol, troponin moves tropomyosin back into position to cover the myosin binding sites on actin. This tropomyosin coverage of the active sites on actin prevents myosin-actin cross-bridge formation and therefore muscle relaxation occurs.

---

muscle, tropomyosin blocks the active sites on the actin molecule where the myosin cross-bridges must attach to produce a contraction. The trigger for contraction to occur is linked to the release of stored calcium (Ca^{2+}) from a region of the sarcoplasmic reticulum termed the **lateral sac,** or sometimes called the *terminal cisternae* (51, 72). In a resting (relaxed) muscle, the concentration of Ca^{2+} in the sarcoplasm is very low. However, when a nerve impulse arrives at the neuromuscular junction, it travels down the transverse tubules to the sarcoplasmic reticulum and causes the release of Ca^{2+}. Much of this Ca^{2+} binds to troponin (see Fig. 8.6), which causes a position change in tropomyosin such that the active sites on the actin are uncovered. This permits the binding of a myosin cross-bridge on the actin molecule. The cross-bridge binding initiates the release of energy stored within the myosin molecule; this produces movement of each cross-bridge, resulting in muscle shortening. This movement of the myosin cross-bridge to pull the actin molecule is often referred to as the "power-stroke." Attachment of "fresh" ATP to the myosin cross-bridges breaks the myosin cross-bridge bound to actin. The enzyme ATPase again hydrolyzes (i.e., breaks down) the ATP attached to the myosin cross-bridge and provides the energy

necessary for "cocking" the myosin cross-bridge for reattachment to another active site on an actin molecule. The breakdown of ATP provides the energy to "cock" the myosin cross-bridge into an energized state; the "cocked" and energized myosin cross-bridge is now ready to bind to another exposed binding site on actin and produce another power stroke. This contraction cycle can be repeated as long as free Ca^{2+} is available to bind to troponin and ATP can be hydrolyzed to provide the energy. Failure of the muscle to maintain homeostasis (e.g., due to inadequate Ca^{2+} levels and high levels of hydrogen ions) results in impaired cross-bridge movement, and the muscle fiber loses the ability to generate force (i.e., muscle fatigue). The causes of exercise-induced muscle fatigue will be introduced in a forthcoming segment. See A Closer Look 8.1 and the associated Figures 8.8 and 8.9 for a step-by-step description of muscle contraction.

Muscle relaxation The signal to stop contraction is the absence of the nerve impulse at the neuromuscular junction. When this occurs, an energy-requiring Ca^{2+} pump located within the sarcoplasmic reticulum begins to move Ca^{2+} back into the sarcoplasmic reticulum. This removal of Ca^{2+} from troponin causes tropomyosin

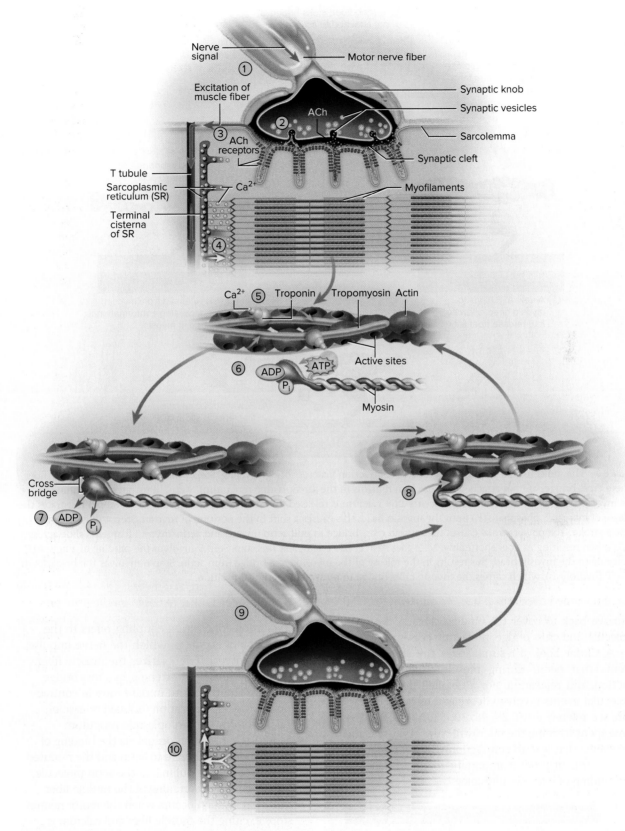

Figure 8.8   The primary events leading muscle excitation, contraction, and relaxation. Steps 1 to 3 illustrate the excitation phase. Steps 4 to 8 represent the events leading to muscle contraction and steps 9 and 10 illustrate muscle relaxation following a contraction. Please see the text and a Closer Look 8.1 for a full explanation of the process of excitation, contraction, and relaxation.

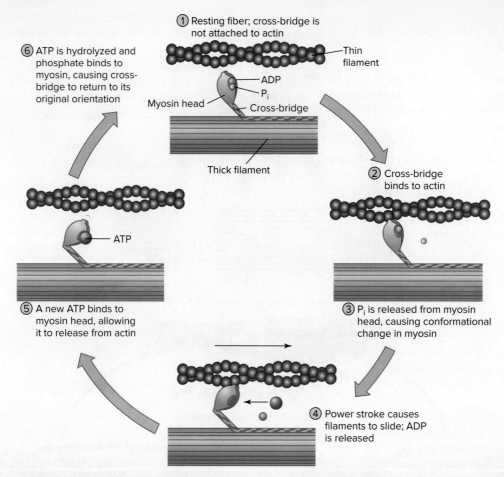

① Resting fiber; cross-bridge is not attached to actin

Thin filament

ADP
P_i

Myosin head
Cross-bridge

Thick filament

⑥ ATP is hydrolyzed and phosphate binds to myosin, causing cross-bridge to return to its original orientation

② Cross-bridge binds to actin

ATP

③ P_i is released from myosin head, causing conformational change in myosin

⑤ A new ATP binds to myosin head, allowing it to release from actin

④ Power stroke causes filaments to slide; ADP is released

Figure 8.9 The molecular steps leading to muscle contraction via cross-bridge cycling. Step 1 illustrates a resting muscle fiber where cross-bridges are not attached (i.e., calcium remains in the sarcoplasmic reticulum). Step 2 illustrates the binding of the myosin cross-bridge to actin, which occurs after calcium is released from the sarcoplasmic reticulum. Step 3 illustrates the release of inorganic phosphate (P_i) from the myosin head; this causes a shift in the position of myosin. Step 4 illustrates the power stroke. The power stroke causes the myosin cross-bridge to pull actin inward and actin/myosin filaments slide across each other, resulting in fiber shortening. Note that ADP is also released at this step. Step 5 involves the binding of a new ATP molecule to the myosin head; this results in the release of the myosin cross-bridge from actin. Step 6 involves the breakdown of ATP (hydrolysis), which causes the myosin cross-bridge to return to its original position.

to move back to cover the binding sites on the actin molecule, and cross-bridge interaction ceases.

A Closer Look 8.1 summarizes the step-by-step events that occur during muscle excitation, contraction, and relaxation. For a detailed discussion of molecular events involved in skeletal muscle contraction, see references (9, 25, 28, 30, 31, 37–39, 47, 75). Time spent learning the microstructure of muscle and the events that lead to contraction will pay dividends later, as this material is important to a thorough understanding of exercise physiology.

IN SUMMARY

■ The process of muscular contraction can be best explained by the sliding filament/swinging cross-bridge model, which proposes that muscle shortening occurs due to movement of the actin filament over the myosin filament.

■ Excitation-contraction coupling refers to the sequence of events in which the nerve impulse (action potential) depolarizes the muscle fiber, leading to muscle shortening by cross-bridge cycling. The trigger to initiate muscle contraction is the depolarization-induced release of calcium from the sarcoplasmic reticulum.

■ Muscular contraction occurs via the binding of the myosin cross-bridge to actin and the repeated cycling of myosin pulling on the actin molecule resulting in the shortening of the muscle fiber.

■ Muscle relaxation occurs when the motor neuron stops exciting the muscle fiber and calcium is pumped backed into the sarcoplasmic reticulum. This removal of calcium from the cytosol causes a position change in tropomyosin, which blocks the myosin cross-bridge binding site on the actin molecule; this action results in muscle relaxation.

EXERCISE AND MUSCLE FATIGUE

High-intensity exercise or prolonged, submaximal exercise results in a decline in the muscle's ability to generate power. This decrease in muscle power output is called fatigue. Specifically, muscle fatigue is defined as a reduction in muscle power output that can result from a decrease in both muscle force generation and shortening velocity. The onset of muscle fatigue during exercise is illustrated in Figure 8.10. Note that muscle fatigue differs from injury to the muscle because muscle fatigue is reversible by a few hours of rest, whereas recovery from muscle damage may take days to weeks to fully recover (30).

The causes of exercise-induced muscle fatigue are complex and not fully understood. Depending upon the type of exercise and the environmental conditions, fatigue may result in disturbances in the central nervous system and/or peripheral factors within skeletal muscle (2). The concept of "central nervous system fatigue" was introduced in Chap. 7, and we will focus on peripheral (i.e., skeletal muscle) fatigue here.

Although the exact causes of muscle fatigue remain under investigation, it is clear that an individual's state of fitness, nutritional status, fiber type composition, and the intensity and duration of exercise all affect the fatigue process (30). Further, regardless of the cause of muscle fatigue, the end result is a decline in muscle force generation due to impaired force production at the cross-bridge level. An overview of the potential contributors to exercise-induced muscle fatigue follows.

The causes of muscle fatigue are complex and vary depending upon the type of exercise performed. For example, muscle fatigue resulting from high-intensity exercise lasting approximately 60 seconds (e.g., sprinting 400 meters) may be due to several factors, including an accumulation of lactate, hydrogen ions, ADP, inorganic phosphate, and free radicals within the active muscle fibers (30). Collectively, the accumulation of these metabolites disrupts muscle

homeostasis and diminishes the number of cross-bridges bound to actin, resulting in diminished force production (24b, 30, 46, 76, 78).

Muscular fatigue that occurs in the later stages of an endurance event lasting two to four hours (i.e., marathon running) may also involve an accumulation of free radicals in the muscle, but other factors such as disturbances in muscle/extracellular electrolyte homeostasis and depletion of muscle glycogen may also contribute to this type of muscle fatigue (30, 55, 56, 58, 59, 78). Muscle fatigue and the limiting factors to exercise performance are discussed in more detail in Chap. 19.

IN SUMMARY

- Muscle fatigue is defined as a reduction in muscle power output that results from decreased muscle force generation and/or decreased shortening velocity.
- The causes of exercise-induced muscle fatigue are complex and vary depending upon the type of exercise performed.

EXERCISE-ASSOCIATED MUSCLE CRAMPS

Almost everyone has experienced muscle cramps at one time or another. Exercise-induced cramps are often associated with prolonged high-intensity exercise. Muscle cramps can be painful and are the result of spasmodic, involuntary muscle contractions. While it is widely agreed that muscle cramps have a nervous system origin, the question remains as to whether the cause of the cramp resides within the peripheral nervous system or central nervous system. These possibilities form the two primary theories to explain exercise-induced muscle cramps. One popular theory is that cramps are caused by dehydration and electrolyte balances. The second theory is that muscle cramps originate in the central nervous system due to increased excitability of motor neurons. Let's discuss each of these potential causes of exercise-associated muscle cramping in more detail.

Exercise-Associated Muscle Cramps Are Not Caused by Dehydration or Electrolyte Imbalance

A popular belief among many coaches and athletes is that muscle cramps result from exercise-induced dehydration and electrolyte imbalance. Supporters of this concept argue that abnormal electrolyte levels (e.g., sodium or magnesium) in the interstitial space surrounding the nerve terminal result in a discharge of acetylcholine from the synaptic knob with the end result being muscle contraction (Figs. 8.4 and 8.8) (7, 8). This uncontrolled release of acetylcholine would

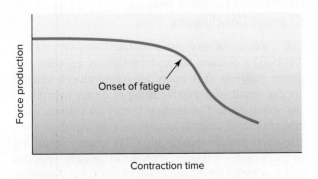

Figure 8.10 Muscular fatigue is characterized by a reduced ability to generate force.

eventually produce widespread, spasmodic muscle contractions (i.e., cramps).

To date, few studies support the concept that exercise-induced muscle cramps result from electrolyte imbalances, and several observations suggest that electrolyte imbalances are not responsible for exercise-associated muscle cramps (66). First, dehydration and electrolyte imbalance affect the entire body, yet the exercising muscles are the only muscles that experience cramps. It follows that, if muscle cramps are caused by dehydration or electrolyte imbalance, cramps would occur in all muscles rather than only the working muscles. Second, repeated electrical stimulation of a small group of skeletal muscles has been shown to induce muscle cramping; this type of contraction-induced muscle cramping occurs without any change in blood electrolyte concentrations (67). Third, static stretching of the cramping muscle often relieves the cramp. If dehydration caused the cramp, stretching would have no effect on cramping because no fluids or electrolytes were added to the body. Finally, athletes that commonly suffer from exercise-induced cramps often have the same blood electrolyte concentrations as athletes that do not experience cramps. Indeed, cramp-prone athletes often drink similar, if not more, fluid than athletes without a history of cramping. In conclusion, limited support exists for the concept that most exercise-associated muscle cramps are the result of dehydration and electrolyte imbalance. Nonetheless, it remains feasible that during some extreme exercise conditions (i.e., prolonged exercise in a hot environment) electrolyte imbalance could result in muscle cramps.

Exercise-Associated Muscle Cramps Are Likely Due to Changes in the Central Nervous System

In contrast to the limited evidence supporting the notion that dehydration/electrolyte imbalances are the most common cause of muscle cramps, experimental evidence suggests that exercise-associated muscle cramps can occur due to exercise-induced changes in the central nervous system that result in increased excitability of motor neurons. Specifically, if motor neurons innervating skeletal muscles become hyperexcited and undergo repeated depolarization, this results in uncontrolled, involuntary muscle contractions (i.e., cramps). Potential causes of increased motor neuron excitability include high levels of excitatory input to the motor neurons and/or the lack of inhibitory input to the motor neurons.

How does prolonged and intense exercise promote increased excitability of motor neurons in the spinal cord? One explanation is that prolonged, intense exercise often results in muscle fatigue and/or

injury, which can promote dysfunction of the muscle spindle and/or the Golgi tendon organ (GTO) (67). Specifically, it is possible that rigorous exercise results in increased afferent signals from the muscle spindle and depressed signals from the GTO. Recall that the GTO provides the central nervous system with feedback about muscle force generation, whereas the muscle spindle functions as a length detector (Chap. 7). Also, remember that stimulation of the GTO sends inhibitory signals to the spinal cord to prevent motor neuron depolarization, whereas stimulation of the muscle spindle sends afferent signals to the spinal cord to promote motor neuron activation. Therefore, in theory, rigorous exercise could promote muscle cramps by decreasing the firing of GTO (i.e., decreased inhibition of motor neuron firing) and increasing the firing of the muscle spindles (i.e., increased motor neuron activation).

Several lines of evidence support the view that exercise can promote dysfunction of muscle sense organs and trigger muscle cramps. First, rigorous exercise can impair Golgi tendon function and reduce the number of afferent signals sent from the GTO to motor neurons (67). Further, electrical stimulation of GTO resulting in increased afferent signals can relieve muscle cramps (67). Similarly, passive stretching of a cramping muscle can often relieve the cramp (67). The mechanism to explain this stretch response is that passive stretching relieves muscle cramps by invoking inverse stretch reflex. Recall that the inverse stretch reflex occurs by stretch-induced activation of the GTO, which inhibits motor neurons in the spinal cord and results in muscle relaxation (Chap. 7). Finally, studies also suggest that prolonged exercise increases muscle spindle firing and that electrical stimulation of muscle spindle afferents induces muscle cramping by sending afferent signals to the spinal cord to activate motor neurons (67). Collectively, these studies provide support for the concept that exercise-induced impairment of muscle sense organs is a potential link to generate muscle cramps via a central nervous system mechanism.

Exercise-Associated Muscle Cramps: Conclusions

The cause(s) of exercise-associated muscle cramps remain(s) a debated topic. Nonetheless, growing evidence suggests that many exercise-induced cramps are the result of excessive firing of motor neurons in the spinal cord. The leading theory to explain exercise-associated muscle cramps is that rigorous exercise alters muscle spindle and GTO function resulting in increased excitatory activity of muscle spindles and a reduced inhibitory effect of the GTO. Together, these actions promote sustained motor neuron activity and the resulting muscle cramp.

Help for People with Muscle Cramps?

As discussed in the text, growing evidence indicates that repetitive firing of motor neurons in the spinal cord is the underlying cause of exercise-induced muscle cramps. Although many common remedies (e.g., sports drinks, bananas, and pickle juice) have been proposed to treat and prevent muscle cramps, none of these interventions has been proven to be consistently effective in the prevention of cramps.

Nonetheless, a recent study provides hope that a treatment plan for muscle cramps is on the horizon. The story of this discovery begins with two scientists who were avid sea kayakers–Rod MacKinnon, MD, Nobel Laureate in Chemistry at Rockefeller University, and Bruce Bean, Ph.D., professor at Harvard Medical School. Both were well-trained and experienced paddlers who carefully monitored both their nutrition and hydration. Yet, during a paddling trip on the ocean, both MacKinnon and Bean developed severe muscle cramps. Battling the persistent muscle cramps, both MacKinnon and Bean eventually made it back to shore. However, this ordeal motivated them to study the mechanisms responsible for muscle cramps.

When MacKinnon found out how little the exercise science community understood about cramping, he became obsessed about developing a treatment plan to prevent muscle cramps. For MacKinnon, a serious athlete who had spent the majority of his professional career investigating ion channels, which appear to play a role in muscle cramps, his two worlds came together, and he began to study the causes of muscle cramps. After several years of research, MacKinnon and his colleagues concluded that muscle cramps do not originate in the muscle itself. Instead, cramps appear to be triggered by a neural mechanism in the central nervous system that promotes excessive firing of the motor neurons in the spinal cord that control muscle contraction. MacKinnon then asked the question, "How do we prevent this excessive firing of motor neurons?"

MacKinnon and colleagues reasoned that a potential treatment to prevent muscle cramps is to suppress the firing of overactive motor neurons by sending a strong inhibitory stimulus into the spinal cord. Further, they predicted that inhibition of motor neuron firing could be achieved by ingestion of natural ingredients that stimulate sensory nerves located in the mouth and throat; importantly these sensory nerves project to the spinal cord and inhibit hyperexcited motor neurons. This mouth to spine connection is not as far-fetched as it sounds. Indeed, we all have experienced the pain associated with drinking icy-cold drinks (commonly called brain freeze). This brain freeze sensation occurs due to the rapid cooling of a cluster of nerves in the roof of the mouth. For similar reasons, ingestion of selected spices and other natural ingredients (e.g., ginger, capsaicin in red peppers) activate specific ion channels in sensory nerves called transient receptor potential (TRP) channels. Activation of these TRP channels switches on nerves that send inhibitory signals to the spinal cord to inhibit the overactive motor neurons that cause cramping.

To test the hypothesis that oral ingestion of natural spices can prevent muscle cramps, MacKinnon and colleagues conducted experiments on volunteer subjects. Their preliminary results indicated that ingestion of these spices activated TRP channels in the mouth and throat, sending inhibitory signals to the spinal cord to block excessive firing of motor neurons. Importantly, these initial results reveal that the frequency and duration of exercise-associated muscle cramps were reduced when subjects ingested a specially formulated spicy beverage before exercise (1). Therefore, it appears that we are moving closer to a scientifically based treatment plan for prevention of exercise-induced muscle cramps. Stay tuned as help to prevent muscle cramps is on the way!

1. Short et al. Orally-administered TRV1 and TRPA1 activators inhibit electrically-induced muscle cramps in normal healthy volunteers. *Neurology.* 84: Supplement S17.003, 2015.

At present, the only known and reliable relief for exercise-induced muscle cramping is passive stretch of the muscle. Nonetheless, over the years, many different "home remedies" have been proposed to prevent and relieve muscle cramping. These include salt tablets, bananas, pickle juice, and sports drinks. Unfortunately, none of these treatments has been scientifically proven to consistently prevent exercise-induced muscle cramps. However, new research suggests that the oral ingestion of one of several natural ingredients has the potential to protect against exercise-induced muscle cramps (see Research Focus 8.1 for details). For more information about exercise and muscle cramps, see Miller (2016) and Minetto et al. (2010) in the Suggested Readings list.

IN SUMMARY

- Muscle cramps are spasmodic and involuntary muscle contractions.
- The cause of exercise-induced muscle cramps continues to be debated and two major theories have emerged: (1) Muscle cramps are caused by dehydration and electrolyte imbalance and (2) muscle cramps originate in the central nervous system.
- Although the exact cause of muscle cramps remains unsettled, it appears that motor neuron hyperexcitability is likely the general underlying cause of many exercise-induced muscle cramps suggesting that muscle cramps originate from the central nervous system.

MUSCLE FIBER TYPES

Human skeletal muscle can be divided into major classes based on the histochemical or biochemical characteristics of the individual fibers. Specifically, muscle fibers are classified into two general categories: (1) slow, type I fibers (also called slow twitch fibers) and (2) fast, type II fibers (also called fast-twitch fibers) (16, 18, 26, 27). Only one type of slow muscle fiber (type I) exists in human muscle, whereas two subcategories of fast, type II fibers exist: (a) type IIa fibers and (b) type IIx fibers. Though some muscles are composed of predominantly fast or slow fibers, most muscles in the body contain a mixture of both slow and fast fiber types. The percentage of the respective fiber types contained in skeletal muscles can be influenced by genetics, blood levels of hormones, and the exercise habits of the individual. From a practical standpoint, the fiber composition of skeletal muscles plays an important role in performance in both power and endurance events (11, 70). How muscle fibers are "typed" is introduced in A Closer Look 8.2.

Overview of Biochemical and Contractile Characteristics of Skeletal Muscle

Before discussing the functional characteristics of specific muscle fiber types, let's discuss the general biochemical and contractile properties of skeletal muscle that are important to muscle function.

Biochemical Properties of Muscle The three primary biochemical characteristics of muscle that are important to muscle function are (1) the oxidative capacity, (2) the type of myosin isoform, and (3) the abundance of contractile protein within the fiber. The oxidative capacity of a muscle fiber is determined by the number of mitochondria, the number of capillaries surrounding the fiber, and the amount of myoglobin within the fiber. A large number of mitochondria provides a greater capacity to produce ATP aerobically. A high number of capillaries surrounding a muscle fiber ensures that the fiber will receive adequate oxygen during periods of contractile activity. Myoglobin is similar to hemoglobin in the blood in that it binds O_2, and it also acts as a "shuttle" mechanism for O_2

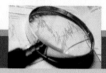

A CLOSER LOOK 8.2

How Are Skeletal Muscle Fibers Typed?

The relative percentage of fast or slow fibers contained in a particular muscle can be estimated by removing a small piece of muscle (via a procedure called a biopsy) and performing histochemical analysis of the individual muscle cells. A common method uses a histochemical procedure that divides muscle fibers into three categories based on the specific "isoform" of myosin found in the fiber. This technique uses selective antibodies that recognize and "tag" each of the different myosin proteins (e.g., type I, type IIa, and type IIx) found in human muscle fibers. Specifically, this method involves the binding of a high-affinity antibody to each unique myosin protein. This technique can then identify different muscle fibers due to color differences across the varying muscle fiber types. Figure 8.11 is an example of a muscle cross-section after immunohistochemical staining for a skeletal muscle membrane protein

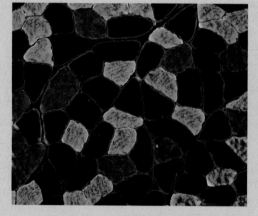

Figure 8.11 Immunohistochemical staining of a cross-sectional area of a skeletal muscle. The red staining is dystrophin protein, which is located within the membrane that surrounds a skeletal muscle fiber. The blue cells are type I fibers, whereas the green cells are type IIa fibers. The cells that appear black are type IIx muscle fibers.
© Scott Powers

(dystrophin), as well as immunohistochemical staining for type I, type IIa, and type IIx skeletal muscle fibers (9, 10, 41, 45).

One of the inherent problems with fiber typing in humans is that a muscle biopsy is usually performed on only one muscle group. Therefore, a single sample from one muscle is not representative of the entire body.

A further complication is that a small sample of fibers taken from a single area of the muscle may not be truly representative of the total fiber population of the muscle biopsied (3, 71). Therefore, it is difficult to make a definitive statement concerning the percentage of muscle fiber types in the whole body based on the staining of a single muscle biopsy.

between the cell membrane and the mitochondria. Therefore, a high myoglobin concentration improves the delivery of oxygen from the capillary to the mitochondria where it will be used. Collectively, the significance of these biochemical characteristics is that a muscle fiber with a high concentration of myoglobin, along with a high number of mitochondria and capillaries, will have a high aerobic capacity and therefore will be fatigue-resistant during prolonged submaximal exercise.

The second important biochemical characteristic of muscle fibers is that the different myosin isoforms differ in their myosin ATPase activity. In humans, three major myosin isoforms exist and these isoforms differ in their activities (i.e., speed that they break down ATP). Muscle fibers that contain ATPase isoforms with high ATPase activity will degrade ATP rapidly; this results in a high speed of muscle shortening. Conversely, muscle fibers with low ATPase activities shorten at slow speeds.

Finally, the third important biochemical characteristic of muscle fibers that influences contractile properties is the abundance of contractile proteins (i.e., actin and myosin) in the muscle fiber. Indeed, large fibers that contain large amounts of actin and myosin generate more force than fibers with low levels of these key contractile proteins. More details about fiber type differences in the levels of actin and myosin will be discussed later in this chapter.

Contractile Properties of Skeletal Muscle In comparing the contractile properties of muscle fiber types, four performance characteristics are important: (1) maximal force production, (2) speed of contraction, (3) maximal power output, and (4) efficiency of contraction. Let's discuss each of these characteristics briefly.

In general, larger muscle fibers produce more force than smaller fibers because they contain more actin and myosin than small fibers. This means more myosin cross-bridges are available for binding to actin and producing force. Also, note that muscle fiber maximal force production is often normalized to how much force the fiber generates per cross-sectional area of the fiber. This property of a skeletal muscle fiber is called the fiber-specific tension or specific force production. In other words, specific tension is the force production divided by the size of the fiber (e.g., specific force = force/fiber cross-sectional area). Muscle fiber-specific force production varies across muscle fiber types and will be discussed in the next segment.

A second key contractile property of muscle fibers is the speed of contraction. The contraction speed of muscle fibers is compared by measuring the maximal shortening velocity (called Vmax) of individual fibers. Vmax represents the highest speed at which

a fiber can shorten. Because muscle fibers shorten by cross-bridge movement (called cross-bridge cycling), Vmax is determined by the rate of cross-bridge cycling. The key biochemical factor that regulates fiber Vmax is the myosin ATPase activity. Therefore, fibers with high myosin ATPase activities (e.g., fast fibers) possess a high Vmax, whereas fibers with low myosin ATPase activities possess a low Vmax (e.g., slow fibers).

A third important contractile property of a muscle fiber is the maximal power output. The power of a muscle fiber is determined by both the force generation and the shortening velocity. Specifically, the maximal power output of a muscle fiber is defined as the product of force generation multiplied by the shortening velocity (i.e., power = force × shortening velocity). Therefore, muscle fibers with a high force generating capacity and a fast shortening velocity can produce a high power output. In contrast, muscle fibers that possess slow shortening velocities and/or a low force generating capacity are not capable of producing extremely high power outputs.

The fourth and final important contractile property of a skeletal muscle fiber is the efficiency of the fiber. The efficiency of a muscle fiber is a measure of the muscle fiber's economy. That is, an efficient fiber would require less energy to perform a certain amount of work compared to a less efficient fiber. In practice, this measurement is made by dividing the amount of energy used (i.e., ATP used) by the amount of force produced. In the next segment, we discuss how individual fiber types differ across these four key contractile properties.

Functional Characteristics of Muscle Fiber Types

Three major muscle fiber types exist in human skeletal muscle (two subtypes of fast fibers–identified as types IIx and IIa; and a slow fiber–identified as type I). Let's begin our discussion of muscle fiber types by examining the biochemical and contractile properties of both slow and fast fibers.

Slow (Type I) Fibers Only one type of slow fiber exists in humans–type I. **Type I fibers** (also called slow-oxidative or **slow-twitch fibers**) contain large numbers of oxidative enzymes (i.e., high mitochondrial volume) and are surrounded by more capillaries than fast, type II fibers. In addition, type I fibers contain higher concentrations of myoglobin than fast fibers. The high concentration of myoglobin, the large number of capillaries, and the high mitochondrial enzyme activities provide type I fibers with a large capacity for aerobic metabolism and a high resistance to fatigue.

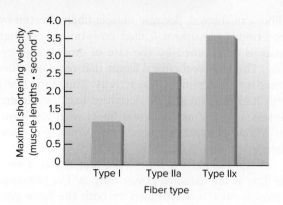

Figure 8.12 Comparison of maximal shortening velocities between fiber types.

Data from Canepari, M., Pellegrino, M. A., D'Antona, G., and Bottinelli, R., "Single Muscle Fiber Properties in Aging and Disuse," *Scandinavian Journal of Medicine & Science in Sports* 20: 10–19, 2010.

In regard to contractile properties (shortening velocity and force generation), type I fibers possess a slower maximal shortening velocity (Vmax) compared to fast fibers (Fig. 8.12) (13, 19, 57). The mechanism to explain this fact was presented earlier (i.e., type I fibers possess a lower myosin ATPase activity compared to fast fibers).

Further, type I fibers produce a lower specific force than fast fibers do (Fig. 8.13(*a*)) (19). The explanation for this observation is that type I fibers contain less actin and myosin per cross-sectional area than fast type II fibers do. This is important because the amount of force generated by a muscle fiber is directly related to the number of myosin cross-bridges bound to actin (i.e., the force generating state) at any given time. Simply stated, the more cross-bridges generating force, the greater the force production. Therefore, fast fibers exert more force than slow fibers because they contain more myosin cross-bridges per cross-sectional area of fiber than do slow fibers.

Finally, type I fibers are more efficient than fast fibers (23). This is important because at any given work rate, highly efficient muscle fibers will require less energy (i.e., ATP) than less efficient fibers. The difference in efficiency between slow and fast fibers is likely due to a lower rate of ATP turnover in slow fibers (23).

Fast (Type IIa and Type IIx) Fibers Two subtypes of fast fibers exist in humans: (1) type IIx and (2) type IIa. **Type IIx fibers** (sometimes called **fast-twitch fibers** or fast-glycolytic fibers) have a relatively small number of mitochondria, have a limited capacity for aerobic metabolism, and have less resistance to fatigue

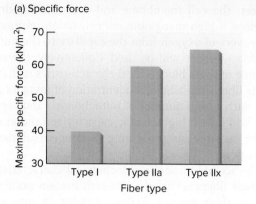

(a) Specific force

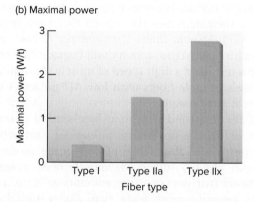

(b) Maximal power

Figure 8.13 Comparison of (*a*) maximal specific force production and (*b*) maximal power output between muscle fiber types.

Data from Canepari, M., Pellegrino, M. A., D'Antona, G., and Bottinelli, R., "Single Muscle Fiber Properties in Aging and Disuse," *Scandinavian Journal of Medicine & Science in Sports* 20: 10–19, 2010.

than slow fibers (33). However, these fibers are rich in glycolytic enzymes, which provide them with a large anaerobic capacity (54).

The fastest skeletal muscle fiber in many small animals (e.g., rats) is the type IIb fiber. For several years, it was believed that the fastest fiber in human skeletal muscle was also a "type IIb" fiber. However, it is now established that the fastest muscle fiber in humans is the type IIx fiber. The story behind this change in scientific thinking follows: In the late 1980s, German and Italian scientists independently discovered a new fast muscle fiber, named type IIx, in rodent skeletal muscle (5, 64). Since the discovery of this type IIx fiber in rodents, it has been determined that this type of myosin is similar in structure to that contained in the fastest muscle fiber in humans (63, 65). Therefore, throughout this textbook, we will refer to type IIx fibers as the fastest skeletal muscle fiber type in humans (24).

The specific force (force per cross-sectional area of the fiber) of type IIx fibers is similar to type IIa fibers, but is greater than type I fibers (Fig. 8.13a) (19).

TABLE 8.1 Characteristics of Human Skeletal Muscle Fiber Types

	FAST FIBERS		SLOW FIBERS
Characteristic	Type IIx	Type IIa	Type I
Number of mitochondria	Low	High/moderate	High
Resistance to fatigue	Low	High/moderate	High
Predominant energy system	Anaerobic	Combination	Aerobic
ATPase activity	Highest	High	Low
Vmax (speed of shortening)	Highest	High	Low
Efficiency	Low	Moderate	High
Specific tension	High	High	Moderate

Further, the myosin ATPase activity in type IIx fibers is higher than other fiber types, resulting in the highest Vmax of all fiber types (Fig. 8.12). It follows that type IIx fibers generate the highest power output of all muscle fiber types (Fig. 8.13(b)) (19).

Type IIx fibers are less efficient than all other fiber types. This low efficiency is due to the high myosin ATPase activity, which results in a greater energy expenditure per unit of work performed (23).

The second type of fast fiber is the **type IIa fiber** (also called **intermediate fibers** or fast-oxidative glycolytic fibers). These fibers contain biochemical and fatigue characteristics that are somewhere between type IIx and type I fibers. Therefore, conceptually, type IIa fibers can be viewed as a mixture of both type I and type IIx fiber characteristics. The comparisons of contractile properties between type IIa and IIx fibers are illustrated in Figures 8.12 and 8.13.

Further, it is important to appreciate that regular exercise training can modify both the biochemical and contractile properties of human muscle fibers and can result in the conversion of fast fibers into slow fibers (12, 35). A detailed discussion of exercise-induced changes in skeletal muscle fibers will be presented in Chap. 13.

Finally, it is important to understand that while the classification of skeletal muscle fibers into three distinct groups is a convenient way to group the functional properties of muscle fibers, each classification exhibits a wide range of contractile and biochemical properties. Indeed, the biochemical and contractile properties of type IIx, type IIa, and type I fibers represent a continuum. Further, an individual muscle fiber can exhibit the blended qualities of more than one single fiber type. For example, some fibers contain more than one type of myosin ATPase (e.g., fibers can contain both types I and IIa myosin ATPases, whereas others may possess both types IIa and IIx myosin ATPases).

IN SUMMARY

- Human skeletal muscle fiber types can be divided into three classes of fibers based on their biochemical and contractile properties. Two categories of fast fibers exist: type IIx and type IIa. One type of slow fiber exists: type I.
- The biochemical and contractile properties characteristic of all muscle fiber types are summarized in Table 8.1.
- Although classifying skeletal muscle fibers into three general groups is a convenient system to study the properties of muscle fibers, human skeletal muscle fibers exhibit a wide range of contractile and biochemical properties. That is, the biochemical and contractile properties of types IIx, IIa, and I fibers represent a continuum instead of three neat packages.

Fiber Types and Performance

Numerous studies have investigated the muscle fiber type makeup of human skeletal muscles, and several interesting facts have emerged. First, there are no apparent sex differences in fiber distribution (54). Second, the average sedentary man or woman possesses approximately 50% slow fibers. Third, highly successful power athletes (e.g., sprinters) typically possess a large percentage of fast fibers, whereas endurance athletes generally have a high percentage of slow fibers (22, 26, 73). Table 8.2 presents some examples of the percentage of slow and fast fibers found in successful athletes and nonathletes.

It is clear from Table 8.2 that considerable variation in the percentage of various fiber types exists even among successful athletes competing in the same event or sport. Indeed, although the percentage of type I (slow) muscle fibers is highly correlated with an individual's $\dot{V}O_2$ max, the percentage of type I fibers can explain only 40% of the variation in $\dot{V}O_2$ max

TABLE 8.2	Typical Muscle Fiber Composition in Elite Athletes	
Sport	% Slow Fibers (Type I)	% Fast Fibers (Types IIx and IIa)
Distance runners	70–80	20–30
Track sprinters	25–30	70–75
Nonathletes	47–53	47–53

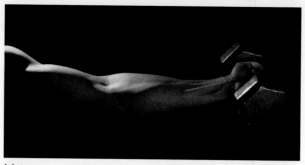

(a)

between individuals (68). Furthermore, two equally successful 10,000-meter runners have been shown to differ in the percentage of slow fibers that each possesses. For example, one runner might be found to possess 70% slow fibers, whereas a similarly successful runner can possess 85% slow fibers. This observation demonstrates that an individual's muscle fiber composition is not the only variable that determines success in athletic events (22). In fact, success in athletic performance is due to a complex interaction of psychological, biochemical, neurological, cardiopulmonary, and biomechanical factors (14, 15).

IN SUMMARY

- Successful power athletes (e.g., sprinters) generally possess a large percentage of fast muscle fibers and therefore a low percentage of slow, type I fibers.
- In contrast to power athletes, endurance athletes (e.g., marathoners) typically possess a high percentage of slow muscle fibers and a low percentage of fast fibers.
- Although muscle fiber types are known to play a role in sport performance, considerable variation exists among successful athletes competing in the same sport.

MUSCLE ACTIONS

The process of skeletal muscle force generation is referred to as a muscle contraction. However, to describe both lengthening and shortening actions of a muscle as a contraction can be confusing. Therefore, the term **muscle action** has been proposed to describe the process of muscle force development. This term is now commonly used to describe different types of muscular contractions (i.e., both lengthening and shortening contractions).

Several types of muscle actions exist. For example, it is possible for skeletal muscle to generate force without a large amount of muscle shortening. This can occur when an individual attempts to perform a "curl" with a dumbbell weight that he or she cannot move (see Fig. 8.14(a)). What happens here is that

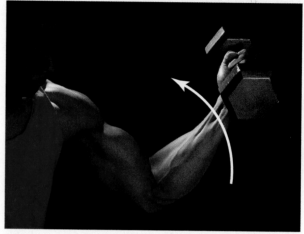

(b)

Figure 8.14 (a) Isometric actions occur when a muscle exerts force but does not shorten. (b) Concentric actions occur when a muscle contracts and shortens.
(A), (B) Courtesy of Stuart Fox

muscle tension increases, but the dumbbell does not move, and therefore neither does the body part that applies the force. This kind of muscle force development is called an **isometric action** and is referred to as a static exercise. Isometric actions are common in the postural muscles of the body, which act to maintain a static body position during periods of standing or sitting.

In contrast to isometric muscle actions, most types of exercise or sports activities require muscle actions that result in the movement of body parts. Exercise that involves movement of body parts is called **dynamic** exercise (formally called isotonic exercise). Two types of muscle actions can occur during dynamic exercise: (1) concentric and (2) eccentric. A muscle action that results in muscular shortening with movement of a body part is called a **concentric action** (Fig. 8.14(b)). An **eccentric action** occurs when a muscle is activated and force is produced, but the muscle lengthens. Table 8.3 summarizes the classifications of exercise and muscle action types.

Note that eccentric muscle actions can result in high stress within the sarcomere. This eccentric action induced stress on the muscle is often associated with

TABLE 8.3	Summary of the Classifications of Exercise and Muscle Action Types	
Type of Exercise	Muscle Action	Muscle Length Change
Dynamic	Concentric	Decreases
	Eccentric	Increases
Static	Isometric	No change

muscle fiber injury, resulting in a loss of muscle force generating capacity and muscle soreness due to inflammation and swelling of the muscle fiber. More details about exercise-induced muscle injury and soreness are presented in Chap. 21.

SPEED OF MUSCLE ACTION AND RELAXATION

If a muscle is given a single stimulus, such as a brief electrical shock applied to the nerve innervating it, the muscle responds with a simple **twitch.** The movement of the muscle can be recorded on a special recording device, and the time periods for contraction and relaxation can be studied. Figure 8.15 illustrates the time course of a simple twitch in an isolated frog muscle. Notice that the twitch can be divided into three phases. First, immediately after the stimulus, there is a brief latent period (lasting a few milliseconds) prior to the beginning of muscle shortening. The second phase of the twitch is the contraction phase, which lasts approximately 40 milliseconds. Finally, the muscle returns to its original length during

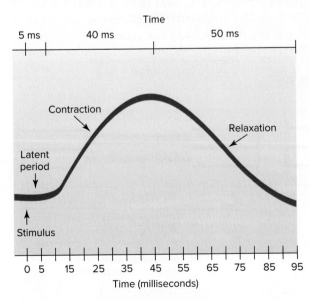

Figure 8.15 A recording of a simple twitch. Note the three time periods (latent period, contraction, and relaxation) following the stimulus.

the relaxation period, which lasts about 50 milliseconds and thus is the longest of the three phases.

The timing of the phases in a simple twitch varies among muscle fiber types. The variability in speed of contraction arises from differences in the responses of the individual fiber types that make up muscles. Individual muscle fibers behave much like individual neurons in that they exhibit all-or-none responses to stimulation. To contract, an individual muscle fiber must receive an appropriate amount of stimulation. However, fast fibers contract in a shorter time period when stimulated than do slow fibers. The explanation for this observation is as follows: The speed of shortening is greater in fast fibers than in slow fibers because the sarcoplasmic reticulum in fast fibers releases Ca^{++} at a faster rate, and fast fibers possess a higher ATPase activity compared to the slow fiber types (19, 26, 29, 62). The higher ATPase activity results in a more rapid splitting of ATP and a quicker release of the energy required for contraction.

FORCE REGULATION IN MUSCLE

As stated earlier, the amount of force generated in a single muscle fiber is related to the number of myosin cross-bridges making contact with actin. However, the amount of force exerted during muscular contraction in a group of muscles is complex and dependent on four primary factors: (1) number and types of motor units recruited, (2) the initial length of the muscle, (3) the nature of the neural stimulation of the motor units, and (4) the contractile history of the muscle (4, 18, 20, 29). A discussion of each of these factors follows.

First, variations in the strength of contraction within an entire muscle depend on both the type and the number of muscle fibers that are stimulated to contract (i.e., recruited). Recall from Chap. 7 that motor units are recruited according to the size principle, and if only a few motor units are recruited, the force is small. It follows that if more motor units are stimulated, the force increases. Figure 8.16 illustrates this point. Note that as the stimulus is increased, the force of contraction is also increased due to the recruitment of additional motor units. Also, recall that fast fibers exert a greater specific force than do slow fibers. Therefore, the types of motor units recruited also influence force production.

A second factor that determines the force exerted by a muscle is the initial length of the muscle at the time of contraction. In regard to force generation, the muscle's ability to generate force changes as a function of muscle length and an "optimal" length exists for maximal force generation. The explanation for the existence of an optimal length is related to the overlap between actin and myosin. For instance,

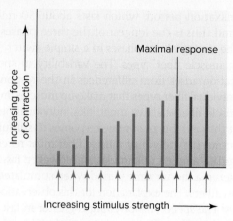

Figure 8.16 The relationship between increasing stimulus strength and the force of contraction. Weak stimuli do not activate many motor units and do not produce great force. In contrast, increasing the stimulus strength recruits more and more motor units and thus produces more force.

myosin, cross-bridges cannot attach and thus tension cannot be developed. At the other extreme, when the muscle is shortened to about 60% of its resting length, the Z lines are very close to the thick myosin filaments; thus, only limited additional shortening can occur.

The third factor that affects the amount of force a muscle exerts upon contraction is the nature of the neural stimulation. Simple muscle twitches studied under experimental conditions reveal some interesting fundamental properties about how muscles function. However, normal body movements involve sustained contractions that are not simple twitches. The sustained contractions involved in normal body movements can be closely replicated in the laboratory if a series of stimulations are applied to the muscle. The recording pictured in Figure 8.18 represents what occurs when successive stimuli are applied to the muscle. The first few contractions represent simple twitches. Note that as the frequency of the neural stimulations is increased, the muscle does not have time to relax between stimuli, and the force produced is additive. This response is called **summation** (addition of successive twitches). If the frequency of stimuli is increased further, individual contractions

when the resting length is longer than optimal, the overlap between actin and myosin is limited and few cross-bridges can attach. This concept is illustrated in Figure 8.17. Note that when the muscle is stretched to the point where there is no overlap of actin and

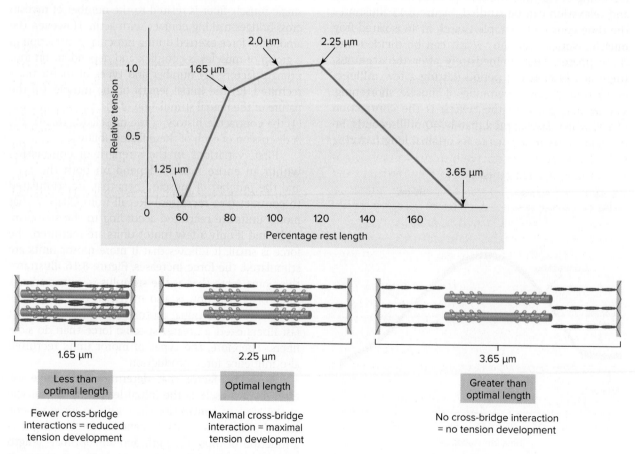

Figure 8.17 Length-tension relationships in skeletal muscle. Note that an optimal length of muscle exists, which will produce maximal force when stimulated. Lengths that are above or below this optimal length result in a reduced amount of force when stimulated.

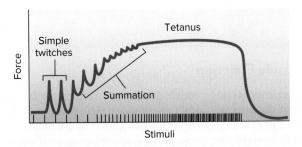

Figure 8.18 Recording showing the change from simple twitches to summation, and finally tetanus. Peaks to the left represent simple twitches, while increasing the frequency of the stimulus (as shown on the x-axis by the closer lines) results in summation of the twitches, and finally tetanus.

are blended in a single, sustained contraction called **tetanus.** A tetanic contraction will continue until the stimuli are stopped or the muscle fatigues.

Muscular contractions that occur during normal body movements are tetanic contractions. These sustained contractions result from a series of rapidly repeated neural impulses conducted by the motor neurons that innervate those motor units involved in the movement. It is important to appreciate that in the body, neural impulses to various motor units do not arrive at the same time as they do in the laboratory-induced tetanic contraction. Instead, various motor units are stimulated to contract at different times. Thus, some motor units are contracting while some are relaxing. This type of tetanic contraction results in a smooth contraction and aids in sustaining a coordinated muscle contraction.

The final factor that influences muscle force production is the prior contractile activity of the muscle. Indeed, the recent contractile history of a muscle can impact muscle force generation in two important and different ways. First, if a muscle performs a bout fatiguing exercise (i.e., prolonged and/or high-intensity contractions), subsequent muscle force production is decreased. The factors that contribute to this fatigue-induced decrement in muscle force generation were discussed earlier in this chapter.

In contrast to the negative effect of fatiguing exercise, a short period of non-fatiguing contractions (e.g., 5 minutes of low-intensity exercise) has been shown to increase muscle force production. This type of low-intensity muscle "warm up" activity results in a phenomenon known as **postactivation potentiation (PAP).** PAP is defined as the increase in muscle force production that occurs following a bout of non-fatiguing, submaximal muscle contractions. The mechanism to explain the positive impact of PAP on muscle performance is that low-intensity muscle contractions results in phosphorylation of myosin light chains (i.e., proteins located at the base of the myosin cross-bridge). This phosphorylation increases the muscle's sensitivity

to calcium released from the sarcoplasmic reticulum, and the end result is increased actin-myosin interaction and improved muscle force production.

In theory, the PAP induced by warm up exercises can improve athletic performance requiring explosive activities such as sprinting, jumping, and throwing. Nonetheless, investigations on PAP are inconsistent with some studies reporting performance improvement, whereas other investigations conclude that PAP does not improve human performance. Therefore, additional research is required to determine if PAP improves athletic performance. For more information on PAP please see Macintosh et al. (2012) and Bouvea et al. (2013) in the Suggested Readings list.

Finally, in addition to the previous discussion of the physiological factors that impact muscle force production, both aging and disease can negatively impact the muscle's ability to generate force. Indeed, aging (>50 years of age) results in a progressive loss of muscle mass, which reduces muscle force production. Also, several chronic diseases (e.g., cancer, muscular dystrophy) result in muscle loss and, therefore, reduce muscle strength. See Clinical Applications 8.1 for more details.

FORCE-VELOCITY/POWER-VELOCITY RELATIONSHIPS

In most physical activities, muscular force is applied through a range of movement. For instance, an athlete performing the shot put applies force against the shot over a specified range of movement prior to release. How far the shot travels is a function of both the speed of the shot upon release and the angle of release. Because success in many athletic events is dependent on speed, it is important to understand the concepts underlying the relationship between muscular force and the speed of movement. The relationship between speed of movement and muscular force is shown in Figure 8.19.

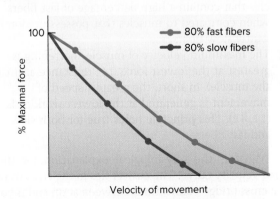

Figure 8.19 Muscle force-velocity relationships. Note that at any given speed of movement, muscle groups with a high percentage of fast fibers exert more *force* than those with muscle groups that contain primarily slow fibers.

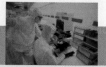

CLINICAL APPLICATIONS 8.1

Both Diseases and Aging Can Negatively Affect Muscle Function

Both old age and disease can have a negative influence on the ability of skeletal muscle to exert force. Let's discuss the impact of old age and several widespread diseases on muscle function.

Aging and Muscle Loss Aging is associated with a loss of muscle mass (called sarcopenia) (48, 77). The age-related decline in muscle mass begins around age 25 and occurs across the lifetime. However, the rate of age-related muscle loss occurs in two distinct phases. The first is a "slow" phase of muscle loss, in which 10% of muscle mass is lost from age 25 to 50 years. Thereafter, there is a rapid loss in muscle mass. In fact, from age 50 to 80 years, an additional 40% of muscle mass is lost. Thus, by age 80, one-half of the total skeletal muscle mass can be lost. Also, aging results in a loss of fast fibers (particularly type IIx) and an increase in slow fibers (52). From a clinical perspective, severe age-related sarcopenia can have negative health consequences because it increases the risk of falls in the elderly and reduces the ability to perform activities of daily living, which results in a loss of independence (52). Researchers are actively studying the mechanisms

to explain age-related sarcopenia in hopes of the discovery of therapeutic treatments. It is important to note that regular bouts of resistance exercise remains one of the most useful and practical means to delay age-related muscle loss. For more details on the impact of aging on skeletal muscle see Mitchell et al. (2012) in Suggested Readings.

Diabetes The incidence of type II diabetes is rapidly increasing worldwide. Unfortunately, uncontrolled diabetes is associated with a progressive loss of muscle mass. Therefore, uncontrolled diabetes combined with aging has the potential to accelerate age-related loss of skeletal muscle mass (17). Notably, both aerobic and resistance exercise training have been shown to be protective against diabetes-induced muscle loss.

Cancer Up to 50% of cancer patients suffer from a rapid loss of skeletal muscle mass (74). This type of disease-related muscle loss is called cachexia (6). Cancer-mediated loss of skeletal muscle results in patient weakness and may account for up to 20% of deaths in cancer patients (34). Indeed, cancer causes wasting of breathing muscles (e.g., diaphragm),

which can lead to respiratory failure and patient death (60). Because of the clinical significance of cachexia, investigators are developing methods to counteract cancer-induced cachexia. Some of the most promising therapies include regular exercise combined with nutritional interventions (44).

Muscular Dystrophy Muscular dystrophy refers to a group of hereditary muscle diseases that weaken skeletal muscles. Collectively, these diseases are characterized by defects in muscle proteins that result in a progressive muscle weakness and a loss of muscle fibers. Although more than 100 different types exist, Duchene muscular dystrophy is the most common childhood form of this disease. The prognosis for people with muscular dystrophy varies with the type. Some forms of muscular dystrophy can be mild and progress slowly over a normal life span. In contrast, other forms of this disorder produce severe muscle weakness along with the loss of the ability to walk and breathe without assistance. Although scientists continue to study muscular dystrophy, there are currently few clinical options to successfully treat the most severe forms of this disease.

Two important points emerge from an examination of Figure 8.19:

1. At any absolute force exerted by the muscle, the velocity or speed of movement is greater in muscles that contain a high percentage of fast fibers when compared to muscles that possess predominantly slow fibers.

2. The maximum velocity of muscle shortening is greatest at the lowest force (i.e., resistance against the muscle). In short, the greatest speed of movement is generated at the lowest workloads (11, 42). This principle holds true for both slow and fast fibers.

What is the physiological explanation for the force-velocity curve? The answer lies in the analysis of the cross-bridge connections between actin and myosin. Recall that the amount of force generated by a muscle is determined by the number of cross-bridges attached between actin and myosin. Also, note that the cross-bridge connections between actin and myosin

require a certain amount of time to make this connection. Therefore, during rapid muscle shortening (i.e., high velocity movement), the actin-myosin filaments move past each other at a fast rate. This rapid shortening restricts the number of cross-bridges that can make a connection and therefore limits muscle force production. Conversely, as muscle shortening velocity decreases, more cross-bridges have time to connect, and muscle force production increases.

The data contained in Figure 8.19 also demonstrate that fast fibers produce greater force and shorten at faster speeds than slow fibers. The biochemical mechanism to explain this observation is related to the fact that fast fibers possess higher ATPase activity than do slow fibers (26, 29). Therefore, ATP is broken down more rapidly in fast fibers when compared to slow fibers. Further, calcium release from the sarcoplasmic reticulum is faster following neural stimulation in fast fibers than in slow fibers (29).

The relationship between force and movement speed has practical importance for the physical

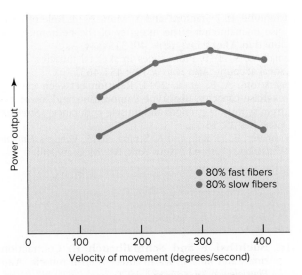

Figure 8.20 Muscle power-velocity relationships. In general, the power produced by a muscle group increases as a function of velocity of movement. At any given speed of movement, muscles that contain a large percentage of fast fibers produce more *power* than those muscles that contain primarily slow fibers.

therapist, athlete, or physical educator. The message is simply that athletes who possess a high percentage of fast fibers have an advantage in power-type athletic events. This explains why successful sprinters and weight lifters typically possess a relatively high percentage of fast fibers.

As might be expected, the fiber-type make-up of a muscle influences the power-velocity curve (see Fig. 8.20). The peak power that can be generated by muscle is greater in muscle that contains a high percentage of fast fibers than in muscle that is largely composed of slow fibers. As with the force-velocity curve, two important points emerge from the examination of the power-velocity curve:

1. At any given velocity of movement, the peak power generated is greater in muscle that contains a high percentage of fast fibers than in muscle with a high percentage of slow fibers. This difference is due to the aforementioned biochemical differences between fast and slow fibers. Again, athletes who possess a high percentage of fast fibers can generate more power than athletes with predominantly slow fibers.

2. The peak power generated by any muscle increases with increasing velocities of movement up to a movement speed of 200 to 300 degrees/second. The reason for the plateau of power output with increasing movement speed is that muscular force decreases with increasing speed of movement (see Fig. 8.19). Therefore, with any given muscle group, there is an optimum speed of movement that will elicit the greatest power output.

IN SUMMARY

- The amount of force generated during muscular contraction is dependent on the following factors: (1) types and number of motor units recruited, (2) the initial muscle length, (3) the nature of the motor units' neural stimulation, and (4) prior contractile activity of the muscle.
- The addition of muscle twitches is termed *summation*. When the frequency of neural stimulation to a motor unit is increased, individual contractions are fused in a sustained contraction called *tetanus*.
- The peak force generated by muscle decreases as the speed of movement increases. However, in general, the amount of power generated by a muscle group increases as a function of movement velocity.

STUDY ACTIVITIES

1. Describe the principal functions of skeletal muscles.
2. List the principal contractile proteins contained in skeletal muscle.
3. Outline the contractile process. Use a step-by-step format illustrating the entire process, beginning with the nerve impulse reaching the neuromuscular junction.
4. Describe the mechanical and biochemical properties of human skeletal muscle fiber types.
5. Discuss those factors thought to be responsible for regulating force during muscular contractions.
6. Define the term *summation*.
7. Graph a simple muscle twitch and a contraction that results in tetanus.
8. Discuss the relationship between force and speed of movement during a muscular contraction.

SUGGESTED READINGS

Fox, S. 2015. *Human Physiology.* New York, NY: McGraw-Hill.

Gouvea, A., I. Fernandes, C. Cesar, W. Silva, and P. Gomes. 2013. The effects of rest intervals on jumping performance: a meta analysis on post-activation potentiation studies. *Journal of Sports Sciences.* 31: 459-467.

Gundersen, K. 2016. Muscle memory and a new cellular model for muscle atrophy and hypertrophy. *Journal of Experimental Biology.* 219: 235-242.

MacIntosh, B.R., R. Holash, and J. Renaud. 2012. Skeletal muscle fatigue-regulation of excitation contraction coupling to avoid metabolic catastrophe. *Journal of Cell Science.* 125: 2105-2114.

Miller, K.C. 2016. Myths and misconceptions about exercise associated muscle cramping. *ACSM's Health and Fitness Journal.* 20: 37-39.

Minetto, M.A., A. Holobar, A. Botter, and D. Farina. 2012. Origin and development of muscle cramps. *Exercise and Sport Science Reviews.* 41: 3-10.

Mitchell, W., J. Williams, P. Atherton, M. Larvin, and M. Narici. 2012. Sarcopenia, dynapenia, and the impact of advancing age on human skeletal muscle size and strength; a quantative review. *Frontiers in Physiology* 3: 1-18.

Nishimune, H. J. Stanford, and Y. Mori. 2014. Role of exercise in maintaining the integrity of the neuromuscular junction. *Muscle and Nerve.* 49: 315-324.

Schiaffino, S. 2010. Fibre types in skeletal muscles: a personal account. *Acta Physiol* 199: 451-463.

Segerstrom, A. B., et al. 2011. Relation between cycling exercise capacity, fiber-type composition, and lower extremity muscle strength and muscle endurance. *J Strength Cond Res* 25: 16-22.

Widmaier, E., H. Raff, and K. Strang. 2015. *Vander's Human Physiology* (10th ed.). New York, NY: McGraw-Hill.

REFERENCES

1. **Allen DL, Roy RR, and Edgerton VR.** Myonuclear domains in muscle adaptation and disease. *Muscle Nerve* 22: 1350-1360, 1999.

2. **Ament W and Verkerke GJ.** Exercise and fatigue. *Sports Medicine* 39: 389-422, 2009.

3. **Armstrong R.** Differential inter- and intramuscular responses to exercise: considerations in use of the biopsy technique. In: *Biochemistry of Exercise,* edited by Knuttgen H, Vogel J, and Poortmans J. Champaign, IL: Human Kinetics, 1983.

4. **Armstrong R and Laughlin H.** Muscle function during locomotion in mammals. In: *Circulation, Respiration, and Metabolism,* edited by Giles R. New York, NY: Springer-Verlag, 1985, pp. 56-63.

5. **Bar A and Pette D.** Three fast myosin heavy chains in adult rat skeletal muscle. *FEBS Lett* 235: 153-155, 1988.

6. **Bennani-Baiti N and Walsh D.** What is cancer anorexia-cachexia syndrome? A historical perspective. *Journal of the Royal College of Physicians of Edinburgh* 39: 257-262, 2009.

7. **Bergeron MF.** Exertional heat cramps: recovery and return to play. *Journal of Sport Rehabilitation* 16: 190-196, 2007.

8. **Bergeron MF.** Heat cramps: fluid and electrolyte challenges during tennis in the heat. *Journal of Science and Medicine in Sport* 6: 19-27, 2003.

9. **Billeter R and Hoppeler H.** Muscular basis of strength. In: *Strength and Power in Sport,* edited by Komi P. Oxford: Blackwell Scientific Publishing, 1992.

10. **Blaauw B, Schiaffino S, and Reggiani C.** Mechanisms modulating skeletal muscle phenotype. *Comprehensive Physiology* 3: 1645-1687, 2013.

11. **Bobbert MF, Ettema GC, and Huijing PA.** The force-length relationship of a muscle-tendon complex: experimental results and model calculations. *European Journal of Applied Physiology and Occupational Physiology* 61: 323-329, 1990.

12. **Booth FW and Thomason DB.** Molecular and cellular adaptation of muscle in response to exercise: perspectives of various models. *Physiological Reviews* 71: 541-585, 1991.

13. **Bottinelli R, Canepari M, Reggiani C, and Stienen GJ.** Myofibrillar ATPase activity during isometric contraction and isomyosin composition in rat single skinned muscle fibres. *The Journal of Physiology* 481 (Pt 3): 663-675, 1994.

14. **Brooks G, Fahey T, White T, and Baldwin KM.** *Exercise Physiology: Human Bioenergetics and Its Applications.* New York, NY: McGraw-Hill, 2004.

15. **Brooks G, Fahey T, White T, and Baldwin KM.** *Fundamentals of Human Performance.* New York, NY: Macmillan, 1987.

16. **Buchthal F and Schmalbruch H.** Contraction times and fibre types in intact human muscle. *Acta Physiologica* 79: 435-452, 1970.

17. **Buford TW, Anton SD, Judge AR, Marzetti E, Wohlgemuth SE, Carter CS, et al.** Models of accelerated sarcopenia: critical pieces for solving the puzzle of age-related muscle atrophy. *Ageing Research Reviews* 9: 369-383, 2010.

18. **Burke R.** The control of muscle force: motor unit recruitment and firing pattern. In: *Human Muscle Power,* edited by Jones N, McCartney N, and McComas A. Champaign, IL: Human Kinetics, 1986.

19. **Canepari M, Pellegrino MA, D'Antona G, and Bottinelli R.** Single muscle fiber properties in aging and disuse. *Scandinavian Journal of Medicine & Science in Sports* 20: 10-19, 2010.

20. **Carlson F and Wilkie D.** *Muscle Physiology.* Englewood Cliffs, NJ: Prentice-Hall, 1974.

21. **Conley KE.** Cellular energetics during exercise. *Advances in Veterinary Science & Comparative Medicine* 38A: 1-39, 1994.

22. **Costill DL, Fink WJ, and Pollock ML.** Muscle fiber composition and enzyme activities of elite distance runners. *Medicine and Science in Sports* 8: 96-100, 1976.

23. **Coyle EF, Sidossis LS, Horowitz JF, and Beltz JD.** Cycling efficiency is related to the percentage of type I muscle fibers. *Medicine & Science in Sports & Exercise* 24: 782-788, 1992.

24. **D'Antona G, Lanfranconi F, Pellegrino MA, Brocca L, Adami R, Rossi R, et al.** Skeletal muscle hypertrophy and structure and function of skeletal muscle fibres in male body builders. *The Journal of Physiology* 570: 611-627, 2006.

24b. **Debold EP.** Potential molecular mechanisms underlying muscle fatigue mediated by reactive oxygen species. *Frontiers in Physiology.* doi: 10.3389/fphys. 6: 239, 2015.

25. **Ebashi S.** Excitation-contraction coupling and the mechanism of muscle contraction. *Annual Review of Physiology* 53: 1-16, 1991.

26. **Edgerton V.** Morphological basis of skeletal muscle power output. In: *Human Muscle Power,* edited by Jones N, McCartney N, and McComas A. Champaign, IL: Human Kinetics, 1986, pp. 43-58.

27. **Edgerton V.** Muscle fiber activation and recruitment. In: *Biochemistry of Exercise,* edited by Knuttgen H, Vogel J, and Poortmans J. Champaign, IL: Human Kinetics, 1983.

28. **Edman K.** Contractile performance of skeletal muscle fibers. In: *Strength and Power in Sport,* edited by

Komi P. Oxford: Blackwell Scientific Publishing, 1992, pp. 96-114.

29. **Faulker J, Claflin D, and McCully K.** Power output of fast and slow fibers from human skeletal muscles. In: *Human Muscle Power*, edited by Jones N, McCartney N, and McComas A. Champaign, IL: Human Kinetics, 1986.

30. **Fitts RH.** The cross-bridge cycle and skeletal muscle fatigue. *Journal of Applied Physiology* 104: 551-558, 2008.

31. **Geeves MA and Holmes KC.** The molecular mechanism of muscle contraction. *Advances in Protein Chemistry* 71: 161-193, 2005.

32. **Gollnick PD and Saltin B.** Significance of skeletal muscle oxidative enzyme enhancement with endurance training. *Clinical Physiology* 2: 1-12, 1982.

33. **Green H.** Muscle power: fiber type recruitment, metabolism, and fatigue. In: *Human Muscle Power*, edited by Jones N, McCartney N, and McComas A. Champaign, IL: Human Kinetics, 1986.

34. **Gullett N, Rossi P, Kucuk O, and Johnstone PA.** Cancer-induced cachexia: a guide for the oncologist. *Journal of the Society for Integrative Oncology* 7: 155-169, 2009.

35. **Gunning P and Hardeman E.** Multiple mechanisms regulate muscle fiber diversity. *The FASEB Journal* 5: 3064-3070, 1991.

36. **Holloszy JO.** Muscle metabolism during exercise. *Archives of Physical Medicine and Rehabilitation* 63: 231-234, 1982.

37. **Holmes KC.** The swinging lever-arm hypothesis of muscle contraction. *Current Biology* 7: R112-118, 1997.

38. **Holmes KC and Geeves MA.** The structural basis of muscle contraction. *Philosophical Transactions of the Royal Society of London* 355: 419-431, 2000.

39. **Holmes KC, Schroder RR, Sweeney HL, and Houdusse A.** The structure of the rigor complex and its implications for the power stroke. *Philosophical Transactions of the Royal Society of London* 359: 1819-1828, 2004.

40. **Huxley HE.** Past, present and future experiments on muscle. *Philosophical Transactions of the Royal Society of London* 355: 539-543, 2000.

41. **Kodama T.** Thermodynamic analysis of muscle ATPase mechanisms. *Physiological Reviews* 65: 467-551, 1985.

42. **Kojima T.** Force-velocity relationship of human elbow flexors in voluntary isotonic contraction under heavy loads. *International Journal of Sports Medicine* 12: 208-213, 1991.

43. **Lieber RL.** *Skeletal Muscle Structure, Function, and Plasticity.* Philadelphia, PA: Lippincott Williams & Wilkins, 2010.

44. **Lowe SS.** Physical activity and palliative cancer care. *Recent Results in Cancer Research (Fortschritte der Krebsforschung)* 186: 349-365, 2011.

45. **Lowey S.** Cardiac and skeletal muscle myosin polymorphism. *Medicine & Science in Sports & Exercise* 18: 284-291, 1986.

46. **MacIntosh BR, Holash R, and Renaud J.** Skeletal muscle fatigue-regulation of excitation contraction coupling to avoid metabolic catastrophe. *Journal of Cell Science* 125: 2105-2114, 2012.

47. **Mansson A, Rassier D, and Tsiavaliaris G.** Poorly understood aspects of striated muscle contraction. *Biomedical Research International.* DOI.org./10.1155/2015/245154, 2015.

48. **Marzetti E, Calvani R, Cesari M, Buford TW, Lorenzi M, Behnke BJ, et al.** Mitochondrial dysfunction and sarcopenia of aging: from signaling pathways to clinical trials. *The International Journal of Biochemistry & Cell Biology* 45: 2288-2301, 2013.

49. **McClung JM, Kavazis AN, DeRuisseau KC, Falk DJ, Deering MA, Lee Y, et al.** Caspase-3 regulation of diaphragm myonuclear domain during mechanical ventilation-induced atrophy. *American Journal of Respiratory and Critical Care Medicine* 175: 150-159, 2007.

50. **Metzger J.** Mechanism of chemomechanical coupling in skeletal muscle during work. In: *Energy Metabolism in Exercise and Sport*, edited by Lamb D, and Gisolfi C. New York, NY: McGraw-Hill, 1992, pp. 1-43.

51. **Moss RL, Diffee GM, and Greaser ML.** Contractile properties of skeletal muscle fibers in relation to myofibrillar protein isoforms. *Reviews of Physiology, Biochemistry and Pharmacology* 126: 1-63, 1995.

52. **Narici MV and Maffulli N.** Sarcopenia: characteristics, mechanisms and functional significance. *British Medical Bulletin* 95: 139-159, 2010.

53. **Nishimune H, Stanford J, and Mori Y.** Role of exercise in maintaining the integrity of the neuromuscular junction. *Muscle and Nerve* 49: 315-324, 2014.

54. **Pette D.** *Plasticity of Muscle.* New York, NY: Walter de Gruyter, 1980.

55. **Powers SK, Talbert EE, and Adhihetty PJ.** Reactive oxygen species as intracellular signals in skeletal muscle. *The Journal of Physiology* 589: 2129-2138, 2011.

56. **Powers SK, Ji LL, Kavazis AN, and Jackson MJ.** Reactive oxygen species: impact on skeletal muscle. *Comprehensive Physiology* 1: 941-969, 2011.

57. **Powers SK, Criswell D, Herb RA, Demirel H, and Dodd S.** Age-related increases in diaphragmatic maximal shortening velocity. *Journal of Applied Physiology* 80: 445-451, 1996.

58. **Powers SK, Nelson WB, and Hudson MB.** Exercise-induced oxidative stress in humans: cause and consequences. *Free Radical Biology & Medicine* 51: 942-950, 2011.

59. **Powers SK and Jackson MJ.** Exercise-induced oxidative stress: cellular mechanisms and impact on muscle force production. *Physiological Reviews* 88: 1243-1276, 2008.

60. **Roberts BM, Ahn B, Smuder AJ, Al-Rajhi M, Gill LC, Beharry AW, et al.** Diaphragm and ventilatory dysfunction during cancer cachexia. *The FASEB Journal* 27: 2600-2610, 2013.

61. **Saladin K.** *Anatomy and Physiology.* Boston, MA: McGraw-Hill, 2014.

62. **Saltin B and Gollnick PD.** Skeletal muscle adaptability: significance for metabolism and performance. In: *Handbook of Physiology*, edited by Peachy L, Adrian R, and Geiger S. Bethesda, MD: American Physiological Society, 1983.

63. **Sant'Ana Pereira J, Ennion S, Moorman A, Goldspink G, and Sargeant A.** The predominant fast myHC's in human skeletal muscle corresponds to the rat IIa and IIx and not IIb (A26). In: *Annual Meeting of Society for Neuroscience*, 1994.

64. **Schiaffino S, Gorza L, Sartore S, Saggin L, Ausoni S, Vianello M, et al.** Three myosin heavy chain isoforms in type 2 skeletal muscle fibres. *Journal of Muscle Research and Cell Motility* 10: 197-205, 1989.

65. **Schiaffino S and Reggiani C.** Fiber types in mammalian skeletal muscles. *Physiology Reviews* 91: 1447-1531, 2011.

66. **Schwellnus MP.** Cause of exercise associated muscle cramps (EAMC)–altered neuromuscular control,

dehydration or electrolyte depletion? *British Journal of Sports Medicine* 43: 401-408, 2009.

67. **Schwellnus MP, Derman EW, and Noakes TD.** Aetiology of skeletal muscle "cramps" during exercise: a novel hypothesis. *Journal of Sports Sciences* 15: 277-285, 1997.

68. **Segerstrom AB, Holmback AM, Hansson O, Elgzyri T, Eriksson KF, Ringsberg K, et al.** Relation between cycling exercise capacity, fiber-type composition, and lower extremity muscle strength and muscle endurance. *The Journal of Strength & Conditioning Research* 25: 16-22, 2011.

69. **Sellers JR.** Fifty years of contractility research post sliding filament hypothesis. *Journal of Muscle Research and Cell Motility* 25: 475-482, 2004.

70. **Simoneau JA, Lortie G, Boulay MR, Marcotte M, Thibault MC, and Bouchard C.** Inheritance of human skeletal muscle and anaerobic capacity adaptation to high-intensity intermittent training. *International Journal of Sports Medicine* 7: 167-171, 1986.

71. **Snow D and Harris R.** Thoroughbreds and greyhounds: biochemical adaptations in creatures of nature and man. In: *Circulation, Respiration, and Metabolism,* edited by Giles R. New York, NY: Springer-Verlag, 1985, pp. 227-239.

72. **Tate CA, Hyek MF, and Taffet GE.** The role of calcium in the energetics of contracting skeletal muscle. *Sports Medicine* 12: 208-217, 1991.

73. **Tesch PA, Thorsson A, and Kaiser P.** Muscle capillary supply and fiber type characteristics in weight and power lifters. *Journal of Applied Physiology* 56: 35-38, 1984.

74. **Tisdale MJ.** Mechanisms of cancer cachexia. *Physiological Reviews* 89: 381-410, 2009.

75. **Vale RD.** Getting a grip on myosin. *Cell* 78: 733-737, 1994.

76. **Vandenboom R.** The myofibrillar complex and fatigue: a review. *Canadian Journal of Applied Physiology* 29: 330-356, 2004.

77. **Vinciguerra M, Musaro A, and Rosenthal N.** Regulation of muscle atrophy in aging and disease. *Advances in Experimental Medicine and Biology* 694: 211-233, 2010.

78. **Westerblad H and Allen DG.** Cellular mechanisms of skeletal muscle fatigue. *Advances in Experimental Medicine and Biology* 538: 563-570, 2003.

79. **White RB, Bierinx AS, Gnocchi VF, and Zammit PS.** Dynamics of muscle fibre growth during postnatal mouse development. *BMC Developmental Biology* 10: 21, 2010.

80. **Wozniak AC, Kong J, Bock E, Pilipowicz O, and Anderson JE.** Signaling satellite-cell activation in skeletal muscle: markers, models, stretch, and potential alternate pathways. *Muscle Nerve* 31: 283-300, 2005.

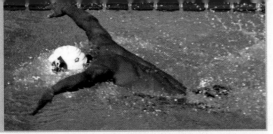

© Action Plus Sports Images/Alamy Stock Photo

9

Circulatory Responses to Exercise

Objectives

By studying this chapter, you should be able to do the following:

1. Provide an overview of the design and function of the circulatory system.

2. Describe the cardiac cycle and the associated electrical activity recorded via the electrocardiogram.

3. Discuss the pattern of redistribution of blood flow during exercise.

4. Outline the circulatory responses to various types of exercise.

5. Identify the factors that regulate local blood flow during exercise.

6. List and discuss those factors responsible for regulation of stroke volume during exercise.

7. Discuss the regulation of cardiac output during exercise.

Outline

Key Terms

arteries
arterioles
atrioventricular node (AV node)
autoregulation
capillaries
cardiac accelerator nerves
cardiac output
cardiovascular control center
central command
diastole
diastolic blood pressure
double product
electrocardiogram (ECG or EKG)
heart rate variability
intercalated discs
mixed venous blood
myocardium
pulmonary circuit
sinoatrial node (SA node)
stroke volume
systole
systolic blood pressure
vagus nerve
veins
venules

One of the major challenges to homeostasis posed by exercise is the increased muscular demand for oxygen; during heavy exercise, the demand may be 15 to 25 times greater than at rest. The primary purpose of the cardiorespiratory system is to deliver adequate amounts of oxygen and remove wastes from body tissues. Further, the circulatory system also transports nutrients and aids in temperature regulation. It is important to remember that the respiratory system and the circulatory system function together as a "coupled unit"; the respiratory system adds oxygen and removes carbon dioxide from the blood, while the circulatory system is responsible for the delivery of oxygenated blood and nutrients to tissues in accordance with their needs. In simple terms, the "cardiorespiratory system" works as a unit to maintain oxygen and carbon dioxide homeostasis in body tissues. A British physician, William Harvey, proposed the first complete theory about how the cardiovascular system works in humans (see A Look Back–Important People in Science).

To meet the increased oxygen demands of muscle during exercise, two major adjustments of blood flow must be made: (1) an increased **cardiac output** (i.e., increased amount of blood pumped per minute by the heart) and (2) a redistribution of blood flow from inactive organs to the active skeletal muscles. However, while the needs of the muscles are being met, other tissues, such as the brain, cannot be denied blood flow. This is accomplished by maintaining blood pressure, the driving force behind blood flow. A thorough understanding of the cardiovascular responses to exercise is important for the student of exercise physiology. Therefore, this chapter describes the design and function of the circulatory system and how it responds during exercise. We begin with a brief review of the anatomy and function of the heart and blood vessels.

ORGANIZATION OF THE CIRCULATORY SYSTEM

The human circulatory system is a closed loop that circulates blood to all body tissues. Circulation of blood requires the action of a muscular pump, the heart, that creates the "pressure head" needed to move blood through the system. Blood travels away from the heart in **arteries** and returns to the heart by way of **veins.** The system is considered "closed" because arteries and veins are continuous with each other through smaller vessels. Arteries branch extensively to form a "tree" of smaller vessels. As the vessels become microscopic, they form **arterioles,** which eventually develop into "beds" of much smaller vessels called **capillaries.** Capillaries are the smallest and most numerous of blood vessels; all exchanges of oxygen, carbon dioxide, and nutrients between tissues and the circulatory system occur across capillary beds. Blood passes from capillary beds to small venous vessels called **venules.** As venules move back toward the heart, they increase in size and become veins. Major veins empty directly into the heart. The mixture of venous blood from both the upper and lower body that accumulates in the right side of the heart is termed **mixed venous blood.** Mixed venous blood, therefore, represents an average of venous blood from the entire body.

Structure of the Heart

The heart is divided into four chambers and is often considered to be two pumps in one. The right atrium and right ventricle form the right pump, and the left atrium and left ventricle combine to make

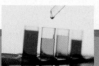

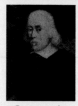

A LOOK BACK—IMPORTANT PEOPLE IN SCIENCE

William Harvey Developed the First Complete Theory of the Circulatory System

William Harvey (1578-1657) was born in England and was educated at both King's College and the University of Cambridge. He later studied medicine at the University of Padua in Italy. After completion of his medical studies, he returned to England and became the personal physician of King James I.

© Bettmann/ Getty Images

Dr. Harvey was fascinated by anatomical studies, and King James I encouraged him to pursue research to improve the practice of medicine. As a researcher, William Harvey made many important discoveries about how the cardiovascular system operates. First, by observing the action of the heart in small animals, Harvey proved that the heart expels blood during each contraction. Further, he also discovered that valves exist in veins and correctly identified them as

restricting the flow of blood in one direction. Dr. Harvey's work on the circulatory system was summarized in a book published in 1628 titled *An Anatomical Study of the Motion of the Heart and of the Blood in Animals.* This text explained Harvey's theories on how the heart propelled blood through a circular course throughout the body and was the first published record to accurately describe how the circulatory system works in humans and other animals.

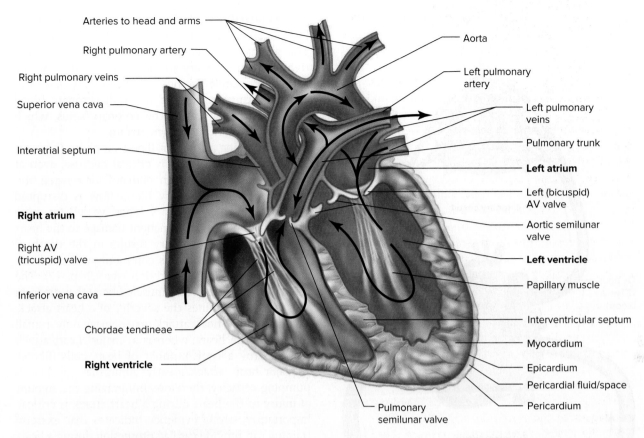

Figure 9.1 Anterior view of the heart.

the left pump (see Fig. 9.1). The right side of the heart is separated from the left side by a muscular wall called the interventricular septum. This septum prevents the mixing of blood from the two sides of the heart.

Blood movement within the heart is from the atria to the ventricles, and from the ventricles, blood is pumped into the arteries. To prevent backward movement of blood, the heart contains four one-way valves. The right and left atrioventricular valves connect the atria with the right and left ventricles, respectively (Fig. 9.1). These valves are also known as the tricuspid valve (right atrioventricular valve) and the bicuspid valve (left atrioventricular valve). Backflow from the arteries into the ventricles is prevented by the pulmonary semilunar valve (right ventricle) and the aortic semilunar valve (left ventricle).

Pulmonary and Systemic Circuits

As mentioned previously, the heart can be considered two pumps in one. The right side of the heart pumps blood that is partially depleted of its oxygen content and contains an elevated carbon dioxide content as a result of gas exchange in the various tissues of the body. This blood is delivered from the right heart into the lungs through the **pulmonary circuit.** At the

lungs, oxygen is loaded into the blood and carbon dioxide is released. This "oxygenated" blood then travels to the left side of the heart and is pumped to the various tissues of the body via the systemic circuit (Fig. 9.2).

> **IN SUMMARY**
>
> - The purposes of the cardiovascular system are the following: (1) the transport of O_2 to tissues and removal of wastes, (2) the transport of nutrients to tissues, and (3) the regulation of body temperature.
> - The heart is two pumps in one. The right side of the heart pumps blood through the pulmonary circulation, and the left side of the heart delivers blood to the systemic circulation.

HEART: MYOCARDIUM AND CARDIAC CYCLE

To better appreciate how the circulatory system adjusts to the stress of exercise, it is important to understand elementary details of heart muscle structure as well as the electrical and mechanical activities of the heart.

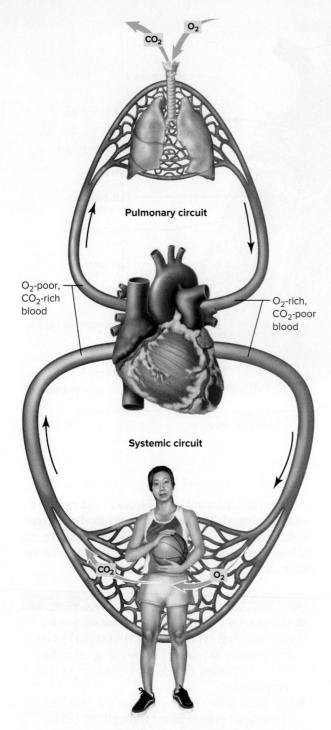

O2

CO2

Pulmonary circuit

O2-poor,
CO2-rich
blood

O2-rich,
CO2-poor
blood

Systemic circuit

CO2

O2

Figure 9.2 Illustration of the systemic and pulmonary circulations. As depicted by the color change from blue to red, blood becomes fully oxygenated as it flows through the lungs and then loses some oxygen (color changes from red to blue) as it flows through the other organs and tissues.

Myocardium

The wall of the heart is composed of three layers: (1) an outer layer called the epicardium, (2) a muscular middle layer, the myocardium, and (3) an inner layer known as the endocardium (see Fig. 9.3). It is

the **myocardium,** or heart muscle, that is responsible for contracting and forcing blood out of the heart. The myocardium receives its blood supply via the right and left coronary arteries, which branch off the aorta and encircle the heart. The coronary veins run alongside the arteries and drain all coronary blood into a larger vein called the coronary sinus, which deposits blood into the right atrium.

Maintaining a constant blood supply to the heart via the coronary arteries is critical because, even at rest, the heart has a high demand for oxygen and nutrients. When coronary blood flow is disrupted (i.e., blockage of a coronary blood vessel) for more than several minutes, permanent damage to the heart occurs. This type of injury results in the death of cardiac muscle cells and is commonly called a heart attack, or myocardial infarction (see Chap. 17). The number of heart cells (i.e., muscle fibers) that die from this insult determines the severity of a heart attack. That is, a "mild" heart attack may damage only a small portion of the heart, whereas a "major" heart attack may destroy a large number of heart cells (fibers). A major heart attack greatly diminishes the heart's pumping capacity; therefore, minimizing the amount of injury to the heart during a heart attack is critical. Importantly, strong evidence indicates that exercise training can provide cardiac protection during a heart attack (see Clinical Applications 9.1).

Heart muscle differs from skeletal muscle in several ways. First, cardiac muscle fibers are shorter than skeletal muscle fibers and are connected in a tight series. Further, cardiac fibers are typically branched, whereas skeletal muscle fibers are elongated and do not branch. Also, cardiac muscle contraction is involuntary, whereas skeletal muscle contractions are under voluntary control.

Another difference between cardiac fibers and skeletal muscle fibers is that, unlike skeletal muscle fibers, heart muscle fibers are all interconnected via **intercalated discs.** These intercellular connections permit the transmission of electrical impulses from one fiber to another. Intercalated discs allow ions to cross from one cardiac muscle fiber to another. Therefore, when one heart fiber is depolarized to contract, all connecting heart fibers also become excited and contract as a unit. This arrangement is called a functional syncytium. Heart muscle cells in the atria are separated from ventricular muscle cells by a layer of connective tissue that does not permit the transmission of electrical impulses. Hence, the atria contract separately from the ventricles.

One more difference between heart and skeletal muscle fibers is that human heart fibers are not divided into different fiber types. The ventricular myocardium is considered to be a homogenous muscle containing one primary fiber type that has similarities to the type I, slow fibers found in skeletal muscle. In

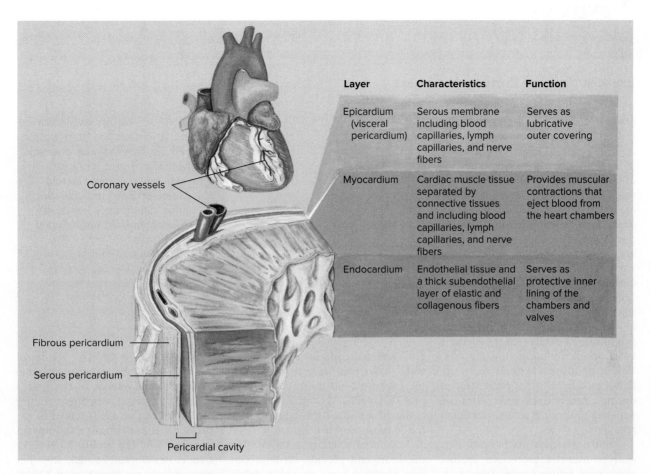

Layer	Characteristics	Function
Epicardium (visceral pericardium)	Serous membrane including blood capillaries, lymph capillaries, and nerve fibers	Serves as lubricative outer covering
Myocardium	Cardiac muscle tissue separated by connective tissues and including blood capillaries, lymph capillaries, and nerve fibers	Provides muscular contractions that eject blood from the heart chambers
Endocardium	Endothelial tissue and a thick subendothelial layer of elastic and collagenous fibers	Serves as protective inner lining of the chambers and valves

Figure 9.3 The heart wall is composed of three distinct layers: (1) epicardium, (2) myocardium, and (3) endocardium.

this regard, heart muscle fibers are highly aerobic and contain large numbers of mitochondria. Note, however, that cardiac muscle fibers contain many more mitochondria than type I, slow skeletal muscle fibers. This fact highlights the importance of continuous aerobic metabolism in the heart.

A final difference between cardiac and skeletal muscle fibers is the ability to recover following an injury to the muscle fibers. Recall from Chap. 8 that skeletal muscle fibers are surrounded by muscle precursor cells called satellite cells. These satellite cells are important because they provide skeletal muscle with the ability to regenerate (i.e., recover) from injury. However, cardiac muscle fibers do not contain satellite cells, and therefore, these heart muscle cells have limited regeneration capacity.

Although heart muscle and skeletal muscle differ in many ways, they are also similar in several ways. For example, both heart and skeletal muscle fibers are striated and contain the same contractile proteins: actin and myosin. Further, both heart and skeletal muscle fibers require calcium to activate the myofilaments (17), and both fibers contract via the sliding filament model of contraction (see Chap. 8). In addition, like skeletal muscle, heart muscle can alter its force of contraction as a function of the degree of overlap of

actin-myosin filaments due to changes in fiber length. Table 9.1 contains a point-by-point comparison of the structural/functional similarities and differences between cardiac and skeletal muscle fibers.

Cardiac Cycle

The cardiac cycle refers to the repeating pattern of contraction and relaxation of the heart. The contraction phase is called **systole** and the relaxation period is called **diastole.** Generally, when these terms are used alone, they refer to contraction and relaxation of the ventricles. However, note that the atria also contract and relax; therefore, there is an atrial systole and diastole. Atrial contraction occurs during ventricular diastole, and atrial relaxation occurs during ventricular systole. The heart thus has a two-step pumping action. The right and left atria contract together, which empties atrial blood into the ventricles. Approximately 0.1 second after the atrial contraction, the ventricles contract and deliver blood into both the systemic and pulmonary circuits.

At rest, contraction of the ventricles during systole ejects about two-thirds of the blood out of the ventricles, leaving about one-third in the ventricles. The ventricles then fill with blood during the next

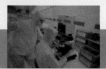

CLINICAL APPLICATIONS 9.1

Exercise Training Protects the Heart

It is now well established that regular exercise training is cardioprotective. Indeed, many epidemiological studies have provided evidence that regular exercise can reduce the incidence of heart attacks and that the survival rate of heart attack victims is greater in active people than in sedentary ones. Recent experiments provide direct evidence that regular endurance exercise training reduces the amount of cardiac damage that occurs during a heart attack (26, 28, 29). The protective effect of exercise is illustrated in Figure 9.4. Notice that exercise training can reduce the magnitude of cardiac injury during a heart attack by approximately 60%. This is significant because the number of cardiac cells that are destroyed during a heart attack determines the patient's chances of a full, functional recovery.

Animal experiments indicate that exercise-induced protection against myocardial injury during a heart attack can be achieved quickly (29).

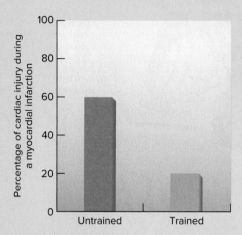

Figure 9.4 Regular endurance exercise protects the heart against cell death during a heart attack. Note that during a myocardial infarction (i.e., heart attack), exercise-trained individuals suffer significantly less cardiac injury compared to untrained individuals.

Data from Powers, S. K., Smuder, A. J., Kavazis, A. N., and Quindry, J. C., "Mechanisms of Exercise-Induced Cardioprotection," *Physiology* 29: 27–38, 2014.

For example, it appears that as few as three to five consecutive days of aerobic exercise (~60 minutes/day) can provide significant cardiac protection against heart attack-mediated damage to the heart muscle (29).

How does exercise training alter the heart and provide cardioprotection during a heart attack? A definitive answer to this question is not available. Nonetheless, evidence suggests that the exercise-training-induced improvement in the heart's ability to resist permanent injury during a heart attack is linked to improvements in the heart's antioxidant capacity (i.e., the ability to remove free radicals) (18, 26, 28, 29). For more details, see Powers et al. (2014) in the Suggested Readings.

TABLE 9.1 A Comparison of the Structural and Functional Differences/Similarities between Heart Muscle and Skeletal Muscle

Structural Comparison	Heart Muscle	Skeletal Muscle
Contractile proteins: actin and myosin	Present	Present
Shape of muscle fibers	Shorter than skeletal muscle fibers and branching	Elongated—no branching
Nuclei	Single	Multiple
Z-discs	Present	Present
Striated	Yes	Yes
Cellular junctions	Yes—intercalated discs	No junctional complexes
Connective tissue	Endomysium	Epimysium, perimysium, and endomysium
Functional Comparison		
Energy production	Aerobic (primarily)	Aerobic and anaerobic
Calcium source (for contraction)	Sarcoplasmic reticulum and extracellular calcium	Sarcoplasmic reticulum
Neural control	Involuntary	Voluntary
Regeneration potential	None—no satellite cells present	Some possibilities via satellite cells

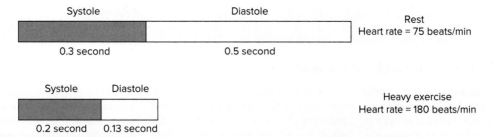

Figure 9.5 Illustration of cardiac cycle at rest and during exercise. Notice that increases in heart rate during exercise are achieved primarily through a decrease in the time spent in diastole; however, at high heart rates, the length of time spent in systole also decreases.

diastole. A healthy 21-year-old female might have an average resting heart rate of 75 beats per minute. This means that the total cardiac cycle lasts 0.8 second, with 0.5 second spent in diastole and the remaining 0.3 second dedicated to systole (17) (see Fig. 9.5). If the heart rate increases from 75 beats per minute to 180 beats per minute (e.g., heavy exercise), there is a reduction in the time spent in both systole and diastole (11). This point is illustrated in Figure 9.5. Note that a rising heart rate results in a greater time reduction in diastole, whereas systole is less affected.

Pressure Changes during the Cardiac Cycle During the cardiac cycle, the pressure within the heart chambers rises and falls. When the atria are relaxed, blood flows into them from the venous circulation. As these chambers fill, the pressure inside gradually increases. Approximately 70% of the blood entering the atria during diastole flows directly into the ventricles through the atrioventricular valves before the atria contract. Upon atrial contraction, atrial pressure rises and forces most of the remaining 30% of the atrial blood into the ventricles.

Pressure in the ventricles is low while they are filling, but when the atria contract, the ventricular pressure increases slightly. Then as the ventricles contract, the pressure rises sharply, which closes the atrioventricular valves and prevents backflow into the atria. As soon as ventricular pressure exceeds the pressure of the pulmonary artery and the aorta, the pulmonary and aortic valves open and blood is forced into both pulmonary and systemic circulations. Figure 9.6 illustrates the changes in ventricular pressure as a function of time during the resting cardiac cycle. Note the occurrence of two heart sounds that are produced by the closing of the atrioventricular valves (first heart sound) and the closing of the aortic and pulmonary valves (second heart sound).

Arterial Blood Pressure

Blood exerts pressure throughout the vascular system but is greatest within the arteries, where it is generally measured and used as an indication of health. Blood pressure is the force exerted by blood against

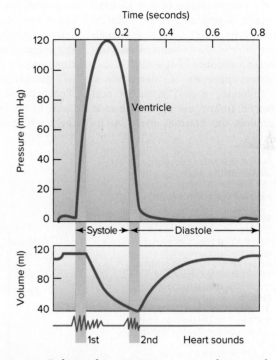

Figure 9.6 Relationship among pressure, volume, and heart sounds during the cardiac cycle. Notice the change in ventricular pressure and volume during the transition from systole to diastole.

the arterial walls and is determined by how much blood is pumped and the resistance to blood flow.

Arterial blood pressure can be estimated by the use of a sphygmomanometer (see A Closer Look 9.1). The normal blood pressure of an adult male is 120/80, while that of adult females tends to be lower (110/70). The larger number in the expression of blood pressure is the systolic pressure expressed in millimeters of mercury (mm Hg). The lower number in the blood pressure ratio is the diastolic pressure, again expressed in mm Hg. **Systolic blood pressure** is the pressure generated as blood is ejected from the heart during ventricular systole. During ventricular relaxation (diastole), the arterial blood pressure decreases and represents **diastolic blood pressure.** The difference between systolic and diastolic blood pressure is called the pulse pressure.

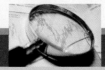
Measurement of Arterial Blood Pressure

Arterial blood pressure is not usually measured directly but is estimated using an instrument called a sphygmomanometer (see Fig. 9.7). This device consists of an inflatable arm cuff connected to a column of mercury. The cuff can be inflated by a bulb pump, with the pressure in the cuff measured by the rising column of mercury. For example, a pressure of 100 mm of mercury (mm Hg) would be enough force to raise the column of mercury upward a distance of 100 mm.

Blood pressure is measured in the following way: The rubber cuff is placed around the upper arm so it surrounds the brachial artery. Air is pumped into the cuff until the pressure around the arm exceeds arterial pressure. Because the pressure applied around the arm is greater than arterial pressure, the brachial artery is squeezed shut and blood flow is stopped. If a stethoscope is placed over the brachial artery (just below the cuff), no sounds are heard, since there is no blood flow. However, if the air control valve is slowly opened to release air, the pressure in the cuff begins to decline, and the pressure around the arm will quickly reach a point that is just slightly below arterial pressure. At this point blood begins to spurt through the artery, producing turbulent flow, and a sharp sound (known as Korotkoff sounds) can be heard through the stethoscope. The pressure (i.e., height of mercury column) at which the first tapping sound is heard represents systolic blood pressure.

As the cuff pressure continues to decline, a series of increasingly louder sounds can be heard. When the pressure in the cuff is equal to or slightly below diastolic blood pressure, the sounds heard through the stethoscope cease because turbulent flow ceases. Therefore, resting diastolic blood pressure represents the height of the mercury column when the sounds disappear.

1. No sound is heard because there is no blood flow when the cuff pressure is high enough to keep the brachial artery closed.

2. **Systolic pressure** is the pressure at which a Korotkoff sound is first heard. When cuff pressure decreases and is no longer able to keep the brachial artery closed during systole, blood is pushed through the partially opened brachial artery to produce turbulent blood flow and a sound. The brachial artery remains closed during diastole.

3. As cuff pressure continues to decrease, the brachial artery opens even more during systole. At first, the artery is closed during diastole, but, as cuff pressure continues to decrease, the brachial artery partially opens during diastole. Turbulent blood flow during systole produces Korotkoff sounds, although the pitch of the sounds changes as the artery becomes more open.

4. **Diastolic pressure** is the pressure at which the sound disappears. Eventually, cuff pressure decreases below the pressure in the brachial artery and it remains open during systole and diastole. Nonturbulent flow is reestablished and no sounds are heard.

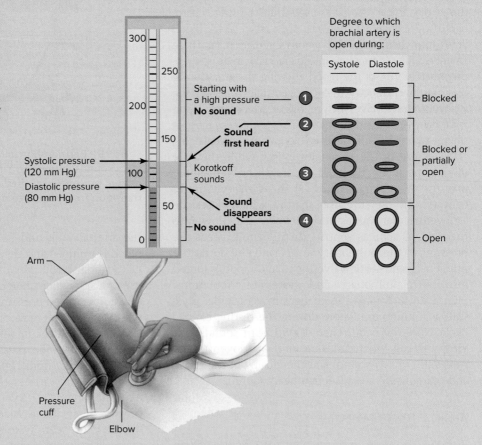

Figure 9.7   A sphygmomanometer is used to measure arterial blood pressure.

The average pressure during a cardiac cycle is called *mean arterial pressure*. Mean arterial blood pressure is important because it determines the rate of blood flow through the systemic circuit.

Determination of mean arterial pressure is not easy. It is not a simple average of systolic and diastolic pressure, because diastole generally lasts longer than systole. However, mean arterial pressure can be estimated at rest in the following way:

Mean arterial pressure = DBP + 0.33 (pulse pressure)

Here, DBP is the diastolic blood pressure, and the pulse pressure is the difference between systolic and diastolic pressures. Let's consider a sample calculation of mean arterial pressure at rest.

For example, suppose an individual has a blood pressure of 120/80 mm Hg. The mean arterial pressure would be:

**Mean arterial pressure = 80 mm Hg
+ 0.33(120 − 80)
= 80 mm Hg + 13
= 93 mm Hg**

Note that this equation cannot be used to compute mean arterial blood pressure during exercise because it is based on the timing of the cardiac cycle at rest. That is, arterial blood pressure rises during systole and falls during diastole across the cardiac cycle. Therefore, to accurately estimate the average arterial blood pressure at any time, systolic and diastolic blood pressure must be measured and the amount of time spent in both systole and diastole must be known. Recall that the time spent in systole and diastole differs between rest and exercise. For example, the formula estimates that the time spent in systole occupies 33% of the total cardiac cycle at rest. However, during maximal exercise, systole may account for 66% of the total cardiac cycle time. Therefore, any formula designed to estimate mean arterial blood pressure must be adjusted to reflect the time spent in systole and diastole.

High blood pressure (called hypertension) is classified as blood pressures above 140/90 mm Hg. Unfortunately, approximately 33% of all adults (>20 years old) in the United States have hypertension (13). Hypertension is generally classified into one of two categories: (1) primary, or essential, hypertension and (2) secondary hypertension. The cause of primary hypertension is multifactorial; that is, there are several factors whose combined effects produce hypertension. This type of hypertension constitutes 95% of all reported cases in the United States. Secondary hypertension is a result of some known disease process, and thus the hypertension is "secondary" to another disease.

Hypertension can lead to a variety of health problems. For example, hypertension increases the workload on the left ventricle, resulting in an adaptive increase in the muscle mass of the left heart (called left ventricular hypertrophy). In the early phases of hypertension-induced left ventricular hypertrophy, the increase in cardiac mass helps to maintain the heart's pumping ability. However, with time, this left ventricular hypertrophy changes the organization and function of cardiac muscle fibers, resulting in diminished pumping capacity of the heart, which can lead to heart failure. Further, the presence of hypertension is a major risk factor for developing arteriosclerosis and heart attacks. Finally, hypertension also increases the risk of kidney damage and the rupture of a cerebral blood vessel resulting in localized brain injury (i.e., a stroke).

Factors That Influence Arterial Blood Pressure

Mean arterial blood pressure is determined by two factors: (1) cardiac output and (2) total vascular resistance. Cardiac output is the amount of blood pumped from the heart, and total vascular resistance is the sum of resistance to blood flow provided by all systemic blood vessels. Mathematically, mean arterial blood pressure is defined as the product of cardiac output times total vascular resistance, as given in the following equation:

**Mean arterial blood pressure = Cardiac output
× Total vascular
resistance**

Therefore, an increase in either cardiac output or vascular resistance results in an increase in mean arterial blood pressure. In the body, mean arterial blood pressure depends on a variety of physiological factors, including cardiac output, blood volume, resistance to flow, and blood viscosity. These relationships are summarized in Figure 9.8. An increase in any of these variables results in an increase in arterial blood pressure. Conversely, a decrease in any of these variables

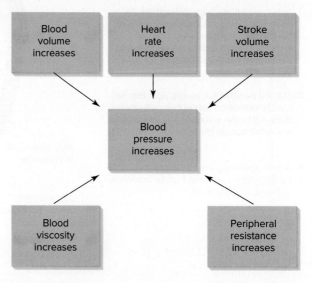

Figure 9.8 Factors that influence arterial blood pressure.

causes a decrease in blood pressure. The relationships between these factors will be discussed in detail in a later section.

How is blood pressure regulated? Acute (short-term) regulation of blood pressure is achieved by the sympathetic nervous system, whereas long-term regulation of blood pressure is primarily a function of the kidneys (4). The kidneys regulate blood pressure by controlling blood volume.

Pressure receptors (called baroreceptors) in the carotid artery and the aorta are sensitive to changes in arterial blood pressure. An increase in arterial pressure triggers these receptors to send impulses to the **cardiovascular control center** (located within the medullar oblongata), which responds by decreasing sympathetic activity. A reduction in sympathetic activity may lower cardiac output and/or reduce vascular resistance, which in turn lowers blood pressure. Conversely, a decrease in blood pressure results in a reduction of baroreceptor activity to the brain. This causes the cardiovascular control center to respond by increasing sympathetic outflow, which raises blood pressure back to normal. For a complete discussion of blood pressure regulation, see Hall (2015) or Fox (2016) in the Suggested Readings.

Electrical Activity of the Heart

Many myocardial cells have the unique potential for spontaneous electrical activity (i.e., each has an intrinsic rhythm). However, in the normal heart, spontaneous electrical activity is limited to a special region located in the right atrium. This region, called the **sinoatrial node (SA node),** serves as the pacemaker for the heart (see Fig. 9.9). Spontaneous electrical activity in the SA node occurs due to a decay of the resting membrane potential via inward diffusion of sodium during diastole. When the SA node reaches the depolarization threshold and "fires," the wave of depolarization spreads over the atria, resulting in atrial contraction. The wave of atrial depolarization cannot directly cross into the ventricles but must be transported by way of specialized conductive tissue. This specialized conductive tissue radiates from a small mass of muscle tissue called the **atrioventricular node (AV node).** This node, located in the floor of the right atrium, connects the atria with the ventricles by a pair of conductive pathways called the *right and left bundle branches* (Fig. 9.9). Note that atrial-mediated depolarization of the AV node is delayed by approximately 0.10 second. This time delay is important because it allows atrial contraction to empty atrial blood into the ventricles prior to ventricular depolarization and contraction. Upon reaching the ventricles, these conductive pathways branch into smaller fibers

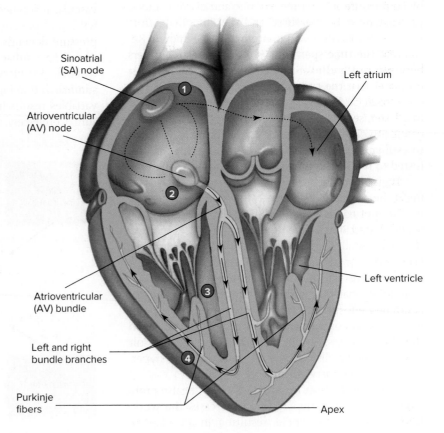

1. Action potentials originate in the sinoatrial (SA) node (the pacemaker) and travel across the wall of the atrium (*arrows*) from the SA node to the atrioventricular (AV) node.

2. Action potentials pass through the AV node and along the atrioventricular (AV) bundle, which extends from the AV node, through the fibrous skeleton, into the interventricular septum.

3. The AV bundle divides into right and left bundle branches, and action potentials descend to the apex of each ventricle along the bundle branches.

4. Action potentials are carried by the Purkinje fibers from the bundle branches to the ventricular walls.

Sinoatrial (SA) node

Left atrium

Atrioventricular (AV) node

Atrioventricular (AV) bundle

Left and right bundle branches

Purkinje fibers

Left ventricle

Apex

Figure 9.9   Conduction system of the heart.

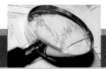

A CLOSER LOOK 9.2

Diagnostic Use of the ECG During Exercise

Cardiologists are physicians who specialize in diseases of the heart and vascular system. One of the diagnostic procedures commonly used to evaluate cardiac function is to make ECG measurements during an incremental exercise test (commonly called a stress test). This allows the physician to observe changes in blood pressure as well as changes in the patient's ECG during periods of exercise-induced stress.

The most common cause of heart disease is the collection of fatty plaque (called atherosclerosis) inside coronary vessels. This collection of plaque reduces blood flow to the myocardium. The adequacy of blood flow to the heart is relative—it depends on the metabolic demand placed on the heart. For example, a small obstruction in a coronary artery may permit adequate blood flow to

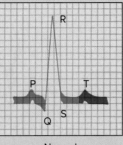
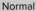

Normal

Ischemia

Figure 9.10 Depression of the S-T segment of the electrocardiogram as a result of myocardial ischemia.

meet the metabolic needs during rest, but a coronary blockage would likely result in inadequate blood flow to the heart during exercise because of the large increase in metabolic demands. Therefore, a graded exercise test may serve as a "stress test" to evaluate cardiac function.

An example of an abnormal exercise ECG is illustrated in Figure 9.10.

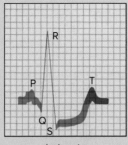

Myocardial ischemia (reduced blood flow) may be detected by changes in the S-T segment of the ECG. Notice the depressed S-T segment in the picture on the right when compared to the normal ECG on the left. This S-T segment depression suggests to the physician that ischemic heart disease may be present and that additional diagnostic procedures may be warranted.

called Purkinje fibers. The Purkinje fibers then spread the wave of depolarization throughout the ventricles.

A recording of the electrical changes that occur in the myocardium during the cardiac cycle is called an **electrocardiogram (ECG or EKG)**. Analysis of ECG waveforms allows the physician to evaluate the heart's ability to conduct impulses and therefore determine if electrical problems exist. Further, analysis of the ECG during exercise is often used in the diagnosis of coronary artery disease (see A Closer Look 9.2). Figure 9.11 illustrates a normal ECG pattern. Notice that the ECG pattern contains several different deflections, or waves, during each cardiac cycle. Each of these distinct waveforms is identified by different letters. The first deflection on the ECG is called the P wave and represents the depolarization of the atria. The second wave, the QRS complex, represents the depolarization of the ventricles and occurs approximately 0.10 second following the P wave. The final deflection, the T wave, is the result of ventricular repolarization. Notice that atrial repolarization is usually not visible on the ECG because it occurs at the same time as the QRS complex (Fig. 9.12). That is, atrial repolarization is "hidden" by the QRS complex.

Finally, Figure 9.13 illustrates the relationship between changes in the intraventricular pressure and the ECG. Note that the QRS complex (i.e., depolarization of the ventricles) occurs at the beginning of systole, whereas the T wave (i.e., repolarization of the

ventricles) occurs at the beginning of diastole. Also, notice that the rise in intraventricular pressure at the beginning of systole results in the first heart sound, due to closure of the atrioventricular valves (AV valves), and that the fall in intraventricular pressure at the end of systole results in the second heart sound, due to the closure of the aortic and pulmonary semi-lunar valves.

IN SUMMARY

- The myocardium is composed of three layers: (1) epicardium (outer layer); (2) myocardium (middle layer composed of cardiac muscle fibers); and (3) endocardium (inner layer).
- The contraction phase of the cardiac cycle is called *systole* and the relaxation period is called *diastole*.
- The average blood pressure during a cardiac cycle is called *mean arterial blood pressure*.
- Blood pressure can be increased by one or all of the following factors:
  a. Increase in blood volume
  b. Increase in heart rate
  c. Increased blood viscosity
  d. Increase in stroke volume
  e. Increased peripheral resistance
- The pacemaker of the heart is the SA node.
- A recording of the electrical activity of the heart during the cardiac cycle is called the *electrocardiogram (ECG or EKG)*.

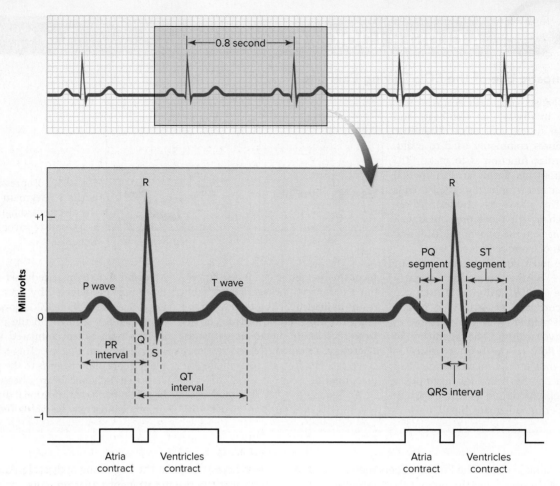

Figure 9.11 The normal electrocardiogram during rest.

CARDIAC OUTPUT

Cardiac output ($\dot{Q}$) is the product of the heart rate (HR) and the **stroke volume** (SV) (amount of blood pumped per heartbeat):

$$\dot{Q} = HR \times SV$$

Thus, cardiac output can be increased due to a rise in either heart rate or stroke volume. During exercise in the upright position (e.g., running, cycling, etc.), the increase in cardiac output is due to an increase in both heart rate and stroke volume. Table 9.2 presents typical values at rest and during maximal exercise for heart rate, stroke volume, and cardiac output in both untrained and highly trained endurance athletes. The gender differences in stroke volume and cardiac output are due mainly to differences in body sizes between men and women (2) (see Table 9.2).

Regulation of Heart Rate

During exercise, the quantity of blood pumped by the heart must change in accordance with the elevated skeletal muscle oxygen demand. Because the SA node controls heart rate, changes in heart rate often involve factors that influence the SA node. The two most prominent factors that influence heart rate are the parasympathetic and sympathetic nervous systems (11).

The parasympathetic fibers that supply the heart arise from neurons in the cardiovascular control center in the medulla oblongata and make up a portion of the **vagus nerve** (4). Upon reaching the heart, these fibers make contact with both the SA node and the AV node (see Fig. 9.14). When stimulated, these nerve endings release acetylcholine, which causes a decrease in the activity of both the SA and AV nodes due to hyperpolarization (i.e., moving the resting membrane potential further from threshold). The end result is a reduction of heart rate. Therefore, the parasympathetic nervous system acts as a braking system to slow down heart rate.

Even at rest, the vagus nerves carry impulses to the SA and AV nodes (11). This is often referred to as parasympathetic tone. As a consequence, changes in parasympathetic activity can cause heart rate to increase or decrease. For instance, a decrease in parasympathetic tone to the heart can elevate heart rate, whereas an increase in parasympathetic activity causes a slowing of heart rate.

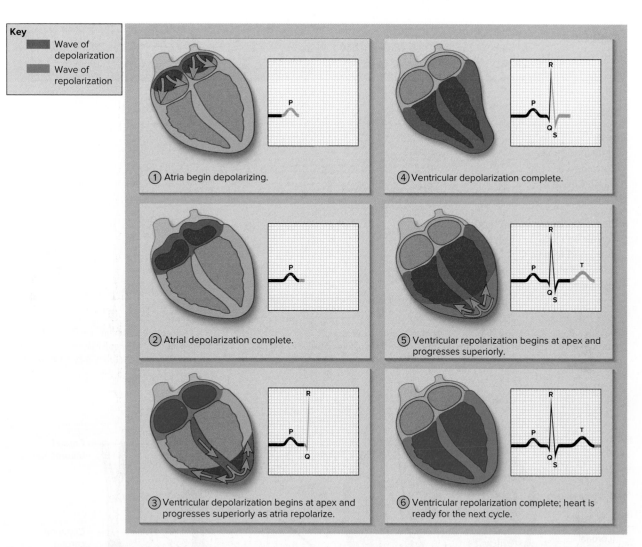

Figure 9.12 An illustration of the relationship between the heart's electrical events and the recording of the ECG. Panels 1–2 illustrate atrial depolarization and the formation of the P wave. Panels 3–4 illustrate ventricular depolarization and formation of the QRS complex. Finally, panels 5–6 illustrate repolarization of the ventricles and formation of the T wave.

Figure 9.13 The relationship between changes in the intraventricular pressure and the ECG. Notice that the QRS complex (i.e., depolarization of the ventricles) occurs at the beginning of systole and the rise in ventricular pressure. Further, note that the T wave (repolarization of the ventricles) occurs at the same time that the ventricles relax at the beginning of diastole.

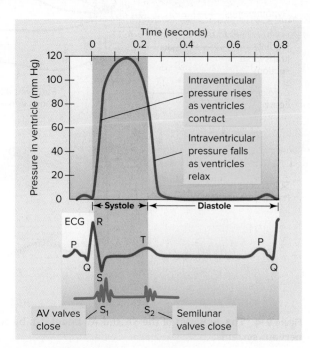

TABLE 9.2	Typical Resting and Maximal Exercise Values for Stroke Volume (SV), Heart Rate (HR), and Cardiac Output (Q̇) for College-Age Untrained Subjects and Trained Endurance Athletes (Body Weights: Male = 70 kg; Female = 50 kg)					
Subject	HR (beats/min)		SV (ml/beat)		Q̇ (l/min)	
Rest						
Untrained male	72	×	70	=	5.00	
Untrained female	75	×	60	=	4.50	
Trained male	50	×	100	=	5.00	
Trained female	55	×	80	=	4.40	
		×				
Max Exercise						
Untrained male	200	×	110	=	22.0	
Untrained female	200	×	90	=	18.0	
Trained male	190	×	180	=	34.2	
Trained female	190	×	125	=	23.8	

Note that values are rounded off.

Data from Borjesson, M., and Pelliccia, A., "Incidence and Aetiology of Sudden Cardiac Death in Young Athletes: An International Perspective," *British Journal of Sports Medicine* 43: 644–648, 2009; Miller, J. D., Pegelow, D. F., Jacques, A. J., and Dempsey, J. A., "Skeletal Muscle Pump Versus Respiratory Muscle Pump: Modulation of Venous Return from the Locomotor Limb in Humans," *Journal of Physiology* 563: 925–943, 2005, p. 68.

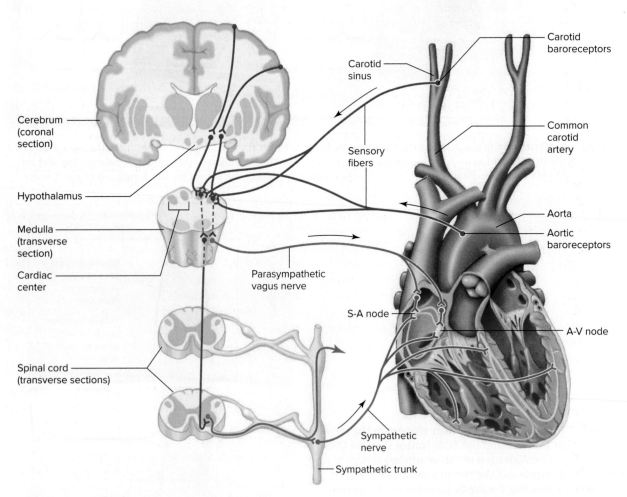

Figure 9.14 The activities of the SA and AV nodes can be altered by both the sympathetic and parasympathetic nervous systems.

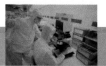
Beta-Blockade and Exercise Heart Rate

Beta-adrenergic blocking medications (beta-blockers) are commonly prescribed for patients with coronary artery disease and/or hypertension. Although there are many different classes of these drugs, all these medications compete with epinephrine and norepinephrine for beta-adrenergic receptors in the heart.

The end result is that beta-blockers reduce heart rate and the vigor of myocardial contraction, thus reducing the oxygen requirement of the heart.

In clinical exercise physiology, it is important to appreciate that all beta-blocking drugs will decrease resting heart rate as well as exercise heart rate.

Indeed, individuals on beta-blocking medications will exhibit lower exercise heart rates during both submaximal and maximal exercise. This is an important fact that should be considered when prescribing exercise and interpreting the exercise test results of individuals using beta-blocking medications.

The initial increase in heart rate during low-intensity exercise, up to approximately 100 beats per minute, is due to a withdrawal of parasympathetic tone (34). This occurs because, without neural input to the SA node, the intrinsic firing rate of the SA node is typically 100 beats per minute. At higher work rates, stimulation of the SA and AV nodes by the sympathetic nervous system is responsible for increases in heart rate (34). Sympathetic fibers reach the heart by means of the **cardiac accelerator nerves,** which innervate both the SA node and the ventricles (Fig. 9.14). Endings of these fibers release norepinephrine upon stimulation, which act on beta receptors in the heart and cause an increase in both heart rate and the force of myocardial contraction. (See Clinical Applications 9.2.)

At rest, a normal balance between parasympathetic tone and sympathetic activity to the heart is maintained by the cardiovascular control center in the medulla oblongata. The cardiovascular control center receives impulses from various parts of the circulatory system relative to changes in important parameters (e.g., blood pressure, blood oxygen tension), and it relays motor impulses to the heart in response to a changing cardiovascular need. For example, an increase in resting blood pressure above normal stimulates pressure receptors in the carotid arteries and the arch of the aorta, which in turn send impulses to the cardiovascular control center (Fig. 9.14). In response, the cardiovascular control center increases parasympathetic activity to the heart to slow the heart rate and reduce cardiac output. This reduction in cardiac output causes blood pressure to decline back toward normal.

Another regulatory reflex involves pressure receptors located in the right atrium. In this case, an increase in right atrial pressure signals the cardiovascular control center that an increase in venous return has occurred; hence, to prevent a backup of blood in the systemic venous system, an increase in cardiac output must result. The cardiovascular control center responds by sending sympathetic accelerator nerve impulses to the heart, which increase heart rate and cardiac output. The end result is that the increase in cardiac output lowers right atrial pressure back to normal, and venous blood pressure is reduced.

Finally, a change in body temperature can influence heart rate. An increase in body temperature above normal results in an increase in heart rate, whereas lowering of body temperature below normal causes a reduction in heart rate (34). For example, exercise in a hot environment results in increased body temperatures and higher heart rates than if the same exercise was performed in a cool environment. This topic is discussed in more detail in Chap. 12.

Heart Rate Variability

As discussed previously, heart rate is regulated by the autonomic nervous system (i.e., balance between the parasympathetic and sympathetic nervous systems). The term **heart rate variability** (HRV) refers to the variation in the time between heartbeats (19). In practice, the time interval (expressed in milliseconds) between two heartbeats can be measured as the R-R time interval using an ECG tracing, as illustrated in Figure 9.11. The HRV is then calculated as the standard deviation of the R-R time interval during a selected time period. A wide variation in HRV is considered to be a good index of a "healthy" balance between the sympathetic and parasympathetic nervous systems, whereas low HRV indicates an imbalance exists in autonomic regulation.

The physiological significance of HRV is that the time variation between heartbeats reflects autonomic balance and is an excellent noninvasive screening tool for many diseases. For example, low HRV has been shown to predict future cardiovascular events, such as sudden cardiac death. Further, low HRV is an independent risk factor for the development of cardiovascular disease, including heart failure, myocardial infarction, and hypertension (20). Epidemiological studies have also established that low HRV is an excellent predictor of increased cardiovascular morbidity and mortality in patients with existing cardiovascular disease.

What is the physiological cause of low HRV variability? Again, the autonomic nervous system regulates many cardiovascular parameters, including both heart rate and HRV. Recall that heart rate can be elevated by increasing sympathetic activity or decreased by increasing parasympathetic (vagal) activity. The balance between the effects of the sympathetic and parasympathetic systems, the two opposite-acting branches of the autonomic nervous system, is referred to as the *sympathovagal balance* and is reflected in the beat-to-beat changes of the cardiac cycle (19).

Numerous factors can influence the sympathovagal balance and thus affect HRV. For example, with advancing age or some disease states, there is a decrease in parasympathetic tone at rest (19) or an increase in sympathetic nervous system outflow (8). This results in a disturbance in sympathovagal balance and a decrease in HRV. Some specific examples of diseases that promote a decrease in HRV are as follows: HRV is decreased in patients suffering from depression, hypertension, and heart disease, and in individuals following a myocardial infarction (19). Importantly, research indicates that physical inactivity promotes a decrease in HRV, whereas regular bouts of aerobic exercise result in increased HRV (19). Therefore, investigation of the types of exercise and specific training programs that have positive influences on HRV has become an important area of research.

Regulation of Stroke Volume

Stroke volume, at rest or during exercise, is regulated by three factors: (1) the end-diastolic volume (EDV), which is the volume of blood in the ventricles at the end of diastole; (2) the average aortic blood pressure; and (3) the strength of ventricular contraction.

EDV is often referred to as "preload," and it influences stroke volume in the following way. Two physiologists, Frank and Starling, demonstrated that the strength of ventricular contraction increased with an enlargement of EDV (i.e., stretch of the ventricles). This relationship has become known as the Frank-Starling law of the heart. The increase in EDV results in a lengthening of cardiac fibers, which improves the force of contraction in a manner similar to that seen in skeletal muscle (discussed in Chap. 8). The mechanism to explain the influence of fiber length on cardiac contractility is that an increase in the length of cardiac fibers increases the number of myosin cross-bridge interactions with actin, resulting in increased force production. A rise in cardiac contractility results in an increase in the amount of blood pumped per beat; the relationship between EDV volume and stroke volume is illustrated in Figure 9.15.

The principal variable that influences EDV is the rate of venous return to the heart. An increase in venous return results in a rise in EDV and, therefore, an increase in stroke volume. Increased venous return and the resulting increase in EDV play a key role in the increase in stroke volume observed during upright exercise.

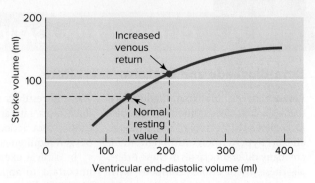

Figure 9.15 An illustration of the relationship between ventricular end-diastolic volume and stroke volume. Notice the increase in stroke volume when venous return increases above the normal resting level.

What factors regulate venous return during exercise? There are three principal mechanisms: (1) constriction of the veins (venoconstriction), (2) pumping action of contracting skeletal muscle (called the muscle pump), and (3) pumping action of the respiratory system (termed the *respiratory pump*).

1. Venoconstriction. Venoconstriction increases venous return by decreasing the diameter of the vessels and increasing the pressure within the vein. The end result of increased venous pressure is to drive blood back toward the heart. Venoconstriction occurs via a reflex sympathetic constriction of smooth muscle in veins draining skeletal muscle, which is controlled by the cardiovascular control center (4).

2. Muscle pump. The muscle pump is a result of the mechanical action of rhythmic skeletal muscle contractions. Therefore, when muscles contract during exercise, they compress veins and push blood back toward the heart. Between contractions, blood refills the veins and the process is repeated. Blood is prevented from flowing away from the heart between contractions by one-way valves located in large veins (Fig. 9.16). During sustained muscular contractions (isometric exercise), the muscle pump cannot operate, and venous return to the heart is reduced.

3. Respiratory pump. The rhythmic pattern of breathing also provides a mechanical pump by which venous return is promoted. The respiratory pump works in the following way. During inspiration, the pressure within the thorax (chest) decreases and abdominal pressure increases. This creates a flow of venous blood from the abdominal region into the thorax and therefore promotes venous return. Although quiet breathing (rest) aids in venous return, the role of the respiratory pump is enhanced during exercise due to the greater respiratory rate and depth. Indeed, recent evidence indicates that the respiratory pump is a dominant factor that promotes venous return to the heart during upright exercise (22).

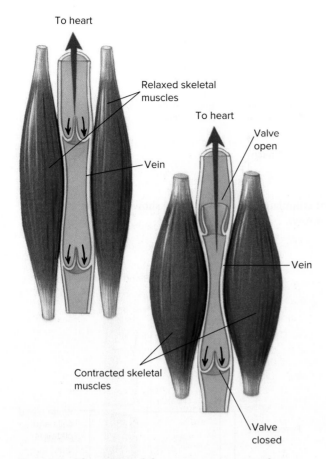

Figure 9.16 The action of the one-way venous valves. Contraction of skeletal muscles helps to pump blood toward the heart, but is prevented from pushing blood away from the heart by closure of the venous valves.

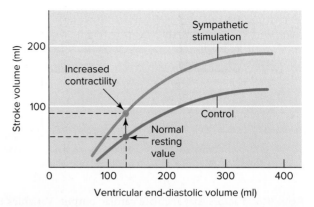

Figure 9.17 Effects of sympathetic stimulation of the heart on stroke volume. Note that sympathetic stimulation results in an increase in stroke volume at any given diastolic volume; that is, sympathetic stimulation increases ventricular contractility via an increased level of intracellular calcium, resulting in a higher myosin cross-bridge interaction with actin.

activation and force production. The relationship between sympathetic stimulation of the heart and stroke volume is illustrated in Figure 9.17. Notice that compared to control conditions (i.e., limited sympathetic stimulation), increased sympathetic stimulation of the heart increases stroke volume at any level of EDV.

To summarize, stroke volume is regulated by three factors: EDV, cardiac contractility, and cardiac afterload. During upright exercise, the exercise-induced increases in stroke volume occur due to both increases in EDV and increased cardiac contractility due to circulating catecholamines and/or sympathetic stimulation. In contrast, an increase in cardiac afterload results in a decrease in stroke volume.

IN SUMMARY

- Cardiac output is the product of heart rate and stroke volume ($\dot{Q} = HR \times SV$). Figure 9.18 summarizes those variables that influence cardiac output during exercise.
- The pacemaker of the heart is the SA node. SA node activity is modified by the parasympathetic nervous system (slows HR) and the sympathetic nervous system (increases HR).
- Heart rate increases at the beginning of exercise due to a withdrawal of parasympathetic tone. At higher work rates, the increase in heart rate is achieved via an increased sympathetic outflow to the SA nodes.
- Stroke volume is regulated via (1) end-diastolic volume, (2) afterload (i.e., aortic blood pressure), and (3) the strength of ventricular contraction.
- Venous return increases during exercise due to (1) venoconstriction, (2) the muscle pump, and (3) the respiratory pump.

A second variable that affects stroke volume is the aortic pressure (mean arterial pressure). In order to eject blood, the pressure generated by the left ventricle must exceed the pressure in the aorta. Therefore, aortic pressure or mean arterial pressure (called afterload) represents a barrier to the ejection of blood from the ventricles. Stroke volume is thus inversely proportional to the afterload; that is, an increase in aortic pressure produces a decrease in stroke volume. However, afterload is minimized during exercise due to arteriole dilation. This arteriole dilation in the working muscles reduces afterload and makes it easier for the heart to pump a large volume of blood.

The final factor that influences stroke volume is the effect of circulating catecholamines (i.e., epinephrine and norepinephrine) and direct sympathetic stimulation of the heart by cardiac accelerator nerves. Both of these mechanisms increase cardiac contractility by increasing the amount of calcium available to the myocardial cell (34). In particular, epinephrine and norepinephrine both increase the entry of extracellular calcium into the cardiac muscle fiber, which increases cross-bridge

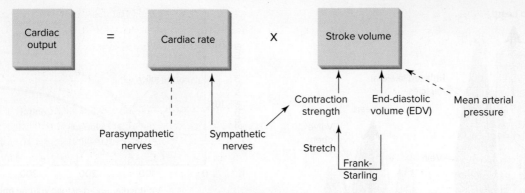

Figure 9.18 Factors that regulate cardiac output. Variables that stimulate cardiac output are shown by solid arrows, and factors that reduce cardiac output are shown by dotted arrows.

HEMODYNAMICS

One of the most important features of the circulatory system is that the system is a continuous "closed loop." Blood flow through the circulatory system results from pressure differences between the two ends of the system. To understand the physical regulation of blood flow to tissues, it is necessary to appreciate the interrelationships between pressure, flow, and resistance. The study of these factors and the physical principles of blood flow is called *hemodynamics*.

Physical Characteristics of Blood

Blood is composed of two principal components: plasma and cells. Plasma is the "watery" portion of blood that contains numerous ions, proteins, and hormones. The cells that make up blood are red blood cells (RBCs), platelets, and white blood cells. Red blood cells contain hemoglobin used for the transport of oxygen (see Chap. 10). Platelets play an important role in blood clotting, and white blood cells are important in preventing infection (Chap. 6).

The percentage of the blood that is composed of cells is called the hematocrit. That is, if 42% of the blood is cells and the remainder is plasma, the hematocrit is 42% (see Fig. 9.19). On a percentage basis, RBCs constitute the largest fraction of cells found in blood. Therefore, the hematocrit is principally influenced by increases or decreases in RBC numbers. The average hematocrit of a normal college-age male is 42%, and the hematocrit of a normal college-age female averages approximately 38%. These values vary among individuals and are dependent on a number of variables.

Blood is several times more viscous than water, and this viscosity increases the difficulty with which blood flows through the circulatory system. One of the major contributors to viscosity is the concentration of RBCs found in the blood. Therefore, during

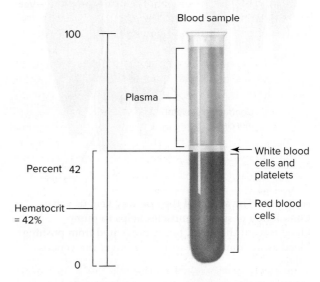

Figure 9.19 Blood cells become packed at the bottom of the test tube when blood is centrifuged; this leaves the plasma at the top of the tube. The percentage of whole blood that is composed of blood cells is termed the *hematocrit*.

periods of anemia (decreased RBCs), the viscosity of blood is lowered. Conversely, an increase in hematocrit results in an elevation in blood viscosity. The potential influence of changing blood viscosity on performance is discussed in Chap. 25.

Relationships among Pressure, Resistance, and Flow

As mentioned earlier, blood flow through the vascular system is dependent upon the difference in pressure at the two ends of the system. For example, if the pressures at the two ends of the vessel are equal, no flow will occur. In contrast, if the pressure is higher at one end of the vessel than the other, blood will flow from the region of higher pressure to the region of lower pressure. The rate of flow is proportional to the pressure difference ($P_1 - P_2$) between the two ends of the tube. In other words, the

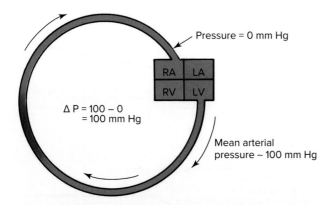

Pressure = 0 mm Hg

RA | LA
RV | LV

ΔP = 100 − 0
= 100 mm Hg

Mean arterial
pressure ~ 100 mm Hg

Figure 9.20 The flow of blood through the systemic circuit is dependent on the pressure difference (ΔP) between the aorta and the right atrium. In this illustration, the mean pressure in the aorta is 100 mm Hg, while the pressure in the right atrium is 0 mm Hg. Therefore, the "driving" pressure across the circuit is 100 mm Hg (100 − 0 = 100).

blood flow is directly related to the pressure differences across the tube, whereby an increase in driving pressure will increase flow. Figure 9.20 illustrates the "pressure head" driving blood flow in the systemic circulatory system under resting conditions. Here, the mean arterial pressure is 100 mm Hg (i.e., this is the pressure of blood in the aorta), while the pressure at the opposite end of the circuit (i.e., pressure in the right atrium) is 0 mm Hg. Therefore, the driving pressure across the circulatory system is 100 mm Hg (100 − 0 = 100).

It should be pointed out that the flow rate of blood through the vascular system is proportional to the pressure difference across the system, but it is inversely proportional to the resistance. In simple terms, this means that when vascular resistance increases, blood flow decreases. Inverse proportionality is expressed mathematically by the placement of this variable in the denominator of a fraction, because a fraction decreases when the denominator increases. Therefore, the relationship between blood flow, pressure, and resistance is given by the equation

$$\textbf{Blood flow} = \frac{\Delta\textbf{Pressure}}{\textbf{Resistance}}$$

where Δ pressure means the difference in pressure between the two ends of the circulatory system. Therefore, blood flow can be increased by either an increase in blood pressure or a decrease in resistance. A fivefold increase in blood flow could be generated by increasing pressure by a factor of five; however, this large increase in blood pressure would be hazardous to health. Fortunately, increases in blood flow during exercise are achieved primarily by a decrease in resistance with a small rise in blood pressure.

What factors contribute to the resistance of blood flow? Resistance to flow is directly proportional to the length of the vessel and the viscosity of blood. However, the most important variable determining

vascular resistance is the diameter of the blood vessel, because vascular resistance is inversely proportional to the fourth power of the radius of the vessel:

$$\textbf{Resistance} = \frac{\textbf{Length} \times \textbf{Viscosity}}{\textbf{Radius}^4}$$

In other words, an increase in either vessel length or blood viscosity results in a proportional increase in resistance. However, reducing the radius of a blood vessel by one-half would increase resistance 16 fold (i.e., $2^4 = 16$)!

Sources of Vascular Resistance

The viscosity of blood and the length of the blood vessels are not manipulated in normal physiology. Therefore, the primary factor regulating blood flow through organs is the diameter of the blood vessel. Indeed, a small decrease in the radius of the blood vessel (vasoconstriction) results in a large increase in vascular resistance and a decrease in blood flow. Specifically, the effect of changes in radius on changes in flow rate are magnified by a power of four and therefore, blood can be diverted from one organ system to another by varying degrees of vasoconstriction and vasodilation. This principle is used during heavy exercise to divert blood toward contracting skeletal muscle and away from less-active tissue. This concept is discussed in detail in the next section, "Changes in Oxygen Delivery to Muscle During Exercise."

The greatest vascular resistance in blood flow occurs in arterioles. This point is illustrated in Figure 9.21. Note the large drop in arterial pressure that occurs

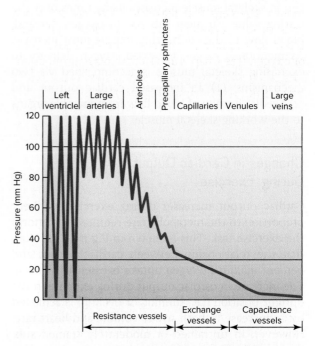

Figure 9.21 Pressure changes across the systemic circulation. Notice the large pressure drop across the arterioles.

across the arterioles; approximately 70% to 80% of the decline in mean arterial pressure occurs across the arterioles.

| IN SUMMARY |

- Blood is composed of two principal components: plasma and cells.
- Blood flow through the vascular system is directly proportional to the pressure at the two ends of the system and inversely proportional to resistance:

$$\text{Blood flow} = \frac{\Delta \text{Pressure}}{\text{Resistance}}$$

- The most important factor determining resistance to blood flow is the radius of the blood vessel. The relationship between vessel radius, vessel length, blood viscosity, and flow is

$$\text{Resistance} = \frac{\text{Length} \times \text{Viscosity}}{\text{Radius}^4}$$

- The greatest vascular resistance to blood flow is offered in the arterioles.

CHANGES IN OXYGEN DELIVERY TO MUSCLE DURING EXERCISE

During intense exercise, the metabolic need for oxygen in skeletal muscle increases many times over the resting value. To meet this rise in oxygen demand, blood flow to the contracting muscle must increase. As mentioned earlier, increased oxygen delivery to exercising skeletal muscle is accomplished via two mechanisms: (1) an increased cardiac output and (2) a redistribution of blood flow from inactive organs to the working skeletal muscle.

Changes in Cardiac Output During Exercise

Cardiac output increases during exercise in direct proportion to the metabolic rate required to perform the exercise task. This is shown in Figure 9.22. Note that the relationship between cardiac output and percent maximal oxygen uptake is essentially linear. The increase in cardiac output during exercise in the upright position (i.e., running or cycling) is achieved by an increase in both stroke volume and heart rate. However, in untrained or moderately trained subjects, stroke volume does not increase beyond a workload of 40% to 60% of $\dot{V}O_2$ max (Figure 9.22).

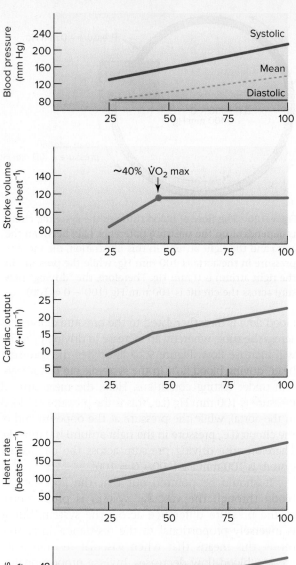

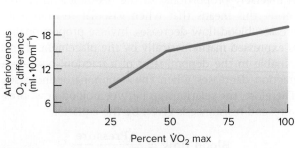

Figure 9.22 Changes in blood pressure, stroke volume, cardiac output, heart rate, and the arterial-mixed venous oxygen difference as a function of relative work rates. See text for details.

Therefore, at work rates greater than 40% to 60% $\dot{V}O_2$ max, the rise in cardiac output in these individuals is achieved by increases in heart rate alone. The examples presented in Figure 9.22 for maximal heart rate, stroke volume, and cardiac output are typical values for a 70-kg, active (but not highly trained) college-age male. See Table 9.2 for examples of maximal stroke volume and cardiac output for trained men and women.

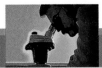
Stroke Volume Does Not Plateau in Endurance Athletes

It is widely accepted that during incremental exercise, stroke volume in active or untrained subjects reaches a plateau at a submaximal work rate (i.e., approximately 40% to 60% $\dot{V}O_2$ max) (Fig. 9.22). The physiological explanation for this plateau in stroke volume is that at high heart rates, the time available for ventricular filling is decreased. Therefore, end-diastolic volume reaches a plateau or may decrease slightly at high-exercise intensities. However, new evidence suggests that during incremental work rates, the stroke volume of endurance athletes (e.g., highly trained distance runners) does not plateau but continues to increase to $\dot{V}O_2$ max (14, 44). What is the explanation for this observation? It appears that compared to untrained subjects, endurance athletes have improved ventricular filling during heavy exercise due to increased venous return. This increase in end-diastolic volume results in an increased force of ventricular contraction (Frank-Starling law) and an increase in stroke volume.

Note that although most experts agree that stroke volume reaches a plateau between 40% and 60% of $\dot{V}O_2$ max during upright exercise in untrained and moderately trained individuals, evidence exists that stroke volume does not plateau in highly trained athletes during running exercise. This point is discussed in more detail in Research Focus 9.1. Further, differences exist in exercise-induced changes in stroke volume between upright exercise (e.g., running) and supine exercise (e.g., swimming). See A Closer Look 9.3 for more details.

Maximal cardiac output tends to decrease in a linear fashion in both men and women after 30 years of age (12). This is primarily due to a decrease in maximal heart rate with age (12). For example, because cardiac output equals heart rate times stroke volume, any decrease in heart rate would result in a decrease in cardiac output. The decrease in maximal heart rate with age in young adults can be estimated by the following formula:

$$\textbf{Max HR} = \textbf{220} - \textbf{age (years)}$$

According to this formula, a 20-year-old subject might have a maximal heart rate of 200 beats per minute (220 − 20 = 200), whereas a 35 year-old would have a maximal heart rate of 185 beats per minute (220 − 35 = 185). However, this is only an estimate, and values can be 20 beats × min^{-1} higher or lower.

The previous formula for adults is not a good predictor of maximal heart rate in older adults or children.

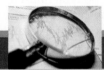

A CLOSER LOOK 9.3

Impact of Body Position on Stroke Volume during Exercise

Body position has a major influence on stroke volume at rest and during exercise because of the effect of gravity on venous return to the heart. Indeed, in the upright position (i.e., standing at rest), gravity promotes blood pooling in the legs. This results in a reduced venous return to the heart and a reduced end-diastolic volume with the outcome being a smaller stroke volume because of the Frank-Starling law of the heart. However, compared to rest, exercise in the upright position (e.g., running or cycling) results in increased venous return, a larger end-diastolic volume, and improved stroke volume. For example, in an untrained individual, stroke volume is typically 60 to 80 ml/beat at rest but stroke volume can increase by 100% during intense exercise due to increased venous return.

In contrast to the exercise in the upright position, intense exercise in a supine position (e.g., swimming) results in only small increases (i.e., 20% to 40%) in stroke volume above resting conditions. The explanation for the difference in stroke volume between exercise in the upright position and supine position is as follows. When the body is resting in the supine position, blood does not pool in the legs, and therefore, venous return to the heart is not impeded. So, compared to the upright position, end-diastolic volumes and stroke volumes are significantly higher in the supine position. Therefore, because stroke volume is already high in the supine position, the increase in stroke volume that occurs during swimming exercise is not as great as the increase in stroke volume that occurs during upright exercise. In summary, differences in the resting end-diastolic volume and stroke volume account for the variations in the exercise-induced increases in stroke volume between swimming and upright exercises such as swimming or cycling.

In adults (>40 years old) and children (ages 7-17), the following formula can be used to predict maximal heart rate (21,39):

$$\text{Max HR} = 208 - 0.7 \times \text{age (years)}$$

According to this formula for children, a 12-year-old child would have a maximal heart rate of 200 beats (208 − 8 = 200). Similar to the formula used to predict maximal heart rates in young adults, the formula for children and older adults provides only an estimate of maximal heart rates, and wide variability in maximal heart rates can exist between different individuals (21,29).

Changes in Arterial-Mixed Venous O_2 Content during Exercise

Figure 9.22 illustrates the exercise-induced changes in the arterial-mixed venous oxygen difference (a − $\bar{v}O_2$ diff). The a − $\bar{v}O_2$ difference represents the amount of O_2 that is taken up from 100 ml of blood by the tissues during one trip around the systemic circuit. An increase in the a − $\bar{v}O_2$ difference during exercise is due to an increase in the amount of O_2 taken up and used for the oxidative production of ATP by skeletal muscle. The relationship between cardiac output ($\dot{Q}$), a − $\bar{v}O_2$ diff, and oxygen uptake is given by the Fick equation:

$$\dot{V}O_2 = \dot{Q} \times (a - \bar{v}O_2 \text{ diff})$$

Simply stated, the Fick equation says that $\dot{V}O_2$ is equal to the product of cardiac output and the a − $\bar{v}O_2$ diff. This means that an increase in either cardiac output or a − $\bar{v}O_2$ diff would elevate $\dot{V}O_2$. Figure 9.22 illustrates that, during exercise, oxygen consumption increases due to both an increase in cardiac output and an increase in the a − $\bar{v}O_2$ difference.

Redistribution of Blood Flow during Exercise

To meet the increased oxygen demand of the skeletal muscles during exercise, it is necessary to increase muscle blood flow while reducing blood flow to less active organs such as the liver, kidneys, and GI tract. Figure 9.23 points out that the change in blood flow to muscle and the splanchnic (pertaining to the viscera) circulation is dictated by the exercise intensity (metabolic rate). That is, the increase in muscle blood flow during exercise and the decrease in splanchnic blood flow change as a linear function of % $\dot{V}O_2$ max (34).

Figure 9.24 illustrates the change in blood flow to various organ systems between resting conditions and during maximal exercise. Several important

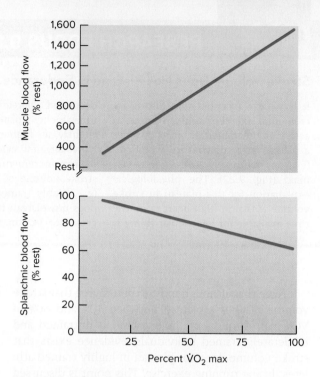

Figure 9.23 Changes in muscle and splanchnic blood flow as a function of exercise intensity. Notice the large increase in muscle blood flow as the work rate increases.

Data from Rowell, L. B., *Human Circulation: Regulation During Physical Stress.* New York, NY: Oxford University Press, 1986.

points need to be stressed. First, at rest, approximately 15% to 20% of total cardiac output is directed toward skeletal muscle (2, 34). However, during maximal exercise, 80% to 85% of total cardiac output goes to contracting skeletal muscle (34). This is necessary to meet the huge increase in muscle oxygen requirements during intense exercise. Second, notice that during heavy exercise, the percentage of total cardiac output that goes to the brain is reduced compared to that during rest. However, the absolute blood flow that reaches the brain is slightly increased above resting values; this is due to the elevated cardiac output during exercise (6, 45). Further, although the percentage of total cardiac output that reaches the myocardium is the same during maximal exercise as it is at rest, the total coronary blood flow is increased due to the increase in cardiac output during heavy exercise. Also, note that skin blood flow increases during both light and moderate exercise but decreases during maximal exercise (6). Finally, compared to rest, blood flow to abdominal organs is also decreased during maximal exercise (Fig. 9.24). This reduction in abdominal blood flow during heavy exercise is an important means of shifting blood flow away from "less active" tissues and toward the working skeletal muscles.

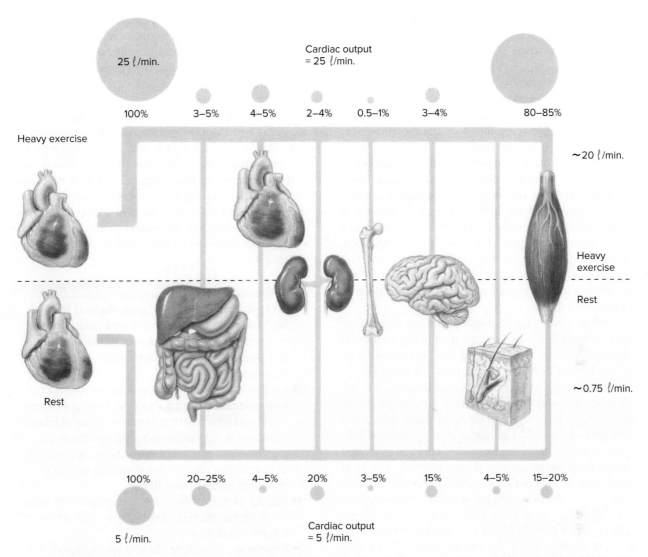

Figure 9.24 Distribution of cardiac output during rest and maximal exercise. At rest, the cardiac output is 5 ℓ/min. (bottom of figure); during maximum exercise, the cardiac output increased five-fold to 25 ℓ/min (top of figure). Note the large increases in blood flow to the skeletal muscle and the reduction in flow to the liver/GI tract.

Reference 2 from Åstrand, P., Rodahl, K., *Textbook of Work Physiology*, 3rd ed. New York: McGraw-Hill, Inc., 1986.

Regulation of Local Blood Flow during Exercise

What regulates blood flow to various organs during exercise? Muscle as well as other body tissues have the unique ability to regulate their own blood flow in direct proportion to their metabolic needs. Blood flow to skeletal muscle during exercise is regulated in the following way. First, the arterioles in skeletal muscle have a high vascular resistance at rest. This is due to adrenergic sympathetic stimulation, which causes arteriole smooth muscle to contract (vasoconstriction)(41). This produces a relatively low blood flow to muscle at rest (4 to 5 ml per minute per 100 grams of muscle), but because to muscles have a large mass,

this accounts for 20% to 25% of total blood flow from the heart.

During exercise, skeletal muscle blood flow increases in direct proportion to the metabolic demand (25). In fact, compared to blood flow at rest, blood delivery to contracting skeletal muscle during intense exercise may rise 100 times (25). This increased muscle blood flow occurs because of a decrease in vascular resistance and is combined with "recruitment" of the capillaries in skeletal muscle. At rest, only 50% to 80% of the capillaries in skeletal muscle are open at any one time. However, during intense exercise, almost all of the capillaries in contracting muscle are open, resulting in increased oxygen delivery to the contracting muscle fibers (34).

The increase in muscle blood flow that occurs during exercise is regulated by several factors that promote vasodilation (25). This type of blood flow regulation is termed **autoregulation** and is the most important factor in regulating blood flow to muscle during exercise. The level of vasodilation that occurs in arterioles and small arteries leading to skeletal muscle is regulated by the metabolic (i.e., oxygen and nutrients) need of the muscle. Specifically, the intensity of exercise and the number of motor units recruited determine the overall need for blood flow to the muscle. For example, during low-intensity exercise, a relatively small number of motor units are recruited into action, resulting in a relatively small demand for blood flow to the contracting muscle. In contrast, high-intensity exercise results in the recruitment of a large number of motor units and, therefore, results in a large increase in muscle blood flow.

What factors are responsible for the autoregulation of muscle blood flow to match the metabolic demand? Skeletal muscle blood flow is controlled by an interaction between several locally formed vasodilators including nitric oxide, prostaglandins, ATP, adenosine, and endothelium derived hyperpolarization factors (25). Further, separate from these substances that promote vasodilation, some locally produced substances inhibit the vasoconstrictor effect of increased sympathetic nerve activity during exercise. The local inhibition of sympathetic-induced vasoconstriction that occurs during exercise is called sympatholysis (25). Although it is clear that sympatholysis occurs and increases muscle blood flow during exercise, the relative importance of this phenomenon on the control of muscle blood flow continues to be a debated topic (25).

Let's discuss the local factors involved in the control of muscle blood flow during exercise in more detail. The increased metabolic rate of skeletal muscle during exercise causes local changes such as increased production of nitric oxide, prostaglandins, ATP, adenosine, and endothelium derived hyperpolarization factors. Each of these factors has been independently shown to promote vasodilation by increasing smooth muscle relaxation in arterioles (25). For example, both nitric oxide and prostaglandins (e.g., prostacyclin) are potent vasodilators. Further, both ATP and adenosine are important vasodilators that increase muscle blood flow during exercise. Finally, endothelium derived hyperpolarization factors act to promote hyperpolarization of smooth muscle cells in arterioles with the end result being smooth muscle relaxation and dilation of the arterioles (25). Current evidence indicates that an interplay between these vasodilatory factors exists so that these elements work together to cause vasodilation of arterioles feeding the contracting skeletal muscle; this vasodilation reduces the vascular resistance and, therefore, increases blood flow (25). To summarize, the exercise-induced increase in local factors result in increased vasodilation of arterioles/small arteries and promote increased blood flow to the contracting muscle in order to match the metabolic demand.

While the vascular resistance in skeletal muscle decreases during exercise, vascular resistance to flow in the visceral organs and other inactivity tissue increases. This occurs due to an increased sympathetic output to these organs, which is regulated by the cardiovascular control center. As a result of the increase in visceral vasoconstriction during exercise (i.e., resistance increases), blood flow to the viscera can decrease to only 20% to 30% of resting values (34).

IN SUMMARY

- Oxygen delivery to exercising skeletal muscle increases due to (1) an increased cardiac output and (2) a redistribution of blood flow from inactive organs to the contracting skeletal muscles.
- Cardiac output increases as a linear function of oxygen uptake during exercise. During exercise in the upright position, stroke volume reaches a plateau at approximately 40% to 60% of $\dot{V}O_2$ max; therefore, at work rates above 40% to 60% $\dot{V}O_2$ max, the rise in cardiac output is due to increases in heart rate alone.
- During exercise, blood flow to contracting muscle is increased, and blood flow to less-active tissues is reduced.
- Regulation of muscle blood flow during exercise is primarily regulated by local factors (called autoregulation). Autoregulation refers to intrinsic control of blood flow by increases in local metabolites (e.g., nitric oxide, prostaglandins, ATP, adenosine, and endothelium-derived hyperpolarization factors). These factors work together to promote vasodilation to increase blood flow to the working muscles.

CIRCULATORY RESPONSES TO EXERCISE

The changes in heart rate and blood pressure that occur during exercise reflect the type and intensity of exercise performed, the duration of exercise, and the environmental conditions under which the work was performed. For example, heart rate and blood pressure are higher during arm work when compared to leg work at a given oxygen uptake. Further, exercise in a hot/humid condition results in higher heart rates when compared to the same exercise in a cool environment. The next several sections discuss the cardiovascular responses to exercise during a variety of exercise conditions.

Emotional Influence

Submaximal exercise in an emotionally charged atmosphere results in higher heart rates and blood pressures when compared to the same work in a psychologically "neutral" environment. This emotional elevation in heart rate and blood pressure response to exercise is mediated by an increase in sympathetic nervous system activity. If the exercise is maximal (e.g., 400-meter dash), high emotion elevates the pre-exercise heart rate and blood pressure but does not generally alter the peak heart rate or blood pressure observed during the exercise itself.

Transition from Rest to Exercise

At the beginning of exercise, there is a rapid increase in heart rate, stroke volume, and cardiac output. It has been demonstrated that heart rate and cardiac output begin to increase within the first second after muscular contraction begins (see Fig. 9.25). If the work rate is constant and below the lactate threshold, a steady-state plateau in heart rate, stroke volume, and cardiac output is reached within two to three minutes. This response is similar to that observed in oxygen uptake at the beginning of exercise (see Chap. 4).

Recovery from Exercise

Recovery from short-term, low-intensity exercise is generally rapid. This is illustrated in Figure 9.25. Notice that heart rate, stroke volume, and cardiac output all decrease rapidly back toward resting levels following this type of exercise. Recovery speed varies from individual to individual, with well-conditioned subjects demonstrating better recuperative powers than untrained subjects. In regard to recovery heart rates, the slopes of heart-rate decay following exercise are generally the same for trained and untrained subjects. However, trained subjects recover faster following exercise because they don't achieve as high a heart rate as untrained subjects during a particular exercise.

Recovery from long-term exercise is much slower than the response depicted in Figure 9.25. This is particularly true when the exercise is performed in hot/humid conditions, because an elevated body temperature delays the fall in heart rate during recovery from exercise (36).

Incremental Exercise

The cardiovascular responses to dynamic incremental exercise were illustrated in Figure 9.22. Heart rate and

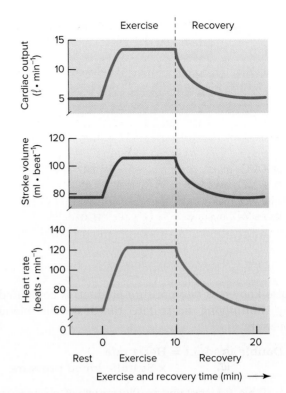

Figure 9.25 Changes in cardiac output, stroke volume, and heart rate during the transition from rest to submaximal constant intensity exercise and during recovery. See text for discussion.

Data from Rowell, L., *Human Circulation: Regulation During Physical Stress.* New York: Oxford University Press, 1986.

cardiac output increase in direct proportion to oxygen uptake. Further, blood flow to muscle increases as a function of oxygen uptake (see Fig. 9.23). This ensures that as the need to synthesize ATP to supply the energy for muscular contraction increases, the supply of O_2 reaching the muscle also increases. However, both cardiac output and heart rate reach a plateau at approximately 100% $\dot{V}O_2$ max (see Fig. 9.22). This point represents a maximal ceiling for oxygen transport to exercising skeletal muscles, and it is thought to occur simultaneously with the attainment of maximal oxygen uptake.

The increase in cardiac output during incremental exercise is achieved via a decrease in vascular resistance to flow and an increase in mean arterial blood pressure. The elevation in mean arterial blood pressure during exercise is due to an increase in systolic pressure, because diastolic pressure remains fairly constant during incremental work (see Fig. 9.22).

As mentioned earlier, the increase in heart rate and systolic blood pressure that occurs during exercise results in an increased workload on the heart. The increased metabolic demand placed on the heart during exercise can be estimated by examining the double product. The **double product**

TABLE 9.3	Changes in the Double Product (i.e., Heart Rate × Systolic Blood Pressure) during an Incremental Exercise Test in a Healthy 21-Year-Old Female Subject		

Note that the double product is a dimensionless term that reflects the relative changes in the workload placed on the heart during exercise and other forms of stress.

Condition	Heart Rate (beats · min⁻¹)	Systolic Blood Pressure (mm Hg)	Double Product
Rest	75	110	8,250
Exercise			
25% $\dot{V}O_2$ max	100	130	13,000
50% $\dot{V}O_2$ max	140	160	22,400
75% $\dot{V}O_2$ max	170	180	30,600
100% $\dot{V}O_2$ max	200	210	42,000

(also known as rate-pressure product) is computed by multiplying heart rate times systolic blood pressure:

Double product = Heart rate × Systolic blood pressure

Table 9.3 contains an illustration of changes in the double product during an incremental exercise test. The take-home message in Table 9.3 is simply that increases in exercise intensity result in an elevation in both heart rate and systolic blood pressure; each of these factors increases the workload placed on the heart.

Careful examination of Table 9.3 reveals that the double product during exercise at $\dot{V}O_2$ max is five times greater than the double product at rest. This implies that maximal exercise increases the workload on the heart by 500% over rest.

The practical application of the double product is that this measure can be used as a guideline to prescribe exercise for patients with coronary artery blockage. For example, suppose a patient develops chest pain (called angina pectoris) at a certain intensity of exercise due to myocardial ischemia at a double product of 30,000. Because chest pain appears at a double product of 30,000, the cardiologist or exercise physiologist would recommend that this patient perform types of exercise that result in a double product of 30,000. This would reduce the risk of the patient developing chest pain due to a high metabolic demand on the heart.

Arm Versus Leg Exercise

As mentioned earlier, at any given level of oxygen consumption, both heart rate and blood pressure are higher during arm work when compared to leg work (1, 24, 33) (see Fig. 9.26). The explanation for

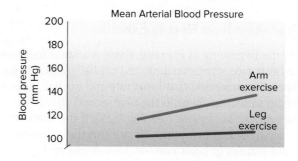

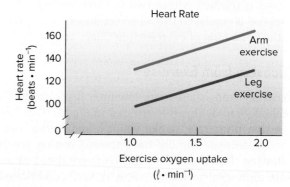

Figure 9.26 Comparison of mean arterial blood pressure and heart rate during submaximal rhythmic arm and leg exercise.

the higher heart rate seems to be linked to a greater sympathetic outflow to the heart during arm work when compared to leg exercise (2). In addition, isometric exercise also increases the heart rate above the expected value based on relative oxygen consumption (1).

The relatively large increase in blood pressure during arm work is due to a vasoconstriction in the inactive muscle groups (2). In contrast, the larger the muscle group (e.g., legs) involved in performing the exercise, the more resistance vessels (arterioles) that are dilated. Therefore, this lower peripheral resistance is reflected in lower blood pressure (because cardiac output × resistance = pressure).

Intermittent Exercise

If exercise is intermittent (e.g., interval training), the extent of the recovery of heart rate and blood pressure between exercise bouts depends on the level of subject fitness, environmental conditions (temperature, humidity), and the duration and intensity of the exercise. With a relatively light effort in a cool environment, there is generally complete recovery between exercise bouts within several minutes. However, if the exercise is intense or the work is performed in a hot/humid environment, there is a cumulative increase in heart rate between efforts, and thus recovery is not complete (38). The practical consequence of performing repeated bouts of light exercise is that many repetitions can be performed. In contrast, the nature of high-intensity exercise dictates that a limited number of efforts can be tolerated.

Prolonged Exercise

Figure 9.27 illustrates the change in heart rate, stroke volume, and cardiac output that occurs during prolonged exercise at a constant work rate. Note that cardiac output is maintained at a constant level throughout the duration of the exercise. However, as the duration of exercise increases, stroke volume declines while heart rate increases (6). Figure 9.27 demonstrates that the ability to maintain a constant cardiac output in the face of declining stroke volume is due to the increase in heart rate being equal in magnitude to the decline in stroke volume.

The increase in heart rate and decrease in stroke volume observed during prolonged exercise is often referred to as *cardiovascular drift* and is due to the influence of rising body temperature on dehydration and a reduction in plasma volume (5, 30, 34). A reduction in plasma volume acts to reduce venous return to the heart and therefore reduce stroke volume. If prolonged exercise is performed in a hot/humid environment, the increase in heart rate and decrease in stroke volume is exaggerated even more than depicted in Figure 9.27 (27, 32). In fact, it is not surprising to find near-maximal heart rates during submaximal exercise in the heat. For example, it has been demonstrated that during a 2.5-hour marathon race at a work rate of 70% to 75% $\dot{V}O_2$ max, maximal

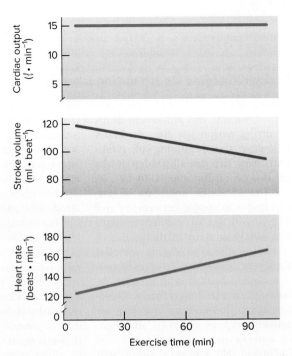

Figure 9.27 Changes in cardiac output, stroke volume, and heart rate during prolonged exercise at a constant intensity. Notice that cardiac output is maintained by an increase in heart rate to offset the fall in stroke volume that occurs during this type of work.

heart rates may be maintained during the last hour of the race (10).

Does prolonged exercise at high heart rates pose a risk for cardiac injury? The answer to this question is almost always "no" for healthy individuals. However, sudden cardiac deaths have occurred in individuals of all ages during exercise. See Clinical Applications 9.3 for more details on sudden cardiac death during exercise.

IN SUMMARY

- The changes in heart rate and blood pressure that occur during exercise are a function of the type and intensity of exercise performed, the duration of exercise, and the environmental conditions.
- The increased metabolic demand placed on the heart during exercise can be estimated by examining the double product.
- At the same level of oxygen consumption, heart rate and blood pressure are greater during arm exercise than during leg exercise.
- The increase in heart rate that occurs during prolonged exercise is called cardiovascular drift.

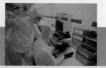
Sudden Cardiac Death during Exercise

Sudden death is defined as an unexpected, natural, and nonviolent death occurring within the first six hours following the beginning of symptoms. Note that not all sudden deaths are due to cardiac events. In fact, in the United States, only 30% of sudden deaths in people between 14 and 21 years of age are cardiac in origin (14, 40). How many of these cases of sudden death occur during exercise? Each year, fewer than 20 cases of sudden cardiac death during exercise are reported in the United States. Therefore, given that millions of people are actively engaged in sports and regular exercise in the United States, the likelihood that a healthy person will die from sudden cardiac death is extremely small. Across the world, it is estimated that sudden cardiac death occurs in 1 out of 200,000 youth athletes (9). Again, the risk of sudden cardiac death in young athletes is limited.

The causes of sudden cardiac death are diverse and vary as a function of age. For example, in children and adolescents, most sudden cardiac deaths occur due to lethal cardiac arrhythmias (abnormal heart rhythm). These arrhythmias can arise from genetic anomalies in coronary arteries, cardiomyopathy (wasting of cardiac muscle due to disease), and/or myocarditis (inflammation of the heart) (3, 9, 40). In adults, coronary heart disease and cardiomyopathy are the most common causes of sudden cardiac death (40). Similar to sudden deaths in children, sudden cardiac deaths in adults are also generally associated with lethal cardiac arrhythmias.

Can a medical exam identify people at risk for sudden cardiac death during exercise? Yes. The combination of a medical history and a complete medical exam by a qualified physician can usually identify individuals with undetected heart disease or genetic defects that would place them at risk for sudden death during exercise. See Semsarian et al. (2015) in the Suggested Readings for more details.

REGULATION OF CARDIOVASCULAR ADJUSTMENTS TO EXERCISE

The cardiovascular adjustments at the beginning of exercise are rapid. Within one second after the commencement of muscular contraction, there is a withdrawal of vagal outflow to the heart, which is followed by an increase in sympathetic stimulation of the heart (34). At the same time, there is a vasodilation of arterioles in active skeletal muscles and a reflex increase in the resistance of vessels in less active areas. The end result is an increase in cardiac output to ensure that blood flow to muscle matches the metabolic needs (see Fig. 9.28). What is the signal to "turn on" the cardiovascular system at the onset of exercise? This question has puzzled physiologists for many years (15). At present, a complete answer is not available. However, recent advances in understanding cardiovascular control have led to the development of the *central command theory* (42).

The term **central command** refers to a motor signal developed within the brain (42). The central command theory of cardiovascular control argues that the initial cardiovascular changes at the beginning of dynamic exercise (e.g., cycle ergometer exercise) are due to centrally generated cardiovascular

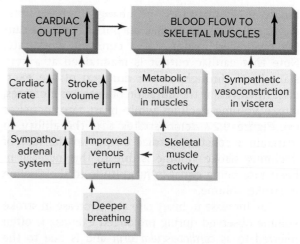

Figure 9.28   A summary of cardiovascular responses to exercise.

motor signals, which set the general pattern of the cardiovascular response. However, it is clear that cardiovascular activity is also regulated by afferent feedback to higher brain centers from heart mechanoreceptors, muscle chemoreceptors, muscle mechanoreceptors, and pressure-sensitive receptors (baroreceptors) located within the carotid arteries and the aortic arch (31, 42). Muscle chemoreceptors are sensitive to increases in muscle metabolites (e.g., potassium, lactic acid) and send messages to higher brain centers to fine-tune the cardiovascular responses to exercise (42). This type of peripheral feedback to the cardiovascular control center (medulla oblongata) is called the *exercise pressor reflex* (7, 23).

Muscle mechanoreceptors (e.g., muscle spindles, Golgi tendon organs) are sensitive to the force and speed of muscular movement. These receptors, like muscle chemoreceptors, send information to higher brain centers to aid in modification of the cardiovascular responses to a given exercise task (34, 35, 43).

Finally, baroreceptors, which are sensitive to changes in arterial blood pressure, may also send afferent information back to the cardiovascular control center to add precision to the cardiovascular activity during exercise. These pressure receptors are important because they regulate arterial blood pressure around an elevated systemic pressure during exercise (34).

In summary, the central command theory proposes that the initial signal to the cardiovascular system at the beginning of exercise comes from higher brain centers. However, fine-tuning of the cardiovascular response to a given exercise test is accomplished via a series of feedback loops from muscle chemoreceptors, muscle mechanoreceptors, and arterial baroreceptors (see Fig. 9.29). The fact that there appears to be some overlap among these three feedback systems during submaximal exercise suggests that redundancy in cardiovascular control exists (34). This is not surprising considering the importance of matching blood flow to the metabolic needs of exercising skeletal muscle. Whether one or many of these feedback loops becomes more important during heavy exercise is not currently

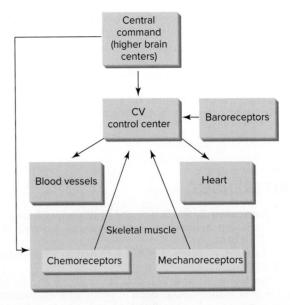

Figure 9.29 A summary of cardiovascular control during exercise. See text for discussion.

known and poses an interesting question for future research.

IN SUMMARY

- The central command theory of cardiovascular control during exercise proposes that the initial signal to "drive" the cardiovascular system at the beginning of exercise comes from higher brain centers.
- Although central command is the primary drive to increase heart rate during exercise, the cardiovascular response to exercise is fine-tuned by feedback from muscle chemoreceptors, muscle mechanoreceptors, and arterial baroreceptors to the cardiovascular control center.

STUDY ACTIVITIES

1. What are the major purposes of the cardiovascular system?
2. Briefly outline the design of the heart. Why is the heart often called "two pumps in one"?
3. Outline the cardiac cycle and the associated electrical activity recorded via the electrocardiogram.
4. Graph the heart rate, stroke volume, and cardiac output response to incremental exercise.
5. What factors regulate heart rate during exercise? Stroke volume?
6. How does exercise influence venous return?
7. What factors determine local blood flow during exercise?
8. Graph the changes that occur in heart rate, stroke volume, and cardiac output during prolonged exercise. What happens to these variables if the exercise is performed in a hot/humid environment?
9. Compare heart rate and blood pressure responses to arm and leg work at the same oxygen uptake. What factors might explain the observed differences?
10. Explain the central command theory of cardiovascular regulation during exercise.

SUGGESTED READINGS

Fadel, P.J. 2015. Reflex control of the circulation during exercise. *Scandavian Journal of Medicine and Science in Sports*. 25:74–82.

Fox, S. 2016. *Human Physiology*. New York, NY: McGraw-Hill Companies.

Hall, J. 2015. *Guyton and Hall Textbook of Medical Physiology*. Philadelphia, PA: Saunders.

Michelina, L., D. O'Leary, P. Raven, and C. Nobrega. 2015. Neural control of circulation and exercise: a translational approach disclosing interactions between central command, arterial baroreflex, and muscle metaboreflex. *American Journal of Physiology: Heart, circulation physiology.* 309:H381-H392.

Mortensen, S. and B. Saltin. 2014. Regulation of the muscle blood flow in humans. *Experimental Physiology.* 99: 1552-1558.

Powers, S.K., A.J. Smuder, A.N. Kavazis, and J.C. Quindry. Mechanisms of exercise-induced cardioprotection. *Physiology.* 29: 27-38, 2014.

Sarelius, I., and U. Pohl. Control of muscle blood flow during exercise: Local factors and integrative mechanisms. *Acta Physiologica (Oxford)* 199: 349-65, 2010.

Semsarian, C., J. Sweeting, and M. Ackerman. 2015. Sudden cardiac death in athletes. *British Medical Journal.* doi:10.1136/bmj.h1218.

REFERENCES

1. **Asmussen E.** Similarities and dissimilarities between static and dynamic exercise. *Circulation Research* 48: 3-10, 1981.

2. **Åstrand P.** *Textbook of Work Physiology.* Champaign, IL: Human Kinetics, 2003.

3. **Borjesson M and Pelliccia A.** Incidence and aetiology of sudden cardiac death in young athletes: an international perspective. *British Journal of Sports Medicine* 43: 644-648, 2009.

4. **Courneya C and Parker M.** *Cardiovascular Physiology: A Clinical Approach.* Philadelphia, PA: Wolters Kluwer, 2010.

5. **Coyle EF and Gonzalez-Alonso J.** Cardiovascular drift during prolonged exercise: new perspectives. *Exercise and Sport Sciences Reviews* 29: 88-92, 2001.

6. **Crandall C and Gonzalez-Alonso J.** Cardiovascular function in the heat-stressed human. *Acta Physiologica (Oxford)* 199: 407-423, 2010.

7. **Duncan G, Johnson RH, and Lambie DG.** Role of sensory nerves in the cardiovascular and respiratory changes with isometric forearm exercise in man. *Clinical Science (London)* 60: 145-155, 1981.

8. **Feldman D, Elton TS, Menachemi DM, and Wexler RK.** Heart rate control with adrenergic blockade: clinical outcomes in cardiovascular medicine. *Vasc Health Risk Management* 6: 387-397, 2010.

9. **Ferreira M.** Sudden cardiac death athletes: a systematic review. *Sports Medicine, Rehabilitation, Therapy, and Technology* 2: 1-6, 2010.

10. **Fox EL and Costill DL.** Estimated cardiorespiratory response during marathon running. *Archives of Environmental Health* 24: 316-324, 1972.

11. **Fox S.** *Human Physiology.* New York, NY: McGraw-Hill, 2016.

12. **Gerstenblith G, Renlund DG, and Lakatta EG.** Cardiovascular response to exercise in younger and older men. *Federation Proceedings* 46: 1834-1839, 1987.

13. **Gillespie C, Kuklina EV, Briss PA, Blair NA, and Hong Y.** Vital signs: prevalence, treatment, and control of hypertension–United States, 1999-2002 and 2005-2008. *Morbidity and Mortality Weekly Report* 60: 103-108, 2011.

14. **Gledhill N, Cox D, and Jamnik R.** Endurance athletes' stroke volume does not plateau: major advantage is diastolic function. *Medicine & Science in Sports & Exercise* 26: 1116-1121, 1994.

15. **Gorman M and Sparks H.** The unanswered question. *News in Physiological Sciences* 6: 191-193, 1991.

16. **Harmon, K, Drezner, J, Maleszewski, J, Lopez-Anderson, M, Owens, M, Prutkin, J, et al.** Pathogenesis of sudden cardiac death in national collegiate athletic association athletes. *Circulation, Arrhythmias and Electrophysiology* 7: 198-201, 2014.

17. **Katz A.** *Physiology of the Heart.* Philadelphia, PA: Wolters Kluwer Lippincott Williams and Wilkins, 2010.

18. **Kavazis AN, McClung JM, Hood DA, and Powers SK.** Exercise induces a cardiac mitochondrial phenotype that resists apoptotic stimuli. *American Journal of Physiology - Heart and Circulatory Physiology* 294: H928-935, 2008.

19. **Levy WC, Cerqueira MD, Harp GD, Johannessen KA, Abrass IB, Schwartz RS, and Stratton JR.** Effect of endurance exercise training on heart rate variability at rest in healthy young and older men. *American Journal of Cardiology* 82: 1236-1241, 1998.

20. **Liew R and Chiam PT.** Risk stratification for sudden cardiac death after acute myocardial infarction. *ANNALS Academy of Medicine Singapore* 39: 237-246, 2010.

21. **Mahon AD, Marjerrison AD, Lee JD, Woodruff ME, and Hanna LE.** Evaluating the prediction of maximal heart rate in children and adolescents. *Research Quarterly for Exercise and Sport* 81: 466-471, 2010.

22. **Miller JD, Pegelow DF, Jacques AJ, and Dempsey JA.** Skeletal muscle pump versus respiratory muscle pump: modulation of venous return from the locomotor limb in humans. *The Journal of Physiology* 563: 925-943, 2005.

23. **Mitchell JH.** J. B. Wolffe memorial lecture. Neural control of the circulation during exercise. *Medicine & Science in Sports & Exercise* 22: 141-154, 1990.

24. **Mitchell JH, Payne FC, Saltin B, and Schibye B.** The role of muscle mass in the cardiovascular response to static contractions. *The Journal of Physiology* 309: 45-54, 1980.

25. **Mortensen S and Saltin B.** Regulation of the muscle blood flow in humans. *Experimental Physiology.* 99: 1552-1558, 2014.

26. **Powers SK, Demirel HA, Vincent HK, Coombes JS, Naito H, Hamilton KL, Shanely RA, and Jessup J.** Exercise training improves myocardial tolerance to in vivo ischemia-reperfusion in the rat. *American Journal of Physiology* 275: R1468-1477, 1998.

27. **Powers SK, Howley ET, and Cox R.** A differential catecholamine response during prolonged exercise and passive heating. *Medicine & Science in Sports & Exercise* 14: 435-439, 1982.

28. **Powers SK, Locke M, and Demirel HA.** Exercise, heat shock proteins, and myocardial protection from I-R injury. *Medicine & Science in Sports & Exercise* 33: 386-392, 2001.

29. **Powers SK, Smuder AJ, Kavazis AN, and Quindry JC.** Mechanisms of exercise-induced cardioprotection. *Physiology* 29: 27-38, 2014.

30. **Raven P and Stevens G.** Cardiovascular function during prolonged exercise. In: *Perspectives in Exercise Science and Sports Medicine: Prolonged Exercise,* edited by Lamb D, and Murray R. Indianapolis: Benchmark Press, 1988, p. 43-71.

31. **Raven PB, Fadel PJ, and Ogoh S.** Arterial baroreflex resetting during exercise: a current perspective. *Experimental Physiology* 91: 37-49, 2006.

32. **Ridge B and Pyke F.** Physiological responses to combinations of exercise and sauna. *Australian Journal of Science and Medicine in Sport* 18: 25-28, 1986.

33. **Rosiello RA, Mahler DA, and Ward JL.** Cardiovascular responses to rowing. *Medicine & Science in Sports & Exercise* 19: 239-245, 1987.

34. **Rowell LB.** *Human Circulation: Regulation During Physical Stress.* New York, NY: Oxford University Press, 1986.

35. **Rowell LB.** What signals govern the cardiovascular responses to exercise? *Medicine & Science in Sports & Exercise* 12: 307-315, 1980.

36. **Rubin SA.** Core temperature regulation of heart rate during exercise in humans. *Journal of Applied Physiology* 62: 1997-2002, 1987.

37. **Sarelius I and Pohl U.** Control of muscle blood flow during exercise: local factors and integrative mechanisms. *Acta physiologica (Oxford)* 199: 349-365, 2010.

38. **Sawka MN, Knowlton RG, and Critz JB.** Thermal and circulatory responses to repeated bouts of prolonged running. *Medicine and Science in Sports* 11: 177-180, 1979.

39. **Tanaka, H, Monahan, K, and Seals, D.** Age-predicted maximal heart rate revisited. *Journal of the American College of Cardiology* 37: 153-156, 2001.

40. **Virmani R, Burke AP, and Farb A.** Sudden cardiac death. *Cardiovascular Pathology* 10: 211-218, 2001.

41. **Whyte J and Laughlin MH.** The effects of acute and chronic exercise on the vasculature. *Acta Physiologica* 199: 441-450, 2010.

42. **Williamson JW, Fadel PJ, and Mitchell JH.** New insights into central cardiovascular control during exercise in humans: a central command update. *Experimental Physiology* 91: 51-58, 2006.

43. **Wyss CR, Ardell JL, Scher AM, and Rowell LB.** Cardiovascular responses to graded reductions in hindlimb perfusion in exercising dogs. *American Journal of Physiology* 245: H481-486, 1983.

44. **Zhou B, Conlee RK, Jensen R, Fellingham GW, George JD, and Fisher AG.** Stroke volume does not plateau during graded exercise in elite male distance runners. *Medicine & Science in Sports & Exercise* 33: 1849-1854, 2001.

45. **Zobl E.** Effect of exercise on the cerebral circulation and metabolism. *Journal of Applied Physiology* 20: 1289-1293, 1965.

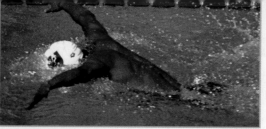

10

Respiration during Exercise

■ Objectives

By studying this chapter, you should be able to do the following:

1. Describe the primary function of the pulmonary system.

2. Outline the major anatomical components of the respiratory system.

3. List the major muscles involved in inspiration and expiration at rest and during exercise.

4. Discuss the importance of matching blood flow to alveolar ventilation in the lung.

5. Explain how gases are transported across the blood-gas interface in the lung.

6. Describe the major transportation modes of O_2 and CO_2 in the blood.

7. Discuss the effects of increasing temperature, decreasing pH, and increasing levels of 2-3 DPG on the oxygen-hemoglobin dissociation curve.

8. Describe the ventilatory response to constant load, steady-state exercise. What happens to ventilation if exercise is prolonged and performed in a hot environment?

9. Describe the ventilatory response to incremental exercise. What factors contribute to the alinear rise in ventilation at work rates above 50% of $\dot{V}O_2$ max?

10. Identify the location and function of chemoreceptors and mechanoreceptors that contribute to the regulation of breathing.

11. Discuss the neural-humoral theory of ventilatory control during exercise.

■ Outline

alveolar ventilation ($\dot{V}_A$)
alveoli
anatomical dead space
aortic bodies
Bohr effect
bulk flow
carotid bodies
cellular respiration
deoxyhemoglobin

diaphragm
diffusion
hemoglobin
myoglobin
oxyhemoglobin
partial pressure
pleura
pulmonary respiration
residual volume (RV)

respiration
spirometry
tidal volume
total lung capacity (TLC)
ventilation
ventilatory threshold (Tvent)
vital capacity (VC)

The word **respiration** is often used in two different contexts in physiology: (1) **pulmonary respiration** and (2) **cellular respiration.** Pulmonary respiration refers to ventilation (breathing) and the exchange of gases (O_2 and CO_2) in the lungs. Cellular respiration relates to O_2 utilization and CO_2 production by the tissues (see Chap. 3). This chapter is concerned with pulmonary respiration, and the term respiration is used in this chapter as a synonym for pulmonary respiration. Because the pulmonary system plays a key role in maintaining blood-gas homeostasis (i.e., O_2 and CO_2 tensions) during exercise, an understanding of lung function during exercise is important. Therefore, this chapter will discuss the design and function of the respiratory system during exercise.

FUNCTION OF THE RESPIRATORY SYSTEM— THE BIG PICTURE

The primary purpose of the respiratory system is to provide a means of gas exchange between the atmosphere and the cells of the body. That is, the respiratory system provides the individual with a means of replacing O_2 and removing CO_2 from the blood. The exchange of O_2 and CO_2 between the lung and blood occurs as a result of two processes: (1) ventilation and (2) diffusion. The term **ventilation** refers to the mechanical process of moving air into and out of the lungs; this process is commonly called breathing. **Diffusion** is the random movement of molecules from an area of high concentration to an area of lower concentration. The big picture summary of the exchange of respiratory gases (i.e., O_2 and CO_2) between the atmosphere and the cells of the body can be described into four continuous and simultaneously occurring processes (Fig. 10.1):

1 **Ventilation:** Ventilation refers to the movement of respiratory gases between the atmosphere and the gas exchange region of the lung (called the alveolar region).
2 **Alveolar gas exchange:** Alveolar gas exchange is the movement of respiratory gases (via

diffusion) between the alveolar region of the lung and the blood. Because the O_2 tension (i.e., O_2 pressure) in the alveolar region of the lungs is higher than the blood, O_2 moves from the lungs to the blood. Similarly, because the tension of CO_2 in the blood is higher than the lung, CO_2 moves from the blood to the lung and is expired.
3 **Circulatory transport:** Circulatory transport refers to the transport of respiratory gases in the blood between the lungs to the cells of the body.
4 **Systemic gas exchange:** Systemic gas exchange is the movement of respiratory gases (via diffusion) from the blood into the cells of the body. Because of the pressure differences, O_2 diffuses from the blood to the cells and CO_2 diffuses from the cells into the venous blood.

The respiratory system also plays an important role in the regulation of the acid-base balance during heavy exercise. This important topic is introduced in this chapter and discussed in more detail in Chap. 11.

IN SUMMARY

- The primary function of the pulmonary system is to provide a means of gas exchange between the atmosphere and the body.
- The respiratory system also plays an important role in the regulation of the acid-base balance during exercise.

STRUCTURE OF THE RESPIRATORY SYSTEM

The human respiratory system is composed of a group of passages that filter air and transport it into the lungs, where gas exchange occurs within tiny air sacs called **alveoli.** The major components of the respiratory system are pictured in Figure 10.2. The organs of the respiratory system include the nose, nasal cavity, pharynx, larynx, trachea, bronchial tree, and the lungs themselves. The upper portion of the respiratory tract includes the nose, nasal cavity, and the pharynx. The lower respiratory zone comprises the trachea,

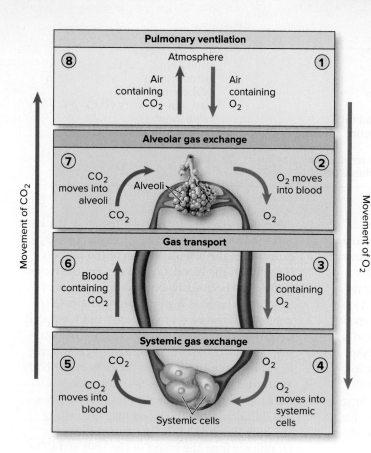

Figure 10.1 Overview of Respiration.
Respiration involves four processes that include pulmonary ventilation, alveolar gas exchange, gas transport, and systemic gas exchange.

McKinley, O'Loughlin, and Bidle, *Anatomy and Physiology: An Integrative Approach*, 2nd ed. New York: McGraw Hill, Inc., 2016.

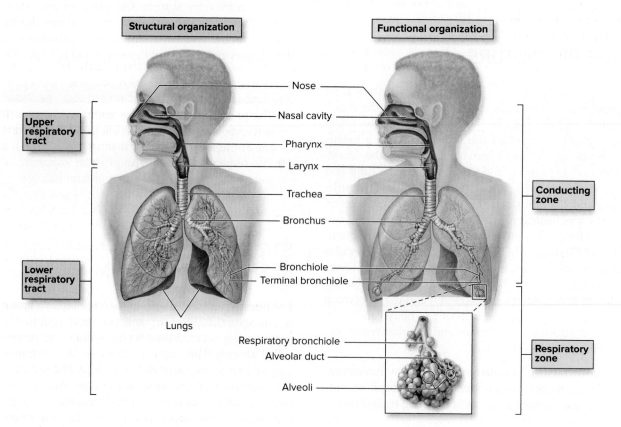

Figure 10.2 Major organs of the respiratory system.

McKinley, O'Loughlin, and Bidle, *Anatomy and Physiology: An Integrative Approach*, 2nd ed. New York: McGraw Hill, Inc., 2016.

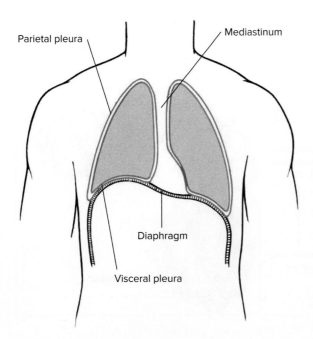

Figure 10.3   Position of the lungs, diaphragm, and pleura.

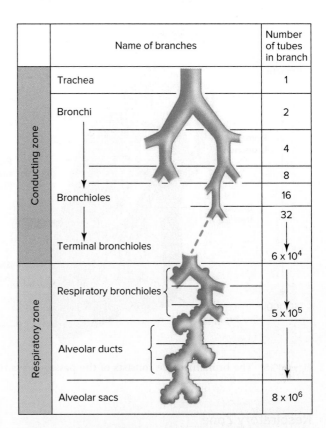

	Name of branches	Number of tubes in branch
Conducting zone	Trachea	1
	Bronchi	2
		4
		8
	Bronchioles	16
		32
	Terminal bronchioles	6×10^4
Respiratory zone	Respiratory bronchioles	5×10^5
	Alveolar ducts	
	Alveolar sacs	8×10^6

Figure 10.4   The conducting zones and respiratory zones of the pulmonary system.

bronchus, and bronchioles; the respiratory bronchioles lead into the alveoli where gas exchange occurs (Fig. 10.2). The anatomical position of the lungs relative to the major muscle of inspiration, the diaphragm, is pictured in Figure 10.3. Notice that both the right and the left lungs are enclosed by a set of membranes called **pleura.** The visceral pleura adheres to the outer surface of the lung, whereas the parietal pleura lines the thoracic walls. These two pleura are separated by a thin layer of fluid that acts as a lubricant, allowing a gliding action of one pleura on the other. The pressure in the pleural cavity (intrapleural pressure) is less than atmospheric and becomes even lower during inspiration, causing air from the environment to move into the lungs. The fact that intrapleural pressure is less than atmospheric is important because it prevents the collapse of the fragile air sacs (i.e., alveoli) within the lungs.

The airways leading to and from the lung are divided into two functional zones: (1) the conducting zone and (2) the respiratory zone (see Fig. 10.2 and Fig. 10.4). The conducting zone includes all those anatomical structures (e.g., trachea, bronchial tree, bronchioles) that air passes through to reach the respiratory zone. The respiratory zone is the region of the lung where gas exchange occurs and includes the respiratory bronchioles, alveolar ducts, and alveolar sacs. Respiratory bronchioles are included in this region because they contain small clusters of alveoli. Let's discuss each of these zones of the respiratory system in more detail.

Conducting Zone

Air enters the trachea from the pharynx (throat), and receives air from both the nasal and oral cavities. At rest, healthy humans breathe through the nose. However, during moderate to heavy exercise, the mouth becomes the major passageway for air (33). For gas to enter or leave the trachea, it must pass through a valve-like opening called the *epiglottis*, which is located between the vocal cords.

The trachea branches into two primary bronchi (right and left) that enter each lung. The bronchial tree then branches several more times before forming bronchioles. Brochioles are small branches of the bronchial tree. The bronchioles then branch several times before they become the alveolar ducts leading to the alveolar sacs and respiratory zone of the lung (see Fig. 10.5).

The conducting zone of the respiratory system not only serves as a passageway for air, but also functions to filter and humidify the air as it moves toward the respiratory zone of the lung. Regardless of the temperature or humidity of the environment, the air that reaches the lung is warmed and is saturated with water vapor (67, 69). This warming and humidification of air prevents the delicate lung tissue from desiccation (drying out) during exercise when breathing is increased (67).

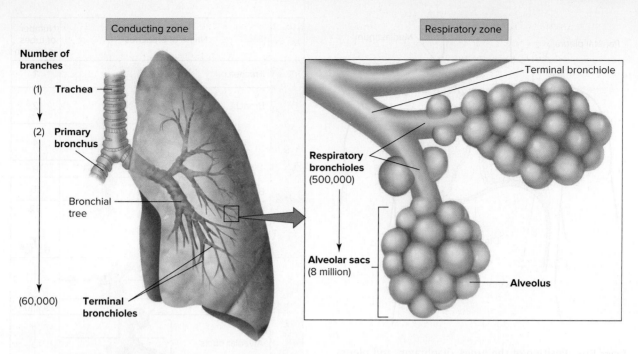

Figure 10.5 The bronchial tree consists of the passageways that connect the trachea and the alveoli.

Respiratory Zone

Gas exchange in the lungs occurs across about 300 million tiny alveoli. The enormous number of these structures provides the lung with a large surface area for diffusion. Indeed, it is estimated that the total surface area available for diffusion in the human lung is 60 to 80 square meters (i.e., size of a tennis court). The rate of gas diffusion is further assisted by the fact that each alveolus is only one cell layer thick, so the total blood–gas barrier is only two cell layers thick (alveolar cell and capillary cell) (see Fig. 10.6).

Although the alveoli provide the ideal structure for gas exchange, the fragility of these tiny "bubbles" presents some problems for the lung. For example, because of the surface tension (pressure exerted due to the properties of water) of the liquid lining the alveoli, relatively large forces develop, which tend to collapse alveoli. Fortunately, some of the alveolar cells (called type II, see Fig. 10.6) synthesize and release a material called *surfactant*, which lowers the surface tension of the alveoli and thus prevents their collapse (60).

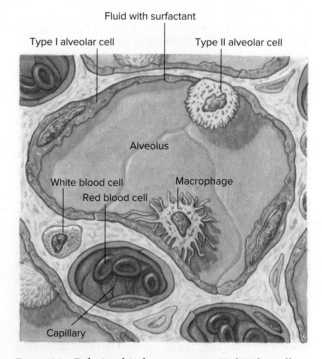

Figure 10.6 Relationship between type II alveolar cells and the alveolus.

IN SUMMARY

- Anatomically, the pulmonary system consists of a group of passages that filter air and transport it into the lungs where gas exchange occurs within tiny air sacs called *alveoli*.
- The air passages of the respiratory system are divided into two functional zones: (1) conducting zone and (2) respiratory zone.

MECHANICS OF BREATHING

Movement of air from the environment to the lungs is called pulmonary ventilation and occurs via a process known as **bulk flow.** Bulk flow refers to the movement of molecules along a passageway due to a pressure difference between the two ends of the passageway. Thus, inspiration occurs due to the pressure in the lungs (intrapulmonary) being reduced below atmospheric pressure. Conversely, expiration occurs when the pressure within the lungs exceeds atmospheric pressure. The process by which this pressure change within the lungs is achieved is discussed within the next several paragraphs.

Inspiration

Any muscle capable of increasing the volume of the chest is considered to be an inspiratory muscle. The **diaphragm** is the most important muscle of inspiration and is essential for normal breathing to occur (33, 66, 67, 89, 91, 93). This thin, dome-shaped muscle attaches to the lower ribs and is innervated by the phrenic nerves. When the diaphragm contracts, it forces the abdominal contents downward and forward. Further, the ribs are lifted outward. The outcome of these two actions is to reduce intrapleural pressure, which in turn causes the lungs to expand. This expansion of the lungs results in a reduction in intrapulmonary pressure below atmospheric, which allows airflow into the lungs (Fig. 10.7).

During normal, quiet breathing, the diaphragm performs most of the work of inspiration. However, during exercise, accessory muscles of inspiration are called into action to assist in breathing (71, 73, 97). These include the external intercostal muscles, pectoralis minor, the scalene muscles, and the sternocleidomastoids (see Fig. 10.8). Collectively, these muscles assist the diaphragm in increasing the dimensions of the chest, which aids in inspiration (see A Closer Look 10.1).

Expiration

Expiration is passive during normal, quiet breathing. That is, no muscular effort is necessary for expiration to occur at rest. This is true because both the lung and chest wall are elastic and return to their equilibrium position after expanding during inspiration (101). However, during exercise, expiration becomes active. The most important muscles involved in expiration are those found in the abdominal wall, which include the rectus abdominus and the external oblique (67). The internal intercostal muscles also assist in expiration by pulling down on the ribs (i.e., depressing the ribs) and decreasing the size of the thoracic cavity. When these muscles contract, the diaphragm is pushed upward (ascends) and the ribs are pulled downward and inward. This results in a decrease in the volume of the chest and expiration occurs.

Airway Resistance

At any rate of airflow into the lungs, the pressure difference that must be developed depends on the resistance of the airways. Airflow through the airways

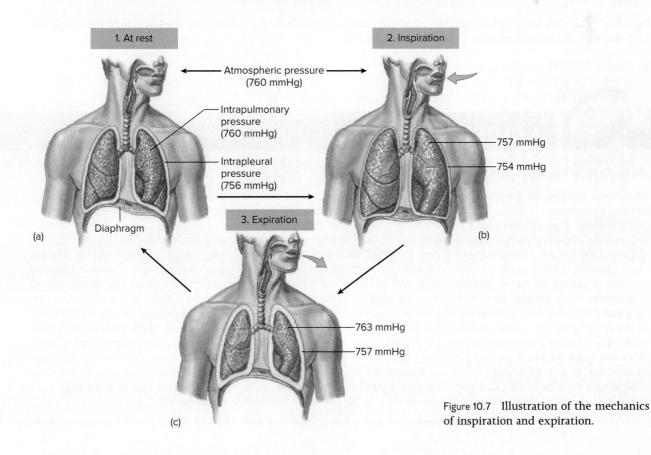

Figure 10.7   Illustration of the mechanics of inspiration and expiration.

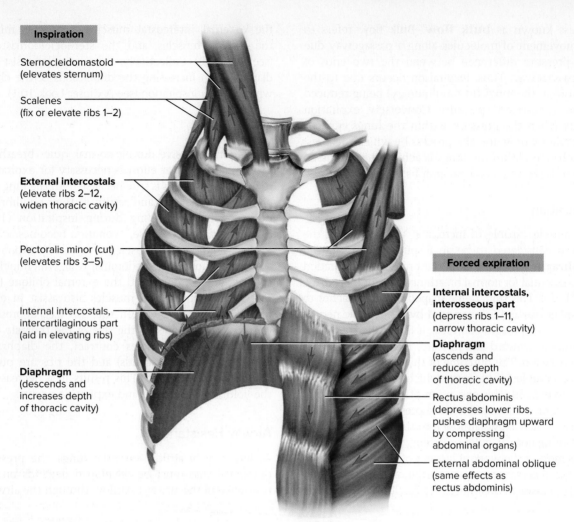

Inspiration

Sternocleidomastoid
(elevates sternum)

Scalenes
(fix or elevate ribs 1–2)

External intercostals
(elevate ribs 2–12,
widen thoracic cavity)

Pectoralis minor (cut)
(elevates ribs 3–5)

Internal intercostals,
intercartilaginous part
(aid in elevating ribs)

Diaphragm
(descends and
increases depth
of thoracic cavity)

Forced expiration

**Internal intercostals,
interosseous part**
(depress ribs 1–11,
narrow thoracic cavity)

Diaphragm
(ascends and
reduces depth
of thoracic cavity)

Rectus abdominis
(depresses lower ribs,
pushes diaphragm upward
by compressing
abdominal organs)

External abdominal oblique
(same effects as
rectus abdominis)

Figure 10.8   The muscles of respiration. The principal muscles of inspiration are shown on the left side of the trunk; the principal muscles of expiration are shown on the right side.

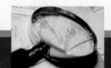

A CLOSER LOOK 10.1

Respiratory Muscles and Exercise

Respiratory muscles are skeletal muscles that are functionally similar to locomotor muscles. Their primary task is to act upon the chest wall to move gas in and out of the lungs to maintain arterial blood gas and pH homeostasis. The importance of normal respiratory muscle function can be appreciated by considering that respiratory muscle failure due to disease or spinal cord injury would result in the inability to ventilate the lungs and maintain blood gas and pH levels within an acceptable range.

Muscular exercise results in an increase in pulmonary ventilation, and therefore an increased workload is placed on respiratory muscles. Historically, it was believed that respiratory muscles do not fatigue during exercise. However, abundant evidence indicates that both prolonged exercise (e.g., 120 minutes) and high-intensity exercise (80% to 100% $\dot{V}O_2$ max) can promote respiratory muscle fatigue (110). The impact of respiratory muscle fatigue on exercise performance is discussed later in this chapter.

Respiratory muscles adapt to regular exercise training in a similar manner to locomotor skeletal muscles. Indeed, endurance exercise training increases respiratory muscle oxidative capacity and improves respiratory muscle endurance (81, 82, 94, 106, 107). Further, exercise training also increases the oxidative capacity and endurance of the upper airway muscles (108). This is important because these muscles play a key role in maintaining open airways to reduce the work of breathing during exercise. For more information on respiratory muscle adaptation to exercise, see McKenzie (2012) in the Suggested Readings.

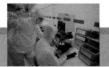
Exercise-Induced Asthma

Asthma is a disease that results in a reversible narrowing of the airways. An asthma "attack" can be caused by both contraction of smooth muscle around the airways (called a bronchospasm) and a collection of mucus within the airway. This reduction in airway diameter results in an increased work of breathing, and individuals suffering from asthma generally report being short of breath (called dyspnea).

Although there are many potential causes of asthma (24, 72), some asthmatic patients develop a bronchospasm during or immediately after exercise.

This is called "exercise-induced bronchospasm" or "exercise-induced asthma" (terms are used interchangeably). When an individual experiences an asthma attack during exercise, breathing becomes labored and a wheezing sound is often heard during expiration. If the asthma attack is severe, it becomes impossible for the individual to exercise at even low intensities because of the dyspnea associated with the increased work of breathing. Asthma is an excellent example of how even a small decrease in airway diameter can result in a large increase in breathing resistance.

Exercise-induced asthma is estimated to occur in more than 10% of elite endurance athletes. However, if asthma is correctly managed in athletes, this problem does not impair performance. Moreover, many of the inhaled asthma drugs do not improve athletic performance and therefore, the doping regulations for these drugs are less strict than in previous times (26). See Del Giacco et al. (2015) in the suggested readings for more details on exercise and asthma. More will be said about exercise-induced asthma in Chap. 17.

---

of the respiratory system can be explained by the following relationship:

$$\text{Airflow} = \frac{P_1 - P_2}{\text{Resistance}}$$

where $P_1 - P_2$ is the pressure difference at the two ends of the airway, and resistance is the resistance to flow offered by the airway. Airflow is increased anytime there is an increase in the pressure gradient across the pulmonary system, or if there is a decrease in airway resistance. This same relationship for blood flow was discussed in Chap. 9.

What factors contribute to airway resistance? By far, the most important variable contributing to airway resistance is the diameter of the airway. Airways that are reduced in size due to disease (chronic obstructive pulmonary disease, asthma, etc.) offer more resistance to flow than healthy, open airways. When the radius of an airway is reduced, the resistance to flow is increased markedly. Therefore, one can easily understand the effect of obstructive lung diseases (e.g., exercise-induced asthma) on increasing the work of breathing, especially during exercise when pulmonary ventilation is 10 to 20 times greater than at rest (see Clinical Applications 10.1 and 10.2).

IN SUMMARY

- The major muscle of inspiration is the diaphragm.
- Air enters the pulmonary system due to intrapulmonary pressure being reduced below atmospheric pressure (bulk flow).
- At rest, expiration is passive. However, during exercise, expiration becomes active, using muscles located in the abdominal wall (e.g., rectus abdominus and external oblique).
- The primary factor that contributes to airflow resistance in the pulmonary system is the diameter of the airway.

PULMONARY VENTILATION

Before beginning a discussion of ventilation, it is helpful to define some commonly used pulmonary physiology symbols:

1. V is used to denote a volume of gas.
2. $\dot{V}$ means volume per unit of time (generally one minute).
3. The subscripts $_{T, D, A, I, E}$ are used to denote tidal ($_T$), dead space ($_D$), alveolar ($_A$), inspired ($_I$), and expired ($_E$), respectively.

Pulmonary ventilation refers to the movement of gas into and out of the lungs. The amount of gas ventilated per minute is the product of the frequency of breathing (f) and the amount of gas moved per breath **(tidal volume):**

$$\dot{V} = V_T \times f$$

In a 70-kg man, the $\dot{V}$ at rest is generally around 7.5 liters/minute, with a tidal volume of 0.5 liter and a frequency of 15 breaths per minute. During maximal exercise, ventilation may reach 120 to 175 liters per minute, with a frequency of 40 to 50 breaths per minute and a tidal volume of approximately 3 to 3.5 liters.

It is important to understand that not all of the air that passes the lips reaches the alveolar gas compartment where gas exchange occurs. Part of each breath remains in conducting airways (trachea, bronchi, etc.) and thus does not participate in gas exchange. This "unused" ventilation is called dead-space ventilation (V_D), and the space it occupies is known as **anatomical dead space.** The volume of inspired gas that reaches the respiratory zone is referred to as **alveolar ventilation ($\dot{V}_A$).** Thus, total

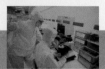
Exercise and Chronic Obstructive Pulmonary Disease

Chronic obstructive pulmonary disease (COPD) is clinically identified by a decreased expiratory airflow resulting from increased airway resistance. Although COPD and asthma both result in blockage of the airways, these diseases differ in one key feature. Asthma is a reversible narrowing of the airways; that is, asthma can come and go. In contrast, COPD is a constant narrowing of the airways. Although COPD patients can experience some variation in airway blockage, these individuals always experience some level of airway obstruction.

Note that COPD is often the result of a combination of two separate lung diseases: (1) chronic bronchitis and (2) emphysema. Each of these individual diseases results in increased airway obstruction. Chronic bronchitis is a lung disorder that results in a constant production of mucus within airways, resulting in airway blockage. Emphysema causes a decreased elastic support of the airways, resulting in airway collapse and increased airway resistance. Two of the greatest risk factors in developing COPD are tobacco smoking and a family history of emphysema (116).

Because COPD patients have a constant narrowing of the airways, this airway resistance places an increased workload on respiratory muscles to move gas in and out of the lung. Recognition of this increased work of breathing leads to the sensation of being short of breath (dyspnea). Because the magnitude of dyspnea is closely linked to the amount of work performed by respiratory muscles, dyspnea in COPD patients is greatly increased during exercise. In patients with severe COPD, dyspnea may become so debilitating that the patient has difficulty in performing routine activities of daily living (e.g., walking to the bathroom, showering, etc.). Treatment guidelines for patients with COPD include a program of pulmonary rehabilitation which includes bouts of regular exercise training (42, 50). Indeed, exercise training (both resistance and aerobic exercise) has been shown to improve the quality of life of patients suffering from COPD (42, 50). See Garvey et al. (2016) and Emtner et al. (2016) in the Suggested Readings for more details on COPD and exercise.

---

minute ventilation can be subdivided into dead space ventilation and alveolar ventilation:

$$\dot{V} = \dot{V}_A + \dot{V}_D$$

Note that pulmonary ventilation is not equally distributed throughout the lung. The bottom of the lung receives more ventilation than the apex (top region), particularly during quiet breathing (67). This changes during exercise, with the apical (top) regions of the lung receiving an increased percentage of the total ventilation (56). More will be said about the regional distribution of ventilation in the lung later in the chapter.

IN SUMMARY

- Pulmonary ventilation refers to the movement of gas into and out of the lungs.
- The volume of gas moved per minute is the product of tidal volume times breathing frequency.

PULMONARY VOLUMES AND CAPACITIES

Pulmonary volumes can be measured via a technique known as **spirometry.** Using this procedure, the subject breathes into a device that is capable of measuring inspired and expired gas volumes. Modern spirometers use computer technology to measure pulmonary volumes and the rate of expired airflow (see Fig. 10.9). Figure 10.10 is a graphic illustration showing the measurement of tidal volumes during quiet breathing and the various lung volumes and capacities that are defined in Table 10.1. Several of these terms require special mention. First, **vital capacity (VC)** is the maximum amount of gas that can be expired after a maximum inspiration. Second, the **residual volume (RV)** is the volume of gas remaining in the lungs after a maximum expiration. Finally, **total lung capacity (TLC)** is the volume of gas in the lungs after a maximum inspiration; it is the sum of the two lung volumes (VC + RV) just mentioned. Note that exercise training does not affect any of these lung volumes or capacities. More will be said about this later on page 249.

Clinically, spirometry is useful in diagnosing lung diseases such as chronic obstructive pulmonary

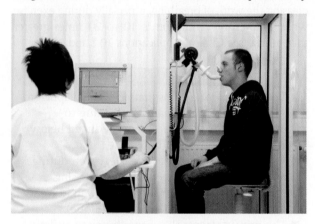

Figure 10.9 Photograph of a computerized spirometer used to measure lung volumes.

© Agencja Fotograficzna Caro/Alamy Stock Photo

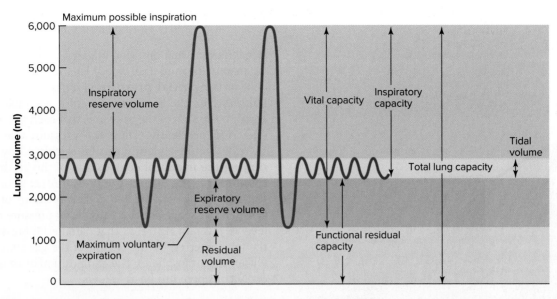

Figure 10.10 A spirogram showing lung volumes and capacities at rest.

disease (COPD). For example, because of increased airway resistance, COPD patients will have a diminished vital capacity and a reduced rate of expired airflow during a maximal expiratory effort. An illustration of how spirometry can detect airway obstruction in patients follows. One of the easiest lung function tests to detect airway blockage is the measurement of forced expiratory volume and vital capacity (VC). The forced expiratory volume (called FEV1) is the volume of gas expired in 1 second during a forced (maximal effort) expiration from a full inspiration. Recall that vital capacity is the total amount of gas that can be expired during a maximal expiration following a full

inspiration. A simple way to make these measures is illustrated in Figure 10.9. The patient is seated in front of the spirometer and breathes through a rubber mouthpiece connected to the spirometer. The patient breathes in maximally and then maximally exhales. The spirometer records the expired volume of gas over time during the expiratory effort.

Figure 10.11 compares the measurements of FEV1 and VC in both a normal, healthy individual and a patient with COPD. Notice, in the normal individual, the vital capacity is 5.0 liters and the FEV1 was 4.0 liters. Therefore, the FEV in this healthy individual is 80% of the VC (i.e., 4.0/5.0 × 100 = 80%).

TABLE 10.1	Respiratory Volumes and Capacities for a 70-Kg Young Adult Male	
Measurement	Typical Value	Definition
Respiratory Volumes		
Tidal volume (TV)	500 ml	Amount of air inhaled or exhaled in one breath during quiet breathing
Inspiratory reserve volume (IRV)	3,000 ml	Amount of air in excess of tidal volume that can be inhaled with maximum effort
Expiratory reserve volume (ERV)	1,200 ml	Amount of air in excess of tidal volume that can be exhaled with maximum effort
Residual volume (RV)	1,300 ml	Amount of air remaining in the lungs after maximum expiration; that is, the amount of air that can never be voluntarily exhaled
Respiratory Capacities		
Vital capacity (VC)	4,700 ml	Amount of air that can be forcefully exhaled following a maximum inspiration VC = (ERV + TV + IRV)
Inspiratory capacity (IC)	3,500 ml	Maximum amount of air that can be inhaled following a normal expiration (IC = TV + IRV)
Functional residual capacity (FRC)	2,500 ml	Amount of air remaining in the lungs following a normal expiration (FRC = RV + ERV)
Total lung capacity (TLC)	6,000 ml	Maximum amount of air in the lungs at the end of a maximum inspiration (TLC = RV + VC)

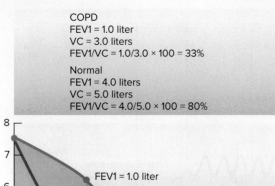

COPD
FEV1 = 1.0 liter
VC = 3.0 liters
FEV1/VC = 1.0/3.0 × 100 = 33%

Normal
FEV1 = 4.0 liters
VC = 5.0 liters
FEV1/VC = 4.0/5.0 × 100 = 80%

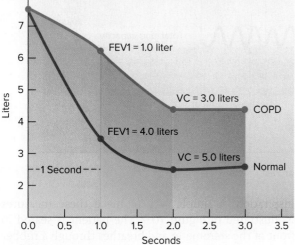

Figure 10.11   A spirogram illustrating the use of forced expired airflow to diagnose airway obstruction. Notice the marked difference in both the forced expired volume in one second (FEV1) and the vital capacity (VC) between the normal individual and the patient with chronic obstructive pulmonary disease (COPD). See text for details.

Indeed, the normal ratio of FEV1 to VC in healthy individuals is 80% or higher.

Now let's analyze the measurement of FEV1 and VC in the patient with COPD. Note that the rate at which air was expired in the COPD patient is much slower than in the healthy subject and only 1.0 liter of air is expired in the first second. Moreover, the vital capacity in the COPD patient is only 3.0 liters. Therefore, in this patient, the ratio of forced expired volume to vital capacity (1.0/3.0 × 100) is 33%. This value is much lower than the normal values for a normal individual (i.e., 80%) and is typical of a COPD patient with severe airway obstruction. For more information on the impact of COPD on exercise tolerance, see Clinical Applications 10.2.

IN SUMMARY

- Pulmonary volumes can be measured using spirometry.
- Vital capacity is the maximum amount of gas that can be expired after a maximal inspiration.
- Residual volume is the amount of gas left in the lungs after a maximal expiration.
- Chronic obstructive pulmonary disease decreases the vital capacity and reduces the rate of expired airflow from the lung during a maximal expiratory effort.

DIFFUSION OF GASES

Prior to discussing diffusion of gases across the alveolar membrane into the blood, let's review the concept of the **partial pressure** of a gas. According to Dalton's law, the total pressure of a gas mixture is equal to the sum of the pressures that each gas would exert independently. Thus, the pressure that each gas exerts independently can be calculated by multiplying the fractional composition of the gas by the absolute pressure (barometric pressure). Let's consider an example calculating the partial pressure of oxygen in air at sea level. The barometric pressure at sea level is 760 mm Hg (recall that barometric pressure is the force exerted by the weight of the gas contained within the atmosphere). The composition of air is generally considered to be as follows:

Gas	Percentage	Fraction
Oxygen	20.93	0.2093
Nitrogen	79.04	0.7904
Carbon dioxide	0.03	0.0003
Total	100.0	

Therefore, the partial pressure of oxygen (PO_2) at sea level can be computed as:

$$PO_2 = 760 \times 0.2093$$
$$PO_2 = 159 \text{ mm Hg}$$

In a similar manner, the partial pressure of nitrogen can be calculated to be:

$$PN_2 = 760 \times 0.7904$$
$$PN_2 = 600.7 \text{ mm Hg}$$

Because O_2, CO_2, and N_2 make up almost 100% of the atmosphere, the total barometric pressure (P) can be computed as:

$$P \text{ (dry atmosphere)} = PO_2 + PN_2 + PCO_2$$

Diffusion of a gas across tissues is described by Fick's law of diffusion, which states that the rate of gas transfer (V gas) is proportional to the tissue area, the diffusion coefficient of the gas (i.e., how easily a molecule diffuses), and the difference in the partial pressure of the gas on the two sides of the tissue, and is inversely proportional to the thickness:

$$V \text{ gas} = \frac{A}{T} \times D \times (P_1 - P_2)$$

where A is the area, T is the thickness of the tissue, D is the diffusion coefficient of the gas, and $P_1 - P_2$ is the difference in the partial pressure between the two sides of the tissue. In simple terms, the rate of diffusion for any single gas is greater when the surface area for diffusion is large and the "driving pressure" between the two sides of the tissue is high. In contrast, an increase in tissue thickness impedes diffusion. The lung is well designed for the diffusion of gases across the alveolar membrane into and out of the blood. First, the total surface area available for diffusion is large. Second, the alveolar membrane is extremely thin. Together, this design makes the lung the ideal organ for gas exchange; this is important because during maximal exercise, the rate of O_2 uptake and CO_2 output can increase 20 to 30 times above rest.

The amount of O_2 or CO_2 dissolved in blood obeys Henry's law and is dependent on the temperature of blood, the partial pressure of the gas, and the solubility of the gas. Because the temperature of the blood does not change a great deal during exercise (i.e., 1–3°C) and the solubility of the gas remains constant, the major factor that determines the amount of dissolved gas is the partial pressure.

Figure 10.12 illustrates gas exchange via diffusion across the alveolar–capillary membranes and at the tissue level. Note that the PCO_2 and PO_2 of blood entering the lung are approximately 46 and 40 mm Hg, respectively. In contrast, the PCO_2 and PO_2 in alveolar gas are around 40 and 105 mm Hg, respectively. As a consequence of the difference in partial pressure

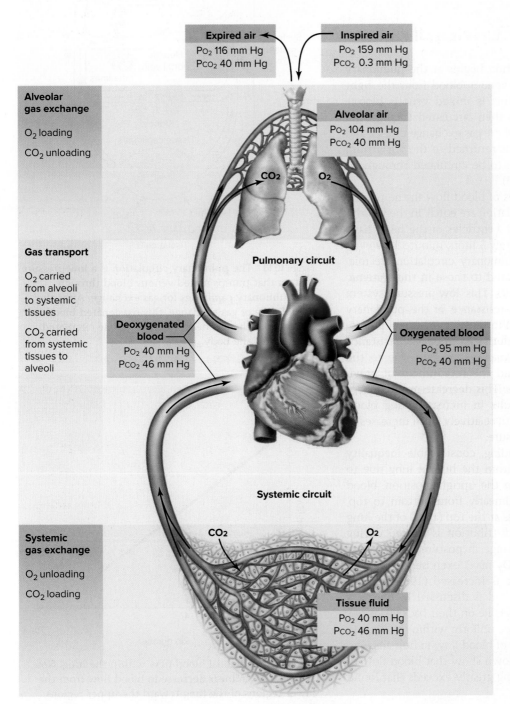

Expired air
PO₂ 116 mm Hg
PCO₂ 40 mm Hg

Inspired air
PO₂ 159 mm Hg
PCO₂ 0.3 mm Hg

Alveolar gas exchange

O₂ loading

CO₂ unloading

Alveolar air
PO₂ 104 mm Hg
PCO₂ 40 mm Hg

CO₂   O₂

Pulmonary circuit

Gas transport

O₂ carried from alveoli to systemic tissues

CO₂ carried from systemic tissues to alveoli

Deoxygenated blood
PO₂ 40 mm Hg
PCO₂ 46 mm Hg

Oxygenated blood
PO₂ 95 mm Hg
PCO₂ 40 mm Hg

Systemic circuit

Systemic gas exchange

O₂ unloading

CO₂ loading

CO₂   O₂

Tissue fluid
PO₂ 40 mm Hg
PCO₂ 46 mm Hg

Figure 10.12 Partial pressures of oxygen (PO₂) and carbon dioxide (PCO₂) in blood as a result of gas exchange in the lung and gas exchange between capillaries and tissues. Note that the alveolar PO₂ of 104 is a result of mixing atmospheric air (i.e., 159 mm Hg at sea level) with existing alveolar gas along with water vapor.

across the blood-gas interface, CO_2 leaves the blood and diffuses into the alveolus, and O_2 diffuses from the alveolus into the blood. Blood leaving the lung has a PO_2 of approximately 95 mm Hg and a PCO_2 of 40 mm Hg.

IN SUMMARY

- Gas moves across the blood-gas interface in the lung due to simple diffusion.
- The rate of diffusion is described by Fick's law, and diffusion is greater when the surface area is large, the tissue thickness is small, and the driving pressure is high.

BLOOD FLOW TO THE LUNG

The pulmonary circulation begins at the pulmonary artery, which receives venous blood from the right ventricle (recall that this is mixed venous blood). Mixed venous blood is then circulated through the pulmonary capillaries where gas exchange occurs, and this oxygenated blood is returned to the left atrium via the pulmonary vein to be circulated throughout the body (see Fig. 10.13).

Recall that the rates of blood flow in the pulmonary and systemic circulation are equal. In the healthy adult, the left and right ventricles of the heart have an output of approximately 5 liters/minute. However, the pressures in the pulmonary circulation are relatively low when compared to those in the systemic circulation (see Chap. 9). This low-pressure system is due to low vascular resistance in the pulmonary circulation (67, 118). An interesting feature of pulmonary circulation is that during exercise, the resistance in the pulmonary vascular system falls due to the distension of vessels and the recruitment of previously unused capillaries. This decrease in pulmonary vascular resistance results in increased lung blood flow during exercise with relatively small increases in pulmonary arterial pressure.

When we are standing, considerable inequality of blood flow exists within the human lung due to gravity. For example, in the upright position, blood flow decreases almost linearly from bottom to top, reaching very low values at the top (apex) of the lung (see Fig. 10.14). This distribution is altered during exercise and with a change in posture. During low-intensity (e.g., ~40% VO_2 max) exercise, blood flow to the top of the lung is increased (19). This will improve gas exchange and is discussed in the next section. When individuals lie on their backs (supine), blood flow becomes more uniform within the lung. In contrast, measurements of blood flow in humans who are suspended upside down show that blood flow to the apex (top) of the lung greatly exceeds that found in the base.

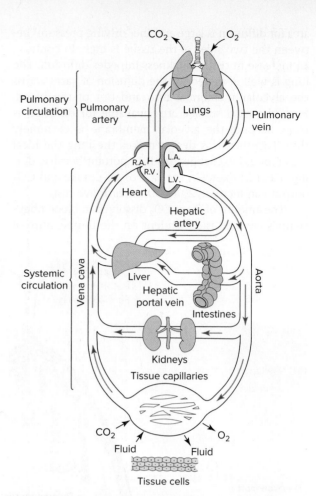

Figure 10.13 The pulmonary circulation is a low-pressure system that pumps mixed venous blood through the pulmonary capillaries for gas exchange. After the completion of gas exchange, this oxygenated blood is returned to the left heart chambers to be circulated throughout the body.

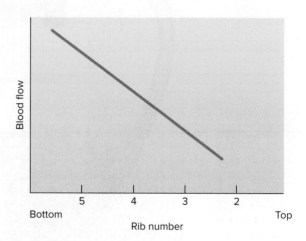

Figure 10.14 Regional blood flow within the lung. Note that there is a linear decrease in blood flow from the lower regions of the lung toward the upper regions.

- The pulmonary circulation is a low-pressure system with a rate of blood flow equal to that in the systemic circuit.
- In a standing position, most of the blood flow to the lung is distributed to the base of the lung due to gravitational force.

VENTILATION–PERFUSION RELATIONSHIPS

Thus far, we have discussed pulmonary ventilation, blood flow to the lungs, and diffusion of gases across the blood-gas barrier in the lung. It seems reasonable to assume that if all these processes were adequate, normal gas exchange would occur in the lung. However, normal gas exchange requires a matching of ventilation to blood flow (perfusion, Q). In other words, an alveolus can be well ventilated, but if blood flow to the alveolus does not adequately match ventilation, gas exchange does not occur. Indeed, mismatching of ventilation and perfusion is responsible for most of the problems of gas exchange that occur due to lung diseases.

The ideal ventilation-to-perfusion ratio (V/Q) is 1.0 or slightly greater. That is, there is a one-to-one matching of ventilation to blood flow, which results in optimum gas exchange. However, the V/Q ratio is generally not equal to 1.0 throughout the lung, but varies depending on the section of the lung being considered (40, 57, 67, 117). This concept is illustrated in Figure 10.15, where the V/Q ratio at the top and the base of the lung is calculated for resting conditions.

Let's discuss the V/Q ratio in the apex of the lung first. Here, the ventilation (at rest) in the upper region of the lung is estimated to be 0.24 liter/minute, whereas the blood flow is predicted to be 0.07 liter/minute. Thus, the V/Q ratio is 3.4 (i.e., 0.24/0.07 = 3.4). A large V/Q ratio represents a disproportionately high ventilation relative to blood flow, which results in poor gas exchange. In contrast, the ventilation at the base of the lung (Fig. 10.15) is 0.82 liter/minute, with a blood flow of 1.29 liters/minute (V/Q ratio = 0.82/1.29 = 0.64). A V/Q ratio less than 1.0 means that blood flow is higher than ventilation to the region in question. Although V/Q ratios less than 1.0 are not indicative of ideal conditions for gas exchange, in most cases, V/Q ratios greater than 0.50 are adequate to meet the gas exchange demands at rest (117).

What effect does exercise have on the V/Q ratio? Light-to-moderate exercise improves the V/Q relationship, whereas heavy exercise may result in a small V/Q inequality and thus, a minor impairment in gas exchange (56). Whether the increase in V/Q inequality is due to low ventilation or low perfusion is not

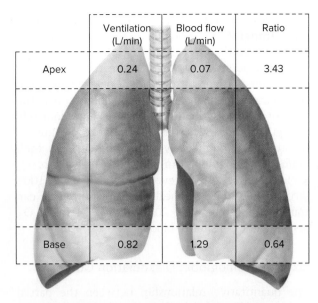

	Ventilation (L/min)	Blood flow (L/min)	Ratio
Apex	0.24	0.07	3.43
Base	0.82	1.29	0.64

Figure 10.15 The relationship between ventilation and blood flow (ventilation/perfusion ratios) at the top (apex) and the base of the lung. The ratios indicate that the base of the lung is overperfused relative to ventilation and that the apex is underperfused relative to ventilation. This uneven matching of blood flow to ventilation results in less-than-perfect gas exchange.

clear. The possible effects of this V/Q mismatch on blood gases will be discussed later in the chapter.

- Efficient gas exchange between the blood and the lung requires proper matching of blood flow to ventilation (called ventilation–perfusion relationships).
- The ideal ratio of ventilation to perfusion is 1.0 or slightly greater, because this ratio implies a perfect matching of blood flow to ventilation.

O_2 AND CO_2 TRANSPORT IN BLOOD

Although some O_2 and CO_2 are transported as dissolved gases in the blood, the major portion of O_2 and CO_2 transported via blood is done by O_2 combining with hemoglobin and CO_2 being transformed into bicarbonate (HCO_3^-). A summary of how O_2 and CO_2 are transported in blood follows.

Hemoglobin and O_2 Transport

Approximately 99% of the O_2 transported in the blood is chemically bound to **hemoglobin,** which is a protein contained in the red blood cells (erythrocytes). Each molecule of hemoglobin can transport four O_2

molecules. The binding of O_2 to hemoglobin forms **oxyhemoglobin;** hemoglobin that is not bound to O_2 is referred to as **deoxyhemoglobin.**

The amount of O_2 that can be transported per unit volume of blood is dependent on the concentration of hemoglobin. Normal hemoglobin concentration for a healthy male and female is approximately 150 grams and 130 grams, respectively, per liter of blood. When completely saturated with O_2, each gram of hemoglobin can transport 1.34 ml of O_2 (67). Therefore, at sea level, if hemoglobin is 100% saturated with O_2, the healthy male and female can transport approximately 200 ml and 174 ml of O_2, respectively, per liter of blood.

Oxygen–Hemoglobin Dissociation Curve

The quantitative relationship between the partial pressure of O_2 (PO_2) and the binding of O_2 to hemoglobin in blood is called the oxygen–hemoglobin disassociation curve (also called the oxyhemoglobin dissociation curve) (Fig. 10.16). Here, the term disassociate means "to separate" O_2 from hemoglobin and therefore, this curve could have also been named the oxygen–hemoglobin association curve. The combination of O_2 with hemoglobin in the lung (alveolar capillaries) is often called loading, and the release of O_2 from hemoglobin at the tissues is commonly called unloading. Thus, loading and unloading are reversible reactions:

$$\text{Deoxyhemoglobin} + O_2 \longleftrightarrow \text{Oxyhemoglobin}$$

The factors that determine the direction of this reaction are (1) the PO_2 of the blood and (2) the affinity or bond strength between hemoglobin and O_2. A high PO_2 drives the reaction to the right (i.e., loading), whereas low PO_2 and a reduced affinity of hemoglobin for O_2 moves the reaction to the left (i.e., unloading). For example, a high PO_2 in the lungs results in

an increase in arterial PO_2 and the formation of oxyhemoglobin (i.e., reaction moves right). In contrast, a low PO_2 in peripheral tissue (e.g., skeletal muscle) results in a decrease of PO_2 in the systemic capillaries and thus O_2 is released from hemoglobin to be used by the tissues (reaction moves left).

The effect of PO_2 on the combination of O_2 with hemoglobin is illustrated by the oxyhemoglobin dissociation curve (Fig. 10.16). This sigmoidal (S-shaped) curve has several interesting features. First, the percent hemoglobin saturated with O_2 (% HbO_2) increases sharply up to an arterial PO_2 of 40 mm Hg. At PO_2 values above 40 mmHg, the increase in % HbO_2 rises slowly to a plateau around 90 to 100 mm Hg, at this point the % HbO_2 is approximately 97%. At rest, the body's O_2 requirements are relatively low, and only about 25% of the O_2 transported in the blood is unloaded to the tissues. In contrast, during intense exercise, the mixed venous PO_2 can be lowered to 18 to 20 mm Hg, and the peripheral tissues can extract up to 90% of the O_2 carried by hemoglobin.

The shape of the oxyhemoglobin dissociation curve is well designed to meet human O_2 transport needs. The relatively flat portion of the curve (above a PO_2 of approximately 90 mm Hg) allows arterial PO_2 to oscillate from 90 to 100 mm Hg without a large drop in % HbO_2. This is important because there is a decline in arterial PO_2 with aging and upon ascent to high altitude. At the other end of the curve (steep portion, 0 to 40 mm Hg), small changes in PO_2 result in a release of large amounts of O_2 from hemoglobin. This is critical during exercise when muscle O_2 consumption is high.

In addition to the effect of blood PO_2 on O_2 binding to hemoglobin, an increase in acidity, temperature, or red blood cell (RBC) levels of 2-3-diphosphoglceric acid (2-3 DPG) can affect the O_2 loading/unloading reaction. This becomes important during exercise and will be discussed in the next segment.

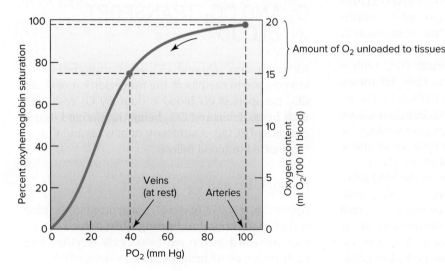

Figure 10.16 The relationship between the partial pressure of O_2 in blood and the relative saturation of hemoglobin with O_2 is pictured here in the oxygen–hemoglobin dissociation curve. Notice the relatively steep portion of the curve up to PO_2 values of 40 mm Hg, after which there is a gradual rise to reach a plateau.

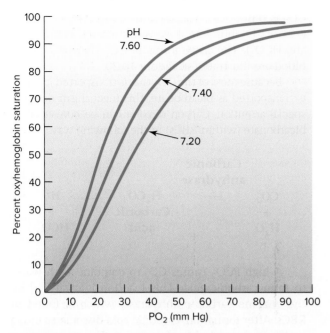

Figure 10.17 The effect of changing blood pH on the shape of the oxygen–hemoglobin dissociation curve. A decrease in pH (increased acidity) results in a rightward shift of the curve (Bohr effect), while an increase in pH (decreased acidity) results in a leftward shift of the curve.

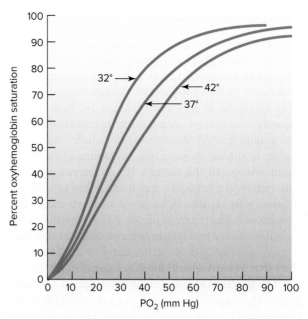

Figure 10.18 The effect of changing blood temperature on the shape of the oxygen–hemoglobin dissociation curve. An increase in temperature results in a rightward shift in the curve, while a decrease in blood temperature results in a leftward shift in the curve.

Effect of pH on O$_2$–Hb Dissociation Curve Let's consider the effect of changing blood acid–base status on hemoglobin's affinity for O$_2$. The strength of the bond between O$_2$ and hemoglobin is weakened by a decrease in blood pH (increased acidity), which results in increased unloading of O$_2$ to the tissues. This is represented by a "right" shift in the oxyhemoglobin curve and is called the **Bohr effect** (see Fig. 10.17). A right shift in the oxyhemoglobin dissociation curve occurs during heavy exercise due to the rise in blood hydrogen ion levels observed in this type of work. The mechanism to explain the Bohr effect is the fact that hydrogen ions bind to hemoglobin, which reduces its O$_2$ transport capacity. Therefore, when there is a higher-than-normal concentration of hydrogen ions in the blood (i.e., acidosis), there is a reduction in hemoglobin affinity for O$_2$. This facilitates the unloading of O$_2$ to the tissues during exercise because the acidity level is higher in muscles.

Temperature Effect on O$_2$–Hb Dissociation Curve Another factor that affects hemoglobin affinity for O$_2$ is temperature. At a constant pH, the affinity of hemoglobin for O$_2$ is inversely related to blood temperature. That is, a decrease in temperature results in a left shift in the oxyhemoglobin curve, whereas an increase in temperature causes a right shift of the curve. This means that an increase in blood temperature weakens the bond between O$_2$ and hemoglobin, which assists in the unloading of O$_2$

to working muscle. Conversely, a decrease in blood temperature results in a stronger bond between O$_2$ and hemoglobin, which hinders O$_2$ release. The effect of increasing blood temperature on the oxyhemoglobin dissociation curve is presented in Figure 10.18. During exercise, increased heat production in the contracting muscle would promote a right shift in the oxyhemoglobin dissociation curve and facilitate unloading of O$_2$ to the tissue.

2-3 DPG and the O$_2$–Hb Dissociation Curve A final factor that can affect the shape of the oxyhemoglobin dissociation curve is the concentration of 2,3 diphosphoglycerate (2-3 DPG) in red blood cells (RBCs). Here's the story on 2-3 DPG's effect on O$_2$ binding to hemoglobin. Red blood cells are unique in that they do not contain a nucleus or mitochondria. Therefore, they must rely on anaerobic glycolysis to meet the cell's energy needs. A by-product of RBC glycolysis is the compound 2-3 DPG, which can combine with hemoglobin and reduce hemoglobin's affinity for O$_2$ (i.e., right shift in oxyhemoglobin dissociation curve).

Red blood cell concentrations of 2-3 DPG increase during exposure to altitude and in anemia (low blood hemoglobin) (67). However, blood 2-3 DPG levels do not increase significantly during exercise at sea level (70, 99). Therefore, the right shift in the oxyhemoglobin curve that occurs during heavy exercise is not due to changes in 2-3 DPG, but to the degree of acidosis and blood temperature elevation.

O₂ Transport in Muscle

Myoglobin is an oxygen-binding protein found in skeletal muscle fibers and cardiac muscle (not in blood) and acts as a "shuttle" to move O_2 from the muscle cell membrane to the mitochondria. Myoglobin is found in large quantities in slow-twitch fibers (i.e., high aerobic capacity), in smaller amounts in intermediate fibers, and in only limited amounts in fast-twitch fibers. Myoglobin is similar in structure to hemoglobin, but is about one-fourth the weight. The difference in structure between myoglobin and hemoglobin results in a difference in O_2 affinity between the two molecules. This point is illustrated in Figure 10.19. Myoglobin has a greater affinity for O_2 than hemoglobin, and therefore the myoglobin–O_2 dissociation curve is much steeper than that of hemoglobin for PO_2 values below 20 mm Hg. The practical implication of the shape of the myoglobin–O_2 dissociation curve is that myoglobin discharges its O_2 at very low PO_2 values. This is important because the PO_2 in the mitochondria of contracting skeletal muscle may be as low as 1 to 2 mm Hg.

Myoglobin O_2 stores may serve as an "O_2 reserve" during transition periods from rest to exercise. At the beginning of exercise, there is a short time lag between the onset of muscular contraction and an increased O_2 delivery to the muscle. Therefore, O_2 bound to myoglobin prior to the initiation of exercise serves to buffer the O_2 needs of the muscle until the cardiopulmonary system can meet the new O_2 requirement. At the conclusion of exercise, myoglobin O_2 stores must be replenished, and this O_2 consumption above rest contributes to the O_2 debt (see Chap. 4).

CO₂ Transport in Blood

Carbon dioxide is transported in the blood in three forms: (1) dissolved CO_2 (about 10% of blood CO_2 is transported this way), (2) CO_2 bound to hemoglobin (called carbaminohemoglobin; about 20% of blood

CO_2 is transported via this form), and (3) bicarbonate (70% of CO_2 found in blood is transported as bicarbonate: HCO_3^-). The three forms of CO_2 transport in the blood are illustrated in Figure 10.20.

Because most of the CO_2 that is transported in blood is transported as bicarbonate, this mechanism deserves special attention. Carbon dioxide can be converted to bicarbonate (within RBCs) in the following way:

$$\underset{\substack{\text{CO}_2 \\ + \\ \text{H}_2\text{O}}}{} \overset{\substack{\textbf{Carbonic} \\ \textbf{anhydrase}}}{\longleftrightarrow} \underset{\substack{\text{H}_2\text{CO}_3 \\ \textbf{Carbonic} \\ \textbf{acid}}}{} \longleftrightarrow \underset{\substack{\text{H}^+ \\ + \\ \text{HCO}_3^-}}{}$$

A high PCO_2 causes CO_2 to combine with water to form carbonic acid. This reaction is catalyzed by the enzyme carbonic anhydrase, which is found in RBCs. After formation, carbonic acid dissociates into a hydrogen ion and a bicarbonate ion. The hydrogen ion then binds to hemoglobin, and the bicarbonate ion diffuses out of the RBC into the plasma (Fig. 10.20). Because bicarbonate carries a negative charge (anion), the removal of a negatively charged molecule from a cell without replacement would result in an electrochemical imbalance across the cell membrane. This problem is avoided by the replacement of bicarbonate by chloride (Cl^-), which diffuses from the plasma into the RBC. This exchange of anions occurs in the RBC as blood moves through the tissue capillaries and is called the chloride shift (Fig. 10.20).

When blood reaches the pulmonary capillaries, the PCO_2 of the blood is greater than that of the alveolus, and thus CO_2 diffuses out of the blood across the blood–gas interface. At the lung, the binding of O_2 to Hb results in a release of the hydrogen ions bound to hemoglobin and promotes the formation of carbonic acid:

$$H^+ + HCO_3^- \longrightarrow H_2CO_3$$

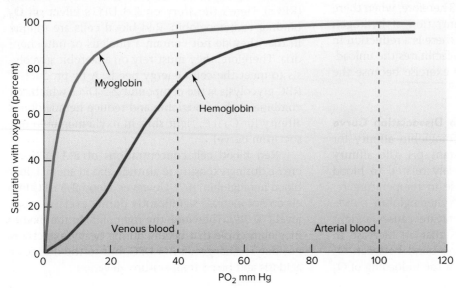

Figure 10.19 Comparison of the dissociation curve for myoglobin and hemoglobin. The steep myoglobin dissociation demonstrates a higher affinity for O_2 than hemoglobin.

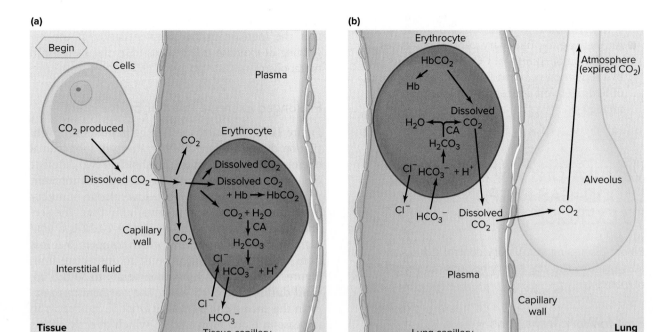

(a)

(b)

Figure 10.20 Summary of carbon dioxide (CO_2) movement from tissues into the blood (*a*) and from the blood into the alveolus of the lung (*b*). Note in Figure 10.20(*a*) that CO_2 is released from the cells and moves into the blood. Carbon dioxide is transported in the blood in three forms: (1) dissolved CO_2, (2) CO_2 combined with hemoglobin ($HbCO_2$), and (3) bicarbonate (HCO_3^-). Notice that as HCO_3^- moves out of red blood cells (erythrocytes), chloride (Cl^-) moves into the erythrocyte (chloride shift) to maintain a balanced charge in the cell. Figure 10.20(*b*) illustrates the movement of CO_2 from the blood into the alveolus of the lung. At the time of CO_2 release into the lung, there is a "reverse chloride shift" and carbonic acid dissociates into CO_2 and H_2O.

Under conditions of low PCO_2 that exist at the alveolus, carbonic acid then dissociates into CO_2 and H_2O:

$$H_2CO_3 \longrightarrow CO_2 + H_2O$$

The release of CO_2 from the blood into the alveoli is removed from the body in the expired gas.

IN SUMMARY

- More than 99% of the O_2 transported in blood is chemically bonded with hemoglobin. The effect of the partial pressure of O_2 on the combination of O_2 with hemoglobin is illustrated by the S-shaped O_2-hemoglobin dissociation curve.
- An increase in body temperature and a reduction in blood pH results in a right shift in the O_2-hemoglobin dissociation curve and a reduced affinity of hemoglobin for O_2.
- Carbon dioxide is transported in blood in three forms: (1) dissolved CO_2 (10% is transported in this way), (2) CO_2 bound to hemoglobin (called carbaminohemoglobin; about 20% of blood CO_2 is transported via this form), and (3) bicarbonate (70% of CO_2 found in blood is transported as bicarbonate [HCO_3^-]).
- Myoglobin is the oxygen-binding protein found in muscle and acts as a shuttle to move O_2 from the muscle cell membrane to the mitochondria.

VENTILATION AND ACID–BASE BALANCE

Pulmonary ventilation can play an important role in removing H^+ from the blood by the HCO_3^- reaction discussed previously (102). For example, an increase in CO_2 in blood or body fluids results in increased hydrogen ion accumulation and thus a decrease in pH. In contrast, removal of CO_2 from blood or body fluids decreases hydrogen ion concentration, and thus an increase in pH results. Recall that the CO_2-carbonic anhydrase reaction occurs as follows:

$$\text{Lung} \longleftarrow$$
$$CO_2 + H_2O \longleftrightarrow H_2CO_3 \longleftrightarrow H^+ + HCO_3^-$$
$$\text{Muscle} \longrightarrow$$

Therefore, an increase in pulmonary ventilation causes exhalation of additional CO_2 and results in a reduction of blood PCO_2 and a lowering of hydrogen ion concentration (i.e., pH would increase in the blood). In contrast, a reduction in pulmonary ventilation would result in a buildup of CO_2 and an increase in hydrogen ion concentration (pH would decrease). The role of the pulmonary system in acid–base balance is discussed again in Chap. 11.

■ An increase in pulmonary ventilation causes exhalation of additional CO_2, which results in a reduction of blood PCO_2 and a lowering of hydrogen ion concentration (i.e., pH increases).

VENTILATORY AND BLOOD–GAS RESPONSES TO EXERCISE

Before discussing ventilatory control during exercise, let's examine the ventilatory response to several types of exercise.

Rest-to-Work Transitions

The change in pulmonary ventilation observed in the transition from rest to constant-load submaximal exercise (i.e., below the lactate threshold) is illustrated in Figure 10.21. Note that pulmonary ventilation (i.e., expired ventilation ($\dot{V}_E$)) increases abruptly at the beginning of exercise, followed by a slower rise toward a steady-state value (8, 21, 22, 38, 53, 80, 87, 120).

Figure 10.21 also points out that arterial pressures of PCO_2 and PO_2 are relatively unchanged during this type of exercise (35, 37, 113). However, note that arterial PO_2 decreases and arterial PCO_2 tends to increase slightly in the transition from rest to steady-state exercise (37). This observation indicates that the increase in alveolar ventilation at the beginning of exercise is not as rapid as the increase in metabolism.

Prolonged Exercise in a Hot Environment

Figure 10.22 illustrates the change in pulmonary ventilation during prolonged, constant-load, submaximal exercise (below the lactate threshold) in two different environmental conditions. The neutral environment represents exercise in a cool, low-relative-humidity environment (19°C, 45% relative humidity). The second condition represented in Figure 10.22 is a hot/high-humidity environment, which hampers heat loss from the body. The major point to appreciate from Figure 10.22 is that ventilation tends to "drift" upward during prolonged work. The mechanism to explain this increase in $\dot{V}_E$ during work in the heat is an increase in blood temperature, which directly affects the respiratory control center (88).

Another interesting point illustrated in Figure 0.22 is that although ventilation is greater during exercise in a hot/humid environment when compared to work in a cool environment, there is little difference in arterial PCO_2 between the two types of exercise. This finding indicates that the increase in ventilation observed during exercise in the heat is due to an increase in breathing frequency and dead-space ventilation.

Incremental Exercise

The ventilatory response for an elite male distance runner and an untrained college student during an incremental exercise test is illustrated in Figure 10.23. In both subjects, ventilation increases as a linear

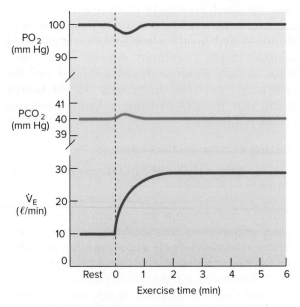

Figure 10.21 The changes in ventilation and partial pressures of O_2 and CO_2 in the transition from rest to steady-state submaximal exercise.

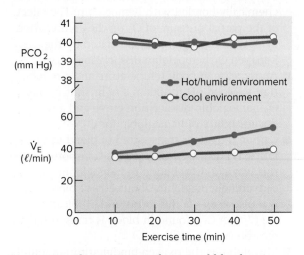

Figure 10.22 Changes in ventilation and blood gas tensions during prolonged, submaximal exercise in a hot/humid environment.

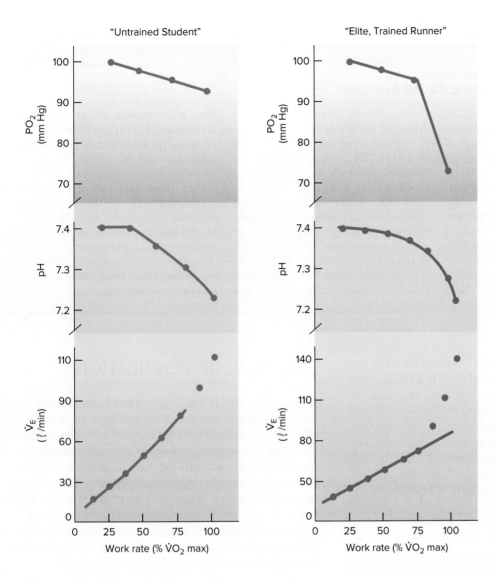

"Untrained Student"

"Elite, Trained Runner"

Figure 10.23 Changes in ventilation, blood-gas tensions, and pH during incremental exercise in a highly trained male distance runner and an untrained male college student.

function of oxygen uptake up to 50% to 75% of O_2 max, where ventilation begins to rise exponentially (114). This V_E "inflection point" has been called the **ventilatory threshold (Tvent)** (7, 55, 77, 78).

An interesting point that emerges from Figure 10.23 is the startling difference between the highly trained elite athlete and the untrained subject in arterial PO_2 during heavy exercise. The untrained subject is able to maintain arterial PO_2 within 10 to 12 mm Hg of the normal resting value, whereas the highly trained distance runner shows a decrease of 30 to 40 mm Hg at near-maximal exercise (30, 33). This drop in arterial PO_2, often observed in the healthy, endurance athlete, is similar to that observed in exercising patients who have severe lung disease. However, not all healthy, elite endurance athletes develop low-arterial PO_2 values (low PO_2 is called *hypoxemia*) during heavy exercise. It appears that only about 40% to 50% of elite highly trained, male endurance athletes ($\dot{V}O_2$ max 4.5 l/min or 68 ml $\cdot$ kg $\cdot$ min^{-1}) show this

marked hypoxemia (85, 93). In addition, the degree of hypoxemia observed in these athletes during heavy work varies considerably among individuals (30, 86, 93, 111). The reason for the subject differences is unclear.

Female endurance athletes also develop exercise-induced hypoxemia (54, 58, 59, 61). In fact, it appears that the incidence of exercise-induced hypoxemia in highly trained and elite female athletes may be greater than males (54, 59, 61). For more information on gender differences in breathing during exercise, see Research Focus 10.1.

Perhaps the most important question concerning exercise-induced hypoxemia in healthy athletes is, what factor(s) accounts for this failure of the pulmonary system? Unfortunately, a complete answer to this question is not available. Nonetheless, it appears that both ventilation-perfusion mismatch and diffusion limitations are likely contributors to exercise-induced hypoxemia in elite athletes (73, 93, 119). Diffusion limitations

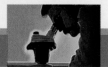

RESEARCH FOCUS 10.1

Sex Differences in Breathing during Exercise

New evidence reveals that sex differences exist in anatomy of the respiratory system and that these anatomical differences impact the breathing response to exercise. Specifically, when matched for age and body weight, women have smaller airways compared to men (98). This is important because a smaller airway results in a greater resistance to airflow, which could limit the maximal ventilatory capacity during high intensity exercise. Further, because women have smaller airways, the energy requirement for breathing during exercise is higher in women compared to men (41). This is significant because an increased work of breathing can accelerate the respiratory muscle fatigue that occurs during prolonged or high-intensity exercise. Moreover, evidence from a growing number of studies suggest that elite female endurance athletes are more likely to experience exercise-induced hypoxemia than their male counterparts (98). It is unclear if the increased incidence of exercise-induced hypoxemia in elite female endurance athletes is due to differences in airway diameter between the sexes. Together, these data indicate that sex differences exist in the ventilatory response to exercise and this could impact the cardiopulmonary response to exercise. For more details on sex differences in the pulmonary system, please see Sheel et al. (2016) in the suggested reading list.

---

during intense exercise in elite athletes could occur due to a reduced amount of time that the RBCs spend in the pulmonary capillary (34). This short RBC transit time in the pulmonary capillaries is due to the high cardiac outputs achieved by these athletes during high-intensity exercise. This high cardiac output during high-intensity exercise results in the rapid movement of RBCs through the lung, which limits the time available for gas equilibrium to be achieved between the lung and blood (30, 96, 121).

IN SUMMARY

- At the beginning of constant-load submaximal exercise, ventilation increases rapidly, followed by a slower rise toward a steady-state value. Arterial PO_2 and PCO_2 are maintained relatively constant during this type of exercise.
- During prolonged exercise in a hot/humid environment, ventilation "drifts" upward due to the influence of rising body temperature on the respiratory control center.
- Incremental exercise results in a linear increase in $\dot{V}_E$ up to approximately 50% to 70% of O_2 max; at higher work rates, ventilation begins to rise exponentially. This ventilatory inflection point is often called the *ventilatory threshold*.
- Exercise-induced hypoxemia occurs in 40% to 50% of elite, highly trained male and female endurance athletes.
- New evidence reveals that women have smaller airways than men, even when matched for lung size. This results in an increased work of breathing during exercise.

CONTROL OF VENTILATION

The precise regulation of pulmonary ventilation at rest and during exercise is an example of a highly efficient control system that maintains blood gas and acid-base homeostasis. Indeed, pulmonary ventilation (i.e., alveolar ventilation) increases during exercise in direct proportion to the intensity of exercise and the increased need for oxygen. This results in a precise control of arterial oxygen content, arterial carbon dioxide levels, and acid-base balance. Let's begin our discussion of ventilatory control during exercise with a review of ventilatory regulation at rest.

Ventilatory Regulation at Rest

As discussed earlier, inspiration and expiration are produced by the contraction and relaxation of the diaphragm during quiet breathing, and by accessory muscles during exercise. Contraction and relaxation of these respiratory muscles are directly controlled by somatic motor neurons in the spinal cord. Motor neuron activity, in turn, is directly controlled by the respiratory control center located in the medulla oblongata.

Respiratory Control Center

The respiratory control center is located in the brain stem within two distinct areas called the medulla oblongata and the pons. The genesis of breathing comes from the firing of several clusters of neurons within the brain stem that serve as pacemakers. Specifically, the stimulus for inspiration comes from three distinct respiratory rhythm centers located within both the medulla oblongata and the pons regions of the brain

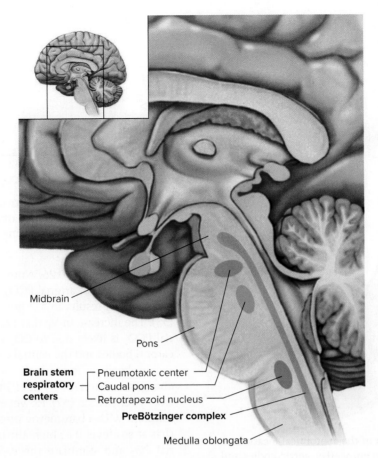

Figure 10.24 Locations of the brain stem respiratory control centers.

Labels in figure:
Midbrain
Pons
Brain stem respiratory centers — Pneumotaxic center / Caudal pons / Retrotrapezoid nucleus
PreBötzinger complex
Medulla oblongata

stem (47). The primary rhythm-generating center in the medulla is called the preBötzinger Complex (preBötC) (32) (Fig. 10.24). Other rhythm-generating centers exist in the pons and are composed of two clusters of neurons called the *pneumotaxic center* and the *caudal pons* (Fig. 10.24). The normal rhythm of breathing occurs due to an interaction between pacemaker neurons in each of these regions (7). At rest, the breathing rhythm is dominated by pacemaker neurons in the preBötC. During exercise, the preBötC interacts with the other respiratory rhythm centers to regulate breathing to match the metabolic demand (100). The interaction between these respiratory pacemakers to control breathing involves both positive and negative feedback to achieve tight regulation.

Input to the Respiratory Control Center

The respiratory control center receives input from both higher brain centers and afferent neural signals from several locations outside of the central nervous system. In general, input to the respiratory control center can be classified into two types: (1) neural and (2) humoral (blood-borne). Neural input refers to signals from higher brain centers or afferent input to the respiratory control center from neurons that are excited by factors other than blood-borne stimuli. Humoral input to the respiratory control center refers to the influence of blood-borne stimuli reaching a specialized chemoreceptor. This receptor reacts to the strength of the stimuli and sends the appropriate message to the medulla. A brief overview of each of these receptors will be presented prior to a discussion of ventilatory control during exercise.

Humoral Chemoreceptors Chemoreceptors are specialized neurons that are capable of responding to changes in the internal environment. Traditionally, respiratory chemoreceptors are classified according to their location as being either *central chemoreceptors* or *peripheral chemoreceptors*.

The central chemoreceptors are located in the medulla (anatomically separate from the respiratory center) and are affected by changes in PCO_2 and H^+ of the cerebrospinal fluid (CSF). An increase in either PCO_2 or H^+ of the CSF results in the central chemoreceptors sending afferent input into the respiratory center to increase ventilation (32, 35).

The primary peripheral chemoreceptors are located in the aortic arch and at the bifurcation of the common carotid artery. The receptors located in the

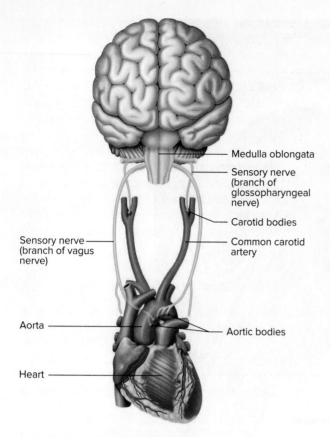

Figure 10.25 Illustration of the anatomical location of the peripheral chemoreceptors (i.e., aortic bodies and carotid bodies). The aortic chemoreceptors respond to arterial changes in arterial H^+ ion concentration (i.e., pH) and PCO_2. The carotid bodies also respond to arterial changes in arterial pH, PCO_2, and also changes in PO_2.

aorta are called **aortic bodies,** and those found in the carotid artery are **carotid bodies** (Fig. 10.25). These peripheral chemoreceptors respond to increases in arterial H^+ concentrations and PCO_2 (1, 4, 10, 49, 109, 116, 122). In addition, the carotid bodies are sensitive to increases in blood potassium levels, norepinephrine, decreases in arterial PO_2, and increased body temperature (17, 32, 49, 75). When comparing these two sets of peripheral chemoreceptors, early studies suggested that the carotid bodies are more important in the control of breathing during exercise (5, 11, 16, 35, 49, 51-52, 67, 103, 105, 113, 115). However, new evidence suggests that the aortic bodies are capable of sensing changes in blood levels of CO_2 (indirectly) and therefore, these chemoreceptors could play an important role in the control of breathing both at rest and during exercise (31). Stay tuned, more research on this topic should be available soon.

How do the central and peripheral chemoreceptors respond to changes in chemical stimuli? The effects of increases in arterial PCO_2 on minute ventilation is

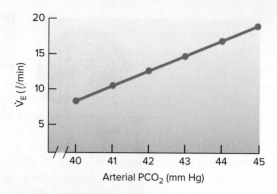

Figure 10.26 Changes in ventilation as a function of increasing arterial PCO_2. Notice that ventilation increases as a linear function of increasing PCO_2.

shown in Figure 10.26. Note that $\dot{V}_E$ increases as a linear function of arterial PCO_2. In general, a 1 mm Hg rise in PCO_2 results in a 2 liter/minute increase in $\dot{V}_E$ (35). The increase in $\dot{V}_E$ that results from a rise in arterial PCO_2 is likely due to CO_2 stimulation of both the carotid bodies and the central chemoreceptors (35, 76).

In healthy individuals breathing at sea level, changes in arterial PO_2 have little effect on the control of ventilation (67). However, exposure to an environment with a barometric pressure much lower than that at sea level (i.e., high altitude) can decrease arterial PO_2 and stimulate the carotid bodies, which in turn signal the respiratory control center to increase ventilation (49). The relationship between arterial PO_2 and $\dot{V}_E$ is illustrated in Figure 10.27. The point on the $PO_2/\dot{V}_E$ curve where $\dot{V}_E$ begins to rise rapidly is called the hypoxic threshold (*hypoxic* means low PO_2) (2). This hypoxic threshold usually occurs around an arterial PO_2 of 60 to 75 mm Hg. The chemoreceptors responsible for the increase in $\dot{V}_E$ following exposure to low PO_2 are the carotid bodies because the aortic and central chemoreceptors in humans do not respond to changes in PO_2 (35, 67).

Increases in blood levels of potassium can also stimulate the carotid bodies and promote an increase in ventilation (17, 75). Because blood potassium levels

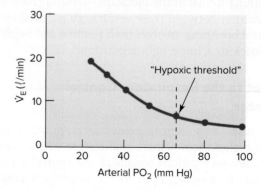

Figure 10.27 Changes in ventilation as a function of decreasing arterial PO_2. Note the existence of a "hypoxic threshold" for ventilation as arterial PO_2 declines.

rise during exercise due to a net potassium efflux from the contracting muscle, potassium may play a role in regulating ventilation during exercise (17, 75). More will be said about this later.

Neural input to the respiratory control center   Neural input to the respiratory control center comes from both higher brain centers and afferent pathways. For example, impulses from the motor cortex (i.e., central command) can activate skeletal muscles to contract and increase ventilation in proportion to the amount of exercise being performed (43). Indeed, neural impulses originating in the motor cortex pass through the medulla and "spill over," causing an increase in $\dot{V}_E$ that reflects the number of muscle motor units being recruited.

Afferent input to the respiratory control center during exercise comes from several peripheral mechanoreceptors, including the muscle spindles, Golgi tendon organs, or joint pressure receptors (25, 27, 65, 104). Growing evidence suggests that this afferent neural feedback from the working muscles is important in regulating breathing during submaximal, steady-state exercise (27, 31). In addition, chemoreceptors located

in muscle may respond to changes in potassium and H^+ concentrations and send afferent information to the respiratory control center to increase breathing. This type of input to the medulla is considered afferent neural information because the stimuli are not humorally mediated. Further, evidence suggests that the right ventricle of the heart contains mechanoreceptors that send afferent information back to the respiratory control center relative to increases in cardiac output (e.g., during exercise) (115). These mechanoreceptors could play important roles in providing afferent input to the respiratory control center at the onset of exercise. Table 10.2 summarizes the major receptors that participate in the control of breathing during exercise.

Ventilatory Control during Submaximal Exercise

In the previous sections, we have discussed several sources of input to the respiratory control center. Let's now discuss how the body regulates breathing during exercise (9, 15, 18, 25, 27, 43, 46, 65, 79, 95, 113, 122). Current evidence suggests that the "initial" drive to increase ventilation during exercise is due to

TABLE 10.2	A Summary of Receptors that Provide Input to the Respiratory Control Center to Regulate Breathing during Exercise	
Receptor	**Stimulus**	**Comments on Control of Breathing**
Chemoreceptors located in medulla oblongata (central chemoreceptor)	$PCO_2 \uparrow$	Central chemoreceptors are sensitive to changes in pH of the cerebrospinal fluid. An increase in arterial PCO_2 results in diffusion of CO_2 from the blood into the brain; this lowers pH and stimulates the central chemoreceptor to send signals to the respiratory control center to increase breathing. This results in increased alveolar ventilation and the elimination of CO_2.
Carotid body (peripheral chemoreceptor)	$PCO_2 \uparrow$ pH $\downarrow$ $PO_2 \downarrow$	The carotid body is sensitive to changes in arterial PO_2, PCO_2, and pH. An increase in arterial PCO_2 stimulates the carotid bodies to send signals to the respiratory control center to increase breathing. Similarly, a decrease in either arterial pH or PO_2 stimulates the carotid bodies to send signals to the respiratory control center to increase ventilation.
Aortic body (peripheral chemoreceptor)	$PCO_2 \uparrow$ pH $\downarrow$	The aortic body is sensitive to changes in arterial PCO_2 and pH. Increased arterial PCO_2 or a decrease in blood pH stimulates the aortic body to send signals to the respiratory control center to increase breathing.
Muscle mechanoreceptors	Muscle contractile activity $\uparrow$	Skeletal muscle contains several mechanoreceptors (e.g., muscle spindle and Golgi tendon organ). Muscle contractile activity stimulates these receptors to send neural signals to the respiratory control center to increase breathing in direct proportion to the exercise intensity.
Muscle chemoreceptors (also called muscle metaboreceptors)	pH $\downarrow$ Potassium $\uparrow$	Skeletal muscle contains chemoreceptors that are sensitive to chemical changes inside and around the muscle fibers. Exercise can decrease muscle pH and increase extracellular potassium concentration; this stimulates these chemoreceptors to send neural signals to the respiratory control center to increase breathing.

neural input from higher brain centers (central command) to the respiratory control center (29). However, the fact that arterial PCO_2 is tightly regulated during most types of submaximal exercise indicates that humoral chemoreceptors and afferent neural feedback from working muscles act to fine-tune breathing to match the metabolic rate and thus maintain a rather constant arterial PCO_2 (13, 14, 27, 49, 74, 113). Indeed, new evidence reveals that during submaximal exercise, 40% to 50% of the drive to breath comes from afferent neural signals sent from exercising muscle to higher brain centers (31). Therefore, ventilation during exercise is regulated by several overlapping factors that provide redundancy to the control system.

During prolonged exercise in a hot environment, ventilation can be influenced by factors other than those discussed previously. For example, the drift upward in $\dot{V}_E$ seen in Figure 10.22 may be due to a direct influence of rising blood temperature on the respiratory control center, and rising blood catecholamines (epinephrine and norepinephrine) stimulating the carotid bodies to increase $\dot{V}_E$ (88).

In summary, the increase in ventilation during submaximal exercise occurs due to an interaction of both neural and chemoreceptor input to the respiratory control center. Efferent neural mechanisms from higher brain centers (central command) provide the initial drive to breathe during exercise, with humoral chemoreceptors and neural feedback from working muscles providing a means of precisely matching ventilation with the amount of CO_2 produced via metabolism. This redundancy in control mechanisms is not surprising when one considers the important role that respiration plays in maintaining a steady state during exercise (48). A summary of respiratory control during submaximal exercise appears in Figure 10.28.

Ventilatory Control during Heavy Exercise

Debate continues regarding the mechanism(s) responsible for the alinear rise in ventilation (ventilatory threshold) that occurs at exercise intensities above the lactate threshold during an incremental exercise test. It appears that several factors contribute to this rise. First, examination of Figure 10.23 suggests that the alinear rise in $\dot{V}_E$ and the decrease in pH often occur simultaneously. Because rising hydrogen ion levels in blood can stimulate the carotid bodies and increase $\dot{V}_E$, it is likely that the rise in blood lactate that occurs during incremental exercise is a key stimulus causing the alinear rise in $\dot{V}_E$ (i.e., ventilatory threshold). Based on this belief, it is common for researchers to estimate the lactate threshold noninvasively by measuring ventilatory threshold (6, 18, 112, 114). Nonetheless, this technique is not perfect; the ventilatory threshold and the lactate threshold do not always occur at the same work rate (44, 78).

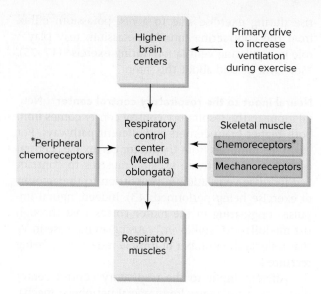

*Act to fine-tune ventilation during exercise

Figure 10.28 A summary of respiratory control during submaximal exercise. See text for details.

What additional factors, other than rising blood lactate, might cause the alinear rise in $\dot{V}_E$ observed during incremental exercise? The close relationship between blood potassium levels and ventilation during heavy exercise has led several investigators to speculate that potassium is an important factor in controlling ventilation during heavy exercise (17, 68, 75). Certainly, other secondary factors, such as rising body temperature and blood catecholamines, can also play a contributory role to the increasing $\dot{V}_E$ during heavy exercise. Further, it is likely that neural input to the respiratory control center influences the ventilatory pattern during incremental exercise. For example, as exercise intensity increases, motor unit recruitment may occur in a nonlinear fashion, and the associated efferent and afferent neural signals to the respiratory control center may promote the alinear rise in $\dot{V}_E$ seen at the ventilatory threshold (78).

To summarize, the rise in blood hydrogen ions observed at the lactate threshold can stimulate ventilation and thus may be a key mechanism to explain the ventilatory threshold. However, secondary factors such as an increase in blood potassium levels, rising body temperature, elevated blood catecholamines, and afferent neural influences might also contribute to ventilatory control during heavy exercise (see A Closer Look 10.2).

Although many investigators, including Jerome Dempsey, H. V. Forster, Brian Whipp, and Karl Wasserman, have all contributed to our understanding of the control of breathing during exercise, we highlight the career of Karl Wasserman for his important contributions to the study of respiratory function during exercise (see Important People in Science).

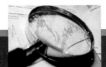
Training Reduces the Ventilatory Response to Exercise

Although exercise training does not alter the structure of the lung, endurance training does promote a decrease in ventilation during submaximal exercise at moderate-to-high-intensity work rates. For example, when comparisons are made at a fixed submaximal work rate, a training program can reduce exercise ventilation by 20% to 30% below pretraining levels (20, 23) (see Fig. 10.29).

What is the mechanism to explain this training-induced reduction in exercise ventilation? A definitive answer is not known. However, this training effect is likely due to changes in the aerobic capacity of the locomotor skeletal muscles. These training-induced changes result in less production of H+ ions and probably less afferent feedback from the working muscles to stimulate breathing (20).

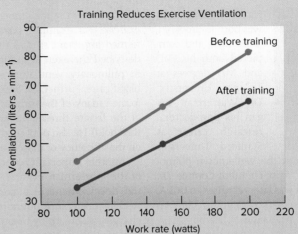

Figure 10.29 Illustration of the effects of endurance training on ventilation during exercise.

IN SUMMARY

- The normal rhythm of breathing is generated by the interaction between separate respiratory rhythm centers located in the medulla oblongata and the pons. At rest, the breathing rhythm is dominated by pacemaker neurons in the preBötzinger Complex.
- During exercise, the respiratory control center receives input from both neural and humoral sources.
- Neural input to the respiratory control center can may come from higher brain centers and from receptors in the exercising muscle.
- Humoral chemoreceptor input to the respiratory control center comes from both central chemoreceptors and peripheral chemoreceptors. The central chemoreceptors are sensitive to increases in PCO_2 and decreases in pH. The peripheral chemoreceptors (carotid bodies are the most important) are sensitive to increases in PCO_2 and decreases in PO_2 or pH.
- A primary drive to increase ventilation during exercise comes from higher brain centers (central command). Importantly, humoral chemoreceptors and neural feedback from working muscles act to fine-tune ventilation and play a significant role in controlling breathing during moderate intensity exercise.

DO THE LUNGS ADAPT TO EXERCISE TRAINING?

It is well known that the muscular–skeletal system and the cardiovascular system are actively engaged during muscular exercise and that both organ systems undergo adaptive changes in response to regular endurance exercise. In contrast, the lungs do not adapt to exercise. Indeed, the lungs in exercise trained individuals are not significantly different from the lungs in a sedentary individual (36, 62). More specifically, endurance exercise training (months to years) has no measurable effect on lung structure and pulmonary function (e.g., diffusion capacity) that will improve pulmonary gas exchange during exercise (36, 62). See McKenzie (2012) for a discussion of the evidence indicating that the lungs do not adapt to exercise training.

If both the cardiovascular system and skeletal muscles adapt to exercise training, why is the adaptability of pulmonary structures substantially less than these other links in the oxygen transport system? The answer is that the structural capacity of the normal lung is "overbuilt" and exceeds the demand for oxygen and carbon dioxide transport in young adults during exercise (36). Therefore, in most individuals, adaptation of the lung to exercise training is not required for the lung to adequately perform the job of maintaining blood-gas homeostasis during exercise. However, one exception to this rule is the highly trained and elite endurance athlete. In a segment of these athletes,

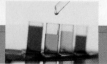
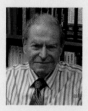
the inability of the lung to increase its gas exchange capabilities in response to exercise training results in a failure of the pulmonary system to match the high requirement for oxygen transfer across the blood–gas barrier during maximal exercise. This failure results in a reduction in the arterial oxygen content (i.e., hypoxemia). The impact of exercise-induced hypoxemia in elite athletes on exercise performance is discussed in the next section.

DOES THE PULMONARY SYSTEM LIMIT MAXIMAL EXERCISE PERFORMANCE?

Although some controversy exists (12), the pulmonary system is not generally considered to be the limiting factor during prolonged submaximal exercise (19, 28, 39, 45). Respiratory muscle failure can occur during certain disease states (e.g., obstructive lung disease), but respiratory muscle fatigue is not thought to limit exercise in healthy humans exercising at low-to-moderate intensity at sea level (28, 39). Indeed, the major muscle of inspiration, the diaphragm, is a highly oxidative muscle that resists fatigue (83, 89, 90). The best evidence that the lungs and respiratory muscles are performing well during prolonged submaximal exercise (e.g., 75% $\dot{V}O_2$ max) is the observation that arterial oxygen content does not decrease during this type of work (84).

Historically, it has not been believed that the pulmonary system limits performance during high-intensity

exercise at sea level (39, 45, 64). However, several studies question this idea. Indeed, growing evidence suggests that the pulmonary system may limit exercise performance during high-intensity exercise (e.g., 95% to 100% $\dot{V}O_2$ max) in trained and untrained healthy subjects. For example, reducing the work of the respiratory muscles (e.g., breathing a low-density helium/oxygen gas) during heavy exercise (90% $\dot{V}O_2$ max) improves exercise performance (63). Breathing this low-density gas decreases the work of breathing and increases the amount of air that can be moved in/out of the lung per minute during heavy exercise. This observation indicates that respiratory muscle fatigue may play a role in limiting human performance at extremely high work rates.

Further, additional research confirms that respiratory muscle fatigue occurs during high-intensity exercise (e.g., ten minutes of exercise at 80% to 85% $\dot{V}O_2$ max) (3). For details on the impact of the respiratory system on exercise performance, see Ask the Expert 10.1. The pulmonary system may also limit performance during high-intensity exercise in the elite endurance athlete who exhibits exercise-induced hypoxemia. Recall that in approximately 40% to 50% of elite endurance athletes, arterial PO_2 declines during heavy exercise to a level that negatively affects their ability to transport oxygen to the working muscles (92, 96, 121) (Fig. 10.22). In these athletes, the pulmonary system cannot keep pace with the need for respiratory gas exchange at workloads near $\dot{V}O_2$ max (30–31, 85, 92, 93). This failure in pulmonary gas exchange may limit exercise performance in these subjects (92).

The Pulmonary System and Exercise Performance Questions and Answers with Dr. Jerome Dempsey

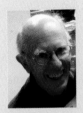

Courtesy of Jerome Dempsey

Jerome Dempsey, Ph.D., a professor emeritus at the University of Wisconsin-Madison, is an internationally known researcher in the field of pulmonary physiology. A significant portion of Dr. Dempsey's research has focused on respiratory gas exchange during exercise and the regulation of pulmonary gas exchange during intense exercise. Without question, Dr. Dempsey's research team has performed many of the "classic" studies that explore the mechanisms responsible for exercise-induced hypoxemia in elite athletes and the effects of exercise on respiratory muscle function. Here, Dr. Dempsey answers questions related to the role that the pulmonary system plays in exercise performance.

QUESTION: Some investigators argue that "specific" training of the respiratory muscles can improve both submaximal and maximal exercise performance. How strong is the evidence to support these claims?

ANSWER: Early research on respiratory muscle training claimed large and unrealistic effects on exercise performance, but these studies did not include placebo controls. When exercise performance is a major outcome variable under consideration, it must be recognized that this has a large volitional component. Therefore, it is essential that the placebo effect be included in the experimental design; i.e., the athletes in both the experimental or control groups must have an "expectation" that their performance will improve as a result of the "treatment." More recently, well-designed studies of respiratory muscle training have shown a small but significant 2% to 3% improvement in time-trial performance (>placebo group) as a result of several weeks of respiratory muscle training, using resistive inspiratory loading. So, if properly done, respiratory muscle training does indeed have a significant, although small, positive influence on endurance performance.

QUESTION: What are the potential mechanism(s) to explain why respiratory muscle training improves exercise performance?

ANSWER: In the absence of direct evidence on this question, we can offer the following possibilities. During heavy-intensity endurance exercise, as the respiratory muscles fatigue (see next) this initiates a metaboreflex from the fatiguing muscles, which increases efferent sympathetic vasoconstrictor activity, which in turn causes a redistribution of blood flow–i.e., reduced blood flow to the limb locomotor muscles and (presumably) increased blood flow to the respiratory muscles. If respiratory muscle training delays the onset of respiratory muscle fatigue during endurance exercise, this will allow less vasoconstriction and therefore greater blood flow and O_2 transport to the exercising limbs, thereby allowing exercise to be sustained longer. We need to add here that highly fit endurance athletes who have not undergone specific respiratory muscle training but who undergo high levels of daily whole-body training also show better conditioned and less fatigable respiratory muscles.

QUESTION: Does whole-body endurance exercise promote respiratory muscle fatigue?

ANSWER: Yes, fatigue of both inspiratory and abdominal expiratory muscles has been demonstrated to result from heavy-intensity endurance exercise in humans of widely varying fitness levels. The method used to quantify this fatigue requires specific electric or magnetic supermaximal stimulation of the motor nerves innervating the diaphragm or expiratory muscles and measurement of a significant reduction in force output of these muscles from pre- to post-exercise, with this fatigue lasting more than 30 to 60 minutes following the exercise. The exercise must be in excess of 80% to 85% of $\dot{V}O_2$ max and be sustained for at least several (>10–15) minutes to the point of volitional exhaustion. It is also known that exercise-induced respiratory muscle fatigue is caused both by the amount of sustained work exerted by the diaphragm (both force production and a high velocity of shortening) and because of the limited amount of blood flow available; i.e., the available total cardiac output must be shared by both the respiratory and limb muscles during heavy exercise.

QUESTION: What are the physiologic effects of respiratory muscle fatigue?

ANSWER: These effects are revealed by the use of a special mechanical ventilator that is capable of unloading the respiratory muscles and substantially reducing the work of breathing during heavy exercise and thereby preventing diaphragm fatigue. Relief of a substantial amount of this high sustained level of respiratory muscle work reduces the rate of development of limb muscle fatigue during whole-body exercise and significantly improves endurance exercise performance. Preventing respiratory muscle fatigue does *not* result in an improvement in ventilation or pulmonary gas exchange, apparently because there is sufficient reserve in the accessory respiratory muscles, and even in the primary inspiratory and expiratory muscles, to provide sufficient alveolar ventilation in healthy subjects. Rather, the major effect of preventing exercise-induced respiratory muscle fatigue is more likely the prevention of the respiratory muscle metaboreflex effects on increasing sympathetically mediated vasoconstriction and an improved vasodilation and blood flow to limb locomotor muscles (see earlier). Please note that these effects of reducing respiratory muscle work on alleviating the development of limb muscle fatigue and increasing exercise performance are present in normal healthy subjects exercising at sea level. These cardiovascular effects of exercise-induced respiratory muscle work are greatly enhanced under conditions of increased ventilation during exercise, such as occurs in healthy subjects in the hypoxia of high altitude and to an even greater extent in patients with chronic heart failure exercising at relatively mild levels at sea level.

IN SUMMARY

■ The pulmonary system does not limit exercise performance in healthy, young subjects during prolonged submaximal exercise (e.g., work rates 90% $\dot{V}O_2$ max).

■ In contrast to submaximal exercise, new evidence indicates that the respiratory system (i.e., respiratory muscle fatigue) may be a limiting factor in exercise performance at work rates >90% $\dot{V}O_2$ max. Further, incomplete pulmonary gas exchange may occur in some elite endurance athletes and limit exercise performance at high exercise intensities.

STUDY ACTIVITIES

1. What is the primary function of the pulmonary system? What secondary functions does it serve?
2. List and discuss the major anatomical components of the respiratory system.
3. What muscle groups are involved in ventilation during rest? During exercise?
4. What is the functional significance of the ventilation-perfusion ratio? How would a high V/Q ratio affect gas exchange in the lung?
5. Discuss those factors that influence the rate of diffusion across the blood-gas interface in the lung.
6. Graph the relationship between hemoglobin-O_2 saturation and the partial pressure of O_2 in the blood. What is the functional significance of the shape of the O_2-hemoglobin dissociation curve? What factors affect the shape of the curve?
7. Discuss the modes of transportation for CO_2 in the blood.
8. Graph the ventilatory response in the transition from rest to constant-load submaximal exercise. What happens to ventilation if the exercise is prolonged and performed in a hot/humid environment? Why?
9. Graph the ventilatory response to incremental exercise. Label the ventilatory threshold. What factor(s) might explain the ventilatory threshold?
10. List and identify the functions of the chemoreceptors that contribute to the control of breathing.
11. What neural afferents might also contribute to the regulation of ventilation during exercise?
12. Discuss the control of ventilation during exercise.

SUGGESTED READINGS

Del Giacco, S., D. Firinu, L. Bjermer, and K. Carlsen. Exercise and asthma: an overview. *European Clinical Respiratory Journal.* 2:27984, 2015.

Dempsey, J. and C. Smith. Pathophysiology of human ventilatory control. *European Respiratory Journal.* 44:495-512, 2014.

Emtner, M. and K. Wadell. Effects of exercise training in patients with chronic obstructive pulmonary disease-a narrative review for FYSS. *British Journal of Sports Medicine.* doi: 10.1136/bjsports-2015-095872, 2016.

Fox, S. *Human Physiology.* New York, NY: McGraw-Hill Companies, 2016.

Garvey, C, M. Bayles, L. Hamm, K. Hill, A. Holland, T. Limberg, and M. Spruit. Pulmonary rehabilitation exercise prescription in chronic obstructive pulmonary disease: Review and selected guidelines: An official statement from the American Association of Cardiovascular and Pulmonary Rehabilitation. *Journal of Cardiopulmonary Rehabilitation Prevention.* 36:75-83, 2016.

McKenzie, D.C. Respiratory physiology: adaptations to high level exercise. *British Journal of Sports Medicine.* 46: 381-384, 2012.

Sheel, A. W., P. Dominelli, and Y. Mogat-Seon. Revisiting dyanapsis: sex-based differences in airways and the mechanics of breathing during exercise. *Experimental Physiology.* 101:213-218, 2016.

West, J. and A. Luks. *Respiratory Physiology–The Essentials.* Philadelphia, PA: Lippincott Williams & Wilkins, 2015.

Widmaier, E., H. Raff, and K. Strang. *Vander's Human Physiology.* New York, NY: McGraw-Hill Companies, 2016.

REFERENCES

1. **Allen CJ and Jones NL.** Rate of change of alveolar carbon dioxide and the control of ventilation during exercise. *Journal of Physiology* 355: 1-9, 1984.
2. **Asmussen E.** Control of ventilation in exercise. In: *Exercise and Sport Science Reviews*, edited by Terjung R. Philadelphia, PA: Franklin Press, 1983.
3. **Babcock MA, Pegelow DF, Harms CA, and Dempsey JA.** Effects of respiratory muscle unloading on exercise-induced diaphragm fatigue. *Journal of Applied Physiology* 93: 201-206, 2002.
4. **Band DM, Wolff CB, Ward J, Cochrane GM, and Prior J.** Respiratory oscillations in arterial carbon dioxide tension as a control signal in exercise. *Nature* 283: 84-85, 1980.
5. **Banzett RB, Coleridge HM, and Coleridge JC.** I. Pulmonary-CO_2 ventilatory reflex in dogs: effective range of CO_2 and results of vagal cooling. *Respiration Physiology* 34: 121-134, 1978.
6. **Beaver WL, Wasserman K, and Whipp BJ.** A new method for detecting anaerobic threshold by gas exchange. *Journal of Applied Physiology* 60: 2020-2027, 1986.
7. **Bellissimo N, Thomas SG, Goode RC, and Anderson GH.** Effect of short-duration physical activity and ventilation threshold on subjective appetite and short-term energy intake in boys. *Appetite* 49: 644-651, 2007.
8. **Bennett FM and Fordyce WE.** Characteristics of the ventilatory exercise stimulus. *Respiration Physiology* 59: 55-63, 1985.
9. **Bennett FM, Tallman RD, Jr., and Grodins FS.** Role of VCO_2 in control of breathing of awake exercising dogs. *Journal of Applied Physiology* 56: 1335-1339, 1984.
10. **Bisgard GE, Forster HV, Mesina J, and Sarazin RG.** Role of the carotid body in hyperpnea of moderate exercise in goats. *Journal of Applied Physiology* 52: 1216-1222, 1982.
11. **Boon JK, Kuhlmann WD, and Fedde MR.** Control of respiration in the chicken: effects of venous CO_2 loading. *Respiration Physiology* 39: 169-181, 1980.

12. **Boutellier U and Piwko P.** The respiratory system as an exercise limiting factor in normal sedentary subjects. *European Journal of Applied Physiology* 64: 145-152, 1992.

13. **Brice AG, Forster HV, Pan LG, Funahashi A, Hoffman MD, Murphy CL, and Lowry TF.** Is the hyperpnea of muscular contractions critically dependent on spinal afferents? *Journal of Applied Physiology* 64: 226-233, 1988.

14. **Brice AG, Forster HV, Pan LG, Funahashi A, Lowry TF, Murphy CL, and Hoffman MD.** Ventilatory and PaCO$_2$ responses to voluntary and electrically induced leg exercise. *Journal of Applied Physiology* 64: 218-225, 1988.

15. **Brown DR, Forster HV, Pan LG, Brice AG, Murphy CL, Lowry TF, Gutting SM, Funahashi A, Hoffman M, and Powers S.** Ventilatory response of spinal cord-lesioned subjects to electrically induced exercise. *Journal of Applied Physiology* 68: 2312-2321, 1990.

16. **Brown HV, Wasserman K, and Whipp BJ.** Effect of beta-adrenergic blockade during exercise on ventilation and gas exchange. *Journal of Applied Physiology* 41: 886-892, 1976.

17. **Busse MW, Maassen N, and Konrad H.** Relation between plasma K+ and ventilation during incremental exercise after glycogen depletion and repletion in man. *Journal of Physiology* 443: 469-476, 1991.

18. **Caiozzo VJ, Davis JA, Ellis JF, Azus JL, Vandagriff R, Prietto CA, and McMaster WC.** A comparison of gas exchange indices used to detect the anaerobic threshold. *Journal of Applied Physiology* 53: 1184-1189, 1982.

19. **Capen RL, Hanson WL, Latham LP, Dawson CA, and Wagner WW, Jr.** Distribution of pulmonary capillary transit times in recruited networks. *Journal of Applied Physiology* 69: 473-478, 1990.

20. **Casaburi R, Storer TW, and Wasserman K.** Mediation of reduced ventilatory response to exercise after endurance training. *Journal of Applied Physiology* 63: 1533-1538, 1987.

21. **Casaburi R, Whipp BJ, Wasserman K, Beaver WL, and Koyal SN.** Ventilatory and gas exchange dynamics in response to sinusoidal work. *Journal of Applied Physiology* 42: 300-301, 1977.

22. **Casaburi R, Whipp BJ, Wasserman K, and Stremel RW.** Ventilatory control characteristics of the exercise hyperpnea as discerned from dynamic forcing techniques. *Chest* 73: 280-283, 1978.

23. **Clanton TL, Dixon GF, Drake J, and Gadek JE.** Effects of swim training on lung volumes and inspiratory muscle conditioning. *Journal of Applied Physiology* 62: 39-46, 1987.

24. **Coleridge H and Coleridge J.** Airway axon reflexes–where now? *News in Physiological Sciences* 10: 91-96, 1995.

25. **Davidson AC, Auyeung V, Luff R, Holland M, Hodgkiss A, and Weinman J.** Prolonged benefit in post-polio syndrome from comprehensive rehabilitation: a pilot study. *Disability and Rehabilitation* 31: 309-317, 2009.

26. **Del Giacco, S., D. Firinu, L. Bjermer, and K. Carlsen.** Exercise and asthma: an overview. *European Clinical Respiratory Journal* 2:27984, 2015.

27. **Dempsey J, Blain G, and Amann M.** Are type II-IV afferents required for a normal steady-state exercise hyperpnea in humans? *Journal of Physiology* 592: 463-474, 2014.

28. **Dempsey J, Aaron E, and Martin B.** Pulmonary function during prolonged exercise. In: *Perspectives in Exercise and Sports Medicine: Prolonged Exercise*, edited by Lamb D, and Murray R. Indianapolis, IN: Benchmark Press, 1988, p. 75-119.

29. **Dempsey J, Forster H, and Ainsworth D.** Regulation of hyperpnea, hyperventilation, and respiratory muscle recruitment during exercise. In: *Regulation of Breathing*, edited by Pack A, and Dempsey J. New York, NY: Marcel Dekker, 1994, p. 1034-1065.

30. **Dempsey J, Hanson P, Pegelow D, Claremont A, and Rankin J.** Limitations to exercise capacity and endurance: pulmonary system. *Canadian Journal of Applied Sport Sciences* 7: 4-13, 1982.

31. **Dempsey, J., G. Blain, and M. Amann.** Are the type III-IV muscle afferents required for normal steady-state exercise hyperpnoea in humans. *Journal of Physiology* 592:463-474, 2014.

32. **Dempsey J and C Smith.** Pathophysiology of human ventilatory control. *European Respiratory Journal* 44:495-512, 2014.

33. **Dempsey JA and Fregosi RF.** Adaptability of the pulmonary system to changing metabolic requirements. *American Journal of Cardiology* 55: 59D-67D, 1985.

34. **Dempsey JA, McKenzie DC, Haverkamp HC, and Eldridge MW.** Update in the understanding of respiratory limitations to exercise performance in fit, active adults. *Chest* 134: 613-622, 2008.

35. **Dempsey JA, Mitchell GS, and Smith CA.** Exercise and chemoreception. *American Review of Respiratory Disease* 129: S31-34, 1984.

36. **Dempsey JA, Sheel AW, Haverkamp HC, Babcock MA, and Harms CA.** [The John Sutton Lecture: CSEP, 2002]. Pulmonary system limitations to exercise in health. *Canadian Journal of Applied Physiology* 28 Suppl: S2-24, 2003.

37. **Dempsey JA, Vidruk EH, and Mitchell GS.** Pulmonary control systems in exercise: update. *Federation Proceedings* 44: 2260-2270, 1985.

38. **Dodd S, Powers S, O'Malley N, Brooks E, and Sommers H.** Effects of beta-adrenergic blockade on ventilation and gas exchange during the rest to work transition. *Aviation, Space, and Environmental Medicine* 59: 255-258, 1988.

39. **Dodd SL, Powers SK, Thompson D, Landry G, and Lawler J.** Exercise performance following intense, short-term ventilatory work. *International Journal of Sports Medicine* 10: 48-52, 1989.

40. **Domino KB, Eisenstein BL, Cheney FW, and Hlastala MP.** Pulmonary blood flow and ventilation-perfusion heterogeneity. *Journal of Applied Physiology* 71: 252-258, 1991.

41. **Dominelli, P., J. Render, Y. molgat-Seon, G. Foster, L. Romer, and A. Sheel.** Oxygen cost of exercise hyperpnoea is greater in women compared with men. *Journal of Physiology* 593: 1965-1979, 2015.

42. **Emtner M and K Wadell.** Effects of exercise training in patients with chronic obstructive pulmonary disease-a narrative review for FYSS. *British Journal of Sports Medicine.* doi:10.1136/bjsports-2015-095872, 2016.

43. **Eldridge FL, Millhorn DE, and Waldrop TG.** Exercise hyperpnea and locomotion: parallel activation from the hypothalamus. *Science* 211: 844-846, 1981.

44. **England P.** The effect of acute thermal dehydration on blood lactate accumulation during incremental exercise. *Journal of Sports Sciences* 2: 105-111, 1985.

45. **Fairbarn MS, Coutts KC, Pardy RL, and McKenzie DC.** Improved respiratory muscle endurance of highly trained cyclists and the effects on maximal exercise performance. *International Journal of Sports Medicine* 12: 66-70, 1991.

46. **Favier R, Desplanches D, Frutoso J, Grandmontagne M, and Flandrois R.** Ventilatory and circulatory transients during exercise: new arguments for a neurohumoral theory. *Journal of Applied Physiology* 54: 647-653, 1983.

47. **Feldman JL and Del Negro CA.** Looking for inspiration: new perspectives on respiratory rhythm. *Nature Reviews Neuroscience* 7: 232-242, 2006.

48. **Forster H and Pan L.** Exercise hyperpnea: characteristics and control. In: *The Lung: Scientific Foundations*, edited by Crystal R, and West J. New York, NY: Raven Press, 1991, p. 1553-1564.

49. **Forster HV and Smith CA.** Contributions of central and peripheral chemoreceptors to the ventilatory response to $CO_2/H+$. *Journal of Applied Physiology* 108: 989-994, 2010.

50. **Garvey, C., M. Bayles, L. Hamm, K. Hill, A. Holland, T. Limberg, and M. Spruit.** Pulmonary rehabilitation exercise prescription in chronic obstructive pulmonary disease: Review and selected guidelines: An official statement from the American Association of Cardiovascular and Pulmonary Rehabilitation. *Journal of Cardiopulmonary Rehabilitation Prevention.* 36:75-83, 2016.

51. **Green JF and Schmidt ND.** Mechanism of hyperpnea induced by changes in pulmonary blood flow. *Journal of Applied Physiology* 56: 1418-1422, 1984.

52. **Green JF and Sheldon MI.** Ventilatory changes associated with changes in pulmonary blood flow in dogs. *Journal of Applied Physiology* 54: 997-1002, 1983.

53. **Grucza R, Miyamoto Y, and Nakazono Y.** Kinetics of cardiorespiratory response to dynamic and rhythmic-static exercise in men. *European Journal of Applied Physiology* 61: 230-236, 1990.

54. **Guenette JA and Sheel AW.** Exercise-induced arterial hypoxaemia in active young women. *Applied Physiology, Nutrition, and Metabolism* 32: 1263-1273, 2007.

55. **Hagberg JM, Coyle EF, Carroll JE, Miller JM, Martin WH, and Brooke MH.** Exercise hyperventilation in patients with McArdle's disease. *Journal of Applied Physiology* 52: 991-994, 1982.

56. **Hammond MD, Gale GE, Kapitan KS, Ries A, and Wagner PD.** Pulmonary gas exchange in humans during exercise at sea level. *Journal of Applied Physiology* 60: 1590-1598, 1986.

57. **Hansen JE, Ulubay G, Chow BF, Sun XG, and Wasserman K.** Mixed-expired and end-tidal CO_2 distinguish between ventilation and perfusion defects during exercise testing in patients with lung and heart diseases. *Chest* 132: 977-983, 2007.

58. **Harms CA, McClaran SR, Nickele GA, Pegelow DF, Nelson WB, and Dempsey JA.** Effect of exercise-induced arterial O_2 desaturation on $\dot{V}O_2$ max in women. *Medicine & Science in Sports & Exercise* 32: 1101-1108, 2000.

59. **Harms CA, McClaran SR, Nickele GA, Pegelow DF, Nelson WB, and Dempsey JA.** Exercise-induced arterial hypoxaemia in healthy young women. *The Journal of Physiology* 507 (Pt 2): 619-628, 1998.

60. **Hawgood S and Shiffer K.** Structures and properties of the surfactant-associated proteins. *Annual Review of Physiology* 53: 375-394, 1991.

61. **Hopkins SR, Barker RC, Brutsaert TD, Gavin TP, Entin P, Olfert IM, Veisel S, and Wagner PD.** Pulmonary gas exchange during exercise in women: effects of exercise type and work increment. *Journal of Applied Physiology* 89: 721-730, 2000.

62. **Hopkins SR and Harms CA.** Gender and pulmonary gas exchange during exercise. *Exercise and Sport Sciences Reviews* 32: 50-56, 2004.

63. **Johnson BD, Aaron EA, Babcock MA, and Dempsey JA.** Respiratory muscle fatigue during exercise: implications for performance. *Medicine & Science in Sports & Exercise* 28: 1129-1137, 1996.

64. **Johnson BD and Dempsey JA.** Demand vs. capacity in the aging pulmonary system. *Exercise and Sport Sciences Reviews* 19: 171-210, 1991.

65. **Kao F.** An experimental study of the pathways involved in exercise hyperpnea employing cross-circulation techniques. In: *The Regulation of Human Respiration*, edited by Cunningham D. Oxford: Blackwell, 1963.

66. **Kavazis AN, DeRuisseau KC, McClung JM, Whidden MA, Falk DJ, Smuder AJ, Sugiura T, and Powers SK.** Diaphragmatic proteasome function is maintained in the ageing Fisher 344 rat. *Experimental Physiology* 92: 895-901, 2007.

67. **Levitzky M.** *Pulmonary Physiology.* New York, NY: McGraw-Hill 2007.

68. **Lindinger MI and Sjogaard G.** Potassium regulation during exercise and recovery. *Sports Medicine* 11: 382-401, 1991.

69. **Lumb AB.** *Nunn's Applied Respiratory Physiology.* Oxford: Butterworth-Heinemann, 2010.

70. **Mairbaurl H, Schobersberger W, Hasibeder W, Schwaberger G, Gaesser G, and Tanaka KR.** Regulation of red cell 2,3-DPG and Hb-O_2-affinity during acute exercise. *European Journal of Applied Physiology* 55: 174-180, 1986.

71. **McParland C, Mink J, and Gallagher CG.** Respiratory adaptations to dead space loading during maximal incremental exercise. *Journal of Applied Physiology* 70: 55-62, 1991.

72. **Moreira A, Delgado L, and Carlsen KH.** Exercise-induced asthma: why is it so frequent in Olympic athletes? *Expert Review of Respiratory Medicine* 5: 1-3, 2011.

73. **Nielsen H.** Arterial desaturation during exercise in man: implications for O_2 uptake and work capacity. *Scandinavian Journal of Medicine in Science and Sports* 13: 339-358, 2003.

74. **Pan LG, Forster HV, Wurster RD, Brice AG, and Lowry TF.** Effect of multiple denervations on the exercise hyperpnea in awake ponies. *Journal of Applied Physiology* 79: 302-311, 1995.

75. **Paterson DJ.** Potassium and ventilation in exercise. *Journal of Applied Physiology* 72: 811-820, 1992.

76. **Paulev PE, Mussell MJ, Miyamoto Y, Nakazono Y, and Sugawara T.** Modeling of alveolar carbon dioxide oscillations with or without exercise. *The Japanese Journal of Physiology* 40: 893-905, 1990.

77. **Powers S.** Ventilatory threshold, running economy, and distance running performance. *Research Quarterly for Exercise and Sport* 54: 179-182, 1983.

78. **Powers S and Beadle R.** Onset of hyperventilation during incremental exercise: a brief review. *Research Quarterly for Exercise and Sport* 56: 352-360, 1985.

79. **Powers SK and Beadle RE.** Control of ventilation during submaximal exercise: a brief review. *Journal of Sports Sciences* 3: 51-65, 1985.

80. **Powers SK, Beadle RE, Thompson D, and Lawler J.** Ventilatory and blood gas dynamics at onset and offset of exercise in the pony. *Journal of Applied Physiology* 62: 141-148, 1987.

81. **Powers SK, Coombes J, and Demirel H.** Exercise training-induced changes in respiratory muscles. *Sports Medicine* 24: 120-131, 1997.

82. **Powers SK and Criswell D.** Adaptive strategies of respiratory muscles in response to endurance exercise. *Medicine & Science in Sports & Exercise* 28: 1115-1122, 1996.

83. **Powers SK, Criswell D, Lawler J, Martin D, Ji LL, Herb RA, and Dudley G.** Regional training-induced alterations in diaphragmatic oxidative and antioxidant enzymes. *Respiration Physiology* 95: 227-237, 1994.

84. **Powers SK, Dodd S, Criswell DD, Lawler J, Martin D, and Grinton S.** Evidence for an alveolar-arterial PO_2 gradient threshold during incremental exercise. *International Journal of Sports Medicine* 12: 313-318, 1991.

85. **Powers SK, Dodd S, Lawler J, Landry G, Kirtley M, McKnight T, and Grinton S.** Incidence of

exercise-induced hypoxemia in elite endurance athletes at sea level. *European Journal of Applied Physiology* 58: 298-302, 1988.

86. **Powers SK, Dodd S, Woodyard J, Beadle RE, and Church G.** Haemoglobin saturation during incremental arm and leg exercise. *British Journal of Sports Medicine* 18: 212-216, 1984.

87. **Powers SK, Dodd S, Woodyard J, and Mangum M.** Caffeine alters ventilatory and gas exchange kinetics during exercise. *Medicine & Science in Sports & Exercise* 18: 101-106, 1986.

88. **Powers SK, Howley ET, and Cox R.** Ventilatory and metabolic reactions to heat stress during prolonged exercise. *The Journal of Sports Medicine and Physical Fitness* 22: 32-36, 1982.

89. **Powers SK, Lawler J, Criswell D, Dodd S, Grinton S, Bagby G, and Silverman H.** Endurance-training-induced cellular adaptations in respiratory muscles. *Journal of Applied Physiology* 68: 2114-2118, 1990.

90. **Powers SK, Lawler J, Criswell D, Lieu FK, and Martin D.** Aging and respiratory muscle metabolic plasticity: effects of endurance training. *Journal of Applied Physiology* 72: 1068-1073, 1992.

91. **Powers SK, Lawler J, Criswell D, Silverman H, Forster HV, Grinton S, and Harkins D.** Regional metabolic differences in the rat diaphragm. *Journal of Applied Physiology* 69: 648-650, 1990.

92. **Powers SK, Lawler J, Dempsey JA, Dodd S, and Landry G.** Effects of incomplete pulmonary gas exchange on $\dot{V}O_2$ max. *Journal of Applied Physiology* 66: 2491-2495, 1989.

93. **Powers SK, Martin D, Cicale M, Collop N, Huang D, and Criswell D.** Exercise-induced hypoxemia in athletes: role of inadequate hyperventilation. *European Journal of Applied Physiology* 65: 37-42, 1992.

94. **Powers SK and Shanely RA.** Exercise-induced changes in diaphragmatic bioenergetic and antioxidant capacity. *Exercise and Sport Sciences Reviews* 30: 69-74, 2002.

95. **Powers SK, Stewart MK, and Landry G.** Ventilatory and gas exchange dynamics in response to head-down tilt with and without venous occlusion. *Aviation, Space, and Environmental Medicine* 59: 239-245, 1988.

96. **Powers SK, and Williams J.** Exercise-induced hypoxemia in highly trained athletes. *Sports Medicine* 4: 46-53, 1987.

97. **Ramonatxo M, Mercier J, Cohendy R, and Prefaut C.** Effect of resistive loads on pattern of respiratory muscle recruitment during exercise. *Journal of Applied Physiology* 71: 1941-1948, 1991.

98. **Sheel, A. W., P. Dominelli, and Y. Mogat-Seon.** Revisiting dyanapsis: sex-based differences in airways and the mechanics of breathing during exercise. *Experimental Physiology.* 101:213-218, 2016.

99. **Spodaryk K and Zoladz JA.** The 2,3-DPG levels of human red blood cells during an incremental exercise test: relationship to the blood acid-base balance. *Physiological Research* 47: 17-22, 1998.

100. **St John WM and Paton JF.** Role of pontile mechanisms in the neurogenesis of eupnea. *Respiratory Physiology & Neurobiology* 143: 321-332, 2004.

101. **Stamenovic D.** Micromechanical foundations of pulmonary elasticity. *Physiological Reviews* 70: 1117-1134, 1990.

102. **Stringer W, Casaburi R, and Wasserman K.** Acid-base regulation during exercise and recovery in humans. *Journal of Applied Physiology* 72: 954-961, 1992.

103. **Suzuki S, Suzuki J, and Okubo T.** Expiratory muscle fatigue in normal subjects. *Journal of Applied Physiology* 70: 2632-2639, 1991.

104. **Tibes U.** Reflex inputs to the cardiovascular and respiratory centers from dynamically working canine muscles.

Some evidence for involvement of group III or IV nerve fibers. *Circulation Research* 41: 332-341, 1977.

105. **Trenchard D, Russell NJ, and Raybould HE.** Non-myelinated vagal lung receptors and their reflex effects on respiration in rabbits. *Respiration Physiology* 55: 63-79, 1984.

106. **Vincent HK, Powers SK, Demirel HA, Coombes JS, and Naito H.** Exercise training protects against contraction-induced lipid peroxidation in the diaphragm. *European Journal of Applied Physiology and Occupational Physiology* 79: 268-273, 1999.

107. **Vincent HK, Powers SK, Stewart DJ, Demirel HA, Shanely RA, and Naito H.** Short-term exercise training improves diaphragm antioxidant capacity and endurance. *European Journal of Applied Physiology* 81: 67-74, 2000.

108. **Vincent HK, Shanely RA, Stewart DJ, Demirel HA, Hamilton KL, Ray AD, Michlin C, Farkas GA, and Powers SK.** Adaptation of upper airway muscles to chronic endurance exercise. *American Journal of Respiratory and Critical Care Medicine* 166: 287-293, 2002.

109. **Virkki A, Polo O, Gyllenberg M, and Aittokallio T.** Can carotid body perfusion act as a respiratory controller? *Journal of Theoretical Biology* 249: 737-748, 2007.

110. **Walker DJ, Walterspacher S, Schlager D, Ertl T, Roecker K, Windisch W, and Kabitz HJ.** Characteristics of diaphragmatic fatigue during exhaustive exercise until task failure. *Respiratory Physiology & Neurobiology* 176: 14-20, 2011.

111. **Warren GL, Cureton KJ, Middendorf WF, Ray CA, and Warren JA.** Red blood cell pulmonary capillary transit time during exercise in athletes. *Medicine & Science in Sports & Exercise* 23: 1353-1361, 1991.

112. **Wasserman K.** The anaerobic threshold measurement to evaluate exercise performance. *American Review of Respiratory Disease* 129: S35-40, 1984.

113. **Wasserman K.** CO_2 flow to the lungs and ventilatory control. In: *Muscular Exercise and the Lung*, edited by Dempsey J, and Reed C. Madison, WI: University of Wisconsin Press, 1977.

114. **Wasserman K, Whipp BJ, Koyl SN, and Beaver WL.** Anaerobic threshold and respiratory gas exchange during exercise. *Journal of Applied Physiology* 35: 236-243, 1973.

115. **Weissman ML, Jones PW, Oren A, Lamarra N, Whipp BJ, and Wasserman K.** Cardiac output increase and gas exchange at start of exercise. *Journal of Applied Physiology* 52: 236-244, 1982.

116. **West J.** *Pulmonary Pathophysiology.* Philadelphia, PA: Lippincott Williams & Wilkins, 2012.

117. **West J and Wagner P.** Ventilation-perfusion relationships. In: *The Lung: Scientific Foundations*, edited by Crystal R, and West J. New York, NY: Raven Press, 1991, p. 1289-1305.

118. **West JB and A. Luks.** *Respiratory Physiology: The Essentials.* Philadelphia, PA: Wolters Kluwer/Lippincott Williams & Wilkins, 2015.

119. **Wetter TJ, Xiang Z, Sonetti DA, Haverkamp HC, Rice AJ, Abbasi AA, Meyer KC, and Dempsey JA.** Role of lung inflammatory mediators as a cause of exercise-induced arterial hypoxemia in young athletes. *Journal of Applied Physiology* 93: 116-126, 2002.

120. **Whipp BJ and Ward SA.** Physiological determinants of pulmonary gas exchange kinetics during exercise. *Medicine & Science in Sports & Exercise* 22: 62-71, 1990.

121. **Williams JH, Powers SK, and Stuart MK.** Hemoglobin desaturation in highly trained athletes during heavy exercise. *Medicine & Science in Sports & Exercise* 18: 168-173, 1986.

122. **Yamamoto WS and Edwards MW, Jr.** Homeostasis of carbon dioxide during intravenous infusion of carbon dioxide. *Journal of Applied Physiology* 15: 807-818, 1960.

11

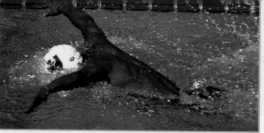

© Action Plus Sports Images/Alamy Stock Photo

Acid-Base Balance during Exercise

■ Objectives

By studying this chapter, you should be able to do the following:

1. Define the terms *acid*, *base*, and *pH*.
2. Discuss the principal ways that hydrogen ions are produced during exercise.
3. Discuss the importance of acid-base regulation to exercise performance.
4. List the principal intracellular and extracellular buffers.

5. Explain the role of respiration in the regulation of acid-base status during exercise.
6. Outline the interaction between intracellular/extracellular buffers and the respiratory system in acid-base regulation during exercise.

■ Outline

■ Key Terms

acid
acidosis
alkalosis
base
buffer
hydrogen ion
ion
pH
respiratory compensation
strong acids
strong bases

An **ion** is any atom that is missing electrons or has gained electrons. A **hydrogen ion** is formed by the loss of the electron; molecules that release hydrogen ions are called *acids*. Substances that readily combine with hydrogen ions are termed *bases*. In physiology, the concentration of hydrogen ions in body fluids is expressed in pH units. The pH of body fluids must be regulated (i.e., normal arterial blood pH = 7.40 ± .02) in order to maintain homeostasis. This regulation of the pH of body fluids is important because changes in hydrogen ion concentrations can alter the rates of enzyme-controlled metabolic reactions and modify numerous other normal body functions. Therefore, acid-base balance is primarily concerned with the regulation of hydrogen ion concentrations. High-intensity exercise can present a serious challenge to hydrogen ion control systems due to hydrogen ion production, and hydrogen ions may limit performance in some types of intense activities (7, 14, 16, 20, 40). Therefore, given the potential detrimental influence of hydrogen ion accumulation on exercise performance, it is important to have an understanding of acid-base regulation.

ACIDS, BASES, AND pH

In biological systems, one of the simplest but most important ions is the hydrogen ion. The concentration of hydrogen ions influences the rates of chemical reactions, the shape and function of enzymes as well as other cellular proteins, and the integrity of the cell itself (10, 46).

An **acid** is defined as a molecule that releases hydrogen ions and thus can raise the hydrogen ion concentration of a solution above that of pure water. In contrast, a **base** is a molecule that is capable of combining with hydrogen ions, which would lower the hydrogen ion concentration of the solution.

Acids that give up hydrogen ions (ionize) more completely are called **strong acids.** For example, sulfuric acid is produced by the metabolism of sulfur-containing amino acids (e.g., cysteine) and is a strong acid. At normal body pH, sulfuric acid liberates almost all of its hydrogen ions and therefore elevates the hydrogen ion concentration of the body.

Bases that ionize more completely are defined as **strong bases.** The bicarbonate ion HCO_3^- is an example of a biologically important strong base. Bicarbonate ions are found in relatively large concentrations in the body. Importantly, bicarbonate ions are capable of combining with hydrogen ions to form a weak acid called carbonic acid. The role of HCO_3^- in the regulation of acid-base balance during exercise will be discussed later in the chapter.

As stated earlier, the concentration of hydrogen ions is expressed in pH units on a scale that runs from 0 to 14. Solutions that contain pH values below 7 are acidic, whereas pH values above 7 are basic. The **pH** of a solution is defined as the negative logarithm of the hydrogen ion concentration (H^+). Recall that a logarithm is the exponent that indicates the power to which one number must be raised to obtain another number. For instance, the logarithm of 100 to the base 10 is 2. Thus, the definition of pH can be written mathematically as:

$$pH = -\log_{10} [H^+]$$

As an example, if the $[H^+] = 40\,nM\,(0.000000040\,M)$, then the pH would be 7.40. A solution is considered neutral in terms of acid-base status if the concentration of H^+ and hydroxyl ions (OH^-) are equal. This is the case for pure water, in which the concentrations for both H^+ and OH^- are 0.00000010 M. Thus, the pH of pure water is:

$$pH \text{ (pure water)} = -\log_{10} [H^+]$$
$$= 7.0$$

Figure 11.1 illustrates the pH scale and highlights that the normal pH of arterial blood is 7.4. Note that as the hydrogen ion concentration increases, pH declines and the acidity of the blood increases, resulting in a condition termed **acidosis.** Conversely, as the hydrogen ion concentration decreases, pH increases and the solution becomes more basic (alkalotic). This condition is termed **alkalosis.** Conditions leading to acidosis or alkalosis are summarized in Figure 11.2.

Again, the normal arterial pH is 7.4, and in healthy people, this value varies less than 0.05 pH unit (42). Failure to maintain acid-base homeostasis in the body can have serious consequences. Indeed, even small changes in blood pH can have negative effects on the function of organ systems. In particular, acidosis can cause dysfunction of both the central nervous system and the cardiovascular system. For example, acidosis can lead to mental confusion and a feeling of fatigue. Further, both increases and decreases in arterial pH can promote abnormal electrical activity in the heart, resulting in rhythm disturbances, and arterial pH values below 7.0 and above 7.8 can have lethal consequences (12, 42). Numerous disease states can result in acid-base disturbances in the body and are introduced in Clinical Applications 11.1.

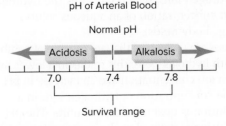

Figure 11.1 The pH scale. If the pH of arterial blood drops below the normal value of 7.4, the resulting condition is termed acidosis. In contrast, if the pH increases above 7.4, blood alkalosis occurs.

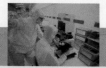

CLINICAL APPLICATIONS 11.1

Conditions and Diseases That Promote Metabolic Acidosis or Alkalosis

As mentioned previously, failure to maintain acid-base homeostasis in the body can have serious consequences and can lead to dysfunction of essential organs. Indeed, even relatively small changes in arterial pH (i.e., 0.1-0.2 pH units) can have a significant negative affect on organ function (12).

Metabolic acidosis occurs due to a gain in the amount of acid in the body. A number of conditions and disease states can promote metabolic acidosis. For example, long-term starvation (i.e., several days without food) can result in metabolic acidosis due to the production of ketoacids in the body as a by-product of high levels of fat metabolism. In extreme circumstances, the type of metabolic acidosis can result in death.

Diabetes is a common metabolic disease that promotes metabolic acidosis. Uncontrolled diabetes can result in a form of metabolic acidosis called diabetic ketoacidosis. Similar to starvation-induced acidosis, this form of acidosis is also due to the overproduction of ketoacids due to high levels of fat metabolism. Worldwide, numerous deaths occur each year from this form of acidosis (12, 42).

Metabolic alkalosis results from a loss of acids from the body. Conditions leading to metabolic alkalosis include severe vomiting and diseases such as kidney disorders that result in a loss of acids (12, 42). In both of these circumstances, the loss of acids results in an overabundance of bases in the body, leading to metabolic alkalosis.

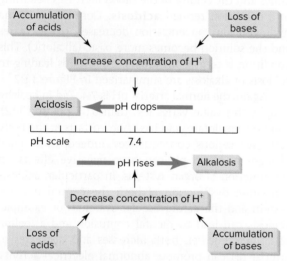

Figure 11.2   Acidosis results from an accumulation of acids or a loss of bases. Alkalosis results from a loss of acids or an accumulation of bases.

IN SUMMARY

- Acids are defined as molecules that release hydrogen ions, which increases the hydrogen ion concentration of an aqueous solution (e.g., body fluids).
- Bases are molecules that are capable of combining with hydrogen ions; this results in a lower hydrogen ion concentration and an increase in pH.
- The concentration of hydrogen ions in a solution is quantified by pH units. The pH of a solution is defined as the negative logarithm of the hydrogen ion concentration:

$$pH = -\log_{10} [H^+]$$

HYDROGEN ION PRODUCTION DURING EXERCISE

Much debate exists regarding the primary sites of hydrogen ion production during exercise (3, 18, 28). Nonetheless, it is clear that high-intensity exercise results in a marked decrease in both muscle and blood pH. Current evidence indicates that the exercise-induced decrease in muscle pH is due to multiple factors. Three important contributors to exercise-induced muscle acidosis are outlined here (11, 25):

1. **Exercise-induced production of carbon dioxide and carbonic acid in the working skeletal muscles.** Carbon dioxide, an end product in the oxidation of carbohydrates, fats, and proteins, is regarded as an acid by virtue of its ability to react with water to form carbonic acid (H_2CO_3), which in turn dissociates to form H^+ and bicarbonate (HCO_3^-):

$$CO_2 + H_2O \longleftrightarrow H^+ + HCO_3^-$$

Because CO_2 is a gas and can be eliminated by the lungs, it is often referred to as a *volatile acid*. During the course of a day, the body produces large amounts of CO_2 due to normal metabolism. During exercise, metabolic production of CO_2 increases and therefore adds a "volatile acid" load on the body.

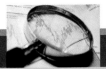

A CLOSER LOOK 11.1

Sport and Exercise-Induced Disturbances in Muscle Acid-Base Balance

What types of sports or exercise promote acid-base disturbances in skeletal muscle? In general, any sport or exercise activity requiring high-intensity muscular contractions that persist for 45 seconds or longer can produce significant amounts of hydrogen ions, resulting in a decrease in muscle and blood pH. Table 11.1 provides a list of popular sports and the risk of developing muscle acid-base disturbances in each sport. Note that the risk of acid-base disturbances is classified as being high, moderate, or low. For sports classified in the low-to-moderate risk category (e.g., soccer), the risk of muscle acid-base disturbance is often connected to effort of the competitor. That is, an aggressive athlete that is constantly playing at 100% effort is more likely to develop an acid-base imbalance compared to the athlete that plays at "half speed" during the game. Also, note that track and field races like the 5,000- and 10,000-meter runs are listed as moderate and low to moderate risks for acid-base disturbances, respectively. In these types of track races, athletes generally produce small amounts of hydrogen ions during most of the race, but a sustained sprint to the finish during the last lap of these events could result in production of relatively large amounts of hydrogen ions and, therefore, result in acid-base disturbances in the muscle and blood.

Because acid-base disturbances can contribute to muscle fatigue and limit exercise performance, it is not surprising that scientists have investigated the possibility that increasing the buffering capacity of the blood results in improved exercise performance. One approach to this problem is to ingest large quantities of a buffer prior to exercise. A discussion of this topic can be found in The Winning Edge 11.1.

2. **Exercise-induced production of lactic acid in the working muscle.** Although controversy exists, it is likely that production of lactic acid (lactate) in the muscle during heavy exercise is a key factor that causes the decrease in muscle pH (3, 28).

3. **Exercise-induced ATP breakdown in the working muscles.** The breakdown of ATP for energy during muscle contraction results in the release of H$^+$ ions (36). For example, the breakdown of ATP results in the following reaction:

$$ATP + H_2O \rightarrow ADP + HPO_4 + H^+$$

Therefore, the breakdown of ATP alone during exercise can be an important source of H$^+$ ions in contracting muscles.

To summarize, debate exists about the primary causes of exercise-induced acidosis. Nonetheless, it is clear that contracting muscles can produce H$^+$ from several sites; therefore, the cause of exercise-induced acidosis is likely due to the production of H$^+$ ions from several different sources. Figure 11.3 provides a summary of the three major metabolic processes that serve as primary sources of hydrogen ions in working skeletal muscle. A discussion of which sports or exercise activities pose the greatest risk of acid-base disturbances is contained in A Closer Look 11.1. Table 11.3 provides an estimate of the risk of developing acidosis in several popular sports.

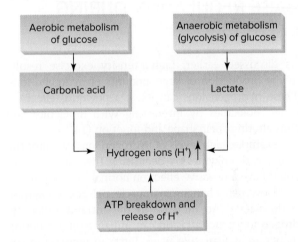

Figure 11.3 Primary sources of hydrogen ions in contracting skeletal muscles.

IN SUMMARY

- High-intensity exercise results in a marked decrease in both muscle and blood pH.
- This exercise-induced decrease in muscle pH is due to multiple factors, including (1) increased production of carbon dioxide; (2) increased production of lactic acid; and (3) the release of H$^+$ ions during the breakdown of ATP.
- Only sporting events that involve high-intensity exercise present a threat to acid-base disturbances during exercise (see Table 11.1).

Sport	Risk of Acid-Base Disturbance
Baseball	Low
Basketball	Low-to-moderate
Boxing	Low-to-moderate
Cross-country skiing	Low
Football (American)	Low
100-meter sprint	Low
100-meter swim	High
400-meter run	High
800-meter run	High
1,500-meter run	Moderate-to-high
5,000-meter run	Moderate
10,000-meter run	Low-to-moderate
Marathon run	Low
Soccer	Low-to-moderate
Weight lifting (low repetitions)	Low
Volleyball	Low

TABLE 11.1 Risk of Developing an Acid-Base Disturbance in Popular Sports

IMPORTANCE OF ACID-BASE REGULATION DURING EXERCISE

As discussed earlier, high-intensity exercise results in the production of large amounts of hydrogen ions. These hydrogen ions can exert a powerful effect on other molecules by interacting with molecules and thus altering their shape and function (14, 16, 33, 41). For example, high levels of hydrogen ions can alter the function of enzymes by decreasing their activity; this could have a negative effect on normal metabolism.

How can changes in muscle pH affect exercise performance? An increase in the intramuscular hydrogen ion concentration can impair exercise performance in at least two ways. First, an increase in the hydrogen ion concentration reduces the muscle cell's ability to produce ATP by inhibiting key enzymes involved in both anaerobic (glycolysis) and aerobic production of ATP (14, 19). Second, hydrogen ions compete with calcium ions for binding sites on troponin, thereby hindering the contractile process (14, 45). This is discussed again in Chap. 19.

IN SUMMARY

- Hydrogen ions can interact with molecules and alter their original size and function.
- Failure to maintain acid-base homeostasis during exercise can impair performance by inhibiting metabolic pathways responsible for the production of ATP or by interfering with the contractile process in the working muscle.

ACID-BASE BUFFER SYSTEMS

From the preceding discussion, it is clear that a rapid accumulation of hydrogen ions during intense exercise can negatively influence muscular performance. Therefore, it is important that the body has control systems capable of regulating acid-base status to prevent drastic decreases or increases in pH. One of the most important means of regulating hydrogen ion concentrations in body fluids is by the aid of buffers. A **buffer** resists pH change by removing hydrogen ions when the hydrogen ion concentration increases, and releasing hydrogen ions when the hydrogen ion concentration falls.

Buffers often consist of a weak acid and its associated base (called a *conjugate base*). The ability of individual buffers to resist pH change is dependent upon two factors. First, individual buffers differ in their intrinsic physiochemical ability to act as buffers. Simply stated, some buffers are better than others. A second factor influencing buffering capacity is the concentration of the buffer present (22, 39). The greater the concentration of a particular buffer, the more effective the buffer can be in preventing pH change.

Intracellular Buffers

The first line of defense in protecting against exercise-induced decreases in pH resides within the muscle fiber itself. Indeed, muscle fibers can protect against the accumulation of hydrogen ions and a decrease in cellular pH in two different ways. First, muscle fibers contain numerous classes of chemical buffers that can eliminate hydrogen ions. Second, the muscle fiber membrane (sarcolemma) contains two major types of hydrogen ion transporters that carry hydrogen ions from inside the muscle fiber into the interstitial space. Let's discuss each of these buffering systems in more detail.

Four major classes of intracellular chemical buffer systems exist in the cytosol of muscle fibers: (1) bicarbonate, (2) phosphates, (3) cellular proteins, and (4) histidine-dipeptides (primarily carnosine) (1, 25, 39). The presence of bicarbonate in skeletal muscle fibers is a useful buffer during exercise (4, 16). Further, several phosphate-containing compounds also serve as intracellular buffers in skeletal muscle fibers, and phosphate buffers are of particular importance at the beginning of exercise (22). Numerous cellular proteins contain the amino acid histidine, which possesses an ionizable group that can accept (i.e., buffer) hydrogen ions. This combination of a hydrogen ion with this cellular protein results in the formation of a weak acid, which protects against a decrease in cellular pH. Finally, muscle fibers also contain several histidine-dipeptides (dipeptides are

TABLE 11.2	Chemical Acid-Base Buffer Systems	
Buffer	Constituents	Actions
Bicarbonate	Bicarbonate (HCO_3^-)	Converts strong acid into weak acid
Phosphates	Phosphates (HPO_4^-)	Converts strong acid into weak acid
Proteins	Proteins containing histidine groups	Accepts hydrogens
Histidine-dipeptides	Primary component is carnosine	Accepts hydrogens

two linked amino acids) that are capable of buffering hydrogen ions. One of the major histidine-dipeptides found in skeletal muscle is carnosine, and growing evidence indicates that carnosine is an important buffer in muscle fibers. Collectively, these four intracellular chemical buffer systems work as unit to provide protection against decreases in muscle pH during intense exercise. A summary of these buffer systems is provided in Table 11.2.

Muscle pH homeostasis is also regulated by the transport of hydrogen ions from muscle fibers into the interstitial space; these hydrogen ions are then buffered by extracellular fluid and blood buffer systems. Two primary transporters that move hydrogen ions across the sarcolemma are the sodium-hydrogen exchanger (NHE) and monocarboxlate transporters (MCTs). The NHE moves sodium ions into the muscle and hydrogen ions out of the muscle into the interstitial space (Fig. 11.4). Specifically, this transporter moves one hydrogen ion out the cell in exchange for one sodium ion. The second hydrogen ion transporter is the MCT. Human skeletal muscles contain two different MCTs that are labeled as MCT1 and MCT4. Both of these molecules mediate a one-to-one co-transport of lactate

and hydrogen ions out of the muscle fiber. In other words, these MCTs carry one lactate molecule and one hydrogen ion across the sarcolemma. Research reveals that these transporters are important in regulating muscle pH during high-intensity exercise.

Influence of Muscle Fiber Type and Exercise Training on Intracellular Buffer Capacity

As discussed in the previous section, muscle fibers can protect against the accumulation of hydrogen ions and a decrease in cellular pH in two different ways: (1) intracellular buffers and (2) hydrogen ion transporters that move hydrogen ions from inside the muscle fiber into the interstitial space. Studies reveal that, compared to slow (i.e., type I) muscle fibers, the intracellular buffering capacity is higher in fast (i.e., type II) muscle fibers (1). Obviously, this higher buffer capacity in fast fibers is advantageous for performance during high-intensity exercise because fast muscle fibers produce high levels of both lactate and hydrogen ions during intense exercise.

Several studies show that high-intensity exercise training improves muscle buffer capacity in both untrained and trained individuals (8, 15). The precise mechanism(s) to explain exercise training-induced improvements in muscle buffer capacity remains a topic of debate. Nonetheless, training has been shown to increase the intracellular content of both carnosine and hydrogen ion transporters (i.e., MCT) in muscle fibers (8, 15). Therefore, it seems likely that a training-induced improvement in muscle buffer capacity is due to increases in both carnosine and hydrogen ion transporters in skeletal muscle.

Extracellular Buffers

The blood contains three principal buffer systems (4, 12, 16, 25): (1) proteins, (2) hemoglobin, and (3) bicarbonate. Blood proteins act as buffers in the

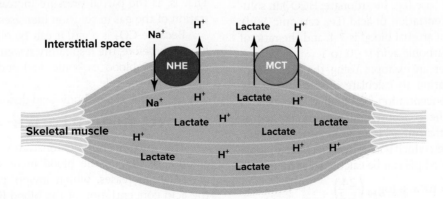

Figure 11.4 Illustration of the two important hydrogen ion (H^+) transporters in skeletal muscle fibers. The sodium-hydrogen exchanger (NHE) moves one sodium (Na^+) molecule into the fiber in exchange for transporting one H^+ outward. The monocarboxlate transporters (MCTs) co-transport one lactate molecule and one H^+ out of the muscle fiber.

extracellular compartment. Like intracellular proteins, these blood proteins contain ionizable groups that are weak acids and therefore act as buffers. However, because blood proteins are found in small quantities, their usefulness as buffers during heavy exercise is limited.

In contrast, hemoglobin is a particularly important protein buffer and is a major blood buffer during resting conditions. In fact, hemoglobin has approximately six times the buffering capacity of plasma proteins due to its high concentration (12, 25). Also contributing to the effectiveness of hemoglobin as a buffer is the fact that deoxygenated hemoglobin is a better buffer than oxygenated hemoglobin. As a result, after hemoglobin becomes deoxygenated in the capillaries, it is better able to bind to hydrogen ions formed when CO_2 enters the blood from the tissues. Thus, hemoglobin helps to minimize pH changes caused by loading of CO_2 into the blood (12).

The bicarbonate buffer system is probably the most important buffer system in the body (4, 25). This fact has been exploited by some investigators who have demonstrated that an increase in blood bicarbonate concentration (ingestion of bicarbonate) results in an improvement in performance in some types of exercise (4, 7, 20, 26) (see The Winning Edge 11.1).

The bicarbonate buffer system involves carbonic acid (H_2CO_3), which undergoes the following dissociation reaction to form bicarbonate (HCO_3^-):

$$CO_2 + H_2O \longleftrightarrow H_2CO_3 \longleftrightarrow H^+ + HCO_3^-$$

The ability of bicarbonate (HCO_3^-) and carbonic acid (H_2CO_3) to act as a buffer system is described mathematically by a relationship known as the Henderson-Hasselbalch equation:

$$pH = pKa + \log_{10}\left(\frac{HCO_3^-}{H_2CO_3}\right)$$

where pKa is the dissociation constant for H_2CO_3 and has a constant value of 6.1. In short, the Henderson-Hasselbalch equation states that the pH of a weak acid solution is determined by the ratio of the concentration of base (i.e., bicarbonate, HCO_3^-) in solution to the concentration of acid (i.e., carbonic acid). The normal pH of arterial blood is 7.4, and the ratio of bicarbonate to carbonic acid is 20 to 1.

Let's consider an example using the Henderson-Hasselbalch equation to calculate arterial blood pH. Normally the concentration of blood bicarbonate is 24 mEq/l and the concentration of carbonic acid is 1.2 mEq/l. Note that mEq/l is an abbreviation for milliequivalent per liter, which is a measure of concentration. Therefore, the blood pH can be calculated as follows:

$$pH = pKa + \log_{10}\left(\frac{24}{1.2}\right)$$
$$= 6.1 + \log_{10} 20$$
$$= 6.1 + 1.3$$
$$pH = 7.4$$

Although the traditional view of acid-base chemistry has considered the levels of bicarbonate and hydrogen ions as two primary determinants of pH, new ideas were advanced in the early 1980s that exposed the complexity of regulating pH balance in the body. These new concepts were launched by Peter Stewart and are introduced in A Look Back–Important People in Science.

IN SUMMARY

- The body maintains acid-base homeostasis by buffer-control systems. A buffer resists pH change by removing hydrogen ions when the pH declines and by releasing hydrogen ions when the pH increases.
- The principal intracellular buffers are proteins, phosphates, bicarbonates, and histidine-dipeptides (i.e., carnosine).
- Muscle fibers possess two important hydrogen ion transporters that carry hydrogen ions from inside the muscle fiber into the interstitial space: (1) sodium/hydrogen exchanger and (2) monocarboxlate transporters.
- Primary extracellular buffers include bicarbonates, hemoglobin, and blood proteins.

RESPIRATORY INFLUENCE ON ACID-BASE BALANCE

The fact that the respiratory system contributes to acid-base balance during exercise was introduced in Chap. 10. However, more details about how the respiratory system contributes to the control of pH will be presented here. Recall that CO_2 is considered a volatile acid because it can be readily changed from CO_2 to carbonic acid (H_2CO_3). Also, remember that it is the partial pressure of CO_2 in the blood that determines the concentration of carbonic acid. For example, according to Henry's law, the concentration of a gas in solution is directly proportional to its partial pressure. That is, as the partial pressure increases, the concentration of the gas in solution increases, and vice versa.

Because CO_2 is a gas, it can be eliminated by the lungs. Therefore, the respiratory system is an important regulator of blood carbonic acid and pH. To better understand the role of the lungs in acid-base balance, let's reexamine the carbonic acid dissociation equation:

$$CO_2 + H_2O \leftrightarrow H_2CO_3 \leftrightarrow H^+ + HCO_3^-$$

This relationship demonstrates that when the amount of CO_2 in the blood increases, the amount of H_2CO_3 increases, which lowers pH by elevating the acid concentration of the blood (i.e., the reaction moves to the right). In contrast, when the CO_2 content of the blood is lowered (i.e., CO_2 is eliminated by the lungs), the pH of the blood increases because

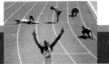
Exercise Physiology Applied to Sports

Nutritional Supplements to Buffer Exercise-Induced Acid-Base Disturbances and Improve Performance

Because intramuscular acidosis is associated with muscle fatigue, numerous studies have explored nutritional supplements to increase buffering capacity in hopes of improving athletic performance during high-intensity exercise. Indeed, it appears that supplements including sodium bicarbonate, sodium citrate, and beta-alanine have the potential to improve buffering capacity and enhance exercise performance during, high-intensity exercise. Let's discuss these supplement strategies to improve muscle buffering capacity in more detail.

Sodium bicarbonate. Bicarbonate is a buffer that plays an important role in maintaining both extracellular and intracellular pH, despite its inability to freely cross the muscle membrane (i.e., sarcolemma). Although controversy exists (2), many studies conclude that performance during high-intensity exercise is improved when athletes ingest sodium bicarbonate prior to exercise (6, 7, 26, 30–32, 34, 37, 40). Specifically, results from numerous studies reveal that boosting the blood-buffering capacity by ingestion of sodium bicarbonate increases time to exhaustion during high-intensity exercise (e.g., 80% to 120% $\dot{V}O_2$ max). For example, a recent survey of the scientific literature reveals that sodium bicarbonate is effective in improving a 60-second "all out" exercise bout by approximately 2% (5). Further, laboratory studies employing repeated bouts of high-intensity exercise (i.e., >100% $\dot{V}O_2$ max) have reported that ingestion of sodium bicarbonate prior to exercise can enhance performance by more than 8% (18). In addition to these laboratory studies, evidence exists that sodium bicarbonate is also beneficial to sport performance in activities where the metabolic demands are primarily anaerobic, such as judo, swimming, and water polo (18).

It appears that sodium bicarbonate improves physical performance by increasing the extracellular buffering capacity, which, in turn, increases the transport of hydrogen ions out of the muscle fibers (38). This would reduce the interference of hydrogen ions on

muscle ATP production and/or the contractile process itself.

In deciding whether to use sodium bicarbonate prior to a sporting event, an athlete should understand the risks associated with this decision. Ingestion of sodium bicarbonate in the doses required to improve blood-buffering capacity can cause gastrointestinal problems, including diarrhea and vomiting (7, 37).

Sodium Citrate. Similar to sodium bicarbonate, sodium citrate is another agent capable of increasing extracellular buffering capacity (18). The question of whether ingestion of sodium citrate can improve exercise performance during high-intensity exercise remains controversial because experimental results are often inconsistent. Nonetheless, a review of the research literature suggests that although low doses of sodium citrate does not improve performance, ingestion of high doses of sodium citrate (i.e., >0.5 grams/kilogram body weight) improves performance during high-intensity cycling exercise lasting 120 to 240 seconds (18).

Unfortunately, similar to sodium bicarbonate, ingestion of high doses of sodium citrate can produce undesired side effects such as nausea, gastrointestinal discomfort, and headaches. Therefore, before deciding whether to use sodium citrate prior to competition, athletes should consider the negative side effects associated with the use of sodium citrate.

Beta-alanine. Recent evidence suggests that supplementation with beta-alanine can play a beneficial role in protecting against exercise-induced acidosis and improve performance during short, high-intensity exercise (39). Beta-alanine is a nonessential amino acid produced in the liver, gut, and kidney. However, fasting blood levels of beta-alanine are low indicating that endogenous synthesis of this amino is limited.

The link between beta-alanine and protection against acidosis is linked to the fact that beta-alanine is an important precursor for the synthesis of carnosine in skeletal muscle. As discussed in the text, carnosine is a

small molecule (dipeptide) found in the cytoplasm of excitable cells (i.e., neurons, skeletal and cardiac muscle fibers) (18). Carnosine has several important physiological functions including the ability to buffer hydrogen ions and protect against exercise-induced decreases in cellular pH (18).

The availability of beta-alanine is the rate limiting factor for carnosine synthesis in muscle fibers. However, supplementation (2 to 3 grams/day) with beta-alanine for >2 weeks results in a 60% to 80% increase in muscle carnosine levels. Importantly, this increase in muscle carnosine levels is associated with a 3% to 5% increase in muscle buffering capacity (18). Theoretically, this increase in intracellular buffering capacity could translate into improvements in performance during high-intensity exercise. In this regard, growing evidence suggests that beta-alanine supplementation improves high-intensity exercise performance in both running and cycling events lasting 1 to 4 minutes (18). Interestingly, some of these studies have recorded performance improvements of 12% to 14% (18).

The only known side effect of beta-alanine supplementation is paraesthesia (tingling of the skin); this sensation begins within 20 minutes after ingestion and lasts up to 60 minutes (18). Although harmless, paraesthesia is unpleasant and, several investigations have reported that paraesthesia can be avoided by staggering dosing throughout the day (18).

Final words of caution on use of "supplement buffers" to improve exercise performance. Regardless of the type of buffer ingested, extremely large doses of any buffer can result in severe alkalosis and pose negative health consequences. Another important consideration in the use of any ergogenic aid is the legality of the drug. In regard to the use of acid-base buffers, some sports regulatory agencies have banned the use of sodium buffers during competition. See Sahlin (2014) and Junior et al. (2015) in Suggested Readings for detailed information about the possible ergogenic effects of sodium bicarbonate, sodium citrate, and beta-alanine.

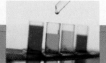

Peter Stewart Challenged Acid-Base Research by Proposing the Concept of "Strong Ion Difference"

Peter Stewart (1921–1993) was born and raised in Winnipeg, Canada. He earned both his Master's and Ph.D. degrees from the University of Minnesota. During a long and productive research career, Dr. Stewart served on the faculty of the University of Illinois, Emory University, and Brown University.

In the 1970s, Dr. Stewart developed a strong interest in acid-base regulation and started to mathematically analyze the variables involved in controlling the pH of body fluids. In 1981, he challenged the traditional concepts of acid-base control by publishing his book titled *How to Understand Acid-Base Balance—A Quantitative Acid-Base Primer for Biology and Medicine*. This book quickly stirred both controversy and debate among researchers in acid-base balance. A brief synopsis of this controversy follows. Historically, it has been believed that the balance between the levels of hydrogen ions and bicarbonate ions determines the pH of body fluids. Dr. Stewart challenged this concept and argued that hydrogen ions and bicarbonate ions are not the independent variables that control acid-base. Instead, he suggested that these variables are dependent variables that are regulated by other factors, including the strong ion difference,° carbon dioxide levels, and the amount of weak and nonvolatile acids in body fluids. So, does this mean that calculating pH using the Henderson-Hasselbalch equation is of no value? The short answer to this question is no. However, Dr. Stewart's work demonstrates that the factors that regulate acid-base balance in the body are probably more complex than originally believed.

Although some physiologists have accepted the science supporting Dr. Stewart's proposal of how acid-base balance is maintained, criticism of his concept of strong ion difference remains. A concern with the strong ion balance concept of acid-base control is the complexity of the chemistry and mathematics behind this model. Moreover, in practice, it is often difficult to measure all the variables required to calculate pH using Dr. Stewart's strong ion difference method. Therefore, in the foreseeable future, the traditional approach to acid-base balance seems certain to prevail.

°In Dr. Stewart's terminology, the strong ion difference is defined as the contrast between the number of strong cations (e.g., sodium, potassium, and calcium) and strong anions (e.g., chloride and lactate) in body fluids (21). You can visit acidbase.org for Stewart's original text. A new edition of Stewart's *Textbook of Clinical Acid-Base Medicine* was recently published and is cited in the references at the end of this chapter (Kellum and Elbers, 2009) (21).

---

less acid is present (reaction moves to the left). Therefore, the respiratory system provides the body with a rapid means of regulating blood pH by controlling the amount of CO_2 present in the blood (17, 27, 44).

IN SUMMARY

- Respiratory control of acid-base balance involves the regulation of blood PCO_2.
- An increase in blood PCO_2 lowers pH, whereas a decrease in blood PCO_2 increases pH.
- Increased pulmonary ventilation can remove CO_2 from the body and thus eliminate hydrogen ions and increase pH.

REGULATION OF ACID-BASE BALANCE VIA THE KIDNEYS

Because the kidneys do not play an important part in acid-base regulation during short-term exercise, only a brief overview of the kidney's role in acid-base balance will be presented here. The principal means by which the kidneys regulate hydrogen ion concentration is by increasing or decreasing the bicarbonate concentration (9–11, 23). When the pH decreases (hydrogen ion concentration increases) in body fluids, the kidney responds by reducing the rate of bicarbonate excretion. This results in an increase in the blood bicarbonate concentration, which assists in buffering the increase in hydrogen ions. Conversely, when the pH of body fluids rises (hydrogen ion concentration decreases), the kidneys increase the rate of bicarbonate excretion. Therefore, by changing the amount of buffer present in body fluids, the kidneys aid in the regulation of the hydrogen ion concentration. The kidney mechanism involved in regulating the bicarbonate concentration is located in a portion of the kidney called the tubule, and acts through a series of complicated reactions and active transport across the tubular wall.

Why is the kidney not an important regulator of acid-base balance during exercise? The answer lies in the amount of time required for the kidney to respond to an acid-base disturbance. It takes several hours for the kidneys to react effectively in response to an increase in blood hydrogen ions (10, 46). Therefore, the kidneys respond too slowly to be of major benefit in the regulation of hydrogen ion concentration during exercise.

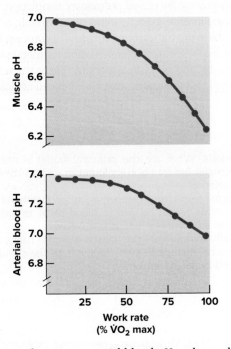

■ Although the kidneys play an important role in the long-term regulation of acid-base balance, the kidneys do not play a major role in the regulation of acid-base balance during exercise.

REGULATION OF ACID-BASE BALANCE DURING EXERCISE

During the final stages of an incremental exercise test or during near-maximal exercise of short duration, there is a decrease in both muscle and blood pH primarily due to the increase in the production of hydrogen ions by the muscle (13, 29). This point is illustrated in Figure 11.5, where the changes in blood and muscle pH during an incremental exercise test are graphed as a function of exercise (i.e., % $\dot{V}O_2$ max). Notice that muscle and blood pH follow similar trends during this type of exercise, but that muscle pH is always 0.4 to 0.6 pH unit lower than blood pH. This ocurrs because muscle hydrogen ion concentration is higher than that of blood, and muscle buffering capacity is lower than that of blood.

The amount of hydrogen ions produced during exercise is dependent on (1) the exercise intensity, (2) the amount of muscle mass involved, and (3) the duration of the exercise (13). Exercise involving high-intensity leg work (e.g., running) may reduce arterial

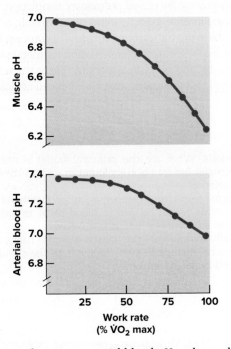

Figure 11.5 Changes in arterial blood pH and muscle pH during incremental exercise. Notice that arterial and muscle pH begin to fall together at work rates above 50% $\dot{V}O_2$ max.

pH from 7.4 to a value of 7.0 within a few minutes (13, 27, 35, 43). Further, repeated bouts of this type of exercise can cause blood pH to decline even further to a value of 6.8 (13). This level of blood pH is the lowest ever recorded and would present a life-threatening situation if it were not corrected within a few minutes.

How does the body regulate acid-base balance during exercise? Because working muscles are the primary source of hydrogen ions during exercise, it is logical that the first line of defense against a rise in acid production resides in the individual muscle fibers. It is estimated that intracellular proteins and histidine dipeptides (i.e., carnosine) contribute as much as 60% of the cell's buffering capacity, with an additional 20% to 30% of the total buffering capacity coming from muscle bicarbonate (25). The final 10% to 20% of muscle buffering capacity comes from intracellular phosphate groups.

Because the muscle's buffering capacity is limited, extracellular fluid (principally the blood) must possess a means of buffering hydrogen ions as well. Therefore, the blood buffering systems become the second line of defense against exercise-induced acidosis. The principal extracellular buffer is blood bicarbonate (25, 39). Hemoglobin and blood proteins assist in this buffer process, but play only a minor role in blood buffering of hydrogen ions during exercise (25). Figure 11.6 illustrates the role of blood bicarbonate as a buffer during incremental exercise (44). Note that at approximately 50% to 60% of $\dot{V}O_2$ max, blood levels of lactate begin to increase and blood pH declines due to the rise in hydrogen ions in the blood. This increase in blood hydrogen ion concentration stimulates the carotid bodies, which then signal the respiratory control center to increase alveolar ventilation (i.e., ventilatory threshold; see Chap. 10). An increase in alveolar ventilation results in the reduction of blood PCO_2 and therefore acts to reduce the acid load produced by exercise (17). The overall process of respiratory assistance in buffering lactic acid during exercise is referred to as **respiratory compensation** for metabolic acidosis.

In summary, the control of acid-base balance during exercise is important. During high-intensity exercise (i.e., work above the lactate threshold), the contracting skeletal muscle produces significant amounts of hydrogen ions. The first line of defense against exercise-induced acidosis resides in the muscle fiber (i.e., bicarbonate, phosphate, and protein buffers). However, because the muscle fiber's buffering capacity is limited, additional buffer systems are required to protect the body against exercise-induced acidosis. In this regard, the second line of defense against pH shifts during exercise is the blood buffer systems (i.e., bicarbonate, phosphate, and protein buffers). Importantly, an increase in pulmonary

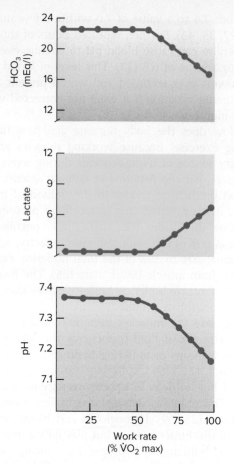

Figure 11.6 Changes in blood concentrations of bicarbonate, lactate, and pH as a function of work rate.

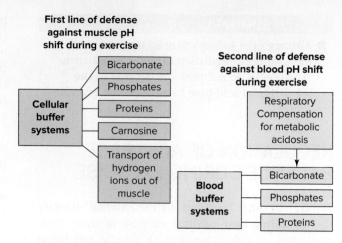

First line of defense against muscle pH shift during exercise

Second line of defense against blood pH shift during exercise

Figure 11.7 The two major lines of defense against pH change during intense exercise.

during intense exercise assists in eliminating carbonic acid by "blowing off carbon dioxide." This respiratory compensation to exercise-induced acidosis plays an important role in the second line of defense against pH change during intense exercise. Together, these first and second lines of defense protect the body against exercise-induced acidosis (Fig. 11.7).

IN SUMMARY

- Figure 11.7 summarizes the "two-stage" process of buffering exercise-induced production of hydrogen ions.
- The first line of defense against hydrogen ions produced in the muscle resides inside the muscle fiber itself. During exercise, muscle buffer systems act rapidly to buffer hydrogen ions and prevent a significant decline in muscle pH.
- The second line of defense against exercise-induced acidosis is the blood buffer systems, which include bicarbonate, phosphate, and protein buffers.
- Importantly, increased pulmonary ventilation during intense exercise eliminates carbonic acid by "blowing off" carbon dioxide. This process is termed "respiratory compensation for metabolic acidosis" and plays an important role in the second line of defense against exercise-induced acidosis.

STUDY ACTIVITIES

1. Define the terms *acid, base, buffer, acidosis, alkalosis,* and *pH*.
2. Graph the pH scale. Label the pH values that represent normal arterial and intracellular pH.
3. List and briefly discuss the major sources of hydrogen ions produced in the muscle during exercise.
4. Why is the maintenance of acid-base homeostasis important to physical performance?
5. Discuss both the intracellular and extracellular buffer mechanisms that protect against exercise-induced

acidosis. What are the principal buffer systems and hydrogen ion transporters found in each of these lines of defense?
6. Discuss respiratory compensation for metabolic acidosis. What would happen to blood pH if an individual began to hyperventilate at rest? Why?
7. Briefly outline how the body resists pH change during exercise. Include in your outline both the cellular and blood buffer systems.

SUGGESTED READINGS

Fox, S. 2015. *Human Physiology.* New York, NY: McGraw-Hill.

Junior, A., V. Painelli, B. Saunders, and G. Artioli. 2015. Nutritional strategies to modulate intracellular and extracellular buffering capacity during high intensity exercise. *Sports Medicine* 45: S71–S81.

Sahlin, K. 2014. Muscle energetics during explosive activities and potential effects of nutrition and training. *Sports Medicine* 44: S167–S173.

Widmaier, E., H. Raff, and K. Strang. 2015. *Vander's Human Physiology,* 10th ed. New York, NY: McGraw-Hill.

REFERENCES

1. **Abe H.** Role of histidine-related compounds as intracellular proton buffering constituents in vertebrae muscle. *Biochemistry* (Moscow) 65: 757-765, 2000.

2. **Aschenbach W, Ocel J, Craft L, Ward C, Spangenburg E, and Williams J.** Effect of oral sodium loading on high-intensity arm ergometry in college wrestlers. *Medicine & Science in Sports & Exercise* 32: 669-675, 2000.

3. **Boning D and Maassen N.** Point: lactic acid is the only physicochemical contributor to the acidosis of exercise. *Journal of Applied Physiology* 105: 358-359, 2008.

4. **Broch-Lips M, Overgaard K, Praetorius HA, and Nielsen OB.** Effects of extracellular HCO₃(–) on fatigue, pHi, and K1 efflux in rat skeletal muscles. *Journal of Applied Physiology* 103: 494-503, 2007.

5. **Carr A, Hopkins W, and Gore C.** Effects of acute alkalosis and acidosis on performance: a meta analysis. *Sports Medicine* 41: 801-814, 2011.

6. **Coombes J and McNaughton L.** The effects of bicarbonate ingestion on leg strength and power during isokinetic knee flexion and extension. *Journal of Strength and Conditioning Research* 7: 241-249, 1993.

7. **Costill DL, Verstappen F, Kuipers H, Janssen E, and Fink W.** Acid-base balance during repeated bouts of exercise: influence of HCO3. *International Journal of Sports and Medicine* 5: 228-231, 1984.

8. **Edge J, Bishop D, and Goodman C.** The effects of training intensity on muscle buffer capacity in females. *European Journal of Applied Physiology* 96: 97-105, 2006.

9. **Fox E, Foss M, and Keteyian S.** *Fox's Physiological Basis for Exercise and Sport.* New York, NY: McGraw-Hill, 1998.

10. **Fox S.** *Human Physiology.* New York, NY: McGraw-Hill, 2015.

11. **Hall JE.** *Guyton and Hall Textbook of Medical Physiology.* Philadelphia, PA: Mosby/Saunders, 2015.

12. **Halperin M, Goldstein M, and Kamel K.** *Fluid, Electrolyte, and Acid-Base Physiology.* Philadelphia, PA: Saunders, 2010.

13. **Hultman E and Sahlin K.** Acid-base balance during exercise. In: *Exercise and Sport Science Reviews*, edited by Hutton R, and Miller D. Philadelphia, PA: Franklin Institute Press, 1980, pp. 41-128.

14. **Hultman E and Sjoholm J.** Biochemical causes of fatigue. In: *Human Muscle Power*, edited by Jones N, McCartney N, and McComas A. Champaign, IL: Human Kinetics, 1986.

15. **Juel C.** Training-induced changes in membrane transport proteins of human skeletal muscle. *European Journal of Applied Physiology* 96: 627-635, 2006.

16. **Jones NL.** Hydrogen ion balance during exercise. *Clinical Science (London)* 59: 85-91, 1980.

17. **Jones NL.** An obsession with CO_2. *Applied Physiology, Nutrition, and Metabolism* 33: 641-650, 2008.

18. **Junior A, Painelli V, Saunders B, and Artioli G.** Nutritional strategies to modulate intracellular and extracellular buffering capacity during high intensity exercise. 45: S71-S81, 2015.

19. **Karlsson J.** Localized muscular fatigue: role of metabolism and substrate depletion. In: *Exercise and Sport Science Reviews*, edited by Hutton R, and Miller D. Philadelphia, PA: Franklin Institute Press, 1979, pp. 1-42.

20. **Katz A, Costill DL, King DS, Hargreaves M, and Fink WJ.** Maximal exercise tolerance after induced alkalosis. *International Journal of Sports and Medicine* 5: 107-110, 1984.

21. **Kellum J and Elbers P,** eds. *Stewart's Textbook of Acid-Base.* acid-base.org, 2009.

22. **Kemp GJ, Tonon C, Malucelli E, Testa C, Liava A, Manners D, et al.** Cytosolic pH buffering during exercise and recovery in skeletal muscle of patients with McArdle's disease. *European Journal of Applied Physiology* 105: 687-694, 2009.

23. **Kiil F.** Mechanisms of transjunctional transport of NaCl and water in proximal tubules of mammalian kidneys. *Acta Physiologica Scandinavia* 175: 55-70, 2002.

24. **Kowalchuk JM, Maltais SA, Yamaji K, and Hughson RL.** The effect of citrate loading on exercise performance, acid-base balance and metabolism. *European Journal of Applied Physiology and Occupational Physiology* 58: 858-864, 1989.

25. **Laiken N and Fanestil D.** Acid-base balance and regulation of hydrogen ion excretion. In: *Physiological Basis of Medical Practice*, edited by West J. Baltimore, MD: Lippincott Williams & Wilkins, 1985.

26. **Linderman J and Fahey TD.** Sodium bicarbonate ingestion and exercise performance. An update. *Sports Medicine* 11: 71-77, 1991.

27. **Lindinger M and Heigenhauser G.** Effects of gas exchange on acid-base balance. *Comprehensive Physiology* 2: 2203-2254, 2012.

28. **Lindinger MI and Heigenhauser GJ.** Counterpoint: lactic acid is not the only physicochemical contributor to the acidosis of exercise. *Journal of Applied Physiology* 105: 359-361; discussion 361-362, 2008.

29. **Marsh GD, Paterson DH, Thompson RT, and Driedger AA.** Coincident thresholds in intracellular phosphorylation potential and pH during progressive exercise. *Journal of Applied Physiology* 71: 1076-1081, 1991.

30. **McNaughton L and Thompson D.** Acute versus chronic sodium bicarbonate ingestion and anaerobic work and power output. *Journal of Sports Medicine and Physical Fitness.* 41: 456-462, 2001.

31. **McNaughton LR, Siegler J, and Midgley A.** Ergogenic effects of sodium bicarbonate. *Current Sports Medicine Reports* 7: 230-236, 2008.

32. **Miller P, Robinson A, Sparks S, Bridge C, Bentley D, and McNaughton, L.** The effects of novel ingestion of sodium bicarbonate on repeated sprint ability. *Journal of Strength and Conditioning Research* 30: 561-568, 2016.

33. **Nattie EE.** The alphastat hypothesis in respiratory control and acid-base balance. *Journal of Applied Physiology* 69: 1201-1207, 1990.

34. **Nielsen HB, Hein L, Svendsen LB, Secher NH, and Quistorff B.** Bicarbonate attenuates intracellular acidosis. *Acta Anaesthesiol Scandinavia* 46: 579-584, 2002.

35. **Robergs RA, Costill DL, Fink WJ, Williams C, Pascoe DD, Chwalbinska-Moneta J, et al.** Effects of warm-up on blood gases, lactate and acid-base status during sprint swimming. *International Journal of Sports and Medicine* 11: 273-278, 1990.

36. **Robergs RA, Ghiasvand F, and Parker D.** Biochemistry of exercise-induced metabolic acidosis. *American Journal of Physiology Regulatory Integrative and Comparative Physiology* 287: R502-516, 2004.

37. **Robertson RJ, Falkel JE, Drash AL, Swank AM, Metz KF, Spungen SA, et al.** Effect of induced alkalosis on physical work capacity during arm and leg exercise. *Ergonomics* 30: 19-31, 1987.

38. **Roth DA and Brooks GA.** Lactate transport is mediated by a membrane-bound carrier in rat skeletal

muscle sarcolemmal vesicles. *Archives Biochemistry Biophysics* 279: 377–385, 1990.

39. **Sale C, Saunders B, and Harris RC.** Effect of beta-alanine supplementation on muscle carnosine concentrations and exercise performance. *Amino Acids* 39: 321–333, 2010.

40. **Siegler JC and Gleadall-Siddall DO.** Sodium bicarbonate ingestion and repeated swim sprint performance. *The Journal of Strength & Conditioning Research* 24: 3105–3111, 2010.

41. **Spriet LL.** Phosphofructokinase activity and acidosis during short-term tetanic contractions. *Canadian Journal of Physiology and Pharmacology* 69: 298–304, 1991.

42. **Stein J.** *Internal Medicine.* St. Louis: Mosby Year-Book, 2002.

43. **Street D, Bangsbo J, and Juel C.** Interstitial pH in human skeletal muscle during and after dynamic graded exercise. *Journal of Physiology* 537: 993–998, 2001.

44. **Strickland M, Lindinger M, Olfert I, Heigenhauser G, and Hopkins S.** Pulmonary gas exchange and acid-base balance during exercise. *Comprehensive Physiology* 3: 693–739, 2013.

45. **Vollestad NK and Sejersted OM.** Biochemical correlates of fatigue. A brief review. *European Journal of Applied Physiology and Occupational Physiology* 57: 336–347, 1988.

46. **Widmaier E, Raff H, and Strang K.** *Vander's Human Physiology.* New York, NY: McGraw-Hill, 2015.

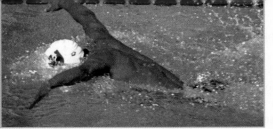

12

Temperature Regulation

■ Objectives

By studying this chapter, you should be able to do the following:

1. Define the term *homeotherm*.
2. Present an overview of heat balance during exercise.
3. Discuss the concept of "core temperature."
4. List the principal means of involuntarily increasing heat production.
5. Define the four processes by which the body can lose heat during exercise.
6. Discuss the role of the preoptic-anterior hypothalamus as the body's thermostat.
7. Explain the thermal events that occur during exercise in both a cool/moderate and hot/humid environment.
8. List the physiological adaptations that occur during acclimatization to heat.
9. Describe the physiological responses to a cold environment.
10. Discuss the physiological changes that occur in response to cold acclimatization.

■ Outline

■ Key Terms

acclimation
acclimatization
conduction
convection
evaporation
homeotherms
hyperthermia
hypothermia
preoptic-anterior
   hypothalamus
radiation
specific heat

Body core temperature regulation is critical because cellular structures and metabolic pathways are affected by temperature. For example, enzymes that regulate metabolic pathways are greatly influenced by temperature changes. Indeed, an increase in body temperature above 45°C (normal core temperature is approximately 37°C) can alter the normal structure of enzymes, resulting in the inability to produce cellular energy (i.e., ATP). Ultimately, an inability to produce cellular energy would result in cell death and eventually death to the organism. Further, a decrease in body temperature below 34°C causes a slowed metabolism and abnormal cardiac function (arrhythmias), which can also lead to death. Hence, people and warm-blooded animals live their entire lives only a few degrees from their thermal death point. Therefore, it is clear that body temperature must be carefully regulated.

Humans and other animals that maintain a rather constant body core temperature are called **homeotherms.** The maintenance of a constant body temperature requires that heat loss must match the rate of heat production. To accomplish thermal regulation, the body is well equipped with both nervous and hormonal mechanisms that regulate metabolic rate as well as the amount of heat loss in response to body temperature changes. The temperature-maintenance strategy of homeotherms uses a "furnace" rather than a "refrigerator" to maintain body temperature at a constant level. That is, the body temperature is set near the high end of the survival range and is held constant by continuous metabolic heat production coupled with a small but continual heat loss. The rationale for this strategy is that temperature regulation by heat generation and conservation is very efficient, whereas the body's cooling capacity is much more limited (5, 20).

Because contracting skeletal muscles produce large amounts of heat, prolonged exercise in a hot/humid environment presents a serious challenge to temperature homeostasis. In fact, many exercise physiologists believe that overheating is the only serious threat to health that exercise presents to a healthy individual. This chapter discusses the principles of temperature regulation during exercise. The cardiovascular and pulmonary responses to exercise in a hot environment have already been discussed in Chaps. 9 and 10, respectively, and the influence of temperature on performance is discussed in Chap. 24.

OVERVIEW OF HEAT BALANCE DURING EXERCISE

D. B. Dill and colleagues performed many of the first studies of heat stress in humans at the Harvard Fatigue Laboratory. This early research provided the scientific foundation for our current understanding

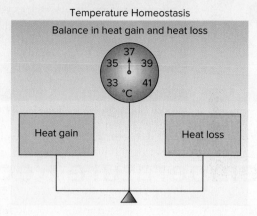

Figure 12.1 During steady-state conditions, temperature homeostasis is maintained by an equal rate of body heat gain and heat loss.

of thermal stress and temperature regulation during exercise. See A Look Back–Important People in Science for a historical overview of the work of D. B. Dill.

The goal of temperature regulation is to maintain a constant core temperature and thus prevent overheating or overcooling. If the core temperature is to remain constant, the amount of heat lost must match the amount of heat gained (see Fig. 12.1). Consistent with that, if heat loss is less than heat production, there is a net gain in body heat and, therefore, body temperature rises; if heat loss exceeds heat production, there is a net loss in body heat, and body temperature decreases.

During exercise, body temperature is regulated by making adjustments in the amount of heat that is lost. In this regard, one of the important functions of the circulatory system is to transport heat. Blood is very effective in this function because it has a high capacity to store heat. When the body is attempting to lose heat, blood flow is increased to the skin as a means of promoting heat loss to the environment. In contrast, when the goal of temperature regulation is to prevent heat loss, blood is directed away from the skin and toward the interior of the body to prevent additional heat loss.

It is important to point out that within the body, temperature varies significantly. That is, there is a gradient between core temperature (i.e., deep central areas, including the heart, lungs, abdominal organs) and the "shell" (skin) temperature. In extreme circumstances (i.e., exposure to very cold temperatures), the core temperature can be 20°C higher than the skin (33). However, such large core-to-shell gradients are rare, and the ideal difference between core and skin temperatures is approximately 4°C (3, 57). Even within the core, temperature varies from one organ to another. Therefore, when discussing body temperature, it is important to be precise as to where the temperature measurements were obtained (i.e., skin temperature or core temperature) (3).

D. B. (Bruce) Dill Was a Pioneer in Environmental and Heat Stress Research

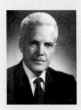

Courtesy of American College of Sports Medicine

After earning his Ph.D. from Stanford University in 1925, **D. B. (Bruce) Dill (1891-1986)** went to Harvard University to work with the renowned physiologist L. J. Henderson. Professor Henderson remains well known today for his contributions to acid-base chemistry, including the Henderson-Hasselbalch equation introduced in Chap. 11.

In 1927, Dr. Dill became one of the founding members of the Harvard Fatigue Laboratory. This important research laboratory was charged with investigating factors that influenced human fatigue, including the impact of extreme environments (i.e., heat, cold, and high altitude), exercise, nutrition, acid-base balance, and aging. During the 20-year existence of the Harvard Fatigue Laboratory, the work completed by Dr. Dill and his colleagues greatly advanced our understanding of both environmental and exercise physiology.

After the closure of the Harvard Fatigue Laboratory, Dr. Dill became the scientific director of the Medical Division of the Army Chemical Center, where he directed research until 1961. Dr. Dill's research at this Army research center produced many important outcomes, including research that led to better methods of cardiopulmonary resuscitation. These same procedures are used today and have saved many lives around the world.

Following his retirement from the Army research center at age 70, Dr. Dill joined the faculty at Indiana University for a five-year research appointment. He then moved to Boulder City, Nevada, to become a research professor at the Desert Research Institute, University of Nevada–Las Vegas. At the Desert Research Institute, Dill continued his work on the physiological impact of heat stress, and he remained active in environmental stress research until his death at age 95. He presented his last lecture at a scientific conference at the age of 93. The topic discussed was the change in D. B. Dill's $\dot{V}O_2$ max during the past 60 years! In fact, at age 93, Bruce Dill was the oldest person to perform a $\dot{V}O_2$ max test. During Dr. Dill's long and productive scientific career, he coauthored numerous books and more than 300 research reports. Many of these studies provided the foundation for our current understanding of the impact of heat stress on human physiology and performance.

IN SUMMARY

- Homeotherms are animals (e.g., humans and other mammals) that maintain a rather constant body core temperature. To maintain a constant core temperature, heat loss must match heat gain.
- Temperature varies markedly within the body. In general, there is a thermal gradient from deep body temperature (core temperature) to the shell (skin) temperature.

TEMPERATURE MEASUREMENT DURING EXERCISE

Measurements of deep-body temperatures can be accomplished with several devices, including mercury thermometers, devices known as thermocouples or thermistors, and/or ingestible core temperature pills (9). In the laboratory setting, a common site of core temperature measurement is the rectum. Although rectal temperature is not the same as the temperature in the brain, where temperature is regulated, it can be used to measure changes in deep-body temperature during exercise. In addition, measuring temperature near the eardrum (called tympanic temperature) is a good estimate of the actual brain temperature.

Another alternative is to measure the temperature of the esophagus as an indication of core temperature. Like rectal temperature, esophageal temperature is not identical to brain temperature, but it provides a measure of deep-body temperature.

Although the measurements of rectal, tympanic, and esophageal temperature can easily be performed in the laboratory setting, each of these techniques has limitations in a field setting. Indeed, it would be difficult to apply these temperature measurement techniques in athletes during an American football or soccer practice session. Nonetheless, the recent development of ingestible temperature sensor telemetry systems has made on-field core temperature measurement possible and allowed the investigation of core temperature changes in athletes during practice sessions (4, 41). These ingestible temperature sensors use low-power radio frequency transmissions to communicate with a temperature monitor. These probes have been shown to be both valid and reliable in measuring core temperature in football players during practice (4). Further, numerous other commercially available devices exist for the measurement of body temperature in the field setting, and the validity of these products has been established (9).

In the laboratory, the measurement of skin temperature provides useful information about the temperature gradient between deep body (i.e., core) temperature and the skin. The magnitude of this core-to-skin temperature gradient is important for body heat loss and will be discussed later in the chapter. Skin temperature can be measured by placing temperature sensors on the skin at various locations. The mean skin temperature can be calculated by measuring skin temperature at several locations and computing the average temperature across these locations. For example, mean skin temperature (T_s) can be estimated by the following formula (27):

$$T_s = (T_{forehead} + T_{chest} + T_{forearm} + T_{thigh} + T_{calf} + T_{abdomen} + T_{back}) \div 7$$

where $T_{forehead}$, T_{chest}, $T_{forearm}$, T_{thigh}, T_{calf}, $T_{abdomen}$, and T_{back} represent skin temperatures measured on the forehead, chest, forearm, thigh, calf, abdomen, and back, respectively.

IN SUMMARY

- Measurements of deep-body temperatures can be accomplished via mercury thermometers or devices known as *thermocouples* or *thermistors*. Common sites of temperature measurement include the rectum, the ear (tympanic temperature), and the esophagus.
- Skin temperature can be measured by placing temperature sensors (thermistors) on the skin at various locations.

OVERVIEW OF HEAT PRODUCTION/HEAT LOSS

As previously stated, the goal of temperature regulation (i.e., thermoregulation) is to maintain a constant core temperature. This regulation is achieved by controlling the rate of heat production and heat loss. When out of balance, the body either gains or loses heat. The temperature control center is an area in the brain called the preoptic-anterior hypothalamus. The **preoptic-anterior hypothalamus** (POAH) works like a thermostat by initiating an increase in heat production when body temperature falls and an increase in the rate of heat loss when body temperature rises. Temperature regulation is controlled by both physical and chemical processes. Let's begin our discussion of temperature regulation by introducing those factors that govern heat production and heat loss.

Heat Production

The body produces internal heat due to normal metabolic processes. At rest or during sleep, metabolic heat production is small; however, during intense exercise, heat production is large. Heat production in the body can be classified as (1) voluntary (exercise) or (2) involuntary (shivering or biochemical heat

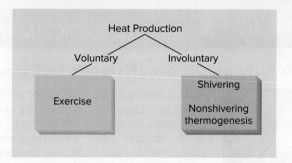

Figure 12.2 The body produces heat due to normal metabolic processes. Heat production can be classified as either voluntary or involuntary.

production caused by the secretion of hormones such as thyroxine and catecholamines) (see Fig. 12.2).

Because the body is, at most, 20% to 30% efficient, 70% to 80% of the energy expended during exercise appears as heat. During intense exercise, this can result in a large heat load. Indeed, prolonged exercise in a hot/humid environment serves as a serious test of the body's ability to lose heat.

Involuntary heat production by shivering is the primary means of increasing heat production during exposure to cold. Maximal shivering can increase the body's heat production by approximately five times the resting value (1, 5). In addition, release of thyroxine from the thyroid gland can also increase metabolic rate. Thyroxine acts by increasing the metabolic rate of all cells in the body (16). Finally, an increase in blood levels of catecholamines (epinephrine and norepinephrine) can increase the rate of cellular metabolism (16). The increase in heat production due to the combined influences of thyroxine and catecholamines is called nonshivering thermogenesis.

Heat Loss

Heat loss from the body may occur by four processes: (1) radiation, (2) conduction, (3) convection, and/or (4) evaporation. The first three of these heat-loss mechanisms require a temperature gradient to exist between the skin and the environment. **Radiation** is heat loss in the form of infrared rays. This involves the transfer of heat from the surface of one object to the surface of another, with no physical contact being involved (e.g., sun transferring heat to the earth via radiation). At rest in a comfortable environment (e.g., room temperature = 21°C), 60% of body heat loss occurs via radiation. This is possible because skin temperature is greater than the temperature of surrounding objects (walls, floor, etc.), and the loss of body heat occurs due to the thermal gradient. Note that on a hot, sunny day when surface temperatures are greater than skin temperature, the body can also gain heat via radiation. To summarize, radiation is heat transfer by infrared rays and can result in either body heat loss or heat gain depending on the environmental conditions.

Conduction is the transfer of heat from the body to the molecules of cooler objects in contact with its surface. In general, the body loses only small amounts of heat due to this process. An example of heat loss due to conduction is the transfer of heat from the body to a metal chair while a person is sitting on it. The heat loss occurs as long as the chair is cooler than the body surface in contact with it.

Convection is a form of heat loss in which heat is transmitted to either air or water molecules in contact with the body. In convective heat loss, air or water molecules are warmed and move away from the source of the heat and are replaced by cooler molecules. An example of forced convection is a fan moving large quantities of cool air past the skin; this would increase the number of cool air molecules coming in contact with the skin and thus promote heat loss. Practically speaking, the amount of heat loss due to convection is dependent on the magnitude of the airflow over the skin. Therefore, under calm wind conditions, cycling at high speeds would improve convective cooling when compared to cycling at slow speeds. Swimming in cool water (water temperature less than skin temperature) also results in convective heat loss. In fact, water's effectiveness in cooling is about 25 times greater than that of air at the same temperature.

The final means of heat loss is evaporation. Evaporation accounts for approximately 25% of the heat loss at rest, but under most environmental conditions, it is the most important means of heat loss during exercise (44). In **evaporation,** heat is transferred from the body to water on the surface of the skin. When this water gains sufficient heat (energy), it is converted to a gas (water vapor), taking the heat away from the body. Evaporation occurs due to a vapor pressure gradient between the skin and the air. Vapor pressure is the pressure exerted by water molecules that have been converted to gas (water vapor). Evaporative cooling during exercise occurs in the following way. When body temperature rises above normal, the nervous system stimulates sweat glands to secrete sweat onto the surface of the skin. As sweat evaporates, heat is lost to the environment, which in turn lowers skin temperature.

Evaporation of sweat from the skin is dependent on three factors: (1) ambient conditions (i.e., air temperature and relative humidity), (2) the convective currents around the body, and (3) the amount of skin surface exposed to the environment (3, 43). At high environmental temperatures, relative humidity is the most important factor influencing the rate of evaporative heat loss. High relative humidity reduces the rate of evaporation. Indeed, when the relative humidity is near 100%, evaporation is lower compared to the level of evaporation that occurs when relative humidity is low (e.g., 30%). Therefore, cooling by way of evaporation is most effective under conditions of low humidity.

Why does high relative humidity reduce the rate of evaporation? The answer is linked to the fact that high relative humidity (RH) reduces the vapor pressure gradient between the skin and the environment. On a hot/humid day (e.g., RH = 80% – 100%), the vapor pressure in the air is close to the vapor pressure on moist skin. Therefore, the rate of evaporation is greatly reduced. High sweat rates during exercise in a hot/high-humidity environment result in useless water loss. That is, sweating per se does not cool the skin; it is evaporation that cools the skin.

Let's explore in more detail those factors that regulate the rate of evaporation. The major point to keep in mind is that evaporation occurs due to a vapor pressure gradient. That is, for evaporative cooling to occur during exercise, the vapor pressure on the skin must be greater than the vapor pressure in the air. Vapor pressure is influenced by both temperature and relative humidity. This relationship is illustrated in Table 12.1. Notice that at any given air temperature, a rise in relative humidity results in increased vapor pressure in the air. Practically speaking, this means that less evaporative cooling occurs during exercise on a hot/humid day when compared to a cool/low-humidity day. For example, an athlete running on a hot/humid day (e.g., air temperature = 30°C; RH = 100%) could have a mean skin temperature between 33°C and 34°C. In this example, the vapor pressure on the skin would be approximately 35 mm Hg, and the air vapor pressure would be approximately 32 mm Hg (Table 12.1). This

TABLE 12.1	The Relationship Between Temperature and Relative Humidity (RH) on Vapor Pressure
50% RH Temperature (°C)	Vapor Pressure (mm Hg)
0	2.3
10	4.6
20	8.8
30	15.9
75% RH Temperature (°C)	Vapor Pressure (mm Hg)
0	3.4
10	6.9
20	13.2
30	23.9
100% RH Temperature (°C)	Vapor Pressure (mm Hg)
0	4.6
10	9.2
20	17.6
30	31.9

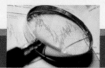
Calculation of Heat Loss via Evaporation

Knowledge that evaporation of 1000 ml of sweat results in 580 kcal of heat loss makes it possible to calculate the sweat and evaporation rate necessary to maintain a specified body temperature during exercise. Consider the following example: John is working on a cycle ergometer at a $\dot{V}O_2$ of 2.0 liters · min^{-1} (energy expenditure of 10.0 kcal · min^{-1}). If he exercises for 20 minutes at this metabolic rate and is 20% efficient, how much

evaporation would be necessary to prevent an increase in core temperature?[1] The total heat produced can be calculated as:

Total energy expenditure
= **20 min × 10 kcal/min**
= **200 kcal**

Total heat produced
= **200 kcal × .80**[1]
= **160 kcal**

The total evaporation necessary to prevent any heat gain would be computed as:

$$\frac{160 \text{ kcal}}{580 \text{ kcal/liter}} = .276 \text{ liter}^2$$
(evaporation necessary to prevent heat gain)

[1]If efficiency is 20%, then 80%, or .80, of the total energy expenditure must be released as heat.
[2]Assumes no other heat-loss mechanism is active.

small vapor pressure gradient between the skin and air (3 mm Hg) would permit only limited evaporation, and therefore little cooling would occur. In contrast, the same athlete running on a cool/low-humidity day (e.g., air temperature = 10°C; RH = 50%) might have a mean skin temperature of 30°C. The vapor pressure gradient between the skin and air under these conditions would be approximately 28 mm Hg (32 − 4 = 28) (Table 12.1). This large skin-to-air vapor pressure gradient would permit a relatively large evaporative rate, and therefore body cooling would occur under these conditions.

How much heat can be lost via evaporation during exercise? Heat loss due to evaporation can be calculated

in the following manner. The body loses 0.58 kcal of heat for each ml of water that evaporates (68). Therefore, evaporation of 1 liter of sweat would result in a heat loss of 580 kcal (1000 ml × 0.58 kcal/ml = 580 kcal). See A Closer Look 12.1 for additional examples of body heat loss calculations.

In summary, most heat loss during exercise (other than swimming) in a cool/moderate environment occurs primarily due to evaporation. In fact, when exercise is performed in a hot environment (where air temperature is greater than skin temperature), evaporation is the only means of losing body heat. The means by which the body gains and loses heat during exercise are summarized in Figure 12.3.

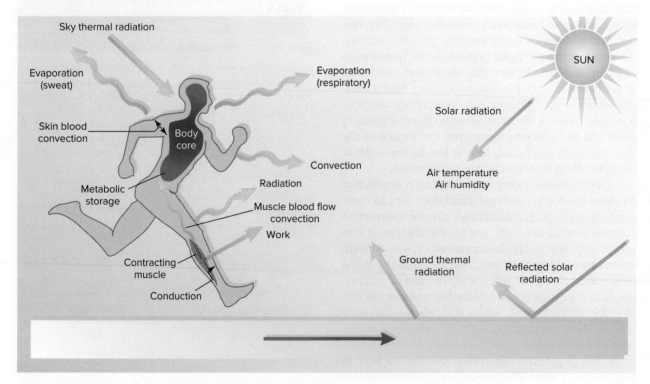

Figure 12.3   A summary of heat exchange mechanisms during exercise.

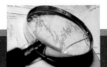

A CLOSER LOOK 12.2

Calculation of Body Temperature Increase during Exercise

Knowledge of the specific heat of the human body, along with information regarding how much heat is produced and lost from the body during exercise, permits the calculation of how much body temperature will increase during an exercise session. To better understand how to perform these calculations, let's consider the following example of an athlete performing an endurance training workout. For example, a well-trained distance runner performs a training session on an outdoor track. The weather on this day is relatively hot (30°C) and humid (60% relative humidity). The runner weighs 60 kg and performs a 40-minute workout at a $\dot{V}O_2$ of 3.0 liters·min^{-1} (i.e., energy expenditure of 15 kcal per minute). If this runner is 20% efficient and can lose only 60% of the heat produced during exercise, how much will her or his body temperature increase during this exercise session?

The total heat storage and body temperature increase during exercise can be calculated in the following steps:

1. **Total energy expenditure**
   = 40 min × 15 kcal/min
   = 600 kcal

2. **Total heat produced**
   = 600 kcal × 0.80[1]
   = 480 kcal

3. **Total heat stored during exercise**
   = 480 kcal × 0.40[2]
   = 192 kcal

4. **Amount of heat storage required to increase body temperature by 1°C**
   = 0.83 kcal/kg × 60 kg[3]
   = 49.8 kcal

The increase in body temperature resulting from this exercise session can now be calculated as follows:

5. **Increase in body temperature (°C) during exercise = Total heat stored during exercise (specific heat × body mass)**
   = 192 kcal/49.8 kcal/°C
   = 3.86°C

In the current example, this exercise bout would result in an increase in body temperature by 3.86°C–that is, 192 kcal/ (0.83 kcal/kg × 60 kg). Therefore, if the athlete began the training session with a body temperature of 37°C, the post-exercise body temperature would increase to 40.86°C (i.e., 37°C + 3.86°C).

[1]If the efficiency is 20%, then 80%, or 0.80, of the total energy expenditure must be released as heat.

[2]If the athlete can lose only 60% of the heat produced during exercise, the remaining 40%, or 0.40, of the heat produced must be stored as heat energy.

[3]The amount of heat required to increase body temperature by 1°C = (specific heat × body mass).

Heat Storage in the Body during Exercise

Now that we have discussed both heat production and heat loss, let's talk about heat storage in the body during exercise. As mentioned earlier, any heat that is produced by the working muscles during exercise and is not lost must be stored in body tissues. Therefore, the amount of heat gain in the body during exercise is computed as the difference between heat production and heat loss:

Body heat gain during exercise = (heat produced − heat loss)

The amount of heat energy required to raise body temperature depends upon the size of the individual (i.e., body weight) and a characteristic of body tissue called **specific heat.** The term *specific heat* refers to the amount of heat energy required to raise 1 kg of body tissue by 1°C. The *specific heat* for the human body is 0.83 kilocalorie (kcal) per kilogram of body mass. Therefore, the amount of heat required to elevate the body temperature by 1°C can be computed as follows:

Heat required to increase body temperature by 1°C = (specific heat × body mass)

For example, using the preceding equation, the amount of heat required to increase body temperature by 1°C in a 70-kg individual can be computed by multiplying the specific heat of the body (0.83 kcal/kg)

by the individual's body weight (70 kg). Therefore, the heat required to increase body temperature by 1°C would be 58.1 kcal (i.e., 0.83 kcal/kg × 70 kg = 58.1 kcal). See A Closer Look 12.2 for an example of body heat gain calculations during exercise.

IN SUMMARY

- Exercise using large muscle groups (i.e., legs) can result in large amounts of heat production. Because the body is, at most, 20% to 30% efficient, 70% to 80% of the energy expended during exercise is released as heat.
- Body heat can be lost by evaporation, convection, conduction, and radiation. During exercise in a cool environment, evaporation is the primary avenue for heat loss.
- The rate of evaporation from the skin is dependent upon three factors: (1) temperature and relative humidity, (2) convective currents around the body, and (3) the amount of skin exposed to the environment.
- Body heat storage is the difference between heat production and heat loss.
- The amount of heat required to elevate body temperature by 1°C is termed the specific heat of the body.

BODY'S THERMOSTAT— PREOPTIC-ANTERIOR HYPOTHALAMUS

Again, the body's temperature regulatory center is located in the preoptic-anterior hypothalamus (POAH). In general, the POAH operates much like a thermostat in your home–that is, it attempts to maintain a relatively constant core temperature around some "set point." The set-point temperature in humans is approximately 37°C.

The input to the temperature-regulating centers in the POAH comes from receptors in both the skin and the core. Changes in environmental temperature are first detected by thermal receptors (both heat and cold) located in the skin. These skin temperature receptors transmit nerve impulses to the POAH, which then initiates the appropriate response in an effort to maintain the body's set-point temperature. Further, heat/cold-sensitive neurons are located in both the spinal cord and the POAH itself, sensing changes in the core temperature.

An increase in core temperature above the set point results in the hypothalamus initiating a series of physiological actions aimed at increasing the amount of heat loss. First, the hypothalamus stimulates the sweat glands, which results in an increase in evaporative heat loss (25, 29). In addition, the vasomotor control center withdraws the normal vasoconstrictor tone to the skin, promoting cutaneous vasodilation and increased skin blood flow and therefore allowing increased heat loss (62). Figure 12.4 illustrates the physiological responses associated with an increase in core temperature. When core temperature returns to normal, the stimulus to promote both sweating and vasodilation is removed. This is an example of a control system using negative feedback (see Chap. 2).

When cold receptors are stimulated in the skin or the POAH, the thermoregulatory control center acts

Physiological responses to Cold

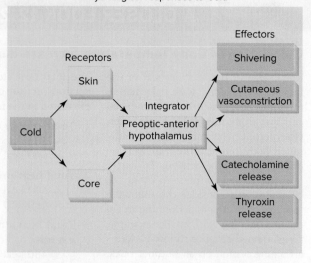

Figure 12.5 An illustration of the physiological responses to cold stress.

to minimize heat loss and increase heat production. To prevent further loss of heat, the body takes several steps of action. First, the vasomotor center directs peripheral blood vessels to vasoconstrict, which reduces heat loss (5, 23). Second, if core temperature drops significantly, involuntary shivering begins (5, 65). Additional responses include stimulation of the pilomotor center, which promotes piloerection (goosebumps). This piloerection reflex is an effective means of increasing the insulation space over the skin in fur-bearing animals but is not an effective means of preventing heat loss in humans. Further, the POAH indirectly increases thyroxine production and release, which increases cellular heat production (5). Finally, the POAH initiates the release of norepinephrine, which increases the rate of cellular metabolism (non-shivering thermogenesis). The physiological responses to a decrease in core temperature are summarized in Figure 12.5.

Shift in the Hypothalamic Thermostat Set Point Due to Fever

A fever is an increase in body temperature above the normal range, and it may be caused by numerous bacterial/viral infections or brain disorders. During a fever, select proteins and toxins secreted by bacteria can cause the set point of the body thermostat to rise above the normal level. Substances that cause this effect are called pyrogens. When the set point of the body thermostat is raised to a higher than normal level, all the mechanisms for raising body temperature are called into play (16). Within a few hours after the thermostat has been set to a higher level, the body core temperature reaches this new level due to heat conservation.

Physiological response to a "heat load"

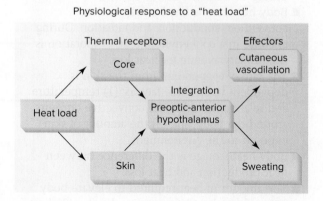

Figure 12.4 A summary illustration of the physiological responses to an increase in "heat load."

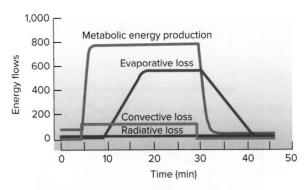

Figure 12.6 Changes in metabolic energy production, evaporative heat loss, convective heat loss, and radiative heat loss during 25 minutes of submaximal exercise in a cool environment.

- The body's thermostat is located in the preoptic-anterior hypothalamus (POAH).
- An increase in core temperature results in the POAH initiating a series of physiological actions aimed at increasing heat loss. These actions include the commencement of sweating and an increase in skin blood flow due to cutaneous vasodilation.
- Cold exposure results in the POAH promoting physiological changes that increase body heat production (shivering) and reduce heat loss (cutaneous vasoconstriction).

THERMAL EVENTS DURING EXERCISE

Now that an overview of how the POAH responds to different thermal challenges has been presented, let's discuss the thermal events that occur during submaximal constant-load exercise in a cool/moderate environment (i.e., low humidity and room temperature). Heat production increases during exercise due to muscular contraction and is directly proportional to the exercise intensity. The venous blood draining the exercising muscle distributes the excess heat throughout the body core. As core temperature increases, thermal sensors in the POAH sense the increase in blood temperature, and the thermal integration center in the POAH compares this increase in temperature with the set-point temperature and finds a difference between the two (18, 43, 46, 66). The response is to direct the nervous system to initiate sweating and to increase blood flow to the skin (45). These acts serve to increase body heat loss and minimize the increase in body temperature. At this point, the internal temperature reaches a new, elevated steady-state level. Note that this new steady-state core temperature does not represent a change in the set-point temperature, as occurs in fever (18, 43, 46, 70). Instead, the thermal regulatory center attempts to return the core temperature back to resting levels but is incapable of doing so in the face of the sustained heat production associated with exercise.

Figure 12.6 illustrates the roles of evaporation, convection, and radiation in heat loss during constant-load exercise in a moderate environment. Notice the constant but small role of convection and radiation in heat loss during this type of exercise. This is due to a constant temperature gradient between the skin and the room. In contrast, evaporation plays the most important role in heat loss during exercise in a cool and low-humidity environment (43, 46, 48).

During constant intensity exercise, the core temperature increase is directly related to the exercise intensity and is independent of ambient temperature over a wide range of conditions (i.e., 8° to 29°C with low relative humidity) (47). This point is illustrated in Figure 12.7. Notice the linear rise in core temperature as the metabolic rate increases. Further, this exercise-induced increase in body core temperature is the same for both arm and leg exercise. The fact that it is the exercise intensity and not the environmental temperature that determines the rise in core temperature during exercise suggests that the method of heat loss during continuous exercise is modified according to ambient conditions (31, 47). This concept is presented in Figure 12.8, which shows heat loss mechanisms during constant-intensity exercise at the same relative humidity but at different environmental (i.e., ambient) temperatures. Note that as the ambient

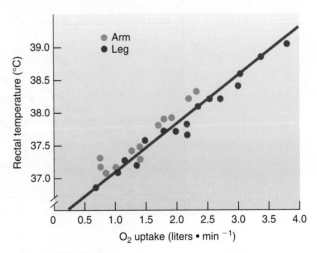

Figure 12.7 The relationship between metabolic rate and rectal temperature during constant-load arm (●) and leg (●) exercise.

Nelson, M., "Die Regulation der Korpertemperatur bei Muskelarbeit," *Scandinavica Archives Physiology* 79: 193. Oxford, England: Blackwell Scientific Publications, Ltd., 1938.

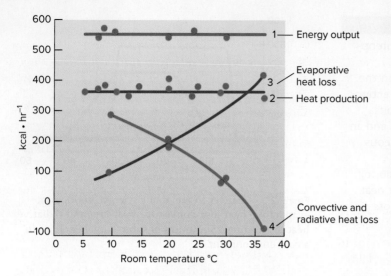

Figure 12.8 Heat exchange during exercise at different environmental temperatures. Notice the change in evaporative and convective/radiative heat loss as the environmental temperature increases. See text for discussion.

Nelson, M., "Die Regulation der Korpertemperatur bei Muskelarbeit," *Scandinavica Archives Physiology* 79: 193. Oxford, England: Blackwell Scientific Publications, Ltd., 1938.

temperature increases, the rate of convective and radiative heat loss decreases due to a decrease in the skin-to-room temperature gradient. This decrease in convective and radiative heat loss is matched by an increase in evaporative heat loss, which allows core temperature to remain the same (see Fig. 12.8).

The relationship between exercise intensity and body heat production is illustrated in Figure 12.9. Notice the linear increase in energy output (expenditure), heat production, and total heat loss as

a function of exercise work rate. Further, note that convective and radiative heat loss are not increased as a function of exercise work rate. This is due to a relatively constant temperature gradient between the skin and the environment. In contrast, there is a consistent rise in evaporative heat loss with increments in exercise intensity. This observation reemphasizes the point that evaporation is the primary means of losing heat during exercise in most environmental conditions.

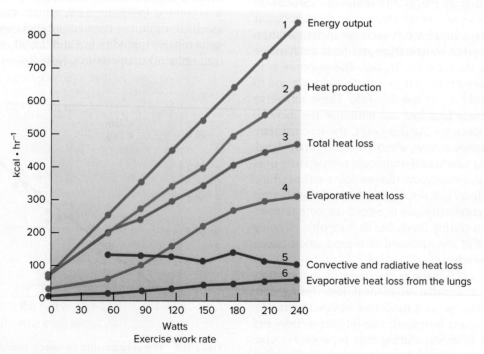

Figure 12.9 Heat exchange at rest and during cycle ergometer exercise at a variety of work rates. Note the steady increase in evaporative heat loss as a function of an increase in power output. In contrast, an increase in metabolic rate has essentially no influence on the rate of convective and radiative heat loss.

Nelson, M., "Die Regulation der Korpertemperatur bei Muskelarbeit," *Scandinavica Archives Physiology* 79: 193. Oxford, England: Blackwell Scientific Publications, Ltd., 1938.

- During constant-intensity exercise, the increase in body temperature is directly related to the exercise intensity.
- Body heat production increases in proportion to exercise intensity.

HEAT INDEX—A MEASURE OF HOW HOT IT FEELS

The Heat Index (HI) is typically expressed in degrees Fahrenheit (F) (or Centigrade) and is a measure of how hot it feels when relative humidity is added to the actual air temperature. In other words, the HI is a measure of the body's perception of how hot it feels. The HI is calculated by combining the air temperature and relative humidity to compute an apparent temperature. As discussed previously, heat loss by evaporation is the most important means of heat loss during exercise (44). However, when the relative humidity is high (i.e., high water vapor saturation in the atmosphere), the evaporation rate of sweat is reduced. This means that heat is removed from the body at a lower rate, resulting in body heat storage and an increase in body temperature. Therefore, high humidity increases an individual's perception of how hot the environment feels. For example, if the air temperature is 82°F and the relative humidity is 80%, the calculated HI is 89°F. In this illustration, the environment feels like 89°F rather than the actual air temperature of 82°F. Figure 12.10 provides the HI over a range of relative humidity (%) values and temperatures.

EXERCISE IN A HOT ENVIRONMENT

Continuous exercise in a hot/humid environment poses a particularly stressful challenge to the maintenance of normal body temperature and fluid homeostasis. High heat and humidity reduce the body's ability to lose heat by radiation/convection and evaporation, respectively. This inability to lose heat during exercise in a hot/humid environment results in a greater core temperature and a higher sweat rate (more fluid loss) when compared to the same exercise in a moderate environment (53–55, 57, 58, 63). This point is illustrated in Figure 12.11. Notice the marked differences in sweat rates and core temperatures during exercise between the hot/humid conditions and the moderate environment. The combined effect of fluid loss and high core temperature increases the risk of **hyperthermia** (large rise in core temperature) and heat injury (see Clinical Applications 12.1 and Chap. 24).

Sweat Rates during Exercise

In an effort to increase evaporative heat loss during exercise, humans rely on their ability to increase sweat production via eccrine sweat glands (i.e., sweat glands under sympathetic cholinergic control) (30). In this regard, exercise in a hot environment greatly increases sweat rates during exercise training or sports competition (4, 19, 30, 61). Note, however, that sweat rates may vary widely across different individuals. For example, heat-accustomed individuals have an earlier onset of sweating and a higher sweat rate during exercise. Further, large individuals (i.e., large body mass) will likely have higher sweat rates compared to smaller individuals. Finally, genetic variations in sweat rates exist such that two individuals with the same body size and level of heat adaptation may also differ in sweat rates.

American football players, wearing full uniforms and practicing in a hot and humid environment, experience some of the largest sweat rates ever recorded for athletes. Although several reasons exist for high sweat loss in these athletes, two major contributors are that many football players possess large body masses and that football uniforms retard heat loss (1, 24). For example, the average sweat loss in football players (body weight range, 180 to 240 pounds) ranges from 4 to 5 liters per hour during a practice session in a hot and humid environment (19). Further, during preseason practice sessions where football athletes are practicing twice a day, the daily sweat loss ranged from 9 to 12 liters of water. Failure to replace this loss of fluid on a daily basis will result in progressive dehydration and increase the risk of heat injury (4, 61, 62). For more information on the importance of fluid replacement during exercise, see The Winning Edge 12.1.

Exercise Performance Is Impaired in a Hot Environment

Performance during prolonged, exercise in a submaximal event (e.g., marathon or long triathlon) is impaired in a hot/humid environment (39). Similarly, hot environmental conditions also decrease athletic performance during high-intensity exercise (e.g., rugby, soccer, or 15-min time trial on cycle) (15, 26, 60). Although the mechanisms responsible for this heat-induced decreased exercise performance continue to be investigated, current evidence indicates that three major factors can contribute to impaired exercise performance in the heat: (1) accelerated muscle fatigue, (2) cardiovascular dysfunction, and/or (3) central nervous system dysfunction (Fig. 12.12). In theory, each of these factors can independently contribute to diminished performance during exercise in a hot environment. However, it is likely that these factors interact to contribute to impaired performance

Temperature °F (°C)	Relative Humidity (%)												
	40	45	50	55	60	65	70	75	80	85	90	95	100
110 (47)	136 (58)												
108 (43)	130 (54)	137 (58)											
106 (41)	124 (51)	130 (54)	137 (58)										
104 (40)	119 (48)	124 (51)	131 (55)	137 (58)									
102 (39)	114 (46)	119 (48)	124 (51)	130 (54)	137 (58)								
100 (38)	109 (43)	114 (46)	118 (48)	124 (51)	129 (54)	136 (58)							
98 (37)	105 (41)	109 (43)	113 (45)	117 (47)	123 (51)	128 (53)	134 (57)						
96 (36)	101 (38)	104 (40)	108 (42)	112 (44)	116 (47)	121 (49)	126 (52)	132 (56)					
94 (34)	97 (36)	100 (38)	103 (39)	106 (41)	110 (43)	114 (46)	119 (48)	124 (51)	129 (54)	135 (57)			
92 (33)	94 (34)	96 (36)	99 (37)	101 (38)	105 (41)	108 (42)	112 (44)	116 (47)	121 (49)	126 (52)	131 (55)		
90 (32)	91 (33)	93 (34)	95 (35)	97 (36)	100 (38)	103 (39)	106 (41)	109 (43)	113 (45)	117 (47)	122 (50)	127 (53)	132 (56)
88 (31)	88 (31)	89 (32)	91 (33)	93 (34)	95 (35)	98 (37)	100 (38)	103 (39)	106 (41)	110 (43)	113 (45)	117 (47)	121 (49)
86 (30)	85 (29)	87 (31)	88 (31)	89 (32)	91 (33)	93 (34)	95 (35)	97 (36)	100 (38)	102 (39)	105 (41)	108 (42)	112 (44)
84 (29)	83 (28)	84 (29)	85 (29)	86 (30)	88 (31)	89 (32)	90 (32)	92 (33)	94 (34)	96 (36)	98 (37)	100 (38)	103 (39)
82 (28)	81 (27)	82 (28)	83 (28)	84 (29)	84 (29)	85 (29)	86 (30)	88 (31)	89 (32)	90 (32)	91 (33)	93 (34)	95 (35)
80 (27)	80 (27)	80 (27)	81 (27)	81 (27)	82 (28)	82 (28)	83 (28)	84 (29)	84 (29)	85 (29)	86 (30)	86 (30)	87 (31)

Category	Heat Index
Extreme Danger	130°F or higher (54°C or higher)
Danger	105–129°F (41–54°C)
Extreme Caution	90–105°F (32–41°C)
Caution	80–90°F (27–32°C)

Figure 12.10 The relationship of relative humidity (%) and temperature and the Heat Index.

Data obtained from National Weather Service–Tulsa.

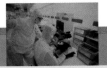
Exercise-Related Heat Injuries Can Be Prevented

Heat injury during exercise can occur when the level of body heat production is high and environmental conditions (e.g., high ambient temperature and humidity) impede heat loss from the body. The primary cause of heat injury is hyperthermia (high body temperature). Increases in body temperature of 2°C to 3°C generally do not have ill effects (3, 7). Nonetheless, increases in body temperature above 40°C to 41°C can be associated with a variety of heat-related problems. Note that heat-related problems during exercise are not "all or none," but form a heat-injury continuum that can extend from a relatively minor problem (i.e., heat syncope) to a life-threatening, major medical emergency (i.e., heat stroke). The general symptoms of heat stress include nausea, headache, dizziness, reduced sweat rate, and the general inability to think rationally.

Each year in the United States, several heat-related problems in American football are reported. Nonetheless, heat-related illness during exercise can be prevented. To prevent overheating during exercise, the following guidelines are useful:

- Exercise during the coolest part of the day.
- Minimize both the intensity and duration of exercise on hot/humid days.
- Expose a maximal surface area of skin for evaporation (i.e., removal of clothing) during exercise.
- When removal of clothing during exercise is not possible (e.g., American football), provide frequent rest/cool-down breaks along with intermittent clothing shed (e.g., removal of helmet and upper clothing).
- To avoid dehydration during exercise, workouts should permit frequent water breaks (coupled with rest/cool-down).
- Rest/cool-down breaks during exercise should remove the athlete from radiant heat gain due to direct sunlight (e.g., sitting under a tent) and offer exposure to circulating, cool air (e.g., fans).
- Measure body weight at the beginning and end of a training (or practice) session to determine the amount of fluid replacement required to restore body water balance before the next training session. Maintaining proper hydration is important because dehydration increases the risk of heat injury.

When an athlete develops symptoms of heat injury, the obvious treatment is to stop exercising and immediately begin cooling the body (e.g., cold water immersion). Cold fluids with electrolytes should also be provided for rehydration. See Chap. 24 for more details on the signs and symptoms of heat injury. Also, see Casa et al. (2015) in Suggested Readings for more information on the prevention and care of exercise-induced heat illness.

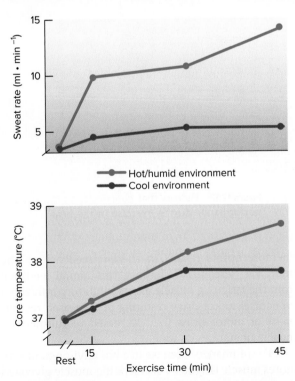

Figure 12.11 Differences in core temperature and sweat rate during 45 minutes of submaximal exercise in a hot/humid environment versus a cool environment.

during exercise in the heat. In this regard, the relative contribution of each of these factors in impaired exercise performance depends upon the exercise intensity and duration. Let's discuss these factors in more detail.

Accelerated Muscle Fatigue During exercise in a hot environment, three major changes occur in muscle metabolism that contribute to muscle fatigue. First, the rate of muscle glycogen breakdown is increased (21). This is important because muscle glycogen depletion contributes to muscle fatigue during prolonged exercise (21). Second, exercise in a hot environment increases muscle lactate production and this exercise-induced increase in muscle lactate levels results in decreased muscle pH, which also contributes to muscle fatigue. Finally, during exercise in a hot environment, skeletal muscle production of free radicals is increased. This is significant because increased production of free radicals in muscles can also contribute to muscle fatigue (72). Recall that free radicals are produced during muscle contraction and that radicals are highly reactive molecules that contain an unpaired electron in their outer orbital (56). This is important because free radicals rapidly react with muscle proteins resulting in oxidative damage

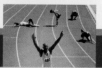

THE WINNING EDGE 12.1

Prevention of Dehydration during Exercise

Athletic performance can be impaired by sweat-induced loss of body water (i.e., dehydration). Indeed, dehydration resulting in loss of 1% to 2% of body weight is sufficient to impair exercise performance (8, 39). Dehydration of greater than 3% of body weight further impairs physiological function and increases the risk of heat injury (8, 38). Therefore, prevention of dehydration during exercise is important to both maximize athletic performance and prevent heat injuries. Dehydration can be avoided by adherence to the following guidelines:

- Athletes should be well hydrated prior to beginning a workout or competition. This can be achieved by drinking 400 to 800 ml of fluid within three hours prior to exercise (37, 39).
- Athletes should consume 150 to 300 ml of fluid every 15 to 20 minutes during exercise (39). The actual volume of fluid ingested during each drinking period should be adjusted to environmental conditions (i.e., rate of sweat loss) and individual tolerances for drinking during exercise.
- To ensure rehydration following exercise, athletes should monitor fluid losses during exercise by recording body weight prior to the workout and then weighing immediately after the workout session. To ensure proper rehydration following exercise, the individual should consume fluids equal to approximately 150% of the weight loss. For example, if an athlete loses 1 kg of body weight during a training session, he/she should consume 1.5 liters of fluid to achieve complete rehydration (39).

- Monitoring the color of urine between workouts is a practical way to judge hydration levels in athletes. For example, in a well-hydrated individual, urine is typically clear or the color of lemonade. In contrast, in dehydrated individuals, urine appears as a dark-yellow fluid.

Which is the optimal rehydration fluid—water or a well-formulated sports drink? The National Athletic Trainers Association has concluded that well-designed sports drinks are superior to water for rehydration following exercise (8). The rationale for this recommendation is that these beverages increase voluntary intake by athletes and allow for more effective rehydration. For more details on fluid replacement during and following exercise, please see Maughan and Shirreffs (2010) and Kenefick and Cheuvront (2012) in Suggested Readings.

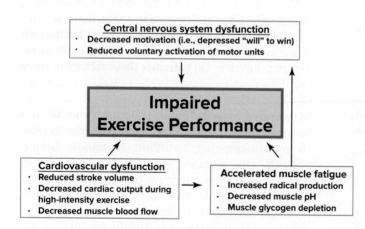

Figure 12.12 Factors that contribute to impaired performance during exercise in the heat.

(i.e., oxidation). This heat-induced increase in muscle radical production can damage contractile proteins (e.g., actin and myosin) resulting in reduced muscle force production (i.e., muscle fatigue) (56).

Further, as illustrated in Figure 12.12, muscle fatigue can contribute to central nervous system dysfunction. This occurs because of peripheral feedback from the fatiguing muscles to the brain resulting in a decreased central motor drive. Specifically, muscle chemoreceptors (also called metaboreceptors) are stimulated during fatiguing exercise. Activation of muscle chemoreceptors results in afferent feedback to the brain via type III/IV afferents; this neural feedback from the fatiguing muscle exerts inhibitory influences on central motor drive resulting in decreased recruitment of motor units (i.e., decreased recruitment of muscle fibers).

To summarize, exercise in a hot environment promotes muscle fatigue by accelerating muscle glycogen depletion, increasing lactate production, and fostering free radical production. In many cases, these three factors interact and contribute to the accelerated muscle fatigue observed during exercise in a hot environment. Further, afferent neural feedback from fatiguing muscles to the brain exerts inhibitory influences on central motor drive resulting in a decrease in the activation of motors units and, consequently, a decrease in muscle force production.

Cardiovascular Dysfunction Cardiovascular dysfunction is another potential contributor to impaired exercise performance in a hot/humid environment. Indeed, heat stress can promote cardiovascular strain (i.e., increased heart rate and decreased stroke volume) and reduced muscle blood flow. Note, however, that reduced muscle blood flow does not contribute to impaired exercise tolerance during light or moderate exercise because muscle blood flow is well maintained during submaximal exercise when dehydration does not occur (12). In contrast, during high-intensity exercise (i.e., near $\dot{V}O_2$ max) performed in a hot/humid environment, there is a progressive decline in muscle blood flow. This reduction in muscle blood flow during exercise in the heat is due to a competition for blood between the working muscles and the skin. That is, as body temperature rises during exercise in a hot environment, blood flow moves away from the contracting muscle toward the skin to assist in cooling the body. Therefore, during high-intensity exercise, reduced muscle blood flow can contribute to impaired exercise performance in the heat; this reduction in muscle blood flow results in reduced oxygen delivery to the muscle and is a contributory factor to the accelerated muscle fatigue that occurs during high-intensity exercise in a hot environment (Fig. 12.12). In contrast, reduced muscle blood flow cannot explain the heat-induced reduction in exercise performance during prolonged submaximal exercise. For more details on how cardiovascular dysfunction contributes to impaired exercise performance in a hot environment, see Nybo et al. (2014) and Sawka et al. (2015) in the Suggested Readings.

Central Nervous System Dysfunction It is well established that both hyperthermia and dehydration can impair exercise performance due to central nervous system dysfunction. Specifically, hyperthermia (high body temperature) acts upon the central nervous system to reduce the mental drive for motor unit recruitment (21, 38, 40). As discussed earlier, activation of muscle chemoreceptors results in afferent feedback to the brain via type III/IV afferents. Again, this neural feedback from the fatiguing muscle exerts inhibitory influences on central motor drive resulting in decreased recruitment of motor units.

To summarize, prolonged exercise in the heat can impede exercise performance due to changes in the central nervous system. This exercise-induced impairment of the central nervous system can arise from hyperthermia, dehydration, and afferent feedback from muscle chemoreceptors. For more details on this topic, see Nybo et al. (2014) in Suggested Readings.

Exercise Performance in a Hot Environment: Summary and Conclusions Exercise in the heat accelerates muscle fatigue and impairs exercise performance. It seems likely that heat-induced fatigue is not due to a single factor but results from a combination of physiological factors (49). Key factors that contribute to heat-induced impairments in exercise performance are accelerated muscle fatigue, impaired cardiovascular function, and central nervous system dysfunction. The relative contribution that each factor plays in heat-induced impaired exercise performance depends upon the duration and intensity of exercise. For example, during prolonged submaximal exercise, central nervous system dysfunction and accelerated muscle fatigue interact to diminish exercise performance. In contrast, cardiovascular dysfunction does not play a major role in impaired exercise performance during prolonged submaximal exercise in the absence of severe dehydration. However, cardiovascular dysfunction (i.e., decreased muscle blood flow) clearly contributes to the diminished exercise performance during high-intensity exercise in a hot environment.

Athletes can use several strategies to improve their exercise performance in a hot environment. For example, athletes can optimize exercise performance in the heat by becoming heat acclimated and consuming fluid before and during exercise. The process of physiological adaptation to heat (heat acclimation) will improve exercise tolerance and will be discussed later in this chapter. Guidelines for the consumption of water before and during athletic performance are presented in The Winning Edge 12.1 and are also discussed in Chap. 23. Further, precooling has been shown to improve exercise performance in a hot environment (see Winning Edge 12.2). Finally, for more details on exercise performance in the heat, see Ask the Expert 12.1.

Gender and Age Differences in Thermoregulation

In the 1960s it was believed that, compared to men, women were less tolerant of exercise in a hot environment. However, these early studies did not match men and women at the same level of heat acclimation and similar body compositions (i.e., equal percent body fat). Indeed, when studies have matched men and women for these characteristics, the gender differences in heat tolerance are small.

Does aging impair one's ability to thermoregulate and exercise in the heat? This issue remains

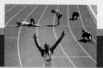

Exercise Physiology Applied to Sports—Precooling the Body Improves Exercise Performance in the Heat

Prolonged exercise in the heat can result in an excessively high body temperature (i.e., hyperthermia) arising from the imbalance between body heat production and heat loss. This is important because a high body temperature negatively impacts many physiological functions and impairs exercise performance. Importantly, sustained high core temperatures can lead to heat illness. Therefore, strategies that prevent excessive body heat storage during prolonged exercise in a hot environment can improve exercise performance and protect against heat injury.

One of the most effective strategies to improve exercise performance in a hot environment is to cool the body prior to exercise (called "precooling"). In short, the purpose of precooling is to lower the body core temperature prior to beginning exercise. The concept is that if an athlete begins exercise with a lower core temperature, induced by precooling, this permits the individual to perform more work prior to reaching an elevated core temperature that limits exercise performance. In this regard, many studies confirm that precooling results in small but significant improvements (i.e., 5% to 7%) in performance during endurance exercise performed in a hot environment (6).

Studies investigating the impact of precooling on exercise performance have used a variety of different cooling techniques including: (1) cold water immersion, (2) cooling (ice) vest, (3) cooling packs, and (4) ingestion of cold drinks (6). Although each of these techniques improves exercise performance in a hot environment, a combination of cooling techniques (e.g., combining cooling pack and cold water immersion) improves performance more than a single cooling technique (6). Using these combined cooling techniques appears to be more effective than a single cooling technique because these "mixed" techniques impact a larger body surface area and result in a lower overall core temperature (6). For more information on precooling and exercise performance, see Bongers et al. (2015) in the Suggested Reading list.

---

controversial, but it does appear that aging results in a reduced ability to regulate body temperature in sedentary individuals (5, 14, 28, 30, 52). However, well-controlled studies have concluded that exercise-conditioned old and young men show little difference in thermoregulation during exercise (52, 64). Further, a recent review of the literature on this subject has concluded that heat tolerance does not appear to be severely compromised by age in healthy and physically active older subjects (28, 30). Based upon the collective evidence, it appears that deconditioning (i.e., decline in $\dot{V}O_2$ max) and a lack of heat acclimatization in older subjects may explain why some of the earlier studies reported a decrease in thermotolerance with age. For more details on the impact of aging on temperature regulation, see Blatteis (2012) in Suggested Readings.

Heat Acclimation

Regular exercise in a hot environment results in a series of physiological adaptations designed to minimize disturbances in homeostasis due to heat stress. The term **acclimatization** refers to physiological adjustments that occur in response to repeated exposure to the natural environment whereas **acclimation** refers to adjustments produced by exposure to artificial conditions in experimental chambers. Nonetheless, the terms acclimation and acclimatization are often used interchangeably to refer to the physiological adaptation that occurs when an individual undergoes repeated exposure to a stressful environment (e.g., hot ambient temperature). In our discussion of exercise and heat tolerance, we will use the term acclimation to denote an improved tolerance to heat stress following repeated exposure (days to weeks) to a hot environment.

Individuals of all ages are capable of acclimating to a hot environment (28, 64). The end result of heat acclimation is a lower heart rate and core temperature during submaximal exercise (14). Although partial heat acclimation can occur by training in a cool environment, it is essential that athletes exercise in a hot environment to obtain maximal heat acclimation (2). Because an elevation in core temperature is the primary stimulus to promote heat acclimation, it is recommended that the athlete perform strenuous interval training or continuous exercise at an intensity exceeding 50% of the athlete's $\dot{V}O_2$ max in order to promote higher core temperatures (50) (see Research Focus 12.1).

The primary adaptations that occur during heat acclimation are an increased plasma volume, earlier onset of sweating, higher sweat rate, reduced salt loss in sweat, a reduced skin blood flow, and increased synthesis of heat shock proteins. It is interesting that heat adaptation occurs rapidly, with almost complete acclimation being achieved by 7 to 14 days

ASK THE EXPERT 12.1

Exercise Performance in a Hot Environment
Questions and Answers with Dr. Michael Sawka

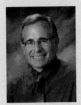

Courtesy of
Dr. Michael
Sawka

Michael Sawka, Ph.D., is Professor of Applied Physiology at the Georgia Institute of Technology.

Dr. Sawka is an internationally recognized expert in both exercise physiology and environmental stress. Indeed, Dr. Sawka has authored more than 200 highly regarded research studies related to both exercise and environmental physiology. In particular, Dr. Sawka and his team have performed many studies investigating the impact of a hot environment on exercise performance.

In this box feature, Dr. Sawka addresses three important questions related to exercise performance in the heat.

QUESTION: Your work has established that environmental heat stress has a negative impact on aerobic exercise performance. However, how does heat stress impact performance in team sports, such as soccer or American football?

ANSWER: The performance of a team is dependent upon the performance of the individual athletes. If the individual athlete's performance is impaired, then it is likely the team's performance will also be suboptimal. In addition, team sports are greatly dependent upon both cohesion and decision making, and there is evidence that heat stress and dehydration can degrade cognitive function, which will have a negative impact on decision making and team cohesion.

QUESTION: Your group has extensively studied the mechanism(s) to explain why environmental heat stress impairs aerobic exercise performance. What are the primary explanations as to why a hot environment impairs aerobic performance?

ANSWER: Heat stress impairs aerobic exercise performance because of two primary reasons: (1) cardiovascular strain needed to support high skin blood flow, and (2) dehydration, which reduces plasma volume and thus increases cardiovascular strain. During exercise in a hot environment, the high skin blood flow and reduced plasma volume both act to reduce venous pressure and thus reduce cardiac filling. Despite a compensatory increase in heart rate and contractility, stroke volume will usually decline and thus make it difficult to maintain blood pressure and to sustain adequate blood flow to skeletal muscle and the brain. In addition, thermal discomfort and perceived exertion are elevated. The net effect is that heat stress degrades maximal aerobic power and that any submaximal work rate is performed at a greater relative work rate (i.e., percent of maximal aerobic power), which also increases perception of effort. Further, heat stress alters skeletal muscle metabolism (increased glycogen use and lactate accumulation) and may modify central nervous system function, which can contribute to impaired exercise performance.

QUESTION: Strong evidence indicates that heat acclimation improves exercise tolerance in hot environments. However, are there other strategies (e.g., precooling or hyperhydration) that athletes can utilize to improve aerobic performance in a hot environment?

ANSWER: By far the most effective strategies to sustain performance during heat stress are to achieve heat acclimation and maintain adequate hydration. In addition, heat acclimation has recently been demonstrated to confer benefits to improve aerobic exercise performance in temperate environments. There is some evidence that precooling and hyperhydration can improve performance in a hot environment, but in my opinion their benefits are marginal and if improperly used might be counterproductive.

Hyperhydration can result in a small increase in blood volume and slightly delay developing dehydration; together, these changes help to support the cardiovascular system during exercise in a hot environment. Nonetheless, these benefits are marginal and, depending upon the methods employed, hyperhydration could increase the likelihood of hyponatremia (i.e., low blood sodium levels), discomfort associated with increased urine output, or elevated risk of headache.

Precooling allows body temperature (skin and core) to be lower at the beginning of exercise, but the small benefits demonstrated in laboratory studies may be lost in real-life competition when athletes are exposed to the hot environment for a significant period before initiating competition. In addition, overcooling the skeletal muscles might initially impair muscle performance.

after the first exposure (51, 70) (Fig. 12.13). A brief discussion of each of these physiological adaptations follows.

Heat acclimation results in a 10% to 12% increase in plasma volume (17, 67). This increased plasma volume maintains central blood volume, stroke volume, and sweating capacity, and allows the body to store more heat with a smaller temperature gain.

A key aspect of heat acclimation is an earlier onset of sweating and an increase in the sweat rate. An earlier onset of sweating simply means that sweating begins rapidly after the commencement of exercise; this translates into less heat storage at the beginning of exercise and a lower core temperature. In addition, heat acclimation can increase the sweating capacity almost threefold above the rate achievable prior to

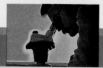

Can Exercise Training in Cool Conditions Promote Heat Acclimation?

Athletes who train in cool environments often travel to warmer climates to compete. Without adequate heat acclimation, these athletes will be at a disadvantage compared to athletes who have developed a high level of heat adaptation by training in a hot/humid environment. Therefore, a key question is, "Can training in heavy clothing in a cool environment promote heat acclimation?" The answer to this question is yes, but the magnitude of the heat acclimation that is obtained by this method is generally less than the maximal level of acclimation that can be achieved by daily training in a hot/humid environment (2, 13).

Nonetheless, "artificial" heat training in heavy clothing in cool conditions appears to be better than attempting no heat acclimation measures (13).

On a related topic, most of us have witnessed individuals exercising in a rubber suit. These exercise suits are typically made of a rubberized vinyl that covers the entire body and prevents evaporative heat loss from the skin. While exercise in these suits will promote increased body temperature and therefore will contribute to heat acclimation, prolonged exercise in a rubber suit is a high-risk endeavor that could lead to high body temperatures and heat injury.

Therefore, wearing a rubber suit during exercise is not recommended because of the risk of hyperthermia associated with the prevention of evaporative heat loss. Also, note that while exercise in a rubber suit will encourage body water loss, exercise in a rubber suit does not necessarily result in the loss of body fat because to lose body fat, you must create an energy (i.e., caloric) deficit. Indeed, while a sweat-induced loss of body water does reduce your body weight, as soon as you replace these fluids by drinking, your body weight will return to normal. See Chap. 18 for details on loss of body fat.

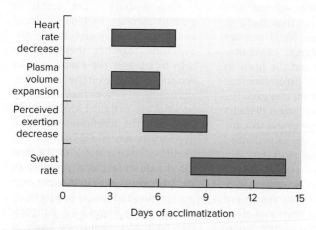

Figure 12.13   The number of days required to reach maximal heat acclimation during consecutive days of heat exposure. Note that maximal heat acclimation is achieved between 7 and 14 days following the initial heat exposure.

heat adaptation (59, 71). Therefore, much more evaporative cooling is possible, which is a major advantage in minimizing heat storage during prolonged work.

Moreover, sweat losses of sodium and chloride are lower following heat acclimation, due to an increased secretion of aldosterone (11). While this adaptation results in a reduction of electrolyte loss and aids in reducing electrolyte disturbances during exercise in the heat, it does not minimize the need to replace the body water loss that occurs during exercise which is higher than normal (see Chaps. 23 and 24).

Moreover, an important part of heat acclimation includes the cellular production of heat shock proteins in skeletal muscle fibers and all other cells of the body. Heat shock proteins are members of a large family of proteins called "stress proteins," which were introduced in Chap. 2. As the name implies, these stress proteins are synthesized in response to stress (e.g., heat) and are designed to prevent cellular damage due to heat or other stresses. Details of how heat shock proteins protect cells against heat stress are located in Research Focus 12.2.

In summary, regular bouts of exercise in a hot environment result in the rapid development of heat acclimation that reaches maximal adaptation within 7 to 14 days. This adaptation results in a reduced heart rate during submaximal exercise in the heat, decreased body core temperature, decreased psychological rating of perceived exertion, and improved exercise performance in a hot environment (34). The days required to reach maximal heat acclimation for these various physiological measures are summarized in Figure 12.13, and an illustration of the impact of heat acclimation on heart rate and core temperature during exercise in the heat is illustrated in Figure 12.14.

Loss of Acclimation

When an individual stops exercising, the loss of heat acclimation is rapid, with reductions in heat tolerance occurring within a few days of inactivity (i.e., no heat exposure) (32). Specifically, heat tolerance decreases significantly within 7 days of no heat exposure, and complete loss of heat tolerance occurs following 28 days of no heat exposure (2). Therefore, repeated exposure to heat is required to maintain heat acclimation (69).

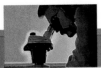

RESEARCH FOCUS 12.2

Heat Acclimation and Heat Shock Proteins

Repeated bouts of prolonged exercise in a warm or hot environment result in many physiological adaptations that minimize disturbances in homeostasis due to heat stress. Collectively, these adaptations improve exercise tolerance in hot environments and reduce the risk of heat injury. Evidence indicates that an important part of this adaptive process is the synthesis of heat shock proteins in numerous tissues, including skeletal muscle and the heart (42). Heat shock proteins represent a family of "stress" proteins that are synthesized in response to cellular stress (i.e., heat, acidosis, tissue injury, etc.). Although heat shock proteins perform a variety of cellular functions, it is clear that these proteins protect cells from thermal injury by stabilizing and refolding damaged proteins. Indeed, heat shock proteins play an important role in the development of thermotolerance and protect body cells from the heat loads associated with prolonged exercise (42).

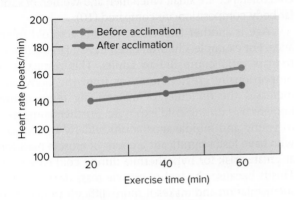

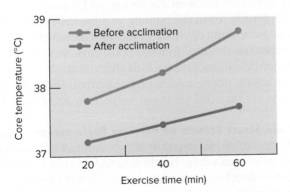

Figure 12.14 Illustration of the impact of heat acclimation on heart rate and core temperature during constant load submaximal (50% $\dot{V}O_2$ max) exercise in a hot environment.

■ Heat acclimation results in (1) an increase in plasma volume, (2) an earlier onset of sweating during exercise, (3) a higher sweat rate, (4) a reduction in the amount of electrolytes lost in sweat, (5) a reduction in skin blood flow, and (6) increased levels of heat shock protein in tissues.

EXERCISE IN A COLD ENVIRONMENT

Exercise in a cold environment enhances an athlete's ability to lose heat and therefore greatly reduces the chance of heat injury. In general, the combination of metabolic heat production and warm clothing prevents the development of **hypothermia** (large decrease in core temperature) during short-term exercise on a cold day. However, exercise in the cold for extended periods of time (e.g., a long triathlon) or swimming in cold water may overpower the body's ability to prevent heat loss, and hypothermia may result. In such cases, heat production during exercise is not able to keep pace with heat loss. This is particularly true during swimming in extremely cold water (e.g., <15°C). Severe hypothermia may result in a loss of judgment, which increases the risk of further cold injury.

Individuals with a high percentage of body fat have an advantage over lean individuals when it comes to cold tolerance (23). Large amounts of subcutaneous fat provide an increased layer of insulation from the cold. This additional insulation reduces the rate of heat loss and therefore improves cold tolerance. For this reason, women generally tolerate mild cold exposure better than men.

Participation in sports activities in the cold may present several other types of problems for the athlete. For example, hands exposed to cold weather become numb due to the reduction in the rate of neural transmission and reduced blood flow due to

IN SUMMARY

■ During prolonged exercise in a moderate environment, core temperature will increase gradually above the normal resting value and will reach a plateau at approximately 30 to 45 minutes.

■ During exercise in a hot/humid environment, core temperature does not reach a plateau, but will continue to rise. Long-term exercise in this type of environment increases the risk of heat injury.

vasoconstriction. This results in a loss of dexterity and affects such skills as throwing and catching. In addition, exposed flesh is susceptible to frostbite, which may present a serious medical condition. Further details of the effects of a cold environment on performance are presented in Chap. 24.

Humans often exercise and work in cold weather environments but, in general, cold weather is not a barrier to performing exercise training or outdoor work. Nonetheless, there are some cases of cold stress (i.e., exercise at low ambient temperatures with high wind or immersion in cold water) that challenge the body's ability to maintain temperature homeostasis (10). Cold stress is defined as any environmental condition that promotes a loss of body heat and threatens temperature homeostasis. In the following sections, we will highlight the physiological responses to exercise in the cold and discuss acclimation to cold. For more details of the effects of exercise in a cold environment, see Chap. 24.

Physiological Responses to Exercise in the Cold

During resting conditions, humans exhibit peripheral vasoconstriction upon exposure to cold. This results in a decrease in skin blood flow that reduces convective heat loss between the skin and the environment; this effectively increases the insulation of the body. In these conditions, heat is lost from the exposed body surface faster than it is replaced and skin temperature decreases (10). During whole body exposure to a cold environment (i.e., individual wearing shorts and short-sleeve shirt), the vasoconstrictor response extends beyond the fingers and spreads throughout the body's peripheral circulation (10). This vasoconstriction response to cold exposure reduces heat loss and protects deep body temperature; however, this occurs at the expense of a decrease in skin temperature (10). Prolonged cold exposure (at rest) can also increase metabolic heat production via both shivering (repeated rhythmic muscle contractions) and increased metabolic heat production by brown adipose tissue (10).

Exercise in a cold environment enhances an athlete's ability to lose heat and therefore greatly reduces the chance of heat injury. In general, the combination of metabolic heat production and warm clothing prevents the development of hypothermia (large decrease in core temperature) during exercise on a cold day. However, exercise in the cold for extended periods of time (e.g., a long triathlon) or swimming in cold water may overpower the body's ability to prevent heat loss, and hypothermia can occur. In such cases, heat production during exercise is not able to keep pace with heat loss. This is particularly true during swimming in extremely cold water (e.g., 15°C or lower).

Factors Affecting Body Heat Loss during Cold Exposure Several factors affect the amount of heat loss that occurs during cold exposure. For example, individuals with a high percentage of body fat have an advantage over lean individuals when it comes to cold tolerance (23, 49). Large amounts of subcutaneous fat provide an increased layer of insulation from the cold. This additional insulation reduces the rate of heat loss and therefore improves cold tolerance. Because women typically possess added subcutaneous fat, women often tolerate mild cold exposure and cold-water immersion better than men (10). Nonetheless, sex differences in cold tolerance are small when men and women of similar body composition are compared (10).

Age is another factor that can impact cold tolerance. For example, children often have a large surface-to-mass ratio compared to adults. This results in a proportionally greater heat loss from the body and increases the difficulty of maintaining temperature homeostasis during cold exposure. Further, compared to young and middle-aged adults, elderly individuals who have lost a significant amount of muscle mass are at greater risk for hypothermia during cold exposure. This is because the loss of muscle mass decreases tissue insulation and makes it more difficult to maintain temperature homeostasis during cold exposure.

Finally, exercise training or physical fitness levels have limited influences on thermoregulatory responses to cold. Indeed, both cross-sectional and longitudinal studies conclude that the ability to tolerate cold is not related to physical fitness levels if subjects are matched for the same percent body fat (10).

Cold Stress Effects on Exercise Performance Cold temperature can impair sports performance in several ways. For example, hands exposed to cold temperatures often become numb due to the reduction in the rate of neural transmission and reduced blood flow due to vasoconstriction. This results in a loss of manual dexterity and affects motor skills such as throwing and catching. The level of cold-induced impairment of manual dexterity is directly correlated with skin temperature. Further, as skin temperature reaches 15°C (i.e., 59°F), manual dexterity begins to decline rapidly with further decreases in temperature (10).

Cold can also impact muscle strength and power output when muscle temperature decreases significantly (10). For example, studies investigating the impact of cold water immersion on muscular strength reveal that reducing muscle by ~8°C can reduce muscle strength and power by 31% to 44% (10). Nonetheless, during exercise in cold air, the temperature of the exercising muscle does not typically decrease and therefore, cold air exposure rarely decreases muscular force production.

To date, only a few studies have investigated the influence of cold air on aerobic exercise performance and unfortunately, there is no consensus about whether aerobic exercise performance is impaired in a cold environment compared to relatively warm temperatures. Similar to the studies of cold air exposure, only a few studies have examined aerobic performance during exercise in cold water. Nonetheless, it is predicted that cold water would potentially have a negative impact on aerobic performance because, compared to air, heat conduction in water is 25 times greater than air resulting in a larger decrease in muscle temperatures (10). See Castellani and Tipton (2016) in the Suggested Readings for more information about the effect of cold stress on exercise performance.

Health Risks during Exercise in the Cold Individuals immersed in cold water (e.g., 15°C or lower) are at risk for hypothermia. In fact, people who accidently fall into rivers or lakes at near freezing temperatures are at risk of death when the body core temperature declines from the normal level of 37°C to 25°C or lower. This level of hypothermia is associated with cardiac arrhythmias and potentially cardiac arrest. Moreover, severe hypothermia also results in a loss of judgment, which increases the risk of further cold injury.

Compared to exercise in cold water, exercise in cold air presents less risk of developing hypothermia. Nonetheless, exposed skin is at risk for frostbite when air temperatures are below freezing. In this regard, if not treated early, frostbite is a serious medical condition that can result in permanent tissue damage (i.e., gangrene) when skin is exposed to cold conditions for long time periods.

Does breathing cold air during exercise pose a risk to the respiratory tract or lungs? The short answer is no. Indeed, the cold air that enters the nose or mouth is rapidly warmed before entering the lungs. However, breathing cold air can trigger exercise-induced asthma in some individuals. This type of exercise-induced asthma is caused by a cooling and drying of the airways, which results in bronchoconstriction. See Chap. 17 for more details on the causes of exercise-induced asthma.

Cold Acclimation

Three major physiological adaptations occur when humans are chronically exposed to cold temperatures (35, 36). First, cold adaptation results in a reduction in the mean skin temperature at which shivering begins. That is, people who are cold acclimated begin shivering at a lower skin temperature when compared to unacclimated individuals. The explanation for this finding is that cold-acclimatized people maintain heat production with less shivering by increasing nonshivering thermogenesis. This is achieved by an increase in the release of norepinephrine, which results in an increase in metabolic heat production (7, 22).

A second physiological adjustment that occurs due to cold acclimation is that cold-adjusted individuals can maintain a higher mean hand-and-foot temperature during cold exposure when compared to unacclimated persons. Cold acclimation apparently results in improved intermittent peripheral vasodilation to increase blood flow (and heat flow) to both the hands and feet (35, 36).

The third and final physiological adaptation to cold is the improved ability to sleep in cold environments. Unacclimated people who try to sleep in cold environments will often shiver so much that sleep is impossible. In contrast, cold-acclimatized individuals can sleep comfortably in cold environments due to their elevated level of nonshivering thermogenesis. The exact time course of complete cold acclimation is not clear. However, subjects placed in a cold chamber begin to show signs of cold acclimation after one week (50).

IN SUMMARY

- During resting conditions, humans exhibit peripheral vasoconstriction upon exposure to cold. This results in a decrease in skin blood flow that reduces convective heat loss between the skin and the environment.
- Exercise in a cold environment enhances an athlete's ability to lose heat and therefore greatly reduces the chance of heat injury.
- Cold acclimation results in three physiological adaptations: (1) increased nonshivering thermogenesis, (2) improved ability to prevent large decreases in skin temperature during cold exposure, and (3) improved ability to sleep in cold environments. The overall goal of these adaptations is to increase heat production and maintain core temperature, which will make the individual more comfortable during cold exposure.

STUDY ACTIVITIES

1. Define the following terms: (1) *homeotherm*, (2) *hyperthermia*, and (3) *hypothermia*.
2. Why does a significant increase in core temperature represent a threat to life?
3. Explain the comment that the term *body temperature* is a misnomer.
4. How is body temperature measured during exercise?

5. Briefly discuss the role of the preoptic-anterior hypothalamus in temperature regulation.
6. List and discuss the four mechanisms of heat loss. Which of these avenues plays the most important part during exercise in a hot/dry environment?
7. Discuss the two general categories of heat production in people.
8. What hormones are involved in biochemical heat production?
9. Briefly outline the thermal events that occur during prolonged exercise in a moderate environment. Include in your discussion information about changes in core temperature, skin blood flow, sweating, and skin temperature.
10. Calculate the amount of evaporation that must occur to remove 400 kcal of heat from the body.
11. How much heat would be removed from the skin if 520 ml of sweat evaporated during a 30-minute period?
12. List and discuss the physiological adaptations that occur during heat acclimation.
13. How might exercise in a cold environment affect dexterity in such skills as throwing and catching?
14. Discuss the physiological changes that occur in response to chronic exposure to cold.

SUGGESTED READINGS

Blatteis, C. 2012. Age-dependent changes in temperature regulation. *Gerontology* 58:289-95.

Bongers, C., D. Thijssen, M. Veltmeijer, M. Hopman, and T. Eijsvogels. 2015. Precooling and percooling both improve performance in the heat: A meta-analysis review. *British Journal of Sports Medicine* 49:377-84.

Casa, D. et al. 2015. National Athletic Trainers' Association position statement: Exertional heat illnesses. *Journal of Athletic Training* 50:986-1000.

Castellani, J., and M. Tipton. 2016. Cold stress effects on exposure tolerance and exercise performance. *Comprehensive Physiology* 6:443-69.

Kenefick, R., and S. Cheuvront. 2012. Hydration for recreational sport and physical activity. *Nutrition Reviews* 70:S137-S142.

Lorenzo, S., J. R. Halliwill, M. N. Sawka, and C. T. Minson. 2010. Heat acclimation improves exercise performance. *Journal of Applied Physiology* 109:1140-47.

Maughan, R. J., and S. M. Shirreffs. 2010. Dehydration and rehydration in competetive sport. *Scandinavian Journal of Medicine & Science in Sports* 20 (Suppl 3):40-47.

Nybo, L., P. Rasmussen, and M. Sawka. 2014. Performance in the heat-physiological factors of importance for hyperthermia-induced fatigue. *Comprehensive Physiology* 4:657-89.

Sawka, M., S. Cheuvront, and R. Kenefick. 2015. Hydration and aerobic performance: Impact of environment. Gatorade Sports Science Institute, Sports Science Exchange. 28: SSE #152.

Sawka, M., J. Perlard, and S. Racinals. 2015. Heat acclimatization to improve athletic performance in warm-hot environments. Gatorade Sports Science Institute, Sports Science Exchange. 28: SSE #153.

REFERENCES

1. **Armstrong LE, Johnson EC, Casa DJ, Ganio MS, McDermott BP, Yamamoto LM, et al.** The American football uniform: uncompensable heat stress and hyperthermic exhaustion. *Journal of Athletic Training* 45: 117-127, 2010.
2. **Armstrong LE and Maresh CM.** The induction and decay of heat acclimatisation in trained athletes. *Sports Medicine* 12: 302-312, 1991.
3. **Åstrand P, Rodahl K, Dahl H, and Stromme S.** *Textbook of Work Physiology.* Champaign, IL: Human Kinetics, 2004.
4. **Bergeron MF, McKeag DB, Casa DJ, Clarkson PM, Dick RW, Eichner ER, et al.** Youth football: heat stress and injury risk. *Medicine & Science in Sports & Exercise* 37: 1421-1430, 2005.
5. **Blatteis CM.** Age-dependent changes in temperature regulation–a mini review. *Gerontology.* 58: 289-295, 2012.
6. **Bongers C, Thijssen D, Veltmeijer M, Hopman M, and Eijsvogels T.** Precooling and percooling both improve performance in the heat: a meta analysis review. *British Journal of Sports Medicine* 49: 377-384, 2015.
7. **Cabanac M.** Temperature regulation. *Annual Review of Physiology* 37: 415-439, 1975.
8. **Casa DJ, Armstrong LE, Hillman SK, Montain SJ, Reiff RV, Rich BS, et al.** National Athletic Trainers' Association position statement: fluid replacement for athletes. *Journal of Athletic Training* 35: 212-224, 2000.
9. **Casa DJ, Becker SM, Ganio MS, Brown CM, Yeargin SW, Roti MW, et al.** Validity of devices that assess body temperature during outdoor exercise in the heat. *Journal of Athletic Training* 42: 333-342, 2007.
10. **Castellani JW and Tipton MJ.** Cold stress effects on exposure tolerance and exercise performance. *Comprehensive Physiology* 6: 443-469, 2016.
11. **Chinevere TD, Kenefick RW, Cheuvront SN, Lukaski HC, and Sawka MN.** Effect of heat acclimation on sweat minerals. *Medicine & Science in Sports & Exercise* 40: 886-891, 2008.
12. **Crandall CG and Gonzalez-Alonso J.** Cardiovascular function in the heat-stressed human. *Acta Physiologica (Oxford)* 199: 407-423, 2010.
13. **Dawson B.** Exercise training in sweat clothing in cool conditions to improve heat tolerance. *Sports Medicine* 17: 233-244, 1994.
14. **Delamarche P, Bittel J, Lacour JR, and Flandrois R.** Thermoregulation at rest and during exercise in prepubertal boys. *European Journal of Applied Physiology and Occupational Physiology* 60: 436-440, 1990.
15. **Ely BR, Cheuvront SN, Kenefick RW, and Sawka MN.** Aerobic performance is degraded, despite modest hyperthermia, in hot environments. *Medicine & Science in Sports & Exercise* 42: 135-141, 2010.
16. **Fox S.** *Human Physiology.* New York, NY: McGraw-Hill, 2012.
17. **Gisolfi C and Cohen J.** Relationships among training, heat acclimation, and heat tolerance in men and women: the controversy revisited. *Medicine and Science in Sports* 11: 56-59, 1979.

18. **Gisolfi C and Wenger C.** Temperature regulation during exercise: old concepts, new ideas. *Exercise and Sport Science Reviews* 12: 339-372, 1984.

19. **Godek SF, Bartolozzi AR, and Godek JJ.** Sweat rate and fluid turnover in American football players compared with runners in a hot and humid environment. *British Journal of Sports Medicine* 39: 205-211; discussion 205-211, 2005.

20. **Gordon CJ.** *Temperature Regulation in Laboratory Rodents.* New York, NY: Oxford Press, 2009.

21. **Hargreaves M.** Physiological limits to exercise performance in the heat. *Journal of Science and Medicine in Sport* 11: 66-71, 2008.

22. **Hong S, Rennie D, and Park Y.** Humans can acclimatize to cold: a lesson from Korean divers. *News in Physiological Sciences* 2: 79-82, 1987.

23. **Horvath SM.** Exercise in a cold environment. *Exercise and Sport Science Reviews* 9: 221-263, 1981.

24. **Johnson EC, Ganio MS, Lee EC, Lopez RM, McDermott BP, Casa DJ, et al.** Perceptual responses while wearing an American football uniform in the heat. *Journal of Athletic Training* 45: 107-116, 2010.

25. **Johnson JM.** Exercise and the cutaneous circulation. *Exercise and Sport Science Reviews* 20: 59-97, 1992.

26. **Kenefick RW, Ely BR, Cheuvront SN, Palombo LJ, Goodman DA, and Sawka MN.** Prior heat stress: effect on subsequent 15-min time trial performance in the heat. *Medicine & Science in Sports & Exercise* 41: 1311-1316, 2009.

27. **Kenney WL.** Control of heat-induced cutaneous vasodilatation in relation to age. *European Journal of Applied Physiology and Occupational Physiology* 57: 120-125, 1988.

28. **Kenney WL.** Thermoregulation at rest and during exercise in healthy older adults. *Exercise and Sport Science Reviews* 25: 41-76, 1997.

29. **Kenney WL and Johnson JM.** Control of skin blood flow during exercise. *Medicine & Science in Sports & Exercise* 24: 303-312, 1992.

30. **Kenney WL and Munce TA.** Invited review: aging and human temperature regulation. *Journal of Applied Physiology* 95: 2598-2603, 2003.

31. **Kruk B, Pekkarinen H, Manninen K, and Hanninen O.** Comparison in men of physiological responses to exercise of increasing intensity at low and moderate ambient temperatures. *European Journal of Applied Physiology and Occupational Physiology* 62: 353-357, 1991.

32. **Lee SM, Williams WJ, and Schneider SM.** Role of skin blood flow and sweating rate in exercise thermoregulation after bed rest. *Journal of Applied Physiology* 92: 2026-2034, 2002.

33. **Lim CL, Byrne C, and Lee JK.** Human thermoregulation and measurement of body temperature in exercise and clinical settings. *ANNALS Academy of Medicine Singapore* 37: 347-353, 2008.

34. **Lorenzo S, Halliwill JR, Sawka MN, and Minson CT.** Heat acclimation improves exercise performance. *Journal of Applied Physiology* 109: 1140-1147, 2010.

35. **Makinen TM.** Different types of cold adaptation in humans. *Frontiers in Bioscience (Scholar Edition)* 2: 1047-1067, 2010.

36. **Makinen TM.** Human cold exposure, adaptation, and performance in high latitude environments. *American Journal of Human Biology* 19: 155-164, 2007.

37. **Maughan R and Murray R.** *Sports Drinks: Basic Science and Practical Aspects.* Boca Raton, FL: CRC Press, 2000.

38. **Maughan RJ.** Distance running in hot environments: a thermal challenge to the elite runner. *Scandinavian Journal of Medicine & Science in Sports* 20 (Suppl 3): 95-102, 2010.

39. **Maughan RJ and Shirreffs SM.** Dehydration and rehydration in competitive sport. *Scandinavian Journal of Medicine & Science in Sports* 20 (Suppl 3): 40-47, 2010.

40. **Maughan RJ, Shirreffs SM, and Watson P.** Exercise, heat, hydration and the brain. *The Journal of the American College of Nutrition* 26: 604S-612S, 2007.

41. **McKenzie J, and Osgood D.** Validation of a new telemetric core temperature monitor. *Journal of Thermal Biology* 29: 605-611, 2004.

42. **Morton JP, Kayani AC, McArdle A, and Drust B.** The exercise-induced stress response of skeletal muscle, with specific emphasis on humans. *Sports Medicine* 39: 643-662, 2009.

43. **Nadel E.** Temperature regulation. In: *Sports Medicine and Physiology,* edited by Strauss R. Philadelphia, PA: W. B. Saunders, 1979.

44. **Nadel E.** Temperature regulation during prolonged exercise. In: *Perspectives in Exercise Science and Sports Medicine: Prolonged Exercise,* edited by Lamb D, and Murray R. Indianapolis, IN: Benchmark Press, 1988, pp. 125-152.

45. **Nielsen B, Savard G, Richter EA, Hargreaves M, and Saltin B.** Muscle blood flow and muscle metabolism during exercise and heat stress. *Journal of Applied Physiology* 69: 1040-1046, 1990.

46. **Nielson B.** Thermoregulation during exercise. *Acta Physiologica Scandinavica* 323 (Suppl): 10-73, 1969.

47. **Nielson M.** Die regulation der korpertemperatur bei muskelarbeit. *Scandinavica Archives Physiology* 79: 193, 1938.

48. **Noble B.** *Physiology of Exercise and Sport.* St. Louis, MO: C. V. Mosby, 1986.

49. **Nybo L, Rasmussen P, and Sawka M.** Performance in the heat-physiological factors of importance for hyperthermia-induced fatigue. *Comprehensive Physiology* 4: 657-689, 2014.

50. **Pandolf KB.** Effects of physical training and cardiorespiratory physical fitness on exercise-heat tolerance: recent observations. *Medicine and Science in Sports* 11: 60-65, 1979.

51. **Pandolf KB.** Time course of heat acclimation and its decay. *International Journal of Sports Medicine* 19 (Suppl 2): S157-160, 1998.

52. **Pandolf KB, Cadarette BS, Sawka MN, Young AJ, Francesconi RP, and Gonzalez RR.** Thermoregulatory responses of middle-aged and young men during dry-heat acclimation. *Journal of Applied Physiology* 65: 65-71, 1988.

53. **Powers SK, Howley ET, and Cox R.** Blood lactate concentrations during submaximal work under differing environmental conditions. *The Journal of Sports Medicine and Physical Fitness* 25: 84-89, 1985.

54. **Powers SK, Howley ET, and Cox R.** A differential catecholamine response during prolonged exercise and passive heating. *Medicine & Science in Sports & Exercise* 14: 435-439, 1982.

55. **Powers SK, Howley ET, and Cox R.** Ventilatory and metabolic reactions to heat stress during prolonged exercise. *The Journal of Sports Medicine and Physical Fitness* 22: 32-36, 1982.

56. **Powers SK, Nelson WB, and Hudson MB.** Exercise-induced oxidative stress: cause and consequences. *Free Radical Biology & Medicine* 51: 942-950, 2011.

57. **Rasch W, Samson P, Cote J, and Cabanac M.** Heat loss from the human head during exercise. *Journal of Applied Physiology* 71: 590-595, 1991.

58. **Robinson S.** Temperature regulation in exercise. *Pediatrics* 32 (Suppl): 691-702, 1963.

59. **Sato F, Owen M, Matthes R, Sato K, and Gisolfi CV.** Functional and morphological changes in the eccrine sweat gland with heat acclimation. *Journal of Applied Physiology* 69: 232-236, 1990.

60. **Shirreffs SM.** Hydration: special issues for playing football in warm and hot environments. *Scandinavian Journal of Medicine & Science in Sports* 20 (Suppl 3): 90-94, 2010.

61. **Shirreffs SM.** The importance of good hydration for work and exercise performance. *Nutrition Reviews* 63: S14-21, 2005.

62. **Simmons G, Wong B, Holowatz L, and Kenney WL.** Changes in the control of skin blood flow with exercise training: where do cutaneous vascular adaptations fit in? *Experimental Physiology* 96:822-828, 2011.

63. **Stolwijk JA, Saltin B, and Gagge AP.** Physiological factors associated with sweating during exercise. *Aerospace Medicine* 39: 1101-1105, 1968.

64. **Thomas CM, Pierzga JM, and Kenney WL.** Aerobic training and cutaneous vasodilation in young and older men. *Journal of Applied Physiology* 86: 1676-1686, 1999.

65. **Tikuisis P, Bell DG, and Jacobs I.** Shivering onset, metabolic response, and convective heat transfer during cold air exposure. *Journal of Applied Physiology* 70: 1996-2002, 1991.

66. **Wanner SP, Guimaraes JB, Rodrigues LO, Marubayashi U, Coimbra CC, and Lima NR.** Muscarinic cholinoceptors in the ventromedial hypothalamic nucleus facilitate tail heat loss during physical exercise. *Brain Research Bulletin* 73: 28-33, 2007.

67. **Wendt D, van Loon LJ, and Lichtenbelt WD.** Thermoregulation during exercise in the heat: strategies for maintaining health and performance. *Sports Medicine* 37: 669-682, 2007.

68. **Wenger CB.** Heat of evaporation of sweat: thermodynamic considerations. *Journal of Applied Physiology* 32: 456-459, 1972.

69. **Williams CG, Wyndham CH, and Morrison JF.** Rate of loss of acclimatization in summer and winter. *Journal of Applied Physiology* 22: 21-26, 1967.

70. **Wyndham CH.** The physiology of exercise under heat stress. *Annual Review of Physiology* 35: 193-220, 1973.

71. **Yanagimoto S, Aoki K, Horikawa N, Shibasaki M, Inoue Y, Nishiyasu T, et al.** Sweating response in physically trained men to sustained handgrip exercise in mildly hyperthermic conditions. *Acta Physiologica Scandinavia* 174: 31-39, 2002.

72. **Zuo L, Christofi FL, Wright VP, Liu CY, Merola AJ, Berliner LJ, et al.** Intra- and extracellular measurement of reactive oxygen species produced during heat stress in diaphragm muscle. *American Journal of Physiology - Cell Physiology* 279: C1058-1066, 2000.

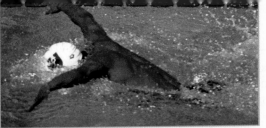

© Action Plus Sports Images/Alamy Stock Photo

13

The Physiology of Training: Effect on $\dot{V}O_2$ Max, Performance, and Strength

■ Objectives

By studying this chapter, you should be able to do the following:

1. Explain the basic principles of training: overload, reversibility, and specificity.

2. Discuss the role that genetics plays in determining $\dot{V}O_2$ max.

3. Describe the typical change in $\dot{V}O_2$ max with endurance-training programs and the effect of the initial (pretraining) value on the magnitude of the increase.

4. Identify typical $\dot{V}O_2$ max values for various sedentary, active, and athletic populations.

5. Understand the contribution of heart rate, stroke volume, and the a-$\bar{v}O_2$ difference in determining $\dot{V}O_2$ max.

6. Discuss how training increases $\dot{V}O_2$ max.

7. Define preload, afterload, and contractility, and discuss the role of each in the increase in the maximal stroke volume that occurs with endurance training.

8. Describe the changes in muscle structure that are responsible for the increase in the maximal a-$\bar{v}O_2$ difference with endurance training.

9. List and discuss the primary changes that occur in skeletal muscle as a result of endurance training.

10. Explain how "high-intensity" endurance training improves acid-base balance during exercise.

11. Outline the "big picture" changes that occur in skeletal muscle as a result of exercise training and discuss the specificity of exercise training responses.

12. List the four primary signal transduction pathways in skeletal muscle.

13. List and define the function of important secondary messengers in skeletal muscle.

14. Outline the signaling events that lead to endurance training-induced muscle adaptation.

15. Discuss how changes in "central command" and "peripheral feedback" following an endurance training program can lower the heart rate, ventilation, and catecholamine responses to a submaximal exercise bout.

16. Describe the underlying causes of the decrease in $\dot{V}O_2$ max that occurs with cessation of endurance training.

17. Contrast the role of neural adaptations with hypertrophy in the increase in strength that occurs with resistance training.

18. Identify the changes that occur in skeletal muscle fibers in response to resistance training.

19. Outline the signaling events that lead to resistance training-induced increases in muscle growth.

20. Discuss how detraining following strength training affects muscle fiber size and strength. Explain how retraining affects muscle fiber size and strength.

21. Explain why concurrent strength and endurance training can impair strength gains.

5'adenosine monophos-
    phate activated protein
    kinase (AMPK)
bradycardia
calciuneurin
CaMK (calmodulin-
    dependent kinase)
IGF-1/Akt/mTOR
    signaling pathway
NFκB (nuclear factor
    kappa B)
overload
PGC-1α (peroxisome
    proliferator-activated
    receptor-gamma
    coactivator 1α)
p38 (mitogen activated
    kinase p38)
reversibility
specificity

A theme throughout this book is that there are regulatory mechanisms (i.e., control systems) operating at rest and during exercise to maintain homeostasis. It is clear that participation in regular endurance exercise increases the cardiovascular system's ability to deliver blood to the working muscles and increases the muscle's capacity to produce ATP aerobically. These parallel changes result in less disruption of the internal environment during exercise. This, of course, leads to improved performance. Further, regular bouts of resistance exercise result in muscular adaptation that increases the muscle's ability to generate force and also improves performance in power events (e.g., weight lifting).

This chapter will discuss the physiological adaptations that occur in response to both endurance exercise training and resistance training. A major objective of this chapter is to tie together much of the physiology that has been presented in earlier chapters, because many tissues and organ systems are either directly or indirectly affected by training programs. In the discussion of endurance training, we consider separately those physiological changes that promote an increase in $\dot{V}O_2$ max from those adaptations associated with improvements in prolonged submaximal performance. This is because $\dot{V}O_2$ max is closely linked to the maximal capacity of the cardiovascular system to deliver blood to the working muscles. The ability to sustain long-term, submaximal exercise is linked more to the maintenance of muscle fiber homeostasis due to specific biochemical properties of the working muscles.

This chapter also explores the physiology of strength development. Further, because endurance training causes adaptations in muscle that may conflict with those adaptations associated with strength training programs, we discuss the issue of whether concurrent resistance and endurance training results in a compromised increase in muscular strength compared to resistance training alone. Let's begin with an introduction to the principles of training.

PRINCIPLES OF TRAINING

The three principles of training are overload, specificity, and reversibility. These principles are introduced here and applied in Chaps. 16 and 17 (training for fitness) and in Chap. 21 (training for performance).

Overload and Reversibility

The **overload** principle refers to the fact that an organ system (e.g., cardiovascular) or tissue (e.g., skeletal muscle) must be exercised at a level beyond which it is accustomed in order to achieve a training adaptation. The system or tissue gradually adapts to this overload. This pattern of progressively overloading a system or tissue as adaptations occur results in improved function over time. The typical variables that constitute the overload include the intensity, duration, and frequency (days per week) of exercise. The corollary of the overload principle is the principle of reversibility. The principle of **reversibility** refers to the fact that the fitness gains by exercising at an overload are quickly lost when training is stopped and the overload is removed.

Specificity

The principle of **specificity** refers to the effect that exercise training is specific to the muscles involved in that activity, the fiber types recruited, the principal energy system involved (aerobic versus anaerobic), the velocity of contraction, and the type of muscle contraction (eccentric, concentric, or isometric). Indeed, the arms do not undergo significant training adaptation during a 10-week running exercise program. Further, this also means that if an individual participates in a low-intensity, distance running program that utilizes the slow-twitch muscle fibers in the legs, there is little or no training effect occurring in fast-twitch fibers in the leg muscles.

Specificity also refers to the types of adaptations occurring in muscle as a result of training. If a muscle is engaged in endurance exercise training, the primary adaptations are increases in capillaries and mitochondria volume, which increase the capacity of the muscle to produce energy aerobically. If a muscle is engaged in heavy resistance training, the primary adaptation is an increase in the quantity of the contractile proteins (59).

IN SUMMARY

- The overload principle reveals that for a training effect to occur, a system or tissue must be challenged with an intensity, duration, or frequency of exercise to which it is unaccustomed. Over time, the tissue or system adapts to this increased load. The reversibility principle is a corollary to the overload principle and refers to the fact that fitness gains are lost when training is stopped.
- The principle of specificity indicates that the training effect is limited to the muscle fibers involved in the activity. In addition, the muscle fiber adapts specifically to the type of activity. Specifically, endurance exercise training promotes an increase in both mitochondria and capillary density in muscle, whereas resistance training results in increased contractile proteins in skeletal muscle.

ENDURANCE TRAINING AND $\dot{V}O_2$ MAX

Maximal oxygen uptake (also called maximal aerobic power or $\dot{V}O_2$ max) is the measure of the maximal capacity of the body to transport and use oxygen during dynamic exercise using large muscle groups (i.e., legs). Chap. 4 introduced this concept, and Chaps. 9 and 10 showed how specific cardiovascular and pulmonary variables respond to graded exercise up to $\dot{V}O_2$ max. The following sections discuss the effect of endurance exercise programs on the increase in $\dot{V}O_2$ max and the physiological changes that are responsible for this increase.

Training Programs and Changes in $\dot{V}O_2$ Max

Endurance training programs that increase $\dot{V}O_2$ max commonly involve continuous dynamic exercise using a large muscle mass (e.g., running, cycling, or swimming) for 20 to 60 minutes per session, three or more times per week at an intensity >50% $\dot{V}O_2$ max. However, abundant evidence also reveals that high-intensity interval training (i.e., 30 seconds all-out efforts) also improves $\dot{V}O_2$ max (34). Details about how to design a training program for the average individual and the athlete are presented in Chaps. 16 and 21, respectively. While endurance training programs of two- to three-months duration typically cause an increase in $\dot{V}O_2$ max between 15% and 20%, the range of improvement can be as low as 2% to 3% for those who start the program with high $\dot{V}O_2$ max values (23), and as high as 50% for individuals with low initial $\dot{V}O_2$ max values or the genetic potential for large improvements in $\dot{V}O_2$ max with training (14, 23, 41, 84). In addition, individuals with a low $\dot{V}O_2$ max prior to training can experience improvements with relatively low training intensities (e.g., 40% to 50% $\dot{V}O_2$ max), whereas individuals with high $\dot{V}O_2$ max values may require higher training intensities (e.g., >70% $\dot{V}O_2$ max) (66).

Relative $\dot{V}O_2$ max (i.e., normalized to body weight) can vary widely in adults depending upon their age, health, and training status. For example, $\dot{V}O_2$ max can be less than 20 ml $\cdot$ kg^{-1} $\cdot$ min^{-1} in patients with severe cardiovascular and pulmonary disease, and more than 80 ml $\cdot$ kg^{-1} $\cdot$ min^{-1} in world-class distance runners and cross-country skiers (Table 13.1). The extremely high $\dot{V}O_2$ max values possessed by elite male and female endurance athletes are the genetic gift of a large cardiovascular capacity and high percentage of slow muscle fibers (5). Indeed, studies have concluded that heritability of $\dot{V}O_2$ max in the untrained state is approximately 50% (12, 13). In other words, about 50% of individual's $\dot{V}O_2$ max is determined by genetics along with environmental influences.

Further, research indicates that the magnitude of improvement in $\dot{V}O_2$ max in response to exercise training is also genetically determined (14). For example, following a standardized training program, there is a wide variation in the level of $\dot{V}O_2$ max improvement among individuals (12, 53). It is estimated that the heritability of training gains in $\dot{V}O_2$ max is approximately 47% (14). Evidence points to differences in mitochondrial DNA as being important in both the individual differences in initial (i.e., untrained) $\dot{V}O_2$ max and the training-induced improvements in $\dot{V}O_2$ max (14). Genetically gifted individuals who show large improvements (e.g., 40% to 50% increase) in $\dot{V}O_2$ max following endurance training are often referred to as "high responders" to exercise training. See A Closer Look 13.1 for more information on this topic.

In addition to genetic factors, both the intensity and duration of endurance training have an important impact on the magnitude in training-induced changes in $\dot{V}O_2$ max. For example, prolonged periods of endurance training (i.e., two to three years) can produce large improvements (e.g., 40% to 50% increases) in $\dot{V}O_2$ max in genetically gifted individuals. Also, high-intensity endurance training can increase $\dot{V}O_2$ max by as much as 50% in individuals with the genetic potential to respond favorably to endurance training (14, 41). For instance, a study revealed a large (e.g. 30% to 50% improvement) and linear increase in $\dot{V}O_2$ max over ten weeks of high-intensity exercise training (41). These results are in contrast with many training studies that show a leveling off of the $\dot{V}O_2$ max values after only a few weeks of training. The much larger increase in $\dot{V}O_2$ max with this ten-week training program was due to a higher intensity, frequency, and duration of training than are commonly employed in endurance exercise programs. We next discuss the physiological adaptations that are responsible for endurance training-induced improvements in $\dot{V}O_2$ max.

TABLE 13.1	$\dot{V}O_2$ Max Values Measured in Healthy and Diseased Populations		
Population		**Males**	**Females**
Healthy			
Cross-country skiers		84	72
Distance runners		83	62
Sedentary: young		45	38
Sedentary: middle-aged adults		35	30
Diseased			
Post-myocardial infarction patients		22	18
Severe pulmonary disease patients		13	13

Values are expressed in ml $\cdot$ kg^{-1} $\cdot$ min^{-1}.

Åstrand, P., and Rodahl, K., Dahl, H., and Stromme, S., *Textbook of Work Physiology*. Champaign, IL Human Kinetics, 2003.

IN SUMMARY

- Endurance training programs that increase $\dot{V}O_2$ max involve a large muscle mass in continuous activity for 20 to 60 minutes per session, three or more times per week, at an intensity of 50% to 85% $\dot{V}O_2$ max. Similiar to continuous endurance training, high-intensity interval training also improves $\dot{V}O_2$ max.
- Although $\dot{V}O_2$ max increases an average of about 15% to 20% as a result of an endurance training program, the largest training-induced increases in $\dot{V}O_2$ max generally occur in those genetically gifted individuals who are often referred to as "high responders" to endurance training adaptations.
- Genetic predisposition accounts for about 50% of one's $\dot{V}O_2$ max value. Very strenuous and/or prolonged endurance training can increase $\dot{V}O_2$ max in normal sedentary individuals by up to 50%.

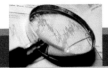
Impact of Genetics on $\dot{V}O_2$ Max and Individual Exercise Training Responses

The link between genetics and $\dot{V}O_2$ max along with the between-subject variations in exercise training responses has been studied for over two decades. An important study investigating genetics and exercise adaptations is known as the HERITAGE Family Study. This investigation has made major contribution to our understanding of the role that genetics plays in determining both $\dot{V}O_2$ max and the biological responses to exercise training. Together, the HERITAGE Family Study and numerous other studies reveal the following information about the role that genetics plays in determining $\dot{V}O_2$ max and the training-induced improvements in $\dot{V}O_2$ max.

■ Heritability determines approximately 50% of $\dot{V}O_2$ max in sedentary adults (13). In other words, 50% of the $\dot{V}O_2$ max of an untrained subject can be explained by genetic differences between individuals.

■ Genetics also plays a key role in determining how individuals respond to training and a large variation exists between people in their ability to improve $\dot{V}O_2$ max in response to training. For example, while the average training-induced improvement in $\dot{V}O_2$ max is 15% to 20%, some individuals are "low responders" to exercise training and achieve only a 2% to 3% improvement in $\dot{V}O_2$ max. In contrast, some individuals are "high responders" to exercise and can achieve a 50% improvement in $\dot{V}O_2$ max. These large variations in the training response illustrate the fact that the heritability of the training adaptation is great and approaches 47% (11,14).

■ Studies reveal that only those individuals with both the genetic makeup for a high $\dot{V}O_2$ max in the untrained state and with the genetic background to be a "high responder" to exercise training have the potential to achieve the high $\dot{V}O_2$ max value required to successfully complete in endurance events (e.g., 5,000 meter run) at the Olympic level.

■ Recent HERITAGE Family studies show that the large variation in the human adaptive response to exercise (i.e., responders vs. nonresponders) is due to 21 different genes that play an important role in training adaptation (14).

Please see Mann et al. (2014) and Tucker and Collins (2012) in the Suggested Reading list to learn more about the impact of genetics on $\dot{V}O_2$ max and the training adaptations to exercise.

WHY DOES EXERCISE TRAINING IMPROVE $\dot{V}O_2$ MAX?

The calculation of oxygen consumption via the Fick equation is illustrated as shown:

$$\dot{V}O_2 \text{ max} = \text{Maximal cardiac output} \times (\text{maximal a-}\bar{v}O_2 \text{ difference})$$

As maximal oxygen uptake is the product of systemic blood flow (cardiac output) and systemic oxygen extraction (arteriovenous [a-$\bar{v}$] oxygen difference), training-induced changes in $\dot{V}O_2$ max occur due to increased maximal cardiac output, increased maximal a-$\bar{v}O_2$ difference, or some combination of both.

Recall from Chap. 9 that cardiac output is determined by the product of heart rate times stroke volume (i.e., amount of blood ejected per heart beat). Also, remember that the a-$\bar{v}O_2$ difference is a measure of how much oxygen is removed from arterial blood and used by the tissues. Again, the Fick equation reveals that training-induced increases in $\dot{V}O_2$ max can be due to increased cardiac output, increased a-$\bar{v}O_2$ difference, or an increase in both. Research reveals that, in untrained subjects, relatively short durations (1 to 4 months) of endurance training increases both

$\dot{V}O_2$ max (+26%) and maximal cardiac output (+10%) but does not significantly increase the maximal a-$\bar{v}O_2$ difference (Fig. 13.1) (69). Therefore, following

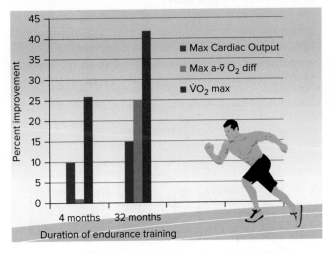

Figure 13.1 Progression of endurance training-induced changes in $\dot{V}O_2$ max, maximal cardiac output, and maximal a-v O_2 difference in healthy, sedentary adults during 4-32 months of training.

Data from Montero, D., Diaz-Canestro, C., and Lundby, C., "Endurance Training and $\dot{V}O_2$ Max: Role of Maximal Cardiac Output and Oxygen Extraction," *Medicine & Science in Sports & Exercise* 47: 2024-2033, 2015.

short-duration training, all of the training-induced improvement in $\dot{V}O_2$ max is due to increases in maximal cardiac output. In contrast, studies reveal that a longer duration of training (i.e., 32 months or more) increases $\dot{V}O_2$ max by increasing both maximal cardiac output (+15%) and the maximal a-$\bar{v}O_2$ difference (+25%) (Fig. 13.1) (69). Note that, following both short- and long-duration endurance training, the exercise-induced increase in maximal cardiac output is entirely due to increases in stroke volume because maximal heart rate either remains constant or slightly decreases.

What causes the maximal stroke volume and the maximal arteriovenous oxygen difference to increase as a result of endurance training? The answers are provided in the next two sections.

Stroke Volume

Recall that stroke volume is the amount of blood ejected from the heart with each beat and is equal to the difference between end diastolic volume (EDV) and end systolic volume (ESV). Note that exercise training does not increase maximal heart rate and, in fact, months of training result in a small decrease in maximal heart rate. Therefore, all training-induced increases in maximal cardiac output must come from increases in stroke volume. Figure 13.2 summarizes the factors that can increase stroke volume in response to endurance training. In brief, an increase in EDV (preload), increased cardiac contractility, or a decrease in total peripheral resistance (afterload) can increase stroke volume. Let's briefly discuss each of these factors relative to the increase in the maximal stroke volume that occurs with endurance training.

End Diastolic Volume (EDV) One of the key factors responsible for training-induced increases in maximal stroke volume is an increase in EDV. An increase in EDV results in stretch of the left ventricle and a corresponding increase in cardiac contractility via the Frank-Starling mechanism (Chap. 9). This increase in EDV in

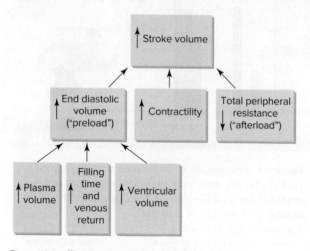

Figure 13.2 Factors increasing stroke volume.

the endurance-trained heart is likely a result of several training-induced changes. A primary mechanism is that plasma volume increases with endurance training, and this contributes to augmented venous return and increased EDV. These training-induced changes in plasma volume and increased stroke volume changes can occur rapidly. For example, a six-day training program (2 hr/day at 65% $\dot{V}O_2$ max) can promote a 7% increase in $\dot{V}O_2$ max, 11% increase in plasma volume, and a 10% increase in stroke volume. This training-induced increase in stroke volume is likely due to an increase in EDV.

Also, note that prolonged endurance training (months to years) increases the volume of the left ventricle with little change in ventricular wall thickness (87). This increase in ventricular volume will accommodate a larger EDV and is predicted to contribute to the training-induced increase in stroke volume (28, 79, 87).

Finally, endurance training not only increases stroke volume during maximal exercise, but also increases stroke volume at rest. The increase in resting stroke volume in endurance-trained athletes is likely due to the increased EDV at rest that results from increased stretch of the myocardium because of the increased ventricular filling time associated with the slower resting heart rate (**bradycardia**) that occurs following endurance training (87).

Cardiac Contractility Cardiac contractility refers to the strength of the cardiac muscle contraction when the fiber length (EDV), afterload (peripheral resistance), and heart rate remain constant. Although an acute exercise bout increases cardiac contractility due to the action of the sympathetic nervous system on the ventricle, it is difficult to determine whether the inherent contractility of the human heart changes with endurance training. This is because the factors that affect contractility (EDV, heart rate, and afterload) are themselves affected by endurance training. Nonetheless, animal studies indicate that high-intensity exercise training increases cardiac pumping ability by increasing the force of ventricular contraction (50, 51, 103). Further, research reveals that endurance exercise training increases left ventricular "twist mechanics" resulting in increased stroke volume (87, 104). Together, these findings indicate that endurance exercise training improves ventricular contractility in both humans and animals.

Afterload The term *afterload* refers to the peripheral resistance against which the ventricle is contracting as it tries to push blood into the aorta. Afterload is important because when the heart contracts against a high peripheral resistance, stroke volume will be reduced (compared to a lower peripheral resistance). Following an endurance-training program, trained muscles offer less resistance to blood flow during maximal exercise due to a reduction in the sympathetic vasoconstrictor activity to the arterioles of the trained muscles.

This decrease in resistance parallels the increase in maximal cardiac output so that mean arterial blood pressure during exercise remains unchanged.

Arteriovenous O$_2$ Difference

As mentioned earlier, endurance training-induced increases in $\dot{V}O_2$ max following many months of training are due to an elevation in both cardiac output (i.e., stroke volume increases) and the a-$\bar{v}O_2$ difference. The training-induced increase in the a-$\bar{v}O_2$ difference is due to increased O$_2$ extraction from the blood. The increased capacity of the muscle to extract O$_2$ following training is primarily due to the increase in capillary density, with an increase in mitochondrial volume being of secondary importance (9, 42). The enlarged capillary density in trained muscle accommodates the increase in muscle blood flow during maximal exercise, decreases the diffusion distance to the mitochondria, and slows the rate of blood flow to allow more time for oxygen diffusion from the capillary to the muscle fiber. Changes in capillary density parallel alterations in leg blood flow and $\dot{V}O_2$ max with training. The increases in mitochondrial number following endurance training increase the muscle fiber's ability to consume oxygen and also contribute to the expanded a-$\bar{v}O_2$ differences. Note, however, the capacity of the mitochondria to use O$_2$ exceeds the capability of the heart to deliver O$_2$, making mitochondrial number not the key factor limiting $\dot{V}O_2$ max (9, 42). Figure 13.3 provides a summary of the factors responsible for the increase in $\dot{V}O_2$ max associated with an endurance training program.

Finally, two scientists who have made major contributions to our understanding of the physiological effects of exercise training are Drs. John O. Holloszy and Bengt Saltin. See A Look Back–Important People in Science for more on these outstanding scientists.

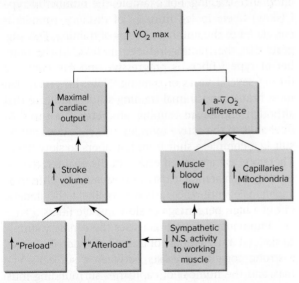

Figure 13.3 Summary of factors causing an increase in $\dot{V}O_2$ max with endurance training.

IN SUMMARY

- In healthy, sedentary subjects, the training-induced improvements in $\dot{V}O_2$ max that occur following short-term training (i.e., ~4 months) are due to increases in maximal cardiac output alone. However, the training-induced improvements in $\dot{V}O_2$ max that occur following long duration training (i.e., 32 months) are the result of both increases in maximal cardiac output (i.e., stroke volume increases) and an increase in the a-$\bar{v}O_2$ difference.

- The training-induced increase in maximal stroke volume is due to both an increase in preload and a decrease in afterload.
  a. The increased preload is primarily due to an increase in end diastolic ventricular volume and the associated increase in plasma volume.
  b. The decreased afterload is due to a decrease in the arteriolar constriction in the trained muscles, increasing maximal muscle blood flow with no change in the mean arterial blood pressure.

- The training-induced increase in the a-$\bar{v}O_2$ difference is due to an increase in the capillary density of the trained muscles, which is needed to accept the increase in maximal muscle blood flow. The greater capillary density allows for a slow red blood cell transit time through the muscle, providing enough time for oxygen diffusion from the capillary into the muscle fiber.

ENDURANCE TRAINING: EFFECTS ON PERFORMANCE AND HOMEOSTASIS

The ability to perform prolonged, submaximal work is dependent on the maintenance of homeostasis during the activity. Endurance training results in a more rapid transition from rest to steady-state exercise, a reduced reliance on the limited liver and muscle glycogen stores, and numerous cardiovascular and thermoregulatory adaptations that assist in maintaining homeostasis. Many of these training-induced adaptations are due to structural and biochemical changes in muscle, and we will discuss those in detail in the next few pages. However, a portion of these adaptations is related to factors external to the muscle. This needs to be stated at the beginning of this section because, while we focus on the link between changes in skeletal muscle and performance, there is evidence that some improvements in performance occur rapidly and might precede structural or biochemical changes in skeletal muscle (36). This suggests that the initial metabolic adaptations to endurance training

Dr. John O. Holloszy, M.D., and Dr. Bengt Saltin, M.D., Ph.D.—Olympic Prize Winners

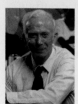

Joe Angeles/
Washington
University in
St. Louis

The International Olympic Committee (IOC) established the IOC Olympic Prize in Sports Sciences to recognize international leaders in research in the sport sciences. The awardee receives $500,000 and an Olympic medal. The prize is awarded every two years.

In 2000, the International Olympic Committee awarded its IOC Prize in Sport Sciences to **Dr. John O. Holloszy**. The prize recognizes his outstanding contributions to our understanding of the effects of endurance training on muscle and metabolism, and how they affect endurance performance, heart disease, diabetes, and aging. That simple sentence cannot do justice to the more than 382 studies he has published in the very best research journals or the impact he has had on the field of exercise science and preventive medicine. Throughout his career, Dr. Holloszy has trained several generations of scientists to follow in his footsteps. His list of post-doctoral fellows, beginning in the 1960s, forms a who's who in exercise physiology; the research contributions of his post-doctoral fellows multiply many times over the effect Dr. Holloszy has had in the field of exercise physiology. Dr. Holloszy continues his active research career at Washington University School of Medicine in the areas of caloric restriction and aging and carbohydrate and fat metabolism.

In 2002, the International Olympic Committee awarded its IOC Prize in Sport Sciences to **Dr. Bengt Saltin**

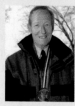

© Harry How/
Pool/Getty
Images

(1935-2014). During a long and productive research career, Dr. Saltin has published more than 451 studies that have broadly expanded our understanding of exercise physiology. More specifically, Dr. Saltin's work has improved our appreciation of training-induced changes in $\dot{V}O_2$ max and the regulation of fuel utilization in skeletal muscle during exercise. Moreover, he performed classic bed-rest studies revealing the important physiological changes that occur following prolonged periods of inactivity. You will note that many of Dr. Saltin's studies are cited throughout this book as a testament to the importance of his research discoveries.

---

might consist of changes in the nervous system or neural-hormonal adaptations, which are followed by biochemical adaptations in muscle fibers.

In the introduction to this chapter, we mentioned that the increase in submaximal performance following an endurance training program is due more to biochemical and structural changes in the trained skeletal muscle than to an increase in $\dot{V}O_2$ max. Common endurance training-induced changes include increases in the percentage of slow muscle fibers (i.e., fast-to-slow fiber type shift), increased mitochondrial volume in fibers, added ability for muscle to metabolize fat, improved muscle antioxidant capacity, and increased capillary density (39). Indeed, these training-induced changes in muscle primarily determine the overall physiological responses to a given submaximal exercise bout. Let's begin our discussion with an overview of endurance training-induced changes in muscle fiber types and capillary number in skeletal muscle.

Endurance Training-Induced Changes in Fiber Type and Capillarity

It is well established that endurance training results in a shift in fast-to-slow muscle fiber type. Recall from Chap. 8 that this exercise-induced shift in muscle fiber type involves a reduction in the amount of fast myosin in the muscle and an increase in slow myosin isoforms. This is significant because slow myosin isoforms have lower myosin ATPase activity but are able to perform more work with less ATP utilization (i.e., more efficient). This fast-to-slow shift in myosin isoforms is physiologically important because it increases mechanical efficiency and therefore can potentially improve endurance performance.

The magnitude of this exercise-induced fiber type shift is dependent upon both the intensity and duration of training sessions along with the total years of endurance training. For example, the number of type I (slow) fibers in leg muscles of distance runners is correlated to the number of years of training. This suggests that the training-induced increase in the number of type I fibers is progressive and can continue during several years of training. Note, however, that most human and animal training studies indicate that although endurance training promotes a fast-to-slow fiber shift in the active muscles, this shift does not result in a complete shift from fast fibers to slow fibers. Therefore, as mentioned earlier in the chapter, the extremely high aerobic capacity possessed by elite male and female endurance athletes is likely the genetic gift of a high percentage of slow muscle fibers.

Endurance training increases the capillary supply to skeletal muscle fibers of trained individuals. In fact, a strong correlation exists between a subject's $\dot{V}O_2$ max and the number of capillaries surrounding muscle fibers in the trained limbs. This exercise-induced capillarization in the skeletal muscle is advantageous

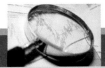
Endurance Exercise Training Increases Mitochondrial Volume and Turnover in Skeletal Muscle

As discussed in the text, both endurance exercise training (i.e., continuous submaximal exercise) and high-intensity interval training promote the synthesis of new mitochondria (called mitochondrial biogenesis), resulting in an increased volume of both subsarcolemmal and intermyofibrillar mitochondria in the trained muscle fibers. Research reveals that the exercise-induced increase in mitochondrial volume is primarily due increased mitochondrial size and not an increased number of mitochondria (58). This exercise-induced increase in mitochondrial volume in muscle fibers results in an improved oxidative capacity and increased ability to use fat

as a fuel source. This improved ability to metabolize fat as a fuel during exercise is advantageous because it spares carbohydrates and prevents depletion of the limited carbohydrate stores in both muscle and liver (58).

In addition to promoting mitochondrial biogenesis, endurance exercise training also increases the removal of damaged mitochondria. Specifically, endurance exercise training promotes the breakdown and removal of "old" and damaged mitochondria; these damaged mitochondria are replaced with "new" and healthy mitochondria that are larger in size. The process of removal and replacement of muscle mitochondria

is commonly referred to as *mitochondrial turnover*. The removal of damaged mitochondria occurs via a process called *mitophagy*. In short, mitophagy is the selective removal of "old" and damaged mitochondria by lysosomes. The end result of exercise-induced increases in mitochondrial turnover is that the muscle mitochondrial population in trained individuals is larger and healthier than the mitochondrial population found in muscle fibers of untrained individuals.

As mentioned earlier, this increase in the volume of healthy mitochondria results in an improved oxidative capacity and increased ability of the muscle fibers to metabolize fats.

because diffusion distances for oxygen and substrate delivery to muscle fibers is reduced. Similarly, the distance for diffusion and removal of metabolic waste from the fiber are also decreased.

Endurance Training Increases Mitochondrial Content in Skeletal Muscle Fibers

Two subpopulations of mitochondria exist in skeletal muscle. One population rests immediately beneath the sarcolemma (subsarcolemmal mitochondria), and the second and larger group of mitochondria (i.e., 80% of total mitochondria) is dispersed around the contractile proteins (intermyofibrillar mitochondria). Endurance training and high-intensity interval training can rapidly increase the volume of both mitochondrial subpopulations in the active skeletal muscle fibers. For example, mitochondrial volume can increase in muscle fibers within the first five days of a training program (102). Prolonged endurance training can typically increase muscle mitochondrial volume by 50% to 100% within the first six weeks of training (16). However, the magnitude of the exercise-induced increase in mitochondria in muscle is dependent upon both the exercise intensity and duration of the exercise sessions. See A Closer Look 13.2 for more details on exercise-induced changes in mitochondrial volume and mitochondrial turnover in muscle fibers. The increased endurance performance that results from mitochondrial biogenesis is due to changes in muscle metabolism during exercise. Let's briefly examine some of these key changes.

At the onset of exercise, ATP is converted to ADP and P_i in the muscle fibers in order to develop tension. The increase in the ADP concentration in the cytoplasm is the immediate stimulus for ATP-producing systems to meet the ATP demands of the cross-bridges. Phosphocreatine responds immediately to this ATP need, followed by glycolysis, and finally mitochondrial oxidative phosphorylation. The latter process becomes the primary source of ATP during the steady-state phase of exercise. How does endurance training affect these oxygen uptake responses at the onset of submaximal steady-state work?

The steady-state $\dot{V}O_2$ measured during a submaximal work test is not affected by endurance training. This means that mitochondria in the working muscles are consuming the same number of O_2 molecules per minute. However, because training results in an increase in the size of mitochondria in muscle, the ATP-producing chore handled by mitochondria differs between untrained and trained skeletal muscles. This point is illustrated in the following example. Suppose an untrained muscle cell has only one small mitochondrion, and a breakdown of 100 units of ATP per minute is needed for the muscle to consume 2.0 liters of O_2 per minute to sustain a constant level of exercise. The breakdown of 100 units of ATP/minute results in the formation of 100 units of ADP/minute in the cytosol of the fiber (see Fig. 13.4). Remember that aerobic formation of ATP requires ADP to be transported into the mitochondria to be combined with P_i to form ATP. After training, when the size of the mitochondria in the cell has doubled, the rate of ADP transportation into the mitochondria has also doubled. Therefore,

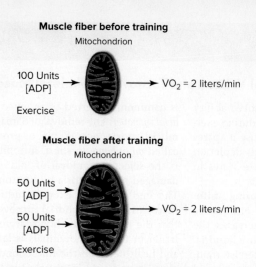

Muscle fiber before training

Mitochondrion

100 Units [ADP] → → VO₂ = 2 liters/min

Exercise

Muscle fiber after training

Mitochondrion

50 Units [ADP] →
50 Units [ADP] → → VO₂ = 2 liters/min

Exercise

Figure 13.4 Influence of mitochondria size on the change in the cytosolic ADP concentration during submaximal exercise. Note that the training-induced increases in mitochondrial size in the muscle improve the rate of ADP transport into the mitochondria, resulting in a lower ADP concentration in the cytosol and less stimulation of glycolysis.

the ADP concentration in the cytosol increases only half as much because of the additional mitochondria present to take up the ADP. This is important for two reasons. First, the lower ADP concentration results in less phosphocreatine depletion because the reaction for this is [ADP] + [PC] → [ATP] + [C]. Second, the lower ADP concentration in the cell also results in less stimulation of glycolysis and, therefore, a reduced production of lactate and H⁺. Collectively, the reduced stimulation of glycolysis due to the lower ADP and higher PC concentrations following endurance training results in less reliance on anaerobic glycolysis to provide ATP at the onset of exercise (30, 37). The net result is a lower oxygen deficit, less depletion of phosphocreatine, and a reduction in lactate and H⁺ formation. Figure 13.5 shows that the biochemical adaptations following endurance training result in a faster rise in the oxygen uptake curve at the onset of work, with less disruption of homeostasis.

Training-Induced Changes in Muscle Fuel Utilization

Plasma glucose is the primary fuel for the nervous system and therefore maintaining plasma glucose levels is vital. Thus, it is not surprising that endurance training promotes biochemical changes in skeletal muscles that assist in maintaining a constant blood glucose concentration during prolonged submaximal exercise. Specifically, endurance training results in a decreased use of glucose (carbohydrate) as fuel and an increase in fat metabolism during prolonged submaximal exercise. Together, these changes spare plasma glucose and increase the reliance on fat as a fuel source

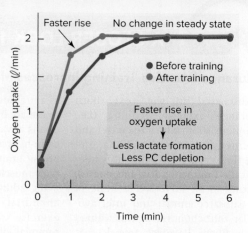

Figure 13.5 Endurance training reduces the O₂ deficit at the onset of work.

in skeletal muscle during exercise. Details of how endurance exercise training alters both carbohydrate and fat metabolism are presented in the next sections.

Endurance Training Results in Decreased Utilization of Plasma Glucose during Prolonged Submaximal Exercise Glucose uptake by contracting skeletal muscles occurs via facilitated diffusion and requires the presence of a glucose transport protein (GLUT4) on the muscle cell membrane (i.e., sarcolemma). Endurance exercise training increases the capacity to transport glucose into skeletal muscle fibers by increasing both the number of GLUT4 glucose transporters and the ability of insulin to promote transport of glucose into the muscle (80). Given these training-induced changes, it is surprising that endurance training results in a decreased reliance on carbohydrate as an energy source during prolonged submaximal exercise. Indeed, uptake and oxidation of glucose from the blood during submaximal exercise is decreased in trained individuals (80). Consequently, trained individuals are better able to maintain blood glucose levels during prolonged exercise.

The mechanisms by which training decreases the utilization of blood glucose are not well known but could be due to a reduced movement of GLUT4 glucose transporters from the cytosol to the muscle membrane (80). Regardless of the mechanism responsible for this training-induced decrease in glucose metabolism during exercise, this slower utilization of glucose during prolonged exercise in trained individuals is a logical adaptation that would decrease the risk of developing hypoglycemia (i.e., low blood glucose levels) during a prolonging exercise bout (e.g., running a marathon).

Endurance Training Increases Fat Metabolism during Exercise Endurance training increases fat metabolism during submaximal exercise by boosting the delivery of fat to the muscle and expanding the

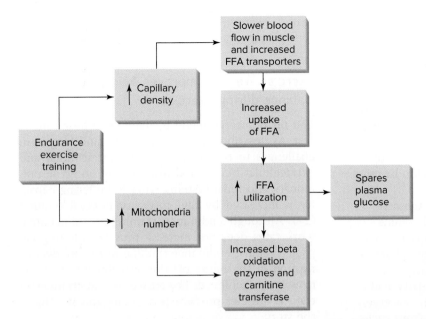

Figure 13.6 Endurance training increases fat metabolism and decreases muscle glucose utilization during prolonged submaximal exercise. This training-induced increase in fat metabolism during submaximal exercise is achieved by increasing capillary density and increasing the number of mitochondria in the muscle fiber.

muscle's ability to metabolize fat (Fig. 13.6). The training-induced increase in fat delivery to the muscle is accomplished by three training-induced adaptations: (1) increased capillary density which enhances the delivery of free fatty acids (FFA) to the muscle; (2) expanded ability to transport FFA across the sarcolemma; and (3) improved capacity to move FFA from the cytoplasm into the mitochondria. Also, endurance exercise training increases the muscle's ability to metabolize fat by increasing the volume of mitochondria in the muscle fiber. This is important because fat metabolism occurs in the mitochondria whereby beta oxidation converts FFA to acetyl-CoA units for metabolism in the Krebs cycle. More details of how endurance training increases fat metabolism follows.

Intramuscular fat provides about 50% of the lipid oxidized during exercise, and plasma FFA provide the rest (45, 101). The uptake of FFA by muscle is proportional to the FFA concentration in the plasma. For FFA to enter the muscle fiber, plasma FFA must be transported across the cell membrane to the cytoplasm and then into the mitochondria before oxidation can occur. Movement of FFA into the muscle cell involves a carrier molecule whose capacity to transport FFA can become saturated at high plasma FFA concentrations (85). However, endurance training increases the capacity to transport FFA across the cell membrane so that, compared to an untrained individual, a trained individual can transport more FFA across the muscle cell membrane (52). This is due to the dramatic training-induced increase in both fatty acid binding protein and fatty acid translocase (FAT) that transport the fatty acids across the sarcolemma into the fiber (48). This increased ability to transport FFA is facilitated by a greater capillary density in the trained muscle, which slows the rate of blood flow past the fiber membrane, allowing more time for the FFA to be transported into the cell (85) (Fig. 13.6).

Endurance exercise training also improves the ability to transport FFA into the mitochondria where fat oxidation occurs. A key step in FFA transport into the mitochondria involves both carnitine palmitoyltransferase I (CPT-I) and FAT. CPT-I and FAT work together to increase FFA entry into the mitochondria, and much of the training-induced increase in fat oxidation is linked to changes in mitochrondrial FAT. The increase in the mitochondrial size with endurance training increases the surface area of the mitochondrial membranes and the amount of CPT-I and FAT such that FFA can be transported at a faster rate from the cytoplasm to the mitochondria for oxidation (86). The faster rate of transport from the cytoplasm to the mitochondria favors the movement of more FFA into the muscle cell from the plasma.

As mentioned previously, endurance training causes an increase in both subpopulations of mitochondria—subsarcolemmal and intermyofibrillar in muscle fibers (54). These increases in mitochondria size elevate the enzymes involved in fatty-acid beta-oxidation. This results in an increased rate at which acetyl-CoA molecules are formed from FFA for entry to the Krebs cycle, where citrate (the first molecule in the cycle) is formed. A high rate of beta oxidation results in increased levels of citrate in the muscle. This is important because high citrate levels inhibit PFK (rate-limiting enzyme in glycolysis), which reduces carbohydrate metabolism (42). The result of all these adaptations is an increase in lipid oxidation and less reliance on carbohydrate metabolism during exercise, thus preserving the limited muscle and liver glycogen stores.

- Endurance training improves the ability of muscle fibers to maintain homeostasis during prolonged exercise.
- Regular bouts of endurance training result in a fast-to-slow shift in muscle fiber types and also increase the number of capillaries surrounding the trained muscle fibers.
- Endurance exercise also increases the size of both subsarcolemmal and intermyofibrillar mitochondria in the exercised muscles.
- The combination of the increase in the density of capillaries and mitochondrial volume in the muscle fiber increases the capacity to transport FFA from the plasma → cytoplasm → mitochondria.
- The increase in the enzymes of the fatty acid cycle increases the rate of formation of acetyl-CoA from FFA for oxidation in the Krebs cycle. This increase in fat oxidation in endurance-trained muscle spares liver and muscle glycogen and plasma glucose. These points are summarized in Figure 13.6.

Endurance Training Improves Muscle Antioxidant Capacity

Free radicals are chemical species or molecules that contain an unpaired electron in their outer orbital. Because of this unpaired electron, radicals are highly reactive and can interact with cellular components to promote damage to proteins, membranes, and DNA.

Therefore, it is not surprising that cells contain a network of molecules that neutralize radicals (i.e., antioxidants) and protect against radical-mediated injury. In general, these cellular antioxidants can be divided into two broad groups. The first set of antioxidants is produced within cells of the body (i.e., endogenous antioxidants), whereas the second group is derived from the diet (i.e., exogenous antioxidants). To provide maximum protection against radicals, these two antioxidant groups work as a team to neutralize radicals and maintain a healthy antioxidant/oxidant balance to prevent radical-mediated cellular damage.

Recall from Chap. 8 that free radicals are produced during muscular contraction, and radical production can disturb cellular homeostasis, promote oxidative damage to muscle contractile proteins, and contribute to muscle fatigue during prolonged endurance events (77, 78). Nonetheless, endurance training can protect muscle fibers against free radical-mediated damage by increasing the levels of endogenous antioxidants in the trained muscles (77). This increase in muscle antioxidant capacity neutralizes free radicals produced during exercise and protects the fiber against free radical-mediated damage during exercise. This protection against exercise-induced oxidative damage can, in turn, protect against radical-mediated muscle fatigue.

Exercise Training Improves Acid-Base Balance during Exercise

The pH of arterial blood is maintained near 7.40 at rest. As described in Chap. 11, acute and long-term challenges to the pH are met by intracellular and extracellular buffers and responses of both the pulmonary and renal systems. Muscle buffering capacity is increased by high-intensity interval training (27). Although endurance training at submaximal work rates does not increase muscle buffering capacity, regular endurance training results in less disruption of the blood pH during submaximal work. How is this achieved? The answer is that endurance-trained muscles produce less lactate and H^+. Here's the story.

Lactate formation occurs when there is an accumulation of NADH and pyruvate in the cytoplasm of the cell where lactate dehydrogenase (LDH) is present:

$$[pyruvate] + [NADH] \rightarrow [lactate] + [NAD]$$

$$LDH$$

Anything that affects the concentration of pyruvate, NADH, or the type of LDH in the cell will affect the rate of lactate formation. We have already seen that the increased size of mitochondria can have a dramatic effect on pyruvate formation; the lower ADP concentration in the cytosol prevents the activation of PFK at the onset of work, and the increased capacity to use fat as a fuel reduces the need for carbohydrate oxidation during prolonged work. If less carbohydrate is used, less pyruvate is formed. In addition, the increase in mitochondria number increases the chance that pyruvate will be taken up by the mitochondria for oxidation in the Krebs cycle, rather than being converted to lactate in the cytoplasm. All of these adaptations favor a lower pyruvate concentration and a reduction in lactate formation.

Two additional biochemical changes in muscle occur due to endurance training that reduces lactate production and, consequently, H^+ formation. The NADH produced during glycolysis can react with pyruvate, as shown in the previous equation, or it can be transported into the mitochondrion to be oxidized in the electron transport chain to form ATP (see Chap. 3). Endurance training increases the number of "shuttles" used to transport electrons associated with NADH from the cytoplasm into the mitochondrion (42). If the NADH formed in glycolysis is more quickly transported to the mitochondria, there will be less lactate and H^+ formation. Last, endurance training causes a change in the type of LDH present in the muscle cell. This enzyme exists in five forms

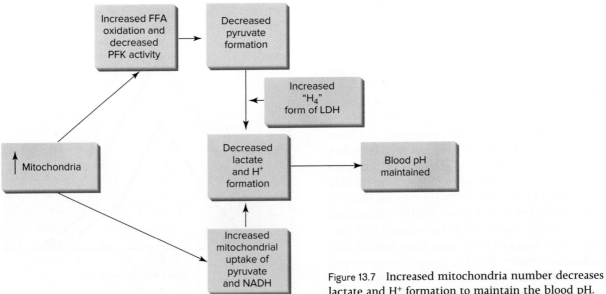

Figure 13.7 Increased mitochondria number decreases lactate and H⁺ formation to maintain the blood pH.

(isozymes): M_4, M_3H, M_2H_2, MH_3, and H_4. The H_4, or heart form of LDH, has a low affinity for the available pyruvate; therefore, the likelihood of lactate production is diminished. Endurance training shifts the LDH toward the H_4 form, making lactate formation less likely and the uptake of pyruvate by the mitochondria more likely. Figure 13.7 summarizes the effects these biochemical changes have on lactate formation and the production of H^+ during submaximal work.

IN SUMMARY

- Endurance training increases endogenous antioxidants in trained muscles, and these changes protect muscle fibers against free-radical mediated damage and fatigue during prolonged endurance exercise.
- High-intensity (interval) exercise training can increase the buffering capacity of the exercised muscles.
- Endurance training does not increase muscle buffering capacity, but regular endurance training results in less disruption of the blood pH during submaximal work because endurance-trained muscles produce less lactate and H^+.

MOLECULAR BASES OF EXERCISE TRAINING ADAPTATION

In the previous segments, we have discussed numerous biochemical changes that occur in skeletal muscle following weeks to months of endurance training. These cellular changes are initiated from an "exercise stimulus" within the active muscles, and the end result is an increased synthesis of specific proteins within muscle fibers. This process of exercise-induced adaptation in skeletal muscle fibers involves many signaling pathways that promote protein synthesis and the formation of new mitochondria (i.e., mitochondrial biogenesis). In the next sections, we present a brief overview of the signaling processes that contribute to exercise-induced muscle adaptation. We begin with a "big picture" view of exercise-induced muscle adaptation to training. This is followed by a brief introduction to both the primary and secondary signaling molecules that participate in muscle adaptation in response to endurance and resistance training. We then highlight the specific signals leading to muscle adaptation due to endurance exercise. Later, we discuss the signaling molecules responsible for muscle adaptation to resistance training.

Training Adaptation—Big Picture

Regardless of whether the training program is endurance exercise or resistance exercise, the exercise-induced adaptation that occurs in muscle fibers is the result of an increase in the amount of specific proteins (39). The process of exercise-induced synthesis of cellular proteins was first introduced in Chap. 2. Recall that the "stress" of exercise stimulates cell signaling pathways in contracting muscle fibers that "switch on" transcriptional activators. These transcriptional activators are responsible for "turning on" specific genes to synthesize new proteins. This gene activation in the cell nucleus results in transcription of messenger RNA (mRNA), which contains the genetic information for a specific protein's amino acid sequence. The newly synthesized mRNA leaves the nucleus and travels to the ribosome where the mRNA message is translated into a specific protein. Remember that individual proteins differ in structure and function and that the specific types of proteins contained in a muscle fiber determine the muscle characteristics and its ability to perform specific types of exercise.

A single bout of endurance exercise is insufficient to produce large changes in proteins within a muscle fiber. Nonetheless, one exercise session promotes transient disturbances in cellular homeostasis that, when repeated over time, result in the specific exercise-induced adaptation associated with long-term training (16, 17). The "big picture" process of exercise-induced training adaptation is as follows. Muscle contraction during a training session generates a signal that promotes muscle adaptation by increasing primary and secondary messengers. These messengers initiate a cascade of coordinated signaling events, resulting in increased expression of specific genes and subsequently the synthesis of new proteins. In short, a bout of exercise generates a transient increase in the quantity of specific mRNAs, which typically peaks during the first four to eight hours post-exercise and returns to basal levels within 24 hours (Fig. 13.8(a)). Also, notice that mRNA levels for specific muscle proteins increase at different rates and peak at varying time periods following an exercise session. This exercise-induced increase in mRNA results in the increased synthesis of specific muscle proteins. Therefore, exercise repeated on a daily basis has a cumulative effect, leading to a progressive increase in specific muscle proteins that improve muscle function (Fig. 13.8(b)). This explains why maintaining a constant level of fitness requires regular bouts of exercise. Further, observe that the training-induced increases in muscle proteins is a gradual process, with large increases in muscle protein levels during the first weeks of training followed by a slower rate of protein accumulation as the training progresses (Fig. 13.8(b)).

Specificity of Exercise Training Responses

As we have seen, skeletal muscle is a very adaptable tissue that responds to exercise training by increasing the expression of multiple genes. The features of exercise-induced muscle adaptation are specific to the training volume, intensity, and frequency. That is, the specific adaptations that occur in skeletal muscle fibers result from the type of exercise stimulus (i.e., resistance vs. endurance exercise). Indeed, dissimilar modes of exercise promote the expression of different genes in the active muscle fibers. Specifically, resistance exercise and endurance exercise promote the activation of different cell signaling pathways; therefore, different genes are activated, resulting in the expression of diverse proteins. For example, prolonged endurance training results in a variety of metabolic

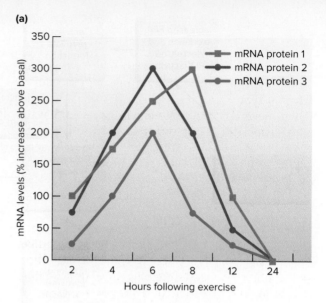

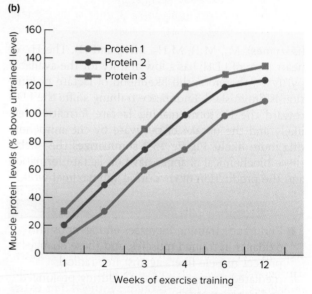

Figure 13.8 (a) An example illustrating the rise and decline of mRNA for three different muscle proteins following an acute bout of exercise. (b) Illustration of the training-induced increase in three different muscle proteins during a 12-week training period.

adaptations (e.g., increased mitochondrial volume) with little change in muscle fiber size. In contrast, heavy resistance exercise results in increased synthesis of contractile proteins and muscle hypertrophy. Consistent with these different functional outcomes induced by these different exercise modes, the signaling pathways and molecular mechanisms responsible for these adaptations are distinct. In the next segment, we introduce the general "primary" signaling pathways that produced exercise-induced training adaptations to both endurance and resistance exercise. This will be followed by a discussion of the secondary signals that are responsible for the increased protein synthesis following different types of exercise training.

Primary Signal Transduction Pathways in Skeletal Muscle

Our understanding of the precise mechanisms that enable skeletal muscle to interpret and respond to different types of exercise remains incomplete. Nonetheless, several primary messengers participate in the exercise-induced adaptation that occurs in skeletal muscle. The four primary signals for muscle adaptation during exercise include mechanical stimuli, increases in cellular calcium, elevated free radicals, and decreases in muscle phosphate/energy levels.

Mechanical Stimuli During resistance exercise training, the mechanical force placed on the muscle fiber triggers signaling processes to promote adaptation. For example, passive stretching of a muscle fiber results in the activation of a mechanoreceptor on the muscle membrane that stimulates biochemical signaling, leading to an increase in contractile protein synthesis (44). Therefore, the signaling events initiated by mechanical load with resistance exercise play an important role in the exercise-induced adaptation of muscle fibers. In this regard, it is clear that muscle fibers can sense differences in the intensity and duration of mechanical stimuli (i.e., resistance exercise vs. endurance exercise) to contribute to the specificity of exercise-induced adaptation (16). In particular, the high levels of mechanical stretch that occur across the muscle membrane during resistance training is the primary signal that promotes contractile protein synthesis, resulting in muscle hypertrophy.

Calcium Calcium is an important signaling mechanism in cells. Indeed, free calcium in the cytoplasm can activate numerous enzymes and other signaling molecules that promote protein synthesis. For example, increased cytosolic levels of calcium activates an important kinase called *calmodulin-dependent kinase*. Calmodulin-dependent kinase is one member of a family of enzymes that promote phosphorylation of various protein substrates. Once activated, calmodulin-dependent kinase initiates a signaling cascade in muscle fibers that contributes to muscle adaptation to exercise training. How does exercise alter muscle calcium levels and control calcium signaling?

Remember from Chap. 8 that neural activation of skeletal muscle contraction promotes calcium release from the sarcoplasmic reticulum, and stoppage of the neural stimulation initiates the reuptake of this calcium from the cytosol back to the sarcoplasmic reticulum via active transport calcium pumps. The level of free calcium in the muscle cytosol is determined by the mode, intensity, and volume of exercise (16). For example, prolonged endurance exercise likely results in long periods of elevated calcium levels in the muscle cytosol, whereas resistance exercise would generate only short cycles of high cytosolic calcium levels (16). Therefore, these exercise-induced differences in cytosolic calcium levels between endurance and resistance exercise determine the downstream calcium-mediated signaling events leading to synthesis of specific muscle proteins. In particular, the sustained high levels of cytosolic calcium that occur during endurance training plays an important signaling role in promoting the adaptations that occur in skeletal muscle in response to this type of training.

Free Radicals Exercise results in the production of free radicals and other oxidants in active skeletal muscles (77). This is important because growing evidence indicates that radicals are important signals for muscle adaptation to exercise training (76, 78). For example, free radical production during exercise can activate nuclear factor kappa B (NFκB) and mitogen-activated kinase p38 (p38). NFκB is an important transcriptional activator that promotes the expression of several muscle proteins, including antioxidant enzymes that protect muscle fibers against exercise-induced oxidative stress (77). p38 is an intracellular kinase that plays a key signaling role in the production of new mitochondria. Note that both p38 and NFκB act as secondary signals involved in exercise-induced muscle adaptation to endurance training and will be discussed in more detail in upcoming sections.

Phosphate/Muscle Energy Levels Muscular exercise accelerates ATP consumption in the working muscle and increases the ratio of AMP/ATP in muscle fibers. Increasing the AMP/ATP ratio can initiate numerous downstream signaling events in skeletal muscle fibers (16). This exercise-induced change in cellular energy state activates numerous signaling molecules, but one of the most important in exercise-induced muscle adaptation is activation of a secondary messenger called **5'adenosine monophosphate activated protein kinase (AMPK).** Indeed, AMPK is an important downstream signaling molecule that senses the energy state of the muscle and is activated by both high-intensity interval training and prolonged endurance exercise. This important kinase regulates numerous muscle signaling processes leading to muscle adaptation in response to endurance training and will be discussed in more detail in the next segment.

Secondary Messengers in Skeletal Muscle

Following the initiation of the primary signal, additional (secondary) signaling pathways are activated to mediate the exercise-induced signal to promote muscle adaptation. Indeed, numerous secondary-signaling pathways exist in skeletal muscle and are regulated at multiple levels. Next, we will provide a "big-picture" overview of seven secondary signaling pathways that play major roles in exercise-induced muscle adaptation. Specifically, we highlight the roles that AMPK, p38, peroxisome proliferator-activated receptor-gamma coactivator 1α (PGC-1α), calmodulin-dependent kinase, calcineurin, NFκB, and mechanistic target of rapamycin (mTOR) play in muscle adaptation to exercise training. Note that the first six of these signaling molecules are involved in muscle adaptation to endurance training whereas the secondary signaling molecule mTOR contributes to muscle adaptation in response to resistance exercise training.

AMPK **AMPK** is an important signaling molecule that is activated during both high-intensity interval training, and submaximal endurance exercise training due to changes in muscle fiber phosphate/energy levels. This key molecule regulates numerous energy-producing pathways in muscle by stimulating glucose uptake and fatty acid oxidation during exercise. AMPK is also linked to the control of muscle gene expression by activating transcription factors associated with fatty acid oxidation and mitochondrial biogenesis. Interestingly, AMPK can inhibit components of the mTOR signaling pathway; the importance of this fact will be discussed later.

P38 Mitogen activated kinase p38 (**p38**) is an important signaling molecule that is activated in muscle fibers during endurance exercise. Although several cellular stresses can activate p38, it seems likely that exercise-induced production of free radicals is a major signal to activate p38 in muscle fibers. Once activated, p38 can contribute to mitochondrial biogenesis by activating PGC-1α.

PGC-1α This key molecule is activated by both high-intensity interval training and submaximal endurance exercise and is considered the master regulator of mitochondrial biogenesis in cells (72). Indeed, **PGC-1α** assists transcriptional activators that promote mitochondrial biogenesis in skeletal muscle following endurance training. Furthermore, PGC-1α regulates many other endurance exercise-mediated changes in skeletal muscle, including the formation of new capillaries (angiogenesis), a fast-to-slow muscle fiber type shift, and synthesis of antioxidant enzymes (72). PGC-1α also plays a role in exercise-induced increases in muscle's ability to metabolize fat and to take up glucose into the muscle fiber. Several factors activate PGC-1α during exercise, including AMPK and p38.

Calmodulin-Dependent Kinase Calmodulin-dependent kinase (**CaMK**) is activated during endurance exercise training (16). This vital kinase exerts influence on exercise-induced muscle adaptation by contributing to the activation of PGC-1α. The primary upstream signal to activate CaMK is increased cytosolic calcium levels.

Calciuneurin **Calciuneurin** is a phosphatase (i.e., enzyme that removes a phosphate group from molecules) activated by increases in cytosolic calcium and participates in several adaptive responses in muscle, including fiber growth/regeneration and the fast-to-slow fiber type transition that occurs as a result of endurance exercise training.

NFκB As mentioned previously, **NFκB** is a transcriptional activator that can be activated by free radicals that are produced in contracting muscles. Active NFκB promotes the expression of several antioxidant enzymes that protect muscle fibers against free radical-mediated injury.

mTOR mTOR is a protein kinase that is the major regulator of protein synthesis and muscle size. Activation of mTOR promotes increased translation that results in increased protein synthesis. Specifically, mTOR is a secondary signaling molecule in muscle adaptation to resistance exercise training that is activated by stimulation of a mechanoreceptor on the sarcolemma of the muscle. More details about mTOR activation and signaling are provided later in the chapter.

IN SUMMARY

- Independent of the type of exercise stimulus (i.e., endurance or resistance exercise), the training-induced adaptation that occurs in muscle fibers is the result of an increase in the amount of specific proteins.
- The exercise-induced adaptations in skeletal muscle fibers are specific to the type of exercise stimulus (i.e., resistance vs. endurance exercise).
- Exercise-induced muscle adaptation occurs due to the coordination between primary and secondary signaling pathways in muscle fibers.
- Four primary signals for exercise-induced muscle adaptation include muscle stretch, increases in cellular free calcium, elevated free radicals, and decreases in muscle phosphate/energy levels. These primary signals then activate downstream secondary signaling pathways to promote gene expression.
- Seven secondary signaling molecules that contribute to exercise-induced muscle adaptation include AMPK, p38, PGC-1α, CaMK, calcineurin, NFκB, and mTOR. These signaling molecules are activated via one of four primary signaling pathways and act directly or indirectly to increase gene expression of specific muscle proteins.

SIGNALING EVENTS LEADING TO ENDURANCE TRAINING-INDUCED MUSCLE ADAPTATION

As we have discussed, endurance training can increase $\dot{V}O_2$ max by 20% to 50% and also improve performance in submaximal endurance events (39). This training-induced improvement is achieved by changes in both cardiac output and capillary density along with alterations at the cellular level in both cardiac and skeletal muscle fibers. In this section, we highlight the major exercise-induced signaling events that promote molecular adaptations in skeletal muscle fibers following both high-intensity interval training and endurance exercise training.

Repeated muscle contractions during submaximal endurance exercise trigger a signaling cascade within the active muscle fibers leading to mitochondrial biogenesis, a shift in muscle fiber type from fast-to-slow, and increased expression of important antioxidant enzymes. As illustrated in Figure 13.9, calcium release, increased AMP/ATP ratio, and production of free radicals are primary signaling

events responsible for activation of the downstream, secondary signaling events (i.e., activation of calcineurin, CaMK, AMPK, p38, NFκB, and PGC-1 α) that lead to mitochondrial biogenesis, fiber type transformation, and increased expression of antioxidant enzymes.

Note in Figure 13.9 that contraction-induced increases in the AMP/ATP ratio activates AMPK in the muscle, whereas increased cellular levels of free calcium are required to activate both CaMK and calcineurin. Active calcineurin acts as a signaling molecule to promote fast-to-slow fiber type transformation. Further, notice that muscle contractions promote an increase in free radicals that serve as the primary signal to activate both p38 and NFκB. Activation of three secondary signals (AMPK, CaMK, and p38) all promote mitochondrial biogenesis by activation of the master regulator of mitochondrial biogenesis, PGC-1α. PGC-1α also contributes to the exercise-induced fast-to-slow fiber type transformation. Finally, note that activation of both PGC-1α and NFκB promote exercise-induced expression of important muscle antioxidant enzymes (76, 77).

Figure 13.10 illustrates the time course of exercise-induced mitochondrial biogenesis. Note that

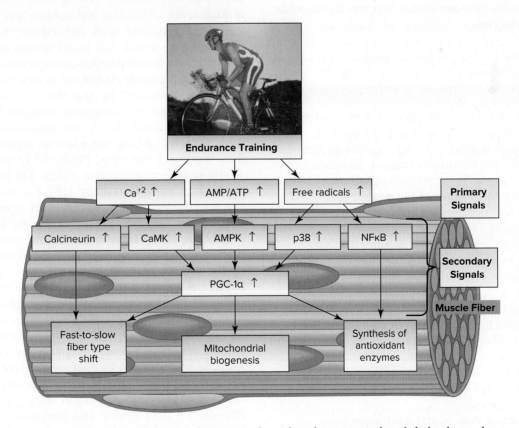

Figure 13.9 Illustration of the intracellular signaling network-mediated exercise-induced skeletal muscle responses to endurance exercise training. Take note that both primary and secondary signals are involved in muscle adaptation to endurance exercise training. See text for more details.

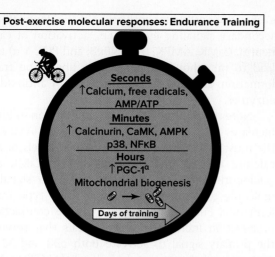

Figure 13.10 Illustration of the time course of molecular responses to endurance exercise training. See text for more details.

a rise in the primary signals to promote mitochondrial biogenesis occurs within the first few seconds after beginning exercise. Within the first few minutes of exercise, the secondary signals involved in exercise-induced muscle adaptation increase within the muscle fibers. Within a few hours following exercise, muscle levels of PGC-1α rise and mitochondrial biogenesis proceeds. Mitochondrial volume in the exercised muscles increases within days and continues as training proceeds.

IN SUMMARY

- Three primary signals involved in endurance exercise-induced muscle adaptation are increases in cellular free calcium, elevated free radicals, and decreases in muscle phosphate/energy levels. These primary signals then activate one or more of the downstream secondary signaling pathways to promote gene expression.
- Six secondary signaling molecules that contribute to endurance exercise-induced muscle adaptation include AMPK, PGC-1α, calcineurin, CaMK, p38, and NFκB.
- Both active calcineurin and PGC-1α play important roles in endurance exercise-induced fast-to-slow fiber transformations.
- Collectively, active CaMK, AMPK, and p38 all participate in activation of PGC-1α. Active PGC-1α is the master regulator for mitochondrial biogenesis.
- Both active PGC-1α and NFκB contribute to the exercise-induced increase in muscle antioxidants.

ENDURANCE TRAINING: LINKS BETWEEN MUSCLE AND SYSTEMIC PHYSIOLOGY

The first portions of this chapter described the importance of the changes occurring in endurance-trained muscle on the maintenance of homeostasis during prolonged submaximal work. Importantly, these exercise-induced adaptations in skeletal muscle are also related to the lower heart rate, ventilation, and catecholamine responses measured during submaximal work following an endurance training program. What is the link between the changes in muscle and the lower heart rate and ventilation responses to exercise?

The following endurance training study illustrates the impact of training-induced adaptations in the body's overall response to a submaximal exercise session. In this study, each subject's left and right legs were tested separately on a cycle ergometer at a submaximal work rate prior to and during an endurance training program. Heart rate and ventilation were measured at the end of the submaximal exercise test, and a blood sample was obtained to monitor changes in lactate, epinephrine, and norepinephrine. During the study, each subject trained only one leg for 13 endurance training sessions. At the end of each week of training, the subject was tested at the same submaximal work rate. Figure 13.11 shows that heart rate, ventilation, blood lactate, and plasma epinephrine and norepinephrine responses decreased throughout the study. At the end of this training program, the "untrained" leg was then trained for five consecutive days at the same submaximal work rate used for the "trained" leg. Physiological measurements were obtained during the exercise session on the first, third, and fifth days. Figure 13.11 shows that all the systems responded as if they had never been exposed to exercise training (15). Therefore, there was no transfer of the training effect from one leg to the other. This example shows that the heart rate, ventilation, and plasma catecholamine responses to prolonged submaximal exercise are determined, not by the specific adaptation of each organ or system, but by the training state of the specific muscle groups engaged in the exercise. How is this possible?

Let's revisit the topic of cardiorespiratory control during exercise to explain why endurance exercise training results in a lower heart rate and ventilatory response to a standard bout of submaximal exercise. Recall from Chaps. 9 and 10 that the control of heart rate and pulmonary ventilation during exercise is achieved by both central and peripheral neural influences that increase heart rate and ventilation to match the increased oxygen demands of exercise. The output of the cardiovascular and respiratory

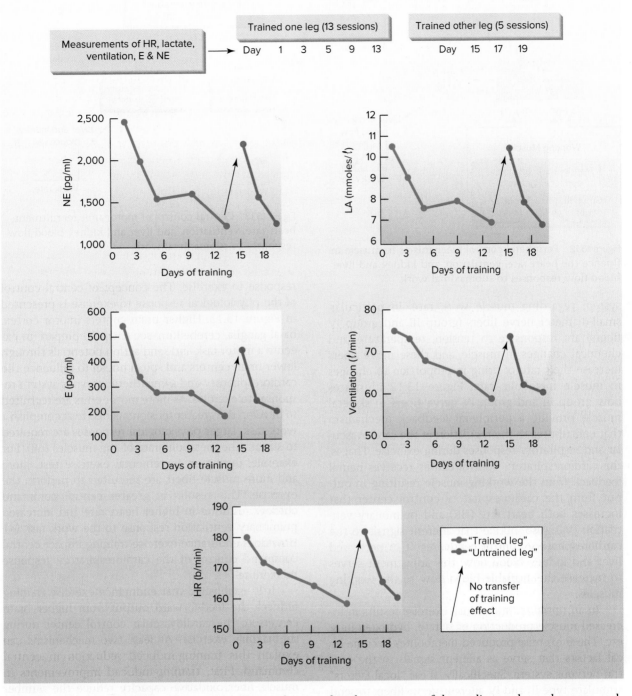

Figure 13.11 The lack of transfer of a training effect, indicating that the responses of the cardiovascular, pulmonary, and sympathetic nervous systems are more dependent on the trained state of the muscles involved in the activity than on some specific adaptation in those systems. Key: norepinephrine = NE; epinephrine = E; heart rate = HR; lactate = LA.

control centers is influenced by neural input from higher brain centers, where the motor task originates, as well as from the muscles carrying out the task. A decrease in motor unit recruitment or a reduction in afferent feedback from the receptors in the working muscles to the brain reduces these cardiorespiratory responses to the work task. Specific details about this issue follow.

Peripheral Feedback

The idea that reflexes in working muscles might control or "drive" cardiovascular or pulmonary systems in proportion to the metabolic rate originated in the early 1900s. Numerous muscle receptors respond to tension and metabolic changes in muscle, and these receptors provide information to the central nervous

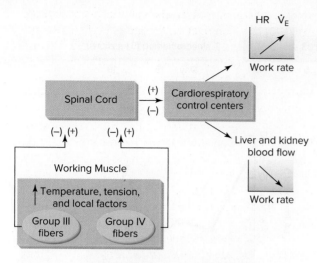

Figure 13.12 Peripheral control mechanisms in muscle influence the heart rate, ventilation, and kidney and liver blood flow responses to submaximal work.

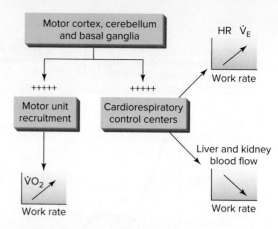

Figure 13.13 Central control of motor unit recruitment, heart rate, ventilation, and liver and kidney blood flow responses to submaximal work.

system regarding muscle work rate. In particular, small-diameter nerve fibers (group III and group IV fibers) are responsive to tension, temperature, and chemical changes in muscle, and these nerve fibers increase their rate of firing in proportion to changes in muscle metabolic rate. Figure 13.12 illustrates how group III and group IV nerve fibers in skeletal muscle provide a peripheral feedback mechanism that contributes to the regulation of the cardiovascular and respiratory responses during exercise. That is, the cardiorespiratory control center receives neural feedback from the working muscle resulting in output from the cardiorespiratory control center that increases both heart rate (HR) and pulmonary ventilation ($\dot{V}_E$). Also, notice that afferent signals to the cardiorespiratory control center result in decreased liver and kidney blood flow; this adjustment serves to increase the available blood flow to the working muscles.

In an untrained individual, exercise results in increased muscle production of lactate, hydrogen ions, etc. These exercise-produced metabolites become local factors that serve as afferent signals to the central nervous system. Specifically, these "local factors" stimulate type III and IV afferent nerve fibers to send afferent signals to the cardiovascular control center to increase both heart rate and pulmonary ventilation. However, following endurance training, the higher mitochondrial volume in the trained muscles results in less production of lactate and hydrogen ions (i.e., fewer local factors) resulting in less chemoreceptor input to the cardiorespiratory control centers.

Central Command

Recall that central command refers to the neural signals originating in higher brain centers that provide a feed forward mechanism to control the cardiorespiratory

response to exercise. The concept of central control of the physiological response to exercise is presented in Figure 13.13. Higher brain centers (motor cortex, basal ganglia, cerebellum–see Chap. 7) prepare to execute a motor task and send action potentials through lower brain centers and spinal nuclei to influence the cardiorespiratory and sympathetic nervous system responses to exercise. As more motor units are recruited to develop the greater tension needed to accomplish a work task, larger physiological responses are required to sustain the metabolic rate of the muscles (68). For example, during an incremental exercise test, more and more muscle fibers are recruited to perform the exercise. This results in greater central command outflow resulting in higher heart rate and increased pulmonary ventilation response to the work task (4). How does endurance exercise training impact central command control of the cardiorespiratory response to exercise?

It is established that endurance exercise training reduces the feed-forward output from higher brain centers to the cardiovascular control center during submaximal exercise. At least two mechanisms can explain this training-induced reduction in central command. First, training-induced improvements in muscle fiber oxidative capacity reduce the number of motor units (i.e., muscle fibers) required to perform a prolonged, submaximal exercise task; this would result in less "central" drive to the cardiorespiratory control center. Second, evidence from one-leg exercise training studies reveals that endurance training also results in direct changes in the central nervous system causing a reduced central command outflow to the cardiorespiratory control center during submaximal exercise. Collectively, this exercise training-induced reduction in feed-forward output from higher brain centers results in lower sympathetic nervous system output, heart rate, and ventilation responses to exercise (68).

- The biochemical changes in muscle due to endurance training influence the heart rate and ventilatory responses to exercise.
- The reduction in "feedback" from chemoreceptors in the trained muscle and a decreased need to recruit motor units to accomplish an exercise task result in reduced sympathetic nervous system, heart rate, and ventilation responses to submaximal exercise.
- Endurance exercise training also reduces central command outflow during submaximal exercise that results in a lower heart rate and ventilatory response during exercise.

DETRAINING FOLLOWING ENDURANCE TRAINING

In the previous sections, we discussed the effects of endurance training on both $\dot{V}O_2$ max and the cellular adaptations that occur in the trained muscle fibers. Let's shift our attention from training adaptations and discuss what happens to $\dot{V}O_2$ max when endurance training ceases. It is well known that when highly trained individuals stop training, $\dot{V}O_2$ max decreases over time. Why? The answer is because both maximal cardiac output and oxygen extraction decline over time with detraining. This point is illustrated in Figure 13.14, which shows changes in maximal oxygen uptake, cardiac output, stroke volume, heart rate, and oxygen extraction over an 84-day period of no training (21). The initial decrease (first 12 days) in $\dot{V}O_2$ max was due entirely to the decrease in stroke volume, because the heart rate and a-$\bar{v}O_2$ difference remained the same or increased. This sudden decrease in maximal stroke volume appears to be due to the rapid loss of plasma volume with detraining (18). When plasma volume was artificially restored by infusion, $\dot{V}O_2$ max increased toward pre-detraining values (18). This was confirmed in a study in which a 200 to 300 ml expansion of plasma volume was shown to increase $\dot{V}O_2$ max, even though the hemoglobin concentration was reduced (19).

Figure 13.14 also reveals that between the 21st and 84th days of detraining, the decrease in $\dot{V}O_2$ max is due to the decrease in the a-$\bar{v}O_2$ difference. This was associated with a decrease in muscle mitochondria, whereas capillary density remained unchanged. The overall oxidative capacity of skeletal muscle was reduced, with the percentage of type IIa fibers decreasing from 43% to 26% and the percentage of type IIx fibers increasing from 5% to 19% (20, 21). This detraining-induced slow-to-fast fiber type shift is opposite to the fast-to-slow shift in muscle fiber type that occurs during endurance exercise training.

Detraining not only decreases $\dot{V}O_2$ max, inactivity can also impair submaximal endurance performance. For example, as few as 14 days of disrupted training (e.g., detraining) can significantly impair submaximal exercise performance (e.g., performance in 10K run). This is due primarily to a decrease in muscle mitochondria (63, 105). Indeed, muscle mitochondrial oxidative capacity undergoes rapid changes at both the onset and termination of exercise training. Figure 13.15

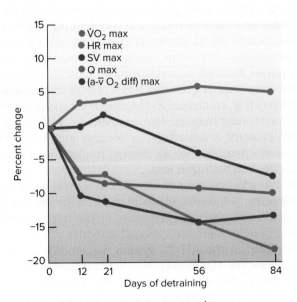

Figure 13.14 Time course of changes in $\dot{V}O_2$ max and associated cardiovascular variables with detraining.

Coyle, E. F., Martin III, W. H., Sinacore, D. R., Joyner, M. J., Hagberg, J. M., and Holloszy, J. O., "Time Course of Loss of Adaptations After Stopping Prolonged Intense Endurance Training," *Journal of Applied Physiology* 57: 1857–1864, 1984.

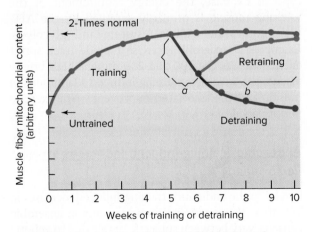

Figure 13.15 Time-course of training/detraining adaptations in mitochondrial content of skeletal muscle. Note that about 50% of the increase in mitochondrial content was lost after one week of detraining (*a*) and that all of the adaptation was lost after five weeks of detraining. Also, it took four weeks of retraining (*b*) to regain the adaptation lost in the first week of detraining.

shows how quickly muscle mitochondria increase at the onset of training, doubling in about five weeks of training. However, only one week of detraining (shown by the letter "a") results in a loss of about 50% of what was gained during the five weeks of training (10, 90). Then three to four weeks of retraining were required to achieve the former levels (shown by the letter "b" in Fig. 13.15).

IN SUMMARY

- After stoppage of exercise training, $\dot{V}O_2$ max begins to decline quickly and can decrease by ~8% within 12 days after cessation of training, and declines by almost 20% following 84 days of detraining.
- The decrease in $\dot{V}O_2$ max with cessation of training is due to a decrease in both maximal stroke volume and oxygen extraction, the reverse of what happens with training.
- Exercise performance during submaximal exercise tasks also declines rapidly in response to detraining, due primarily to a decrease in the number of mitochondria in muscle fibers.

MUSCLE ADAPTATIONS TO ANAEROBIC EXERCISE TRAINING

Anaerobic exercise refers to short-duration (i.e., 10 to 30 seconds), high-intensity (i.e., all-out effort) exercise bouts. This type of "all-out" exercise is often called "sprint training" and is performed at exercise intensities above $\dot{V}O_2$ max. Recall that during this type of exercise, the energy requirement of the working muscle is primarily supplied by the ATP-phosphocreatine (ATP-PC) system and glycolysis. Examples of anaerobic exercise include track sprint events such as the 100 and 200 meters. Let's briefly discuss the anaerobic training-induced adaptations in muscle and the associated improvement in exercise performance.

Anaerobic Training-Induced Increases in Performance

Similar to the endurance training-induced increases in $\dot{V}O_2$ max, sprint training improvements in anaerobic capacity vary between subjects, largely due to genetic differences. For example, following 4 to 10 weeks of anaerobic training, the percent improvement in both peak anaerobic power and capacity varies from 3% to 25% across individuals (81). Regardless of the size of the increase in anaerobic power, this training-induced increase in anaerobic power output translates into performance improvements during high-intensity exercise lasting less than 30 seconds.

Anaerobic Training-Induced Changes in Skeletal Muscles

It is important to appreciate that the adaptations in muscle that occur following sprint training are due to the time of the exercise interval (81). Indeed, the energy systems used during high-intensity exercise differ markedly depending upon the duration of exercise. For example, during maximal exercise lasting 10 seconds or less, almost all of the energy is derived from the ATP-PC system. However, when sprint exercise lasts for 20 to 30 seconds, the relative contribution of anaerobic energy production decreases and approximately 20% of the energy is produced aerobically (81). This is a reminder that no form of exercise is purely anaerobic or aerobic. Therefore, because the metabolic demands of short- and long-duration sprint exercise are different, it follows that the intramuscular adaptations depend on the makeup of the exercise training program. Following this review about the interactions between aerobic and anaerobic energy production in muscle, let's discuss sprint training-stimulated adaptations to skeletal muscle.

As introduced in Chap. 11, muscle fibers are protected against exercise-induced decreases in pH by both intracellular buffers and hydrogen ion transporters that move hydrogen ions from inside of the muscle across the sarcolemma. Studies show that both sprint training (exercise duration = 10 to 30 seconds) and high-intensity interval training (interval duration = 30 to 60 seconds) improve muscle buffer capacity (81). The mechanisms responsible for exercise-induced improvements in muscle buffering capacity include increased levels of both intracellular buffers (e.g., carnosine) and hydrogen ion transporters. This training-induced improvement in muscle buffer capacity is advantageous because high-intensity exercise results in an accelerated production of both lactate and hydrogen ions.

In addition to improvements in muscle buffering capacity, >4 weeks of sprint training in untrained subjects results in hypertrophy of fast (type IIa and IIx) muscle fibers and elevated activities of enzymes involved in the ATP-PC system (i.e., myokinase and creatine phosphokinase) (81). Not surprisingly, this increase in fiber size is associated with a rise in muscle strength. The improved activity of enzymes involved in the ATP-PC system results in an improved ability to rapidly breakdown phosphocreatine for energy during high-intensity exercise. Additionally, sprint training also increases the activities of key glycolytic enzymes, which raise the muscle's capacity to produce ATP via glycolysis (29, 81).

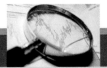
Aging, Strength, and Training

Aging is associated with a decline in strength, with most of the decline occurring after age 50. The loss of strength is due, in part, to a loss of muscle mass (sarcopenia), which is related to the loss of both type I and II fibers, atrophy of existing type II fibers, and an increase in intramuscular fat and connective tissue (46). This age-related loss of muscle fibers appears to occur as a result of losing motor neurons. Therefore, entire motor units are lost during aging. In addition, the remaining type I or type II muscle fibers cluster in homogeneous groups, in contrast to the heterogeneous distribution of fiber types seen in a muscle cross-section from younger individuals (46).

That is the bad news. The good news is that a progressive resistance-training program causes muscle hypertrophy and gains in strength in older individuals, including those in their 90s (31, 32). Such strength training programs are important, not only for being able to carry out activities of daily living, but also for improved balance and reducing the risk of falls (43, 46).

Although resistance exercise training can produce muscle hypertrophy and strength gains in limb muscles of old people, muscle fibers do not typically develop hypertrophy to the same extent in old individuals compared to young even if they perform the same training program (3,46). This age-related difference in the ability of older individuals to respond to resistance training may be related to an aging-suppressed satellite cell function (3). More details about this issue will be provided later in the chapter.

Also, it is common for many older adults to use over-the-counter nonsteroidal anti-inflammatory drugs (e.g., ibuprofen and acetaminophen) to combat both arthritis and sore muscles. Both of these drugs inhibit the activity of cyclooxygenase, which is an enzyme that produces prostaglandins and is involved in inflammatory processes in cells. However, several animal studies suggest that these cyclooxygenase inhibitors can interfere with resistance training-induced muscle hypertrophy (71, 89). These findings suggest that use of these drugs concurrently with strength training would be counterproductive. Nonetheless, two recent human studies have demonstrated that these commonly used pain killers do not impede strength gains in older people engaged in resistance exercise training (57, 99). In fact, one of these studies suggests that concurrent strength training and use of either ibuprofen or acetaminophen may actually enhance muscle hypertrophy and suggests that the cyclooxygenase pathways may be involved in the regulation of muscle protein content in humans (99). These findings are good news for older adults engaged in regular strength training.

Finally, as mentioned earlier in this chapter, high-intensity interval training (i.e., exercising at or near $\dot{V}O_2$ max for 30 seconds or more) promotes mitochondrial biogenesis. In contrast, short bouts of sprint exercise training (i.e., 5 to 10 seconds duration) do not generally increase mitochondrial volume in muscle fibers as these training adaptations are limited to changes in the ATP-PC system and glycolysis.

IN SUMMARY

- Muscle adaptations that occur in response to sprint training vary depending upon the duration of exercise.
- Short-duration (10 to 30 seconds) sprint exercise training results in increased muscle buffer capacity, increases in the size of fast (type II) muscle fibers, and an improved ability to generate ATP via anaerobic energy systems.
- High-intensity exercise training involving intervals of 30 seconds or more promotes adaptations in both anaerobic and aerobic energy systems (i.e., increased mitochondrial biogenesis).

PHYSIOLOGICAL EFFECTS OF STRENGTH TRAINING

The basic principles of training related to improving strength have been around for many years, and Morpurgo's observation that gains in strength were associated with increases in muscle size was made more than 100 years ago (6). Despite this history, most recent research on the effects of training has focused on $\dot{V}O_2$ max and endurance performance, possibly because of their link to the prevention and treatment of heart disease. However, it is now recognized that resistance training has many health benefits and becomes even more important with advancing age. See A Closer Look 13.3 for background on why strength training is important as we age.

Before we begin, some terms and basic principles need to be introduced. Muscular strength refers to the maximal force that a muscle or muscle group can generate and is commonly expressed as the one-repetition maximum, or 1-RM, which is the maximum load that can be moved through a full range of motion. Muscular endurance refers to the ability to make repeated contractions against a submaximal load. Consistent with our earlier discussion of training and $\dot{V}O_2$ max, large individual differences exist in the response to strength-training programs, and the percent gain in strength is inversely related to the initial strength (55). These observations imply a genetic limitation to the gains that can be achieved with training, similar to those observed for training-induced increases in $\dot{V}O_2$ max. Finally, the basic principles of training, overload, and specificity apply here as well. For example, high-load resistance training (8 to 12 reps/set) results primarily in gains in muscular strength; in contrast, low-load resistance training (>20 reps/set) results in gains in muscular endurance, with less increases in strength (55). What physiological changes occur with resistance training that result in improvements in muscular strength? The next segments will address this question by providing the details of how the body adapts to resistance training.

MECHANISMS RESPONSIBLE FOR RESISTANCE TRAINING-INDUCED INCREASES IN STRENGTH

Chapters 7 and 8 described the roles that motor unit recruitment, stimulus frequency, and synchronous firing of motor units play in the development of muscle tension, as well as the fact that type II motor units develop more tension than type I motor units. These factors are very much involved in the improvement

of strength with training. That is, resistance training increases muscular strength by changes in both the nervous system and an increase in muscle mass. In the next two segments, we will discuss the roles that both the nervous system and muscular growth play in the development of strength resulting from a resistance training program. Figure 13.16 provides a schematic to follow that will facilitate our discussion of both neural and muscular factors related to gains in strength (33, 82). In training studies of short duration (8 to 20 weeks), neural adaptations related to learning, coordination, and the ability to recruit the primary muscles (i.e., prime movers) play a major role in the gain in strength. In contrast, during long-term training programs, an increase in muscle size plays the major role in strength development. Let's discuss these resistance training-induced changes in the nervous system and muscle in more detail.

Resistance Training-Induced Changes in the Nervous System

A significant portion of the strength gains that occur with resistance training, especially early in a program, is due to neural adaptations and not an enlargement of muscle (82). This point is illustrated in Figure 13.16. Also, note that the neural adaptations to strength training are different from those that occur with endurance exercise training. Recall that Figure 13.11 illustrated the point that when one leg was trained on a cycle ergometer, the endurance training effect did not "carry over" to the untrained leg. In contrast, when one arm

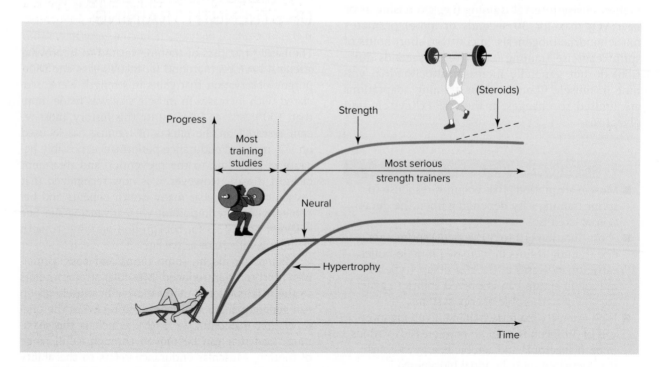

Figure 13.16 Relative roles of neural and muscular adaptations to resistance training.

is exposed to resistance training, a portion of the training effect is "transferred" to the other arm. In this case, the gain in strength in the trained arm was due to both muscle hypertrophy and an increased ability to activate motor units, whereas the strength gain in the untrained arm was due solely to neural adaptation (82). Similar results have been reported in a study using a one-leg resistance-training model. In this study, one leg was exposed to resistance training and the gains of muscular strength and endurance of the trained leg were also partially realized in the untrained leg (49). These neural adaptations that occur in response to resistance training result in an improved ability to recruit motor units, alter motor neuron firing rates, enhance motor unit synchronization during a particular movement pattern, and result in the removal of neural inhibition (33, 82). Collectively, these changes result in an increase in muscle force production.

Resistance Training-Induced Increases in Skeletal Muscle Size

Recall from Chap. 8 that the amount of force produced by a muscle is directly linked to the amount of actin and myosin within the muscle fibers. The explanation for this observation is that the more myosin cross-bridges that are attached to actin and engaged in the power stroke, the more force produced. This simple principle explains why larger muscles containing more actin and myosin generate more force than smaller muscles. In response to resistance training, skeletal muscles can increase their size by increasing the size of existing fibers (hypertrophy) or increasing their number of total fibers (hyperplasia) in the muscle. Let's discuss these two types of muscle growth separately.

Hyperplasia As mentioned previously, hyperplasia refers to an increase in the total number of muscle fibers within a specific muscle (e.g., biceps brachii). The question of whether resistance training-induced increases in muscle size are achieved by hyperplasia has been raised by animal studies indicating that resistance training can promote an increased number of fibers in the trained muscles (67, 93). However, whether resistance training promotes the generation of new muscle fibers in humans remains controversial, as studies that both support (64) and deny this concept exist in the literature (61). Nonetheless, even if hyperplasia does occur in humans, current evidence indicates that most (90% to 95%) of the increase in muscle size following resistance training occurs due to an increase in muscle fiber size (hypertrophy) and not hyperplasia (22, 33).

Hypertrophy As discussed previously, an increase in muscle fiber cross-sectional area (fiber hypertrophy) is regarded as the primary means to increase muscle size during long-term strength training (33). In general, the resistance training-induced increase in muscle fiber size is a gradual process that occurs during months to years of training. However, there is evidence that with high-intensity resistance training, changes in muscle size are detectable by three weeks (~10 sessions) of training (88). Further, although resistance training increases the size of both type I and II fibers, weight training elicits a greater degree of hypertrophy in type II fibers (55, 97). This is physiologically significant because type II fibers generate a greater specific force (i.e., force per cross-sectional area) than type I fibers. The mechanisms to explain why type II fibers are more prone to hypertrophy than type I fibers remains unclear, and additional research is needed to resolve this issue.

This resistance training-induced increase in fiber cross-sectional area results from an increase in myofibrillar proteins (i.e., actin and myosin). This increase in actin/myosin filaments in the fiber occurs due to the addition of sarcomeres in parallel to the existing sarcomeres, resulting in muscle fiber hypertrophy (33). The addition of additional contractile proteins increases the number of myosin cross-bridges in the fiber and therefore increases the fiber's ability to generate force.

Resistance Training-Induced Changes in Muscle Fiber Type

Similar to endurance training, prolonged periods of resistance training have also been shown to promote a fast-to-slow shift in muscle fiber types within the trained muscles (91, 92). However, strength training-induced shifts in muscle fiber types appear to be less prominent than endurance training-induced transformations because all of the change in fiber type is a movement from type IIx to type IIa, with no increase in the percentage of type I fibers. For example, it has been reported that 20 weeks of resistance training can decrease the percentage of type IIx fibers by 5% to 11%, with a corresponding rise in type IIa fibers in the trained muscles (92). At present, there are no long-term (i.e., several years) resistance-training studies, so it is unknown if this type IIx to IIa fiber transformation will continue over a prolonged period.

Can Resistance Training Improve Muscle Oxidative Capacity and Increase Capillary Number?

As discussed earlier in this chapter, endurance exercise training increases the oxidative capacity (i.e., mitochondrial number increases) and the antioxidant capacity in the exercised muscle fibers. Endurance training also promotes the formation of new capillaries and therefore increases muscle capillarization. Does resistance training also promote these changes in the trained muscle? The answer to this question remains unclear because longitudinal investigations of the effect of resistance training on muscle oxidative capacity have been inconsistent with studies reporting that resistance training decreases mitochondrial content in muscle (62); other studies indicate no change in muscle oxidative capacity (98), and still other investigations conclude that resistance training can promote small increases in muscle oxidative capacity (94). Similarly, investigations about the effect of resistance training on muscle capillarization have failed to provide consistent results, with some studies reporting no formation of new capillaries with training and other reports indicating that strength training can promote small increases in capillary number. What is the explanation for these divergent results? Numerous factors could explain these divergent findings, including the frequency of training, the duration of training, and the number of repetitions performed during training. In fact, studies that incorporated long-duration resistance training programs and high frequencies of training (three days/week) and high volume (i.e., high number of repetitions) of exercise reported small improvements in muscle oxidative capacity and capillarization. Therefore, it appears that whether resistance training improves muscle oxidative properties is dependent upon the duration of the training period and the volume of exercise performed.

Resistance Training Improves Muscle Antioxidant Enzyme Activity

Although limited evidence exists, it appears that resistance exercise training can improve muscle antioxidant capacity. Indeed, a recent study investigated the effects of 12 weeks of strength training on the activities of key antioxidant enzymes in the trained muscles. The results revealed that resistance training increased the activities of two important muscle antioxidant enzymes by almost 100% (73). Therefore, similar to endurance exercise, resistance exercise training improves the muscle's antioxidant capacity, which should provide cellular protection against the oxidative damage associated with exercise-induced production of free radicals.

IN SUMMARY

- Increases in strength due to short-term (8 to 20 weeks) resistance training are largely the result of changes in the nervous system, whereas gains in strength during long-term training programs are due to an increase in the size of the muscle.
- Whether or not hyperplasia occurs in response to resistance training remains controversial. Nonetheless, current evidence suggests that most (90% to 95%) of the increase in muscle size following resistance training occurs due to an increase in muscle hypertrophy and not hyperplasia.

- Prolonged periods of resistance training can promote a fast-to-slow shift in muscle fiber types. Most of this training-induced fiber shift is the conversion of type IIx to type IIa fibers, with no increase in the number of type I fibers.
- Whether resistance training improves muscle oxidative properties remains controversial. However, it is possible that long-term and high-volume resistance training programs can improve muscle oxidative capacity and increase capillary number around the trained fibers.
- Resistance training improves the antioxidant capacity of the trained muscle fibers.

TIME COURSE AND SIGNALING EVENTS LEADING TO RESISTANCE TRAINING-INDUCED MUSCLE GROWTH

An increase in muscle fiber size (hypertrophy) occurs when the rate of protein synthesis exceeds the rate of protein breakdown. Resistance exercise induces muscle hypertrophy by triggering a cascade of chemical signaling events that increases protein synthesis in the exercised muscle fibers. In this section, we will discuss the time course of exercise-induced protein synthesis and highlight the differences in muscle protein synthesis between trained and untrained subjects. We will also discuss how mechanical loading (i.e., resistance exercise training) regulates the signaling events that increase muscle protein synthesis. Finally, we will also examine the role that satellite cells play in resistance training-induced muscle hypertrophy. Let's begin with a discussion of the time course of exercise-induced increases in muscle protein synthesis in both trained and untrained individuals.

Time Course of Muscle Protein Synthesis

A single bout of resistance exercise promotes an increase in both muscle protein synthesis and protein breakdown following exercise. However, muscle growth results because the exercise-induced increase in muscle protein synthesis exceeds the rate of protein breakdown. Nonetheless, resistance training-induced muscle growth occurs at a relatively slow rate because protein synthesis must exceed protein breakdown for several weeks to achieve significant muscle growth.

Muscle protein synthesis increases rapidly following a resistance training session. Indeed, a single bout of resistance exercise increases muscle protein synthesis

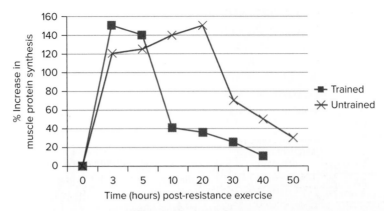

Figure 13.17 Time course of muscle protein synthesis following a single bout of resistance exercise training.

Data are compiled from Damas, F., Phillips, S., Vechin, F., and Ugrinowitch, C., "A Review of Resistance Training Changes in Skeletal Muscle Protein Synthesis and Their Contribution to Hypertrophy," *Sports Medicine* 45: 801-807, 2015; MacDougall, J. D., Gibala, M. J., Tarnopolsky, M. A., MacDonald, J. R., Interisano, S. A., and Yarasheski, K. E., "The Time Course for Elevated Muscle Protein Synthesis Following Heavy Resistance Exercise," *Canadian Journal of Applied Physiology* 20: 480–486, 1995; Tang, J. E., Perco, J. G., Moore, D. R., Wilkinson, S. B., and Phillips, S. M., "Resistance Training Alters the Response of Fed State Mixed Muscle Protein Synthesis in Young Men," *American Journal of Physiology: Regulatory, Integrative and Comparative Physiology* 294: R172–178, 2008.

by 50% to 150% within 1 to 4 hours following exercise in both trained and untrained individuals (Figure 13.17) (24, 60, 95). This exercise-induced increase in protein synthesis remains elevated for 30 to 48 hours depending upon the training status of the individual (24, 60, 95). Specifically, post-exercise protein synthesis remains elevated for a longer period in untrained individuals (Figure 13.17) (24). This means that, following a single bout of resistance exercise, the total amount of muscle protein synthesis is greater in untrained subjects compared to trained individuals. This observation explains why the rate of exercise-induced muscle hypertrophy typically occurs more rapidly in untrained subjects compared to trained ones (24).

Signaling Events Leading to Resistance Training-Induced Muscle Growth

While resistance exercise increases the mRNA levels of muscle contractile proteins, the exercise-induced increase in muscle protein synthesis is largely due to an increase in the amount of protein synthesized per molecule of mRNA rather than an increase in total mRNA (39). In other words, resistance exercise primarily elevates muscle protein synthesis by increasing the efficiency of translation.

What are the molecular signals that stimulate muscle protein synthesis following a bout of resistance exercise? Key steps in the intracellular signaling pathway that increase muscle protein synthesis are illustrated in Figure 13.18. Notice that the initial (i.e., primary) signal for resistance exercise-induced protein synthesis is the contraction-induced activation of a mechanoreceptor on the sarcolemma; this triggers a series of downstream signaling events leading to increased protein synthesis and muscle growth (i.e., hypertrophy). Let's discuss this process in more detail.

As mentioned earlier in this chapter, a protein kinase called the mechanistic target of rapamycin (mTOR) is the major regulator of protein synthesis and muscle size (39, 47). Indeed, activation of mTOR promotes protein synthesis by increasing translation, which results in increased protein synthesis (39). Understanding of how mTOR is regulated by exercise remains a hot topic of research. Historically, it was believed that resistance exercise training-induced increases in insulin-like growth factor 1 (IGF-1) was required to promote muscle hypertrophy. However, this is not the case as new evidence reveals that other signaling molecules are likely responsible for the exercise-induced activation of mTOR. Specifically, two signaling molecules that directly activate mTOR include a lipid molecule called phosphatidic acid (PA) and a second molecule known as Rheb which is short for Ras homolog enriched in brain. Let's now discuss how resistance exercise activates mTOR to increase muscle protein synthesis.

The cellular site for regulation of mTOR activation is an organelle known as the late endosome/lysosomal complex; for simplicity, we will refer to this complex as the lysosome. Notice in Figure 13.18 that mTOR, PA, and Rheb are all connected to the lysosome. At rest, mTOR remains inactive because only low levels of PA exist in the muscle fiber. Further, in inactive muscle, Rheb activation of mTOR is inhibited by a molecule called tuberous sclerosis complex 2 (TSC2). Therefore, in order to activate mTOR, one of the following events needs to occur: (1) muscle levels of PA must increase, and/or (2) TSC2 blockade of Rheb must be eliminated. Interestingly, resistance exercise results in an increase in muscle levels of PA and the removal of TSC2 inhibition of Rheb. A summary of how this is accomplished follows.

Muscle contractions during resistance exercise activate a mechanoreceptor on the sarcolemma that

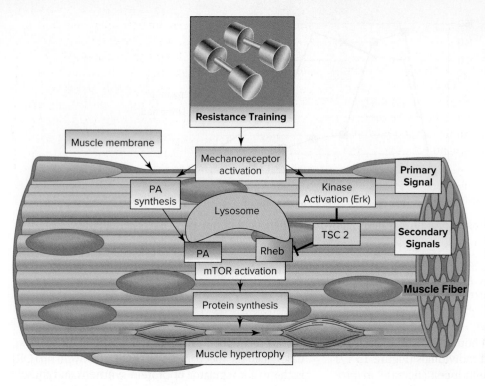

Figure 13.18 Illustration of the intracellular signaling network mediating exercise-induced skeletal muscle responses to resistance training. Notice that both primary and secondary signals are involved in muscle adaptation to resistance exercise training. See text for more details.

stimulates the enzymes responsible for the synthesis of PA. This exercise-induced rise in muscle levels of PA results in PA molecules binding to mTOR leading to mTOR activation. Moreover, contraction-induced activation of mechanoreceptors also activates an enzyme called extracellular signal-regulated kinase (Erk) that phosphorylates and inhibits TSC2. It follows that exercise-induced activation of Erk blocks TSC2's ability to inhibit Rheb and therefore Rheb remains free to activate mTOR.

In summary, mTOR is the primary activator of muscle protein synthesis. Resistance exercise triggers muscle signaling events that activate mTOR leading to increased protein synthesis. This process begins with contraction-induced activation of a mechanoreceptor on the fiber membrane that can activate mTOR in two ways. First, exercise-mediated mechanoreceptor signaling promotes the synthesis of PA, which is an mTOR activator. Second, contraction-mediated mechanoreceptor signaling activates another mTOR activator, Rheb. This occurs because muscle contractions activate the enzyme, Erk, which phosphorylates the Rheb inhibitor, TSC2; this phosphorylation removes TSC2's inhibition of Rheb, which enables Rheb to activate mTOR. Together, these exercise-mediated signaling actions activate mTOR and promote muscle protein synthesis.

Figure 13.19 illustrates the time-dependent changes in resistance exercise-induced signaling in skeletal muscles. Note that within seconds after beginning exercise, muscle levels of activated Rheb and phosphatidic acid begin to rise. Further, within minutes after the initiation of exercise, mTOR activation begins and within 1 to 4 hours, muscle protein

synthesis increases. However, because protein synthesis must exceed protein breakdown for several days to several weeks to achieve significant muscle growth, exercise-induced gain in both muscle hypertrophy and strength is a relatively slow process.

Finally, it is important to note that an exercise-induced increase in muscle protein synthesis requires that all essential amino acids be present in the muscle. Therefore, adequate ingestion of high-quality protein prior to or following a workout is essential to optimize muscle growth during resistance training. For more details on the amount and timing of protein ingestion on protein synthesis in athletes, see Phillips (2012) in the Suggested Readings.

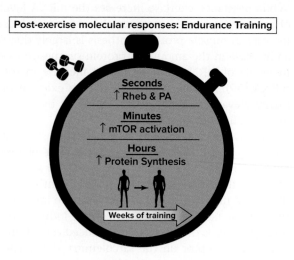

Figure 13.19 Illustration of the time course of molecular responses to resistance exercise training. See text for more details.

Role of Satellite Cells in Resistance Training-Induced Hypertrophy

Research reveals that the initial hypertrophy of skeletal muscle fibers during the first few weeks of a resistance training program can occur without the addition of new myonuclei. However, as muscle fibers continue to increase in size in response to resistance training, these growing fibers begin to add new nuclei (myonuclei) within the fiber. Indeed, it appears that the addition of new nuclei to the muscle is required to increase muscle size after the initial growth that occurs early in the training process. This process is illustrated in Figure 13.20. Recall from Chap. 8 that the source of these additional myonuclei is the satellite cell, which is a type of adult stem cell located between the sarcolemma and the outer layer of connective tissue (i.e., basal lamina) around the fiber (8). In healthy young subjects, resistance training activates satellite cells to divide and fuse with the adjacent muscle fiber to increase the number of nuclei in the fiber (1, 3). This increase in the number of myonuclei in growing fibers results in a constant ratio between the number of myonuclei and the size of the fiber. Importantly, the addition of these myonuclei to a growing fiber appears to be a requirement to support the increased size and continued growth of muscle fibers in response to strength training. In fact, evidence indicates that the removal of satellite cells from skeletal muscle limits the fibers' ability to grow in response to overload (1, 2, 74).

Why are additional myonuclei required to achieve the maximal level of muscle hypertrophy in response to resistance training? A possible explanation is that the addition of myonuclei to growing muscle fibers is a requirement to maintain the high level of translational capacity required to synthesize muscle proteins at a high rate following a strength training session (1). That is, a single myonucleus can only manage to produce mRNAs for a specific volume of muscle; therefore, as the muscle fiber increases in size, the addition of new myonuclei is required to manage the new growth (i.e., increased volume).

As discussed in A Closer Look 13.3, skeletal muscle fibers do not hypertrophy to the same level in older individuals compared to young adults even if they perform the same resistance training program (3,46). This age-related difference in the ability of older individuals to respond to resistance training is likely linked to an age-related suppression of satellite cell number and function (3). For example, the number of satellite cells is lower in muscle of old individuals compared to young adults (3). Further, research reveals that exercise-induced satellite cell activation is impaired by aging (3). The mechanism to explain why satellite cell activation is reduced in older people remains a topic of debate. Nonetheless, current evidence suggests that the age-related impairment in satellite cell function is likely due to a reduction in growth factors (i.e., IGF-1) available to activate satellite cells along with increased systemic inflammation that has a negative impact on satellite cell function.

To conclude, satellite cells are the source of additional nuclei in muscle fibers, and the addition of myonuclei to growing fibers appears to be essential for optimal fiber hypertrophy in response to resistance training (2). Further, although resistance training results in hypertrophy of muscle fibers in older individuals, muscle fibers do not hypertrophy to the same extent in old individuals compared to young. This reduced ability to achieve resistance training-induced hypertrophy in muscles in older individuals appears to be due to an age-related suppression of satellite cell number and function. For more details on satellite cell function in muscles, see Always et al. (2014) and Snijders et al. (2015) in the Suggested Reading list.

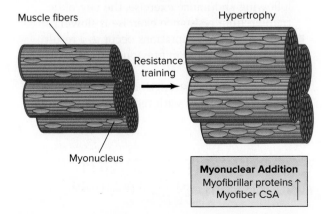

Figure 13.20 Resistance training-induced fiber hypertrophy results in a parallel increase in myonuclei, myofibrillar proteins, and fiber cross-sectional area (CSA).

IN SUMMARY

- Resistance training increases the synthesis of contractile proteins in muscle; this results in an increase in the cross-sectional area of the fiber.
- Resistance training-induced increases in protein synthesis occur via an increase in translation, which is controlled by the mTOR signaling pathway.
- Resistance exercise increases muscle levels of phosphatidic acid and Rheb. Both of these molecules are capable of activating mTOR signaling, which subsequently increases muscle protein synthesis.
- Resistance training results in parallel increases in muscle fiber cross-sectional area and increased numbers of myonuclei.
- Satellite cells are the source of additional myonuclei in muscle fibers, and the addition of myonuclei to muscle fibers is a requirement to achieve maximal fiber hypertrophy in response to resistance training.

DETRAINING FOLLOWING STRENGTH TRAINING

Similar to detraining following endurance training, the "use it or lose it" adage also applies to a resistance training program. Indeed, it is well established that stoppage of resistance training results in a loss of muscular strength and in muscle atrophy. However, compared to endurance training, the rate of detraining (i.e., loss of strength) after a resistance training program is slower. This point is illustrated in Figure 13.21. Specifically, Figure 13.21(*a*) illustrates the impact of 30 weeks of detraining on muscle strength and muscle fiber size and also shows the impact of six weeks of retraining after the prolonged period of detraining (91). In this study, subjects engaged in a 20-week program of resistance training. This rigorous training program resulted in a 60% increase in maximal dynamic strength (leg extension) and hypertrophy in all three major fiber types in the extensor muscles of the legs. Following 30 weeks of detraining, the subjects experienced a 31% decrease in maximal dynamic muscle strength. However, this detraining-induced loss of dynamic strength was associated with a relatively small degree of muscle atrophy. For example, type I fibers atrophied approximately −2%, type IIa fibers atrophied 210%, and type IIx fibers atrophied −13% (Fig. 13.21(*b*)). This finding suggests that much of the loss of strength associated with detraining is associated with changes in the nervous system. Collectively, these data indicate that resistance training-induced muscular adaptations (i.e., dynamic strength and muscle hypertrophy) can be retained for relatively long periods during detraining.

Also, notice that six weeks of retraining resulted in a rapid regaining of dynamic muscular strength and a complete restoration of muscle fiber size back to the peak training levels (Fig. 13.21) (91). These results reveal that rapid muscular adaptations occur as a result of the reinstatement of strength training in previously trained individuals. This speedy improvement in muscle strength during retraining explains how power athletes can often return to "competitive form" quickly after long periods of detraining.

Finally, studies also reveal that after dynamic muscular strength has been increased by resistance training, a reduced-frequency maintenance program of weight lifting can sustain strength for an extended period. For instance, it has been shown that following a 12-week period of rigorous strength training (three days/week), as few as one training day per week can maintain maximal dynamic strength for up to 12 weeks (35). Further, another study reported that maximal dynamic strength of lower back muscles can be maintained for 12 weeks by only one training day every 2 weeks (100). Collectively, these studies indicate that strength can be maintained for up to 12 weeks with reduced resistance training frequency.

(a)

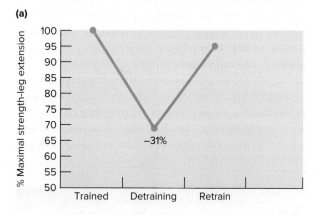

(b)

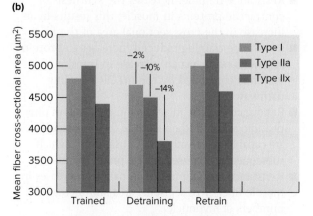

Figure 13.21 (*a*) Changes in dynamic muscle strength following 30 weeks of detraining and at the completion of six weeks of resistance exercise retraining. (*b*) Changes in muscle fiber cross-sectional area following 30 weeks of detraining followed by six weeks of resistance exercise retraining.

IN SUMMARY

- The stoppage of resistance training results in a loss of muscular strength and muscle atrophy. However, compared to the rate of detraining following endurance exercise, the rate of detraining from resistance exercise is slower.
- Rapid muscular adaptations occur as a result of strength training in previously trained individuals.
- Maximal dynamic strength can be maintained for up to 12 weeks with reduced training frequency.

CONCURRENT STRENGTH AND ENDURANCE TRAINING

At this point in the chapter, it may have occurred to you that concurrent resistance and endurance training might interfere with the adaptations associated with resistance training alone. For example, resistance training results in an increase in muscle fiber size, whereas endurance training does not increase fiber size. Does one type of training really interfere with the effects of the other? Although this topic remains controversial, a growing number of studies have demonstrated that performing concurrent resistance and endurance exercise training results in impaired strength gains when compared to resistance training alone. Let's take a closer look at this issue.

In 1980, Hickson reported that a ten-week combined strength and endurance training program resulted in similar gains in $\dot{V}O_2$ max compared to an endurance-only group, but concurrent training (strength + endurance) results in an interference with the gains in strength (40). The strength-only group increased strength throughout the entire ten weeks, but the combined strength and endurance group showed a leveling off and a decrease in strength at the end of the training program.

Since this early study of Hickson and colleagues, numerous other investigations have supported or disagreed with the notion that strength development is impaired during concurrent training. Many of the differences in these studies appear to arise from variations in training programs. For example, Sale et al. suggest that the effectiveness of concurrent training may depend on a variety of factors, such as the intensity, volume, and frequency of training, and how the training modes are integrated (83). Indeed, clearly, the frequency and intensity of training has an impact on the potential for one type of training to interfere with the other (65). That is, studies that combine frequent training sessions and high-intensity endurance exercise often report that concurrent training impairs strength gains (26, 56). In fact, a recent review of the literature reveals that whether or not concurrent resistance/endurance training impairs strength gains is directly dependent upon both the duration of endurance exercise training (minutes/training session) and the frequency of training (days/week) (106). Specifically, concurrent training studies where subjects performed endurance training on >2 days per week and >30 minutes/day consistently concluded that concurrent training impairs strength gains and muscular hypertrophy compared to subjects performing resistance training alone (106). Potential mechanisms to explain why concurrent training impairs strength gains are addressed in the next section.

Mechanisms Responsible for the Impairment of Strength Development during Concurrent Strength and Endurance Training

Over the years, several mechanisms have been proposed to explain why concurrent endurance and strength training impedes strength development compared to strength training alone. These include neural components, glycogen depletion, fiber-type transition, overtraining, and impaired protein synthesis. A brief discussion of each of these possibilities follows.

Neural Factors It has been proposed that concurrent strength and endurance training impairs strength development because of neural factors. Specifically, some investigators have suggested that concurrent training impairs motor unit recruitment and therefore decreases muscle force production (26). However, limited evidence exists to support this possibility (38). Therefore, it is currently unclear if changes in motor unit recruitment contribute to the impairment of strength gains when concurrent resistance and endurance training is performed.

Low Muscle Glycogen Content Successive bouts of either strength or endurance training can produce chronically low levels of muscle glycogen (70). That is, repeated endurance training and/or repeated bouts of resistance exercise can result in low resting levels of muscle glycogen. Therefore, beginning a training session with low muscle glycogen can reduce the ability to perform subsequent resistance training sessions and impair the magnitude of the strength-training adaptations.

Overtraining Overtraining is often defined as an imbalance between training and recovery. In theory, overtraining could contribute to the inability to attain optimal strength gains when concurrent strength and endurance exercise training is performed. Nonetheless, no experimental studies provide direct evidence that overtraining is a major factor that contributes to the inhibition of strength gains when both resistance and endurance exercise are performed.

Depressed Protein Synthesis Concurrent resistance and endurance exercise bouts could result in impaired protein synthesis following resistance exercise training (7, 39, 70). The science behind this concept is as follows. Recall that resistance exercise training increases muscle contractile protein synthesis by activation of the mTOR signaling pathway (Fig. 13.22). In contrast, endurance exercise training increases AMPK activation and promotes mitochondrial biogenesis. Further, active AMPK can activate a signaling molecule called tuberous sclerosis complex 2 (TSC2). Active TSC 2 inhibits mTOR activity and therefore impairs protein synthesis (39). Hence, the AMPK/TSC 2 pathway provides a biochemical link to explain why concurrent endurance/resistance training may impair strength gains. Although the activation of TSC 2 in skeletal muscle during endurance training is a plausible explanation for why endurance training impedes strength gains, additional research is needed to determine if this biochemical signaling path is the sole explanation for why this occurs.

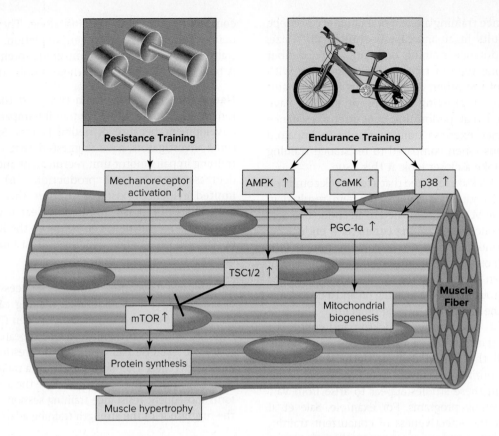

Figure 13.22 Intracellular signaling networks mediating exercise-induced skeletal muscle responses to resistance and endurance exercise training programs. Resistance exercise training activates the mTOR pathway that promotes protein synthesis by increasing translation. Endurance exercise training activates several secondary signals to promote an increase in PGC-1α and increased mitochondrial biogenesis. Note that activation of AMPK by endurance training can inhibit mTOR signaling via the tuberous sclerosis complex 2 (TSC 2) and suppress resistance training-induced protein synthesis. The interaction between these two intracellular signaling networks can potentially explain why concurrent resistance and endurance training programs can reduce strength gains observed with resistance training alone.

IN SUMMARY

- Individuals who engage in concurrent resistance training and high-intensity endurance exercise training often report that concurrent training impairs strength gains.
- Several mechanisms can potentially explain why concurrent training may impair strength gains. These include neural factors, low muscle glycogen content, overtraining, and depressed protein synthesis.
- Concurrent resistance and endurance exercise bouts can theoretically impair protein synthesis following resistance exercise training. The science behind this prediction is illustrated in Figure 13.22.

STUDY ACTIVITIES

1. Explain the basic principles of training: overload, specificity, and reversibility.
2. Discuss the role that genetics plays in determining $\dot{V}O_2$ max.
3. Indicate the typical change in $\dot{V}O_2$ max with endurance-training programs and the effect of the initial (pretraining) value on the magnitude of the increase.
4. State typical $\dot{V}O_2$ max values for various sedentary, active, and athletic populations.
5. Understand the contribution of heart rate, stroke volume, and the a-$\bar{v}O_2$ difference in determining $\dot{V}O_2$ max.
6. Discuss how training increases $\dot{V}O_2$ max.
7. Define preload, afterload, and contractility, and discuss the role of each in the increase in the maximal stroke volume that occurs with endurance training.
8. Describe the changes in muscle structure that are responsible for the increase in the maximal a-$\bar{v}O_2$ difference with endurance training.
9. List and discuss the primary changes that occur in skeletal muscle as a result of endurance training.
10. Explain how endurance training improves acid-base balance during exercise.

11. Outline the "big picture" changes that occur in skeletal muscle as a result of exercise training and discuss the specificity of exercise-training responses.
12. List the four primary signal transduction pathways in skeletal muscle.
13. List and define the function of six important secondary messengers in skeletal muscle.
14. Outline the signaling events that lead to endurance training-induced muscle adaptation.
15. Discuss how changes in "central command" and "peripheral feedback" following an endurance training program can lower the heart rate, ventilation, and catecholamine responses to a submaximal exercise bout.
16. Describe the underlying causes of the decrease in $\dot{V}O_2$ max that occurs with cessation of endurance training.
17. Contrast the role of neural adaptations with hypertrophy in the increase in strength that occurs with resistance training.
18. Identify the primary changes that occur in skeletal muscle fibers in response to resistance training.
19. Outline the signaling events that lead to resistance training-induced increases in muscle growth.
20. Discuss how detraining following strength training affects muscle fiber size and strength.
21. How does retraining influence muscle fiber size and strength?
22. Explain why concurrent strength and endurance training can impair strength gains.

SUGGESTED READINGS

Alway, S.E., M. J. Myers, and J. S. Mohamed. Regulation of satellite cell function in sarcopenia. *Frontiers in Aging Neuroscience* 6: 1-15, 2014.

Bouchard, C. Genomic predictors of trainability. *Experimental Physiology* 97: 347-352, 2012.

Camera, D., W. Smiles, and J. Hawley. 2016. Exercise-induced skeletal muscle signaling pathways and human performance. Free Radic Biol Med. http://hx.doi.org/10.1016/j.freeradbiomed.2016.02.007.

Fiuza-Luces, C., N. Garatachea, N. Burger, and A. Lucia. Exercise is the real polypill. *Physiology.* 28: 330-358, 2013.

Folland, J. P., and A. G. Williams. The adaptations to strength training: methodological and neurological contributions to increased strength. *Sports Medicine* 37: 145-68, 2007.

Hawley, J. A. Molecular responses to strength and endurance training: are they incompatible? *Applied Physiology, Nutrition, and Metabolism* 34:355-61, 2009.

Lundby, C., and R. Jacobs. Adaptations of skeletal muscle mitochondria to exercise training. *Experimental Physiology* 101: 17-22, 2016

Mann, T., and R. Lamberts. High responders and low responders: Factors associated with individual variation in response to standardized training. 44: 1113-1124, 2014.

Olasunkanmi, A., A. Abdullahi, and P. Tavajohi-Fini. mTORC1 and the regulation of skeletal muscle anabolism and mass. *Applied Physiology, Nutrition, and Metabolism* 37:395-406, 2012.

Phillips, S.M. Dietary protein requirements and adaptive advantages in athletes. *British Journal of Nutrition* 108: S158-S167, 2012.

Powers, S. K., E. E. Talbert, and P. J. Adhihetty. Reactive oxygen and nitrogen species as intracellular signals in skeletal muscle. *Journal of Physiology* 589: 2129-2138, 2011.

Snijders, T., J. P. Nederveen, B. R. McKay, S. Joanisse, L. B. Verdijk, L. van Loon, and G. Parise. Satellite cells in human skeletal muscle plasticity. *Frontiers in Physiology* 6: 1-21, 2015.

Tucker, R., and M. Collins. What makes champions? A review of the relative contribution of genes and training to sporting success. *British Journal of Sports Medicine*, 2012. doi:10.1136/bjsports-2011-090548.

Wackerhage, H. 2014. *Molecular Exercise Physiology.* New York, NY: Routledge.

REFERENCES

1. **Adams GR.** Satellite cell proliferation and skeletal muscle hypertrophy. *Applied Physiology, Nutrition, and Metabolism* 31: 782-790, 2006.
2. **Adams GR, Caiozzo VJ, Haddad F, and Baldwin KM.** Cellular and molecular responses to increased skeletal muscle loading after irradiation. *American Journal of Physiology - Cell Physiology* 283: C1182-1195, 2002.
3. **Alway SE, Myers, MJ, and Mohamed JS.** Regulation of satellite cell function in sarcopenia. *Fronters in Aging Neuroscience* 6: 1-15, 2014.
4. **Asmussen E, Johansen SH, Jorgensen M, and Nielsen M.** On the nervous factors controlling respiration and circulation during exercise. Experiments with curarization. *Acta Physiologica Scandinavia* 63: 343-350, 1965.
5. **Åstrand P, Rodahl K., H. Dahl, and S. Stromme.** *Textbook of Work Physiology.* Champaign, IL Human Kinetics, 2003.
6. **Atha J.** Strengthening muscle. In: *Exercise and Sport Science Reviews*, edited by Miller D. Philadelphia, PA: The Franklin Institute Press, 1981, pp. 1-73.
7. **Baar K.** Using molecular biology to maximize concurrent training. *Sports Medicine* 44:S117-S125, 2014.
8. **Biressi S and Rando TA.** Heterogeneity in the muscle satellite cell population. *Seminars in Cell and Developmental Biology* 21: 845-854, 2010.
9. **Blomqvist CG and Saltin B.** Cardiovascular adaptations to physical training. *Annual Review of Physiology* 45: 169-189, 1983.
10. **Booth F.** Effects of endurance exercise on cytochrome C turnover in skeletal muscle. *Annals of the New York Academy of Sciences* 301: 431-439, 1977.
11. **Bouchard C, An P, Rice T, Skinner JS, Wilmore JH, Gagnon J, et al.** Familial aggregation of $\dot{V}O(2max)$ response to exercise training: results from the HERITAGE Family Study. *Journal of Applied Physiology* 87: 1003-1008, 1999.
12. **Bouchard C.** Genomic predictors of trainability. *Experimental Physiology* 97:347-352, 2012.
13. **Bouchard C, Daw EW, Rice T, Perusse L, Gagnon J, Province MA, et al.** Familial resemblance for $\dot{V}O_2$ max in the sedentary state: the HERITAGE family study. *Medicine & Science in Sports & Exercise* 30: 252-258, 1998.
14. **Bouchard C, Sarzynski MA, Rice TK, Kraus WE, Church TS, Sung YJ, et al.** Genomic predictors of

maximal oxygen uptake response to standardized exercise training programs. *Journal of Applied Physiology* 110: 1160-1170, 2011.

15. **Camera D, Smiles W, and Hawley JA.** Exercise-induced skeletal muscle signaling pathways and human athletic performance. http://hx.doi.org/10.1016/j.freeradbiomed.2016.02.007. 2016.

16. **Coffey VG and Hawley JA.** The molecular bases of training adaptation. *Sports Medicine* 37: 737-763, 2007.

17. **Coffey VG, Pilegaard H, Garnham AP, O'Brien BJ, and Hawley JA.** Consecutive bouts of diverse contractile activity alter acute responses in human skeletal muscle. *Journal of Applied Physiology* 106: 1187-1197, 2009.

18. **Coyle EF, Hemmert MK, and Coggan AR.** Effects of detraining on cardiovascular responses to exercise: role of blood volume. *Journal of Applied Physiology* 60: 95-99, 1986.

19. **Coyle EF, Hopper MK, and Coggan AR.** Maximal oxygen uptake relative to plasma volume expansion. *International Journal of Sports Medicine* 11: 116-119, 1990.

20. **Coyle EF, Martin WH, III, Bloomfield SA, Lowry OH, and Holloszy JO.** Effects of detraining on responses to submaximal exercise. *Journal of Applied Physiology* 59: 853-859, 1985.

21. **Coyle EF, Martin WH, III, Sinacore DR, Joyner MJ, Hagberg JM, and Holloszy JO.** Time course of loss of adaptations after stopping prolonged intense endurance training. *Journal of Applied Physiology* 57: 1857-1864, 1984.

22. **Craig B.** Hyperplasia: Scientific fact or fiction? *Strength & Conditioning Journal* 23: 42-44, 2001.

23. **Cronan TL III and Howley ET.** The effect of training on epinephrine and norepinephrine excretion. *Medicine and Science in Sports* 6: 122-125, 1974.

24. **Damas F, Phillips S, Vechin F, and Ugrinowitch C.** A review of resistance training changes in skeletal muscle protein synthesis and their contribution to hypertrophy. *Sports Medcine* 45: 801-807, 2015.

25. **Dudley GA, Abraham WM, and Terjung RL.** Influence of exercise intensity and duration on biochemical adaptations in skeletal muscle. *Journal of Applied Physiology* 53: 844-850, 1982.

26. **Dudley GA and Djamil R.** Incompatibility of endurance- and strength-training modes of exercise. *Journal of Applied Physiology* 59: 1446-1451, 1985.

27. **Edge J, Bishop D, and Goodman C.** The effects of training intensity on muscle buffer capacity in females. *European Journal of Applied Physiology* 96: 97-105, 2006.

28. **Ehsani AA, Hagberg JM, and Hickson RC.** Rapid changes in left ventricular dimensions and mass in response to physical conditioning and deconditioning. *American Journal of Cardiology* 42: 52-56, 1978.

29. **Esbjornsson Liljedahl M, Holm I, Sylven C, and Jansson E.** Different responses of skeletal muscle following sprint training in men and women. *European Journal of Applied Physiology and Occupational Physiology* 74:375-383, 1996.

30. **Favier RJ, Constable SH, Chen M, and Holloszy JO.** Endurance exercise training reduces lactate production. *Journal of Applied Physiology* 61: 885-889, 1986.

31. **Fiatarone MA, Marks EC, Ryan ND, Meredith CN, Lipsitz LA, and Evans WJ.** High-intensity strength training in nonagenarians: effects on skeletal muscle. *JAMA* 263: 3029-3034, 1990.

32. **Fiatarone MA, O'Neill EF, Ryan ND, Clements KM, Solares GR, Nelson ME, et al.** Exercise training and nutritional supplementation for physical frailty in very elderly people. *The New England Journal of Medicine* 330: 1769-1775, 1994.

33. **Folland JP and Williams AG.** The adaptations to strength training: morphological and neurological contributions to increased strength. *Sports Medicine* 37: 145-168, 2007.

34. **Gist N, Fedewa M, Dishman R, and Cureton K.** Sprint interval training effects on aerobic capacity: A systematic review and meta-analysis. *Sports Medicine* 44:269-279, 2014.

35. **Graves JE, Pollock ML, Leggett SH, Braith RW, Carpenter DM, and Bishop LE.** Effect of reduced training frequency on muscular strength. *International Journal of Sports Medicine* 9: 316-319, 1988.

36. **Green HJ, Jones S, Ball-Burnett ME, Smith D, Livesey J, and Farrance BW.** Early muscular and metabolic adaptations to prolonged exercise training in humans. *Journal of Applied Physiology* 70: 2032-2038, 1991.

37. **Hagberg JM, Hickson RC, Ehsani AA, and Holloszy JO.** Faster adjustment to and recovery from submaximal exercise in the trained state. *Journal of Applied Physiology* 48: 218-224, 1980.

38. **Hakkinen K, Alen M, Kraemer WJ, Gorostiaga E, Izquierdo M, Rusko H, et al.** Neuromuscular adaptations during concurrent strength and endurance training versus strength training. *European Journal of Applied Physiology* 89: 42-52, 2003.

39. **Hawley JA.** Molecular responses to strength and endurance training: are they incompatible? *Applied Physiology, Nutrition, and Metabolism* 34: 355-361, 2009.

40. **Hickson RC.** Interference of strength development by simultaneously training for strength and endurance. *European Journal of Applied Physiology and Occupational Physiology* 45: 255-263, 1980.

41. **Hickson RC, Dvorak BA, Gorostiaga EM, Kurowski TT, and Foster C.** Potential for strength and endurance training to amplify endurance performance. *Journal of Applied Physiology* 65: 2285-2290, 1988.

42. **Holloszy JO and Coyle EF.** Adaptations of skeletal muscle to endurance exercise and their metabolic consequences. *Journal of Applied Physiology* 56: 831-838, 1984.

43. **Holviala JH, Sallinen JM, Kraemer WJ, Alen MJ, and Hakkinen KK.** Effects of strength training on muscle strength characteristics, functional capabilities, and balance in middle-aged and older women. *Journal of Strength and Conditioning Research* 20: 336-344, 2006.

44. **Hornberger TA, Armstrong DD, Koh TJ, Burkholder TJ, and Esser KA.** Intracellular signaling specificity in response to uniaxial vs. multiaxial stretch: implications for mechanotransduction. *American Journal of Physiology - Cell Physiology* 288: C185-194, 2005.

45. **Horowitz JF.** Fatty acid mobilization from adipose tissue during exercise. *Trends in Endocrinology & Metabolism* 14: 386-392, 2003.

46. **Hunter GR, McCarthy JP, and Bamman MM.** Effects of resistance training on older adults. *Sports Medicine* 34: 329-348, 2004.

47. **Jacobs B, Goodman C, and Hornberger T.** The mechanical activation of mTOR signaling: an emerging role for late endosome/lysosomal targeting. *Journal of Muscle Research and Cell Motility* 35:11-21, 2014.

48. **Juel C.** Training-induced changes in membrane transport proteins of human skeletal muscle. *European Journal of Applied Physiology* 96: 627-635, 2006.

49. **Kannus P, Alosa D, Cook L, Johnson RJ, Renstrom P, Pope M, Beynnon B, et al.** Effect of one-legged exercise on the strength, power and endurance of the contralateral leg: a randomized, controlled study using isometric and concentric isokinetic training. *European Journal of Applied Physiology and Occupational Physiology* 64: 117-126, 1992.

50. **Kemi OJ, Hoydal MA, Macquaide N, Haram PM, Koch LG, Britton SL, et al.** The effect of exercise training on transverse tubules in normal, remodeled, and reverse remodeled hearts. *Journal of Cellular Physiology* 2010.

51. **Kemi OJ and Wisloff U.** Mechanisms of exercise-induced improvements in the contractile apparatus of the mammalian myocardium. *Acta Physiologica (Oxford)* 199: 425-439, 2010.

52. **Kiens B, Essen-Gustavsson B, Christensen NJ, and Saltin B.** Skeletal muscle substrate utilization during submaximal exercise in man: effect of endurance training. *Journal Physiology* 469: 459-478, 1993.

53. **Klissouras V.** Heritability of adaptive variation. *Journal of Applied Physiology* 31: 338-344, 1971.

54. **Koves TR, Noland RC, Bates AL, Henes ST, Muoio DM, and Cortright RN.** Subsarcolemmal and intermyofibrillar mitochondria play distinct roles in regulating skeletal muscle fatty acid metabolism. *American Journal of Physiology - Cell Physiology* 288: C1074-1082, 2005.

55. **Kraemer WJ, Deschenes MR, and Fleck SJ.** Physiological adaptations to resistance exercise: implications for athletic conditioning. *Sports Medicine* 6: 246-256, 1988.

56. **Kraemer WJ, Patton JF, Gordon SE, Harman EA, Deschenes MR, Reynolds K, et al.** Compatibility of high-intensity strength and endurance training on hormonal and skeletal muscle adaptations. *Journal of Applied Physiology* 78: 976-989, 1995.

57. **Krentz JR, Quest B, Farthing JP, Quest DW, and Chilibeck PD.** The effects of ibuprofen on muscle hypertrophy, strength, and soreness during resistance training. *Applied Physiology, Nutrition, and Metabolism* 33: 470-475, 2008.

58. **Lundby C and Jacobs R.** Adaptations of skeletal muscle mitochondria to exercise training. *Experimental Physiology* 101.1: 17-22, 2016.

59. **MacDougall JD.** Morphological changes in human skeletal muscle following strength training and immobilization. In: *Human Muscle Power*, edited by Jones N, McCartney N, and McComas A. Champaign, IL: Human Kinetics, 1986, pp. 269-285.

60. **MacDougall JD, Gibala MJ, Tarnopolsky MA, MacDonald JR, Interisano SA, and Yarasheski KE.** The time course for elevated muscle protein synthesis following heavy resistance exercise. *Canadian Journal of Applied Physiology* 20: 480-486, 1995.

61. **MacDougall JD, Sale DG, Alway SE, and Sutton JR.** Muscle fiber number in biceps brachii in bodybuilders and control subjects. *Journal of Applied Physiology* 57: 1399-1403, 1984.

62. **MacDougall JD, Sale DG, Elder GC, and Sutton JR.** Muscle ultrastructural characteristics of elite powerlifters and bodybuilders. *European Journal of Applied Physiology* 48: 117-126, 1982.

63. **Madsen K, Pedersen PK, Djurhuus MS, and Klitgaard NA.** Effects of detraining on endurance capacity and metabolic changes during prolonged exhaustive exercise. *Journal of Applied Physiology* 75: 1444-1451, 1993.

64. **McCall GE, Byrnes WC, Dickinson A, Pattany PM, and Fleck SJ.** Muscle fiber hypertrophy, hyperplasia, and capillary density in college men after resistance training. *Journal of Applied Physiology* 81: 2004-2012, 1996.

65. **McCarthy JP, Pozniak MA, and Agre JC.** Neuromuscular adaptations to concurrent strength and endurance training. *Medicine & Science in Sports & Exercise* 34: 511-519, 2002.

66. **Midgley AW, McNaughton LR, and Wilkinson M.** Is there an optimal training intensity for enhancing the maximal oxygen uptake of distance runners?: empirical research findings, current opinions, physiological rationale and practical recommendations. *Sports Medicine* 36: 117-132, 2006.

67. **Mikesky AE, Giddings CJ, Matthews W, and Gonyea WJ.** Changes in muscle fiber size and composition in response to heavy-resistance exercise. *Medicine & Science in Sports & Exercise* 23: 1042-1049, 1991.

68. **Mitchell JH.** J.B. Wolffe memorial lecture. Neural control of the circulation during exercise. *Medicine & Science in Sports & Exercise* 22: 141-154, 1990.

69. **Montero D, Diaz-Canestro C, and Lundby C.** Endurance training and VO$_2$ max: Role of maximal cardiac output and oxygen extraction. *Medicine & Science in Sports & Exercise* 47:2024-2033, 2015.

70. **Nader GA.** Concurrent strength and endurance training: from molecules to man. *Medicine & Science in Sports & Exercise* 38: 1965-1970, 2006.

71. **Novak ML, Billich W, Smith SM, Sukhija KB, McLoughlin TJ, Hornberger TA, et al.** COX-2 inhibitor reduces skeletal muscle hypertrophy in mice. *American Journal of Physiology Regulatory Integrative and Comparative Physiology* 296: R1132-1139, 2009.

72. **Olesen J, Kiilerich K, and Pilegaard H.** PGC-1αlpha-mediated adaptations in skeletal muscle. *Pflügers Archiv* 460: 153-162, 2010.

73. **Parise G, Phillips SM, Kaczor JJ, and Tarnopolsky MA.** Antioxidant enzyme activity is up-regulated after unilateral resistance exercise training in older adults. *Free Radical Biology & Medicine* 39: 289-295, 2005.

74. **Petrella, J, Kim J, Cross J, Kosek D, and Bamman M.** Efficacy of myonuclear addition may explain differential myofiber growth among resistance-trained young and older men and women. *American Journal of Physiology* 291:E937-E946, 2006.

75. **Powers SK, KJ Sollanek, MP Wiggs, HA Demirel, and AJ Smuder.** Exercise-induced improvements in myocardial antioxidant capacity: the antioxidant players and cardioprotection. *Free Radical Research* 48:43-51, 2014.

76. **Powers SK, Duarte J, Kavazis AN, and Talbert EE.** Reactive oxygen species are signalling molecules for skeletal muscle adaptation. *Experimental Physiology* 95: 1-9, 2010.

77. **Powers SK, Nelson WB, and Hudson MB.** Exercise-induced oxidative stress in humans: cause and consequences. *Free Radical Biology & Medicine* 51(5): 942-950, 2011.

78. **Powers SK, Talbert EE, and Adhihetty PJ.** Reactive oxygen and nitrogen species as intracellular signals in skeletal muscle. *Journal of Physiology* 589: 2129-2138, 2011.

79. **Rerych SK, Scholz PM, Sabiston DC, Jr., and Jones RH.** Effects of exercise training on left ventricular function in normal subjects: a longitudinal

study by radionuclide angiography. *American Journal of Cardiology* 45: 244-252, 1980.

80. **Richter E and Hargreaves M.** Exercise, GLUT 4, and skeletal muscle glucose uptake. *Physiological Reviews* 93: 993-1017, 2013.

81. **Ross A and Leveritt M.** Long-term metabolic and skeletal muscle adaptations to short-sprint training. *Sports Medicine* 15:1063-1082, 2001.

82. **Sale DG.** Neural adaptation to resistance training. *Medicine & Science in Sports & Exercise* 20: S135-145, 1988.

83. **Sale DG, Jacobs I, MacDougall JD, and Garner S.** Comparison of two regimens of concurrent strength and endurance training. *Medicine & Science in Sports & Exercise* 22: 348-356, 1990.

84. **Saltin B.** Physiological effects of physical conditioning. *Medicine and Science in Sports* 1: 50-56, 1969.

85. **Saltin B and Astrand PO.** Free fatty acids and exercise. *The American Journal of Clinical Nutrition* 57: 752S-757S; discussion 757S-758S, 1993.

86. **Saltin B and Gollnick P.** Skeletal muscle adaptability: Significance for metabolism and performance. In: *Handbook of Physiology*, edited by Peachey L, Adrian R, and Geiger S. Baltimore, MD: Lippincott Williams & Wilkins, 1983.

87. **Schiros CG, Ahmed MI, Sangala T, Zha W, McGriffin DC, Bamman MM, et al.** Importance of three-dimension geometric analysis in the assessment of the athlete's heart. *American Journal of Cardiology* 111: 1067-1072, 2013.

88. **Seynnes OR, de Boer M, and Narici MV.** Early skeletal muscle hypertrophy and architectural changes in response to high-intensity resistance training. *Journal of Applied Physiology* 102: 368-373, 2007.

89. **Soltow QA, Betters JL, Sellman JE, Lira VA, Long JH, and Criswell DS.** Ibuprofen inhibits skeletal muscle hypertrophy in rats. *Medicine & Science in Sports & Exercise* 38: 840-846, 2006.

90. **Spina RJ, Ogawa T, Kohrt WM, Martin WH, III, Holloszy JO, and Ehsani AA.** Differences in cardiovascular adaptations to endurance exercise training between older men and women. *Journal of Applied Physiology* 75: 849-855, 1993.

91. **Staron RS, Leonardi MJ, Karapondo DL, Malicky ES, Falkel JE, Hagerman FC, et al.** Strength and skeletal muscle adaptations in heavy-resistance-trained women after detraining and retraining. *Journal of Applied Physiology* 70: 631-640, 1991.

92. **Staron RS, Malicky ES, Leonardi MJ, Falkel JE, Hagerman FC, and Dudley GA.** Muscle hypertrophy and fast fiber type conversions in heavy resistance-trained women. *European Journal of Applied Physiology and Occupational Physiology* 60: 71-79, 1990.

93. **Tamaki T, Uchiyama S, and Nakano S.** A weight-lifting exercise model for inducing hypertrophy in the hindlimb muscles of rats. *Medicine & Science in Sports & Exercise* 24: 881-886, 1992.

94. **Tang JE, Hartman JW, and Phillips SM.** Increased muscle oxidative potential following resistance training induced fibre hypertrophy in young men. *Applied Physiology, Nutrition, and Metabolism* 31: 495-501, 2006.

95. **Tang JE, Perco JG, Moore DR, Wilkinson SB, and Phillips SM.** Resistance training alters the response of fed state mixed muscle protein synthesis in young men. *American Journal of Physiology Regulatory Integrative and Comparative Physiology* 294: R172-178, 2008.

96. **Terjung RL.** Muscle adaptations to aerobic training. In: *Sports Science Exchange.* Barrington, IL: Gatorade Sports Science Institute, 1995.

97. **Tesch PA.** Skeletal muscle adaptations consequent to long-term heavy resistance exercise. *Medicine & Science in Sports & Exercise* 20: S132-134, 1988.

98. **Tesch PA, Komi PV, and Hakkinen K.** Enzymatic adaptations consequent to long-term strength training. *International Journal of Sports Medicine* 8 (Suppl 1): 66-69, 1987.

99. **Trappe TA, Carroll CC, Dickinson JM, LeMoine JK, Haus JM, Sullivan BE, et al.** Influence of acetaminophen and ibuprofen on skeletal muscle adaptations to resistance exercise in older adults. *American Journal of Physiology Regulatory Integrative and Comparative Physiology* 300: R655-662, 2011.

100. **Tucci JT, Carpenter DM, Pollock ML, Graves JE, and Leggett SH.** Effect of reduced frequency of training and detraining on lumbar extension strength. *Spine* (Phila Pa 1976) 17: 1497-1501, 1992.

101. **Van Loon L.** Use of intramuscular triacylglycerol as a substrate source during exercise in humans. *Journal of Applied Physiology* 97: 1170-1187, 2004.

102. **Vincent HK, Powers SK, Stewart DJ, Demirel HA, Shanely RA, and Naito H.** Short-term exercise training improves diaphragm antioxidant capacity and endurance. *European Journal of Applied Physiology* 81: 67-74, 2000.

103. **Wang Y, Wisloff U, and Kemi OJ.** Animal models in the study of exercise-induced cardiac hypertrophy. *Physiological Research* 59: 633-644, 2010.

104. **Weiner RB, Hutter AM, Wang F, Kim J, Weyman AE, Wood MJ, et al.** The impact of endurance exercise training on left ventricle torsion. *JACC Cardiovasc Imaging* 3: 1001-1009, 2010.

105. **Wibom R, Hultman E, Johansson M, Matherei K, Constantin-Teodosiu D, and Schantz PG.** Adaptation of mitochondrial ATP production in human skeletal muscle to endurance training and detraining. *Journal of Applied Physiology* 73: 2004-2010, 1992.

106. **Wilson JM, Marin PJ, Rhea MR, Wilson SM, Loenneke JP, and Anderson JC.** Concurrent training: a meta-analysis examining interference of aerobic and resistance exercises. *Journal of Strength and Conditioning Research* 26: 2293-2307, 2012.

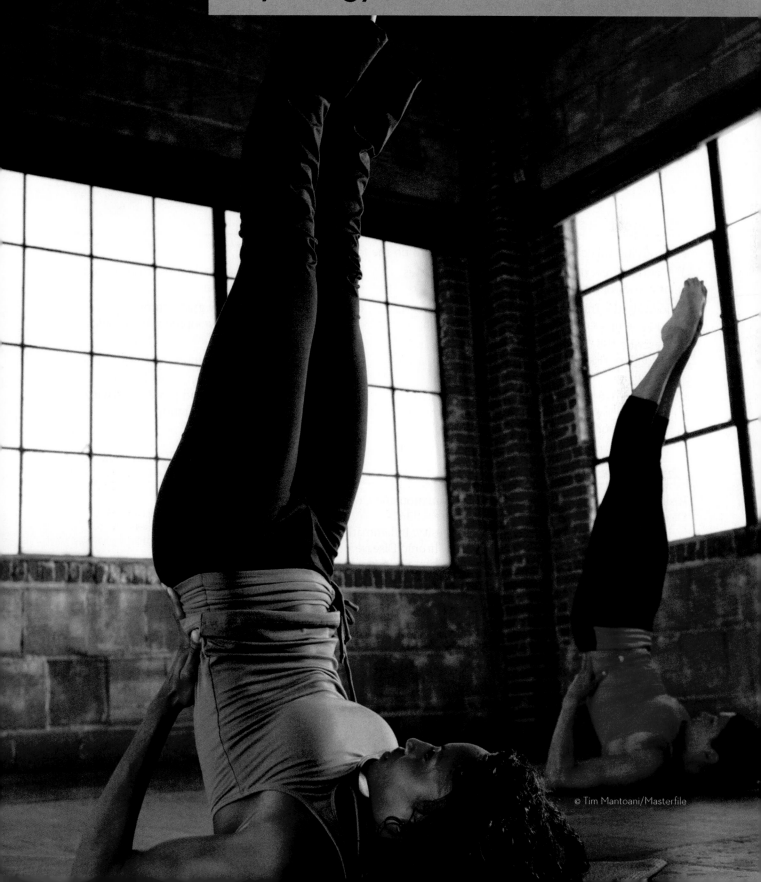

SECTION 2

Physiology of Health and Fitness

© Tim Mantoani/Masterfile

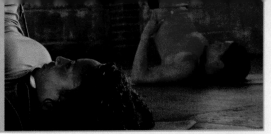

14

Preventing Chronic Disease: Physical Activity and Healthy Eating

■ Objectives

By studying this chapter, you should be able to do the following:

1. Contrast infectious with degenerative diseases as causes of death.

2. Identify the three major categories of risk factors and examples of specific risk factors in each.

3. Describe the difference between primary and secondary risk factors for coronary heart disease (CHD).

4. Characterize physical inactivity as a coronary heart disease risk factor comparable to smoking, hypertension, and high serum cholesterol.

5. Describe the process of atherosclerosis related to coronary heart disease.

6. Describe the role of low-grade chronic inflammation in the development of chronic diseases.

7. Describe the metabolic syndrome and possible causes.

8. Describe the role of diet and physical activity from an anti-inflammatory standpoint.

■ Outline

■ Key Terms

atherosclerosis
degenerative diseases
infectious diseases
low-grade chronic inflammation
primary risk factor
secondary risk factor
web of causation

In this section of the textbook, the Physiology of Health and Fitness, we focus on the importance of two major variables, physical activity (Chaps. 15, 16, and 17) and healthy eating (Chap. 18), as crucial ingredients to a healthy lifestyle. There is absolutely no question that physical inactivity is a major risk factor for numerous chronic diseases including heart disease, type 2 diabetes, and cancer (65). In like manner, choosing healthy foods to obtain essential nutrients, while matching caloric intake with caloric expenditure, goes a long way in dealing with our obesity epidemic and its dire consequences. In this chapter, we begin with a discussion of risk factors for chronic diseases that examines the environmental, genetic, and behavioral links to health and disease. These risk factors direct public health interventions to reduce the overall risk to the population (e.g., stop-smoking campaigns). Although risk factors describe the causes of disease from a macro level, they don't address the underlying physiological causes of these chronic diseases. We will try to do that by exploring the proposition that it is a low-level systemic inflammation (see Chap. 6) that is causing many of these chronic diseases. Finally, we will bring the discussion back to physical activity and healthy eating as ways of dealing with chronic disease.

RISK FACTORS FOR CHRONIC DISEASES

Over the past 100 years, attention has shifted from **infectious diseases** (e.g., tuberculosis and pneumonia) as the major causes of death to chronic **degenerative diseases,** such as cancer and cardiovascular diseases. The *leading* causes of death describe the specific diseases linked to that outcome. In 2013, the top five leading causes of death were diseases of the heart, malignant neoplasms (cancer), chronic lower respiratory diseases, accidents (unintentional injuries), and cerebrovascular diseases (stroke) (71). The onset of most of the leading causes of death can be delayed or prevented by addressing the risk factors for these diseases. Epidemiologists are the scientists

who play a major role in exploring the distribution of diseases in the population and the factors that have an impact on those diseases. Figure 14.1 shows that risk factors associated with chronic diseases can be divided into three categories (68).

Inherited/Biological

These factors include the following:

- Age–Older individuals have more chronic diseases than younger individuals.
- Gender–Men develop cardiovascular disease at an earlier age than women, but women experience more strokes than men (4).
- Race–African Americans develop about 30% more heart disease than non-Hispanic whites (67).
- Susceptibility to disease–Several diseases have a genetic component that increases the potential for having a disease.

Environmental

Environmental factors that affect health and disease include the following:

- Physical factors (e.g., climate, water, altitude, pollution)
- Socioeconomic factors (e.g., income, housing, education, workplace characteristics)
- Family (e.g., parental values, divorce, and extended family and friends)

Behavioral

The *actual* causes of death describe which behaviors (e.g., smoking) are linked to death (see the right side of Fig. 14.1). That smoking is at the top of the list should be no surprise given its connection to both lung cancer and cardiovascular diseases. In fact, it is the number one actual cause of deaths, accounting for 18% of all deaths. The existence of smoking-cessation programs and laws

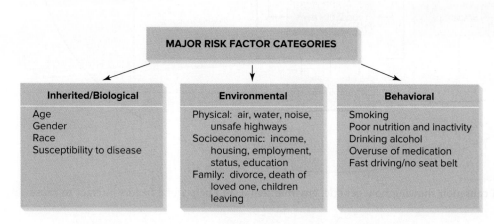

Figure 14.1 Major categories of risk factors with examples of each.

U.S. Department of Health Education and Welfare, *Healthy People: The Surgeon General's Report on Health Promotion and Disease Prevention.* Washington, D.C.: U.S. Government Printing Office, 1979.

that restrict areas in which one can smoke speak to the seriousness with which our society takes that risk to our health. The number two actual cause of death is poor diet and physical inactivity (15.2%), with alcohol consumption being number three (3.5%) (39, 40). The emphasis on healthy eating at work and in schools, the creation of new parks and bike trails to enhance opportunities to be physically active, and "don't drink and drive" campaigns are examples of some systematic attempts to help alter these behaviors.

In contrast to infectious disease, in which a single pathogen may be the cause of a disease, establishing the cause of a disease is much more difficult when dealing with chronic, degenerative diseases such as cardiovascular disease. The reason is that genetic, environmental, and behavioral factors interact in a complex manner to cause the disease. The difficulty of establishing "cause" for these complex diseases is best described by an epidemiologic model called the **web of causation** (37, 62).

In an oversimplification, Figure 14.2 shows links among three major classes of risk factors: genetic

(e.g., gender, race), environmental (e.g., access to inexpensive high-fat foods; access to convenient places to walk, cycle, and play), and behavioral (e.g., diet, smoking, inadequate physical activity, too much physical inactivity [TV, video, computer]) (62, 63). They act alone and interact with each other to cause **atherosclerosis,** a condition in which a fatty plaque builds up in (not on) the inner wall of an artery. Many of the risk factors interact to cause overweight, obesity, and type 2 diabetes–problems that are connected to cardiovascular disease. Trying to tease out the effect that one factor has on another and on the final disease process is a difficult task that makes work in epidemiology interesting and challenging. The factors in the web of causation are positively associated with the development of cardiovascular diseases but are not sufficient in and of themselves to cause them. These are called risk factors, and they play a major role in developing prevention programs aimed at reducing disease and premature death associated with degenerative diseases. To expand on this risk factor concept, we will focus on coronary heart disease.

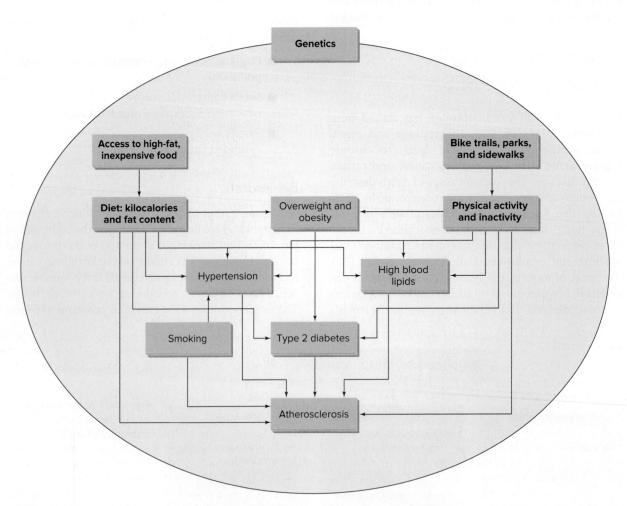

Figure 14.2 Simplified web of causation showing how genetic, environmental, and behavioral factors interact to cause atherosclerosis.

RISK FACTORS FOR CORONARY HEART DISEASE

Coronary heart disease (CHD) is associated with a gradual narrowing of the arteries serving the heart due to a thickening of the inner lining of the artery. This process, called atherosclerosis, is the leading contributor to heart attack and stroke deaths (20). It is now widely accepted that some people are at a greater risk of developing CHD than others.

Historically, **risk factors** for CHD were divided into **primary,** or major, and **secondary,** or contributing. *Primary* meant that a factor in and of itself increased the risk of CHD, and *secondary* meant that a certain factor increased the risk of CHD only if one of the primary factors was already present, or that its significance had not been precisely determined (15). Lists of risk factors have evolved over time as more epidemiological evidence has accumulated, showing the association between various behaviors (e.g., physical inactivity) or characteristics (e.g., obesity) and CHD. Consequently, a practical approach used to classify risk factors is to list those that can be changed and those that can't, no matter whether they are primary or secondary.

Currently, the American College of Sports Medicine (ACSM) lists eight risk factors (2):

- Age
- Family history
- Cigarette smoking
- Sedentary lifestyle
- Obesity
- Hypertension
- Dyslipidemia
- Prediabetes

Some of these risk factors, like age and family history, cannot be changed, but most can. An analysis of modifiable risk factors highlighted the impact that intervention programs have had on specific risk factors such as smoking and hypertension (19); however, interventions, in general, have not resulted in much of a reduction in the risk of CHD (22). This has been taken as a call to action to develop better behavior-change interventions to achieve better results.

You may have noticed that a high-fat diet was not listed in the above list of risk factors. In part, that is due to the fact that the impact of a high-fat diet is represented in the dyslipidemia and obesity risk factors. That said, there is clear evidence that high dietary salt and transfat intake and low omega-3-fatty acid intake are implicated as risk factors in chronic disease (19). In fact, dietary factors have an impact on a wide variety of the risk factors: obesity, hypertension, dyslipidemia, and prediabetes. Characteristics of a healthy diet will be addressed in Chap. 18. Finally, and important from the standpoint of this text, there exists a substantial body of evidence that physical inactivity is a major cause of many chronic diseases, including different cancers and various cardiovascular and metabolic diseases (11, 12, 65). We will see more on this in the next section and in Chaps. 16 and 17. To estimate your or your parent's ten-year risk of having a heart attack, go to **http://cvdrisk.nhlbi.nih.gov.**

IN SUMMARY

- Risk factors can be divided into three categories: genetic/biological, environmental, and behavioral.
- The risk factors for CHD include some you cannot change (e.g., age and family history) and many you can (cigarette smoking, inactivity, obesity, hypertension, dyslipidemia, and prediabetes).

Physical Inactivity as a Risk Factor

After looking at the web of causation for cardiovascular disease in Figure 14.2, one can understand how difficult it is to determine whether an observed association between a risk factor and a disease is a causal one or is due simply to chance. To facilitate the process of determining cause, epidemiologists apply the following guidelines (6):

- Temporal association–Does the cause precede the effect?
- Plausibility–Is the association consistent with other knowledge?
- Consistency–Have similar results been shown in other studies?
- Strength–What is the strength of the association (relative risk) between the cause and the effect? Relative risk is sometimes expressed as the ratio of the risk of disease among those exposed to the factor to the risk of those unexposed. The greater the ratio, the stronger the association.
- Dose-response relationship–Is increased exposure to the possible cause associated with increased effect?
- Reversibility–Does the removal of the possible cause lead to a reduction of the disease risk?
- Study design–Is the evidence based on strong study design?
- Judging the evidence–How many lines of evidence lead to the conclusion?

The concern about whether a risk factor is causally related to cardiovascular disease has special significance for physical activity. For many years, physical inactivity was believed to be only weakly associated with heart disease and was not given much attention as a public health concern. However, in the late 1980s and early 1990s, that view changed rather dramatically. In 1987, Powell et al. (54) did a systematic review of the literature dealing with the role of physical activity in the primary prevention of coronary heart disease, applying the just-listed guidelines to establish causation. They found that the majority of studies indicated that the level of physical inactivity predated the onset of CHD, thus meeting the temporal requirement. They also found a dose-response relationship in that as physical activity increased, the risk of CHD decreased, and the association was stronger in the better studies. The latter results met the consistency and study design criteria for causality. The review found the association to be plausible given the role of physical activity in improving glucose tolerance, increasing fibrinolysis (breaking of clots), and reducing blood pressure. The investigators calculated the relative risk of CHD due to inactivity to be about 1.9, meaning that sedentary people had about twice the chance of experiencing CHD that physically active people had. The relative risk was similar to smoking (2.5), high serum cholesterol (2.4), and high blood pressure (2.1). When the authors controlled for smoking, blood pressure, cholesterol, age, and sex (all of which are associated with CHD), the association of physical activity and CHD remained, indicating that physical activity was an independent risk factor for CHD (54). In 1992, the American Heart Association added physical inactivity to its list of primary or major risk factors for cardiovascular disease (3).

To estimate the real impact a risk factor may have on a population, epidemiologists try to balance the relative risk with the number of people in the population that have the risk factor. This balancing act is summed up in the calculation of the population-attributable risk for each risk factor (16). Figure 14.3 describes the relative risk for selected risk factors and the percentage of the population affected. Given the large number of people who are inactive, changes in physical activity habits have a great potential to reduce CHD and other chronic diseases (11, 65).

IN SUMMARY

- Physical inactivity is an independent risk factor for CHD.
- The relative risk of CHD due to inactivity (1.9) is similar to that of hypertension (2.1) and high cholesterol (2.4). The fact that a large percentage of the population is inactive indicates the enormous impact a change in physical activity habits can have on the nation's risk for CHD.

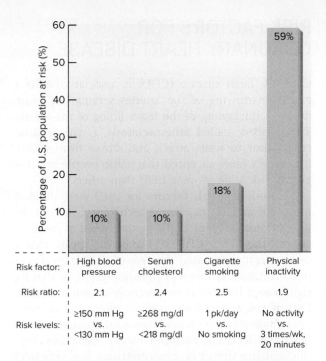

Risk factor:	High blood pressure	Serum cholesterol	Cigarette smoking	Physical inactivity
Risk ratio:	2.1	2.4	2.5	1.9
Risk levels:	≥150 mm Hg vs. <130 mm Hg	≥268 mg/dl vs. <218 mg/dl	1 pk/day vs. No smoking	No activity vs. 3 times/wk, 20 minutes

Figure 14.3 Percentages of U.S. population at risk for recognized risk factors related to coronary heart disease and risk ratio for each risk factor.

Physical Activity and Health

Regular participation in physical activity has a positive impact on our health. In 2001, a special symposium examined whether a dose-response relationship existed between physical activity and a variety of health outcomes (31). At the end of that decade, another systematic review of the literature (66) was conducted on this same topic prior to the publication of the first set of national physical activity guidelines: *2008 U.S. Physical Activity Guidelines* (65). This review supported the vast majority of the findings in the earlier report. Regular participation in physical activity was associated with:

- Lower rates of all-cause mortality, total cardiovascular disease (CVD), and coronary heart disease incidence and mortality
- Increased weight loss and reduced amount of weight regain after weight loss
- A lower incidence of obesity, type 2 diabetes, and metabolic syndrome
- A lower risk of colon and breast cancer
- An improvement in the ability of older adults to do activities of daily living
- Reduced risk of falls in older adults at risk of falling
- A reduction in depression and cognitive decline in adults and older adults

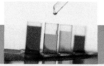

A LOOK BACK—IMPORTANT PEOPLE IN SCIENCE

Jeremy N. Morris and Ralph S. Paffenbarger, Jr.—Olympic Prize Winners

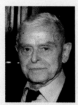

© Ed Howley

In 1996, the International Olympic Committee (IOC) awarded its first IOC Olympic Prize in sport sciences to Drs. Jeremy N. Morris and Ralph S. Paffenbarger, Jr., for their pioneering studies showing how exercise reduces the risk of heart disease.

Dr. Jeremy N. Morris, D.Sc., D.P.H, Fellow of the Royal College of Physicians, was professor of public health at the University of London, England. He was one of the first epidemiologists to provide scientific support showing the impact of occupational and leisure-time physical activity on the risk of heart disease. In one study, he compared conductors on London's double-decker buses who climbed 500 to 750 stairs per work day with drivers who sat for 90% of their shift. In another study, postal letter carriers who walked or cycled their routes were compared to sedentary telephonists and clerks. In both cases, those in the more active occupations had fewer heart attacks (43). In another set of studies, he examined the effect of different amounts and types of leisure-time physical activities on the risk of CHD in those who held naturally sedentary jobs. He found that only those

doing vigorous activity during their leisure time experienced protection against CHD (42). For more information on Dr. Morris, see Paffenbarger et al. (47) and Blair et al. (10).

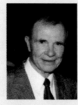

© Ed Howley

Dr. Ralph S. Paffenbarger, Jr., received his medical degree from Northwestern University in Chicago in 1947 and became a commissioned officer in the U.S. Public Health Service. During this time, he completed his M.P.H. and Dr.P.H. degrees at Johns Hopkins. He worked on the polio epidemic until the first vaccine became available in 1955 and then shifted his attention to issues related to physical activity and health. The findings of one of Dr. Paffenbarger's studies on longshoremen (49) confirmed the findings of Dr. Morris, showing that strenuous occupational physical activity was associated with a lower risk of CHD. However, Dr. Paffenbarger is best known for the Harvard Alumni Study (begun in 1960), which tracked alumni who matriculated between 1916 and 1950. The investigators had access to medical and other records when the alumni were students, and they were able to follow the alumni over the

years with questionnaires to obtain information about current behaviors (e.g., physical activity, diet, smoking) and examine the link between those behaviors and health problems (e.g., heart disease, hypertension, stroke) and cause of death. More than 100 publications have resulted from this study. Dr. Paffenbarger's research showed that alumni who participated in greater amounts of physical activity had a lower risk of heart attack (50). In addition, he was able to show that those who increased physical activity from one time period to the next had a 23% reduction in death from all causes—showing that it is never too late to begin an exercise program (48).

Dr. Paffenbarger practiced what he preached, being a successful marathon and ultramarathon runner. He had a major impact on the 1995 public health physical activity recommendation from the Centers for Disease Control and Prevention (52), and in the development of "Physical Activity and Health: A Report of the Surgeon General" (64). Dr. Paffenbarger died in 2007 and Dr. Morris in 2009, but their legacies as scientists, mentors, and role models will live on for years to come.

Information for this biographical sketch is taken from cited articles and publicly available curricula vita.

- Favorable changes in cardiovascular risk factors, including blood pressure and blood lipid profile

In general, the review found that:

- The volume of physical activity done was the most important variable tied to health outcomes.

- The risk of many chronic diseases was reduced about 20% to 40% by regular participation in physical activity, with the greatest gains made by those moving from doing no activity to doing some activity (55).

- Some physical activity is better than none and there is no lower threshold for benefits. Individuals are encouraged to be active

even if they cannot meet the minimum intensity or duration recommendations (55, 65).

- A dose-response relationship existed for most health outcomes, meaning that "more is better." See Figure 14.4 as an example for the health outcome "death from all causes."

That last finding, "more is better," had to be balanced by the increased risk of adverse outcomes when too much was done or when the exercise was a major change from what was currently being done. See more on this in Chap. 16. For information on two individuals who have had a major impact on our understanding of physical activity and heart disease, see A Look Back–Important People in Science.

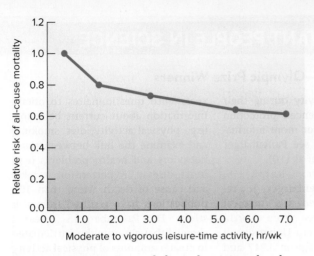

Figure 14.4   Dose-response of physical activity related to all-cause mortality.

U.S. Department of Health and Human Services, *Physical Activity Guidelines Advisory Committee Report 2008*, Figure G1.3, p.G1-19. www.health.gov/paguidelines/committeereport.aspx.

INFLAMMATION AND CORONARY HEART DISEASE

We have just seen that a wide variety of risk factors are linked to heart disease. But how are these risk factors connected physiologically to the actual appearance of the disease? In atherosclerosis, the narrowing of the coronary artery can result in a reduction in blood flow that may ultimately lead to a heart attack. The decrease in the diameter of the lumen is due to a buildup of lipid and fibrous materials (plaque) in the inner lining of the artery, called the *intima* (see Fig. 14.5). In many ways, atherosclerosis has been viewed as a plumbing issue, and procedures to flatten the plaque back to the arterial wall (angioplasty) or change out the pipe (coronary artery bypass graft) have been used to correct the problem (see Chap.17 for more on those procedures). However, most of the heart attacks and many strokes occur, not from a gradual occlusion of an artery, but from a sudden rupture of the plaque that triggers a blood clot and blocks blood flow. Let's look at this in more detail (35, 36).

It has become clear that atherosclerosis is caused by the process of inflammation initiated in the inner lining of the artery (35, 36). Inflammation is a response of a tissue to injury that involves the recruitment of white blood cells (leukocytes) to the site of the injury (see Chap. 6). Normally, the endothelial cells (endothelium) that line the inner surface of the artery do not support the binding of leukocytes; however, when the endothelium is activated by risk factors such as smoking, high blood pressure, a high-fat diet, or obesity, the endothelium generates

adhesion molecules on its surface that can bind readily to leukocytes (especially monocytes and T cells) in the blood (see Fig. 14.5) (34, 35, 36)

- Once bound to the adhesion molecules, the endothelial cells secrete chemokines that attract the monocytes to enter the intima, where they mature into macrophages (see Fig. 14.5A).
- The macrophages develop scavenger receptors on their surface that help them ingest large amounts of modified LDL cholesterol.
- The macrophages become loaded with fatty droplets and develop into foam cells (see right side of Fig. 14.5A). These foam cells and the T cells make up the "fatty streak," the earliest form of atherosclerotic plaque.
- As the process continues, the macrophages multiply due to growth factors they produce, and the size of the plaque increases.
- As this is developing, some of the smooth muscle cells in the middle layer (media) of the artery move to the top layer of the intima (near the lumen) where they multiply and, with connective tissue, form a fibrous matrix cap over the fatty core of the plaque (see Fig. 14.5B).

At some point, the foam cells release inflammatory signals that lead to the digestion and weakening of the fibrous matrix cap. If the cap ruptures, the chemicals from the foam cell interact with factors in the blood to form a clot (thrombus) that might be large enough to completely block an artery (see Fig. 14.5C). It is this process that causes most heart attacks (35, 36).

Obesity, Inflammation, and Chronic Disease

It is now recognized that a **low-grade chronic inflammation** is linked to a wide variety of chronic diseases, including hypertension, heart disease and stroke, some cancers, respiratory conditions, type 2 diabetes, and the metabolic syndrome (to be discussed in more detail in the next section) (38, 60). The chronic low-grade inflammation is characterized by a two- to threefold increase in inflammatory cytokines (e.g., tumor necrosis factor alpha [TNF-α], interleukin-6 [IL-6], and C-reactive protein [CRP]).

Of interest to the readers of this text is the impact of obesity on inflammation and chronic disease. Currently in the United States, 35.7% of adults are obese (46). Obesity is linked to a variety of chronic diseases, including CHD, hypertension, and type 2 diabetes, to name a few. The physiological connection between having too much adipose tissue and

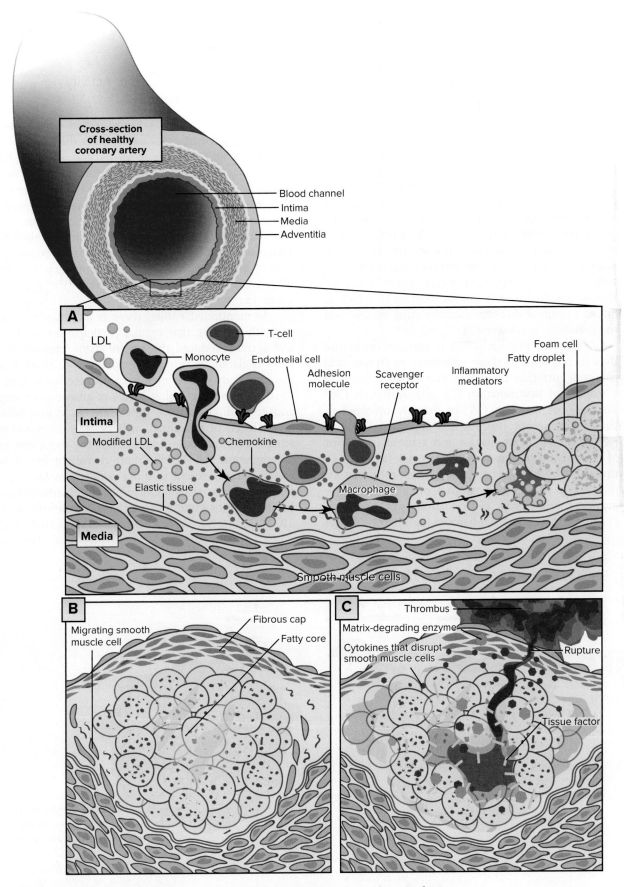

Figure 14.5 Process of inflammation leading to the rupture of an atherosclerotic plaque.

Adapted from Libby, P., "Atherosclerosis: The New View," *Scientific American*, May 2002, p. 46–55.

the inflammation related to chronic disease includes the hormones and inflammatory cytokines released by adipose tissue (27, 69).

Under normal conditions, adipocytes synthesize and store lipids and release anti-inflammatory hormones (e.g., adiponectin–see A Closer Look 5.2). However, the adipocytes have the capacity to secrete a variety of inflammatory cytokines (e.g., IL-6). When the adipocytes, especially those in the visceral area, increase in size, as seen in obesity, they secrete more IL-6 and less adiponectin (27). In addition, macrophages infiltrate the enlarged visceral adipose tissue, promote a local inflammation, and secrete TNF-α, a potent inflammatory cytokine (69). Increased amounts of free fatty acids (FFA), IL-6, and TNF-a (and reduced amounts of adiponectin) are released from the visceral adipose tissue into the liver and then the general circulation. In combination, they interfere with the action of insulin (causing insulin resistance), which is linked to type 2 diabetes, cardiovascular disease, and the metabolic syndrome (21, 27, 60, 69).

C-reactive protein (CRP) is released from the liver in response to these inflammatory factors, and the concentration of CRP in the blood is used as a marker of inflammation (35, 36). Although CRP may (69) or may not (35) be directly involved in the atherosclerotic process, it is clear that CRP is a risk factor for heart disease and a useful predictor of disease risk in those with other risk factors (14). Investigators have used it and other inflammatory markers to evaluate the impact of different strategies on the low-grade inflammation associated with chronic diseases. Both pharmacological (i.e., drugs)

and nonpharmacological (i.e., diet and exercise) interventions have been used to try to reduce this systemic inflammation.

Healthy Eating and Physical Activity to Combat Inflammation

In terms of healthy eating, Esposito et al. have shown that eating a Mediterranean-style diet (high in fruits, vegetables, legumes, whole grains, and olive oil) for two years resulted in a dramatic reduction in CRP and IL-6, with no changes observed in the control group (23). Further, such results were observed even without weight loss (58). This dietary-induced reduction in inflammatory markers is believed to be linked to suppression of pathways that stimulates the transcription of genes involved in the inflammation process (28). We will see more on healthy eating plans in Chap. 18.

As mentioned earlier, there is an abundance of research showing that regular participation in physical activity reduces the risk of many chronic diseases. Related to systemic inflammation, there is a growing body of evidence from prospective longitudinal studies that higher levels of physical activity and/or cardiorespiratory fitness are associated with lower levels of inflammation (8, 9, 33). Intervention studies confirm these findings, but the reduction in inflammation may be due more to weight loss than exercise itself, except in those populations (e. g., patients in cardiac rehabilitation, obese individuals) that have higher baseline levels of inflammation (7, 8, 9, 18, 29, 33, 45, 51, 59, 73). Figure 14.6 shows potential

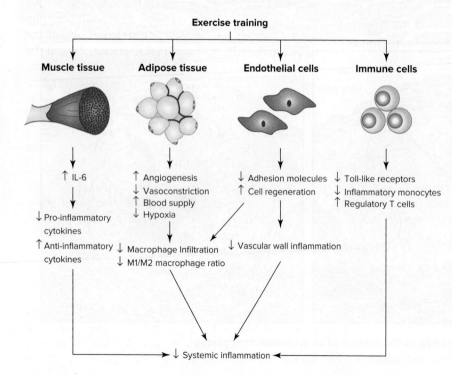

Figure 14.6 Potential mechanisms through which exercise training reduces chronic inflammation in obesity.

Adapted from You T., Arsenis, N. C., Disanzo, B. L., and LaMonte, M. J., "Effects of Exercise Training on Chronic Inflammation in Obesity," *Sports Medicine* 43: 243–256, 2013.

mechanisms through which exercise training might reduce chronic inflammation in obesity (73):

- Acute exercise stimulates IL-6 release from skeletal muscle, which suppresses pro-inflammatory cytokines.

- Exercise training may increase angiogenesis (creation of new blood vessels) in adipose tissue to result in an increase in blood flow and a reduction in hypoxia and associated chronic inflammation in adipose tissue.

- Exercise also reduces adhesion molecule production in endothelial cells and lowers vascular wall inflammation.

- Exercise training may reduce the expression of toll-like receptors (that recognize molecules tied to pathogens) and the number of pro-inflammatory monocytes.

It is clear that anti-inflammatory activity is not the only mechanism responsible for the health benefits of exercise (13, 24, 38, 53). Exercise affects a wide variety of risk factors (e.g., blood pressure, abdominal fat, HDL-C), and the evidence is overwhelming that exercise training is very important in reducing the risk of many chronic diseases (11). Given all this, it is clear that to reduce the risks of chronic diseases, we should use a combination of dietary change to the Mediterranean style, a reduction in body weight to an appropriate level, and an increase in physical activity and/or cardiorespiratory fitness to achieve that goal, since each has an independent effect (see Chaps. 16, 17, and 18 for more on each of these).

THE METABOLIC SYNDROME

We end this chapter with a discussion of the metabolic syndrome as a way of pulling together all of what we have seen and emphasizing, again, the importance of healthy eating and physical activity in the prevention and treatment of chronic diseases. Epidemiologists are not the only scientists interested in examining potential relationships between variables in order to have a greater understanding of what causes chronic diseases. Physiologists study how tissues and organs function to maintain homeostasis and try to uncover the source of a problem when homeostasis is not maintained. A good example of a failure to maintain homeostasis is hypertension, a problem that affects more than 28% of adult Americans (72). Interestingly, investigators have found that hypertension does not generally occur in isolation. It is not uncommon for hypertensive individuals to also have multiple metabolic abnormalities, such as

- Obesity—especially abdominal obesity
- Insulin resistance—a condition in which tissues do not take up glucose easily when

stimulated with insulin; muscle is the primary site of insulin resistance

- Dyslipidemia—abnormal levels of triglycerides and other lipids

The fact that these abnormalities often occur as a group suggests a common underlying cause that might give us a better understanding of the disease processes associated with hypertension. The coexistence of insulin resistance, dyslipidemia, and hypertension has been called Syndrome X (57); those who add obesity to the model call it the Deadly Quartet (30). However, metabolic syndrome is currently the preferred term. To establish the prevalence of metabolic syndrome in the population, scientists first established an operational definition of the syndrome—a person has to have three or more of the following to be considered as having the syndrome (44):

- Abdominal obesity: waist circumference >102 cm in men and >88 cm in women
- Hypertriglyceridemia: ≥150 mg/dl
- Low high-density lipoprotein (HDL) cholesterol: <40 mg/dl in men and <50 mg/dl in women
- High blood pressure: ≥130/85 mm Hg
- High fasting blood glucose: ≥100 mg/dl

The overall prevalence of metabolic syndrome in the United States from 2003 to 2012 was 33%, with a greater prevalence for women (35.6%) than men (30.3%) (1).

What causes the metabolic syndrome? Two theories have been advanced, and they are not mutually exclusive. One theory is that the cause of metabolic syndrome is a low-grade chronic inflammation, similar to what we have just seen for atherosclerosis. Figure 14.7 shows the complex interrelationships of the various metabolic disorders that these authors call the *cardiovascular metabolic syndrome* because of its obvious connection to cardiovascular disease (56, 70). The double arrows in the figure indicate that each of the disorders can affect the others. The sheer complexity of this web of causation makes it difficult to identify a single cause of metabolic syndrome. Two potential interpretations include the following:

- The increased levels of inflammatory cytokines (e.g., TNF-α, IL-6, CRP) cause the insulin resistance that leads to obesity and type 2 diabetes (56).
- The central obesity leads to an increase in inflammatory cytokines and FFA that, in turn, cause the insulin resistance (41).

Obviously, there are other interpretations, and the inflammation theory is not alone in suggesting cause. The other theory is that an elevated level of oxidative stress causes metabolic syndrome. Oxidative

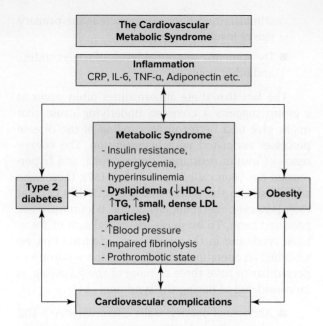

Figure 14.7 The cardiovascular metabolic syndrome. The figure shows the complex interrelationships of the various metabolic disorders. The double arrows indicate that each disorder can affect the others, creating a complex web of causation.

From Rana, J. S., Nieuwdorp, M., Jukema, J. W., and Kastelein, J. J. P., "Cardiovascular Metabolic Syndrome—An Interplay of Obesity, Inflammation, Diabetes and Coronary Heart Disease," *Diabetes, Obesity and Metabolism* 9: 218-232, 2007.

stress exists when free radicals (highly reactive molecules that are missing an electron) accumulate because they are being produced faster than our antioxidant systems can neutralize them, or because the level of antioxidants is inadequate, or both. These highly reactive free radicals react with and can damage lipids, enzymes, and DNA. This can lead, in turn, to altered

cellular function and to an inflammation response to deal with the cell damage. A growing body of evidence links oxidative stress to hypertension, insulin resistance, cardiovascular disease, type 2 diabetes, and metabolic syndrome (26, 61). We are sure to hear more about these theories in the years ahead. What can we do about these chronic diseases?

Figure 14.8 provides some clear suggestions that make it a nice wrap-up of what we have just seen and points the way for what is ahead (32). There is a large body of evidence showing that endurance exercise training favorably affects a majority of the risk factors making up metabolic syndrome (25), with less support for resistance training (5, 17). You will read more about exercise programming in Chaps. 16 and 17. In addition, the importance of diet in achieving a healthy body composition will be explained in detail in Chap. 18. Not surprisingly, diet and exercise are the principal nonpharmacological interventions used to prevent and treat a variety of chronic diseases. See Suggested Readings for the most current guidelines for both diet and physical activity.

IN SUMMARY

- The metabolic syndrome model describes connections between and among obesity, peripheral insulin resistance, hypertension, and dyslipidemia.
- Potential underlying causes of metabolic syndrome include a low-grade chronic inflammation and an increase in oxidative stress.
- Exercising, eating a healthy diet, and maintaining a healthy weight are strategies to both prevent and treat these chronic diseases.

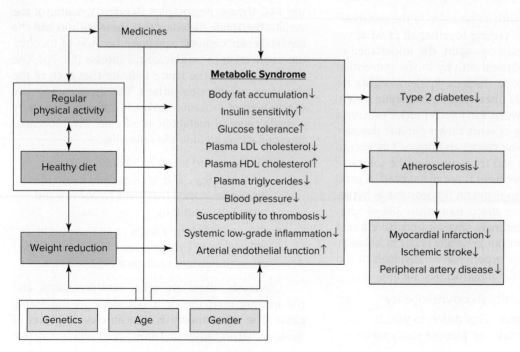

Figure 14.8 Interventions used to prevent and treat metabolic syndrome, type 2 diabetes, and cardiovascular disease. The focus is on regular physical activity and a healthy diet.

Lakka, T. A., and Laaksonen, D. E., "Physical Activity in Prevention and Treatment of the Metabolic Syndrome," *Applied Physiology, Nutrition, and Metabolism* 32: 76–88, 2007.

STUDY ACTIVITIES

1. What are the leading causes of death? How about the top three actual causes of death?
2. List the major categories of risk factors and give examples of some in each category.
3. In the web of causation for atherosclerosis, are the various risk factors directly linked to the disease? How do the risk factors interact?
4. Physical inactivity was long considered only a secondary risk factor. What "proof" did investigators have to offer to convince the scientific community otherwise?
5. List the steps (beginning with activation of epithelial cells on the intima) leading to the rupture of plaque that can result in a clot that can cause a heart attack.
6. Discuss the role that enlarged adipose tissue cells (seen in obesity) play in the inflammation response related to numerous chronic diseases.
7. What is metabolic syndrome and what are its potential underlying causes?
8. What two behaviors should be the focus of attention to minimize the systemic inflammation that is linked to chronic disease?

SUGGESTED READINGS

Oppenheimer, G.M. 2010. Framingham Heart Study: the first 20 years. *Progress in Cardiovascular Diseases* 53: 55-61.

Stone, N. J., J. Robinson, A. H. Lichtenstein, C. N. B. Merz, C. B. Blum, R. H. Eckel, et al. 2013. ACC/AHA guidelines on the treatment of blood cholesterol to reduce atherosclerotic cardiovascular risk in adults: a report of the American College of Cardiology/American Heart Association Task Force on Practice Guidelines. http://circ.ahajournals.org /content/early/2013/ 11/11/01.cir.0000437738.63853.7a

U.S. Department of Agriculture. 2015. *Dietary Guidelines for Americans.* www.cnpp.usda.gov/dietaryguidelines.htm

U.S. Department of Health and Human Services. 2008. *2008 Physical Activity Guidelines for Americans.* www.health.gov/PAGuidelines/

U.S. Department of Health and Human Services. 2010. *Healthy People 2020.* www.healthypeople.gov/2020/default.aspx

REFERENCES

1. **Aguilar M, Bhuket T, Torres S, Liu B, and Wong RJ.** Prevalence of the metabolic syndrome in the Unites States, 2003-2012. *JAMA* 313: 1973-1974.
2. **American College of Sports Medicine.** *ACSM's Guidelines for Exercise Testing and Prescription.* Philadelphia, PA: Lippincott Williams & Wilkins, 2014.
3. **American Heart Association.** Statement on exercise. Benefits and recommendations for physical activity programs for all Americans. A statement for health professionals by the Committee on Exercise and Cardiac Rehabilitation of the Council on Clinical Cardiology, American Heart Association. *Circulation* 86: 340-344, 1992.
4. **American Heart Association.** Women and cardiovascular diseases–statistics. http://americanheart.org/presenter.jhtml?identifier=3000941, 2010.
5. **Bateman LA, Slentz CA, Willis LH, Shields AT, Piner LW, Bales CW, et al.** Comparison of aerobic versus resistance exercise training effects on metabolic syndrome (from the Studies of a Targeted Risk Reduction Intervention Through Defined Exercise-STRRIDEAT/RT). *American Journal of Cardiology* 108: 838-844, 2011.
6. **Beaglehole R, Bonita R, and Kjellström T.** *Basic Epidemiology.* Geneva: World Health Organization, 1993.
7. **Beavers KM, Ambrosius WT, Nicklas, BJ, and Rejeski WJ.** Independent and combined effects of physical activity and weight loss on inflammatory biomarkers in overweight and obese older adults. *Journal of the American Geriatrics Society* 61: 1089-1094, 2013.
8. **Beavers KM, Brinkly TE, and Nicklas BJ.** Effect of exercise training on chronic inflammation. *Clinica Chemica Acta* 411: 785-793, 2010.
9. **Beavers KM, Hsu F-C, Isom S, Kritchevsky SB, Church T, Goodpaster B, et al.** Long-term physical activity and inflammatory biomarkers in older adults. *Medicine & Science in Sports & Exercise* 42: 2189-2196, 2010.
10. **Blair SN, Smith GD, Lee IM, Fox K, Hillsdon M, McKeown RE, et al.** A tribute to Professor Jeremiah Morris: the man who invented the field of physical activity epidemiology. *Annals of Epidemiology* 20: 651-660, 2010.
11. **Booth, FW, Roberts CK, and Laye MJ.** Lack of exercise is a major cause of chronic diseases. *Journal of Comparative Physiology* 2: 1143-1211, 2012.
12. **Bouchard C, Shephard R, Stevens T, Sutton J, and McPherson B.** Exercise, fitness, and health: the consensus statement. In *Exercise, Fitness, and Health,* edited by Bouchard C, Shephard RJ, Stevens T, Sutton JR, and McPherson BD. Champaign, IL: Human Kinetics, 1990, pp. 3-28.
13. **Brandt C and Pedersen BK.** The role of exercise-induced myokines in muscle homeostasis and the defense against chronic disease. *Journal of Biomedicine and Biotechnology* Article ID: 520258, 2010.
14. **Buckley DI, Fu R, Freeman M, Rogers K, and Helfand M.** C-reactive protein as a risk factor for coronary heart disease: a systematic review and meta-analysis for the U. S. Preventive Services Task Force. *Annals of Internal Medicine* 151: 483-495, 2009.
15. **Caspersen C and Heath G.** The risk factor concept of coronary heart disease. In *Resource Manual for Guidelines for Graded Exercise Testing and Prescription,* edited by Blair SN, Painter P, Pate R, Smith L, and Taylor C. Philadelphia, PA: Lea & Febiger, 1988, pp. 111-125.
16. **Caspersen CJ.** Physical activity epidemiology: concepts, methods, and applications to exercise science. *Exercise and Sport Science Reviews* 17: 423-473, 1989.
17. **Church TS.** Exercise in obesity, metabolic syndrome, and diabetes *Progress in Cardiovascular Diseases* 53: 412-418, 2011.

18. **Church TS, Earnest CP, Thompson AM, Priest EL, Rodarte RQ, Saunders T, et al.** Exercise without weight loss does not reduce c-reactive protein: the INFLAME study. *Medicine & Science in Sports & Exercise* 42: 708-716, 2010.

19. **Danaei G, Ding EL, Mozaffarian D, Taylor B, Rehm J, Murray CJL, et al.** The preventable causes of death in the United States: comparative risk assessment of dietary, lifestyle, and metabolic factors. *PLOS Medicine* 6: e1000058, doi:10.1371, 2009.

20. **Dawber T.** *The Framingham Study.* Cambridge: Harvard University Press, 1980.

21. **Després J-P.** Abdominal obesity and cardiovascular disease: is inflammation the missing link? *Canadian Journal of Cardiology* 28: 642-652, 2012.

22. **Ebrahim S, Taylor F, Ward K, Beswick A, Burke M, and Smith GD.** Multiple risk factor interventions for primary prevention of coronary heart disease. *Cochrane Database Systym Reviews* 1: CD001561, 2011.

23. **Esposito K, Marfella R, Ciotola M, Di Palo C, Giugliano F, Giugliano G, et al.** Effect of a Mediterranean-style diet on endothelial dysfunction and markers of vascular inflammation in the metabolic syndrome. *JAMA* 292: 1440-1446, 2004.

24. **Gleeson M, Bishop NC, Stensel DJ, Lindley MR, Mastana SS, and Nimmo MA.** The anti-inflammatory effects of exercise: mechanisms and implications for the prevention and treatment of disease. *Nature Reviews Immunology* 11: 607-615, 2011.

25. **Golbidi S, Mesdaghinia A, and Laher I.** Exercise and the metabolic syndrome. *Oxidative Medicine and Cellular Longevity* Volume 2012, No. 349710.

26. **Grattagliano I, Palmieri VO, Portincasa P, Moschetta A, and Palasciano G.** Oxidative stress-induced risk factors associated with the metabolic syndrome: a unifying hypothesis. *The Journal of Nutritional Biochemistry* 19: 491-504, 2008.

27. **Gustafson B.** Adipose tissue, inflammation and atherosclerosis. *Journal of Atherosclerosis and Thrombosis* 17: 332-341, 2010.

28. **Hardman WE.** Diet components can suppress inflammation and reduce cancer risk. *Nutrition Research and Practice* 8(3): 233-240, June 2014; doi: 10.4162/nrp.2014.8.3.233. Epub 2014 May 15

29. **Imayama I, Ulrich CM, Alfano CM, Wang CC, Xiao LR, Wener MH, et al.** Effects of a caloric restriction weight loss diet and exercise on inflammatory biomarkers in overweight/obese postmenopausal women: a randomized controlled trial. *Cancer Research* 72: 2314-2326, 2012.

30. **Kaplan NM.** The deadly quartet: upper-body obesity, glucose intolerance, hypertriglyceridemia, and hypertension. *Archives of Internal Medicine* 149: 1514-1520, 1989.

31. **Kasaniemi YA, Danforth JE, Jensen MD, Kopelman PG, Lefebvre P, and Reeder BA.** Dose-response issues concerning physical activity and health: an evidence-based symposium. *Medicine & Science in Sports & Exercise* 33 (Suppl): S351-358, 2001.

32. **Lakka TA and Laaksonen DE.** Physical activity in prevention and treatment of the metabolic syndrome. *Applied Physiology, Nutrition, and Metabolism* 32: 76-88, 2007.

33. **Lavie CJ, Church TS, Milani RV, and Earnest CP.** Impact of physical activity, cardiorespiratory fitness, and exercise training on markers of inflammation. *Journal of Cardiopulmonary Rehabilitation and Prevention* 31: 137-145, 2011.

34. **Libby P.** Atherosclerosis: the new view. *Scientific American* May 2002: 46-55, 2002.

35. **Libby P, Okamoto Y, Rocha VZ, and Folco E.** Inflammation in atherosclerosis. *Circ J* 74: 213-220, 2010.

36. **Libby P, Ridker PM, and Maseri A.** Inflammation and atherosclerosis. *Circulation Journal* 105: 1135-1143, 2002.

37. **MacMahon B and Pugh T.** *Epidemiology.* Boston, MA: Little, Brown, 1970.

38. **Mathur N and Pedersen BK.** Exercise as a means to control low-grade systemic inflammation. *Mediators of Inflammation* 2008: 1-6, 2008.

39. **Mokdad AH, Marks JS, Stroup DF, and Gerberding JL.** Actual causes of death in the United States, 2000. *JAMA* 291: 1238-1245, 2004.

40. **Mokdad AH, Marks JS, Stroup DF, and Gerberding JL.** Correction: actual causes of death in the United States, 2000. *JAMA* 293: 293-294, 2005.

41. **Monteiro R and Azavedo I.** Chronic inflammation in obesity and the metabolic syndrome. *Mediators of Inflammation* Article ID 289645, 2010.

42. **Morris JN, Chave SP, Adam C, Sirey C, Epstein L, and Sheehan DJ.** Vigorous exercise in leisure-time and the incidence of coronary heart-disease. *Lancet* 1: 333-339, 1973.

43. **Morris JN, Heady JA, Raffle PA, Roberts CG, and Parks JW.** Coronary heart disease and physical activity of work. *Lancet* 265: 1111-1120; concl, 1953.

44. **National Heart Blood and Lung Institute.** *Third Report of the National Cholesterol Education Program (NCEP) Expert Panel.* Detection, evaluation, and treatment of high blood cholesterol in adults (Adult Treatment Panel III) executive summary. NIH Publication No. 02-5285, 2002.

45. **Nimmo MA, Leggate M, Viana JL, and King JA.** The effect of physical activity on mediators of inflammation. *Diabetes, Obesity and Metabolism* 15 (Suppl. 3): 51-60, 2013.

46. **Ogden CL, Carroll MD, Kit BK, and Flegal KM.** Prevalence of obesity in the United States 2009-2010. *National Center for Health Statistics Data Brief.* No. 82, 2012.

47. **Paffenbarger RS, Jr., Blair SN, and Lee I-M.** A history of physical activity, cardiovascular health and longevity: the scientific contributions of Jeremy N. Morris, DSc, DPH, FRCP. *International Journal of Epidemiology* 30: 1184-1192, 2001.

48. **Paffenbarger RS, Jr., Hyde RT, Wing AL, Lee IM, Jung DL, and Kampert JB.** The association of changes in physical-activity level and other lifestyle characteristics with mortality among men. *The New England Journal of Medicine* 328: 538-545, 1993.

49. **Paffenbarger RS, Jr., Laughlin ME, Gima AS, and Black RA.** Work activity of longshoremen as related to death from coronary heart disease and stroke. *The New England Journal of Medicine* 282: 1109-1114, 1970.

50. **Paffenbarger RS, Jr., Wing AL, and Hyde RT.** Physical activity as an index of heart attack risk in college alumni. *American Journal of Epidemiology* 108: 161-175, 1978.

51. **Palmefors H, DuttaRoy S, Rundqvist B, and Borjesson M.** The effect of physical activity or exercise on key biomarkers in atherosclerosis–A systematic review. *Atherosclerosis* 235: 150-161, 2014.

52. **Pate RR, Pratt M, Blair SN, Haskell WL, Macera CA, Bouchard C, et al.** Physical activity and public health. A recommendation from the Centers for Disease Control and Prevention and the American College of Sports Medicine. *JAMA* 273: 402-407, 1995.

53. **Pedersen BK.** Edward F. Adolph distinguished lecture: muscle as an endocrine organ: IL-6 and other myokines. *Journal of Applied Physiology* 107: 1006-1014, 2009.

54. **Powell KE, Thompson PD, Caspersen CJ, and Kendrick JS.** Physical activity and the incidence of coronary heart disease. *Annual Review of Public Health* 8: 253-287, 1987.

55. **Powell KE, Paluch AE, and Blair SN.** Physical activity for health: what kind? How much? How intense? On top of what? *Annual Review of Public Health* 32: 349-365, 2011.

56. **Rana JS, Nieuwdorp M, Jukema JW, and Kastelein JJP.** Cardiovascular metabolic syndrome–an interplay of obesity, inflammation, diabetes and coronary heart disease. *Diabetes, Obesity and Metabolism* 9: 218-232, 2007.

57. **Reaven GM.** Banting lecture 1988. Role of insulin resistance in human disease. *Diabetes* 37: 1595-1607, 1988.

58. **Richard C, Couture P, Desroches S, and Lamarche B.** Effect of the Mediterranean diet with and without weight loss on markers of inflammation in men with metabolic syndrome. *Obesity* 21: 541-557, 2013.

59. **Ringseis R, Eder K, Mooren FC, Krüger K.** Metabolic signals and innate immune activation in obesity and exercise. *Exercise Immunology Review* 21: 58-68, 2015.

60. **Rizvi AA.** Hypertension, obesity, and inflammation: the complex designs of the deadly trio. *Metabolic Syndrome and Related Disorders* 8: 287-294, 2010.

61. **Roberts CK and Sindhu KK.** Oxidative stress and the metabolic syndrome. *Life Sciences* 84: 705-712, 2009.

62. **Rockett I.** Population and health: an introduction to epidemiology. *Population Bulletin Journal* 49: 1-48, 1994.

63. **Stallones R.** *Public Health Monograph 76.* Washington, DC: U.S. Government Printing Office, 1966.

64. **U. S. Department of Health and Human Services.** *Physical Activity and Health: A Report of the Surgeon General.* Washington, DC: U.S. Government Printing Office, 1996.

65. **U.S. Department of Health and Human Services.** 2008 Physical activity guidelines for Americans. www.health.gov/paguidelines/guidelines/, 2008

66. **U.S. Department of Health and Human Services.** Physical Activity Guidelines Advisory Committee Report 2008. wwwhealthgov/paguidelines/committeereportaspx, 2008.

67. **U.S. Department of Health and Human Services.** Heart disease and African Americans. http://minorityhealthhhsgov/templates/contentaspx?ID=3018, 2010.

68. **U.S. Department of Health Education and Welfare.** *Healthy People: The Surgeon General's Report on Health Promotion and Disease Prevention.* Washington, DC: U.S. Government Printing Office, 1979.

69. **Wang Z and Nakayama T.** Inflammation, a link between obesity and cardiovascular disease. *Mediators of Inflammation* Article ID 535918, 2010.

70. **Wassink AM, Olijhoek JK, and Visseren FL.** The metabolic syndrome: metabolic changes with vascular consequences. *European Journal of Clinical Investigation* 37: 8-17, 2007.

71. **Xu J, Murphy SL, Kochanek KD, and Bastian BA.** Deaths: final data for 2013. *National Vital Statistics Reports* 64: 1-118, 2016.

72. **Yoon SS, Burt V, Louis T, and Carroll, MD.** Hypertension among adults in the United States, 2009-2010. *National Center for Health Statistics Data Brief.* No. 107, 2012.

73. **You T, Arsenis NC, Disanzo BL, and LaMonte MJ.** Effects of exercise training on chronic inflammation in obesity. *Sports Medicine* 43: 243-256, 2013.

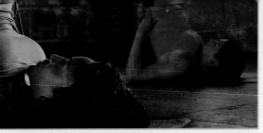

15

Exercise Tests to Evaluate Cardiorespiratory Fitness

© Tim Mantoani/Masterfile

■ Objectives

By studying this chapter, you should be able to do the following:

1. Identify the sequence of steps in the procedures for evaluating cardiorespiratory fitness (CRF).

2. Describe one maximal and one submaximal field test used to evaluate CRF.

3. Explain the rationale underlying the use of distance runs as estimates of CRF.

4. Identify the common measures taken during a graded exercise test (GXT).

5. Describe changes in the ECG that may take place during a GXT in subjects with ischemic heart disease.

6. Describe the primary and secondary criteria for having achieved $\dot{V}O_2$ max.

7. Estimate $\dot{V}O_2$ max from the last stage of a GXT and list the concerns about the protocol that may affect that estimate.

8. Estimate $\dot{V}O_2$ max by extrapolating the HR/$\dot{V}O_2$ relationship to the person's age-predicted maximal HR.

9. Describe the problems with the assumptions made in the extrapolation procedure used in Objective 8, and name the environmental and subject variables that must be controlled to improve such estimates.

10. Identify the criteria used to terminate the GXT.

11. Explain why there are so many different GXT protocols and why the rate of progression through the test is important.

12. Describe the YMCA's procedure to set the rate of progression on a cycle ergometer test.

13. Estimate $\dot{V}O_2$ max with the Åstrand and Ryhming nomogram given a data set for the cycle ergometer or step test.

■ Key Terms

angina pectoris
arrhythmia
conduction disturbances
double product
dyspnea
field test
myocardial ischemia
ST segment depression

In Chap. 14, we discussed the risk factors that limit health and contribute to coronary heart disease (CHD). One of those risk factors was a sedentary lifestyle. There is no question that by increasing our physical activity and cardiorespiratory function (fitness) (CRF), we can reduce the risk of many chronic diseases and death from all causes (110). You are already familiar with the use of a graded exercise test (GXT) to measure $\dot{V}O_2$ max; this chapter picks up on that theme and discusses the types of tests used to evaluate CRF. The type of test used depends on the fitness of the person being tested; the purpose of the test (experimental or epidemiological investigation); and the facilities, equipment, and personnel available to conduct the test. The choice of the GXT is different for a young healthy child compared to a 60-year-old person with CHD risk factors. The GXT might be used as a CRF test prior to entry into a fitness program, or it could be used as a diagnostic test by a cardiologist who evaluates a 12-lead electrocardiogram for evidence of heart disease. Clearly, the type of personnel and equipment, and, of course, the cost would be very different in these two situations. See texts by Heyward, Nieman, Howley and Thompson, and the American College of Sports Medicine in Suggested Readings for a more complete treatment of testing procedures to evaluate CRF.

TESTING PROCEDURES

Part of the reason for such diversity in exercise testing procedures is the risk associated with exercise testing. The risk of cardiac events during exercise testing is low in apparently healthy individuals, but increases as the number of risk factors increases. In general, the overall risk of severe cardiovascular complications or death is about 6/10,000 symptom-limited tests in a mixed population (2). The risk is lower for submaximal tests. How is risk assessed?

Screening

One of the most common tools used to estimate the risk associated with exercise testing or engaging in regular exercise has been the Canadian government's *Physical Activity Readiness Questionnaire (PAR-Q)*. Answering seven simple yes/no questions provided guidance about this risk, and about 50 million people per year completed this questionnaire (113). If all responses were "no," the person was directed to an exercise test and an appropriate physical activity program. However, a single "yes" response directed the person to a physician for follow-up before engaging in activity. Recently, the *PAR-Q* was revised to address concerns that too many people (~20%) were being inappropriately directed to medical personnel for clearance, and

that the original questionnaire was not based on a systematic review of the evidence relating physical activity to health (112). See Figure 15.1 for the first page of the PAR-Q+.

In contrast to the original version, anyone checking a "yes" response on the *PAR-Q+* is directed to additional questions dealing with chronic disease issues (e.g., cancer, cardiovascular diseases, diabetes) on pages 2 and 3 of the questionnaire to clarify the nature of the problem. If all responses are "no" to the additional questions, the person is directed to an appropriate exercise test and physical activity program. A single "yes" response to these additional questions directs the individual to a qualified exercise professional and/or the *ePARmed-X+*, an online questionnaire, to further clarify the risk associated with participation in exercise. Using these new procedures, only ~1% of individuals taking the *PAR-Q+* are directed to seek help from medical personnel, while the rest are encouraged to participate in appropriate physical activity (18). This is an excellent outcome given the many substantial health benefits and the general low risk associated with participation in physical activity. The *PAR-Q+* is available in both a paper and online version (http://eparmedx.com/?page_id=75), and we encourage you to print out a paper version for your records. In addition, we suggest that you complete both of the online versions of the *PAR-Q+* and the *ePARmed-X+* for experience. To understand how both of these questionnaires work, you should respond "yes" to one question in both sections of the *PAR-Q+*.

The American College of Sports Medicine has also changed its approach to screening participants for physical activity based, in part, on the same concerns mentioned earlier for the PAR-Q+—excessive physician referrals (95). ACSM's previous screening process used the number of risk factors for cardiovascular disease (CVD), and the presence of signs or symptoms and/or known cardiovascular, metabolic, renal, and/or pulmonary diseases to establish risk classifications: low risk, moderate risk, and high risk. These risk classification were used to direct the individual to obtain a medical examination and/or exercise test prior to exercise participation. In contrast, the new ACSM exercise health screening process is based on (a) the individual's current level of physical activity, (b) presence of signs or symptoms, and/or known cardiovascular, metabolic, or renal disease, and (c) the desired exercise intensity. Figure 15.2 shows ACSM's new decision-making algorithm. The absence of risk factors from this model does not mean that information on CVD risk factors is not important. In fact, they state that identifying and controlling CVD risk factors is an important objective of overall cardiovascular and metabolic disease prevention and management (95); it is just not as important in screening participants for physical activity as was once believed. Further,

2015 PAR-Q+

The Physical Activity Readiness Questionnarie for Everyone

The health benefits of regular physical activity are clear; more people should engage in physical activity every day of the week. Participating in physical activity is very safe for MOST people. This questionnaire will tell you whether it is necessary for you to seek further advice from your doctor OR a qualified exercise professional before becoming more physically active.

GENERAL HEALTH QUESTIONS

Please read the seven questions below carefully and answer each one honestly: check YES or NO.	YES	NO
1) Has your doctor ever said that you have a heart condition ☐ OR high blood pressure ☐ ?	☐	☐
2) Do you feel pain in your chest at rest, during your daily activities of living, **OR** when you do physical activity?	☐	☐
3) Do you lose balance because of dizziness **OR** have you lost consciousness in the last 12 months? Please answer **NO** if your dizziness was associated with over breathing (including during vigorous exercise).	☐	☐
4) Have you ever been diagnosed with another chronic medical condition (other than heart disease or high blood pressure)? **PLEASE LIST CONDITION(S) HERE:** _____	☐	☐
5) Are you currently taking prescribed medications for a chronic medical condition? **PLEASE LIST CONDITION(S) AND MEDICATIONS HERE:** _____	☐	☐
6) Do you currently have (or have had within the past 12 months) a bone, joint, or soft tissue (muscle, ligament, or tenson) problem that could be made worse by becoming more physically active? Please answer **NO** if you had a problem in the past, but it *does not limit your current ability* to be physically active. **PLEASE LIST CONDITION(S) HERE:** _____	☐	☐
7) Has your doctor ever said that you should only do medically supervised physical activity?	☐	☐

☑ **If you answered NO to all of the questions above, you are cleared for physical activity. GO to Page 4 to sign the PARTICIPANT DECLARATION. You do not need to completed Pages 2 and 3.**

- ▶ Start becoming much more physically active – start slowly and build up gradually.
- ▶ Follow International Physical Activity Guidelines for your age (www.who.int/dietphysicalactivity/en/).
- ▶ You may take part in a health and fitness appraisal.
- ▶ If you are over the age of 45 years and **NOT** accustomed to regular vigorous to maximal effort exercise, consult a qualified exercise professional before engaging in this intensity of exercise.
- ▶ If you have any further questions, contact a qualified exercise professional.

⬤ **If you answered YES to one or more of the questions above, COMPLETE PAGES 2 AND 3.**

⚠ **Delay becoming more active it:**
- ✔ You have a temporary illness such a cold or fever; it is best to wait until you feel better.
- ✔ You are pregnant - talk to your healthcare practitioner, your physician, a qualified exercise professional, and/or complete the ePARmed-X+ at **www.eparmedx.com** before becoming more physically active.
- ✔ Your health changes - answer the questions on Pages 2 and 3 of this document and/or talk to your doctor or a qualified exercise professional before continuing with any physical activity program.

✝OSHF
Ontario Society for Health and Fitness

Copyright 2015 PAR-Q+ Collaboration
01-01-2015

Figure 15.1   Physical Activity Readiness Questionnaire for Everyone (PAR-Q+).

Warburton DER, Gledhill N, Jamnik VK, Bredin SSD, McKenzie DC, Stone J, Charlesworth S, Shephard RJ, on behalf of the PAR-Q+ Collaboration. The Physical Activity Readiness Questionnaire for Everyone (PAR-Q+) and electronic Physical Activity Readiness Medical Examination (ePARmed-X+): Summary of consensus panel recommendations. *Health & Fitness Journal of Canada* 2011;4:26-37. Reprinted with permission from the PAR-Q+ Collaboration and the authors of the PAR-Q+ (Dr. Darren Warburton, Dr. Norman Gledhill, Dr. Veronica Jamnik, Dr. Roy Shephard, and Dr. Shannon Bredin)..

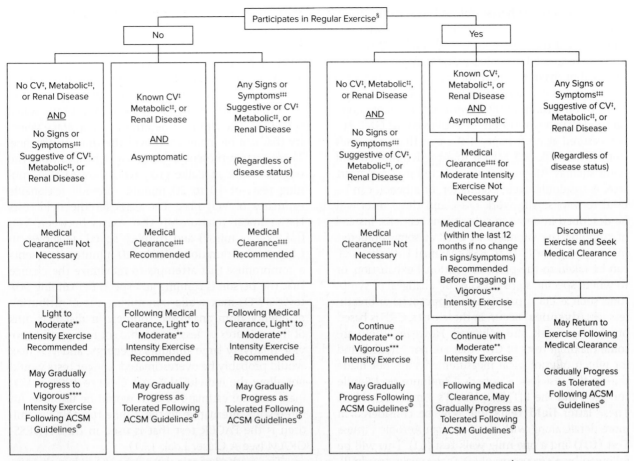

§Exercise participation, performing planned, structured physical activity at least 30 min at moderate intensity on at least 3 d·wk⁻¹ for at least the last 3 months.
*Light-intensity exercise, 30% to <40% HRR or $\dot{V}O_2R$, 2 to <3 METs, 9–11 RPE, an intensity that causes slight increases in HR and breathing.
**Moderate-intensity exercise, 40% to <60% HRR or $\dot{V}O_2R$, 3 to <6 METs, 12–13 RPE, an intensity that causes noticeable increases in HR and breathing.
***Vigorous-intensity exercise ≥60% HRR or $\dot{V}O_2R$, ≥6 METs, ≥14 RPE, an intensity that causes substantial increases in HR and breathing.
‡CVD, cardiac, peripheral vascular, or cerebrovascular disease.
‡‡Metabolic disease, type 1 and 2 diabetes mellitus.
‡‡‡Signs and symptoms, at rest or during activity; includes pain, discomfort in the chest, neck, jaw, arms, or other areas that may result from ischemia; shortness of breath at rest or with mild exertion; dizziness or syncope; orthopnea or paroxysmal nocturnal dyspnea; ankle edema; palpitations or tachycardia; intermittent claudication; known heart murmur; or unusual fatigue or shortness of breath with usual activities.
‡‡‡‡Medical clearance, approval from a health care professional to engage in exercise.
ΦACSM Guidelines, see *ACSM's Guidelines for Exercise Testing and Prescription, 9th edition*, 2014.

Figure 15.2 Exercise preparticipation health screening logic model for aerobic exercise participation.

instead of the screening process making a specific recommendation for an individual to have an exercise test or a medical examination, the new algorithm simply refers the individual to a health care professional to obtain medical clearance prior to participation. The aim is to reduce barriers to participation while addressing the risks to those with known or suspected chronic diseases.

The following provides some insights into how to interpret figure 15.2 (102):

■ Participants who have not been diagnosed with CV, metabolic, or renal disease and who don't have signs or symptoms of these diseases do not require medical clearance, whether they are current regular exercisers or not.

■ Participants with signs and symptoms indicative of CV, metabolic, or renal disease

are always recommended to receive medical clearance, regardless of their disease status or whether they are current regular exercisers.

■ Participants with established CV, metabolic, or renal disease and who are asymptomatic need medical clearance prior to exercise participation if they are not regular exercisers. In contrast, participants with these same characteristics, but who are regular exercisers, only need medical clearance if they plan to pursue vigorous intensity aerobic exercise.

Resting and Exercise Measures

Following the screening, measurements of heart rate and blood pressure are taken at rest prior to the exercise test. Additional measurements, such as a blood sample for serum cholesterol and an electrocardiogram (ECG), may also be obtained, with the latter one a necessity if the GXT is to be a diagnostic test. The exercise tests used to evaluate CRF may require a submaximal or maximal effort by the subject. They may be conducted in a lab containing sophisticated equipment or on a running track with nothing more complicated than a stopwatch. In a submaximal GXT, HR is measured at each stage of the test that progresses from light work (<3 METs) to a predetermined end point such as 70% to 85% of predicted maximal heart rate. A treadmill, cycle ergometer, or a bench can be used to impose the work rates, and these tests will be described in detail in subsequent sections. Instead of stopping the submaximal GXT at some predetermined end point (70% to 85% maximal HR), the GXT can be taken to the point of volitional exhaustion, or to where specific signs (ECG or BP changes) or symptoms such as chest pain (**angina pectoris**) or breathlessness (**dyspnea**) occur. In these cases, CRF is based on the last work rate achieved. However, there are some maximal tests of CRF that are not "graded" and for which physiological measurements are not made during the test [e.g., Cooper's 12-minute or 1.5-mile run (26), and the FITNESSGRAM's 1-mile run (114)]. These latter **field tests** will now be considered in more detail, along with the Canadian Aerobic Fitness Test (101) and a one-mile walk test (61). This will be followed by a discussion of GXTs using the treadmill, cycle ergometer, and bench step.

IN SUMMARY

- The steps to follow before conducting an exercise test to evaluate CRF include the following:
- Review the health history for known diseases, signs and symptoms, and risk factors.
- Stratify the level of risk.
- Determine the type of test and level of supervision needed.

FIELD TESTS FOR ESTIMATING CRF

Maximal Run Tests

Some field tests for CRF involve a measurement of how far a person can run in a set time (12 to 15 minutes) or how fast a person can run a set distance (1 to 2 miles). The advantages of such field tests include their moderately high correlation with $\dot{V}O_2$ max, the use of a natural activity, the large numbers of people who can be tested at one time, and the low cost. The disadvantages of using field tests include the difficulty of monitoring physiological responses,

the importance that motivation plays in the outcome, and the fact that the test is not graded but is a maximal effort. These field tests should be used only after a person has progressed through a program of exercise at lower intensities. The most popular field test for adults is Cooper's 12-minute or 1.5-mile run (26), and for school children, the FITNESSGRAM's 1-mile walk/run (114). The aim is to determine the average velocity that can be maintained over the time or distance. These tests represent evolutionary changes from the original work of Balke (10), who showed that running tests of 10 to 20 minutes provide reasonable estimates of $\dot{V}O_2$ max. The basis for the field tests is the linear relationship that exists between $\dot{V}O_2$ $(ml \cdot kg^{-1} \cdot min^{-1})$ and running speed, as shown in Chap. 1. The duration of 10 to 20 minutes represents a compromise that attempts to maximize the chance that the person is running at a speed demanding 90% to 95% $\dot{V}O_2$ max while minimizing the contribution of energy from anaerobic sources. In distance runs of five minutes or less, anaerobic sources would provide relatively large amounts of energy, and $\dot{V}O_2$ max would probably be overestimated. Longer tests would not allow the individual to run close to 100% of $\dot{V}O_2$ max, and the estimate of CRF would be too low. An interesting alternative to the 1-mile run test for children is the PACER test that is used in the FITNESSGRAM (see A Closer Look 15.1).

The method of calculating the $\dot{V}O_2$ when the running speed is known was described in detail in A Closer Look 1.1, and the formula is presented here again:

$$\dot{V}O_2 = 0.2 \ ml \cdot kg^{-1} \cdot min^{-1}/m \cdot min^{-1} + 3.5 \ ml \cdot kg^{-1} \cdot min^{-1}$$

This formula provides reasonable estimates of $\dot{V}O_2$ max for adults, but would underestimate values for young children because of their relatively poor economy of running (31). On the other hand, this formula would overestimate the value for $\dot{V}O_2$ max for those who walk because the net cost of walking is half that of running (see A Closer Look 1.1):

$$\dot{V}O_2 = 0.1 \ ml \cdot kg^{-1} \cdot min^{-1} \ per \ m \cdot min^{-1} + 3.5 \ ml \cdot kg^{-1} \cdot min^{-1}$$

Although percentile rankings of $\dot{V}O_2$ max by age and sex are available (see Table 15.1), estimates of $\dot{V}O_2$ max based on distance runs are most useful when compared over time for the same individual rather than between individuals. Variation in economy of running, motivation, and other factors makes such comparisons of estimated $\dot{V}O_2$ max values between individuals unreasonable (6, 100). In this light, distance swim and bicycle riding tests provide useful information about changes in an individual's CRF over time, even though estimates of $\dot{V}O_2$ max are not available (25, 27).

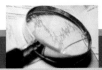

A CLOSER LOOK 15.1

Progressive Aerobic Cardiovascular Endurance Run (PACER)

An alternative test of aerobic fitness for schoolchildren is the Progressive Aerobic Cardiovascular Endurance Run, or PACER. The PACER test is part of the fitness testing battery in the FITNESSGRAM developed by the Cooper Institute (114). This test, developed by Léger et al. (65, 66), is a 20-meter shuttle run test done to the sound of a "beep" as the student moves between the boundary lines. The speed required at the start is 5.3 mph (8.5 km/hr), and it increases 0.3 mph (0.5 km/hr) each minute. Three rapid beeps signal progression to the next level, where the

time between beeps becomes shorter. The test is terminated when the student cannot keep up with the beeps, and the number of 20-meter laps completed is used to estimate aerobic fitness. Verbal feedback during the test appears to improve performance (77). In a recent study of a group of 10- to 15-year-old youth (98) $\dot{V}O_2$ max values measured on the PACER test were identical to those measured on a standard treadmill test. In addition, there were no differences in the maximal heart rate or RER values, lending additional validity to the PACER test as an

excellent indicator of CRF in children. Criterion-referenced standards for aerobic fitness (see A Closer Look 15.2) have been validated for this test (24).

This protocol has also been used as a field test to estimate $\dot{V}O_2$ max in adults (76, 107), with evidence that a practice test might be needed for improved reliability (64). In another version, called the square shuttle run test, subjects run around a 15-meter square in a gym. Based on directly measured $\dot{V}O_2$ during the run, it has been shown to have good validity and reliability when testing adults (37).

TABLE 15.1	Percentile Rankings for $\dot{V}O_2$ Max by Age and Gender											
	Men [Age Group (y)]						Women [Age Group (y)]					
Percentile	20–29	30–39	40–49	50–59	60–69	70–79	20–29	30–39	40–49	50–59	60–69	70–79
95	66.3	59.8	55.6	50.7	43.0	39.7	56.0	45.8	41.7	35.9	29.4	24.1
90	61.8	56.5	52.1	45.6	40.3	36.6	51.3	41.4	38.4	32.0	27.0	23.1
85	59.3	54.2	49.3	43.2	38.2	35.5	48.3	39.3	36.0	30.2	25.6	22.2
80	57.1	51.6	46.7	41.2	36.1	31.4	46.5	37.5	34.0	28.6	24.6	21.3
75	55.2	49.2	45.0	39.7	34.5	30.4	44.7	36.1	32.4	27.6	23.8	20.8
70	53.7	48.0	43.9	38.2	32.9	28.4	43.2	34.6	31.1	26.8	23.1	20.5
65	52.1	46.6	42.1	36.3	31.6	27.6	41.6	33.5	30.0	26.0	22.0	19.9
60	50.2	45.2	40.3	35.1	30.5	26.9	40.6	32.2	28.7	25.2	21.2	19.4
55	49.0	43.8	38.9	33.8	29.1	25.6	38.9	31.2	27.7	24.4	20.5	19.2
50	48.0	42.4	37.8	32.6	28.2	24.4	37.6	30.2	26.7	23.4	20.0	18.3
45	46.5	41.3	36.7	31.6	27.2	24.0	35.9	29.3	25.9	22.7	19.6	17.8
40	44.9	39.6	35.7	30.7	26.6	22.8	34.6	28.2	24.9	21.8	18.9	17.0
35	43.5	38.5	34.6	29.5	25.7	22.4	33.6	27.4	24.1	21.2	18.4	16.8
30	41.9	37.4	33.3	28.4	24.6	21.2	32.0	26.4	23.3	20.6	17.9	15.9
25	40.1	35.9	31.9	27.1	23.7	20.4	30.5	25.3	22.1	19.9	17.2	15.6
20	38.1	34.1	30.5	26.1	22.4	19.2	28.6	24.1	21.3	19.1	16.5	15.1
15	35.4	32.7	29.0	24.4	21.2	18.2	26.2	22.5	20.0	18.3	15.6	14.6
10	32.1	30.2	26.8	22.8	19.8	17.1	23.9	20.9	18.8	17.3	14.6	13.6
5	29.0	27.2	24.2	20.9	17.4	16.3	21.7	19.0	17.0	16.0	13.4	13.1

Values are in ml · kg⁻¹ · min⁻¹; M = men; W = women.

Fitness categories (percentile): Superior = 95; Excellent = 80–90; Good = 60–75; Fair = 40–55; Poor = 20–35; Very Poor = 5–15.

The formulas used for estimating $\dot{V}O_2$ max from a 12-minute run are not very useful for prepubescent children because their economy of running is less than that of an adult (31). Investigators (63) addressed this problem by testing first-, second-, and third-grade boys and girls with 800-, 1,200-, and 1,600-meter runs, and related performance to the measured $\dot{V}O_2$

max scores. They found the 1,600-meter run was the best predictor with good test/retest reliability (r = 0.82 to 0.92) in children who were given instruction on paced running (63). Although performance in a run test is obviously a function of $\dot{V}O_2$ max, both running economy and the ability to run at a high % $\dot{V}O_2$ max also play a role (13, 14). It has been shown in young

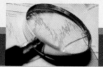
Cardiovascular Fitness Standards for Children

The best way to evaluate fitness in children has been a concern for educators and scientists for the past century (90). The most recent controversy has revolved around the question of what kind of standards to use in making judgments about a child's level of fitness. Normative standards such as percentile scores have traditionally been used to describe where a child stands relative to his or her peers. (e.g., 75th percentile). The current thinking, especially for health-related fitness tests (one-mile walk/run test and the skinfold test), is that criterion-reference standards might be more appropriate. Criterion-reference standards attempt to describe the minimum level of fitness consistent with good health, independent of what percentile that might be in a normative data set. For example, Blair (16) showed that in adults, $\dot{V}O_2$ max values associated with a low risk of disease were not that high; e.g., ≥ 35 ml $\cdot$ kg^{-1} $\cdot$ min^{-1} for men and ≥ 30 ml $\cdot$ kg^{-1} $\cdot$ min^{-1} for women 20 to 39 years of age. This information was used in setting the criterion-reference standards for the FITNESSGRAM, the fitness evaluation program developed by the Cooper Institute (114). $\dot{V}O_2$ max standards were set at 42 ml $\cdot$ kg^{-1} $\cdot$ min^{-1} for boys 5 to 17 years of age. For girls, the values were set at 40 ml $\cdot$ kg^{-1} $\cdot$ min^{-1} for ages 5 to 9 years of age, with a decrease of 1 ml $\cdot$ kg^{-1} $\cdot$ min^{-1} per year until age 14, where the 35 ml $\cdot$ kg^{-1} $\cdot$ min^{-1} value held until age 17 years. After the criterion-reference standards were set, the designers of the test had to translate those ml $\cdot$ kg^{-1} $\cdot$ min^{-1} values into equivalent one-mile run times–the actual test the children would take. The test designers had to consider the % $\dot{V}O_2$ max at which the children would perform during the run, and the fact that economy of running improves with age. These steps, although complicated, have led to standards that are now used nationwide to classify children as to whether they have a sufficient level of cardiorespiratory fitness consistent with a low risk of disease (30). A recent study (67) and a major review (22) confirmed the validity of the criterion-referenced standards. In addition, the FITNESSGRAM was shown to be valid and reliable when administered by teachers in a typical school setting (83). For those interested in the history of the FITNESSGRAM, see the article by Plowman et al. in Suggested Readings.

---

children of 6 to 11 years of age that % $\dot{V}O_2$ max is more closely related to performance of the 1-mile walk/run than is $\dot{V}O_2$ max (75). (See A Closer Look 15.2.)

$\dot{V}O_2$ max (ml $\cdot$ kg^{-1} $\cdot$ min^{-1}) estimated in an endurance run test is influenced by cardiovascular function and body fatness. It has been shown that differences in estimated $\dot{V}O_2$ max values between males and females can be explained, in part, by differences in % body fat (28, 31, 104). In a 12-minute run test, performance was decreased 89 meters when body weight was experimentally increased to simulate an additional 5% fat (29). One should expect, then, that with a combined exercise and weight reduction program, CRF assessed using a running test will increase due to both an increase in cardiovascular function and a decrease in % body fat. In Table 15.1, categories for $\dot{V}O_2$ max values are adjusted for age due to the observation that in the general population $\dot{V}O_2$ max decreases with age. However, studies (111) have shown that $\dot{V}O_2$ max does not decrease as fast in males who maintain their physical activity program and body weight. This observation provides additional rationale for a regular evaluation of CRF to keep track of small changes before they become big changes.

Walk Tests

An alternative to the maximal run tests used to evaluate CRF is a one-mile walk test in which the HR is monitored during the test (61). The equation used to predict $\dot{V}O_2$ max was based on one population of men and women, aged 30 to 69, and was then validated on another comparable population. The subject walks as fast as possible for one mile on a flat, measured track, and HR is measured at the end of the last lap. The following equation can be used to estimate $\dot{V}O_2$ max (ml $\cdot$ kg^{-1} $\cdot$ min^{-1}):

$$\dot{V}O_2 \text{ max} = 132.853 - 0.0769 \text{ (wt)} \\ - 0.3877 \text{ (age)} + 6.315 \text{ (sex)} \\ - 3.2649 \text{ (time)} - 0.1565 \text{ (HR)}$$

where (wt) is body weight in pounds, (age) is in years, (sex) equals 0 for female and 1 for male, (time) is in minutes and hundredths of minutes, and (HR) is in beats $\cdot$ min^{-1} measured at the end of the last quarter-mile.

Let's calculate the CRF of a 25-year-old man who weighs 170 lb (77.1 kg) and who walked the mile in 20.0 minutes with a postexercise HR of 140 b $\cdot$ min^{-1}.

$$\dot{V}O_2 \text{ max} = 132.853 - 0.0769 \text{ (170)} \\ - 0.3877 \text{ (25)} + 6.315 \text{ (1)} \\ - 3.2649 \text{ (20.0)} - 0.1565 \text{ (140)} \\ = 29.2 \text{ ml} \cdot \text{kg}^{-1} \cdot \text{min}^{-1}.$$

This man's CRF lies between the 5th and 10th percentile (see Table 15.1), indicating a need for additional exercise to improve CRF (see Chap. 16 for details on how to go about this).

This test appears to fill a void in the field tests available to estimate $\dot{V}O_2$ max because it uses a common activity and requires the simple measurement of HR. As a participant's fitness improves, the time required for

TABLE 15.2A	Starting Stage for Men and Women of Different Age Groups for the Modified Canadian Aerobic Fitness Test	
	STARTING STAGE	
Age Group (Year)	Males	Females
15–19	4	3
20–29	4	3
30–39	3	3
40–49	3	2
50–59	2	1
60–69	1	1

TABLE 15.2B	Stepping Cadence and Oxygen Cost of Each Stage for the Modified Canadian Aerobic Fitness Test (mCAFT) for Men and Women			
mCAFT Stage Completed	**FEMALES**		**MALES**	
	Stepping Cadence	O_2 Cost	Stepping Cadence	O_2 Cost
1	66	15.9	66	15.9
2	84	18.0	84	18.0
3	102	22.0	102	22.0
4	114	24.5	114	24.5
5	120	26.3	132	29.5
6	132	29.5	144	33.6
7	144	33.6	118*	36.2
8	118*	36.2	132*	40.1

*Single-step test. The O_2 cost is in $ml \cdot kg^{-1} \cdot min^{-1}$.
From the Canadian Society of Exercise Physiology.

the mile and/or the HR response decreases, increasing the estimated $\dot{V}O_2$ max. A similar study using a two-kilometer walk test supports this proposition (88).

Modified Canadian Aerobic Fitness Test

In contrast to the Cooper 1.5-mile run test and the one-mile walk test, which require an all-out effort, the Modified Canadian Aerobic Fitness Test (mCAFT) is a submaximal step test that uses the lowest two eight-inch (20 cm) steps found in a conventional staircase (101). The six-count stepping cadence in this test is maintained by a recording. Prior to the test, the person completes the PAR-Q+ to determine if he or she should proceed. The original CAFT (101) was modified in 1993 to improve its reliability and the test's estimate of $\dot{V}O_2$ max, especially for fit subjects (115, 116). The first three-minute stage of the mCAFT

is based on the age of the subject (see Table 15.2a), with each stage having a specified cadence (steps/min) for males and females (see Table 15.2b). Note that stages were added to the original test to address the need to challenge the most fit subjects. The subject steps for three minutes at the specified step rate, and an immediate post exercise ten-second pulse rate is measured. The subject continues on through the stages of the test until the pulse rate is close to 85% of age-predicted maximal heart rate (220 − age). $\dot{V}O_2$ max can be estimated from these results using the following equation (20):

$$\text{Estimated } \dot{V}O_2 \text{ max} = 17.2 + (1.29 \times \dot{V}O_2) - (0.09 \times \text{Mass}) - (0.18 \times \text{Age})$$

where $\dot{V}O_2$ = energy cost of the final stage in ml (see Table 15.2b), mass is in kilograms, and age is in years.

For example, if a 30 year old woman, who weighs 130 lbs (59.0 kg), completes stage 5 of the mCAFT, her estimated $\dot{V}O_2$ max would be:

$$\dot{V}O_2 \text{ max} = 17.2 + (1.29 \times 26.5) - (0.09 \times 59) - (0.18 \times 30) = 40.4 \text{ ml} \cdot kg^{-1} \cdot min^{-1}.$$

This woman's CRF lies between the 85th and 90th percentile, indicating an excellent value (see Table 15.1).

IN SUMMARY

- Field tests for CRF use natural activities such as walking, running, and stepping, in which large numbers of people can be tested at low cost. However, for some, physiological responses are difficult to measure, and motivation plays an important role in the outcome.
- $\dot{V}O_2$ max estimates from all-out run tests are based on the linear relationship between running speed and the oxygen cost of running.
- The Modified Canadian Aerobic Fitness Test is a step test that uses conventional eight-inch steps to evaluate cardiorespiratory fitness.
- Criterion-referenced standards for $\dot{V}O_2$ max are available. They are preferable to percentile rankings because they focus attention on health-related goals rather than comparisons with others.

GRADED EXERCISE TESTS: MEASUREMENTS

Cardiorespiratory fitness is commonly measured using a treadmill, a cycle ergometer, or a stepping bench. These tests are usually incremental, in which the work rate changes every two to three minutes until the subject reaches some predetermined end point or when some pathological sign or symptom occurs. These GXTs can be maximal or submaximal, and the variables measured during the test can be as simple as HR and BP, or as complex as $\dot{V}O_2$; it depends on the purpose of the test and the facilities, equipment, and personnel involved (50). What follows is a brief summary of common measurements made during a GXT.

Heart Rate

Heart rate can be measured by palpation of the radial or carotid artery, using surface electrodes that transmit the signal to an electrocardiograph, or using a heart watch. In palpating the carotid artery, care must be taken not to use too much pressure because this could slow the HR by way of the baroreceptor reflex. However, when people are trained in this procedure, reliable measurements can be obtained (89, 99). Heart rate is measured over a 15- to 30-second time period *during* steady-state exercise to obtain a reliable estimate of the HR. If using a *post exercise* HR as an indication of the HR during exercise, the HR should be measured for ten seconds within the first 15 seconds after stopping exercise because the HR changes rapidly at this time. The ten-second count is multiplied by 6 to express the HR in beats · min⁻¹ (99).

Blood Pressure

Blood pressure is measured by auscultation as described in Chap. 9. It is important to use the proper cuff size and a sensitive stethoscope to obtain accurate values at rest and during exercise. In addition, if using an aneroid sphygmomanometer, it is important to calibrate it on a regular basis against the mercury sphygmomanometer (59). During the walking or cycling exercise test (BP cannot be reliably measured during a running test), the microphone of the stethoscope is placed below the cuff and over an area where the sound is the loudest (in many cases, this will be over the brachial artery in the intramuscular space on the medial side of the arm). The subject should not be holding onto the handlebar of the cycle or the railings of the treadmill during the measurement. The first Korotkoff sound is taken as systolic BP, and the fourth sound (change in tone or muffling) is taken as diastolic BP (92).

ECG

GXTs are used to diagnose CHD because exercise causes the heart to work harder and challenges the coronary arteries' ability to deliver sufficient blood to meet the oxygen demand of the myocardium. An estimate of the work (and O_2 demand) of the heart is the **double product**–the product of the HR and the systolic BP (60, 86). As you already know, HR and systolic BP increase with exercise intensity such that myocardial oxygen demand increases throughout the test. The electrocardiogram (ECG) is used as an indicator of the ability of the heart to function normally during these times of imposed work. During exercise, the ECG can be measured with a single bipolar lead (e.g., CM₅), but a full 12-lead arrangement is preferred (2). The ECG is evaluated for arrhythmias, conduction disturbances, and myocardial ischemia. **Arrhythmias** are irregularities in the normal electrical rhythm of the heart that can be localized to the atria (e.g., atrial fibrillation), the AV node (e.g., premature junctional contraction), or in the ventricles (e.g., premature ventricular contractions–PVCs). **Conduction disturbances** describe a defect in which depolarization is slowed or completely blocked (e.g., first-degree AV block or bundle branch block). **Myocardial ischemia** is defined as an inadequate perfusion of the myocardium relative to the metabolic demand of the heart. Because oxygen uptake by the myocardium is almost completely flow dependent, a flow limitation causes an oxygen insufficiency. A *symptom* of myocardial ischemia is angina pectoris, which is pain or discomfort caused by a temporary ischemia; the pain could be located in the center of the chest, neck, jaw, or shoulders, or could radiate to the arms and hands (12). However, angina symptoms in women may include nausea, breathlessness, abdominal pain, or extreme fatigue. A *sign* associated with myocardial ischemia is a depression of the ST segment **(ST segment depression)** on the electrocardiogram (see Chap. 9). Interested readers are referred to Dubin's introductory text on ECG analysis (see Suggested Readings) and Ellestad's text on exercise electrocardiography (33).

Rating of Perceived Exertion

Another common measurement made at each stage of the GXT is Borg's (17) Rating of Perceived Exertion (RPE). Table 15.3 lists his original and revised scales. The original scale used the rankings 6 to 20 to approximate the HR values from rest to maximum (60–200). The revised scale represents an attempt to provide a ratio scale of the RPE values. The RPE scores can be used as indicators of subjective effort and provide a quantitative way to track a person's progress through a GXT or an exercise session (21, 23, 43). This is helpful in knowing when a subject is approaching exhaustion, and the values can be used to predict $\dot{V}O_2$ max (34) and prescribe exercise intensity (see Chap. 16). However, large between-subject variability in RPE ratings has been noted at the same heart rate, suggesting caution in using the scales (2). What follows is a suggested statement from the

TABLE 15.3 Rating of Perceived Exertion Scales	
Original Rating Scale	Revised Rating Scale
6	0 Nothing at all
7 Very, very light	0.5 Very, very light (just noticeable)
8	1 Very light
9 Very light	2 Light (weak)
10	3 Moderate
11 Fairly light	4 Somewhat hard
12	5 Heavy (strong)
13 Somewhat hard	6
14	7 Very heavy
15 Hard	8
16	9
17 Very hard	10 Very, very heavy (almost max)
18	• Maximal
19 Very, very hard	
20	

Indianapolis, IN: American College of Sports Medicine, 1982, reference 17.

ACSM Guidelines to read to the subject before testing (3) (p. 78):

> During the exercise test we want you to pay close attention to how hard you feel the exercise work rate is. This feeling should reflect your total amount of exertion and fatigue, combining all sensations and feelings of physical stress, effort, and fatigue. Don't concern yourself with any one factor such as leg pain, shortness of breath, or exercise intensity, but try to concentrate on your total, inner feeling of exertion. Try not to underestimate or overestimate your feeling of exertion; be as accurate as you can.

Termination Criteria

The reasons for stopping a GXT vary with the type of population being tested and the purpose of the test. Table 15.4, from the *ACSM's Guidelines for Exercise Testing and Prescription,* is appropriate for nondiagnostic GXTs in apparently healthy adults (2).

IN SUMMARY

- Typical measurements obtained during a GXT include heart rate, blood pressure, ECG, and rating of perceived exertion.
- Specific signs (e.g., fall in systolic pressure with an increase in work rate) and symptoms (e.g., dizziness) are used to stop GXTs.

$\dot{V}O_2$ MAX

The measurement of $\dot{V}O_2$ max represents the standard against which any estimate of CRF is compared. In fact, a recent policy statement from the AHA emphasized the importance of both measuring $\dot{V}O_2$ max and developing a national database of $\dot{V}O_2$ max values, across age and sex, with which to compare individuals (56). Table 15.1 in this chapter represents the achievement of the latter goal (57). As described in Chap. 4, $\dot{V}O_2$ increases with increasing loads on a GXT until the maximal capacity of the cardiorespiratory system is reached; attention to detail is crucial if one is to obtain accurate values (73). The primary criterion for having achieved a true $\dot{V}O_2$ max is that the $\dot{V}O_2$ fails to increase when the workload is increased—yielding a plateau in the $\dot{V}O_2$ (49, 109). However, a plateau is observed in only about 50% of healthy adult subjects. As a result, a number of secondary criteria were developed to provide some objective evidence

TABLE 15.4 General Indications for Stopping an Exercise Test in Low-Risk Adults*
• Onset of angina or angina-like symptoms
• Drop in systolic blood pressure (SBP) of >10 mm Hg with an increase in work rate or if SBP decreases below the value obtained in the same position prior to testing
• Excessive rise in blood pressure: systolic pressure >250 mm Hg and/or diastolic pressure >115 mm Hg
• Shortness of breath, wheezing, leg cramps, or claudication
• Signs of poor perfusion: light headedness, confusion, ataxia, pallor, cyanosis, nausea, or cold and clammy skin
• Failure of heart rate to increase with increased exercise intensity
• Noticeable change in heart rhythm by palpation or auscultation
• Subject requests to stop
• Physical or verbal manifestations of severe fatigue
• Failure of the testing equipment

*Assumes that testing is nondiagnostic and is being performed without direct physician involvement or ECG monitoring.

From American College of Sports Medicine. *ACSM's Guidelines for Exercise Testing and Prescription.* Baltimore, MD: Lippincott Williams & Wilkins, 2014.

that the highest $\dot{V}O_2$ measured was $\dot{V}O_2$ max. These secondary criteria included:

- A post exercise blood lactate concentration of >8 mmoles. L^{-1} (5)
- An R exceeding 1.15 (54)

All of the secondary criteria were developed using discontinuous GXT protocols using predominately healthy adult males as subjects. In a discontinuous GXT, the subject completes only one stage of the test and then returns to the lab hours or days later to do the next stage. Perhaps it is not surprising that when these secondary criteria are applied to the typical continuous GXT protocols in which all stages are completed in one visit to the lab and across diverse populations, their usefulness is called into question (78, 79, 93). Although many subjects will meet these secondary criteria (32), some, especially the elderly (103), children (5), and postcoronary subjects (58), will not. In addition, one should not expect a subject to meet all of these standards (58, 103). For example, in one study (103), 20% of the women subjects who met the "leveling off" criterion did not even achieve an R of 1.00! The R values have been shown to vary with age and the training status of the subjects (1). In general, these criteria are useful because they give the investigator an objective indicator of the subject's effort. However, subjects should not be expected to meet all the criteria on any single test (32, 51). Some investigators use heart rate (e.g., a value within 10 b/min of age-predicted maximal heart rate) as a criterion for having achieved $\dot{V}O_2$ max. However, due to the relatively large potential error (1 SD = 10-12 b/min) in estimating maximal heart rate with the age-predicted formulas (e.g., 220 − age), there is little or no support for its use as a criterion for having achieved $\dot{V}O_2$ max (51). Given the concerns raised about the secondary criteria, there has been a renewed focus (39, 46, 78) on the primary variable–verification of the $\dot{V}O_2$ max value on the same test day (see A Closer Look 4.2 for more on this).

$\dot{V}O_2$ max is a very reproducible measure on subjects tested with the same test protocol on the same piece of equipment. The value for $\dot{V}O_2$ max does not seem to be dependent on whether the test is a continuous GXT or a discontinuous GXT, as long as it is conducted with the same work instrument (32, 35, 72, 106). However, when $\dot{V}O_2$ max values are compared across protocols, some systematic differences appear (9). The highest value for $\dot{V}O_2$ max is usually measured with a running test up a grade on a treadmill, followed by a walking test up a grade on a treadmill, and then on a cycle ergometer. In American populations, walk test protocols yield values about 6% lower than those for a run test (72), while cycle test protocols yield values about 10% to 11% lower than those for a run test (32, 36, 62). Europeans show only

a 5% to 7% difference in this latter comparison (9, 48). An arm ergometer test will yield values equal to about 70% of the $\dot{V}O_2$ max measured with the legs (40, 97). It is important to recognize these differences when comparing one test to another, or when comparing the same subject over time with different modes of exercise. These differences among tests have led to the convention to call $\dot{V}O_2$ *max* the value measured on a graded running test; $\dot{V}O_2$ *peak* is the term used to describe the highest $\dot{V}O_2$ achieved on walk, cycle, or arm ergometer protocol (96). However, these terms can cause confusion when applied to highly trained athletes, such as cyclists, because they have higher $\dot{V}O_2$ max values when measured on a cycle, compared to a treadmill (108). The actual measurement of $\dot{V}O_2$ max is crucial for research studies and in some clinical settings. However, it is unreasonable to expect the actual measurement of $\dot{V}O_2$ max to be used as the CRF standard in fitness programs.

Estimation of $\dot{V}O_2$ Max from Last Work Rate

Given the complexity and cost of the procedures involved in the measurement of $\dot{V}O_2$ max, it is no surprise that in many fitness and clinical settings, $\dot{V}O_2$ max is estimated with equations that allow the calculation of $\dot{V}O_2$ max from the last work rate achieved on the GXT. The equations for estimating the oxygen cost of running and walking outlined in Chap. 1 allow such calculations and, in general, the estimates are reasonable (81, 82). What is important in the use of these equations is that the work test is suited to the individual. If the increments in the GXT from one stage to the next are too large relative to a person's CRF, or if the time for each stage is so short that a person might not be able to achieve the steady-state oxygen requirement for that stage, then the equations will overestimate the person's $\dot{V}O_2$ max (38, 45, 81). As described in Chap. 4, poorly fit individuals take longer to achieve the steady state at moderate to heavy work rates, and this increases the chance of an overestimation of $\dot{V}O_2$ max when using these formulas. This suggests that a more conservative protocol be used for low-fit individuals to allow them to reach a steady state at each stage. A recommended procedure is to use only the last completed stage of a test. However, independent of the proper matching of the protocol with the individual, it must be remembered that these are only estimations (see A Closer Look 15.3).

Estimation of $\dot{V}O_2$ Max from Submaximal HR Response

Another common procedure used with GXT protocols is to estimate $\dot{V}O_2$ max on the basis of the subject's HR response to a variety of submaximal work

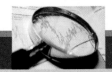

A CLOSER LOOK 15.3

Error in Estimating V̇O₂ Max

It is important to remember that the estimation of V̇O₂ max by any of the methods described in this chapter is associated with an inherent "error" compared to the directly measured V̇O₂ max value. When investigators try to determine the validity of an exercise test to estimate V̇O₂ max, they must first test large numbers of subjects in the laboratory to actually measure each subject's V̇O₂ max. On another day, the investigators may have the subjects complete a distance run for time, or a standardized graded treadmill or cycle ergometer test to determine the highest percent grade/speed or work rate that the subject can achieve. That information is then used to develop an equation to predict the measured V̇O₂ max value from the time of the distance run, the last grade/speed achieved on a

treadmill test, or the final work rate on the cycle ergometer test.

The predicted value will not usually equal the measured V̇O₂ max value, and a term called the standard error (SE) is used to describe how far off (higher or lower) the predicted value might be from the true value when using the prediction equation. One standard error (±SE) describes where 68% of the estimates are compared to the true value. If the SE were ±1 ml · kg⁻¹ · min⁻¹, then 68% of the predicted V̇O₂ max values would fall within ±1 ml · kg⁻¹ · min⁻¹ of the true value. Typically, the SE is larger than that (2, 92). For example:

- If V̇O₂ max is estimated from the last stage of a maximal test, the SE = ±3 ml · kg⁻¹ · min⁻¹.

- If V̇O₂ max is estimated from heart rate values measured during a submaximal test, the SE = ±4-5 ml · kg⁻¹ · min⁻¹.

- If V̇O₂ max is estimated from the 1-mile walk test or the 12-minute run test described earlier, the SE = ±5 ml · kg⁻¹ · min⁻¹.

The relatively large standard errors might suggest that these tests have little value, but that is not the case. The tests are reliable, and when the same individual takes the same test over time, the change in estimated V̇O₂ max monitored by the test is a reasonable reflection of improvements in cardiorespiratory fitness. This can serve as both a motivational and educational tool when working with fitness clients.

---

rates (42). In these tests, the HR is plotted against work rate (or estimated V̇O₂) until the termination criterion of 70% to 85% of age-predicted maximal HR is reached. Figure 15.3 shows the HR response for a 20-year-old who has completed a submaximal GXT on a cycle ergometer. Heart rate was measured at each work rate until a value equal to 85% of estimated maximal HR was reached (170 b · min⁻¹). A line was

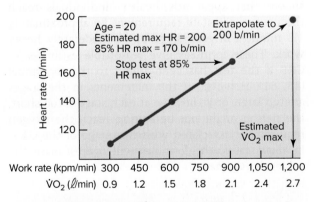

Figure 15.3 Estimation of V̇O₂ max from heart rate values measured during a series of submaximal work rates on a cycle ergometer. The test was stopped when the subject reached 85% of maximal HR. A line is drawn through the HR points measured during the test and is extrapolated to the age-predicted estimate of maximal HR. Another line is dropped from that point to the x-axis, and the V̇O₂ max is identified.

drawn through the HR points and extrapolated to the estimated maximal HR, which is calculated by subtracting age from 220. Another line is dropped from that point to the x-axis, and the work rate or V̇O₂ (in this case, 2.7 L · min⁻¹) that would have been achieved if the individual had worked until maximal HR was reached is recorded (42). Although this is a simple and commonly used procedure to estimate V̇O₂ max, it has several potential problems.

The first problem relates to the formula used for estimating the maximal HR. These estimates have a standard deviation (SD) of about ±11 b · min⁻¹ (68). A 20-year-old's maximal HR might be estimated to be 200 b · min⁻¹, but if a person were at ±2 SD, the value would be 178 or 222 b · min⁻¹. For those who do maximal testing, one will occasionally observe subjects having *measured* maximal HRs ±20 b · min⁻¹ away from their age-predicted estimate of maximal heart rate. Taking this as an example, what if the subject in Figure 15.3 had a true measured maximal HR of only 180 b · min⁻¹ instead of the estimated 200 b · min⁻¹? The estimated V̇O₂ max would be an overestimation of the correct value.

Further, a submaximal end point, such as 85% of estimated maximal heart rate, may be very light work for one person but maximal work for another. The reason for this is related to the estimate of maximal heart rate (220 – age) mentioned earlier. If a 30-year-old has a real maximum heart rate of 160 b min⁻¹ and the GXT takes the person to 85% of estimated maximal HR ($220 - 30 = 190$; 85% of $190 = 161$ b $\cdot$ min^{-1}), then the person would be taken to maximal HR.

Another problem with submaximal GXT protocols using the HR response as the primary indicator of fitness is that any variable that affects submaximal heart rate will affect the slope of the HR/$\dot{V}O_2$ line and, of course, the estimate of $\dot{V}O_2$ max. These variables include eating prior to the test, dehydration, elevated body temperature, temperature and humidity of the testing area, emotional state of the subject, medications that affect HR, and previous physical activity (7, 100). Clearly, many environmental variables must be controlled if one is to use such protocols to estimate $\dot{V}O_2$ max.

Despite these problems, this estimate of $\dot{V}O_2$ max is useful in providing appropriate feedback to participants in fitness programs. Following training, the HR response to any fixed submaximal work rate is lower, suggesting an increase in $\dot{V}O_2$ max when the HR/$\dot{V}O_2$ line is drawn through those HR points to the age-predicted maximal HR. In this case, because the same individual is being tested over time, the $220 -$ age formula introduces only a constant and unknown error that will not affect the projection of the HR/$\dot{V}O_2$ line. Further, the low cost, ease of measurement, and high reliability make it a good test that can be used for education and motivation.

IN SUMMARY

- The measurement of $\dot{V}O_2$ max is the gold standard measure of cardiorespiratory fitness.
- $\dot{V}O_2$ max can be estimated based on the final work rate achieved in a graded exercise test.
- $\dot{V}O_2$ max can be estimated from heart rate responses to submaximal exercise by extrapolating the relationship to the subject's age-predicted estimate of maximal heart rate. Careful attention to environmental factors that can affect the heart rate response to submaximal exercise is an important aspect of the procedures for these tests.

GRADED EXERCISE TEST PROTOCOLS

The GXT protocols can be either submaximal or maximal, depending on the end points used to stop the test. The choice of the GXT should be based on the population (athletes, cardiac patients, children), purpose (estimate CRF, measure $\dot{V}O_2$ max, diagnose CHD), and cost (equipment and personnel) (50, 53). This section will discuss the selection of the test based on these factors and provide examples of common GXT protocols.

When choosing a GXT protocol, the population being tested must be considered, given that the last stage in a GXT for cardiac patients might not even be a warm-up for a young, athletic subject. Test protocols should vary in terms of the initial work rate, how large the increment in work rate will be between stages, and the duration of each stage. In general, the GXT for a sedentary subject might start at 2 to 3 METs (1 MET = 3.5 ml $\cdot$ kg^{-1} $\cdot$ min^{-1}) and progress at about 1 MET per stage, with each stage lasting two to three minutes to allow enough time for a steady state to be reached. For young, active subjects, the initial work rate might be 5 METs, with increments of 2 to 3 METs per stage (92). Table 15.5 shows four well-known treadmill protocols and the populations for which they are suited. The National Exercise and Heart Disease protocol (85) is usually used with poorly fit subjects, with the work rate increasing only 1 MET each three minutes. The Standard Balke protocol (11) starts at about 4 METs and progresses 1 MET each two minutes, and is suitable for most average sedentary adults. The Bruce protocol for young, active subjects (19) starts at about 5 METs and progresses at 2 to 3 METs per stage. This protocol includes walking and running up a grade, and may not be suitable for those at the low end of the fitness continuum. The last protocol shown is used by the fit and athletic populations, with the speed (e.g., 7 or 10 mph) dependent on the fitness of the subject (7).

As mentioned earlier, one of the most common approaches used in estimating $\dot{V}O_2$ max is to take the final stage in the test and apply the formula for converting grade and speed to $\dot{V}O_2$ in ml $\cdot$ kg^{-1} $\cdot$ min^{-1}. Nagle et al. (84) and Montoye et al. (81) have shown that apparently healthy individuals reach the new steady-state requirement by approximately 1.5 minutes of each stage up to moderately heavy work. These formulas give reasonable estimates of CRF if the test has been suited to the individual (45, 81). However, if the increments in the stages are too large, or if the time at each stage is too short, the person might not be able to reach the oxygen requirement associated with that stage of the GXT. In these cases, the formulas will overestimate the subject's $\dot{V}O_2$ max.

IN SUMMARY

- When selecting a GXT, the population being tested must be considered. The initial work rate and the rate of change of work rate need to accommodate the capabilities of the population.

TABLE 15.5 Treadmill Protocols

A—NATIONAL EXERCISE AND HEART DISEASE PROTOCOL FOR POORLY FIT SUBJECTS (84)

Stage*	METs	Speed (mph)	% Grade
1	2.5	2	0
2	3.5	2	3.5
3	4.5	2	7.0
4	5.5	2	10.5
5	6.5	2	14.0
6	7.5	2	17.5
7	8.5	3	12.5
8	9.5	3	15.0
9	10.5	3	17.5

*Stage lasts three minutes.

B—STANDARD BALKE PROTOCOL FOR NORMAL SEDENTARY SUBJECTS (11)

Stage*	METs	Speed (mph)	% Grade
1	4.3	3	2.5
2	5.4	3	5.0
3	6.4	3	7.5
4	7.4	3	10.0
5	8.5	3	12.5
6	9.5	3	15.0
7	10.5	3	17.5
8	11.6	3	20.0
9	12.6	3	22.5

*Stage lasts two minutes.

C—BRUCE PROTOCOL FOR YOUNG, ACTIVE SUBJECTS (19)

Stage*	METs	Speed (mph)	% Grade
1	5	1.7	10
2	7	2.5	12
3	9.5	3.4	14
4	13	4.2	16
5	16	5.0	18

*Stage lasts three minutes.

D—ÅSTRAND AND RODAHL PROTOCOL FOR VERY FIT SUBJECTS (7)

Stage*	METs	Speed (mph)	% Grade
1	12.9/18	7/10	2.5
2	14.1/19.8	7/10	5.0
3	15.3/21.5	7/10	7.5
4	16.5/23.2	7/10	10.0
5	17.7/24.9	7/10	12.5

*Stage lasts two minutes; vigorous warm-up precedes test.

Treadmill

Treadmill GXT protocols can accommodate most people, from those least fit to those most fit, and use the natural activities of walking and running. Treadmills set the pace for the subject and provide the greatest potential load on the cardiovascular system. However, they are expensive, not portable, and make some measurements (BP and blood sampling) difficult (100). As mentioned previously, the type of treadmill test does influence the magnitude of the measured $\dot{V}O_2$ max, with the graded running test giving the highest value, the running test at 0% grade the next highest, and the walking test protocols the lowest (9, 72). There are also some limitations in the types of measurements that can be made, depending on whether walking or running is used. For example, during running tests, the measurement of BP is not convenient and may be less accurate, and there is more potential for artifact in the ECG tracing.

For estimates of $\dot{V}O_2$ to be obtained from grade and speed considerations, the grade and speed settings must be correct (50). In addition, the subject must follow instructions carefully and not hold onto the treadmill railing during the test. If this is not done, estimates of $\dot{V}O_2$ max based on either the HR/$\dot{V}O_2$ extrapolation procedure or the formula that uses the last speed/grade combination achieved will not be accurate (6, 94). For example, when a subject who was walking on a treadmill at 3.4 mph and 14% grade held onto the railing, the HR decreased 17 b · min^{-1} (6). This would result in an overestimation of the $\dot{V}O_2$ max using either of the submaximal procedures just mentioned, and special equations would have to be developed if holding onto the handrail were allowed (74). Finally, with the treadmill, there is no need to make adjustments to the $\dot{V}O_2$ calculation due to differences in body weight. Treadmill tests require the subject to carry his or her own weight, and the $\dot{V}O_2$ is therefore proportional to body weight (80).

In the following example of a submaximal GXT, a 45-year-old male completes a Balke Standard Protocol (3 mph, 2.5% each two minutes), and the test is terminated at 85% of age-predicted maximal HR (149 b · min^{-1}). Heart rate was measured in the last 30 seconds of each stage, and $\dot{V}O_2$ max was estimated by the HR/$\dot{V}O_2$ extrapolation to age-predicted maximal HR (175 b · min^{-1}). Figure 15.4 shows the plot of the HR response at each stage and the extrapolation to the person's estimated maximal heart rate. In the early stages of the test, the HR did not increase in a predictable manner with increasing grade. This may be due to the changes in stroke volume that occur early in upright work (see Chap. 9). The beginning stages also act as a warm-up and adjustment period for the subject. The HR response is usually quite linear, between 110 b · min^{-1} and 85% maximal HR (8).

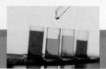
Bruno Balke, M.D., Ph.D.—The "Father" of ACSM Certification Programs

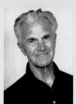

Courtesy of Monterey Bay Video Productions (MBVP)

As we mentioned in Chap. 0, the history of exercise physiology in the United States during the twentieth century had a very strong European flavor. This was certainly the case for the development of fitness testing and cardiac rehabilitation. **Dr. Bruno Balke** (1907-1999) received his training in physical education, medicine, and physiology in Germany and was invited to this country by Dr. Ulrich Luft in 1950.

During the 1950s, Dr. Balke conducted research on high-altitude tolerance and high-speed flight for the U.S. Air Force at the School of Aviation Medicine in San Antonio, Texas, and later, for the Federal Aviation Agency in Oklahoma City. His research on work-capacity testing on the treadmill led to the development of the exercise test protocols that bear his name

(discussed earlier in this chapter). In addition, his distance-run field test to evaluate cardiovascular fitness (maximal aerobic power) was modified by Dr. Ken Cooper for use in his well-known aerobics books (see "Field Tests for Estimating CRF" in this chapter).

Dr. Balke left government service in 1963 to create the Biodynamics Laboratory at the University of Wisconsin, Madison. Francis J. Nagle, Ph.D., whom he had worked with in Oklahoma City, followed in 1964, and both had joint appointments with the physical education and physiology departments. Dr. Balke's quantitative approach to exercise physiology questions, especially as they related to fitness and performance, set the standard for other graduate exercise physiology programs. He regarded his time in Madison as the most productive in his career.

Dr. Balke left Wisconsin for Aspen, Colorado, in 1973. During this time, he invested himself in the development of American College of Sports

Medicine (ACSM) certification programs for exercise leaders of fitness and cardiac rehabilitation programs. Special meetings were held in Aspen to develop the certification programs and *ACSM's Guidelines for Exercise Testing and Prescription*. The first workshops associated with these certification programs were held in Aspen as well. Many consider him the "father" of ACSM certification programs.

Dr. Balke was active in the early days of the ACSM and served as its president in 1966. Balke also took the lead in the creation of ACSM's research journal, then known as *Medicine and Science in Sports*, and was its first editor-in-chief. He enjoyed teaching others how to do things, and he viewed as his greatest accomplishment the graduation of the Ph.D. students from his lab who would now teach others. Dr. Balke died in 1999 at the age of 92, but his legacy will live on for years to come. For more on this interesting man, see his autobiography in Suggested Readings.

The HR/$\dot{V}O_2$ line is extrapolated to 175 b · min⁻¹, and a vertical line is dropped to the x-axis where the estimated $\dot{V}O_2$ max is identified: 11.6 METs, or 40.6 ml ·

kg⁻¹ · min⁻¹. In a recent study in which subjects ran on a treadmill at several submaximal speeds, the HR extrapolation method estimated $\dot{V}O_2$ max well using the ACSM equation for running (69).

Finally, investigators have adapted the one-mile walk test mentioned earlier under "field test" so it could be done on a treadmill. Subjects completed a questionnaire to rate their level of physical activity and then walked on the treadmill at a self-selected speed that they classified as "brisk." The investigators had to develop a new prediction equation, different from the outdoor test, and it was shown to provide a valid estimate of $\dot{V}O_2$ max (91). To learn more about an individual who had a major impact on fitness testing, see A Look Back–Important People in Science.

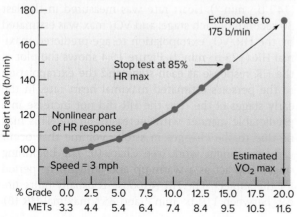

Figure 15.4 Estimation of $\dot{V}O_2$ max from the heart rate values measured during different stages of a treadmill test.

From Howley, E. T., and Franks, B. D., *Health/Fitness Instructor's Handbook*. Champaign, IL: Human Kinetics Publishers, Inc., 1986.

Cycle Ergometer

Cycle ergometers are portable, moderately priced work instruments that allow measurements to be made easily. However, they are self-paced and can result in some localized leg fatigue (100). On mechanically braked cycle ergometers (e.g., Monark), the work rate can be increased by increasing the pedal rate and/or the resistance on the flywheel. Generally, the pedal rate is maintained constant during a GXT at a rate suitable to the populations being tested: 50 to 60 rpm for the low to average fit, and 70 to 100 for the highly fit and competitive cyclists (44). The pedal rate is maintained by having the subject pedal to a metronome or by providing some other source of feedback (e.g., digital display of the rpm). The load on the wheel is increased in a sequential fashion to systematically overload the cardiovascular system. The starting work rate and the increment from one stage to the next depend on the fitness of the subject and the purpose of the test. The $\dot{V}O_2$ can be estimated from an equation that gives reasonable estimates of the $\dot{V}O_2$ up to work rates of about 1200 kpm · min^{-1} (2):

$$\dot{V}O_2 \text{ (ml} \cdot \text{kg}^{-1} \cdot \text{min}^{-1}) = 1.8 \text{ ml} \cdot \text{kpm}^{-1} \text{ (work rate)}$$
$$\times \text{ M}^{-1} + 7 \text{ ml} \cdot \text{kg}^{-1} \cdot \text{min}^{-1}$$

The cycle ergometer is different from the treadmill in that the body weight is supported by the seat, and the work rate is dependent primarily on the crank speed and the load on the wheel. This means that for a small person, the relative $\dot{V}O_2$ at any work rate is higher than that for a big person. For example, if a work rate requires a $\dot{V}O_2$ of 2100 ml · min^{-1}, this represents a relative $\dot{V}O_2$ of 35 ml · kg^{-1} · min^{-1} for a 60-kg person, and only 23 ml · kg^{-1} · min^{-1} for a 90-kg person. In addition, the increments in the work rate, by demanding a fixed increase in the $\dot{V}O_2$ (e.g., an increment of 150 kpm · min^{-1} is equal to a $\dot{V}O_2$ change of 270 ml · min^{-1}), force a small and unfit subject to make larger cardiovascular adjustments than a large or high-fit subject. These factors have been taken into consideration by the YMCA (42) in recommending submaximal GXT protocols. The idea is to provide a means of obtaining a variety of HR responses to several submaximal work rates in a way that reduces the duration of the test.

Figure 15.5 shows the different "routes" followed in the YMCA protocol depending on the subject's HR response to a work rate of 150 kpm · min^{-1}. The YMCA protocol makes use of the observation that the relationship between $\dot{V}O_2$ and HR is a linear one between 110 and 150 b · min^{-1}. For this reason, the YMCA protocol requires the subject to exercise at only one more work rate past the one that yields an HR $\geq$ 110 b · min^{-1}. As a general recommendation for all cycle ergometer tests, seat height is adjusted so that the knee is slightly bent when the foot is at the bottom of the pedal swing and parallel to the floor; the seat height is recorded for later testing. In the YMCA protocol, each stage lasts three minutes and heart rate values are obtained in the last 30 seconds of the second and third minutes. If the difference in HR is <5 b · min^{-1} between the two time periods, a steady state is assumed; if not, an additional minute is added to that stage. A line then connects the two HR values and is extrapolated to the subject's estimated maximal HR. A vertical line is dropped to the x-axis, and the estimated $\dot{V}O_2$ max value is obtained as described for the submaximal treadmill protocol.

Figure 15.6 shows the YMCA protocol for a 30-year-old female who weighs 60 kg. The first work rate was 150 kpm · min^{-1}, and a heart rate of 103 b · min^{-1} was measured. Following the YMCA protocol, the next loads were 300 and then 450 kpm · min^{-1}, and the measured HR values were 115 and

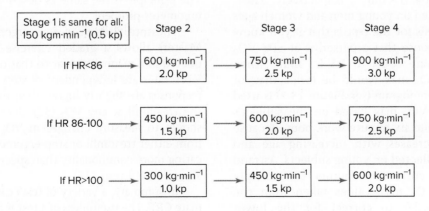

Figure 15.5 YMCA protocol used to select work rates for submaximal cycle ergometer tests.

Golding, L. A., *YMCA Fitness Testing and Assessment Manual.* Champaign, IL: Human Kinetics, 2000.

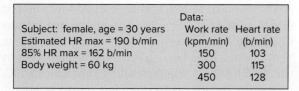

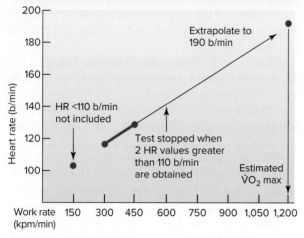

Figure 15.6 Example of the YMCA protocol used to estimate $\dot{V}O_2$ max.

From Howley, E. T., and Franks, B. D., *Health/Fitness Instructor's Handbook*. Champaign, IL: Human Kinetics Publishers, Inc., 1986.

128 b · min⁻¹, respectively. A line was drawn through the two HR points greater than 110 b · min⁻¹ and extrapolated to age-predicted max HR (190 b · min⁻¹). The estimated $\dot{V}O_2$ max for this woman was approximately 2.58 L · min⁻¹ or 43 ml · kg⁻¹ · min⁻¹, using the previous equation.

In addition to this extrapolation procedure for estimating $\dot{V}O_2$ max, Åstrand and Ryhming (8) provide a method that requires the subject to complete one work bout of approximately six minutes, demanding an HR between 125 and 170 b · min⁻¹. These investigators observed that at 50% $\dot{V}O_2$ max, males had an average HR of 128, and females, 138 b · min⁻¹, and at 70% $\dot{V}O_2$ max, the average HRs were 154 and 164 b · min⁻¹, respectively. These data were collected on young men and women ages 18 to 30. The basis for the test is that if you know from an HR response that a person is at 50% $\dot{V}O_2$ max at a work rate equal to 1.5 L · min⁻¹, then the estimated $\dot{V}O_2$ max would be twice that, or 3.0 L · min⁻¹. A nomogram (see Figure 15.7) is used to estimate the $\dot{V}O_2$ max based on the subject's HR response to one six-minute work bout. Because maximal HR decreases with increasing age and the data were collected on young subjects, Åstrand (4) established correction factors to multiply the estimated $\dot{V}O_2$ max values taken from the nomogram in order to correct for the lower maximal HR.

Step Test

A step-test protocol is used to estimate $\dot{V}O_2$ max in the same way that treadmill and cycle ergometer protocols are used. The step test does not require expensive equipment, the step height does not have to be calibrated, everyone is familiar with the stepping exercise, and the energy requirement is proportional to body weight, as with the treadmill (70). The work rate can be increased by increasing the step height while keeping the cadence the same, or by increasing the cadence while keeping the step height the same, or both. The step height can be varied with a hand-cranking device (84) or by using a series of steps with increments in step height of 10 cm. The rate of stepping is established with a metronome, and the stepping cadence has four counts: up, up, down, down. The subjects must step all the way up and down in time with the metronome. Figure 15.8 shows the results of a step test on a 60-year-old female. In this step test, the height of the step was kept constant at 16 cm and the rate of stepping increased 6 lifts · min⁻¹ each two minutes. The line drawn through the HR points is extrapolated to the estimated maximal HR, 160 b · min⁻¹, and a line is dropped to the horizontal axis to estimate the $\dot{V}O_2$ max using the following equation (2):

$$\dot{V}O_2 = 0.2 \text{ (step rate)} + [1.33 \times 1.8 \\ \times \text{ (step height [m])} \times \text{ (step rate)}] + 3.5$$

The equation yields values in ml · kg⁻¹ · min⁻¹, which are converted to METs by dividing by 3.5. Please note that the mCAFT step test was presented earlier in this chapter under *field tests* because it was originally designed to be used in one's home. However, it is a perfectly suitable test for a fitness setting.

The Åstrand and Ryhming (8) nomogram (Figure 5.6) also accommodates a step test, using a rate of 22.5 lifts per minute (metronome = 90) and step heights of 40 cm for men and 33 cm for women. The principle is the same as described for their cycle ergometer protocol.

The introduction of step ergometers (i.e., StairMaster) allows a graded exercise test to be conducted in a manner similar to that of a treadmill. The work rates are independent of step rate, and the HR responses are slightly higher than those measured on the treadmill at any $\dot{V}O_2$ (52). Such a test has been shown to measure changes in $\dot{V}O_2$ max that result from either treadmill or step-ergometer training, indicating more commonality than specificity among step and treadmill tests (15).

In summary, a variety of tests can be used to estimate CRF. The usefulness of a test is a function of both the accuracy of the measurement and the ability to

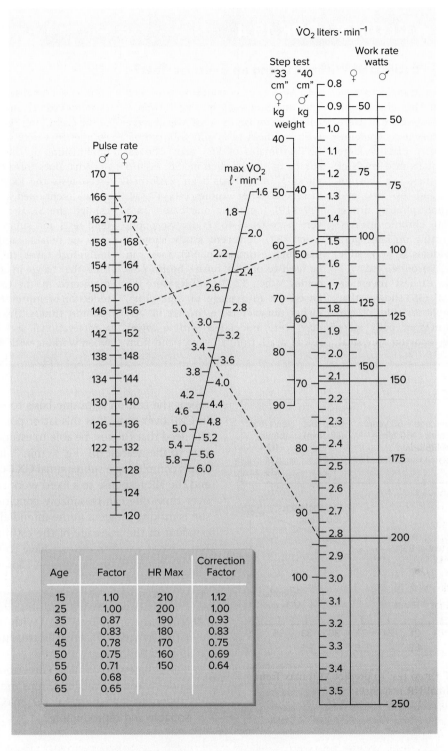

Figure 15.7 Nomogram for the estimation of $\dot{V}O_2$ max from submaximal HR values measured on either a cycle ergometer or step test. For the cycle ergometer, the work rate in watts (1 watt = 6.1 kpm · min⁻¹) is shown on the two rightmost columns, one for men and one for women. The results of a cycle ergometer test for a man who worked at 200 watts is shown. A dashed line is drawn between the 200-watt work rate and the HR value of 166 measured during the test. The estimated $\dot{V}O_2$ max is 3.6 L · min⁻¹. The step test uses a rate of 22.5 lifts · min⁻¹, and two different step heights: 33 cm for women and 40 cm for men. The step test scale lists body weight for the subject, and the results of a test on a 61-kg woman are shown. A dashed line is drawn between the 61 kg on the 33-cm scale and the HR value of 156 b · min⁻¹ measured during the test. The estimated $\dot{V}O_2$ max is 2.4 L · min⁻¹. These estimates of $\dot{V}O_2$ max are influenced by the person's maximal HR, which is known to decrease with age. A correction factor chosen from the accompanying table corrects these $\dot{V}O_2$ max values when either the maximal HR or age is known. Simply multiply the $\dot{V}O_2$ value by the correction factor.

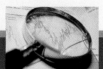

A CLOSER LOOK 15.4

Can $\dot{V}O_2$ Max Be Estimated Without Doing an Exercise Test?

This may seem like a strange question given the focus of this chapter on exercise testing. However, if it were possible, investigators (e.g., epidemiologists) could easily classify large numbers of individuals into levels of cardiorespiratory fitness (e.g., bottom 20%, middle 20%, and top 20%), and determine if cardiorespiratory fitness is linked to various chronic diseases. Doing exercise testing on large populations of individuals is impossible due to time, cost, personnel, etc.

In one of the earliest investigations, Jackson et al. (55) showed that by using the simple variables of age, gender, body fatness or body mass index, and self-reported physical activity, $\dot{V}O_2$ max could be estimated with an SE of ~ ±5 ml · kg^{-1} · min^{-1}, an error similar to what we observe with our field tests and submaximal GXT estimates of $\dot{V}O_2$ max. The accuracy of the prediction (SE ~ ±4-6 ml/kg^{-1} · min^{-1}) has been confirmed in several other studies (40, 47, 71, 117-119), including one based on a very large (N = 4637) diverse population (87). A recent study showed that such estimates of $\dot{V}O_2$ max can be used to predict future health outcomes. When 32,391 adults were followed for an average of nine years, higher nonexercise estimates of $\dot{V}O_2$ max were associated with a lower risk of death from all causes and from cardiovascular disease. Further, these estimates of $\dot{V}O_2$ max were much better at classifying risk than any of the components (e.g., age, body mass index) making up the estimate (105).

What does this say about doing exercise tests–the focus of this chapter? As we mentioned at the outset, even though the SE is relatively large for field tests and submaximal GXTs, the tests are reliable, and when the same individual takes the same test over time, the change in estimated $\dot{V}O_2$ max monitored by the test is a reasonable reflection of improvements in cardiorespiratory fitness. This can serve as both a motivational and educational tool when working with fitness clients.

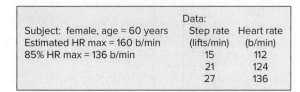

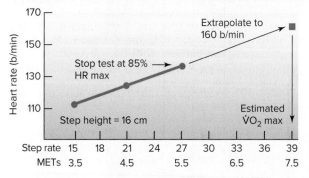

Figure 15.8 Use of a step test to predict $\dot{V}O_2$ max from a series of submaximal HR responses.

From Howley, E. T., and Franks, B. D., *Health/Fitness Instructor's Handbook*. Champaign, IL: Human Kinetics Publishers, Inc., 1986.

repeat the test on a routine basis to evaluate changes in CRF over time. It is this latter point that decreases the need that the test be able to estimate the true $\dot{V}O_2$ max to the nearest ml · kg^{-1} · min^{-1}. In effect, if a person is completing a submaximal GXT on a regular basis and the HR response to a fixed work rate is decreasing over time, one can reasonably conclude that the person is making progress in the intended direction, independent of the accuracy of the estimate of $\dot{V}O_2$ max. But what if a person did not have to take an exercise test to estimate $\dot{V}O_2$ max? See A Closer Look 15.4.

IN SUMMARY

- $\dot{V}O_2$ max can be estimated with the extrapolation procedure using the treadmill, cycle ergometer, or step.
- The subject must follow directions carefully and environmental conditions must be controlled if the estimate of $\dot{V}O_2$ max is to be reasonable and reproducible.

STUDY ACTIVITIES

1. Go online (http://eparmedx.com/?page_id=75) and complete the PAR-Q+ and ePARMed-X+ for a friend or family member who has one or more risk factors for heart disease.
2. What procedure does the American College of Sports Medicine recommend to estimate an individual's risk associated with exercise testing or participation in exercise?
3. Describe one maximal and one submaximal field test to estimate $\dot{V}O_2$ max.
4. A 40-year-old man runs 1.5 miles (2,415 meters) in ten minutes. What is his estimated $\dot{V}O_2$ max? Is his value "normal"?
5. Because many subjects do not exhibit a plateau in oxygen consumption in the last stages of a maximal GXT,

what other criteria could be used to show that the person was exercising maximally when the highest $\dot{V}O_2$ was measured?

6. Given the following information collected during a treadmill test on a 50-year-old man, estimate his $\dot{V}O_2$ max.

Work Rate	Heart Rate
3 METs	110
5 METs	125
7 METs	140

7. Given the assumption that the formula 220 – age can be used to estimate maximal heart rate, how far off could you be in your estimate of $\dot{V}O_2$ max in Question 6?

8. What information do you gain by monitoring the RPE during a GXT?

9. List five reasons for stopping a GXT for low-risk adults.

10. Should you use the same GXT protocol on all subjects? Why or why not?

SUGGESTED READINGS

American College of Sports Medicine. 2014. *ACSM's Guidelines for Exercise Testing and Prescription*, 9th ed. Baltimore, MD: Lippincott Williams & Wilkins.

Balke, B. 2007. *Matters of the Heart: Adventures in Sports Medicine* (H. Marg, ed.). Monterey, CA: Healthy Learning.

Dubin, D. 2000. *Rapid Interpretation of EKGs: A Programmed Course*, 6th ed. Tampa, FL: Cover.

Heyward, V. H. 2014. *Advanced Fitness Assessment and Exercise Prescription*, 7th ed. Champaign, IL: Human Kinetics.

Howley, E. T., and D. L. Thompson. 2017. *Fitness Professional's Handbook*. 7th ed. Champaign, IL: Human Kinetics.

Nieman, D. 2011. *Fitness Testing and Prescription*, 7th ed. New York, NY: McGraw-Hill.

Plowman, S. A., C. L. Sterling, C. B. Corbin, M. D. Meredith, G. J. Welk, and J. R. Morrow. 2006. The history of the FITNESSGRAM®. *Journal of Physical Activity and Health*. 3 (Supple 2): S5–S20.

REFERENCES

1. **Aitken JC and Thompson J.** The respiratory V̇ CO2/V̇O2 exchange ratio during maximum exercise and its use as a predictor of maximum oxygen uptake. *European Journal of Applied Physiology and Occupational Physiology* 57: 714–719, 1988.

2. **American College of Sports Medicine.** *ACSM's Guidelines for Exercise Testing and Prescription*. Baltimore, MD: Lippincott Williams & Wilkins, 2014.

3. **American College of Sports Medicine.** *Guidelines for Exercise Testing and Prescription*. Baltimore, MD: Lippincott Williams & Wilkins, 2006.

4. **Åstrand I.** Aerobic work capacity in men and women with special reference to age. *Acta Physiologica Scandinavica* 49: 1–92, 1960.

5. **Åstrand PO.** *Experimental Studies of Physical Working Capacity in Relation to Sex and Age.* Copenhagen: Manksgaard, 1952.

6. **Åstrand PO.** Principles of ergometry and their implications in sports practice. *International Journal of Sports Medicine* 5: 102–105, 1984.

7. **Åstrand PO and Rodahl K.** *Textbook of Work Physiology.* New York, NY: McGraw-Hill, 1986.

8. **Åstrand PO and Ryhming I.** A nomogram for calculation of aerobic capacity (physical fitness) from pulse rate during sub-maximal work. *Journal of Applied Physiology* 7: 218–221, 1954.

9. **Åstrand PO and Saltin B.** Maximal oxygen uptake and heart rate in various types of muscular activity. *Journal of Applied Physiology* 16: 977–981, 1961.

10. **Balke B.** *A Simple Field Test for Assessment of Physical Fitness.* Civil Aeromedical Research Institute Report 63–66, 1963.

11. **Balke B.** *Advanced Exercise Procedures for Evaluation of the Cardiovascular System. Monograph.* Milton: The Burdick Corporation, 1970.

12. **Bassett DR, Jr.** Exercise related to ECG and medications. In ET Howley and DL Thompson, *Fitness Professional's Handbook*, Champaign, IL: Human Kinetics, 2017.

13. **Bassett DR Jr. and Howley ET.** Limiting factors for maximum oxygen uptake and determinants of endurance performance. *Medicine & Science in Sports & Exercise* 32: 70–84, 2000.

14. **Bassett DR Jr. and Howley ET.** Maximal oxygen uptake: "classical" versus "contemporary" viewpoints. *Medicine & Science in Sports & Exercise* 29: 591–603, 1997.

15. **Ben-Ezra V and Verstraete R.** Step ergometry: is it task-specific training? *European Journal of Applied Physiology and Occupational Physiology* 63: 261–264, 1991.

16. **Blair SN, Kohl HW, III, Paffenbarger RS, Jr., Clark DG, Cooper KH, and Gibbons LW.** Physical fitness and all-cause mortality: a prospective study of healthy men and women. *JAMA* 262: 2395–2401, 1989.

17. **Borg GA.** Psychophysical bases of perceived exertion. *Medicine & Science in Sports & Exercise* 14: 377–381, 1982.

18. **Bredin S. S. D.** PAR-Q+ and ePARmed-X+. New risk stratification and physical activity clearance strategy for physicians and patients alike. *Canadian Family Physician.* 59: 273–277, 2013.

19. **Bruce RA.** Multi-stage treadmill tests of maximal and submaximal exercise. In *Exercise Testing and Training of Apparently Healthy Individuals: A Handbook for Physicians.* New York, NY: American Heart Association, 1972, pp. 32–34.

20. **Canadian Society for Exercise Physiology.** *Canadian Society for Exercise Physiology-Physical Activity Training for Health.* Ottawa: Canada, 2013

21. **Carton RL and Rhodes EC.** A critical review of the literature on ratings scales for perceived exertion. *Sports Medicine* 2: 198–222, 1985.

22. **Castro-Piñero J, Artero EG, España-Romero V, Ortega FB, Sjöström M, Suni J, et al.** Criterion-related validity of field-based fitness tests in youth: a systematic review. *British Journal of Sports Medicine* 44: 934–943, 2010.

23. **Chow RJ and Wilmore JH.** The regulation of exercise intensity by ratings of perceived exertion. *Journal of Cardiac Rehabilitation* 4: 382–387, 1984.

24. **Chun DM, Corbin CB, and Pangrazi RP.** Validation of criterion-referenced standards for the mile run and progressive aerobic cardiovascular endurance tests. *Research Quarterly for Exercise and Sport* 71: 125-134, 2000.

25. **Conley DS, Cureton KJ, Dengel DR, and Weyand PG.** Validation of the 12-min swim as a field test of peak aerobic power in young men. *Medicine & Science in Sports & Exercise* 23: 766-773, 1991.

26. **Cooper KH.** *The Aerobics Way.* New York, NY: Bantam, 1977.

27. **Cooper M and Cooper KH.** *Aerobics for Women.* New York, NY: Evans, 1972.

28. **Cureton KJ, Hensley LD, and Tiburzi A.** Body fatness and performance differences between men and women. *Research Quarterly* 50: 333-340, 1979.

29. **Cureton KJ, Sparling PB, Evans BW, Johnson SM, Kong UD, and Purvis JW.** Effect of experimental alterations in excess weight on aerobic capacity and distance running performance. *Medicine and Science in Sports* 10: 194-199, 1978.

30. **Cureton KJ and Warren GL.** Criterion-referenced standards for youth health-related fitness tests: a tutorial. *Research Quarterly for Exercise and Sport* 61: 7-19, 1990.

31. **Daniels J, Oldridge N, Nagle F, and White B.** Differences and changes in $\dot{V}O_2$ among young runners 10 to 18 years of age. *Medicine and Science in Sports* 10: 200-203, 1978.

32. **Duncan GE, Howley ET, and Johnson BN.** Applicability of $\dot{V}O_2$ max criteria: discontinuous versus continuous protocols. *Medicine & Science in Sports & Exercise* 29: 273-278, 1997.

33. **Ellestad M.** *Stress Testing: Principles and Practice.* Philadelphia, PA: F. A. Davis, 2003.

34. **Eston RG, Faulkner JA, Mason EA, and Parfitt G.** The validity of predicting maximal oxygen uptake from perceptually regulated graded exercise tests of different durations. *European Journal of Applied Physiology* 97: 535-541, 2006.

35. **Falls HB and Humphrey LD.** A comparison of methods for eliciting maximum oxygen uptake from college women during treadmill walking. *Medicine and Science in Sports* 5: 239-241, 1973.

36. **Faulkner JA, Roberts DE, Elk RL, and Conway J.** Cardiovascular responses to submaximum and maximum effort cycling and running. *Journal of Applied Physiology* 30: 457-461, 1971.

37. **Flouris AD, Metsios GS, Famisis K, Geladas N, and Koutedakis Y.** Prediction of $\dot{V}O_2$ max from a new field test based on portable indirect calorimetry. *Journal of Science and Medicine in Sport* 13:70-73, 2010.

38. **Foster C.** Prediction of oxygen uptake during exercise testing in cardiac patients and health volunteers. *Journal of Cardiac Rehabilitation* 4: 537-542, 1984.

39. **Foster C, Kuffel E, Bradley N, Battista RA, Wright G, Porcari JP, et al.** $\dot{V}O_2$ max during successive maximal efforts. *European Journal of Applied Physiology* 102: 67-72, 2007.

40. **Franklin BA.** Exercise testing, training and arm ergometry. *Sports Medicine* 2: 100-119, 1985.

41. **George JD, Stone WJ, and Burkett LN.** Nonexercise $\dot{V}O_2$ max estimation for physcially active college students. *Medicine & Science in Sports & Exercise* 29: 415-423, 1997.

42. **Golding LA.** YMCA *Fitness Testing and Assessment Manual.* Champaign, IL: Human Kinetics, 2000.

43. **Gutmann M.** Perceived exertion-heart rate relationship during exercise testing and training of cardiac patients. *Journal of Cardiac Rehabilitation* 1: 52-59, 1981.

44. **Hagberg JM, Mullin JP, Giese MD, and Spitznagel E.** Effect of pedaling rate on submaximal exercise responses of competitive cyclists. *Journal of Applied Physiology* 51: 447-451, 1981.

45. **Haskell WL, Savin W, Oldridge N, and DeBusk R.** Factors influencing estimated oxygen uptake during exercise testing soon after myocardial infarction. *American Journal of Cardiology* 50: 299-304, 1982.

46. **Hawkins MN, Raven PB, Snell PG, Stray-Gundersen J, and Levine BD.** Maximal oxygen uptake as a parametric measure of cardiorespiratory capacity. *Medicine & Science in Sports & Exercise* 39: 103-107, 2007.

47. **Heil DP, Freedson PS, Ahlquist LE, Price J, and Rippe JM.** Nonexercise regression models to estimate peak oxygen consumption. *Medicine & Science in Sports & Exercise* 27: 599-606, 1995.

48. **Hermansen L, and Saltin B.** Oxygen uptake during maximal treadmill and bicycle exercise. *Journal of Applied Physiology* 26: 31-37, 1969.

49. **Hill A and Lupton H.** Muscular exercise, lactic acid, and the supply and utilization of oxygen. *Q J Med* 16: 135-171, 1923.

50. **Howley ET.** Exercise testing laboratory. In *Resource Manual for Guidelines for Exercise Testing and Prescription,* edited by Blair SN. Philadelphia, PA: Lea & Febiger, 1988.

51. **Howley ET, Bassett DR Jr., and Welch HG.** Criteria for maximal oxygen uptake: review and commentary. *Medicine & Science in Sports & Exercise* 27: 1292-1301, 1995.

52. **Howley ET, Colacino DL, and Swensen TC.** Factors affecting the oxygen cost of stepping on an electronic stepping ergometer. *Medicine & Science in Sports & Exercise* 24: 1055-1058, 1992.

53. **Howley ET and Thompson, DL.** *Fitness Professional's Handbook,* 7th ed. Champaign, IL: Human Kinetics, 2017.

54. **Issekutz B, Birkhead NC, and Rodahl K.** The use of respiratory quotients in assessment of aerobic power capacity. *Journal of Applied Physiology* 17: 47-50, 1962.

55. **Jackson AS, Blair SN, Mahar MT, Wier LT, Ross RM, and Stuteville JE.** Prediction of functional aerobic capacity without exercise testing. *Medicine & Science in Sports & Exercise* 22: 863-870, 1990.

56. **Kaminsky LA, Arena R, Beckie TM, Brubaker PH, Church TS, Forman DE, Franklin BA, Gulati M, Lavie CJ, Myers J, Patel MJ, Piña IL, Weintraub WS, and Williams MA.** The importance of cardiorespiratory fitness in the United States: the need for a national registry. A policy statement from the American Heart Association. *Circulation* 127: 652-662, 2013.

57. **Kaminsky LA, Arena R, and Myers J.** Reference standards for cardiorespiratory fitness measured with cardiopulmonary exercise testing: data from the Fitness Registry and the Importance of Exercise National Database. *Mayo Clinic Proceedings* 90: 1515-1523, 2015.

58. **Kavanagh T and Shephard RJ.** Maximum exercise tests on "postcoronary" patients. *Journal of Applied Physiology* 40: 611-618, 1976.

59. **Kirkendall WM, Feinleib M, Freis ED, and Mark AL.** Recommendations for human blood pressure determination by sphygmomanometers: subcommittee of the AHA Postgraduate Education Committee. *Circulation* 62: 1146A-1155A, 1980.

60. **Kitamura K, Jorgensen CR, Gobel FL, Taylor HL, and Wang Y.** Hemodynamic correlates of myocardial

oxygen consumption during upright exercise. *Journal of Applied Physiology* 32: 516-522, 1972.

61. **Kline GM, Porcari JP, Hintermeister R, Freedson PS, Ward A, McCarron RF, et al.** Estimation of $\dot{V}O_2$ max from a one-mile track walk, gender, age, and body weight. *Medicine & Science in Sports & Exercise* 19: 253-259, 1987.

62. **Kohl HW, Gibbons LW, Gordon NF, and Blair SN.** An empirical evaluation of the ACSM guidelines for exercise testing. *Medicine & Science in Sports & Exercise* 22: 533-539, 1990.

63. **Krahenbuhl GS, Pangrazi RP, Petersen GW, Burkett LN, and Schneider MJ.** Field testing of cardiorespiratory fitness in primary school children. *Medicine and Science in Sports* 10: 208-213, 1978.

64. **Lamb KL and Rogers L.** A re-appraisal of the reliability of the 20 m multi-stage shuttle run test. *European Journal of Applied Physiology* 100: 287-292, 2007.

65. **Léger LA and Lambert J.** A maximal multistage 20-m shuttle run test to predict $\dot{V}O_2$ max. *European Journal of Applied Physiology and Occupational Physiology* 49: 1-12, 1982.

66. **Léger LA, Mercier D, Gadoury C, and Lambert J.** The multistage 20 metre shuttle run test for aerobic fitness. *Journal of Sports Sciences* 6: 93-101, 1988.

67. **Lobelo F, Pate RR, Dowda M, Liese AD, and Ruiz JR.** Validity of cardiorespiratory fitness criterion-referenced standards for adolescents. *Medicine and Science in Sports and Exercise* 41: 1222-1229, 2009.

68. **Londeree BR and Moeschberger ML.** Influence of age and other factors on maximal heart rate. *Journal of Cardiac Rehabilitation* 4: 44-49, 1984.

69. **Marsh CE.** Evaluation of the American College of Sports Medicine submaximal treadmill running test for predicting $\dot{V}O_2$ max. *Journal of Strength and Conditioning Research.* 26: 548-554, 2012.

70. **Margaria R, Aghemo P, and Rovelli E.** Indirect determination of maximal O_2 consumption in man. *Journal of Applied Physiology* 20: 1070-1073, 1965.

71. **Matthews CE, Heil DP, Freedson PS, and Pastides H.** Classification of cardiorespiratory fitness without exercise testing. *Medicine & Science in Sports & Exercise* 31: 486-493, 1999.

72. **McArdle WD, Katch FI, and Pechar GS.** Comparison of continuous and discontinuous treadmill and bicycle tests for max $\dot{V}O_2$. *Medicine and Science in Sports* 5: 156-160, 1973.

73. **McConnell TR.** Practical considerations in the testing of $\dot{V}O_2$ max in runners. *Sports Medicine* 5: 57-68, 1988.

74. **McConnell TR and Clark BA.** Prediction of maximal oxygen consumption during handrail supported treadmill exercise. *Journal of Cardiopulmonary Rehabilitation* 7: 324-331, 1987.

75. **McCormack WP, Cureton KJ, Bullock TA, and Weyand PG.** Metabolic determinants of 1-mile run/walk performance in children. *Medicine and Science in Sports and Exercise* 23: 611-617, 1991.

76. **McNaughton L, Hall P, and Cooley D.** Validation of several methods of estimating maximal oxygen uptake in young men. *Perceptual and Motor Skills* 87: 575-584, 1998.

77. **Metsios GS, Flouris AD, Koutedakis Y, and Theodorakis Y.** The effect of performance feedback on cardiorespiratory fitness field tests. *Journal of Science and Medicine in Sport/Sports Medicine Australia* 9: 263-266, 2006.

78. **Midgley AW and Carroll S.** Emergence of the verification phase procedure for confirming "true" $\dot{V}O_2$ max. *Scandinavian Journal of Medicine and Science in Sports* 19: 313-322, 2009.

79. **Midgley AW, McNaughton LR, Polman R, and Marchant D.** Criteria for determination of maximal oxygen uptake. *Sports Medicine* 37: 1019-1028, 2007.

80. **Montoye HJ and Ayen T.** Body size adjustment for oxygen requirement in treadmill walking. *Research Quarterly for Exercise and Sport* 57: 82-84, 1986.

81. **Montoye HJ, Ayen T, Nagle F, and Howley ET.** The oxygen requirement for horizontal and grade walking on a motor-driven treadmill. *Medicine & Science in Sports & Exercise* 17: 640-645, 1985.

82. **Montoye HJ, Ayen T, and Washburn RA.** The estimation of $\dot{V}O_2$ max from maximal and sub-maximal measurements in males, age 10-39. *Research Quarterly for Exercise and Sport* 57: 250-253, 1986.

83. **Morrow JR, Jr., Martin SB, and Jackson AW.** Reliability and validity of the FITNESSGRAM®: quality of teacher-collected health-related fitness surveillance data. *Research Quarterly for Exercise and Sport* 81: S24-S30, 2010.

84. **Nagle FJ, Balke B, and Naughton JP.** Gradational step tests for assessing work capacity. *Journal of Applied Physiology* 20: 745-748, 1965.

85. **Naughton JP and Haider R.** Methods of exercise testing. In *Exercise Testing and Exercise Training in Coronary Heart Disease,* edited by Naughton JP, Hellerstein HK, and Mohler LC. New York, NY: Academic Press, 1973, pp. 79-91.

86. **Nelson RR, Gobel FL, Jorgensen CR, Wang K, Wang Y, and Taylor HL.** Hemodynamic predictors of myocardial oxygen consumption during static and dynamic exercise. *Circulation* 50: 1179-1189, 1974.

87. **Nes BM, Janszky I, Vatten LJ, Nilsen TIL, Aspenes ST, and Wisloff U.** Estimating $\dot{V}O_2$ peak from a non-exercise prediction model: the HUNT Study, Norway. *Medicine & Science in Sports & Exercise* 43: 2024-2030, 2011.

88. **Oja P, Laukkanen R, Pasanen M, Tyry T, and Vuori I.** A 2-km walking test for assessing the cardiorespiratory fitness of healthy adults. *International Journal of Sports Medicine* 12: 356-362, 1991.

89. **Oldridge NB, Haskell WL, and Single P.** Carotid palpation, coronary heart disease and exercise rehabilitation. *Medicine & Science in Sports & Exercise* 13: 6-8, 1981.

90. **Park RJ.** Measurement of physical fitness: a historical perspective. edited by U.S. Department of Health and Human Services, Public Health Service, 1989.

91. **Pober DM, Freedson PS, Kline GM, McInnis KJ, and Rippe JM.** Development and validation of a one-mile treadmill walk test to predict peak oxygen uptake in healthy adults ages 40 to 79 years. *Canadian Journal of Applied Physiology = Revue Canadienne de Physiologie Appliquee* 27: 575-589, 2002.

92. **Pollock ML and Wilmore JH.** *Exercise in Health and Disease.* Philadelphia, PA: W. B. Saunders, 1990.

93. **Poole DC, Wilkerson DP, and Jones AM.** Validity of criteria for establishing maximal O_2 uptake during ramp exercise tests. *European Journal of Applied Physiology.* 102: 403-410, 2008.

94. **Ragg KE, Murray TP, Karbonit LM, and Jump DA.** Errors in predicting functional capacity from a treadmill exercise stress test. *American Heart Journal* 100: 581-583, 1980.

95. **Riebe D, Franklin BA, Thompson PD, Ewing-Garber C, Whitfield GP, Magal M, and Pescatello LS.** Updating ACSM's recommendations for

exercise preparticipation health screening. *Medicine & Science in Sports & Exercise.* 47: 2473-2479, 2015.

96. **Rowell LB.** Human cardiovascular adjustments to exercise and thermal stress. *Physiological Reviews* 54: 75-159, 1974.

97. **Sawka MN, Foley ME, Pimental NA, Toner MM, and Pandolf KB.** Determination of maximal aerobic power during upper-body exercise. *Journal of Applied Physiology* 54: 113-117, 1983.

98. **Scott SN, Thompson DL, and Coe DP.** The ability of the PACER to elicit peak exercise response in the youth. *Medicine & Science in Sports & Exercise* 45:1139-1143, 2013.

99. **Sedlock D.** Accuracy of subject-palpated carotid pulse after exercise. *The Physician and Sports Medicine* 11: 106-116, 1983.

100. **Shephard RJ.** Tests of maximum oxygen intake: a critical review. *Sports Medicine* 1: 99-124, 1984.

101. **Shephard RJ, Bailey DA, and Mirwald RL.** Development of the Canadian home fitness test. *Canadian Medical Association Journal* 114: 675-679, 1976.

102. **Shipe M.** Health risk appraisal. In *Fitness Professional's Handbook,* edited by Howley ET and Thompson DL. Champaign, IL: Human Kinetics Publishers, 2016, pp. 48-76

103. **Sidney KH and Shephard RJ.** Maximum and sub-maximum exercise tests in men and women in the seventh, eighth, and ninth decades of life. *Journal of Applied Physiology* 43: 280-287, 1977.

104. **Sparling PB and Cureton KJ.** Biological determinants of the sex difference in 12-min run performance. *Medicine & Science in Sports & Exercise* 15: 218-223, 1983.

105. **Stamatakis E, Hamer M, O'Donovan G, Batty GD, and Kivimaki M.** A non-exercise testing method for estimating cardiorespiratory fitness: associations with all-cause and cardiovascular mortality in a pooled analysis of eight population-based cohorts. *European Heart Journal* 34: 750-758, 2013.

106. **Stamford BA.** Step increment versus constant load tests for determination of maximal oxygen uptake. *European Journal of Applied Physiology and Occupational Physiology* 35: 89-93, 1976.

107. **Stickland MK, Petersen SR, and Bouffard M.** Prediction of maximal aerobic power from the 20-m multi-stage shuttle run test. *Canadian Journal of Applied Physiology = Revue Canadienne de Physiologie Appliquee* 28: 272-282, 2003.

108. **Stromme SB, Ingjer F, and Meen HD.** Assessment of maximal aerobic power in specifically trained athletes. *Journal of Applied Physiology* 42: 833-837, 1977.

109. **Taylor HL, Buskirk E, and Henschel A.** Maximal oxygen intake as an objective measure of cardio-respiratory performance. *Journal of Applied Physiology* 8: 73-80, 1955.

110. **U.S. Department of Health and Human Services.** 2008 Physcial activity guidelines for Americans. www.healthgov/paguidelines/guidelines/defaultaspx, 2008.

111. **Wallace JP.** Physical conditioning: intervention in aging cardiovascular function: part A: quantitation, epidemiology, and clinical research. In *Intervention in the Aging Process,* edited by Liss AR,1983, pp. 307-323.

112. **Warburton DER, Gledhill N, Jamnik VK, Bredin SSD, McKenzie DC, Stone J, et al.** Evidence-based risk assessment and recommendations for physical activity clearance: Consensus Document 2011. *Applied Physiology, Nutrition, and Metabolism* 36: S266-S298, 2011.

113. **Warburton DER, Jamnik VK, Bredin SSD, McKenzie DC, Stone J, Shephard RJ, et al.** Evidence-based risk assessment and recommendations for physical activity clearance: an introduction. *Applied Physiology, Nutrition, and Metabolism* 36: S1-S2, 2011.

114. **Welk GJ and Meredith MD.** *FITNESSGRAM/ ACTIVITYGRAM Reference Guide.* Dallas, TX: The Cooper Institute, 2008.

115. **Weller IM, Thomas SG, Corey PN, and Cox MH.** Prediction of maximal oxygen uptake from a modified Canadian aerobic fitness test. *Canadian Journal of Applied Physiology = Revue Canadienne de Physiologie Appliquee* 18: 175-188, 1993.

116. **Weller IMR, Thomas SG, Gledhill N, Paterson D, and Quinney A.** A study to validate the modified Canadian aerobic fitness test. *Canadian Journal of Applied Physiology* 20: 211-221, 1995.

117. **Whaley MH, Kaminsky LA, SDwyer GB, and Getchell LH.** Failure of predicted $\dot{V}O_2$ peak to discriminate physical fitness in epidemiological studies. *Medicine & Science in Sports & Exercise* 27: 85-91, 1995.

118. **Wier LT, Jackson AS, Ayers GW, and Arenare B.** Nonexercise models for estimating $\dot{V}O_2$ max with waist girth, percent fat, or BMI. *Medicine & Science in Sports & Exercise* 38: 555-561, 2006.

119. **Williford HN, Scharff-Olson M, Wang N, Blessing DL, Smith FH, and Duey WJ.** Cross-validation of non-exercise predictions of $\dot{V}O_2$ peak in women. *Medicine & Science in Sports & Exercise* 28: 926-930, 1996.

16

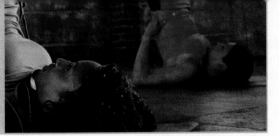

© Tim Mantoani/Masterfile

Exercise Prescriptions for Health and Fitness

■ Objectives

By studying this chapter, you should be able to do the following:

1. Contrast exercise with physical activity; explain how both relate to a lower risk of CHD and improvement in cardiorespiratory fitness (CRF).

2. Describe the current public health physical activity recommendation from the *U.S. Physical Activity Guidelines* to improve the health status of sedentary U.S. adults.

3. Explain what screening and progression mean for a person wanting to initiate an exercise program.

4. Identify the optimal range of frequency, intensity, time (duration), and type (FITT) of activity associated with improvements in CRF.

5. Calculate a target heart rate range by either the heart rate reserve or percent of maximal HR method.

6. Discuss guidelines related to progression that facilitate the transition from easy to more demanding exercise programs.

7. Explain how the target heart rate (THR) helps adjust exercise intensity in times of high heat, humidity, or while at altitude.

8. Describe the health benefits of resistance training and summarize recommended resistance-training and stretching programs for adults.

■ Key Terms

dose
effect (response)
exercise
physical activity (PA)
physical fitness
target heart rate (THR) range

In Chap. 14, we discussed a variety of risk factors related to cardiovascular and other diseases. Physical inactivity had long been considered only a secondary risk factor in the development of CHD–that is, an inactive lifestyle would increase a person's risk for CHD only if other primary risk factors were present. However, as explained in Chap. 14, this is no longer the case. Numerous studies (57, 59, 70, 75) confirm that physical inactivity is a primary risk factor for coronary heart disease (CHD), similar to smoking, hypertension, and high serum cholesterol. These studies also show that regular vigorous physical activity is instrumental in reducing the risk of CHD in those who smoke or are hypertensive (50, 58). Based on this growing body of evidence, the American Heart Association (AHA) recognized physical inactivity as a primary or major risk factor (7). Finally, epidemiological studies show that increases in physical activity (60) and fitness (11) are associated with a reduced death rate from all causes as well as from CHD. This means that physical activity should be used along with other therapies to reduce the risk of CHD in those possessing other risk factors. Consequently, there is little disagreement that regular physical activity is a necessary part of a healthy lifestyle (85). The only question is, how much?

Before we answer this question, we need to distinguish among the terms *physical activity, exercise,* and *physical fitness*. **Physical activity (PA)** is defined as any form of muscular activity. Therefore, physical activity results in the expenditure of energy proportional to muscular work and is related to physical fitness. **Physical fitness** is defined as a set of attributes that people have or develop that relate to the ability to perform physical activity. **Exercise** represents a subset of physical activity that is planned, with a goal of improving or maintaining fitness (16). These distinctions, while subtle, are important to understand in our discussion of the role of physical activity as part of a healthy lifestyle. For example, there is no question that a planned exercise program will improve $\dot{V}O_2$ max and that a higher $\dot{V}O_2$ max is associated with a lower death rate (12). However, we must emphasize that physical activity, including that done at a moderate intensity, results in substantial health benefits (34, 83). The reduction in the risks of CHD due to the latter types of activity may be mediated through changes in the distribution of cholesterol, an increase in fibrinolysis (clot dissolving) activity (32), or a reduction in systemic low-grade inflammations (see Chap. 14). It should be no surprise that the American College of Sports Medicine (in the *ACSM's Guidelines for Exercise Testing and Prescription*) and *Physical Activity and Health: A Report of the Surgeon General* state the need for increased participation in moderate-intensity exercise (e.g., brisk walking) throughout the life span (3, 83). Such a recommendation is consistent with

exposing the general population to low-risk physical activity to achieve health-related benefits aimed at reducing cardiovascular and metabolic diseases. In contrast to this general recommendation for everyone, there is a need to follow a variety of guidelines in prescribing moderate to strenuous exercise that is aimed at improving $\dot{V}O_2$ max. We will address both concerns in this chapter. For information on training for performance, see Chap. 21.

IN SUMMARY

- Physical inactivity has been classified as a primary risk factor for coronary heart disease.
- Regular participation in physical activity can reduce the overall risk for those who smoke or who are hypertensive.
- Those who increase their physical activity and/or cardiorespiratory fitness have a lower death rate from all causes compared to those who remain sedentary.

PRESCRIPTION OF EXERCISE

The concern about the proper **dose** of exercise needed to bring about a desired **effect (response)** is similar to the physician's need to know the type and quantity of a drug, as well as the time frame over which it must be taken, to cure a disease. Clearly, there is a difference in what is needed to cure a headache compared to what is needed to cure tuberculosis. In the same way, there is no question that the dose of physical activity needed to achieve high-level running performance is different from that required to improve a health-related outcome (e.g., lower blood pressure) or fitness (e.g., an increase in $\dot{V}O_2$ max). This dose-response relationship for medications is described in Figure 16.1 (27).

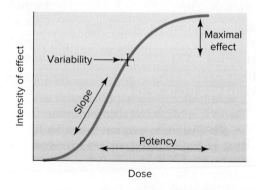

Figure 16.1 The relationship between the dose of a drug (expressed as the log of the dose) and the effect.

Data from Goodman, L. S., and Gilman, A., *The Pharmacological Basis of Therapeutics.* New York, NY: Macmillan, 1975.

- *Potency.* The potency of a drug is a relatively unimportant characteristic in that it makes little difference whether the effective dose of a drug is 1 μg or 100 mg as long as it can be administered in an appropriate dosage. Applied to exercise, walking four miles is as effective in expending calories as running two miles.

- *Slope.* The slope of the curve gives some information about how much of a change in effect is obtained from a change in dose. Some physiological measures change quickly for a given dose of exercise, while some health-related effects require the application of exercise over many months to see a desired outcome.

- *Maximal effect.* The maximal effect (efficacy) of a drug varies with the type of drug. For example, morphine can relieve pain of all intensities, while aspirin is effective against only mild-to-moderate pain. Similarly, strenuous exercise can cause an increase in $\dot{V}O_2$ max as well as modify risk factors, while light-to-moderate exercise can change risk factors with a smaller impact on $\dot{V}O_2$ max (an important point we will return to later).

- *Variability.* The effect of a drug varies between individuals–and within individuals–depending on the circumstances. The intersecting brackets in Figure 16.1 indicate the variability in the dose required to bring about a particular effect and the variability in the effect associated with a given dose. For example, gains in $\dot{V}O_2$ max due to endurance training show considerable variation, even when the initial $\dot{V}O_2$ max value is controlled for (21).

- *Side effect.* A last point worth mentioning that can also be applied to our discussion of exercise prescription is that no drug produces a single effect. The spectrum of effects might include adverse (side) effects that limit the usefulness of the drug. For exercise, the side effects might include increased risk of injury.

In contrast to drugs that individuals stop taking when a disease is cured, there is a need to engage in some form of physical activity throughout one's life to experience the health-related and fitness effects.

Dose-Response

The dose of physical activity and exercise is usually characterized by the FITT principle, which contains the following factors:

- *Frequency (F)*–how often an activity is done. This could be expressed in days per week or the number of times per day.

- *Intensity (I)*–how hard the activity is. Intensity can be described in terms of % $\dot{V}O_2$ max, % maximal heart rate, rating of perceived exertion, and the lactate threshold

- *Time (T)*–the duration of the activity. This is typically expressed as the number of minutes of activity.

- *Type (T)*–the mode or kind of activity done. This could simply refer to whether the exercise is a resistance vs. cardiovascular endurance type, or within the latter, swimming vs. running vs. rowing.

The FITT principle allows all of the major elements of an exercise intervention to be individually prescribed. In addition, the product of Frequency × Intensity × Time yields the volume (V) of exercise, which is directly related to health benefits (47, 83, 84). Another element of an exercise prescription, called progression (P), describes how to transition an individual from easier to harder exercise over the course of a training program. We will address that in the context of general guidelines for exercise later in the chapter. Lastly, the *ACSM Guidelines for Exercise Testing and Prescription* (3) incorporates all of these variables to yield the acronym FITT-VP as a reminder of what to address in an exercise prescription.

The responses (effects) resulting from an exercise intervention could include an increase in cardiorespiratory fitness ($\dot{V}O_2$ max) and a variety of health outcomes as described in Chapter 14; however, it is clear that the latter health-related effects are not dependent on an increase in $\dot{V}O_2$ max (31, 32, 83). This is important and provides a transition to our next section.

IN SUMMARY

- An exercise dose reflects the interaction of the intensity, frequency, and duration to yield the volume of exercise.
- The response to an exercise intervention can include both functional changes (e.g., an increase in $\dot{V}O_2$ max) and health outcomes (e.g., lower blood pressure), independent of each other.

Physical Activity and Health

The issue of the proper dose of exercise to bring about a desired effect is a crucial one in the prescription of exercise for both prevention and rehabilitation. Over the past three decades, we have learned that the proper dose differs greatly, depending on the outcome. For example, an improvement in some health-related variable (e.g., resting blood pressure) might be accomplished with an exercise intensity lower than that required to achieve an increase in $\dot{V}O_2$ max. In addition, the frequency with which the exercise must be taken to have the desired effect varies with the intensity and the duration of the session (see later discussion).

Certain physiological variables respond quickly to a "dose" of exercise. For example, the sympathetic nervous system, blood lactate, and heart rate adapt rapidly to exercise training, taking only days to see changes in response. In contrast to these rapid responses to exercise training, a variety of physiological variables, such as the capillary number, change more slowly (76). Similarly, when Haskell describes the potential association between physical activity and health, he distinguishes between short-term (acute) and long-term (training) responses (31). The following terms are used to describe the patterns of responses in the weeks following the initiation of a dose of exercise:

- Acute responses—occur with one or several exercise bouts but do not improve further
- Rapid responses—benefits occur early and plateau
- Linear—gains are made continuously over time
- Delayed—occur only after weeks of training

The need for such distinctions can be seen in Figure 16.2, which shows proposed dose-response relationships between physical activity, defined as minutes of exercise per week at 60% to 70% of maximal work capacity, and a variety of physiological responses (42): (a) blood pressure and insulin sensitivity are most responsive to exercise, (b) changes in $\dot{V}O_2$ max and resting heart rate are intermediate, and (c) serum lipid changes such as high-density lipoprotein (HDL) are delayed.

In 1995, in an attempt to deal with the epidemic of physical inactivity and its impact on health, the American College of Sports Medicine and the Centers for Disease Control and Prevention (CDC) published guidelines that were based on a comprehensive review of the literature dealing with the health-related aspects of physical activity (61). Their recommendation was that every U.S. adult should accumulate 30 minutes or more of moderate-intensity (3 to 5.9 METs) physical activity on most, preferably all, days of the week. This recommendation was based on the finding that caloric expenditure and total time (the volume) of physical activity were associated with reduced cardiovascular disease and mortality. Further, doing the activity in intermittent bouts as short as 10 minutes was a suitable way of meeting the 30-minute goal (6, 61, 83).

In 2007, the ACSM and AHA released an update to the 1995 public health physical activity

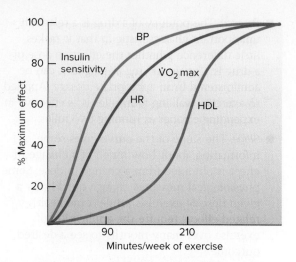

Figure 16.2 Proposed dose-response relationships between amount of exercise performed per week at 60% to 70% maximum work capacity and changes in several variables. Blood pressure (BP) and insulin sensitivity (curve to the left side) appear to be most sensitive to exercise. Maximum oxygen consumption ($\dot{V}O_2$ max) and resting heart rate, which are parameters of physical fitness (middle curve), are next in sensitivity, and lipid changes such as high-density lipoprotein (HDL) (right-hand curve) are least sensitive.

guidelines (33), and in 2008, the first edition of the *U.S. Physical Activity Guidelines* was released (83). Both guidelines supported the original statement but attempted to provide more clarity about the roles of moderate versus strenuous physical activity in meeting the recommendation (33, 83). Because of the similarity between the two, we will present only the *U.S. Physical Activity Guidelines*.

- Individuals can realize the substantial health-related benefits of physical activity by doing between 150 and 300 minutes of moderate-intensity physical activity per week, or 75 to 150 minutes of vigorous-intensity physical activity per week, or some combination of the two.
  - 150 minutes of moderate-intensity physical activity or 75 minutes of vigorous-intensity physical activity is the minimum goal.
  - The range of physical activity (150 to 300 minutes) indicates that more health-related benefits are realized by doing additional activity (i.e., more is better).

The health-related gains associated with physical activity are realized when the volume of PA is between about 500 and 1000 MET-min per week (83). Moderate-intensity PA is defined as absolute intensities of 3.0 to 5.9 METs, and vigorous-intensity PA is defined as intensities of 6.0 METs or more.

- For example, walking at 3 mph requires ~3.3 METs, an activity at the low end of the moderate-intensity range. If the person walks at this speed for 30 minutes, an energy expenditure of 99 MET-min (3.3 METs times 30 min) is achieved. If done five days per week, the volume of PA is 495 MET-min per week.

- If an individual were to jog at 5 mph (~8 METs) for 25 minutes, the PA volume would be 200 MET-min (8 METs × 25 min). If done three days per week, the energy expenditure would be 600 MET-min per week.

- The fact that it takes about twice the time when doing moderate-intensity PA to achieve the same energy expenditure (volume of exercise) as when doing vigorous-intensity PA leads to the 2:1 ratio when comparing the time it takes to meet the PA guidelines for these different intensities (150 min for moderate intensity vs. 75 min for vigorous intensity).

- In addition, and consistent with existing *ACSM Guidelines*, the new federal guidelines recommended resistance training (at least one set, or 8 to 12 repetitions, of 8 to 10 exercises) on two or more days per week to improve or maintain muscular strength and endurance (33, 83).

These new guidelines only spell out the number of minutes per week, without listing the number of days per week to exercise. That does not mean that one should do the 150 minutes of moderate-intensity physical activity on one day and rest for six days. For reasons that will be discussed later, spreading out the physical activity and exercise over the course of the week makes it easier to schedule and reduces the risk of adverse events (83). Even though there is an emphasis on moderate-intensity PA, because this is the type of activity most frequently done by adults (e.g., a brisk walk), much can be gained from participation in vigorous-intensity PA (see Clinical Applications 16.1).

IN SUMMARY

- To realize the health-related benefits of physical activity, adults should do between 150 and 300 minutes of moderate-intensity physical activity per week, or 75 to 150 minutes of vigorous-intensity physical activity per week, or some combination of the two.

- Resistance training (8 to 10 exercises, 8 to 12 repetitions) should be done on two or more nonconsecutive days per week).

GENERAL GUIDELINES FOR IMPROVING FITNESS

An increase in moderate-intensity physical activity is an important goal for reducing health-related problems in sedentary individuals. These benefits occur at a point where the overall risk associated with physical activity is relatively small. However, even though the risk of cardiac arrest in habitually active men is higher during vigorous activity, the overall (rest + exercise) risk of cardiac arrest in vigorously active men is only 40% of the risk in sedentary men (78). Figure 16.3 shows that the relative risk of death from all causes decreases as cardiorespiratory fitness ($\dot{V}O_2$ max) increases, with the largest decrease occurring when the least fit (lowest 20% or quintile) moves up one category (55). This relationship also is true when applied to the risk of chronic diseases (49, 69, 84). Based on a meta-analysis of such studies it has been estimated that for each 1 MET increase in cardiorespiratory fitness, the risk of death from all causes decreases 13% (49). The strength of these data has resulted in a recommendation from the American Heart Association to develop a national database (registry) of carefully measured $\dot{V}O_2$ max values to use as a

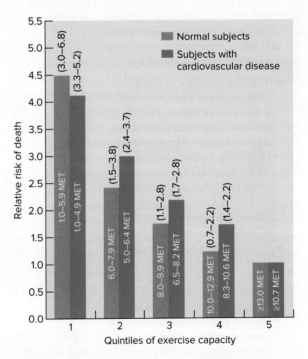

Figure 16.3 Age-adjusted relative risks of death from any cause according to quintile of exercise capacity among normal subjects and subjects with cardiovascular disease.

From Myers, J., Prakash, M., Froelicher, V., Do, D., Partington, S., and Atwood, J. E., "Exercise Capacity and Mortality Among Men Referred for Exercise Testing," *New England Journal of Medicine* 346: 793–801, 2002.

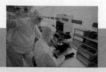

Achieving Health-Related Outcomes: Is Vigorous Exercise Better Than Moderate Activity?

There has been an ongoing debate over this question since the ACSM/CDC released their public health PA recommendation in 1995, with its emphasis on moderate-intensity PA. Prior to that, the emphasis was on vigorous-intensity exercise as described in the classic position stands of the ACSM (1). It must be noted that although moderate-intensity PA was emphasized, the 1995 statement also indicated that more exercise was better and encouraged vigorous exercise. Therefore, the question remains: is vigorous-intensity PA better than moderate-intensity PA for health-related outcomes?

Swain and Franklin (80) addressed this question in a systematic review of the literature examining the relationship of PA to the incidence of CHD and risk factors for CHD. It was important in this review that the total energy expenditure associated with the PA was controlled for to allow a fair comparison of moderate-intensity versus vigorous-intensity PA (since for any duration of vigorous PA, more energy would be expended compared to moderate-intensity PA). Their findings follow:

■ The vast majority of epidemiological studies observed a greater reduction in the risk of cardiovascular disease with vigorous-intensity PA (≥6 METs) than with moderate-intensity PA (3 to 5.9 METs). In addition, more favorable risk factor profiles were found for those doing vigorous-intensity vs. moderate-intensity PA.

■ Clinical intervention studies showed, generally, greater improvements in diastolic blood pressure, glucose control, and cardiorespiratory fitness after vigorous-intensity PA, compared to moderate-intensity PA. However, there was no difference between the two intensity categories for improvements in systolic blood pressure, the blood lipid profile, or loss of body fat.

Clearly, more health-related benefits are realized, independent of the larger gains in $\dot{V}O_2$ max, through participating in vigorous-intensity exercise. O'Donovan et al. (56) supported these findings by showing that even when training groups are doing vigorous-intensity exercise, the higher the intensity, the better the impact on CHD risk factors. In addition, regular participation in vigorous-intensity PA was shown to be associated with less sick leave, whereas moderate-intensity PA appeared to have no effect (71). This raises other questions: what is moderate-intensity PA? Vigorous-intensity PA?

Public health PA recommendations define moderate-intensity PA as being equal to an *absolute intensity* of 3 to 5.9 METs, but surprising as it may seem, moderate-intensity exercise may actually be vigorous-intensity PA for a large segment of the population. Figure 16.4 shows the *relative intensity* for two fixed exercises (walking at 3 or 4 mph) to vary considerably across the range of $\dot{V}O_2$ max values (39, 84). Consequently, individuals with low $\dot{V}O_2$ max values who are doing moderate-intensity physical activity (3 to 5.9 METs) may actually be working at a relative intensity equivalent to vigorous exercise (≥60% $\dot{V}O_2$ max), consistent with achieving gains in $\dot{V}O_2$ max. This example emphasizes the need to consider measures of the relative exercise intensity (e.g., % HR max, %$\dot{V}O_2$ max) when developing PA programs, rather than relying solely on the absolute intensities (e.g., METs). Therefore, "moderate" activities, coupled with the lower threshold of training in deconditioned individuals, may be sufficient to elevate the metabolic rate and heart rate to the appropriate levels needed to achieve the various fitness ($\dot{V}O_2$ max) and health benefits that were a part of the original ACSM fitness recommendation.

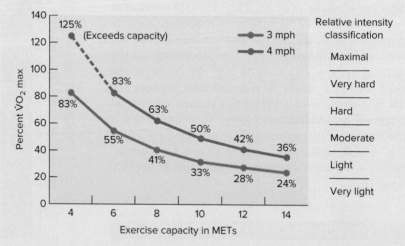

Figure 16.4 The relative exercise intensity for walking at 3.0 mph (3.3 METs) and 4.0 mph (5.0 METs) expressed as a percent of $\dot{V}O_2$ max for adults with an exercise capacity ranging from 4 to 14 METs. From U.S. Department of Health and Human Services. Physical Activity Guidelines Advisory Committee Report 2008.

Figure D.1 from U.S. Department of Health and Human Services, *Physical Activity Guidelines Advisory Committee Report 2008*, p. D-7. www.health.gov/paguidelines/committeereport.aspx.

reference in making decisions about risk (43). The data on $\dot{V}O_2$ max in Table 15.1 represent the fruits of that endeavor (44). In addition to the lower risk of death and disease, a higher $\dot{V}O_2$ max increases one's ability to engage in a broad range of recreational activities. The purpose of this section is to review the general guidelines for exercise programs aimed at increasing $\dot{V}O_2$ max. In Chap. 13, the concepts of overload and specificity were presented relative to the adaptations that take place with different training programs. Although these principles apply here, it is important to remember that little exercise is needed to achieve a health-related effect. This stands in marked contrast to the intensity of exercise needed to achieve performance goals (see Chap. 21).

IN SUMMARY

- In previously sedentary subjects, small changes in physical activity result in a large number of health benefits with only minimal risk.
- Strenuous exercise increases the risk of a heart attack during the activity, but reduces the overall (rest + exercise) risk of such an event.
- Moderate-to-high levels of cardiorespiratory fitness confers additional health benefits and increases one's ability to engage in recreational activities.

Screening

The first thing to do, if not already done in the evaluation of CRF, is to carry out some form of health status screening to decide who should begin an exercise program and who should obtain further consultation with a medical professional (see Chap. 15 for details). The risk of cardiovascular complications during exercise is directly related to the degree of pre-existing cardiac disease. In young people, the risk of sudden death is about 1/133,000 and 1/769,000 per year in men and women, respectively, due primarily to congenital or acquired heart disease. In adults, the risk of sudden death during vigorous-intensity physical activity is one per year for every 15,000 to 18,000 individuals (3).

Progression

A major point made throughout the *U.S. Physical Activity Guidelines* (83) is to use progression when introducing someone to physical activity or helping an individual move from moderate-intensity to vigorous-intensity activity. Further, this approach is used across populations, from children to older adults. General recommendations include:

- Using the relative intensity to guide the level of effort
- Transitioning from light- to moderate- to vigorous-intensity activity, not the reverse (e.g., walk before you jog/run)
- Starting with light- to moderate-intensity activity and increasing the number of minutes per day or days per week before increasing intensity
- The increase should be approximately 10% (e.g., 10 minutes more for someone doing 100 minutes per week)
- The rate of increase is lower for older, less fit, and those unaccustomed to exercise

The emphasis on moderate-intensity activities, such as walking at 3 to 4 mph, early in the fitness program is consistent with this recommendation, and the participant must be educated not to move too quickly into the more demanding activities. For more on this, see the section "Sequence of Physical Activities."

Warm-Up, Stretch, and Cool-Down, Stretch

Prior to beginning the actual exercise session, a variety of very light exercises and stretches are done to improve the transition from rest to the exercise state. The emphasis at the onset of an exercise session is to gradually increase the level of activity until the proper intensity is reached. Stretching exercises to increase the range of motion of the joints involved in the activity, as well as specific stretches to increase the flexibility of the lower back, are included in the warm-up. At the end of the activity session, about five minutes of cool-down activities–slow walking and stretching exercises–are recommended to gradually return HR and BP toward normal. This part of the exercise session is viewed as important in reducing the chance of a hypotensive episode after the exercise session (40).

EXERCISE PRESCRIPTION FOR CRF

The exercise program includes dynamic, large-muscle activities such as walking, jogging, running, swimming, cycling, rowing, and dancing. The CRF training effect of exercise programs is dependent on the proper frequency, duration, and intensity of the exercise sessions to generate an appropriate energy

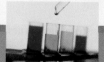
Michael L. Pollock, Ph.D., Laid the Foundation for Exercise Prescription

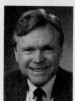

Courtesy of American College of Sports Medicine

Michael L. Pollock received his Ph.D. at the University of Illinois under the direction of Dr. Thomas K. Cureton (see Chap. 0's A Look Back—Important People in Science). In so many ways, Dr. Pollock built on Dr. Cureton's commitment to fitness but raised it to a much higher level. Mike Pollock's research laid the foundation for much of the quantitative aspects of exercise prescription that were established in the 1970s and are little changed today. When we read about the optimal intensity, frequency, and duration of exercise to achieve fitness goals and health benefits, we have Dr. Pollock to thank for providing the foundation for much of that. In 1972, he published a chapter, "Quantification of Endurance Training Programs," in the first volume of Exercise and Sports Sciences Reviews. This chapter led the way

for the American College of Sports Medicine's first position stand in 1978: "Recommended Quantity and Quality of Exercise for Developing and Maintaining Fitness," of which Dr. Pollock was the lead author. His research on the importance of strength training was instrumental in including resistance training in a later revision of that position stand. In addition, Mike Pollock's name is attached to one of the most popular equations for converting the sum of skinfolds into percentage of body fat. The fact that these equations are still used on a daily basis, many years after their development, speaks well of the quality of his work in so many areas.

Dr. Pollock also had a major impact on the development, maturation, and recognition of cardiopulmonary exercise testing and training. His research publications and textbooks (Heart Disease and Rehabilitation and Exercise in Health and Disease) in this area provided clear guidance for the delivery of

safe and effective exercise programs in the cardiopulmonary rehabilitation environment (see Suggested Readings for a textbook written in his honor: Pollock's Textbook of Cardiovascular Disease and Rehabilitation). He was a founding member of the American Association of Cardiovascular and Pulmonary Rehabilitation (AACVPR) and was the founder of the Journal of Cardiopulmonary Rehabilitation. In addition to these valuable contributions, Dr. Pollock served as president of the American College of Sports Medicine.

Mike Pollock accomplished all this work while suffering (quietly) from ankylosing spondylitis–a degenerative inflammatory disease that impairs the mobility of the spinal column. He died of a stroke in 1998, but his legacy is with us each day we do exercise testing, write an exercise prescription, and talk about "how much exercise is enough?"

Special thanks to Barry Franklin and William Haskell for information for this box.

---

expenditure (exercise volume). Historically, the relative intensity has been used to structure exercise programs to increase CRF. The ACSM recommends three to five sessions per week, for 20 to 60 minutes per session, at an intensity of about 40% to 89% heart rate reserve (HRR) or oxygen uptake reserve ($\dot{V}O_2R$) (3). This relative intensity range accommodates both moderate intensity (40% to 59% HRR) and vigorous intensity (60% to 89% HRR). The term, % $\dot{V}O_2R$, is being used in place of the traditional % $\dot{V}O_2$ max, but for those of average to high fitness, the terms are quite similar (40). The combination of the frequency, intensity, and duration should result in a volume of 500 to 1000 MET-min per week (1, 3). See A Look Back–Important People in Science for information on someone who had a major impact on exercise testing and prescription.

Frequency

The frequency of exercise is higher for moderate-intensity exercise ($\geq$5 days/wk) than vigorous-intensity exercise ($\geq$3 days/wk) in order to achieve the

recommended volume of exercise (1, 3, 83). Improvements in CRF increase with the frequency of exercise sessions, with two sessions being the minimum, and the gains in CRF leveling off after three to four sessions per week (3, 86). Gains in CRF can be achieved with a two-day-per-week program, but the intensity has to be higher than the three-day-per-week program, and participants might not achieve weight-loss goals (64). In addition, the high-intensity exercise associated with a two-day-per-week frequency is inappropriate for previously sedentary individuals. If one is doing vigorous-intensity exercise, a schedule of three to four days per week includes a day off between sessions and reduces the scheduling problems associated with planned exercise programs. Figure 16.5 shows that higher frequencies are associated with higher rates of injuries (63, 65, 66, 84).

Intensity

Intensity describes the overload on the cardiovascular system that is needed to bring about a training effect. It should be no surprise that the intensity

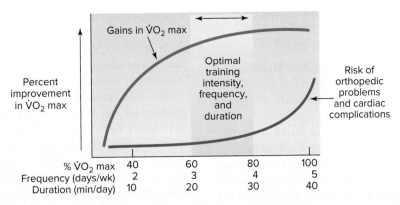

Figure 16.5 Effects of increasing the frequency, duration, and intensity of exercise on the increase in $\dot{V}O_2$ max in a training program. This figure demonstrates the increasing risk of orthopedic problems due to exercise sessions that are too long or conducted too many times per week. The probability of cardiac complications increases with exercise intensity beyond that recommended for improvements in cardiorespiratory fitness.

threshold for a CRF training effect is lower for the less fit and higher for the more fit. Swain and Franklin (81) found that the threshold for an improvement in $\dot{V}O_2$ max was only 30% of oxygen uptake reserve ($\dot{V}O_2R$) for those with $\dot{V}O_2$ max values less than 40 ml · kg^{-1} · min^{-1}, and only 46% $\dot{V}O_2R$ for those with a $\dot{V}O_2$ max greater than 40 ml · kg^{-1} · min^{-1}. However, in general, they found that higher-intensity exercise was better for increasing $\dot{V}O_2$ max. As mentioned at the beginning of this section, the range of exercise intensities associated with an increase in $\dot{V}O_2$ max is 40% to 89% $\dot{V}O_2R$, which is similar to 40% to 89% $\dot{V}O_2$ max for people of average or better fitness. However, for most people, 60% to 80% $\dot{V}O_2$ max seems to be a range sufficient to achieve CRF goals (40). It appears that for this information to be useful, the exercise leader has to know the energy requirements ($\dot{V}O_2$) of all the fitness activities so that a correct match can be made between the activity and the participant. Fortunately, because of the linear relationship between exercise intensity and HR, the exercise intensity can be set by using the HR values equivalent to 60% to 80% $\dot{V}O_2$ max. The range of heart rate values associated with the exercise intensity needed to have a CRF training effect is called the **target heart rate (THR) range.** How do you determine the THR range?

Direct Method Figure 16.6 shows the HR response of a 20-year-old subject during a maximal GXT on a treadmill. The subject's $\dot{V}O_2$ max was 12 METs so that 60% and 80% $\dot{V}O_2$ max is equal to about 7.2 and 9.6 METs, respectively. A line is drawn from each of these work rates up to the HR/$\dot{V}O_2$ line and over to the y-axis, where the HR values equivalent to these work rates are obtained. These HR values, 138 to 164 b · min^{-1}, represent the THR range, the proper intensity for a CRF training effect (1, 40).

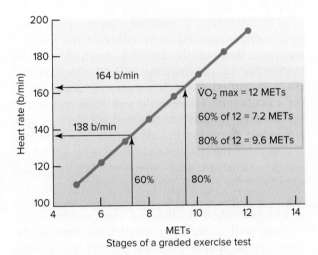

Figure 16.6 Target heart rate range determined from the results of an exercise stress test. The heart rate values measured at work rates equal to 60% and 80% $\dot{V}O_2$ max constitute the THR range.

Indirect Methods The THR range can also be estimated by some simple calculations, knowing that the relationship between HR and $\dot{V}O_2$ is linear. The heart rate reserve, or Karvonen, method of calculating a THR range has three simple steps (45, 46):

1. Subtract resting HR from maximal HR to obtain HR reserve (HRR).
2. Take 60% and 80% of the HRR.
3. Add each HRR value to resting HR to obtain the THR range.

For example:

1. If a subject has a maximal HR of 200 b · min^{-1} and a resting HR of 60 b · min^{-1}, then the HRR is 140 b · min^{-1} (200 − 60).
2. 60% × 140 b · min^{-1} = 84 b · min^{-1} and 80% × 140 b · min^{-1} = 112 b · min^{-1}

3. $84 \text{ b} \cdot \text{min}^{-1} + 60 \text{ b} \cdot \text{min}^{-1} = 144 \text{ b} \cdot \text{min}^{-1}$
   $112 \text{ b} \cdot \text{min}^{-1} + 60 \text{ b} \cdot \text{min}^{-1} = 172 \text{ b} \cdot \text{min}^{-1}$
   The THR range is 144 to 172 $\text{b} \cdot \text{min}^{-1}$.

This method gives reasonable estimates of the exercise intensity because 60% to 80% of the HRR is equal to about 60% to 80% $\dot{V}O_2$ max for those with average or high fitness.

The other indirect method of calculating the THR range is the *percentage of maximal* HR method. In this method, you simply take 70% and 85% of maximal HR to obtain the THR range. In the following example, the subject has a maximal HR of 200 $\text{b} \cdot \text{min}^{-1}$. The THR range for this person is 140 to 170 $\text{b} \cdot \text{min}^{-1}$ (70% × 200 = 140 $\text{b} \cdot \text{min}^{-1}$; 85% × 200 = 170 $\text{b} \cdot \text{min}^{-1}$). Seventy percent of maximal HR is equal to about 55% $\dot{V}O_2$ max, and 85% of maximal HR is equal to about 75% $\dot{V}O_2$ max, both within the intensity range needed for CRF gains, but slightly more conservative than the 60% to 80% HHR (35–37, 52).

The intensity of exercise can be prescribed by the direct method or by either of the indirect methods. Both of the indirect methods require knowledge of the maximal HR. If the maximal HR is measured during a maximal GXT, use it in the calculations. However, if you have to use the age-adjusted estimate of maximal HR (220 − age), remember the potential error with the standard deviation of the estimate equal to ±11 $\text{b} \cdot \text{min}^{-1}$. Tanaka, Monahan, and Seals (82) evaluated the validity of the classic "220 − age" equation to estimate maximal HR. They carried out an analysis of 351 published studies and cross-validated the findings with a well-controlled laboratory study. They found almost identical results using both approaches: HR max = 208 − 0.7 × age. This new equation yields maximal heart rate values that are 6 $\text{b} \cdot \text{min}^{-1}$ lower for 20-year-olds and 6 $\text{b} \cdot \text{min}^{-1}$ higher for 60-year-olds. A recent longitudinal study confirmed this with their equation being HR max = 207 − 0.7 × age (24). Although the new formulas yield better estimates of HR max *on average*, the investigators emphasize the fact that the estimated HR max for a given individual is still associated with a standard deviation of ±10 $\text{b} \cdot \text{min}^{-1}$.

- When using an exercise heart rate value to estimate the % $\dot{V}O_2$ max or % $\dot{V}O_2R$ at which the individual is working, the error is about 6 6% (i.e., 60% HRR = 60 ± 6% $\dot{V}O_2R$) for two-thirds of the population when the *measured* maximal heart rate is known.

- If we use an age-predicted *estimate of* maximal heart rate to set the target heart rate range, the error involved in estimating the maximal heart rate value (one standard deviation is ± 10 $\text{b} \cdot \text{min}^{-1}$) adds to the error in estimating % $\dot{V}O_2$ max or % $\dot{V}O_2R$.

Consequently, the estimated THR range is a *guideline* for exercise intensity and is meant to be used with other information (e.g., degree of effort, abnormal symptoms or signs) to determine if the exercise intensity is reasonable.

In this regard, Borg's RPE scale can be used as an adjunct to HR in prescribing exercise intensity for apparently healthy individuals. The RPE range of 12 to 17 on the original Borg scale covers the range of exercise intensities similar to 40% to 89% HRR (1, 3, 10, 19, 29, 30, 67). The RPE scale is helpful because the participant learns to associate the THR range with a certain whole-body perception of effort, decreasing the need for frequent pulse rate measurements. The RPE scale has been shown to have a high test-retest reliability (18), and it is closely linked to the % $\dot{V}O_2$ max and lactate threshold, independent of the mode of exercise and fitness of the subject (38, 74, 77). Remember, the intensity threshold needed to achieve CRF goals is lower for the less fit, and vice versa. In contrast to using continuous exercise at a specified intensity to achieve one's goals, there is heightened interest in the use of high-intensity intermittent exercise to achieve the same goals in a shorter period of time (see Clinical Applications 16.2).

Time (Duration)

The duration or time has to be viewed together with intensity, in that the volume of exercise is an important variable associated with improvements in CRF after the minimal threshold of intensity is achieved (3). For those working at lower intensities, a greater duration will be needed to achieve the same energy expenditure of someone working at a higher intensity. A good example showing the role that duration and volume play (at constant exercise intensity) in the increase in CRF is a study by Church et al. (20). Sedentary, postmenopausal overweight or obese women were randomly assigned into either a control group or one of three moderate-intensity (~50% $\dot{V}O_2$ peak) physical activity groups to achieve an energy expenditure of 4, 8, or 12 kcal/kg per week. The increase in $\dot{V}O_2$ peak was 4.2%, 6%, and 8.2% in these groups, respectively, indicating a dose-response relationship with exercise duration (20). This is important, given that many sedentary persons can more easily accomplish an exercise session of low intensity and long duration than the reverse, and achieve the health-related benefits of physical activity with minimal risk. Obviously, if participants choose to exercise at higher intensities, it would take less time to achieve an energy expenditure goal. Figure 16.5 shows that doing strenuous exercise (75% $\dot{V}O_2$ max) for more than 30 minutes per session increases the risk of orthopedic problems.

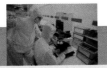
High-Intensity Interval Training (HIIT)

The physical activity guidelines presented thus far have focused on continuous aerobic activity done at either a moderate (e.g., 3 to 5.9 METs for 30 min/day, 5 days per week) or vigorous intensity ($\geq$6 METs, 25 min/day, 3 days per week). However, a mode of training that has been used by a variety of endurance athletes for more than 100 years has grown in popularity in fitness programs. That mode is interval training, now commonly called high-intensity interval (intermittent) training (HIIT). HIIT programs usually begin with a warm-up, followed by a series of brief bouts of high-intensity exercise, with each bout separated by a recovery period of rest or exercise at a lower intensity. The "high/low" interval is repeated a specified number of times (e.g., a series of 3 to 10 intervals), and is followed by a recovery period before the series is repeated. Consequently, the number of variables included in a HIIT exercise prescription include at least the following (13, 14):

- Type of exercise (e.g., run, cycle)
- Intensity settings and durations of both the high and low parts of an interval
- Number of intervals done per series
- Intensity and duration of recovery between series

Although HIIT programs are more complicated to structure than the typical physical activity recommendations mentioned above, the renewed interest in them has been stimulated by research showing that these programs result in very large physiological changes in a very short period of time. For example, after only six sessions of four to seven "all-out" 30-s Wingate tests with 4 minutes of recovery between each, there were increases in oxidative capacity, the capacity for fat oxidation, intramuscular glucose transporters, resting muscle glycogen levels, and exercise performance (e.g., time to exhaustion at a fixed workload) (15, 25, 26, 51).

Because this supra maximal Wingate HIIT protocol was so demanding and potentially dangerous for some individuals, an alternative HIIT protocol was tested. In this protocol subjects did ten 60-s work bouts at an intensity that demanded ~90% maximal HR, followed by 60s of recovery. The results were similar to the more strenuous Wingate HIIT protocol (26). Interestingly, HIIT protocols like this alternative version are perceived as being more enjoyable compared to 50 minutes of continuous exercise at 70% $\dot{V}O_2$ max, even though the RPE was higher in the HIIT protocol (9). Systematic reviews of the research in this area continue to support these observations (53), including the impact of HIIT on patients with cardiovascular disease (23, 28, 48).

Not all interval training programs require one to exercise at near-maximal or supra-maximal levels. As shown in Table 16.1, the use of a jog/walk interval is a good way to help someone transition from moderate-intensity to vigorous-intensity physical activity.

Lastly, we recommend reading the classic studies by Åstrand et al. and Christensen et al. in Suggested Readings to see the impact that variations in the length of the exercise and/or rest interval have on HR, $\dot{V}O_2$, and lactate responses, compared to continuous exercise.

IN SUMMARY

- A sedentary person needs to go through a health status screening before participating in exercise.
- Exercise programs for previously sedentary persons should start with moderate-intensity activities (walking) and focus on increasing frequency and duration to gain additional health benefits before intensity is increased.
- The optimal characteristics of a vigorous-intensity exercise program to increase $\dot{V}O_2$ max are intensity = 60% to 80% $\dot{V}O_2$ max; frequency = three to four times per week; duration = minutes needed to achieve a volume of 500 to 1000 MET-min per week.
- The THR range, taken as 60% to 80% HRR, or 70% to 85% of maximal HR, is a reasonable estimate of the proper exercise intensity.

To determine if the subject is in the THR range during the activity, HR should be checked immediately after stopping, taking a 10-second pulse count within the first 15 seconds. The pulse can be taken at the radial artery or the carotid artery; if the latter is used, the participant should use only light pressure, since heavy pressure can actually slow the HR (40, 67). However, when possible, a "heart watch" should be used for greater accuracy.

As mentioned earlier, it is important that sedentary individuals start slowly before exercising at the recommended intensities specified in the THR range. The next section provides some suggestions on how to make that transition.

SEQUENCE OF PHYSICAL ACTIVITY

The old adage that you should "walk before you run" is consistent with the way exercise should be recommended to sedentary persons, be they young or old (83).

After the person demonstrates an ability to do prolonged walking without fatigue, then controlled fitness exercises conducted at a reasonable intensity (THR) can be introduced. After that, and depending on the interest of the participant, a variety of fitness activities that are more game-like can be included. This section will deal with this sequence of activities that can lead to a fit life (40).

Walking

The primary activity to recommend to someone who has been sedentary for a long time is walking, or its equivalent if orthopedic problems exist. This recommendation is consistent with the introductory material on health benefits described in Chap. 14, and it deals with the issue of injuries associated with more strenuous physical activity. In addition, there is good reason to believe that some (many) individuals may use walking as their primary or only form of exercise. The emphasis at this stage is to simply get people active by providing an activity that can be done anywhere, anytime, and with anyone, young or old. In this way, the number of possible interfering factors that can result in the discontinuance of the exercise is reduced.

The person should choose comfortable shoes that are flexible, offer a wide base of support, and have a fitted heel cup. There are a great number of "walking" shoes available, but a special pair of shoes is not usually required. The emphasis is on getting started; if walking becomes a "serious" activity or leads to hiking, then the investment would be reasonable. If weather is not to interfere with the activity, then proper selection of clothing is necessary. The participant should wear light, loose-fitting clothing in warm weather, and layers of wool or polypropylene in cold weather. For those who cannot bear the extremes in temperature and humidity out of doors, various shopping malls provide a controlled environment with a smooth surface. Walkers should choose the areas in which they walk with care in order to avoid damaged streets, high traffic zones, and poorly lighted areas. Safety is important in any health-related exercise program (40, 83). A walking program is presented in Table 16.1 (40). The steps are rather simple in that progression to the next stage does not occur unless the individual feels comfortable at the current stage. The HR should be recorded as described previously, but the emphasis is not on achieving the THR. Later on in the walking program, if higher walking speeds are used, the THR zone will be attained. Remember that walking, in spite of not being very strenuous by the THR zone scale, when combined with long duration is an effective part of a weight-control and CHD risk factor reduction program (59, 68, 83). Walking is an activity that many people find they can do every day, providing many opportunities to expend calories.

Jogging

Jogging begins when a person moves at a speed and form that results in a period of flight between foot strikes; this may be 3 or 4 mph, or 6 or 7 mph, depending on the fitness of the individual. As described in Chap. 1, the net energy cost of jogging/running is about twice that of walking at slow to moderate speeds and requires a greater cardiovascular response. This is not the only reason for the jogging program to follow a walking program; there is also more stress on joints and muscles due to the impact forces that must be tolerated during the push off and landing while jogging (17).

The emphasis at the start of a jogging program is to make the transition from the walking program in such a way as to minimize the discomfort associated with the introduction of any new activity. This is accomplished by beginning with a jog-walk-jog program that eases the person into jogging by mixing in the lower energy cost and trauma associated with walking. The jogging speed is set according to the THR, with the aim to stay at the low end of the THR zone at the beginning of the program. As the participant adapts to jogging, the HR response for any jogging speed will decrease, and jogging speed will have to be increased to stay in the THR zone. This is the primary marker that a training effect is taking place. Table 16.1 also presents a jogging program with some simple rules to follow. Special attention is made to completing the walking program first, staying in the THR zone, and not progressing to the next level if the participant is not comfortable with the current level. Jogging is not for everyone, and for those who are obese, or have ankle, knee, or hip problems, it might be a good activity to avoid. Two activities that reduce such stress are cycling (stationary or outdoor) and swimming (40). More on exercise for special populations will be presented in Chap. 17.

Games and Sports

As a person becomes accustomed to exercising in the THR range while jogging, swimming, or cycling, more uncontrolled activities can be introduced that require higher levels of energy expenditure, but do so in a more intermittent fashion. Games (paddleball, racquetball, squash), sports (basketball, soccer), and various forms of group exercise can keep a person's interest and make it more likely that the person will maintain a physically active life. These activities should be built on a walk-and-jogging base to reduce the chance that the participant will make poor adjustments to the activity. In addition, by having the habit of walking or jogging (swimming or cycling), the participant will still be able to maintain his or her habit of physical activity when there is no one to play with or lead the class. In contrast to jogging, cycling, or swimming, it will be more difficult to stay in the THR range with these intermittent

TABLE 16.1 Examples of Walking and Jogging Programs

Walking Program			Jogging/ Running Program	
Rules			**Rules**	
1. Start at a level that feels comfortable			1. Complete walking program first.	
2. Stretch before each session			2. Walk and stretch before each session	
3. Be aware of aches and pains			3. Be aware of aches and pains	
4. Progress one stage when comfortable			4. Progress one stage when comfortable	
5. Monitor HR, but do not be concerned about being in the THR zone			5. Stay at low-end of the THR zone by varying time of walk/jog interval or jogging pace	
6. Walk at least five days per week			6. Do program on every-other day basis	
Stage	**Time (min)**	**Comments**	**Stage**	
1	10	Walk at a comfortable pace	1	Jog ten steps, walk ten steps; repeat five times and check HR. Do for 20–30 minutes.
2	15		2	Jog 20 steps, walk ten steps; repeat five times and check HR. Do for 20–30 minutes.
3	20	Split into two ten-minute walks if needed	3	Jog 30 steps, walk ten steps; repeat five times and check HR. Do for 20–30 minutes.
4	25		4	Jog one minute, walk ten steps; repeat five times and check HR. Do for 20–30 minutes.
5	30	Do two 15-minute walks if preferred	5	Jog two minutes, walk ten steps; repeat five times and check HR. Do for 20–30 minutes.
6	35		6	Jog one lap and check HR. Walk briefly and complete four to six laps
7	40	Two 20-minute walks will meet goal	7	Jog two laps and check HR. Walk briefly and complete four to six laps
8	45		8	Jog one mile and check HR. Walk briefly and do 1.5 to 2 miles.
9	50	You can do 25 minutes in the A.M. and P.M.	9	Jog continuously for 20–40 minutes and check HR.

Adapted from Walking and Jogging programs listed on pages 410 and 412 of Howley, E. T., and Thompson, D. L., *Fitness Professional's Handbook*, 7th ed. Champaign, IL: Human Kinetics, 2017.

activities. It is more likely that the HR will move from below the threshold value to above the top end of the THR from time to time. This is a normal response to activities that are intermittent in nature. It must be stressed, however, that when playing games, it is important that the participants have some degree of skill and be reasonably well matched. If one is much better than the other, neither will have a good workout (54).

STRENGTH AND FLEXIBILITY TRAINING

The focus in this chapter has been on training to improve cardiorespiratory fitness. However, both the ACSM position stand on fitness (1) and the updates on the public health PA guidelines (33, 83) recommend both strength and flexibility exercises as part of the complete fitness program. Table 16.2 shows

that resistance training has a variety of health benefits in addition to increasing or maintaining strength (8). Collectively, these health-related findings point to the need for resistance training to be a part of a regular exercise program. The ACSM recommendation emphasizes dynamic exercises done on a routine basis, but early on there was some debate about how much is enough (see Clinical Applications 16.3).

Flexibility usually refers to the ability to move a joint through its normal range of motion. Current ACSM recommendations for static stretching include (2):

- Stretching to the point of mild discomfort and holding for 10 to 30s
- Doing each stretch two to four times
- Doing stretching exercises ≥2 days per week

In addition, dynamic, ballistic, and proprioceptive neuromuscular facilitation (PNF) methods are appropriate for improving flexibility.

Variable	Aerobic Exercise	Resistance Exercise
TABLE 16.2 Comparison of Effects of Aerobic Exercise with Resistance Exercise on Health and Fitness Variables[a]		
Total body fat	↓↓	↓
Intra-abdominal fat	↓↓	↓↔
Lean body mass	↔	↑↑
Body weight	↓	↔
Resting metabolic rate	↑	↑↑
Muscular strength	↔	↑↑↑
Muscular mass	↔	↑↑
Muscular power	↔	↑
Capillary density	↑	↔
Mitochondrial volume	↑↑	↓↔
Mitochondrial density	↑↑	↓↔
Basal insulin levels	↓	↓
Insulin sensitivity	↑↑	↑↑
Insulin response to glucose challenge	↓↓	↓↓
Resting heart rate	↓↓	↔
SBP at rest	↓↓	↓
DBP at rest	↓↓	↓
Peak VO$_2$	↑↑↑	↑↔
Submaximal and maximal endurance time	↑↑↑	↑↑
Submaximal exercise rate-pressure product	↓↓↓	↓↓

Abbreviations: DBP, diastolic blood pressure; SBP, systolic blood pressure.

[a]↑ Indicates increased; ↓, decreased; ↔, negligible effect; 1 arrow, small effect; 2 arrows, moderate effect; 3 arrows, large effect.

It is beyond the scope of this text to go into detail regarding strength and flexibility programs aimed at improving or maintaining these fitness components. We recommend the works by Faigenbaum and McInnis, for muscular strength and endurance, and by Liemohn, for flexibility and low-back function, as good starting points. These can be found in Suggested Readings.

IN SUMMARY

- A logical progression of physical activities is from walking to jogging to games. The progression addresses issues of intensity, as well as the risk of injury. For many, walking may be their only aerobic activity.
- Strength and flexibility activities should be included as a regular part of an exercise program.

ENVIRONMENTAL CONCERNS

It is important that the participant be educated about the effects of extreme heat and humidity, altitude, and cold on the adaptation to exercise. The THR range acts as a guide in that it provides feedback to the participant about the interaction of the environment and the exercise intensity. As the heat and humidity increase, there is an increased need to circulate additional blood to the skin to dissipate the heat. As altitude increases, there is less oxygen bound to hemoglobin, and the person must pump more blood to the muscles to have the same oxygen delivery. In both of these situations, the HR response to a fixed exercise bout will be higher. To counter this tendency and stay in the THR range, the subject should decrease the work rate. Exercise in most cold environments can be refreshing and safe if a person plans in advance and dresses accordingly. However, there are some temperature/wind combinations that should be avoided because of the inability to adapt to them. As mentioned previously, some people simply plan exercise indoors (shopping malls, health spas, home exercise) during those occasions so that their routine is not interrupted. These environmental factors will be considered in more detail in Chap. 24.

IN SUMMARY

- The THR acts as a guide to adjust exercise intensity in adverse environments such as high temperature and humidity or altitude.
- A decrease in exercise intensity will counter the effects of high environmental temperature and humidity to allow one to stay in the target HR zone.

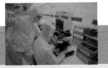
Strength Training: Single Versus Multiple Sets

It wasn't until 1998 that the ACSM recommended resistance training as part of a well-rounded fitness program. The goals were to increase or maintain muscular strength and endurance, the fat-free mass, and bone mineral density (1). To accomplish this, the ACSM recommended:

- A minimum of one set of eight to ten exercises that conditions the major muscle groups
- Eight to twelve reps per set (10 to 15 for older individuals)
- Two or more nonconsecutive sessions per week

Although the position stand acknowledges that "multiple-set regimes may provide greater benefits," the review of literature supported the use of one set to achieve the health-related and fitness goals.

Not all agreed with that interpretation of the literature. The debate about one set versus multiple sets was raised to a higher level when the ACSM published a second position stand in 2002 with a focus on progression models of resistance training for improving strength (5). This position stand recommended a variety of approaches to achieve strength goals, including using multiple sets. Since the appearance of that position stand, a number of systematic analyses of the research literature dealing with the issue of single set versus multiple sets have been published (22, 72, 75, 87).

These review articles, as well as other studies (41, 76), indicate rather convincingly that multiple sets are better than one set at increasing strength. However, "when maximal strength gain is not the principal goal of the training program, a single-set protocol may be sufficient to significantly improve upper- and lower-body strength as well as being time efficient" (22). This would appear to support both the "one-set" recommendation for improving and maintaining muscular fitness in the average individual as well as the "multiple-set" recommendation for those interested in achieving higher strength goals.

The issue of dose-response was discussed earlier in this chapter relative to health-related outcomes and increases in $\dot{V}O_2$ max. For strength and conditioning programs, it became clear that what was required for *maximal gains* in strength in untrained subjects was less than that required for trained subejcts and athletes (62, 73):

- For untrained subjects: do four sets at 60% 1-RM, three days a week (73).
- For trained subjects: do four sets at 80% 1-RM, two days a week (73).
- For athletes: do eight sets at 85% 1-RM, two days a week (62).

This growing body of research prompted the American College of Sports Medicine to update its 2002 position stand on progression models in resistance training for healthy adults (4). What follows is a brief summary of the position stand for gains in strength. Additional guidelines are provided in the position stand for gains in hypertrophy, power, and local muscular endurance.

- For novice (untrained individuals): loads should correspond to 60% to 70% of 1-RM for 8 to 12 repetitions; do one to three sets at slow and moderate velocities of contraction, with at least two- to three-minute rest between sets; train two to three days per week.
- For intermediate (~six months training) individuals: loads should correspond to 60% to 70% of 1-RM for 8 to 12 repetitions; use multiple sets with variations in volume and intensity over time; do at moderate velocities of contraction with three- to five-minute rest between sets; train three to four days a week.
- For advanced (years of training) individuals: loads should correspond to 80% to 100% of 1-RM; do multiple sets with variations in volume and intensity over time, using variable velocities of contraction (relative to intensity), with at least two- to three-minute rest between sets; train four to six days a week.

These guidelines were incorporated in both the ACSM 2011 position stand on fitness (2) and in the 2014 edition of *Guidelines for Exercise Testing and Prescription* (3).

STUDY ACTIVITIES

1. What are the practical implications of classifying physical inactivity as a primary risk factor?
2. From a public health standpoint, why is there so much attention paid to increasing a sedentary person's physical activity by a small amount rather than recommending strenuous exercise?
3. What is the risk of cardiac arrest for someone who participates in a regular physical activity program?
4. What is the difference between "exercise" and "physical activity"?
5. List the optimal frequency, intensity, and duration of exercise needed to achieve an increase in cardiorespiratory function.
6. For a person with a maximal heart rate of 180 b · min^{-1} and a resting heart rate of 70 b · min^{-1}, calculate a target

heart rate range by the Karvonen method and the percent of maximal HR method.

7. Recommend an appropriate progression of activities for a sedentary person wanting to become fit.

8. Why is it important to monitor heart rate frequently during exercise in heat, in humidity, and at altitude?

9. How does resistance training compare with aerobic training in reducing risk of disease?

10. What is the recommended resistance-training program for untrained adults?

SUGGESTED READINGS

American College of Sports Medicine. 2013. *ACSM's Resource Manual for Guidelines for Exercise Testing and Prescription.* 7th ed. Baltimore, MD: Lippincott Williams & Wilkins.

Åstrand, I., P-O. Åstrand, E. H. Christensen, and R. Hedman. 1960. Intermittent muscular work. *Acta Physiologica Scandinavia.* 48: 448-453.

Baechle, T. R., and R. W. Earle. 2016. *Essentials of Strength Training and Conditioning.* 4th ed. Champaign, IL: Human Kinetics.

Christensen, E. H., R. Hedman, and B. Saltin. 1960. Intermittent and continuous running. *Acta Physiologica Scandinavica.* 50: 269-286.

Durstine, J. L., G. E. Moore, M. J. LaMonte, and B. A. Franklin. 2008. *Pollock's Textbook of Cardiovascular Disease and Rehabilitation.* Champaign, IL: Human Kinetics.

Faigenbaum, A. D. 2017. Exercise prescription for muscular fitness. In *Fitness Professional's Handbook,* 7th ed. E. T. Howley and D. L. Thompson (eds). Champaign, IL: Human Kinetics.

Howley, E. T., and D. L. Thompson. 2017. *Fitness Professional's Handbook.* 7th ed. Champaign, IL: Human Kinetics.

Gagnon, L. H. 2017. Exercise prescription for flexibility and low-back function. In *Fitness Professional's Handbook.* 7th ed. E. T. Howley and D. L. Thompson (eds). Champaign, IL: Human Kinetics.

U.S. Department of Health and Human Services. 1996. *Physical Activity and Health: A Report of the Surgeon General.* Atlanta, GA: U.S. Department of Health and Human Services, Centers for Disease Control and Prevention, National Center for Chronic Disease Prevention and Health Promotion.

REFERENCES

1. **American College of Sports Medicine.** American College of Sports Medicine position stand: the recommended quantity and quality of exercise for developing and maintaining cardiorespiratory and muscular fitness, and flexibility in healthy adults. *Medicine & Science in Sports & Exercise* 30: 975-991, 1998.

2. **American College of Sports Medicine.** Quantity and quality of exercise for developing and maintaining cardiorespiratory, musculoskeletal, and neuromotor fitness in apparently healthy adults: guidance for prescribing exercise. *Medicine & Science in Sports & Exercise* 43:1334-1359, 2011.

3. **American College of Sports Medicine.** *Guidelines for Exercise Testing and Prescription.* Baltimore, MD: Lippincott Williams & Wilkins, 2014.

4. **American College of Sports Medicine.** Progression models in resistance training for healthy adults. *Medicine & Science in Sports & Exercise* 41: 1510-1530, 2009.

5. **American College of Sports Medicine.** Progression models in resistance training for healthy adults. *Medicine & Science in Sports & Exercise* 34: 364-380, 2002.

6. **American College of Sports Medicine.** Summary statement: workshop on physical activity and public health. *Sports Medicine Bulletin* 28: 7, 1993.

7. **American Heart Association.** Statement on exercise: benefits and recommendations for physical activity programs for all Americans. A statement for health professionals by the Committee on Exercise and Cardiac Rehabilitation of the Council on Clinical Cardiology, American Heart Association. *Circulation* 86: 340-344, 1992.

8. **Artero EG, Lee D-C, Lavie CJ, España-Romero V, Sui X, Church TS, et al.** Effects of muscular strength on cardiovascular risk factors and prognosis. *Journal of Cardiopulmonary Rehabilitation and Prevention* 32: 351-358, 2012.

9. **Bartlett JD, Close GL, Maclaren DPM, Gregson W, Drust B, and Morton JP.** High-intensity running is perceived to be more enjoyable than moderate-intensity continuous exercise: implications for exercise adherence. *Journal of Sport Sciences* 29: 547-553, 2011.

10. **Birk TJ and Birk CA.** Use of ratings of perceived exertion for exercise prescription. *Sports Medicine* 4: 1-8, 1987.

11. **Blair SN, Kohl HW, III, Barlow CE, Paffenbarger RS, Jr., Gibbons LW, and Macera CA.** Changes in physical fitness and all-cause mortality: a prospective study of healthy and unhealthy men. JAMA 273: 1093-1098, 1995.

12. **Blair SN, Kohl HW, III, Paffenbarger RS, Jr., Clark DG, Cooper KH, and Gibbons LW.** Physical fitness and all-cause mortality: a prospective study of healthy men and women. JAMA 262: 2395-2401, 1989.

13. **Buchheit M and Laursen PB.** High-intensity interval training, solutions to the programming puzzle. Part I: Cardiopulmonary emphasis. *Sports Medicine* 43: 313-338, 2013.

14. **Buchheit M and Laursen PB.** High-intensity interval training, solutions to the programming puzzle. Part II: Anaerobic energy, neuromuscular load and practical applications. *Sports Medicine* 43: 927-954, 2013.

15. **Burgomaster KA, Hughes SC, Heigenhauser GJF, Bradwell SN, and Gibala MJ.** Six sessions of sprint interval training increases muscle oxidative potential and cycle endurance capacity in humans. *Journal of Applied Physiology* 98: 1985-1990, 2005.

16. **Caspersen CJ, Powell KE, and Christenson GM.** Physical activity, exercise, and physical fitness: definitions and distinctions for health-related research. *Public Health Reports* 100: 126-131, 1985.

17. **Cavanagh PR.** *The Running Shoe Book.* Mountain View, CA: Anderson World, 1980.

18. **Ceci R and Hassmen P.** Self-monitored exercise at three different RPE intensities in treadmill vs field running. *Medicine & Science in Sports & Exercise* 23: 732-738, 1991.

19. **Chow RJ and Wilmore JH.** The regulation of exercise intensity by ratings of perceived exertion. *Journal of Cardiac Rehabilitation* 4: 382-387, 1984.

20. **Church TS, Earnest CP, Skinner JS, and Blair SN.** Effects of different doses of physical activity on cardiorespiratory fitness among sedentary, overweight or obese postmenopausal women with elevated blood pressure: a randomized controlled trial. *JAMA* 297: 2081-2091, 2007.

21. **Dionne FT, Turcotte L, Thibault MC, Boulay MR, Skinner JS, and Bouchard C.** Mitochondrial DNA sequence polymorphism, $\dot{V}O_2$ max, and response to endurance training. *Medicine & Science in Sports & Exercise* 23: 177-185, 1991.

22. **Galvao DA and Taaffe DR.** Single- vs. multiple-set resistance training: recent developments in the controversy. *Journal of Strength and Conditioning Research/National Strength & Conditioning Association* 18: 660-667, 2004.

23. **Gayda M, Ribeiro PAB, Juneau M, and Nigam A.** Comparison of different forms of exercise training in patients with cardiac disease: where does high-intensity interval training fit? *Canadian Journal of Cardiology* 32: 485-494, 2016.

24. **Gellish RL, Goslin BR, Olson RE, McDonald A, Russi GD, and Moudgil VK.** Longitudinal modeling of the relationship between age and maximal heart rate. *Medicine & Science in Sports & Exercise* 39: 822-829, 2007.

25. **Gibala MJ and McGee SL.** Metabolic adaptations to short-term high-intensity interval training a little pain for a lot of gain? *Exercise and Sport Science Review* 36: 58-63, 2008.

26. **Gibala MJ, Little JP, MacDonald J, and Hawley JA.** Physiological adaptations to low-volume, high-intensity interval training in health and disease. *Journal of Physiology* 590(5): 1077-1084, 2012.

27. **Goodman LS and Gilman A.** *The Pharmacological Basis of Therapeutics.* New York, NY: Macmillan, 1975.

28. **Guiraud T, Nigam A, Gremeaux V, Meyer P, Juneau M, and Bosquet L.** High-intensity interval training in cardiac rehabilitation. *Sports Medicine* 42: 587-605, 2012.

29. **Gutmann M.** Perceived exertion-heart rate relationship during exercise testing and training in cardiac patients. *Journal of Cardiac Rehabilitation* 1: 52-59, 1981.

30. **Hage P.** Perceived exertion: one measure of exercise intensity. *Physician and Sportsmedicine* 9: 136-143, 1981.

31. **Haskell WL.** Dose-response issues from a biological perspective. In *Physical Activity, Fitness, and Health*, edited by Bouchard C, Shephard RJ, and Stevens T. Champaign, IL: Human Kinetics, 1994, pp. 1030-1039.

32. **Haskell WL.** Physical activity and health: need to define the required stimulus. *The American Journal of Cardiology* 55: 4D-9D, 1985.

33. **Haskell WL, Lee IM, Pate RR, Powell KE, Blair SN, Franklin BA, et al.** Physical activity and public health: updated recommendation for adults from the American College of Sports Medicine and the American Heart Association. *Medicine & Science in Sports & Exercise* 39: 1423-1434, 2007.

34. **Haskell WL, Montoye HJ, and Orenstein D.** Physical activity and exercise to achieve health-related physical fitness components. *Public Health Report* 100: 202-212, 1985.

35. **Hellerstein H.** Principles of exercise prescription for normals and cardiac subjects. In *Exercise Training in Coronary Heart Disease*, edited by Naughton JP, and Hellerstein HK. New York, NY: Academic Press, 1973, pp. 129-167.

36. **Hellerstein HK and Ader R.** Relationship between percent maximal oxygen uptake (% max $\dot{V}O_2$) and percent maximal heart rate (% MHR) in normals and cardiacs (ASHD). *Circulation* 43-44 (Suppl II): 76, 1971.

37. **Hellerstein HK and Franklin BA.** Exercise testing and prescription. In *Rehabilitation of the Coronary Patient*, edited by Wenger NK, and Hellerstein HK. New York, NY: Wiley, 1984, pp. 197-284.

38. **Hetzler RK, Seip RL, Boutcher SH, Pierce E, Snead D, and Weltman A.** Effect of exercise modality on ratings of perceived exertion at various lactate concentrations. *Medicine & Science in Sports & Exercise* 23: 88-92, 1991.

39. **Howley ET.** Type of activity: resistance, aerobic and leisure versus occupational physical activity. *Medicine & Science in Sports & Exercise* 33: S364-369; discussion S419-320, 2001.

40. **Howley ET and Thompson DL.** *Fitness Professional's Handbook.* 7th ed. Champaign, IL: Human Kinetics, 2017.

41. **Humburg H, Baars H, Schroder J, Reer R, and Braumann KM.** 1-set vs. 3-set resistance training: a crossover study. *Journal of Strength and Conditioning Research/National Strength & Conditioning Association* 21: 578-582, 2007.

42. **Jennings GL, Deakin G, Korner P, Meredith I, Kingwell B, and Nelson L.** What is the dose-response relationship between exercise training and blood pressure? *Annals of Medicine* 23: 313-318, 1991.

43. **Kaminsky LA, Arena R, Beckie TM, Brubaker PH, Church TS, Forman DE, et al.** The importance of cardiorespiratory fitness in the United States: the need for a national registry. A policy statement from

the American Heart Association. *Circulation* 127: 652-662, 2012.

44. **Kaminsky LA, Arena R, and Myers J.** Reference standards for cardiorespiratory fitness measured with cardiopulmonary exercise testing: data from the Fitness Registry and the Importance of Exercise National Database. *Mayo Clinic Proceedings* 90: 1515-1523, 2015.

45. **Karvonen J and Vuorimaa T.** Heart rate and exercise intensity during sports activities: practical application. *Sports Medicine* 5: 303-311, 1988.

46. **Karvonen MJ, Kentala E, and Mustala O.** The effects of training on heart rate; a longitudinal study. *Annales Medicinae Experimentalis et Biologiae Fenniae* 35: 307-315, 1957.

47. **Kasaniemi YA, Danforth JE, Jensen MD, Kopelman PG, Lefebvre P, and Reeder BA.** Dose-response issues concerning physical activity and health: an evidenced-based symposium. *Medicine & Science in Sports & Exercise* 33 (Suppl): S351-358, 2001.

48. **Kessler HS, Sisson SB, and Short KR.** The Potential for high-intensity interval training to reduce cardio-metabolic disease risk. *Sports Medicine* 42: 489-509, 2012.

49. **Kodama S, Saito K, Tanaka S, Maki M, Yachi Y, Asumi M, et al.** Cardiorespiratory fitness as a quantitative predictor of all-cause mortality and cardiovascular events in healthy men and women. *Journal of the American Medical Association* 301: 2024-2035, 2009.

50. **Lee IM, Hsieh CC, and Paffenbarger RS, Jr.** Exercise intensity and longevity in men. The Harvard alumni health study. *JAMA* 273: 1179-1184, 1995.

51. **Little JP, Safdar A, Wilkin GP, Tarnopolsky MA, and Gibala MJ.** A practical model of low-volume high-intensity interval training induces mitochondrial biogenesis in human skeletal muscle: potential mechanisms. *Journal of Physiology* 588(6): 1011-1022, 2010.

52. **Londeree BR and Ames SA.** Trend analysis of the % VO2 max-HR regression. *Medicine and Science in Sports* 8: 123-125, 1976.

53. **Milanovic, Z, Sporis G, and Weston M.** Effectiveness of high-intensity interval training (HIT) and continuous endurance training for VO$_{2max}$ improvements: a systematic review and meta-analysis of controlled trials. *Sports Medicine.* 45: 1469-1481, 2015.

54. **Morgans L.** Heart rate responses during singles and doubles tennis competition. *Physician and Sportsmedicine* 15: 67-74, 1987.

55. **Myers J, Prakash M, Froelicher V, Do D, Partington S, and Atwood JE.** Exercise capacity and mortality among men referred for exercise testing. *New England Journal of Medicine* 346: 793-801, 2002.

56. **O'Donovan G, Owen A, Bird SR, Kearney EM, Nevill AM, Jones DW, et al.** Changes in cardiorespiratory fitness and coronary heart disease risk factors following 24 wk of moderate- or high-intensity exercise of equal energy cost. *Journal of Applied Physiology* 98: 1619-1625, 2005.

57. **Paffenbarger RS and Hale WE.** Work activity and coronary heart mortality. *New England Journal of Medicine* 292: 545-550, 1975.

58. **Paffenbarger RS, Hyde RT, and Wing AL.** Physical activity and physical fitness as determinants of health and longevity. In *Exercise, Fitness and Health*, edited by Bouchard C, Shephard RJ, Stevens T, Sutton JR, and McPherson BD. Champaign, IL: Human Kinetics, 1990, pp. 33-48.

59. **Paffenbarger RS, Jr., Hyde RT, Wing AL, and Hsieh CC.** Physical activity, all-cause mortality, and longevity of college alumni. *New England Journal of Medicine* 314: 605-613, 1986.

60. **Paffenbarger RS, Jr., Hyde RT, Wing AL, Lee IM, Jung DL, and Kampert JB.** The association of changes in physical-activity level and other lifestyle characteristics with mortality among men. *New England Journal of Medicine* 328: 538-545, 1993.

61. **Pate RR, Pratt M, Blair SN, Haskell WL, Macera CA, Bouchard C, et al.** Physical activity and public health: a recommendation from the Centers for Disease Control and Prevention and the American College of Sports Medicine. *JAMA* 273: 402-407, 1995.

62. **Peterson MD, Rhea MR, and Alvar BA.** Maximizing strength development in athletes: a meta-analysis to determine the dose-response relationship. *Journal of Strength and Conditioning Research/National Strength & Conditioning Association* 18: 377-382, 2004.

63. **Pollock ML.** How much exercise is enough? *Physician and Sportsmedicine* 6: 50-64, 1978.

64. **Pollock ML, Broida J, Kendrick Z, Miller HS, Jr., Janeway R, and Linnerud AC.** Effects of training two days per week at different intensities on middle-aged men. *Medicine and Science in Sports* 4: 192-197, 1972.

65. **Pollock ML, Dimmick J, Miller HS, Jr., Kendrick Z, and Linnerud AC.** Effects of mode of training on cardiovascular function and body composition of adult men. *Medicine and Science in Sports* 7: 139-145, 1975.

66. **Pollock ML, Gettman LR, Milesis CA, Bah MD, Durstine L, and Johnson RB.** Effects of frequency and duration of training on attrition and incidence of injury. *Medicine and Science in Sports* 9: 31-36, 1977.

67. **Pollock ML, and Wilmore JH.** *Exercise in Health and Disease.* Philadelphia, IL: W. B. Saunders, 1990.

68. **Porcari JP, Ebbeling CB, Ward A, Freedson PS, and Rippe JM.** Walking for exercise testing and training. *Sports Medicine* 8: 189-200, 1989.

69. **Powell KE, Paluch AE, and Blair SN.** Physical activity for health:What kind? How much? How intense? On top of what? *Annual Review of Public Health* 2011 32: 349-365.

70. **Powell KE, Thompson PD, Caspersen CJ, and Kendrick JS.** Physical activity and the incidence of coronary heart disease. *Annual Review of Public Health* 8: 253-287, 1987.

71. **Proper KI, van den Heuvel SG, De Vroome EM, Hildebrandt VH, and Van der Beek AJ.** Dose-response relation between physical activity and sick leave. *British Journal of Sports Medicine* 40: 173-178, 2006.

72. **Rhea MR, Alvar BA, and Burkett LN.** Single versus multiple sets for strength: a meta-analysis to address the controversy. *Research Quarterly for Exercise and Sport* 73: 485-488, 2002.

73. **Rhea MR, Alvar BA, Burkett LN, and Ball SD.** A meta-analysis to determine the dose response for strength development. *Medicine & Science in Sports & Exercise* 35: 456-464, 2003.

74. **Robertson RJ, Goss FL, Auble TE, Cassinelli DA, Spina RJ, Glickman EL, et al.** Cross-modal exercise prescription at absolute and relative oxygen uptake using perceived exertion. *Medicine & Science in Sports & Exercise* 22: 653-659, 1990.

75. **Ronnestad BR, Egeland W, Kvamme NH, Refsnes PE, Kadi F, and Raastad T.** Dissimilar effects of one- and three-set strength training on strength and muscle mass gains in upper and lower body in untrained subjects. *Journal of Strength and Conditioning Research/National Strength & Conditioning Association* 21: 157-163, 2007.

76. **Saltin B, and Gollnick PD.** Skeletal muscle adaptability: significance for metabolism and performance. In *Handbook of Physiology–Section 10: Skeletal Muscle*, edited by Peachey LD, Adrian RH, and Geiger SR. Baltimore, MD: Lippincott Williams & Wilkins, 1983.

77. **Seip RL, Snead D, Pierce EF, Stein P, and Weltman A.** Perceptual responses and blood lactate concentration: effect of training state. *Medicine & Science in Sports & Exercise* 23: 80-87, 1991.

78. **Siscovick DS, Weiss NS, Fletcher RH, and Lasky T.** The incidence of primary cardiac arrest during vigorous exercise. *New England Journal of Medicine* 311: 874-877, 1984.

79. **Siscovick DS, Weiss NS, Fletcher RH, Schoenbach VJ, and Wagner EH.** Habitual vigorous exercise and primary cardiac arrest: effect of other risk factors on the relationship. *Journal of Chronic Diseases* 37: 625-631, 1984.

80. **Swain DP and Franklin BA.** Comparison of cardioprotective benefits of vigorous versus moderate intensity aerobic exercise. *American Journal of Cardiology* 97: 141-147, 2006.

81. **Swain DP and Franklin BA.** $\dot{V}O_{(2)}$ reserve and the minimal intensity for improving cardiorespiratory fitness. *Medicine & Science in Sports & Exercise* 34: 152-157, 2002.

82. **Tanaka H, Monahan KD, and Seals DR.** Age-predicted maximal heart rate revisited. *Journal of the American College of Cardiology* 37: 153-156, 2001.

83. **U.S. Department of Health and Human Services.** 2008 Physcial activity guidelines for Americans. www.health.gov/paguidelines/guidelines/

84. **U.S. Department of Health and Human Services.** Physical Activity Guidelines Advisory Committee Report 2008. www.healthgov/paguidelines/committeereportaspx 2008.

85. **U.S. Department of Health and Human Services.** *Healthy People 2000: National Health Promotion and Disease Prevention Objectives.* U.S. Government Printing Office, 1990.

86. **Wenger HA and Bell GJ.** The interactions of intensity, frequency and duration of exercise training in altering cardiorespiratory fitness. *Sports Medicine* 3: 346-356, 1986.

87. **Wolfe BL, LeMura LM, and Cole PJ.** Quantitative analysis of single- vs. multiple-set programs in resistance training. *Journal of Strength and Conditioning Research/National Strength & Conditioning Association* 18: 35-47, 2004.

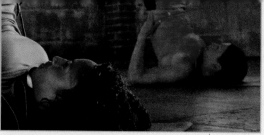

© Tim Mantoani/Masterfile

17

Exercise for Special Populations

■ Objectives

By studying this chapter, you should be able to do the following:

1. Describe the difference between type 1 and type 2 diabetes.

2. Explain why exercise may complicate the life of a person with type 1 diabetes, while being a recommended and primary part of a program for someone with type 2 diabetes.

3. Describe the changes in diet and insulin that might be made prior to a person with diabetes doing exercise.

4. Describe the cause of exercise-induced asthma, and how one may deal with this problem as part of an exercise prescription.

5. Contrast chronic obstructive pulmonary disease (COPD) with asthma in terms of

causes, prognosis, and the role of rehabilitation programs in a return to "normal" function.

6. Identify the types of patient populations that one might see in a cardiac rehabilitation program.

7. Contrast Phase I with Phase II and Phase III cardiac rehabilitation programs.

8. Describe the physiological changes in older adults that result from an endurance-training program.

9. Outline the physical activity recommendations for older adults who cannot do the regular adult program.

10. Describe the guidelines for exercise programs for pregnant women.

■ Outline

■ Key Terms

arrhythmias
beta-receptor agonist
    (β_2-agonist)
coronary artery bypass graft
    surgery (CABGS)
cromolyn sodium
diabetic coma
immunotherapy
insulin shock
ketosis
mast cell
myocardial infarction (MI)
nitroglycerin
percutaneous transluminal
    coronary angioplasty (PTCA)

Chapter 16 presented some recommendations for planning an appropriate exercise program for the apparently healthy individual. Exercise has also been used as a primary nonpharmacological intervention for a variety of problems, such as obesity and mild hypertension, and as a normal part of therapy for the treatment of diabetes and coronary heart disease. This chapter discusses the special concerns that must be addressed when exercise is used for populations with specific diseases, disabilities, or limitations. However, the student of exercise science should recognize that this information is introductory in nature. See *ACSM's Exercise Management for Persons with Chronic Diseases and Disabilities* in Suggested Readings for a comprehensive look at this topic.

DIABETES

Diabetes is a disease characterized by hyperglycemia (elevated blood glucose) resulting from inadequate insulin secretion (type 1), reduced insulin action (type 2), or both (8). Diabetes is a major health problem and leading cause of death in the United States, representing a total (direct and indirect) annual cost of $245 billion in 2012. Of the more than 29.1 million individuals with diabetes, only 21.0 million are diagnosed. Further, the number with prediabetes (see later) is a staggering 86 million (**www.cdc.gov/diabetes/data/statistics/2014StatisticsReport.html**). Diabetes is diagnosed on the basis of plasma glucose (PG) criteria, either based on a fasting plasma glucose (PG $\geq$126 mg $\cdot$ dl^{-1} [7.0 mmol $\cdot$ L^{-1}]) or a two-hour plasma glucose value after a 75-g oral glucose tolerance test (PG $\geq$200 mg $\cdot$ dl^{-1}) or glycosylated hemoglobin (HbA1C) criteria (A1C $\geq$6.5%) (8). Those with diabetes are divided into two distinct groups on the basis of whether the diabetes is caused by lack of insulin (type 1) or a resistance to insulin (type 2). Type 1, insulin-dependent diabetes, develops primarily in young persons and is associated with viral (flulike) infections. The warning signs, which develop quickly, consist of (25):

- Frequent urination/unusual thirst
- Extreme hunger
- Rapid weight loss, weakness, and fatigue
- Irritability, nausea, and vomiting

Because those with type 1 diabetes do not produce insulin, they are dependent on exogenous (injected) insulin to maintain the blood glucose concentration within normal limits. Type 2, noninsulin-dependent, diabetes typically develops more slowly and later in life than does type 1 diabetes; however, some overweight children are diagnosed with this disease. Type 2 diabetes represents about 90% to 95% of all diabetes cases (8), and it is linked to upper-body or android obesity and physical inactivity. The increased mass of fat tissue increases the production of proinflammatory cytokines like TNF-α and decreases the production of anti-inflammatory hormones like adiponectin (see Chaps. 5 and 14). These changes result in a resistance to insulin, which is usually available in adequate amounts within the body. However, some individuals with type 2 diabetes may require injectable insulin or an oral medication that stimulates the pancreas to produce additional insulin. Not surprisingly, the treatment of type 2 diabetes includes diet (9) and exercise (7, 11) to reduce body weight and to help control plasma glucose. Table 17.1 summarizes the differences between type 1 and type 2 diabetes (49).

TABLE 17.1	Comparison of Type 1 and Type 2 Diabetes Mellitus	
Feature	Type 1	Type 2
Usual age at onset	Under 20 years	Over 40 years
Development of symptoms	Rapid	Slow
Percentage of diabetic population	About 5%	About 95%
Development of ketoacidosis	Common	Rare
Association with obesity	Rare	Common
Beta cells of islets (at onset of disease)	Destroyed	Not destroyed
Insulin secretion	Decreased	Normal or increased
Autoantibodies to islet cells	Present	Absent
Associated with particular MHC antigens*	Yes	Unclear
Treatment	Insulin injections	Diet and exercise; oral stimulators of insulin sensitivity

*MHC refers to the major histocompatibility complex on chromosome 6 that is linked to transplant rejection and to autoimmune diseases in which the immune system attacks the host's tissues—in this case the islets of Langerhans that produce insulin.

- Type 1, or insulin-dependent, diabetes develops early in life and represents 5% of those with diabetes.
- Type 2, or insulin-resistant, diabetes occurs later in life and is associated with upper-body or android obesity and physical inactivity. Diet and exercise are important parts of the treatment program for type 2 diabetes to achieve weight loss and improved insulin sensitivity.

Exercise and Diabetes

In Chaps. 4 and 5, we described how exercise increases the rate at which muscle removes glucose from the blood to provide energy for contraction. This effect makes exercise a useful part of the treatment of diabetes because it helps regulate the blood glucose concentration. However, this beneficial effect of exercise is dependent on whether the individual with diabetes is in reasonable "control" before exercise begins. Control means that the blood glucose concentration is close to normal. Figure 17.1 shows the effect of a prolonged exercise bout on individuals with diabetes who were in control versus those who had not taken an adequate amount of insulin. A lack of insulin causes **ketosis,** a metabolic acidosis resulting from the accumulation of too many ketone bodies (due to excessive fat metabolism). An individual with type 1 diabetes who is in control shows a decrease in plasma glucose toward normal values during exercise, suggesting better control. On the other hand, those with type 1 diabetes who do not inject an adequate amount of insulin before exercise show an increase in the plasma glucose concentration (7, 10). Why the difference in response? Those in control have sufficient insulin such that glucose can be taken up into muscle during exercise and can counter the normal increase in glucose release from the liver due to the action of catecholamines and glucagon (see Chap. 5). In contrast, those with inadequate insulin experience only a small increase in glucose utilization by muscle but have the normal increase in glucose release from the liver. This, of course, causes an elevation of the plasma glucose, resulting in hyperglycemia.

Figure 17.2 summarizes these effects and adds one more (63). If an individual with insulin-dependent diabetes starts exercise with too much insulin, the rate at which plasma glucose is used by muscle is accelerated, while glucose release from the liver is decreased. This causes a dangerous hypoglycemic response. This information is crucial to understanding how to prescribe exercise for those with diabetes. Because the importance of exercise as part of a treatment plan is different for type 1 and type 2 diabetes, we will discuss each type separately.

Type 1 Diabetes   For many years, exercise was one part of the treatment for type 1 diabetes, with insulin and diet being the other two (64). However, as mentioned earlier, if an individual with diabetes is not

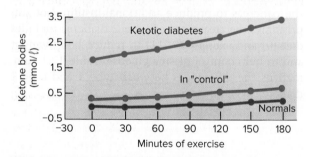

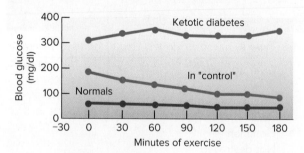

Figure 17.1   **Effect of prolonged exercise on blood glucose and ketone body levels in normal subjects, those with diabetes in "control," and those with diabetes taking an inadequate amount of insulin (ketosis).**

Berger, M., et al., "Metabolic and Hormonal Effects of Muscular Exercise in Juvenile Type Diabetics," *Diabetologia* 13: 355–365. New York: Springer-Verlag, 1977.

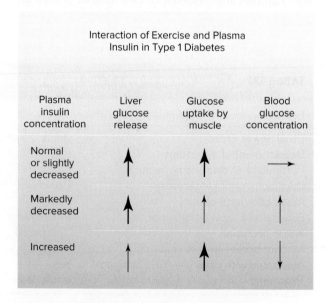

Figure 17.2   **Effect of varied plasma insulin levels in type 1 diabetes on glucose homeostasis during exercise.**

in control prior to exercise, the ability to maintain a reasonable plasma glucose concentration may be compromised. Further, exercise programs, by themselves, have not been shown to improve control of blood glucose (9). The greatest concern is not the hyperglycemia and ketosis that can lead to **diabetic coma** when too little insulin is present; rather, it is the possibility of hypoglycemia, which can lead to **insulin shock.** Richter and Galbo (92) and Kemmer and Berger (64) point out the difficulties those with type 1 diabetes have starting an exercise program: They must maintain a regular exercise schedule in terms of intensity, frequency, and duration, as well as altering diet and insulin. Such regimentation is difficult for some to follow, and given the variability in how blood glucose might respond to exercise on a day-to-day basis, the use of exercise as a primary tool in maintaining metabolic control has been diminished (9). Because metabolic control can be achieved by altering insulin and diet based on self-monitored blood glucose, exercise complicates this picture (64, 94). However, considering the importance of physical activity in an individual's life, and the effect of regular activity on coronary heart disease (CHD) risk factors, those with type 1 diabetes should not be discouraged from participation in regular exercise–if there are no complications (9). What kind of clearance is needed?

As described in Chap. 15, the need for medical clearance is based on the individual's current pattern of physical activity; the presence of signs, symptoms, or known cardiovascular, metabolic, or renal diseases; and the desired intensity of the exercise training program. Those diagnosed with diabetes who are currently doing a moderate-intensity (40% to <60% HRR) physical activity program for 30 minutes on at least three days a week can continue with that program without medical clearance. That said, medical clearance is needed if these individuals want to do vigorous-intensity (≥60% HRR) exercise. However, for individuals with diabetes who are inactive, medical clearance is recommended independent of the desired intensity of the exercise program.

These recommendations are based on the elevated risk individuals with diabetes have and the observation that strenuous exercise may accelerate or worsen retina, kidney, or peripheral nerve damage that is already present. The concern for the retina is related to the higher blood pressures developed during exercise, whereas the concern for the kidney is related to the decrease in blood flow to that organ with increasing intensities of exercise. The peripheral nerve damage may block signals coming from the foot such that serious damage may occur before it is perceived. Proper shoes for exercise, as well as the choice of the activity, are important (10, 35, 70).

The primary concern to address when exercise is prescribed for individuals with type 1 diabetes is the avoidance of hypoglycemia. This is achieved through careful self-monitoring of the blood glucose concentration before, during, and after exercise, and varying carbohydrate intake and insulin, depending on the exercise intensity and duration, and the fitness of the individual (10):

- Metabolic control before physical activity
  - Avoid physical activity if fasting glucose levels are >250 mg/dl and ketosis is present. Use caution if glucose levels are <300 mg/dl without ketosis.
  - Ingest added carbohydrate if glucose levels are <100 mg/dl.
- Blood glucose monitoring before and after physical activity
  - Identify when changes in insulin or food intake are needed.
  - Learn how blood glucose responds to different types of physical activity.
- Food intake
  - Consume added carbohydrate as needed to prevent hypoglycemia.
  - Carbohydrate-based foods should be readily available during and after physical activity.

Variability exists in how those with type 1 diabetes respond to exercise and hypoglycemia (21). Consequently, frequent and consistent monitoring of blood glucose and fine-tuning of the insulin dose and carbohydrate intake are essential for long-term success in preventing hypoglycemia.

The exercise prescription for those with type 1 diabetes must also consider other problems associated with this disease: autonomic neuropathy, peripheral neuropathy, retinopathy, and nephropathy. Individuals with autonomic nervous system dysfunction may have abnormal heart rate and blood pressure responses to exercise. Those with peripheral nerve damage may experience pain, impaired balance, weakness, and decreased proprioception. Damage to the retina is common with diabetes and is aggravated by increased blood pressure or any jarring action directed at the head. Finally, kidney damage is also a common experience for those with type 1 diabetes. This can lead to altered blood pressure responses that can affect the retina (10, 70, 110). It should be no surprise that the exercise prescription for those with diabetes must address these problems if they are present. Recommendations from the American College of Sports Medicine include the following (5, 7, 35):

Aerobic exercise training:

- Exercise three to seven days per week

- Work at 40% to 85% heart rate reserve or 12 to 16 on the 6 to 20 RPE scale
- Do 20 to 60 minutes per session to accumulate at least 150 minutes of moderate-intensity or 75 minutes of vigorous-intensity physical activity per week
- Use nonweight-bearing, low-impact activities (bicycle or stationary cycle, swimming, water exercise), if weight-bearing activities are contraindicated

Resistance exercise training:

- Exercise two to three days per week
- Work at 60% to 80% 1-RM; ~11 to 15 on 6 to 20 RPE scale
- Do one to three sets of 8 to 12 repetitions (10 to 15 to start) for major muscle groups, avoiding the Valsalva maneuver.

Other:

- Follow a progression schedule for both aerobic and resistance training programs.
- Drink more fluid and carry a readily available form of carbohydrate and adequate identification.
- Exercise with someone who can help in an emergency.

In conclusion, although exercise may not have a major impact on long-term measures of blood glucose control (i.e., glycosylated hemoglobin [HbA1C]) in those with type 1 diabetes (65), the fact that those who stay physically active have fewer complications is reason enough to pursue the active life.

IN SUMMARY

- A sedentary individual with type 1 diabetes has to juggle diet and insulin to achieve control of the blood glucose concentration. An exercise program may complicate matters, and therefore exercise is not viewed as a primary means of achieving "control." In spite of this, those with diabetes are encouraged to participate in a regular exercise program to experience its health-related benefits.
- Those with diabetes may have to increase carbohydrate intake and/or decrease the amount of insulin prior to activity to maintain the glucose concentration close to normal during the exercise. The extent of these alterations is dependent on a number of factors, including the intensity and duration of the physical activity, the blood glucose concentration prior to the exercise, and the physical fitness of the individual.

Type 2 Diabetes　As mentioned earlier, type 2 diabetes occurs later in life, and people with this condition have a variety of risk factors in addition to their diabetes: hypertension, high cholesterol, obesity, and inactivity (see Chap. 14). Given the rate at which type 2 diabetes is increasing, more attention is being paid to identifying persons early in the disease process to delay or prevent the problem (see Research Focus 17.1). There is convincing evidence that type 2 diabetes is linked to a lack of physical activity, independent of obesity (7). In addition, current research supports the benefits of exercise training in the prevention and treatment of insulin resistance and type 2 diabetes (5, 7, 11). In contrast to an individual with type 1 diabetes whose life may be more complicated (in terms of blood glucose control) at the start of an exercise program, exercise is a primary recommendation for those with type 2 diabetes, both to help deal with the obesity that is usually present and to help control blood glucose. The combination of exercise and diet may be sufficient and eliminate the need for insulin or the oral medication used to stimulate insulin secretion (7, 11). Because those with type 2 diabetes represent more than 90% of all those with diabetes, and because type 2 diabetes occurs later in life (after 40 years of age), it is not uncommon to see such individuals in adult fitness programs. It is important for clear communication to exist between the participant and the exercise leader to reduce the chance of a "surprise" hypoglycemic response.

Individuals with type 2 diabetes do not experience the same fluctuations in blood glucose during exercise as do those with type 1 diabetes; however, those taking oral medication to stimulate insulin secretion may have to decrease their dosage to maintain a normal blood glucose concentration during exercise (7). The exercise prescription for those with type 2 diabetes is similar to what was just presented for type 1 diabetes (5, 35), including the resistance training, which, when combined with aerobic training, results in benefits greater than either type alone (31). Exercise volume appears to be the most important variable in achieving blood glucose control as measured by HbA1C (108). However, given that many individuals with type 2 diabetes are also overweight or obese (7):

- The focus should be on moderate-intensity physical activity (e.g., brisk walking) in which individuals can begin with ten-minute bouts, with the goal of at least 150 minutes per week. More is gained by walking for longer periods.
- The frequency of aerobic activity should be as high as four to seven times per week to promote a sustained increase in insulin sensitivity in muscle and to facilitate weight loss and weight maintenance.

Prevention or Delay of Type 2 Diabetes

Over the past decade, there has been an increase in the prevalence of type 2 diabetes that is linked to the increased prevalence of obesity. A great deal of research has been under way to try to understand how to prevent or slow down the development of type 2 diabetes. One of the first things is earlier identification of people at risk of type 2 diabetes with the use of the fasting blood glucose and the oral glucose tolerance test (person drinks 75 g of glucose and blood samples are taken at 30 minutes and one, two, and three hours to track how fast glucose is taken up into tissues). These tests are used to identify those with (8):

■ Impaired fasting glucose (IFG): if fasting blood glucose values are ≥100 mg/dl (5.6 mmol/l) but <126 mg/dl (7.0 mmol/l).

■ Impaired glucose tolerance (IGT): Two-hour value in an oral glucose tolerance test is ≥140 mg/dl (7.8 mmol/l) but <200 mg/dl (11.1 mmol/l).

Those with IFG or IGT are said to be "prediabetic" (8). As mentioned earlier, approximately 86 million Americans age 20 or older are classified as being prediabetic (**www.cdc.gov/diabetes/data/ statistics/2014StatisticsReport .html**). Studies have shown that both drugs and lifestyle modifications can slow down or prevent the development of type 2 diabetes. However, lifestyle changes–increasing physical activity by 150 minutes per week and losing 5% to 10% of body weight– seem to be a better approach than using drugs. In a now-classic study, lifestyle modifications reduced the risk of type 2 diabetes by 58%, better than metformin, one of the best drugs available (68). A recent review of all of the clinical trials in this area confirmed the findings that nonpharmacological therapy is a crucial part of the prevention process (107). In addition to dealing with the prediabetes problems, the loss of weight and increased physical activity reduce the risk of several cardiovascular risk factors (10). This "good news" must be balanced by the reality that we need better and cheaper ways to change the eating and physical activity behaviors of the average person.

As with all exercise programs for deconditioned individuals, it is more important to do too little than too much at the start of a program. By starting with moderate activity and gradually increasing the duration, exercise can be done each day. This will provide an opportunity to learn how to maintain adequate control of blood glucose while minimizing the chance of a hypoglycemic response. In addition, a "habit" of exercise will develop that is crucial if one is to realize the benefits, because the exercise-induced increase in insulin sensitivity does not last long (7). Further, the combination of intensity, frequency, and duration mentioned previously has been shown to directly benefit those with borderline hypertension, a condition often associated with type 2 diabetes. Consistent with the recommendations for type 1 diabetes, clear identification and a readily available source of carbohydrate should be carried along in any exercise session. In addition, it would be much safer for an individual with diabetes to exercise with someone who could help out if a problem occurred.

Exercise is only one part of the treatment; diet is the other. The American Diabetes Association (9) states that there are four goals related to nutrition therapy for all people with diabetes:

■ To achieve and maintain
  ● Blood glucose levels in the normal range or as close to normal as is safely possible
  ● A lipid and lipoprotein profile that reduces the risk for vascular disease
  ● Blood pressure levels in the normal range or as close to normal as is safely possible

■ To prevent, or at least slow, the rate of development of the chronic complications of diabetes by modifying nutrient intake and lifestyle

■ To address individual nutrition needs, taking into account personal and cultural preferences and willingness to change

■ To maintain the pleasure of eating by limiting food choices only when indicated by scientific evidence

The emphasis in achieving optimal nutrition is through a high-carbohydrate diet (with little processed sugars) to achieve nutrient goals for protein, vitamins, and minerals. The low-fat diet has been shown to be useful in achieving weight-loss and blood lipid goals as well as blood glucose control (9). Those with type 2 diabetes secure a variety of benefits from proper exercise and dietary practices: lower body fat and weight (see Chap. 18), increased high-density-lipoprotein (HDL) cholesterol, increased sensitivity to insulin (decreasing the need), improved capacity for work, and an improved self-concept (7). These changes should not only improve the prognosis as far as control of blood glucose is concerned, but also reduce the overall risk of CHD.

■ Those with type 2 diabetes have a variety of risk factors in addition to their diabetes, including hypertension, high cholesterol, obesity, and inactivity.

■ An exercise prescription emphasizing low-intensity, long-duration activity that is done almost every day will maximize the benefits related to insulin sensitivity and weight loss.

■ The dietary recommendation is for a low-fat diet, similar to what is recommended for all Americans for good health, with the additional goals of achieving normal serum glucose and lipid levels.

ASTHMA

Asthma is a respiratory problem characterized by a chronic inflammation of the airways and a reversible airway obstruction. An asthma attack is associated with a shortness of breath accompanied by a wheezing sound. It is due to a contraction of the smooth muscle around the airways, a swelling of the mucosal cells, and a hypersecretion of mucus. Asthma can be caused by an allergic reaction, exercise, aspirin, dust, pollutants, and emotion (85).

Asthma is a common disease in the United States. In 2014, it was estimated that 17.7 million Americans have asthma, including 6.3 million children. A total of 1.8 million emergency room visits and 3,630 deaths were attributed to asthma. Estimated direct and indirect costs were more than $50 billion (**www.cdc.gov/nchs/fastats/asthma.htm**).

Diagnosis and Causes

The diagnosis of asthma is made using pulmonary-function testing. If an obstruction to airflow (e.g., low maximal expiratory flow rate) is corrected by administration of a bronchodilator, then asthma is suspected. An asthma attack is the result of an orderly sequence of events that can be initiated by a variety of factors such as dust, chemicals, or exercise. These events are important if we are to understand how certain medications prevent or relieve the asthma attack.

In acquired immunity (see Chap. 6), an antigen (or allergen) stimulates the B-cells to produce antibodies (immunoglobulins [Ig]) to protect against a subsequent exposure to that allergen. However, in those who are genetically predisposed to have allergies, the B-cells produce IgE antibodies rather than IgG antibodies, which attach to the surface of mast cells lining the bronchial tubes. Upon re-exposure, the allergen binds to these IgE antibodies on the mast cell, and large amounts of various inflammatory mediators are released from the mast cell. These mediators include histamine, prostaglandins, and leukotrienes, and cause the following early-phase reactions (see Fig. 17.3):

■ Increased secretion of mucus

■ Increased blood flow

■ Swelling of the epithelial lining

■ Contraction of smooth muscle surrounding the airway

These early-phase reactions may lead to late-phase reactions involving release of additional mediators from eosinophils that prolong the inflammation process (49, 114). In short, these events cause an immediate, and possibly sustained, reduction in one's ability to breathe.

Prevention/Relief of Asthma

A variety of steps can be taken to prevent the occurrence of an asthma attack and to provide relief should one occur. If a person is sensitive (allergic) to something, then simple avoidance of the allergen will prevent the problem. If a person cannot avoid contact with the allergen, **immunotherapy** may be helpful in making the person less sensitive to the allergen while being treated.

Drugs have been developed to deal with the mast cell, which is a focal point in the asthmatic response, as well as the bronchiolar smooth muscle that causes the decrease in airway diameter. **Cromolyn sodium** inhibits the chemical mediator release from the mast cell. **Beta-receptor agonists (β_2-agonists)** also decrease chemical mediator release and cause the relaxation of bronchiolar smooth muscle. These effects are brought about through increased adenylate cyclase activity leading to an elevation of cytoplasmic cyclic AMP (see Chap. 5). However, daily use of β_2-agonists should be avoided because a desensitization of the β_2 receptor on the mast cells may occur (less of a response for the same level of drug). A physician can change the medication to achieve better control (12, 91). Corticosteroids and leukotriene antagonists are used to reduce the inflammation response, which is central to dealing with the long-term management of asthma (33, 78, 85, 91). Treatment with corticosteroids has been shown to increase arterial blood oxygenation and time to exhaustion from 9.9 minutes to 14.8 minutes in a treadmill test done at 90% of $\dot{V}O_2$ max (56). The net result of the medications is that both the inflammation response and the constriction of bronchiolar smooth muscle are blocked.

Exercise-Induced Asthma

A form of asthma that may be of particular interest to the reader is exercise-induced asthma (EIA). The asthma attack is caused by exercise and can occur

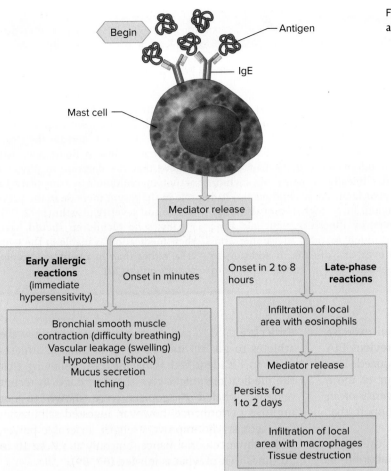

Figure 17.3   Proposed mechanism by which an asthma attack is initiated.

Begin

Antigen

IgE

Mast cell

Mediator release

Early allergic reactions (immediate hypersensitivity)

Onset in minutes

Onset in 2 to 8 hours

Late-phase reactions

Bronchial smooth muscle contraction (difficulty breathing)
Vascular leakage (swelling)
Hypotension (shock)
Mucus secretion
Itching

Infiltration of local area with eosinophils

Mediator release

Persists for 1 to 2 days

Infiltration of local area with macrophages
Tissue destruction

5 to 15 minutes (early phase) or 4 to 6 hours (late phase) after exercise. The prevalence of EIA varies from 7% to 20% in the general population, to 30% to 70% in elite winter athletes and elite athletes in summer endurance sports, and 70% to 90% in individuals with persistent asthma (91, 113). What is interesting is that 61% of the 1984 U.S. Olympic team members with EIA won an Olympic medal (111). Furthermore, if one compares 1988 Olympic athletes who experienced EIA with the athletes who did not, one finds no difference in the percentage who won medals (78). Similar success was noted through the 2008 Olympics (91). Clearly, if anyone wondered whether EIA can be controlled, those results should dispel any doubts.

Many causes of EIA have been identified over the past 100 years. These include cold air, hypocapnia (low PCO_2), respiratory alkalosis, and specific intensities and durations of exercise. The focus of attention is now on the *cooling and drying* of the respiratory tract that occurs when large volumes of dry air are breathed during the exercise session (1, 27). Respiratory heat loss is related primarily to the rate of ventilation, with the humidity and the temperature of the inspired air being of secondary and tertiary importance. As you remember from Chap. 10, when dry air is taken into the lungs, it is moistened and warmed as it moves throught the respiratory airways. In this way, moisture is evaporated from the surface of the airways, which is therefore cooled.

The proposed mechanism for how EIA is initiated takes us back to the mast cell mentioned earlier. When dry air removes water from the surface of the mast cell, an increase in osmolarity occurs. This increase in osmolarity triggers the release of chemical mediators and the narrowing of the airways (78, 85, 91).

The probability of an exercise-induced bronchospasm is related to the type of exercise, the time since the previous bout of exercise, the interval since medication was taken, and the temperature and humidity of the inspired air. It has been known since the late 1600s that certain types of exercise cause an attack more readily than others. Running was observed to cause more attacks than cycling or walking, which, in turn, caused more than swimming (78, 85, 91). However, in elite athletes, asthma is diagnosed more frequently in swimmers than in other sports. It may be that these elite swimmers self-selected the sport which is less likely to trigger EIA (91).

Generally, EIA is precipitated more with strenuous, long-duration exercise compared to short-term, moderate-intensity exercise. One way to deal with this is to do short-duration exercise (<5 min) at low

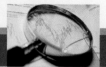

Screening for Asthma in Children

Asthma is the leading cause of chronic illness and the most common respiratory disorder in children (39). Concern has been expressed about the need for screening programs early in life to identify those with a high risk of developing asthma. Jones and Bowen (59) measured peak expiratory flow rate before and after an all-out run in children from ten primary schools. Over a six-year follow-up period, they compared children who had a negative result with those who had a positive result (a decrease in peak expiratory flow rate of $\geq 15\%$) due to the exercise test. Of the 864 children not known to have asthma, 60 had a positive test result. A follow-up of 55 of these 60 children showed 32 had developed clinically recognizable asthma six years later. These children also had a significantly higher prevalence of respiratory illnesses. Such field tests have much to offer in gaining control over this disease. In addition to screening, there is strong support to not back away from physical activity for asthmatic children. Most studies show that children with asthma can exercise safely and increase their cardiorespiratory fitness. Some scientists believe that the decrease in physical activity in children may have played a role in the recent increase in the prevalence and severity of asthma (72, 97). Finally, scho olchildren should have their medication available in the gym area, rather than in a central administrator's office (78).

to moderate intensities. Further, when an exercise session occurs within 60 minutes of a previous EIA attack, the degree of bronchospasm is reduced. This suggests that a warm-up within an hour of more strenuous exercise would reduce the severity of an attack, and there is good evidence to support that proposition (75, 78, 85, 91).

There was special concern for the athletes of the 1984 Olympic Games, given the pollution in Los Angeles, which can aggravate an EIA attack (88). As mentioned before, the fact that 61% of the athletes who experienced EIA won Olympic medals suggests that procedures for preventing EIA with medication are generally established. Voy (111) reports that a simple questionnaire identified 90% of the athletes with EIA, even though only 52% were receiving treatment prior to the Olympics. However, there is abundant evidence that self-reported symptoms of asthma and/ or EIA are not reliable for evaluating EIA in competitive athletes (91, 113). Typically, a strenuous exercise challenge (e.g., running at 85% to 90% of maximal heart rate on a treadmill) lasting six to eight minutes is used to evaluate the presence of EIA (5). Some recommend that the air they breathe should be cool and dry during the test, or that the athlete should perform the exercise challenge in the environment that triggers it (113). In addition, a nonexercise test can be used in which the subject breathes cool, dry air containing 5% CO_2 (to maintain the blood's CO_2 level) for six minutes at 85% of predicted maximum voluntary ventilation. It is a test of choice for screening elite athletes (42, 113), but it is much too complicated to use on a general basis, especially for children where a field test may be sufficient (see A Closer Look 17.1). In any case, a 10% or greater decrease in forced expiratory flow rate in one second (FEV_1) is classified as a positive test (113). The medications mentioned

earlier are used to manage the condition to allow the athletes to go "all out." Some nonasthmatic athletes want to be identified as having EIA, believing that the medications might give them an edge. In recent reviews, inhaled β_2-agonists were shown to not improve performance; however, ingested salbutamol (a β_2-agonist) did improve strength, anaerobic power, and endurance performance, but only at a dose 10 to 20 times that of what is inhaled (67, 89).

A growing body of evidence suggests that specific nutritional factors may be helpful in managing EIA. The strategies include a reduction in salt intake and an increased intake of omega-3 fatty acids and caffeine (76). As more research supports these findings, the message will be clear to those with asthma, as it has been for those with high blood pressure, blood lipid abnormalities, and diabetes—that diet really does matter.

In a majority of cases, EIA can be prevented with the medications mentioned earlier, used alone or in combination (23, 73, 85, 91, 103). The person with asthma who is participating in a fitness program should also follow a medication plan to *prevent* the occurrence of an EIA attack. The exercise session should include the conventional warm-up, with mild-to-moderate activity planned in five-minute segments. For those new to exercise, the person should be introduced to the program in a progressive manner to titrate the intensity and build up the endurance needed to do the full exercise prescription. The aerobic exercise program recommendations for those with asthma include (5):

■ Frequency: at least 2 to 3 days/week,
■ Intensity: 60% of $\dot{V}O_2$ peak or the work rate at the ventilatory threshold,
■ Time: at least 20 to 30 minute/day

Swimming is better than other types of exercise, given that air above the water contains more moisture. A scarf or face mask can be used when exercising outdoors in cold weather to help trap moisture. The participant should carry an inhaler with a β_2-agonist and use it at the first sign of wheezing (78, 85). As with the person with diabetes, the buddy system is a good plan to follow in case a major attack occurs.

IN SUMMARY

- An asthma attack is brought on when an agent triggers a mast cell in the respiratory tract to release chemical mediators. These chemical mediators cause a constriction of bronchiolar smooth muscle along with an increase in secretions into the airways.
- Cromolyn sodium and β_2-adrenergic agonists act to prevent this by reducing mediator release from the mast cell and causing relaxation of smooth muscle surrounding the airways.
- After the routine of exercise has been introduced, the person may progress toward the exercise prescription of 2 to 3 days/week, 20 to 30 minute/day at about 60% $\dot{V}O_2$ peak or the ventilatory threshold. Drugs should be used prior to exercise to prevent an attack, and β_2-adrenergic agonists should be carried along in case one occurs.

CHRONIC OBSTRUCTIVE PULMONARY DISEASE

Chronic obstructive pulmonary diseases (COPD) cause a reduction in airflow that can have a dramatic effect on daily activities. These diseases, found primarily in smokers and ex-smokers, include chronic bronchitis, emphysema, and bronchial asthma, either alone or in combination. COPD is distinct from the exercise-induced asthma discussed earlier in that the airway obstruction remains in spite of continuous medication (36, 37, 95). Chronic bronchitis is characterized by a persistent production of sputum due primarily to a thickened bronchial wall with excess secretions. In emphysema, the elastic recoil of alveoli and bronchioles is reduced and those pulmonary structures are enlarged (37). The patient with developing COPD cannot perform normal activities without experiencing dyspnea, but, tragically, by the time this occurs, the disease is already well advanced. COPD is characterized by a decreased ability to exhale, and because of the narrowed airways, a "wheezing" sound is made. The person with COPD experiences a decreased capacity for work, which may influence employment, but he/she may also experience an increase in psychological problems, including anxiety (regarding the simple act of breathing) and depression (related to a loss of sense of self-worth) (95).

It should be no surprise then that treatment of COPD includes more than simple medication and oxygen-inhalation therapy. A typical COPD rehabilitation program focuses on the goal of the patient's ability for self-care. To achieve that goal, a number of medical and support personnel are recruited to deal with the various manifestations of the disease process (24, 102). The COPD patient receives education about the different ways to deal with the disease, including breathing exercises, ways to approach the activities of daily living at home, and how to handle work-related problems. The latter can be so affected that new on-the-job responsibilities may have to be assigned, or if the person cannot meet the requirements, retirement may be the only outcome. To help deal with these problems, counseling by psychologists and clergy may be needed for the patient and family. The extent of these problems is directly related to the severity of the disease. Those with minimal disease may require the help of only a few of the professionals just mentioned, whereas others with severe disease may require the assistance of all. It is therefore important to understand that the rehabilitation program is very individualized (36, 37, 102).

Testing and Training

The consistent recommendation for anyone with known disease is to have a complete medical exam, including exercise testing, prior to beginning an exercise program (see Chap. 15) (5, 26). This is especially true for COPD patients because the severity of the disease varies greatly. A common test used to classify COPD patients is the FEV_1. Because the FEV_1 test is not a good predictor of exercise performance, Cooper (36) emphasizes a need to focus on the hyperinflation of the lung, which results from air trapping due to the person's inability to exhale completely. Hyperinflation is linked more directly to patients' outcomes, including exercise performance (26, 36, 37). A graded exercise test (GXT) to evaluate $\dot{V}O_2$ max, maximum exercise ventilation, and changes in the arterial blood gases, PO_2 and PCO_2, is also recommended. The results of this GXT are helpful in developing the exercise prescription, especially when selecting the appropriate exercise intensity (37). However, because the FEV_1 test is the most common, guidelines have been established to screen patients with this test. The Global Initiatives for Chronic Obstructive Lung Disease **(www.goldcopd.org)** provides guidelines to use in working with patients with COPD. They classify patients into the following four categories based on post-bronchodilator FEV_1:

- GOLD I–Mild COPD: $FEV_1 \geq 80\%$ predicted
- GOLD II–Moderate COPD: $50\% \leq FEV_1 < 80\%$ predicted
- GOLD III–Severe COPD: $30\% \leq FEV_1 < 50\%$ predicted
- GOLD IV–Very severe COPD: $FEV_1 < 30\%$ predicted.

Individuals in GOLD I are usually unaware that their lung function is abnormal. In contrast, within GOLD categories II through IV, the health status of patients varies from very poor to being relatively well preserved. Consequently, a formal assessment of symptoms is also required (26, 52).

Even though exercise training does not reverse the disease process, it can interrupt the steady increase in symptoms of fatigue and breathlessness and the decline in quality of life. In general, the physical activity guidelines for older adults (see later in this chapter) are recommended for COPD patients (5). This includes both aerobic and resistance components, the latter dealing with local muscle fatigue issues in both the lower and upper body.

However, due to the wide range of symptoms within each GOLD category, GXT results can be most helpful. During the GXT, the O_2 saturation of arterial blood is monitored, and the patient is asked to rate the level of breathlessness using a dyspnea scale of 1 to 4:

- 1. Light, barely noticeable
- 2. Moderate, bothersome
- 3. Moderately severe, very uncomfortable
- 4. Most severe or intense dyspnea ever experienced

These results can help define an appropriate intensity to use in the aerobic portion of the exercise program and determine whether supplemental oxygen is needed (5, 37, 102). Both moderate-intensity and high-intensity exercises are used, depending on patient status. High-intensity interval training (HIIT) is also used because it allows the patient to work at a higher intensity (for a shorter duration) than conventional continuous training. There appear to be clear benefits to this approach, including a reduction in the respiratory load due to the short duration of the activity (see more on HIIT in Clinical Application 16.2) (5, 102). Respiratory muscle training may be used, depending on the patient, but it is not a standard part of pulmonary rehabilitation (5, 37, 102).

Generally, COPD patients achieve an increase in exercise tolerance without dyspnea and an increase in the sense of well-being, but without a reversal of the disease process (24, 37, 102). The changes in the

psychological variables are very important in the long run, given that the person's willingness to continue the exercise program is a major factor in determining the rate of decline during the course of the disease (19, 24).

IN SUMMARY

- Chronic obstructive pulmonary diseases (COPD) include chronic asthma, emphysema, and bronchitis. These latter two diseases create changes in the lung that are irreversible and result in a gradual deterioration of function.
- Rehabilitation is a multidisciplinary approach involving medication, breathing exercises, dietary therapy, exercise, and counseling. The programs are individually designed due to the severity of the illness, and the goals are pragmatic in terms of the events of daily living and work.

HYPERTENSION

As mentioned in Chap. 14, the risk of CHD increases with increases in resting values of systolic and diastolic blood pressure (60). Blood pressure (BP) classifications have changed over the years, with normal BP being <120/<80 mm Hg. Prehypertension exists when either the systolic BP is 120 to 139 mm Hg or the diastolic BP is 80 to 89 mm Hg. The prehypertension category is not unlike the prediabetes category mentioned earlier in the chapter. The idea is to identify potential problems early and try to prevent or delay the development of hypertension. Stage 1 hypertension is a systolic BP of 140 to 159 mm Hg or a diastolic BP of 90 to 99 mm Hg. Approximately one-third of all U.S. adults have hypertension (**www.cdc.gov/nchs/fastats/hypertension.htm**). Stage 1 individuals represent the majority of all people with hypertension, and they account for most of the morbidity and mortality associated with hypertension (53). Although there is little disagreement that medication should be used to treat hypertension, many believe that nonpharmacological approaches should be used for those with mild or borderline hypertension (5, 17, 54, 60, 61, 118). The reasons nonpharmacological approaches are recommended include the possibility of side effects due to medication and the counterproductive behavioral changes associated with classifying a person as a "patient" (54).

Generally, the person with mild hypertension should have a physical exam to identify potential underlying problems, as well as the presence of other risk factors. Kannel (60) indicates that while medication might be used to control blood pressure when multiple risk factors (smoking, high cholesterol, inactivity, etc.) are present, the simple act of stopping smoking confers more immediate benefit against the overall risk of CHD than any medication. It is within this context that a non-pharmacological intervention program focuses on the use of exercise and diet to control blood pressure and establish behaviors that favorably influence other aspects of health (17, 54).

Dietary recommendations to control blood pressure include a reduction in sodium intake for those sensitive to excess sodium, and in caloric intake for those who are overweight (30). Kaplan's (61) review indicates that salt restriction results in an average reduction in systolic and diastolic blood pressures of 5 and 3 mm Hg, and a 1-kg weight loss is associated with a 1.6 and 1.3 mm Hg reduction, respectively. Both fitness and physical activity are inversely related to the development of hypertension (28). Endurance exercise is associated with a 5 to 7 mm Hg reduction in resting blood pressure in people with hypertension; however, the magnitude of the reduction is inversely related to the pretraining blood pressure (5, 53). Although not all hypertensive individuals respond to endurance exercise in this way, exercise is recommended for all because other changes occur to reduce the risk of CHD, even if blood pressure is not reduced (53).

The standard American College of Sports Medicine exercise prescription for improving $\dot{V}O_2$ max (see Chap. 16) is also effective in reducing blood pressure in people with hypertension. However, exercise in the moderate-intensity range (i.e., 40% to 59% of heart rate reserve) is effective and can be accomplished with lifestyle activities and structured exercise programs. The recommendation is to do at least 30 minutes on most, preferably all, days of the week, supplemented by resistance training at 60% to 80% 1-RM (3, 5, 53, 100, 112). In addition to using exercise to lower elevated blood pressure, it is recommended that individuals (44, 53, 69):

- Lose weight if overweight
- Limit alcohol intake (no more than 2 drinks/day for most men and 1 drink/day for women)
- Reduce sodium intake, ideally to 1.5 g/day
- Eat a diet rich in fruits, vegetables, low-fat dairy products (see DASH diet in Chap. 18)
- Stop smoking.

For recreational athletes who need medication to control blood pressure, the preferred drugs are the angiotensin-converting enzyme (ACE) inhibitors and calcium channel blockers (3, 5, 112). Blood pressure should be checked frequently so that the medication regimen can be altered by the physician, if necessary.

IN SUMMARY

- Exercise can be used as a nonpharmacological intervention for those with hypertension. Exercise recommendations include not only the standard ACSM model for improving $\dot{V}O_2$ max, but also moderate-intensity physical activity (40% to 59% $\dot{V}O_2$ max), done most days per week, and for 30 minutes per session. For those on medication, blood pressure should be checked frequently.

CARDIAC REHABILITATION

Exercise training is now an accepted part of the therapy used to restore an individual who has some form of CHD. The details of how to structure such programs, from the first steps taken after being confined to a bed to the time of returning to work and beyond, are spelled out clearly in books such as *ACSM's Guidelines for Exercise Testing and Prescription* (5), *ACSM's Exercise Management for Persons with Chronic Diseases and Disabilities*, and *ACSM's Resource Manual for Guidelines for Exercise Testing and Prescription* (see Suggested Readings). This brief section will comment on various aspects of such programs.

Population

The persons served by cardiac rehabilitation programs include those who have experienced angina pectoris, myocardial infarctions (MI), coronary artery bypass graft surgery (CABGS), and angioplasty (50, 51). Angina pectoris is the chest pain related to ischemia of the ventricle due to occlusion of one or more of the coronary arteries. The symptoms occur when the work of the heart (estimated by the double product: systolic blood pressure × HR) exceeds a certain value. **Nitroglycerin** is used to prevent an attack and/or relieve the pain by relaxing the smooth muscle in veins to reduce venous return and the work of the heart. People with angina may also be treated with a beta blocker to reduce the HR and/or blood pressure so that the angina symptoms occur at a later stage into work. Exercise training supports this drug effect: As the person becomes trained, the HR response at any work rate is reduced. This allows the individual to take on more tasks without experiencing the chest pain.

Myocardial infarction (MI) patients have actual heart damage (loss of ventricular muscle) due to a prolonged occlusion of one or more of the coronary arteries. The degree to which left ventricular function is compromised is dependent on the mass of the ventricle permanently damaged. These patients are usually on medications to reduce the work of the heart (β-blockers) and control the irritability of the heart tissue so that dangerous **arrhythmias** (irregular heart rhythms) do not occur. Generally, these patients experience a training effect similar to those who do not have an MI (50).

Coronary artery bypass graft surgery (CABGS) patients have had surgery to bypass one or more blocked coronary arteries. In this procedure, either a saphenous vein or an internal mammary artery from the patient is sutured onto the existing coronary arteries above and below the blockage. Sixty percent of those with saphenous vein grafts experience an occlusion by year 11, while the mammary artery graft is still patent in 93% of patients by year 10 (51). The success of the surgery is dependent on the amount of heart damage that existed prior to surgery, as well as the success of the revascularization itself. In those who had chronic angina pectoris prior to CABGS, most find a relief of symptoms, with 70% having no more pain at five-year follow-up. Generally, with an increased blood flow to the ventricle, there is an improvement in both left ventricular function and the capacity for work (51). These patients benefit from systematic exercise training because most are deconditioned prior to surgery as a result of activity restrictions related to chest pain. In addition, exercise improves the chance that the blood vessel graft will remain open (90). Finally, the cardiac rehabilitation program helps the patient to differentiate angina pain from chest wall pain related to the surgery. The overall result is a smoother and less traumatic transition back to normal function.

Some CHD patients undergo **percutaneous transluminal coronary angioplasty (PTCA)** to open occluded arteries. In this procedure, the chest is not opened; instead, a balloon-tipped catheter (a long, slender tube) is inserted into the coronary artery, where the balloon is inflated to push the plaque back toward the arterial wall (51, 105). "Stents" may be used in the PTCA procedure to help keep the artery open. Unfortunately, 30% of clients undergoing a PTCA will show an occlusion within six months, versus only 5% to 8% of those receiving a drug-eluting stent that reduces the chance of inflammation of the blood vessel (51). For more on who should and should not be referred to cardiac rehabilitation programs, see Thomas et al. in Suggested Readings.

Testing

The testing of patients with CHD is much more involved than that presented for the apparently healthy person in Chap. 15 (45). There are classes of CHD patients for whom exercise or exercise testing is inappropriate and dangerous. To help make that judgment, the ACSM provides list of absolute and relative contraindications to exercise testing (5). For

those who can be tested, a 12-lead ECG is monitored at discrete intervals during the GXT, while a variety of leads are displayed continuously. Blood pressure, RPE, and various signs or symptoms are also noted. The criteria for terminating the GXT go well beyond achieving a certain percentage of maximal HR, focusing instead on various pathological signs (e.g., ST-segment depression) and symptoms, such as angina pectoris. On the basis of the response to the GXT, the person may be referred for additional testing, such as the use of radioactive molecules (e.g., ^{99m}technetium sestamibi) to evaluate heart function at rest and during exercise, or direct angiography, in which a dye that is opaque to X-rays is injected into the coronary arteries to determine the blockage directly (74). The results of all the tests are used to classify the individual as a low-, intermediate-, or high-risk patient. The resulting classification has a major impact on deciding whether to use exercise as a part of the rehabilitation process and, if exercise is appropriate, determines the type and format of the exercise program (5). In addition, the results of diagnostic clinical exercise testing can be used for disability assessment (55).

Exercise Programs

Cardiac rehabilitation includes a "Phase I" inpatient exercise program that is used to help the patients make the transition from the cardiovascular event (e.g., an MI that put them in the hospital) to the time of discharge from the hospital. The specific signs and symptoms exhibited by the patient are used to determine whether the patient should be placed in an exercise program and, if so, when to terminate the exercise session (5). After the patient is discharged from the hospital, a "Phase II" program can be started. This program resembles the one mentioned earlier for apparently healthy persons in that warm-up with stretching, endurance, and strengthening exercises and cool-down activities are included. However, the CHD patients, who are generally very deconditioned ($\dot{V}O_2$ max of ~20 ml · kg^{-1} · min^{-1}), require only light exercise to achieve their target heart rate (THR). In addition, because these patients are on a variety of medications that may decrease maximal heart rate, the THR zone is determined from their GXT results; the 220 − age formula cannot be used. The patients usually begin with intermittent low-intensity exercise (one minute on, one minute off) using a variety of exercises to distribute the total work output over a larger muscle mass. In time, the patient increases the duration of the work period for each exercise. The strengthening exercises emphasize a low-resistance and high-repetition format to involve the major muscle groups; free and machine weights, bands, and wall pulleys can be used in a circuit program format. Initial loads should allow 12 to 15 repetitions that can be done comfortably. Loads should be gradually increased as strength increases. A series of eight to ten exercises should be done to involve the major muscle groups on two to three days a week (5). Given that CABGS and post-MI patients have had direct damage to their hearts, the exercise should facilitate, not interfere with, the healing process. As you might guess, given the nature of the patient and the risk involved, cardiac rehabilitation programs take place in hospitals and clinics where there is direct medical supervision and the capacity to deal with emergencies, should they occur. After a patient completes an 8- to 12-week "Phase II" program, the person may continue in a "Phase III" program away from the hospital where there is less supervision, except for the ability to respond to an emergency (5). The frequency of major cardiovascular complications associated with doing exercise in cardiac rehabilitation programs is quite low (84, 104). What are the benefits of such programs to the patient with CHD?

Effects There is no question that people with CHD have improved cardiovascular function as a result of an exercise program. This is shown in higher $\dot{V}O_2$ max values, higher work rates achieved without ischemia as shown by angina pectoris or ST-segment changes, and an increased capacity for prolonged submaximal work (50, 51, 66, 97). The improved lipid profile (lower total cholesterol and higher HDL cholesterol) is a function of more than the exercise alone, given that weight loss and the saturated fat content of the diet can modify these variables (see Chap. 18). There is evidence that home-based cardiac rehabilitation programs for low-risk patients generate outcomes similar to hospital-based programs, but because only a limited number of patients have been involved in these home-based programs, more work needs to be done (58). It must be mentioned that a cardiac rehabilitation program should not be viewed simply as an exercise program. It is a multi-intervention effort involving exercise, medication, diet, and counseling. The latter characteristics are what make these programs "secondary prevention programs" aimed at reducing the risk of a subsequent cardiac event in high-risk patient populations. See Hamm et al. in Suggested Readings for information on the core competencies of cardiac rehabilitation/secondary prevention professionals.

What is surprising, given the documented success of cardiac rehabilitation programs, is that they are underutilized. A variety of studies over the past ten years have shown that following discharge from a hospital after treatment for an MI, PCTA, or CABG only about 60% of the patients were referred for cardiac rehabilitation, despite the recognized benefits (13, 20, 22, 43). Clearly, more needs to be done to increase the use of cardiac rehabilitation programs—the patients would be the winners.

IN SUMMARY

■ Cardiac rehabilitation programs serve a variety of patients, including those having angina pectoris, bypass surgery, myocardial infarctions, and angioplasty. These patients may be taking nitroglycerin to control angina symptoms, β-blockers to reduce the work of the heart, or anti-arrhythmia medications to control dangerous heart rhythms.

■ The exercise tests for CHD patients include a 12-lead ECG and are used for referral to other tests. Exercise programs bring about large changes in functional capacity in these populations due to their low starting point. The programs are gradual and are based on their entry-level exercise tests and other clinical findings.

EXERCISE FOR OLDER ADULTS

The number of older individuals (over age 65) in the United States will double between 2000 and 2040 as the "baby boom" generation comes to full maturity (**www.aoa.acl.gov/aging statistics/profile/2014/docs/2014-profile.pdf**). Older individuals are a special challenge from the standpoint of exercise prescription due to the usual presence of chronic disease and physical activity limitations. However, participation in physical activity and exercise will go a long way in preventing the progress of diseases and in extending the years of independent living (4, 80, 109).

Maximal Aerobic Power

Figure 17.4 shows that maximal aerobic power decreases at the rate of about 1% per year from its peak value, which occurs at age 20 to 40 years, depending on the population (57, 106). The dotted line on the figure represents the dividing line between the ability to live independently and being dependent on others. Further, $\dot{V}O_2$ max values below this cutoff are also associated with much higher rates of all-cause mortality (see Fig. 16.3). A report by Kasch et al. (62) shows that not only can this decline be interrupted by a physical activity program, but middle-aged men who maintain their activity and body weight show half the expected decrease in $\dot{V}O_2$ max over a 20-year period. The same is apparently not the case for women (see A Closer Look 17.2). Consistent with Kasch et al. (62), cross-sectional and longitudinal data show that the decrease in $\dot{V}O_2$ max with age is influenced by decreases in physical activity and increases in percent body fat, as well as any true "aging" effect (57). Because the vast majority of people experience a steady decline in $\dot{V}O_2$ max over time, by 60 years of age, their ability to engage comfortably in normal activities is reduced. This initiates

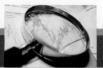

A CLOSER LOOK 17.2

Changes in $\dot{V}O_2$ Max with Age in Women

A study (48) has called into question some of our accepted wisdom about the change in $\dot{V}O_2$ max with age and the effect of fitness on that response. The authors' systematic and analytical review of the literature (a meta-analysis) showed that in endurance-trained women, $\dot{V}O_2$ max fell 6.2 ml·kg^{-1}·min^{-1} per decade, in contrast to 4.4 ml·kg^{-1}·min^{-1} and 3.5 ml·kg^{-1}·min^{-1} for active and sedentary women, respectively. This was different from what had been observed in men, and about whom most of the "accepted wisdom" had been based. It must be noted, however, that when these absolute changes (ml·kg^{-1}·min^{-1}) were expressed as a percentage of their respective $\dot{V}O_2$ max values, the percent decline was about 10% per decade for all groups, which is similar to what has been measured in sedentary men. Why did the most highly fit female subjects experience the largest change in $\dot{V}O_2$ max with age?

The investigators examined the decreases in maximal heart rate with age in these three groups to see if it might help explain why $\dot{V}O_2$ max decreased fastest in the most-fit group. It didn't. The decline in maximal heart rate was similar across the three groups (7.0 to 7.9 b·min^{-1} per decade) and could not explain why the most-fit group had the fastest decline in $\dot{V}O_2$ max. The authors suggested the following possibilities:

- Baseline effect. Those with the highest $\dot{V}O_2$ max values had the greatest decline. A parallel observation was found in comparisons between men and women. On average, young men have higher $\dot{V}O_2$ max values than do young women; the men also have a greater decrease in $\dot{V}O_2$ max with age. However, the percent decline is about 10% per decade for both genders, similar to what has been observed for the three groups of women.

- The most-fit women were found to have a greater decrease in their training stimulus with age, compared with sedentary women (since the sedentary women were just that, sedentar; their "change" would have been modest at best). The large reduction in training volume as they aged would help explain why the most-fit women had the greatest loss in $\dot{V}O_2$ max.

- An increase in body weight in adults with age is associated with a decline in $\dot{V}O_2$ max (ml·kg^{-1}·min^{-1}). The authors wondered if a difference in weight gain could help explain why the most-fit (least-fat) subjects had the greatest decrease in $\dot{V}O_2$ max. Interestingly, they found no support for this in their data analysis.

The authors remind us that, in spite of these observations, men and women of any age who participate regularly in endurance training have higher $\dot{V}O_2$ max values than their less active counterparts.

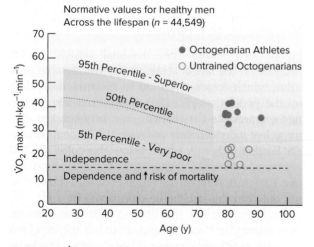

Figure 17.4 $\dot{V}O_2$ max values of octogenarian lifelong endurance athletes and healthy untrained octogenarians. The dotted line represents the prognostic $\dot{V}O_2$ max (5 METs or 17.5 ml·kg^{-1}·min^{-1}) generally necessary for an independent lifestyle and associated risk for mortality.

a vicious cycle that leads to lower and lower levels of cardiorespiratory fitness, which may not allow them to perform daily tasks. In turn, this affects quality of life and independence, which may necessitate reliance on others

(5). See A Look Back–Important People in Science for an individual who helped shape our understanding of the role of exercise in slowing the physiological changes we typically see with aging. A physical activity program is useful in dealing not only with this downward spiral of cardiorespiratory fitness, but also with the osteoporosis that is related to the sudden hip fractures that can lead to more inactivity and death (4, 6, 80, 109).

Response to Training

Over the past 30 years, a substantial body of knowledge has accumulated, documenting the capacity of older individuals to experience a training effect similar to what has been observed in younger men and women (4, 80). This has major ramifications when one considers the increase in the number of older individuals in our population and the need to maintain their health status and independence for as long as possible. Data on the effect of exercise on older individuals have been obtained from cross-sectional studies comparing older athletes to their sedentary counterparts and from longitudinal studies in which training programs have been carried out over many months. A brief summary of each follows (54, 83).

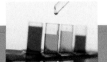

Dr. Fred W. Kasch's Adult Fitness Program Studied Patients Over 40 Years

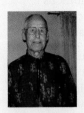

Courtesy of Dr. Lindsay Carter

Dr. Fred W. Kasch received his B.S. and M.S. degrees at the University of Illinois, Urbana, and his Ph.D. at New York University. Dr. Kasch was hired at San Diego State University in 1948 and within ten years established one of the first adult fitness programs in the country–a unique thing to do at a time when the medical community did not view the combination of exercise and adults as anything but risky business. His adult fitness program recruited cardiac patients, as well as those with high blood pressure and those who simply wanted to become fit. Dr. John Boyer, a cardiologist, began to work with Dr. Kasch in the early 1960s, and together, with their students, they collected data on the participants at regular intervals over the next 40 years to allow them to study changes over time. Measurements included an ECG, blood pressure, weight, body fatness, and measured $\dot{V}O_2$ max (using classical techniques that involved a Douglas bag and Scholander gas analyzer). At regular intervals over the 40 years, Dr. Kasch and his colleagues published research papers updating the changes (or lack thereof) that occurred in the program's participants. These reports showed that, compared with sedentary adults, regular participation in Kasch's program resulted in:

- Decreases in blood pressure in those who were hypertensive
- Maintenance of normal resting blood pressure over the years when inactive peers were experiencing an "age-related" increase in resting blood pressure values
- Decreases in body fatness and the maintenance of lower percent fat values over time

- A much slower decrease in $\dot{V}O_2$ max over the years

Dr. Kasch's reports provided clear evidence to the medical community that regular participation in exercise provided excellent health-related benefits in adults of various ages, including those with diagnosed disease. His adult fitness program became a model that was emulated by others throughout the 1970s and beyond. Dr. Kasch published more than 100 articles over his career.

Dr. Kasch practiced what he preached throughout his entire life, remaining active as an archer and deer hunter into his nineties. He made his own long bow and arrows and began each day with a regimen of exercise that each of us would do well to follow. Dr. Kasch passed away on April 8, 2008, a few days short of his 95th birthday. His memory and influence will live on.

Cross-sectional studies have shown that, in contrast to older sedentary individuals, endurance-trained older athletes have:

- Higher $\dot{V}O_2$ max values
- Higher HDL cholesterol, and lower triglycerides, total, and LDL cholesterol
- Enhanced glucose tolerance and insulin sensitivity
- Greater strength, quicker reaction time, and a lower risk of falling

These comparisons could be biased due to the potential for a strong genetic factor that might drive an individual to pursue an active life. In contrast, longitudinal studies compare a trained group to a control group over many months to see how each changes; this minimizes the concerns raised in the cross-sectional studies. The results from these studies parallel those mentioned previously. Endurance training:

- Increases $\dot{V}O_2$ max and the kinetics of oxygen uptake in a manner similar to younger individuals, but more time may be required for the training effect to occur (14). In men, the increase in $\dot{V}O_2$ max is due to both peripheral (skeletal muscle) and central

(cardiovascular) adaptations. However, the increase in $\dot{V}O_2$ max in older women is due solely to peripheral adaptations (101).

- Causes favorable changes in blood lipids, but the changes seem to be linked to a reduction in body fatness, rather than exercise, per se.
- Lowers blood pressure to the same degree as shown for younger people with hypertension.
- Improves glucose tolerance and insulin sensitivity.
- Increases or maintains muscular strength and bone density. It must be added that resistance training results in large increases in strength, which may play an important role in reducing the risk of falls.

We currently have a variety of physical activity recommendations for older adults (4, 80, 109). What follows is a compilation, based primarily on the *U.S. Physical Activity Guidelines*:

- The following PA guidelines are the same for adults and older adults:
  - All older adults should avoid inactivity; some PA is better than none, and older

adults who participate in any amount of PA gain some health benefits.

- For substantial health benefits, older adults should do at least 150 minutes a week of moderate-intensity PA or 75 minutes per week of vigorous-intensity aerobic PA, or an appropriate combination of both. The PA should be done in bouts of at least ten minutes, and the total amount should be spread throughout the week.
  - On a scale of 0 to 10 for a level of physical exertion, use 5 to 6 for moderate-intensity PA and 7 to 8 for vigorous-intensity PA.
- For additional and more extensive health benefits, older adults should increase their aerobic physical activity to 300 minutes per week of moderate-intensity PA or 150 minutes per week of vigorous-intensity PA. Additional health benefits can be gained by going beyond this amount.
- Older adults should also perform 8 to 10 muscle-strengthening exercises on at least two days per week using the major muscle groups. A resistance should be used that allows 8 to 12 repetitions for each exercise. The strength training program helps with the typical loss of muscle/strength, bone mass, and balance seen in this population (see later discussion).
- Perform flexibility exercises for at least ten minutes on at least two days per week. Recent evidence shows that flexibility exercise can improve the walking ability of older adults (faster speed, longer stride) (38).

■ The following guidelines are just for older adults:
- If older adults cannot do 150 minutes of moderate-intensity PA per week because of chronic conditions, they should be as active as their abilities and conditions allow.
- Older adults should determine their level of effort for physical activity relative to their level of fitness.
- Older adults should do exercises that maintain or improve balance if they are at risk of falling. In that regard, exercise programs using multiple modes appear to have an advantage in fall prevention (16). Balance exercises may include backward walking, sideways walking, heel walking, toe walking, and standing from a seated position. The difficulty (and risk) of the exercises can be increased by (a) progressing from a wide to narrow base of support and (b) moving the center of

mass side to side, or doing crossover or sideways walking. To control risk, supervision may be needed until the older adult can demonstrate independence (34).
- Older adults with chronic conditions should understand how their conditions affect their ability to do regular PA safely.

An important point made throughout the *U.S. Physical Activity Guidelines* is the importance of progression, and this is certainly the case when working with older adults (109). Visit the following website to see exercise programs for older adults: **www.nia.nih.gov/ health/publication/exercise-physical-activity**.

Bone Health and Osteoporosis

Bone is a dynamic tissue that is able to increase in size and strength in response to increased demands through the action of osteoblasts that cause bone deposition. In contrast, when bone is not challenged (e.g., lack of gravity, inactivity), it is resorbed by the action of osteoclasts, resulting in a loss of strength, size, and density (49). The latter is a major concern for older adults. Osteoporosis is a loss of bone mass that primarily affects women over 50 years of age and is responsible for 1.5 million fractures annually (87, 99). Type I osteoporosis is related to vertebral and distal radius fractures in 50- to 65-year-olds and is eight times more common in women than men. Type II osteoporosis, found in those aged 70 and above, results in hip, pelvic, and distal humerus fractures and is twice as common in women (18). The problem is more common in women over age 50 due to menopause and the lack of estrogen. Hormone replacement therapy (HRT) initiated early in menopause prevents bone loss and can increase bone mineral density and reduce fracture risk (18, 87). However, such treatments are not without risks. HRT has been associated with an increase in cardiovascular disease and mortality and an increased risk of certain cancers (81). Given that prevention is better than treatment, attention is focused on the primary environmental factors that impact bone growth: adequate dietary calcium and vitamin D, and exercise throughout life (6, 87, 99).

Dietary calcium and vitamin D are important in preventing and treating osteoporosis. Although dietary intake of calcium for females is inadequate, when supplements are included and the average intake of calcium is considered, only adolescent girls fell dramatically short of achieving the recommendation (15). This is a major concern for the latter age group because it is during this time that bone mass should be built up. Vitamin D intakes were better across the board for all but the oldest age group, in part because their vitamin D requirement is higher than for other age groups (see Chap. 18) (15).

Bone structure is maintained by the force of gravity (upright posture) and the lateral forces associated with muscle contraction. Even though the best exercise prescription for bone health in adults is a work in progress, we have guidance from both the ACSM and the *U.S. Physical Activity Guidelines* (4, 6, 80, 87, 109):

- Frequency: weight-bearing activities 3 to 5 times/week; resistance exercise 2 to 3 times/week

- Intensity: Aerobic: moderate (40% to <60% HRR) to vigorous (>60% HRR); Resistance: moderate (60% to 80% 1RM; 8 to 12 repetitions) to vigorous (>80% 1RM; 5 to 6 repetitions)

- Duration: 30 to 60 min/day of a combination of weight-bearing endurance activities, activities that involve jumping, and resistance exercise that targets all the muscle groups

- Modes: weight-bearing endurance activities (tennis, stair climbing, jogging, at least intermittently during walking); activities that involve jumping (volleyball, basketball); and resistance exercise

Clearly, as age increases, one would have to use additional care to ensure that exercises can be done safely. For some special insights into what is needed for bone health, see Ask the Expert 17.1.

Strength

Strength declines only about 10% between 20 and 50 years of age, but decreases at a much faster rate after that. The loss of strength is due, in part, to the lower level of physical activity in older individuals, but the large decrease in strength between 60 and 80 years of age is due to the actual loss of muscle mass, a condition known as sarcopenia. The Clinical Applications in Chap. 8 provides a good overview of this problem and is worth rereading at this point. The good news is that strength training can increase strength in older individuals by about 30%, much like that seen in younger individuals (4, 86). Following the resistance training program mentioned earlier in this section will accomplish that goal.

There is no question that older adults, like their younger counterparts, exhibit a specificity and an adaptability to training, be it for strength or endurance. Consequently, the exercise program should provide endurance, flexibility, and strength activities within the capacity of the population being served in order to make improvements in these fitness components. A combination of strength training and balance training has been shown to reduce the risk of falls (4, 80, 109). This combination of exercises has been packaged into what has become known as *neuromotor exercise training or functional fitness training*

(5). Although the specific parameters for the exercise prescription (i.e., FITT) are not known, programs exist for those across the fitness spectrum, from very fit to those with chronic disease.

In conclusion, the use of exercise programs for older adults improves cardiorespiratory fitness and strength and helps to maintain the integrity of bone. When this is coupled with the opportunity for socialization, it is easy to see why exercise is an important part of life from youth to old age. See Clinical Application 17.1 for physical activity recommendations for a population of patients that does not receive much attention.

IN SUMMARY

- The "normal" deterioration of physiological function with age can be attenuated or reversed with regular endurance and strength training. The benefits of participation in a regular exercise program include an improved risk factor profile (e.g., higher HDL and lower LDL cholesterol, improved insulin sensitivity, higher $\dot{V}O_2$ max, and lower blood pressure), but the training effects may take longer to realize.

- The guidelines for exercise training programs for older adults are similar to those for younger people, emphasizing the need for a medical exam and screening for risk factors. The effort required to bring about the training effect may be less than for younger individuals.

EXERCISE DURING PREGNANCY

Pregnancy places special demands on a woman due to the developing fetus's needs for calories, protein, minerals, vitamins, and, of course, the physiologically stable environment needed to process these nutrients. It is against this background that the implementation of a physical activity program must be evaluated. A pregnant woman should begin with a thorough medical examination by her physician to rule out complications that would make exercise inappropriate, and to provide specific information about signs or symptoms to watch for during the course of the pregnancy. Absolute contraindications for aerobic exercise during pregnancy include hemodynamically significant heart disease, restrictive lung disease, incompetent cervix/cerclage, multiple gestation at risk for premature labor, persistent second- and third-trimester bleeding, placenta previa after 26 weeks of gestation, premature labor during the current pregnancy, ruptured membranes, preeclampsia or pregnancy-induced hypertension, and severe anemia. Relative contraindications include anemia, unevaluated maternal cardiac arrhythmias, chronic bronchitis, poorly controlled type

Exercise and Bone Health Questions and Answers with Dr. Susan A. Bloomfield

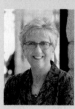

Courtesy of Susan Bloomfield

Dr. Susan Bloomfield *is Professor in the Department of Health and Kinesiology, a member of the Graduate Faculty in Nutrition & Food Science, and Associate Dean for Research in the College of Education and Human Development at Texas A&M University. Her research utilizes animal models to study the integrative physiology driving bone adaptation to modeled microgravity, prolonged caloric restriction, and exercise, as well as functional relationships of bone and muscle in these models. She lives in College Station with her a rowdy Lab mix named Beau and two cats, and can be found competing at U.S. Masters swim meets several times each year.*

QUESTION: What are the primary factors affecting bone health?

ANSWER: Optimal bone health depends on adequate nutritional intake of calcium, vitamin D, energy, and protein as well as regular exercise in the context of a normal reproductive hormonal profile. If serum levels of estrogen or testosterone are low, bone mass (usually measured by bone mineral density, or BMD) tends to decline. Interestingly, the primary effect of estrogen is to suppress activity of osteoclasts (bone-resorbing cells). Hence, estrogen deficiency, whether occurring at menopause or after prolonged amenorrhea in a young woman, "takes the brakes off" bone resorption and bone loss results. Growth hormone and, in adults, IGF-I and leptin are endocrine factors that vary with nutritional status. Declines in any of these "metabolic" hormones also have a negative impact on bone balance. It is important to get adequate energy and protein to support optimal bone health. Interestingly, there is good evidence that regular physical activity is critical to maximizing the beneficial impact of calcium intake on bone mass. And there is very clear evidence that if all weight-bearing physical activity is removed, the skeleton will "downsize" itself to match that reduced loadbearing. For example, unless they are diligent with their exercise regimes and nutritional intake, ISS astronauts lose bone mass ten-fold faster while in space than do post menopausal women!

QUESTION: Is exercise and good nutrition more important later in life when bone loss most often occurs?

ANSWER: As important as exercise and good nutrition are after the age of 50, when age-related or menopause-induced bone loss becomes more apparent, the most critical years from a public health viewpoint actually fall right around puberty. We gain an incredible 30% of our eventual peak bone mass in the three years surrounding puberty; further increases in BMD occur until at least the age of 25. The greatest impact of exercise on BMD and optimal bone geometry occurs during these years of rapid growth, with the result that the active child grows into an adult with a high peak bone mass before age-related loss begins. High calcium intakes (1200 to 1500 mg/day) at this age help ensure the maximal benefit. However, calcium intake is declining among American children and, ironically, most dramatically in adolescent girls who stand to benefit the most in terms of reducing their risk of osteoporotic fractures later in life. The clear public health message here is that we need to promote more consumption of calcium-rich foods (especially milk!) and more physical activity for American children and teens. This translates to the removal of soda machines from our schools' hallways and the promotion of regular physical education classes through high school. On a population-wide basis, the prevention of osteoporosis, rather than attention to treating established bone loss, is likely to be far more effective. That said, those of us on the other end of the aging span need to pay attention to good nutrition and exercise, particularly to maintain adequate (and toned) muscle mass to minimize aging-related bone loss and our risk of fragility fractures.

QUESTION: What are the general characteristics of exercise programs that produce increments in bone mass and decrease the risk of osteoporotic fractures later in life?

ANSWER: There are important lessons to learn from key experiments done in animal models, with results being more and more frequently applied to the human condition. For example, experiments by Rubin and Lanyon (96) on the ulnas of turkeys revealed the importance of the magnitude of force applied to bone (as opposed to many loading cycles) as well as a unique distribution of loading. Hence, we have the current emphasis on either weight-training or weight-bearing activities that involve impact forces to provide adequate stimulus to the skeleton. In addition, a diversified exercise program that uses a wide variety of muscle groups with frequent and varied movement patterns is better than a monotonous signal to bone like running or cycling. More recent findings from Robling and fellow researchers (93), using external loading of rat tibiae, suggest that two four shorter exercise bouts spread over the day might be more osteogenic (promoting gain in bone mass) than one long bout. Interestingly, this approach agrees well with the recommendations we're hearing from exercise epidemiologists that activity accumulated over the day provides significant health benefits. Incorporating more activity into our daily life (commuting by bicycle, physical work at home, more walking as well as planned exercise) holds much promise for improving bone health across the life span.

Physical Activity and Cancer

As mentioned in Chap. 14, cancer is the second leading cause of death in the United States. We have become accustomed to seeing physical activity recommendations for chronic diseases like diabetes, heart disease, and COPD, but cancer does not receive as much attention. However, the *2008 Physical Activity Guidelines for Americans* indicated that there was strong evidence that regular physical activity was linked to a lower risk of colon and breast cancer and moderate evidence for a lower risk of lung and endometrial cancer (109). Eight years later the study by Moore, et al, (77) provides clear evidence that regular participation in physical activity is associated with a lower risk of 13 different types of cancer–even more reason to promote the message about physical activity and the *prevention* of chronic diseases like cancer (77). But what about those who have cancer and are undergoing treatment for it? What exercise prescription is recommended?

That is not an easy question to answer because of differences among patients in the tumor site (e.g., brain, breast, blood), the cancer stage (e.g., Stage 1 [localized] vs. Stage 4 [spread to distant tissue]), the type of treatment (e.g., chemotherapy, radiation, surgery), and the response of the patient to the treatment (e.g., minimal vs. many side effects). Further, knowing that some

of these factors change throughout a treatment regime, the consistent recommendation across various agencies serving patients with cancer is to *avoid inactivity* (5, 98). Needless to say, the patient should work with his/her doctors to determine what kinds of exercises to do *and* avoid, as well as to plan an appropriate course of action that might include a physical therapist, a qualified fitness professional (see **http://certification.acsm.org/acsm-cancer-exercise-trainer**), or a program that can be done with minimal or no assistance.

Exercise progression is the key, taking the patients from their current level of physical activity to the goals described in the *Physical Activity Guidelines* for older adults presented in this chapter. Progression should be applied to (5, 98):

- Frequency: begin with every other day, with goal of most/all days per week
- Intensity: start at light intensity using the HR (<60% HRR), MET scale (<3 METs), or perceived exertion (<12 on original Borg RPE scale), and work up to moderate intensity
- Time: begin with several short sessions per day, and increase the duration of the sessions until one continuous session of 30 minutes can be done. If more

than 150 minutes per week of moderate-intensity activity can be done, they should be encouraged to do so.

- Flexibility and strengthening exercises, which should also be done at least two days per week.

Patients should be educated to be aware that how they respond to their routine exercises might dictate reducing or stopping exercise, or seeking immediate help. For example, intensity should be reduced if the degree of effort becomes "very hard;" assistance may be needed if chest discomfort, shortness of breath, cramping, or excessive fatigue are experienced; and exercise should be skipped if a fever (>101 °F/38.3 °C) is present (82). See Schmitz's chapter for more on this important topic (98). Research in this area is ongoing and will certainly lead to new insights on physical activity in cancer prevention and recommendations for cancer treatment. In the meantime, regular physical activity should be encouraged as a way to help prevent the disease and improve cancer treatment outcomes. One closing note, the study by Moore et al. (77) also found that the risk of malignant melanoma was increased with leisure-time physical activity–probably linked to sun exposure–additional motivation to use sun block.

---

1 diabetes, extreme morbid obesity, extreme underweight (BMI <12), history of extremely sedentary lifestyle, intrauterine growth restriction in current pregnancy, poorly controlled hypertension, orthopedic limitations, poorly controlled seizure disorder, poorly controlled hyperthyroidism, and heavy smoking (2). Clearly, to protect mother and fetus, a consultation with a physician is an appropriate recommendation prior to the initiation of an exercise program.

Interestingly, compared to our knowledge of how diabetic, asthmatic, and cardiac patients respond to exercise training, we are now only beginning to understand how the mother and fetus respond to such a program (29, 116, 117). In general, the following describe the major cardiovascular and metabolic

adaptations to pregnancy compared to the nonpregnant state (115, 116):

- Blood volume increases 40% to 50%.
- Oxygen uptake is slightly higher at rest and during submaximal exercise.
- The oxygen cost of weight-bearing exercise is markedly increased.
- Heart rates are higher at rest and during submaximal exercise.
- Cardiac output is higher at rest and during submaximal exercise for the first two trimesters; in the third trimester, cardiac output is lower and the potential for arterial hypotension is greater.

In spite of all these changes, moderate exercise does not appear to interfere with oxygen delivery to the fetus, and the heart rate response of the fetus shows no signs of distress. The fetal heart rate increases with the intensity and duration of exercise, and it gradually returns to normal during postexercise recovery (115–117). Cardiac output has been shown to be higher at 26 weeks' gestation during submaximal exercise than at 8 weeks following delivery. The fact that the a-$\bar{v}O_2$ difference was lower suggests that the higher cardiac output was distributed to other vascular beds (e.g., the uterus) and muscle blood flow was maintained (117). Since absolute $\dot{V}O_2$ max (L/min) doesn't change much over the course of a pregnancy (71), what happens when exercise training is done during pregnancy?

In general, there is evidence that estimated $\dot{V}O_2$ max (in L/min) is increased as a result of training in previously sedentary pregnant women, while relative $\dot{V}O_2$ max (ml $\cdot$ kg^{-1} $\cdot$ min^{-1}) is maintained or increased slightly, despite the weight gain (117). What is interesting is that when well-conditioned recreational athletes trained throughout and following their pregnancy, absolute $\dot{V}O_2$ max was increased as long as 36 to 44 weeks after delivery compared to a "control" group of women who maintained training and did not become pregnant (32). This suggests that the combination of pregnancy and training resulted in adaptations greater than what could be achieved by training alone. What are reasonable recommendations to follow when a pregnant woman wants to exercise?

Guidelines have been developing over the past two decades. In an earlier set of guidelines from the American College of Obstetricians and Gynecologists (ACOG), fixed criteria (e.g., don't exercise over an HR of 140 b/min) were provided, with the emphasis on taking a conservative approach to exercise prescription. Current guidelines emphasize the need to avoid doing exercise in the supine position to avoid a reduction in venous return and orthostatic hypotension (2). Weight-supported activities are encouraged due to the lower risk of injury, and attention is focused on the need for hydration to maintain body temperature in the normal range associated with exercise. Research suggests that normal exercise-induced increases in body temperatures carry little risk to the fetus (2, 29, 116).

The American College of Obstetricians and Gynecologists states that in the absence of either medical or obstetric complications, pregnant women can follow the public health recommendation of doing 150 minutes of moderate-intensity physical activity per week. Individuals should use a progression format beginning, for example, with 15 minutes, three days per week until the 150 minutes per week goal is reached. This recommendation was supported in a recent review of the literature (79).

- Recreational and competitive athletes with uncomplicated pregnancies can remain active during pregnancy and modify activities as medically indicated. Pregnant women who engage in strenuous exercise require close medical supervision.

- Previously inactive women and those with medical or obstetric complications should be evaluated by a physician before exercise recommendations are made.

- A physically active woman with a history of, or at risk for, preterm labor or fetal growth restriction should reduce her activity in the second and third trimesters.

Mudd, L. M., Owe, K. M., Mottola, M. F., and Pivarnik, J. M., "Health Benefits of Physical Activity During Pregnancy: An International Perspective," *Medicine and Science in Sports and Exercise* 45:268–277, 2013.

For those doing structured exercise programs, the *Canadian Guidelines* (41) suggest using the "talk test" (reduce intensity when conversation cannot be continued without pauses to catch one's breath) or the RPE (12–14 on the original Borg scale) to set exercise intensity. This has been endorsed in the current ACOG recommendations (2). However, the following heart rate ranges were offered for additional guidance in the PARmed-X for Pregnancy (**www.csep.ca/cmfiles/publications/parq/parmed-xpreg.pdf**):

- Less than 20 years of age, 140–155
- 20–29 years of age
  - Low fit: 129–144
  - Active: 135–150
  - Fit: 145–160
  - BMI>25 kg $\cdot$ m^{-2}: 102–124
- 30–39 years of age
  - Low fit: 128–144
  - Active: 130–145
  - Fit: 140–156
  - BMI > 25 kg $\cdot$ m^{-2}: 101–120

Source: www.csep.ca/cmfiles/publications/parq/parmed-xpreg.pdf.

In spite of the growing body of knowledge supporting the appropriateness of recommending exercise during pregnancy, only about 50% of private/small group practice obstetricians recommend physical activity during pregnancy (46). This is unfortunate given that regular physical activity during pregnancy is associated with a reduced risk of both gestational diabetes and preeclampsia, growing problems in an overweight and obese society (40). A recent study emphasized the need to disseminate current recommendations and information about the risks and benefits of physical activity during pregnancy to obstetricians in order to overcome the gap between science and practice (47).

STUDY ACTIVITIES

1. What is the difference between type 1 and type 2 diabetes?
2. If a person with type 1 diabetes does not take an adequate amount of insulin, what happens to the blood glucose concentration during prolonged exercise? Why?
3. If exercise is helpful in controlling blood glucose in those with type 2 diabetes, how could it complicate the life of a person with type 1 diabetes?
4. Provide general recommendations regarding changes in insulin and diet for those with diabetes who engage in exercise.
5. How is exercise-induced asthma triggered, and how can the exercise prescription be modified to reduce the potential for an exercise-induced asthma attack?
6. What are exercise and diet recommendations for the nonpharmacological treatment of those with borderline hypertension?
7. What is COPD, and where does exercise fit in as part of a rehabilitation program?
8. What are angina pectoris, CABGS, and angioplasty?
9. Contrast Phase I cardiac rehabilitation programs with the Phase II and Phase III programs.
10. How do older adults respond to exercise training compared to younger subjects?
11. Older adult strength training programs focus on more than muscle and strength. Explain.
12. What are the recommended guidelines for a pregnant woman who wants to begin an exercise program?

SUGGESTED READINGS

American College of Sports Medicine. 2016. *ACSM's Exercise Management for Persons with Chronic Diseases and Disabilities.* Champaign, IL: Human Kinetics.

American College of Sports Medicine. 2014. *ACSM's Resource Manual for Guidelines for Exercise Testing and Prescription* 6th ed. Baltimore, MD: Lippincott Williams & Wilkins.

Hamm, L. F., B. K. Sanderson, P. A. Ades, K. Berra, L. A. Kaminsky, J. L. Roitman, et al. 2011. Core competencies for cardiac rehabilitation/secondary prevention professionals: 2010 update. *Journal of Cardiopulmonary Rehabilitation and Prevention* 31: 2-10.

Thomas, R. J., M. King, K. Lui, N. Oldridge, I. L. Piña, and J. Spertus. 2010. ACC/AHA 2010 update: performance measures on cardiac rehabilitation for referral to cardiac rehabilitation/secondary prevention services. *Journal of the American College of Cardiology* 56: 1159-67.

REFERENCES

1. **Ali Z, Norsk P, and Ulrik CS.** Mechanisms and management of exercise-induced asthma in elite athletes. *Journal of Asthma* 49: 480-486, 2012.
2. **American College of Obstetricians and Gynecologists.** Physical activity and exercise during pregnancy and the postpartum period. (Committee Opinion No. 650). *Obstetrics & Gynecology* 126: e135-42, 2015.
3. **American College of Sports Medicine.** Exercise and hypertension. *Medicine & Science in Sports & Exercise* 25: i-x, 2004.
4. **American College of Sports Medicine.** Exercise and physical activity for the older adult. *Medicine & Science in Sports & Exercise* 41: 1510-1530, 2009.
5. **American College of Sports Medicine.** *Guidelines for Exercise Testing and Prescription.* Baltimore, MD: Lippincott Williams & Wlikins, 2014.
6. **American College of Sports Medicine.** Physcial activity and bone health. *Medicine & Science in Sports & Exercise* 36: 1985-1996, 2004.
7. **American College of Sports Medicine and American Diabetes Association.** Exercise and type 2 diabetes. *Medicine & Science in Sports & Exercise* 42: 2282-2303, 2010.
8. **American Diabetes Association.** Classification and diagnosis of diabetes. *Diabetes Care* 39: S13-S22, 2016.
9. **American Diabetes Association.** Nutrition recommendations and interventions for diabetes. *Diabetes Care* 30 (Suppl 1): S48-65, 2007.
10. **American Diabetes Association.** Physical activity/exercise and diabetes. *Diabetes Care* 27: S58-62, 2004.
11. **American Diabetes Association.** Prevention or delay of type 2 diabetes. *Diabetes Care* 27: S47-54, 2004.
12. **Anderson SD, Caillaud C, and Brannan JD.** Beta2-agonists and exercise-induced asthma. *Clinical Reviews in Allergy & Immunology* 31: 163-180, 2006.
13. **Aragam KG, Dai D, Neely ML, Bhatt DL, Roe MT, Rumsfeld JS, et al.** Gaps in referral to cardiac rehabilitation of patients undergoing percutaneous coronary intervention in the United States. *Journal of the American College of Cardiology* 65: 2079-2088, 2015.
14. **Babcock MA, Paterson DH, and Cunningham DA.** Effects of aerobic endurance training on gas exchange kinetics of older men. *Medicine & Science in Sports & Exercise* 26: 447-452, 1994.
15. **Bailey RL, Dodd KW, Goldman JA, Gahche JJ, Dwyer JT, Moshfegh AJ, et al.** Estimation of total usual calcium and vitamin D intakes in the United States. *Journal of Nutrition* 140: 817-822, 2010.
16. **Baker MK, Atlantis E, and Fiatarone Singh MA.** Multi-modal exercise programs for older adults. *Age and Ageing* 36: 375-381, 2007.

17. **Bassett DR and Zweifler AJ.** Risk factors and risk factor management. In *Clinical Ischemic Syndromes*, edited by Zelenock GB, D'Alecy LG, Fantone III JC, Shlafer M, and Stanley JC. St. Louis, MO: C. V. Mosby, 1990, pp. 15-46.

18. **Bloomfield SA and Smith SS.** Osteoporosis. In *ACSM's Exercise Management for Persons with Chronic Diseases and Disabilities*. Champaign, IL: Human Kinetics, 2003, pp. 222-229.

19. **Booker R.** Chronic obstructive pulmonary disease: non-pharmacological approaches. *British Journal of Nursing* 14: 14-18, 2005.

20. **Boyden T, Rubenfire M, and Franklin B.** Will increasing referral to cardiac rehabilitatation improve participation? *Preventive Cardiology* 13: 192-201, 2010.

21. **Briscoe VJ, Tate DB, and Davis SN.** Type 1 diabetes: exercise and hypoglycemia. *Applied Physiology, Nutrition, and Metabolism = Physiologie Appliquee, Nutrition et Metabolisme* 32: 576-582, 2007.

22. **Brown TM, Hernandez AF, Bittner V, Cannon CP, Ellrodt G, Liang L, et al.** Predictors of cardiac rehabilitation referral in coronary artery disease patients: finding from the American Heart Association Get With the Guidelines Program. *Journal of the American College of Cardiology* 54: 515-521, 2009.

23. **Brusasco V and Crimi E.** Allergy and sports: exercise-induced asthma. *International Journal of Sports Medicine* 15 (Suppl 3): S184-186, 1994.

24. **Butts JF, Belfer MH, and Gebke KB.** Exercise for patients with COPD: an integral yet underutilized intervention. *Physician and Sportsmedicine* 41: 49-57, 2013.

25. **Campaign BN.** Exercise and diabetes mellitus. In *ACSM's Resource Manual for Guidelines for Graded Exercise Testing and Prescription*. Baltimore, MD: Lippincott Williams & Wilkins, 2001, pp. 277-284.

26. **Carlin BW.** Diagnostic procedures in patients with pulmonary diseases. In *ACSM's Resource Manual for Guidelines for Exercise Testing and Prescription*, 7th ed. Baltimore, MD: Lippincott Williams & Wilkins, 2014, pp. 397-412.

27. **Carlsen KH.** Sports in extreme conditions: the impact of exercise in cold temperatures on asthma and bronchial hyper-responsiveness in athletes. *British Journal of Sports Medicine* 46: 796-799, 2012.

28. **Carnethon MR, Evans NS, Church TS, Lewis CE, Schreiner PJ, Jacobs DR, et al.** Joint associations of physical activity and aerobic fitness on the development of incident hypertension: coronary artery disease risk development in young adults. *Hypertension* 56: 49-55, 2010.

29. **Carpenter MW.** Physical activity, fitness, and health of the pregnant mother and fetus. In *Physical Activity, Fitness, and Health*, edited by Bouchard C, Shephard RJ, and Stephens T. Champaign, IL: Human Kinetics, 1994, pp. 967-979.

30. **Chobanian AV, Bakris GL, Black HR, Cushman WC, Green LA, Izzo JL, Jr., et al.** Seventh report of the Joint National Committee on Prevention, Detection, Evaluation, and Treatment of High Blood Pressure. *Hypertension* 42: 1206-1252, 2003.

31. **Church T.** Exercise in obesity, metabolic syndrome, and diabetes. *Progress in Cardiovascular Disease* 53: 412-418, 2011.

32. **Clapp JF III and Capeless E.** The $\dot{V}O_{2max}$ of recreational athletes before and after pregnancy. *Medicine & Science in Sports & Exercise* 23: 1128-1133, 1991.

33. **Clark CJ.** Asthma. In *ACSM's Exercise Management for Persons with Chronic Diseases and Disabilities*. Champaign, IL: Human Kinetics, 2003, pp. 105-110.

34. **Coe DP and Fiatarone Singh M.** Exercise prescription in special populations: women, pregnancy, children, and older adults. In *ACSM's Resource Manual for Guidelines for Exercise Testing and Prescription*, edited by Swain DP. Baltimore: Wolters Kluwer/Lippincott Williams & Wilkins, 2014, pp. 565-595.

35. **Colberg SR.** Exercise Prescription for patients with diabetes. In *ACSM's Resource Manual for Guidelines for Exercise Testing and Prescription.*, edited by Swain DP. Baltimore, MD: Lippincott Williams & Wilkins, 2014, pp. 661-681.

36. **Cooper CB.** Airflow obstruction and exercise. *Respiratory Medicine* 103: 325-334, 2009.

37. **Cooper CB and Storer TW.** Exercise prescription in patients with pulmonary disease. In *ACSM's Resource Manual for Guidelines for Exercise Testing and Prescription*, edited by Ehrman JK. Baltimore, MD: Lippincott Williams & Wilkins, 2010, pp. 575-599.

38. **Cristopoliski F, Barela JA, Leite N, Fowler NE, and Rodacki ALF.** Stretching exercise programs improve gait in the elderly. *Gerontology* 55: 614-620, 2009.

39. **Cypcar D and Lemanske RF, Jr.** Asthma and exercise. *Clinics in Chest Medicine* 15: 351-368, 1994.

40. **Damm P, Breitowicz B, and Hegaard H.** Exercise, pregnancy, and insulin sensitivity–what is new? *Applied Physiology, Nutrition, and Metabolism = Physiologie Appliquee, Nutrition et Metabolisme* 32: 537-540, 2007.

41. **Davies GA, Wolfe LA, Mottola MF, and MacKinnon C.** Joint SOGC/CSEP clinical practice guideline: exercise in pregnancy and the postpartum period. *Canadian Journal of Applied Physiology = Revue Canadienne de Physiologie Appliquee* 28: 330-341, 2003.

42. **Dickinson JW, Whyte GP, McConnell AK, and Harries MG.** Screening elite winter athletes for exercise induced asthma: a comparison of three challenge methods. *British Journal of Sports Medicine* 40: 179-182; discussion 179-182, 2006.

43. **Doll JA, Hellkamp A, Ho MP, Kontos MC, Whooley MA, Peterson ED, and Wang TY.** Participation in cardiac rehabilitation programs among older patients after acute myocardial infarction. *JAMA Internal Medicine* 175: 1700-1701, 2015.

44. **Durstine JL, Moore GE, Painter PL, Macko R, Gordon BT, and Kraus WE.** Chronic conditions strongly associated with physical inactivity. In *ACSM's Exercise Management for Persons with Chronic Diseases and Disabilities*, edited by Moore GE, Durstine JL, and Painter PL. Champaign IL: Human Kinetics, 2016, pp. 71-94.

45. **Ehrman JK and Schairer JR.** Diagnostic procedures for cardiovascular disease. In *ACSM's Resource Manual for Guidelines for Exercise Testing and Prescription*. Baltimore, MD: Lippincott Williams & Wilkins, 2006, pp. 277-288.

46. **Entin PL and Munhall KM.** Recommendations regarding exercise during pregnancy made by private/small group practice obstetricians in the USA. *Journal of Sports Science and Medicine* 5: 449-458, 2006.

47. **Everson KR and Pompeii LA.** Obstetrician practice patterns and recommendations for physcial activity during pregnancy. *Journal of Women's Health* 19: 1733-1740, 2010.

48. **Fitzgerald MD, Tanaka H, Tran ZV, and Seals DR.** Age-related declines in maximal aerobic capacity in regularly exercising vs. sedentary women: a meta-analysis. *Journal of Applied Physiology* 83: 160-165, 1997.

49. **Fox, SI.** *Human Physiology.* New York, NY: McGraw-Hill, 2011.

50. **Franklin BA.** Myocardial infarction. In *ACSM's Exercise Management for Persons with Chronic Disease and*

Disabilities, edited by Durstine JL, Moore GE, Painter PL, and Roberts SO. Champaign, IL: Human Kinetics, 2009, p. 49-57.

51. **Franklin BA.** Revascularization: CABGS abd PTCA or PCI. In *ACSM's Exercise Management for Persons with Chronic Disease and Disabilities*, edited by Durstine JL, Moore GE, Painter PL, and Roberts SO. Champaign, IL: 2009.

52. **Global Initiative for Chronic Obstructive Lung Disease (GOLD).** *Global Strategy for Diagnosis, Management, and Prevention of COPD.* www.goldcopd.org, 2013.

53. **Gordon NF.** Hypertension. In *ACSM's Exercise Management for Persons with Chronic Disease and Disabilities*, edited by Durstine JL, Moore GE, Painter PL, and Roberts SO. Champaign, IL: Human Kinetics, 2009, pp. 107-113.

54. **Hagberg JM.** Exercise, fitness, and hypertension. In *Exercise, Fitness, and Health*, edited by Bouchard C, Shephard RJ, Stephens T, Sutton JR, and McPherson BD. Champaign, IL: Human Kinetics, 1990, pp. 455-466.

55. **Hamm LF, Wenger NK, Arena R, Forman DE, Lavie CJ, Miller TD, et al.** Cardiac rehabilitation and cardiovascular disability: role of assessment and improving functional capacity. *Journal of Cardiopulmonary Rehabilitation and Prevention* 33: 1-11, 2013.

56. **Haverkamp HC, Dempsey JA, Pegelow DF, Miller JD, Romer LM, Santana M, et al.** Treatment of airway inflammation improves exercise pulmonary gas exchange and performance in asthmatic subjects. *The Journal of Allergy and Clinical Immunology* 120: 39-47, 2007.

57. **Jackson AS, Sui X, Hebert JR, Church TS, and Blair SN.** Role of lifestyle and aging on the longitudinal change in cardiorespiratory fitness. *Archives of Internal Medicine Journal* 169: 1781-1787, 2009.

58. **Jolly K, Taylor RS, Lip GY, and Stevens A.** Home-based cardiac rehabilitation compared with centre-based rehabilitation and usual care: a systematic review and meta-analysis. *International Journal of Cardiology* 111: 343-351, 2006.

59. **Jones A and Bowen M.** Screening for childhood asthma using an exercise test. *British Journal of General Practice* 44: 127-131, 1994.

60. **Kannel WB.** Bishop lecture. Contribution of the Framingham Study to preventive cardiology. *Journal of the American College of Cardiology* 15: 206-211, 1990.

61. **Kaplan NM.** *Clinical Hypertension.* Baltimore, MD: Lippincott Williams & Wilkins, 1998.

62. **Kasch FW, Boyer JL, Van Camp SP, Verity LS, and Wallace JP.** The effect of physical activity and inactivity on aerobic power in older men (a longitudinal study). *Physician and Sportsmedicine* 18: 73-83, 1990.

63. **Katz RM.** Coping with exercise-induced asthma in sports. *Physician and Sportsmedicine* 15: 100-112, 1987.

64. **Kemmer FW and Berger M.** Exercise and diabetes mellitus: physical activity as a part of daily life and its role in the treatment of diabetic patients. *International Journal of Sports Medicine* 4: 77-88, 1983.

65. **Kennedy A, Nirantharakumar K, Chimen M, Pang TT, Hemming K, Andrews RC, et al.** Does exercise improve glycaemic control in type 1 diabetics? A systematic review and meta-analysis. *PLOS ONE* 8: e58861, 2013.

66. **Keteyian SJ.** Exercise prescription for patients with cardiovascular disease. In *ACSM's Resource Manual for Guidelines for Exercise Testing and Prescription*, 7th ed. Baltimore, MD: Lippincott Williams & Wilkins, 2014, pp. 619-634.

67. **Kindermann W.** Do inhaled β_2-agonists have an ergogenic potential in non-asthmatic competitive athletes? *Sports Medicine* 37: 95-102, 2007.

68. **Knowler WC, Barrett-Connor E, Fowler SE, Hamman RF, Lachin JM, Walker EA, et al.** Reduction in the incidence of type 2 diabetes with lifestyle intervention or Metformin. *New England Journal of Medicine* 346: 393-403, 2002.

69. **Koliaki C and Katsilambros N.** Dietary sodium, potassium, and alcohol: key players in the pathophysiology, prevention, and treatment of dietary hypertension. *Nutrition Reviews* 71: 402-411, 2013.

70. **Lampman RM and Campaign BN.** Exercise testing in patients with diabetes. In *ACSM's Resource Manual for Guidelines for Exercise Testing and Prescription.* Baltimore, MD: Lippincott Williams & Wilkins, 2006, pp. 245-254.

71. **Lotgering FK, van Doorn MB, Struijk PC, Pool J, and Wallenburg HC.** Maximal aerobic exercise in pregnant women: heart rate, O_2 consumption, CO_2 production, and ventilation. *Journal of Applied Physiology* 70: 1016-1023, 1991.

72. **Lucas SR and Platts-Mills TA.** Physical activity and exercise in asthma: relevance to etiology and treatment. *Journal of Allergy and Clinical Immunology* 115: 928-934, 2005.

73. **Mahler DA.** Exercise-induced asthma. *Medicine & Science in Sports & Exercis* 25: 554-561, 1993.

74. **McCullough PA.** Diagnostic procedures for cardiovascular disease. In *ACSM's Resource Manual for Guidelines for Exercise Testing and Prescription*, edited by Ehrman JK. Baltimore, MD: Lippincott Williams & Wilkins, 2010, pp. 360-374.

75. **McKenzie DC, McLuckie SL, and Stirling DR.** The protective effects of continuous and interval exercise in athletes with exercise-induced asthma. *Medicine & Science in Sports & Exercise* 26: 951-956, 1994.

76. **Mickleborough TD, Head SK, and Lindley MR.** Exercise-induced asthma: nutritional management. *Current Sports Medicine Reports* 10: 197-202, 2011.

77. **Moore SC, Lee I-M, Weiderpass E, et al.** Association of leisure-time physical activity with risk of 26 types of cancer in 1.44 million adults. *JAMA Internal Medicine* 176: 816-825, 2016.

78. **Morton AR and Fitch KD.** *Exercise Testing and Exercise Prescription for Special Cases.* Baltimore, MD: Lippincott Williams & Wilkins, 2005.

79. **Mudd LM, Owe KM, Mottola MF, and Pivarnik JM.** Health benefits of physical activity during pregnancy: an international perspective. *Medicine & Science in Sports & Exercise* 45:268-277, 2013.

80. **Nelson ME, Rejeski WJ, Blair SN, Duncan PW, Judge JO, King AC, et al.** Physical activity and public health in older adults: recommendations from the American College of Sports Medicine and the American Heart Association. *Medicine & Science in Sports & Exercise* 39: 1435-1445, 2007.

81. **Nichols DL and Essery EV.** Osteoporosis and exercise. In *ACSM's Resource Manual for Guidelines for Exercise Testing and Prescription.* Baltimore, MD: Lippincott Williams & Wilkins, 2006, pp. 489-499.

82. **Painter PL and Moore GE.** Art of clinical exercise programming. In *ACSM's Exercise Management for Persons with Chronic Diseases and Disabilities*, edited by Moore GE, Durstine JL, and Painter PL. Champaign IL: Human Kinetics, 2016, pp. 33-46.

83. **Paterson DH, Jones GR, and Rice CL.** Ageing and physical activity: evidence to develop exercise recommendations for older adults. *Canadian Journal of Public Health* 98 (Suppl 2): S69-108, 2007.

84. **Pavy B, Iliou MC, Meurin P, Tabet JY, and Corone S.** Safety of exercise training for cardiac patients: results of the French registry of complications during cardiac rehabilitation. *Archives of Internal Medicine* 166: 2329-2334, 2006.

85. **Peno-Green LA and Cooper CB.** Treatment and rehabilitation of pulmonary diseases. In *ACSM's Resource Manual for Guidelines for Exercise Testing and Prescription.* Baltimore, MD: Lippincott Williams & Wilkins, 2006, pp. 452-469.

86. **Peterson MD, Rhea MR, Sen A, and Gordon PM.** Resistance exercise for muscular strength in older adults: a meta analysis. *Ageing Research Reviews* 9: 226-237, 2010.

87. **Petit MA, Hughes JM, and Warpeha JM.** Exercise prescription for people with osteoporosis. In *ACSM's Resource Manual for Guidelines for Exercise Testing and Prescription,* edited by Ehrman JK. Baltimore, MD: Lippincott Williams & Wilkins, 2010, pp. 635-650.

88. **Pierson WE, Covert DS, Koenig JQ, Namekata T, and Kim YS.** Implications of air pollution effects on athletic performance. *Medicine & Science in Sports & Exercise* 18: 322-327, 1986.

89. **Pluim BM, de Hon O, Staal JB, Limpens J, Kuipers H, Overbeek SE, et al.** Beta 2-agonists and physical performance: a systematic review and meta-analysis of randomized control trials. *Sports Medicine* 41: 39-57, 2011.

90. **Quaglietti S and Froelicher VF.** Physical activity and cardiac rehabilitation for patients with coronary heart disease. In *Physical Activity, Fitness, and Health,* edited by Bouchard C, Shephard RJ, and Stephens T. Champaign, IL: Human Kinetics, 1994, pp. 591-608.

91. **Randolph C.** An update on exercise-induced bronchoconstriction with and without asthma. *Current Allergy and Asthma Reports* 9: 433-438, 2009.

92. **Richter EA and Galbo H.** Diabetes, insulin and exercise. *Sports Medicine* 3: 275-288, 1986.

93. **Robling AG, Burr DB, and Turner CH.** Partitioning a daily mechanical stimulus into discrete loading bouts improves the osteogenic response to loading. *Journal of Bone and Mineral Research* 15: 1596-1602, 2000.

94. **Rogers MA.** Acute effects of exercise on glucose tolerance in non-insulin-dependent diabetes. *Medicine & Science in Sports & Exercise* 21: 362-368, 1989.

95. **Romer L.** Pathophysiology and treatment of pulmonary disease. In *ACSM's Resource Manual for Guidelines for Exercise Testing and Prescription,* 7th ed. Baltimore, MD: Lippincott Williams & Wilkins, 2014, pp. 121-137.

96. **Rubin CT and Lanyon LE.** Regulation of bone mass by mechanical strain magnitude. *Calcified Tissue International* 37: 411-417, 1985.

97. **Schairer JS and Keteyian SJ.** Exercise testing in patients with cardiovascular disease. In *ACSM's Resource Manual for Guidelines for Exercise Testing and Prescription.* Baltimore, MD: Lippincott Williams & Wilkins, 2006, pp. 439-451.

98. **Schmitz K. Cancer.** In *ACSM's Exercise Management for Persons with Chronic Diseases and Disabilities,* edited by Moore GE, Durstine JL, and Painter PL. Champaign IL: Human Kinetics, 2016, pp. 115-123.

99. **Scibora L.** Exercise prescription for patients with osteoporosis. In *ACSM's Resource Manual for Guidelines for Exercise Testing and Prescription.* Baltimore, MD: Lippincott Williams & Wilkins, 2014, pp. 699-712.

100. **Skinner JS.** Hypertension. In *Exercise Testing and Exercise Prescription for Special Cases,* edited by Skinner JS. Baltimore, MD: Lippincott Williams & Wilkins, 2005, pp. 305-312.

101. **Spina RJ.** Cardiovascular adaptations to endurance exercise training in older men and women. *Exercise and Sport Sciences Reviews* 27: 317-332, 1999.

102. **Storer TW.** Exercise prescription for patients with pulmonary disease. In *ACSM's Resource Manual for Guidelines for Exercise Testing and Prescription,* 7th ed. Baltimore, MD: Lippincott Williams & Wilkins, 2014, pp. 635-660.

103. **Storms WW.** Review of exercise-induced asthma. *Medicine & Science in Sports & Exercise* 35: 1464-1470, 2003.

104. **Thompson PD, Franklin BA, Balady GJ, Blair SN, Corrado D, Estes NA, III, et al.** Exercise and acute cardiovascular events placing the risks into perspective: a scientific statement from the American Heart Association Council on Nutrition, Physical Activity, and Metabolism and the Council on Clinical Cardiology. *Circulation* 115: 2358-2368, 2007.

105. **Tommaso CL, Lesch M, and Sonnenblick EH.** Alterations in cardiac function in coronary heart disease, myocardial infarction, and coronary bypass surgery. In *Rehabilitation of the Coronary Patient,* edited by Wenger NK, and Hellerstein HK. New York, NY: Wiley, 1984, pp. 41-66.

106. **Trappe S, Hayes E, Galpin A, Kaminsky L, Jemiolo B, Fink W, et al.** New records in aerobic power among octogenarian lifelong endurance athletes. *Journal of Applied Physiology* 114: 3-10, 2013.

107. **Tuomilehto J.** Nonpharmacoligcal therapy and exercise in the prevention of type 2 diabetes. *Diabetes Care* 32: S189-S193, 2009.

108. **Umpierre D, Ribeiro PAB, Schaan BD, and Ribeiro JP.** Volume of supervised exercise training impacts glycaemic control in patients with type 2 diabetes: a systematic review with meta-regression analysis. *Diabetologia.* 56: 242-251, 2013.

109. **U.S. Department of Health and Human Services.** *2008 Physcial Activity Guideliens for Americans.* Washington, DC: U.S. Department of Health and Human Services, 2008.

110. **Verity LS.** Exercise testing in patients with cardiovascular disease. In *Diabetes and Exercise.* Baltimore, MD: Lippincott Williams & Wilkins, 2006, pp. 470-479.

111. **Voy RO.** The U.S. Olympic Committee experience with exercise-induced bronchospasm, 1984. *Medicine and Science in Sports and Exercise* 18: 328-330, 1986.

112. **Wallace JP.** Exercise in hypertension: a clinical review. *Sports Medicine* 33: 585-598, 2003.

113. **Weiler JM, Bonini S, Coifman R, Craig T, Delgado L, Capao-Filipe M, et al.** American Academy of Allergy, Asthma & Immunology Work Group report: exercise-induced asthma. *Journal of Allergy and Clinical Immunology* 119: 1349-1358, 2007.

114. **Widmaier EP, Raff H, and Strang KT.** *Vander's Human Physiology.* 13th ed. New York, NY: McGraw-Hill, 2014.

115. **Wolfe LA.** Pregnancy. In *Exercise Testing and Exercise Prescription for Special Cases,* edited by Skinner JS. Baltimore, MD: Lippincott Williams & Wilkins, 2005, pp. 377-391.

116. **Wolfe LA, Brenner IK, and Mottola MF.** Maternal exercise, fetal well-being and pregnancy outcome. *Exercise and Sport Sciences Reviews* 22: 145-194, 1994.

117. **Wolfe LA, Ohtake PJ, Mottola MF, and McGrath MJ.** Physiological interactions between pregnancy and aerobic exercise. *Exercise and Sport Sciences Reviews* 17: 295-351, 1989.

118. **World Hypertension League.** Physical exercise in the management of hypertension: a consensus statement by the World Hypertension League. *Journal of Hypertension* 9: 283-287, 1991.

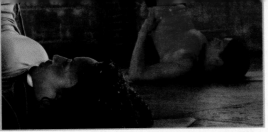

© Tim Mantoani/Masterfile

18

Nutrition and Body Composition for Health

■ Objectives

By studying this chapter, you should be able to do the following:

1. Describe what is meant by the terms *Recommended Dietary Allowance (RDA)* and *Adequate Intake (IA)*, and how they relate to the *Daily Value (DV)* used in food labeling.

2. List the six classes of nutrients.

3. Identify the fat- and water-soluble vitamins.

4. Describe why there is concern about the levels of intake of calcium, iron, and sodium in terms of health and disease.

5. Identify the two major classes of carbohydrates, and describe what the glycemic index is.

6. Identify the recommended changes in fat intake to improve health status.

7. List the nutrients that should be limited according to the 2015 *Dietary Guidelines for Americans*.

8. Identify the five food groups in the U.S. Style Healthy Eating Plan.

9. Describe the limitation of height/weight tables and the Body Mass Index in determining overweight and obesity.

10. Describe the two-component model of body composition and the assumptions made about the density values for the fat-free mass and the fat mass.

11. Explain the principle underlying the measurement of whole-body density with underwater weighing and why one must correct for residual volume.

12. Explain the principle by which bioelectrical impedance analysis (BIA) can be used to estimate the fat-free mass.

13. Explain how a sum of skinfolds can be used to estimate a percentage of body fatness value.

14. List the recommended percentage of body fatness values for health and fitness for males and females, and explain the concern for both high and low values.

15. Describe the roles of genetics and environment in the development of obesity.

16. Describe the pattern of change in body weight and caloric intake over the adult years.

17. Discuss the changes in body composition when weight is lost by diet alone versus diet plus exercise.

18. Describe the relationship of the fat-free mass to the BMR.

19. Define and give an example of thermogenesis.

20. Describe physical activity recommendations for preventing overweight and obesity, and for the prevention of weight regain in those who were previously obese.

C hap. 14 described factors that limit health and fitness. These included hypertension, obesity, and elevated serum cholesterol. These three risk factors are linked to an excessive consumption of salt, total calories, and dietary fat, respectively. Clearly, knowledge of nutrition is essential to our understanding of health-related fitness. Whereas Chaps. 3 and 4 described the metabolism of carbohydrates, fats, and proteins, this chapter focuses on the type of diet that should provide them. The first part of the chapter presents nutrition standards and what they mean, a summary of the six classes of nutrients, dietary guidelines, and eating patterns (diets) to help meet those guidelines. The second part of the chapter discusses methods for measuring body composition, and the third part examines the role of exercise and diet in weight control. Nutrition related to athletic performance is covered in Chap. 23.

STANDARDS OF NUTRITION

Food provides the carbohydrates, fats, proteins, minerals, vitamins, and water needed for life. The quantity of each nutrient needed for proper function and health is defined in one of the **Dietary Reference Intakes (DRIs),** an umbrella term encompassing specific standards for dietary intake. The DRIs include the following (61, 62, 63):

- **Recommended Dietary Allowance (RDA).** The average daily dietary nutrient intake level sufficient to meet the nutrient requirements of nearly all (97%-98%) healthy individuals in a particular group.

- **Adequate Intakes (AIs).** The AI describes levels that are assumed to be adequate when an RDA cannot be determined.

- **Tolerable Upper Intake Level (UL).** The highest average daily nutrient intake level likely to pose no risk of adverse health effects.

- **Acceptable Macronutrient Distribution Ranges (AMDRs).** These are defined as ranges of intakes for a particular energy source that is associated with a reduced risk of chronic disease, while providing adequate intake of essential nutrients. The ranges are 20% to 35% for fat, 45% to 65% carbohydrate, and the balance, 10% to 35%, is protein.

- **Estimated Energy Requirement (EER).** The average dietary energy intake that is predicted to maintain energy balance in a healthy adult of a defined age, gender, weight, height, and level of physical activity, consistent with good health (see appendix B for the EERs for males and females across various age groups).

- **Daily Value (DV).** Standard used in nutritional labeling to indicate how much of various nutrients is contained in the food we eat based on a 2000-calorie diet. For example, if one serving of a product provides 11% of the DV for fat, it contains 11% of the total amount of fat recommended for one day. Figure 18.1 provides an example of a food label.

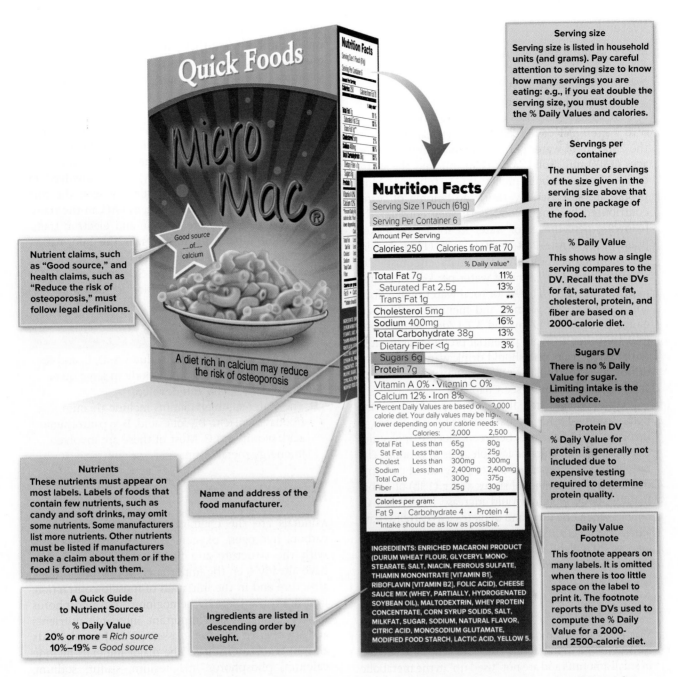

Serving size

Serving size is listed in household units (and grams). Pay careful attention to serving size to know how many servings you are eating: e.g., if you eat double the serving size, you must double the % Daily Values and calories.

Servings per container

The number of servings of the size given in the serving size above that are in one package of the food.

% Daily Value

This shows how a single serving compares to the DV. Recall that the DVs for fat, saturated fat, cholesterol, protein, and fiber are based on a 2000-calorie diet.

Sugars DV

There is no % Daily Value for sugar. Limiting intake is the best advice.

Protein DV

% Daily Value for protein is generally not included due to expensive testing required to determine protein quality.

Daily Value Footnote

This footnote appears on many labels. It is omitted when there is too little space on the label to print it. The footnote reports the DVs used to compute the % Daily Value for a 2000- and 2500-calorie diet.

Nutrient claims, such as "Good source," and **health claims,** such as "Reduce the risk of osteoporosis," must follow legal definitions.

Nutrients

These nutrients must appear on most labels. Labels of foods that contain few nutrients, such as candy and soft drinks, may omit some nutrients. Some manufacturers list more nutrients. Other nutrients must be listed if manufacturers make a claim about them or if the food is fortified with them.

Name and address of the food manufacturer.

A Quick Guide to Nutrient Sources

% Daily Value
20% or more = *Rich source*
10%–19% = *Good source*

Ingredients are listed in descending order by weight.

Nutrition Facts

Serving Size 1 Pouch (61g)
Serving Per Container 6

Amount Per Serving	
Calories 250	Calories from Fat 70

	% Daily value*
Total Fat 7g	11%
Saturated Fat 2.5g	13%
Trans Fat 1g	**
Cholesterol 5mg	2%
Sodium 400mg	16%
Total Carbohydrate 38g	13%
Dietary Fiber <1g	3%
Sugars 6g	
Protein 7g	

Vitamin A 0% • Vitamin C 0%
Calcium 12% • Iron 8%

*Percent Daily Values are based on a 2,000 calorie diet. Your daily values may be higher or lower depending on your calorie needs:

		Calories:	2,000	2,500
Total Fat	Less than		65g	80g
Sat Fat	Less than		20g	25g
Cholest	Less than		300mg	300mg
Sodium	Less than		2,400mg	2,400mg
Total Carb			300g	375g
Fiber			25g	30g

Calories per gram:
Fat 9 • Carbohydrate 4 • Protein 4

**Intake should be as low as possible.

INGREDIENTS: ENRICHED MACARONI PRODUCT (DURUM WHEAT FLOUR, GLYCERYL MONO-STEARATE, SALT, NIACIN, FERROUS SULFATE, THIAMIN MONONITRATE [VITAMIN B1], RIBOFLAVIN [VITAMIN B2], FOLIC ACID), CHEESE SAUCE MIX (WHEY, PARTIALLY, HYDROGENATED SOYBEAN OIL), MALTODEXTRIN, WHEY PROTEIN CONCENTRATE, CORN SYRUP SOLIDS, SALT, MILKFAT, SUGAR, SODIUM, NATURAL FLAVOR, CITRIC ACID, MONOSODIUM GLUTAMATE, MODIFIED FOOD STARCH, LACTIC ACID, YELLOW 5.

Figure 18.1 Food packages must list product name, name and address of the manufacturer, amount of product in the package, and ingredients. The Nutrition Facts panel is required on virtually all packaged food products. The % Daily Value listed on the label is the percent of the amount of a nutrient needed daily that is provided by a single serving of the product.

- Dietary Reference Intakes include a collection of standards (e.g., RDA) for levels of specific nutrients (e.g., vitamins) and the ranges of macronutrient intake (e.g., carbohydrates) consistent with good health.
- The Daily Value (DV) is a standard used in nutritional labeling.

CLASSES OF NUTRIENTS

There are six classes of nutrients: water, vitamins, minerals, carbohydrates, fats, and proteins. In the following sections, each nutrient is described briefly, and the primary food sources of each are identified.

Water

Water is absolutely essential for life. Under normal conditions without exercise, water loss equals about 2500 ml/day, with most lost in urine. However, as higher environmental temperatures and heavy exercise are added, water loss can increase dramatically to 6 to 7 liters per day (165). Under normal conditions the 2500 ml of water per day is replaced with beverages (1500 ml), "solid" food (750 ml), and the water derived from metabolic processes (250 ml) (161). Most people are surprised by the large volume of water contributed by "solid" food until they consider the following percentages of water in solid food: baked potato–75%, apple–75%, lettuce–96% (161). A general recommendation under ordinary circumstances is to consume 1 to 1.5 ml of water per kcal of energy expenditure (107). The AI for total water intake (food and beverages) for women and men 19 to 70 years of age is set at 2.7 L/day and 3.7 L/day, respectively (62). However, to avoid potential problems associated with dehydration, one should drink water before and during exercise; thirst is not an adequate stimulus to achieve water balance (see Chap. 23).

Water weight can fluctuate depending on the body stores of carbohydrate and protein. Water is involved in the linkage between glucose molecules in glycogen and amino acid molecules in protein. The ratio is about 2.7 grams of water per gram of carbohydrate, and if an individual stores 454 g (1 lb) of carbohydrate, body weight would increase by 3.7 lbs. Of course, when one diets and depletes this carbohydrate store, the reverse occurs. This results in an apparent (and rapid) weight loss of 3.7 lbs when only 1816 kcal (454 g of carbohydrate times 4 kcal/g) have been lost.

Vitamins

Vitamins were introduced in Chap. 3 as organic catalysts involved in metabolic reactions. They are needed in small amounts and are not "used up" in the metabolic reactions. However, they are degraded (metabolized) like any biological molecule and must be replaced on a regular basis to maintain body stores. Several vitamins are in a precursor, or **provitamin,** form in foods and are converted to the active form in the body. Beta-carotene, the most important of the provitamin A compounds, is a good example. A chronic lack of certain vitamins can lead to **deficiency** diseases, and an excess of others can lead to a **toxicity** condition (161). In our presentation, vitamins will be divided into the fat-soluble and water-soluble groups.

Fat-Soluble Vitamins The fat-soluble vitamins include A, D, E, and K. These vitamins can be stored in large quantities in the body; thus, a deficiency state takes longer to develop than for water-soluble vitamins. However, because of their solubility, so much can be stored that a toxicity condition can occur. Table 18.1 summarizes the information on these vitamins, including the RDA/AI standards, dietary sources, and functions.

Water-Soluble Vitamins The water-soluble vitamins include vitamin C and the B vitamins: thiamin (B_1), riboflavin (B_2), niacin, pyridoxine (B_6), folic acid, B_{12}, pantothenic acid, and biotin. Most are involved in energy metabolism. You have already seen the role of niacin, as NAD, and riboflavin, as FAD, in the transfer of energy in the Krebs cycle and electron transport chain. Table 18.1 summarizes the information on these vitamins, including the RDA/AI standards, dietary sources, and functions. See Appendix C for recommended intakes of vitamins for males and females across various age groups.

IN SUMMARY

- The fat-soluble vitamins include A, D, E, and K. These can be stored in the body in large quantities and toxicity can develop.
- The water-soluble vitamins include thiamin, riboflavin, niacin, B_6, folic acid, B_{12}, pantothenic acid, biotin, and C. Most of these are involved in energy metabolism.

Minerals

Minerals are the chemical **elements,** other than carbon, hydrogen, oxygen, and nitrogen, associated with the structure and function of the body. We have already seen the importance of calcium in bone structure and in the initiation of muscle contraction, iron in O_2 transport by hemoglobin, and phosphorus in ATP. Minerals are important inorganic nutrients and are divided into two classes: (a) **major minerals** and (b) **trace elements.** The major minerals include calcium, phosphorus, magnesium, sulfur, sodium, potassium, and chloride, with whole-body quantities ranging from 35 g for magnesium to 1200 g for calcium in a 70-kg man (161). The trace elements include iron, iodine, fluoride, zinc, selenium, copper, cobalt, chromium, manganese, molybdenum, arsenic, nickel, and vanadium. There are only 4 g of iron and 0.0009 g of vanadium in a 70-kg man. Like vitamins, some minerals taken in excess (e.g., iron and zinc) can be toxic. The following sections focus attention on calcium, iron, and sodium.

Calcium Calcium (Ca^{++}) and phosphorus combine with organic molecules to form the teeth and bones. The bones are a "store" of calcium that helps to maintain the plasma Ca^{++} concentration when dietary intake is inadequate (see parathyroid hormone in

TABLE 18.1   A Summary of Vitamins

Vitamin	Major Functions	Dietary Sources*	RDA or AI*

Vitamin A (retinoids) and provitamin A (carotenoids)	Promote vision: light and color
	Promote growth
	Prevent drying of skin and eyes
	Promote resistance to bacterial infection
		Vitamin A
		  Liver
		  Fortified milk
		  Fortified breakfast cereals
		Provitamin A
		  Sweet potatoes, spinach, greens, carrots, cantaloupe, apricots, broccoli
			Men: 900 micrograms
			Women: 700 micrograms

D (chole- and ergocalciferol) micrograms)	Facilitate absorption of calcium and phosphorus Maintain optimal calcification of bone	Vitamin D-fortified milk Fortified breakfast cereals Fish oils Sardines Salmon	15 micrograms
E (tocopherols)	Act as an antioxidant: prevent breakdown of vitamin A and unsaturated fatty acids	Vegetable oils Some greens Some fruits Fortified breakfast cereals	15 milligrams
K (phyilo- and menaquinone)	Help form prothrombin and other factors for blood clotting and contribute to bone metabolism	Green vegetables Liver	Men: 120 micrograms* Women: 90 micrograms*

Vitamin	Major Functions	Dietary Sources*	RDA or AI*
Thiamin	Coenzyme involved in carbohydrate metabolism; nerve function	Sunflower seeds, pork, whole and enriched grains, dried beans, peas, brewers yeast	Men: 1.2 milligrams Women: 1.1 milligrams
Riboflavin	Coenzyme involved in energy metabolism	Milk, mushrooms, spinach, liver, enriched grains	Men: 1.3 milligrams Women: 1.1 milligrams
Niacin	Coenzyme involved in energy metabolism, fat synthesis, fat breakdown	Mushrooms, bran, tuna, salmon, chicken, beef, liver, peanuts, enriched grains	Men: 16 milligrams Women: 14 milligrams
Pantothenic acid	Coenzyme involved in energy metabolism, fat synthesis, fat breakdown	Mushrooms, liver, broccoli, eggs; most foods have some	5 milligrams*
Biotin	Coenzyme involved in glucose production, fat synthesis	Cheese, egg yolks, cauliflower, peanut butter, liver	30 micrograms
Vitamin B$_6$, pyridoxine, and other forms	Coenzyme involved in protein metabolism, neurotransmitter synthesis, hemoglobin synthesis, many other functions	Animal protein foods, spinach, broccoli, bananas, salmon, sunflower seeds	1.3 milligrams
Folate (folic acid)	Coenzyme involved in DNA synthesis, other functions	Green leafy vegetables, orange juice, organ meats, sprouts, sunflower seeds	400 micrograms
Vitamin B$_{12}$ (cobalamins)	Coenzyme involved in folate metabolism, nerve function, other functions	Animal foods, especially organ meats, oysters, clams (not natural in plants)	2.4 micrograms
Vitamin C (ascorbic acid)	Connective tissue synthesis, hormone synthesis, neurotransmitter synthesis	Citrus fruits, strawberries, broccoli, greens	Men: 90 milligrams Women: 75 milligrams

Note: Values are the Recommended Dietary Allowances (RDAs) for adults 19 to 50 years, unless marked by an asterisk (*), in which case they represent the Adequate Intakes (AIs). The Tolerable Upper Intake Levels (ULs) are listed under toxicity; intakes above these values can lead to negative health consequences.

Chap.5). Bone is constantly turning over its calcium and phosphorus, so diet must replace what is lost. If the diet is deficient in calcium for a long time, loss of bone, or **osteoporosis,** can occur. Three major factors are implicated: dietary calcium intake, inadequate estrogen, and lack of physical activity (see Chap. 17 for more on this) (3).

There is concern that the increase in osteoporosis in our society is related to an inadequate calcium intake. The adult RDA for calcium is 1000 mg/day, and although many men come close to meeting the standard, few women do (161). Given that the RDA is higher for 9–18-year-olds (1300 mg/day) and for females 51 to 70 years of age (1200 mg/day), the concern is greater for those age groups. Although menopause is the usual cause of a reduced secretion of estrogen, young, extremely active female athletes are experiencing this problem associated with amenorrhea (4). The decrease in estrogen secretion is associated with the acceleration of osteoporosis. Because exercise has been shown to slow the rate of bone loss, we now have physical activity recommendations to build bone mass in early childhood and to hold on to it as we age (2, 3, 153) (see Ask the Expert 17.1 in Chap. 17).

Iron   The majority of iron is found in hemoglobin in the red blood cells, which is involved with oxygen transport to cells (see Chap. 10). Other iron-containing molecules include myoglobin in muscle and the cytochromes in mitochondria, accounting for about 25% of the body's iron. A large portion of the remaining iron is bound to **ferritin** in the liver, with the serum ferritin concentration being a sensitive measure of iron status (161, 165).

To remain in iron balance, the RDA is set at 8 mg/day for an adult male and 18 mg/day for an adult female; the higher amount is needed to replace that which is lost in the menses. In spite of the higher need for iron, American women take in only 13.2 mg/day, whereas men take in 17.5 mg/day (150). This is due to higher caloric intakes in males than females. The diet provides iron in two forms, heme (ferrous) and nonheme (ferric). Heme iron, found primarily in meats, fish, and organ meats, is absorbed better than nonheme iron, which is found in vegetables. However, the absorption of nonheme iron can be increased by the presence of meat, fish, and vitamin C (55, 161, 165).

Anemia is a condition in which the hemoglobin concentration is low: less than 13 g/dl in men and less than 12 g/dl in women. This can be the result of blood loss (e.g., blood donation or bleeding) or a lack of vitamins or minerals in the diet. The most common cause of anemia in North America is a lack of dietary iron (161, 165). In fact, iron deficiency is the most common nutrient deficiency. In iron-deficiency anemia, the iron bound to **transferrin** in the plasma is reduced, and serum ferritin (an indicator of iron stores) is low (55). Although children aged one to five years, adolescents, young adult women, and the elderly are more apt to develop anemia, it also occurs in competitive athletes. This latter point is discussed in detail in Chap. 23.

Sodium   Sodium is directly involved in the maintenance of the resting membrane potential and the generation of action potential in nerves (see Chap. 7) and muscles (see Chap. 8). In addition, sodium is the primary electrolyte determining the extracellular fluid volume. If sodium stores fall, the extracellular volume, including plasma, decreases. This could cause major problems with the maintenance of the mean arterial blood pressure (see Chap. 9) and body temperature (see Chap. 12).

The problem in our society is not with sodium stores that are too small, but just the opposite. The estimated average intake of sodium for Americans ages two years and older is about 3400 mg/day. This is considerably more than the AI for adults (1500 mg/day) and exceeds the UL for adults (2300 mg/day) (152). There is no question about the link between sodium intake and blood pressure, with evidence showing that reducing salt intake is feasible and will result in a reduction in cardiovascular morbidity and mortality (70, 162). The **Dietary Guidelines for Americans** have consistently supported the need to reduce sodium intake, and they recommend eating patterns (see later) to accomplish that goal. Those involved in athletic competition or strenuous exercise or who work in the heat must be concerned about adequate sodium replacement. Generally, because these individuals consume more kcal of food (containing more sodium), this is usually not a problem. More on this is in Chap. 23.

The previous sections have focused attention on three minerals–calcium, iron, and sodium–because of their relationship to current medical and health-related problems. A summary of the minerals, including the RDA/AI values, functions, and food sources is presented in Table 18.2. See Appendix D for recommended intakes of minerals (elements) for males and females across various age groups.

IN SUMMARY

- The major minerals include calcium, phosphorus, magnesium, sulfur, sodium, potassium, and chloride. The trace elements include iron, iodine, fluoride, zinc, selenium, copper, cobalt, chromium, manganese, molybdenum, arsenic, nickel, and vanadium.
- Inadequate calcium and iron intake has been linked with osteoporosis and anemia, respectively. The *Dietary Guidelines for Americans* recommends eating patterns to address these concerns.

TABLE 18.2   A Summary of Minerals

Mineral	Major Functions	Dietary Sources	RDA or AI*
Sodium	Functions as a major ion of the extra-cellular fluid; aids nerve impulse transmission	Table salt, processed foods, condiments, sauces, soups, chips	1500 milligrams*
Potassium	Functions as a major ion of intra-cellular fluid; aids nerve impulse transmission	Spinach, squash, bananas, orange juice other vegetables and fruits, milk, meat, legumes, whole grains	4700 milligrams*
Chloride	Functions as a major ion of the extra-cellular fl uid; participates in acid production in stomach; aids nerve transmission	Table salt, some vegetables, processed foods	2300 milligrams*
Calcium	Provides bone and tooth strength; helps blood clotting; aids nerve impulse transmission; required for muscle contractions	Dairy products, canned fish, leafy vegetables, tofu, fortified orange juice (and other forti-fied foods)	1000 milligrams
Phosphorus	Required for bone and tooth strength; serves as part of various metabolic compounds; functions as major ion of intracellular fluid	Dairy products, processed foods, fish, soft drinks, bakery products, meats	700 milligrams
Magnesium	Provides bone strength; aids enzyme function; aids nerve and heart function	Wheat bran, green vegetables, nuts, chocolate, legumes	Men: 420 milligrams Women: 320 milligrams
Mineral	**Major Functions**	**Dietary Sources**	**RDA or AI***
Iron	Used for hemoglobin and other key compounds used in respiration; used for immune function	Meats, spinach, seafood, broccoli peas, bran, enriched breads	Men: 8 milligrams Women: 18 milligrams
Zinc	Required for enzymes, involved in growth, immunity, alcohol metabolism sexual development, and reproduction	Seafoods, meats, greens, whole grains	Men: 11 milligrams Women: 8 milligrams
Selenium	Aids antioxidant system	Meats, eggs, fish, seafoods, whole grains	55 micrograms
Iodide	Iodide Aids thyroid hormone	Iodized salt, white bread, salt-water fish, dairy products	150 micrograms
Copper	Aids in iron metabolism; works with many enzymes, such as those involved in protein metabolism and hormone synthesis	Liver, cocoa, beans, nuts, whole grains, dried fruits	900 micrograms
Fluoride	Increases resistance of tooth enamel to dental caries	Fluoridated water, toothpaste, dental treatments, tea, seaweed	Men: 4 milligrams* Women: 3 milligrams*
Chromium	Enhances blood glucose control	Egg yolks, whole grains, pork, nuts, mushrooms, beer	Men: 30–35 micrograms* Women: 20–25 micrograms*
Manganese	Manganese Aids action of some enzymes, such as those involved in carbohydrate metabolism	Nuts, oats, beans, tea	Men: 2.3 milligrams* Women: 1.8 milligrams*
Molybdenum	Aids action of some enzymes	Beans, grains, nuts	45 micrograms

Note: Values are the Recommended Dietary Allowances (RDAs) for adults 19 to 50 years, unless marked by an asterisk (*), in which case they represent the Adequate Intakes (AIs). The Tolerable Upper Intake Levels (ULs) are listed under toxicity; intakes above these values can lead to negative health consequences.

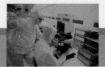
Glycemic Index—What Is It and Is It Important?

We all know that when we eat, insulin secretion increases to promote the uptake, use, and storage of carbohydrates. The degree to which the blood glucose concentration increases and remains elevated depends on the kinds and amounts of carbohydrate ingested, as well as the person's insulin response and tissue sensitivity to the insulin (133).

It is well known that certain carbohydrates elicit a more rapid blood glucose response than others. The glycemic index (GI) has been used to describe the magnitude of those differences and help those who have difficulty processing glucose make better decisions in planning meals. The GI quantifies the blood glucose response (above fasting) to a specific carbohydrate food over a two-hour period following ingestion. This response is compared to a reference food (glucose or white bread) of the same weight. Those foods with a low GI would provide less of a challenge to someone with a reduced capacity to take up and use glucose (e.g., a person with type 2 diabetes). However, because these carbohydrates are compared on a "per gram" basis, the GI does not consider the impact that the actual amount of carbohydrate in the meal has on the response. The "glycemic load (GL)" attempts to do that by multiplying the GI by the amount of carbohydrate in the serving (133). The simplicity of the GI and GL is complicated by the fact that most meals do not contain a single carbohydrate. Factors such as the amount of protein and fat in the diet will affect the blood glucose response to the carbohydrate ingested.

Although there is support for using the GI to help with food selection to manage both metabolic and cardiovascular disease, there is a growing body of evidence that low GI/GL diets have inconsistent results in terms of changing cardiovascular risk factors (76, 127), and that benefits are observed primarily in women and not men (41, 88, 93). Finally, where positive effects have been observed, the GL, not the GI, appears to be the most important factor (41). However, there is a new twist to this tale of the GI and GL.

Fructose makes up a substantial part of total carbohydrate intake in the average American's diet. Concern was raised several years ago when it was found that there was a parallel increase in the intake of high-fructose corn syrup and obesity prevalence in this country. The reason for the concern is that, in contrast to glucose, fructose does not increase the insulin and leptin responses as much, and consequently, it provides less input to the brain centers associated with feeding and body weight (16). In concert with this, when fructose is administered directly into the brain, food intake actually increases, opposite of the effect of glucose (28, 77). It should be no surprise that some investigators suggest that we examine the role of the "fructose index" (FI) and "fructose load" (FL) on the development of cardiometabolic disease, rather than limit it to GI and GL alone (131). That said, the most recent evidence based on controlled feeding studies suggests that increased cardiometabolic risk is observed only when fructose and sugar-sweetened beverages are consumed at high levels or when they supplement a diet with excess energy (54). We are sure to hear more about this in the future.

Carbohydrates

Carbohydrates and fats are the primary sources of energy in the average American diet. The Acceptable Macronutrient Distribution Range (AMDR) for carbohydrate is 45% to 65% (63). Carbohydrates suffer a bad reputation from those trying to lose weight, especially when you consider that you would have to eat more than twice as much carbohydrate as fat to consume the same number of calories (4 kcal/g versus 9 kcal/g). Carbohydrates can be divided into two classes: those that can be digested and metabolized for energy (sugars and starches), and those that are indigestible (fiber). The sugars are found in jellies, jams, fruits, soft drinks, honey, syrups, and milk, whereas the starches are found in cereals, flour, potatoes, and other vegetables (161).

Sugars and Starches Carbohydrate is a major energy source for all tissues and a crucial source for two: red blood cells and neurons. The red blood cells depend exclusively on anaerobic glycolysis for energy, and the nervous system functions well only on carbohydrate. These two tissues can consume 180 grams of glucose per day (31). Given this need, it is no surprise that the plasma glucose concentration is maintained within narrow limits by hormonal control mechanisms (see Chap. 5). During strenuous exercise, the muscle can use 180 grams of glucose in less than one hour. As a result of these needs, one might expect that carbohydrate would make up a large fraction of our energy intake. Currently, about 50% of energy intake is derived from carbohydrate (150), within the AMDR carbohydrate intakes (63). There is great interest not only in the amount of carbohydrate in the diet but also in the type of carbohydrate as it relates to the prevention and management of diabetes (see Clinical Applications 18.1). The *Dietary Guidelines for Americans* have consistently stressed the need to avoid too much sugar (152), and the recommended eating patterns that will be presented later address this need.

Dietary Fiber Dietary fiber is divided into the following classes (63):

- *Dietary fiber* consists of nondigestible carbohydrates and lignin that are *intrinsic and intact* in plants. Examples of dietary fiber include plant nonstarch polysaccharides such as cellulose, pectin, gums, hemicellulose, and fibers in oat and wheat bran.

- *Functional fiber* consists of *isolated, nondigestible carbohydrates* that have beneficial physiological effects in humans. Examples include isolated, nondigestible plants (e.g., resistant starches, pectin, and gums) and animal (e.g., chitin and chitosan) or commercially produced (e.g., resistant starch, inulin, and indigestible dextrins) carbohydrates.

- *Total fiber* is the sum of dietary fiber and functional fiber.

Dietary fiber cannot be digested and metabolized, and consequently it provides a sense of fullness (satiation) during a meal without adding calories (38). This fact has been used by bakeries that lower the number of calories per slice of bread. Pectin and gum are used in food processing to thicken, stabilize, or emulsify the constituents of various food products (161).

Dietary fiber has long been linked to optimal health. Fiber acts as a hydrated sponge as it moves along the large intestine, making constipation less likely by reducing transit time (5, 38, 161). Vegetarian diets high in soluble fiber have been linked to lower serum cholesterol due to the loss of more cholesterol-containing bile acids in the feces. However, the fact that vegetarian diets are also lower in the percentage of calories from fat, which can also lower serum cholesterol, makes the interpretation of the data more complicated (38). Although a high-fiber diet reduces the incidence of diverticulosis, a condition in which outpouchings (diverticula) occur in the colon wall, the role of fiber in preventing colon cancer is mixed (5, 38).

Given the broad role of dietary fiber in normal health, it is no surprise that it has long been recommend that Americans increase their intake of fiber. The AI for total fiber, based on an intake level observed to protect against coronary heart disease, has been set at 38 and 25 g/day for men and women, 19 to 50 years of age, respectively (63). Each of the recommended eating patterns from the Dietary Guidelines for Americans (see later) include food groups to help meet this goal.

Fats

Dietary lipids include triglycerides, phospholipids, and **cholesterol.** The Acceptable Macronutrient Distribution Range for fat is 20% to 35%. If solid at room temperature, lipids are fats; if liquid, oils. Lipids contain 9 kcal/g and represent about 33% of the American diet, within the AMDR range, and lower than the 42% recorded in 1977 (29, 53, 100, 150, 154, 161). However, part of the decrease in this percentage was due to an increase in total calorie consumption, primarily from carbohydrate (27).

Fat not only provides fuel for energy but it is also important in the absorption of fat-soluble vitamins and for cell membrane structure, hormone synthesis (steroids), insulation, and the protection of vital organs. Most fat is stored in adipose tissue for subsequent release into the bloodstream as free fatty acids (see Chap. 4). Because of fat's caloric density (9 kcal/g), we are able to carry a large energy reserve, with little weight. In fact, the energy content of one pound of adipose tissue, 3500 kcal, is sufficient to cover the energy cost of running a marathon. The other side of this coin is that because of this very high caloric density, it takes a long time to decrease the mass of adipose tissue when on a diet.

The focus of attention in the medical community has been on the role of dietary fat in the development of atherosclerosis (see Chap. 14). Dietary recommendations from many health organizations include a reduction in salt intake to control blood pressure (see minerals) and a reduction in fat intake, especially saturated fat and *trans* fat, to alter cholesterol levels. Usually, the cholesterol concentration in the serum is divided into two classes on the basis of what type of **lipoprotein** is carrying the cholesterol. **Low-density lipoproteins (LDLs)** carry more cholesterol than do the **high-density lipoproteins (HDLs).** High levels of **LDL cholesterol** are directly related to cardiovascular risk, whereas high levels of **HDL cholesterol** offer protection from heart disease. The concentration of HDL cholesterol is influenced by heredity, gender, exercise, and diet. Diets high in saturated fats and *trans* fats increase LDL cholesterol. A reduction in the sources of saturated fats would reduce LDL cholesterol. In fact, just substituting unsaturated fats for saturated fats (and not changing the percentage of fat in the diet) will lower serum cholesterol. Past and current *Dietary Guidelines for Americans* have promoted eating patterns to reduce the saturated fat intake to no more than 10% of caloric intake (see later). In addition, systematic steps are being taken to reduce or eliminate *trans* fats from the diet. These fats rival saturated fats as a contributor to heart disease, and substituting polyunsaturated fats should reduce cholesterol levels (75).

Protein

Even though protein has the same energy density as carbohydrate (4 kcal/g), it is not viewed as a primary energy source, as are fats and carbohydrates.

Rather, it is important because it contains the nine essential (indispensable) amino acids, without which the body cannot synthesize all the proteins needed for tissues, enzymes, and hormones. The *quality* of protein in a diet is based on how well these essential amino acids are represented. In terms of quality, the best sources for protein are eggs, milk, and fish, with *good* sources being meat, poultry, cheese, and soybeans. *Fair* sources of protein include grains, vegetables, seeds and nuts, and other legumes. Given that a meal contains a variety of foods, one food of higher-quality protein tends to complement another of lower-quality protein to result in an adequate intake of essential amino acids (161). The Acceptable Macronutrient Distribution Range for protein is 10% to 35%.

The adult RDA protein requirement of 0.8 g/kg is easily met with diets that include a variety of the aforementioned foods. Although the vast majority of Americans meet this recommendation, an athlete's protein requirement is higher than this level. The protein requirement for athletes is discussed in Chap. 23.

IN SUMMARY

- Carbohydrate is a primary source of energy in the American diet and is divided into two classes: that which can be metabolized (sugars and starches) and dietary fiber.
- Americans consume too much saturated fat, and the recommended change is to reduce this to no more than 10% of the total calories. *Trans* fat intake should be reduced as much as possible.
- The protein requirement of 0.8 g/kg can be met with low-fat selections to minimize fat intake.

DIETARY GUIDELINES FOR AMERICANS

We are all familiar with the work of the American Heart Association (AHA), the American Cancer Society (ACS), and the American Diabetes Association (ADA) that brings special attention to the importance of diet in the prevention and treatment of cardiovascular diseases, cancers, and diabetes, respectively. As mentioned in Chap. 14, an underlying component associated with these chronic diseases is a chronic low-grade systemic inflammation, which can be altered with diet and physical activity. Foods recommended for good health have a high **nutrient density,** meaning they contain more nutrients (e.g., vitamins, protein) per calorie, and increase the

chance of meeting nutrition standards and achieving a healthy body weight (161).

The *Dietary Guidelines for Americans* (152) is an evidence-based document that is published every five years by the Department of Health and Human Services and the U.S. Department of Agriculture. The primary purpose of the *Guidelines* is to inform the development of food, nutrition, and health policy and programs at the national level.

The five overarching Guidelines of the 2015–2020 report are the following:

1. **Follow a healthy eating pattern across the lifespan.** All food and beverages choices matter. Choose a healthy eating pattern at an appropriate calorie level to help achieve and maintain a healthy body weight, support nutrient adequacy, and reduce the risk of chronic disease.
2. **Focus on variety, nutrient density, and amount.** To meet nutrient needs within calorie limits, choose a variety of nutrient-dense foods across and within all food groups in recommended amounts.
3. **Limit calories from added sugars and saturated fats and reduce sodium intake.** Consume an eating pattern low in added sugars, saturated fats, and sodium. Cut back on foods and beverages higher in these components to amounts that fit within healthy eating patterns.
4. **Shift to healthier food and beverage choices.** Choose nutrient-dense foods and beverages across and within all food groups in place of less healthy choices. Consider cultural and personal preferences to make these shifts easier to accomplish and maintain.
5. **Support healthy eating patterns for all.** Everyone has a role in helping to create and support healthy eating patterns in multiple settings and support healthy eating patterns in multiple settings nationwide, from home to school to work to communities.

Key Recommendations

Select a healthy eating pattern that accounts for all foods and beverages within an appropriate calorie level.

A healthy eating patterns includes the following:

- A variety of vegetables from all of the subgroups–dark green, red and orange, legumes (beans and peas), starchy, and other
- Fruits, especially whole fruits
- Grains, at least half of which are whole grains
- Fat-free or low-fat dairy, including milk, yogurt, cheese, and/or fortified soy beverages

- A variety of protein foods, including seafood, lean meats and poultry, eggs, legumes (beans and peas), and nuts, seeds, and soy products
- Oils

A healthy eating patterns limits:

- Saturated fats, *trans* fats, added sugars, and sodium.

Some key recommendations have quantitative goals associated with dietary components that should be limited. These components are of particular public health concern in the United States, and the specified limits can help individuals achieve healthy eating patterns within calorie limits:

- Consume less than 10% of calories per day from added sugars
- Consume less than 10% of calories per day from saturated fats
- If alcohol is consumed, it should be consumed in moderation–up to one drink per day for women and up to two drinks per day for men–and only by adults of legal drinking age.

Americans should aim to achieve and maintain a healthy body weight. The relationship between diet and physical activity contributes to calorie balance and managing body weight. As such, the *Dietary Guidelines* includes a Key Recommendation to:

- Meet the *Physical Activity Guidelines for Americans* (see Chap. 16).

A good diet would allow an individual to achieve the RDA/AI for protein, minerals, and vitamins, while emphasizing healthy carbohydrates and minimizing unhealthy fats. Beginning with the 2010 *Dietary*

Guidelines for Americans a variety of food group plans were developed to help individuals meet the *Dietary Guidelines*.

Healthy Eating Plans

The 2010 *Dietary Guidelines for Americans* (151) provided eating plans that had abundant vegetables and fruits, whole grains, moderate amounts of foods high in protein (seafood, beans and peas, nuts, seeds, soy products, meat, poultry, and eggs), limited amounts of foods high in added sugars, more oils than solid fats, with some having substantial amounts of low-fat milk and milk products. These diets had a high unsaturated-to-saturated fat ratio, more fiber, and a high potassium content. At the beginning of this section we indicated that various organizations (e.g., AHA) emphasize the importance of diet in the prevention and treatment of various chronic diseases. Table 18.3 shows the consistency in dietary and physical activity recommendations across these organizations (146). These recommendations are clearly in tune with the eating plans described in the 2015-2020 *Dietary Guidelines for Americans*.

Healthy U.S.-Style Eating Pattern   This food plan is the same as the **USDA Food Pattern** from the 2010 *Dietary Guidelines for Americans*. This plan identified daily amounts of foods with a focus on nutrient density from the five major food groups (and *subgroups*):

- Vegetables–includes *dark green* (broccoli and spinach) and *red and orange* (carrots and sweet potatoes) vegetables; *beans and peas, starchy vegetables* (corn, potatoes), and *others* (onions, iceberg lettuce)
- Fruits–fresh, frozen, canned, or dried

TABLE 18.3	Consistency of Dietary and Physical Activity Recommendations Among Chronic Disease Organizations		
Lifestyle Factor	American Diabetes Association	American Heart Association	American Cancer Society/ American Institute for Cancer Research
Weight control	+++	+++	+++
Increase fiber	+	++	++
Increase plant food	+	++	+++
Decrease total fat	NA	+++	+++
Decrease saturated fat	++	++	+
Avoid *trans*-fatty acids	++	+++	+
Increase omega-3 fatty acids	++	++	++
Alcohol	moderation	moderation	moderation
Daily physical activity	++.	+++	++

NA—not addressed

Thompson, C. A., and Thompson, P. A., "Healthy Lifestyle and Cancer Prevention," *ACSM's Health & Fitness Journal* 12: 18–26, 2008.

- Grains–including *whole-grain* products (whole-wheat bread) and *enriched grains* (white bread and pasta)
- Dairy products–with the emphasis on low-fat choices
- Protein foods–all meat, poultry, seafood, eggs, nuts, seeds, and processed soy products, with an emphasis on low-fat choices

Details for this plan can be found at **http://health.gov/dietaryguidelines/2015/guidelines/appendix-3/.**

Healthy Mediterranean-Style Eating Pattern This eating plan was developed by modifying the Healthy U.S.-Style Eating Pattern. Its development took into account research examining the effect of the Mediterranean style diet on health outcomes. This eating pattern contains more fruit and seafood and less dairy than does the Healthy U.S.-Style Eating Pattern and, as a result, calcium and vitamin D are a little lower. Details for this eating plan can be found at **http://health.gov/dietaryguidelines/2015/guidelines/appendix-4/.**

Healthy Vegetarian Eating Pattern This plan was developed by modifying the Healthy U.S.-Style Eating Pattern. This vegetarian plan has more legumes (beans and peas), soy products, nuts and seeds, and whole grains. It is somewhat higher in calcium and dietary fiber and lower in vitamin D due to differences in foods in the protein food group. Details can be found at **http://health.gov/dietaryguidelines/2015/guidelines/appendix-5/.**

Dietary Approaches to Stop Hypertension (DASH) The DASH eating plan is an example of a healthy eating plan and has many of the same characteristics as the Healthy U.S.-Style Eating Pattern. The DASH plan was developed (as indicated in the title) to deal with hypertension, both to prevent it and to lower blood pressure in those with the problem. The DASH eating plan has been recognized for some time as an excellent approach to healthy eating consistent with reducing cardiovascular risk factors and achieving and maintaining a normal body weight. In addition, use of the DASH eating plan in a weight-loss program conveys more benefits to patients with metabolic syndrome than does a regular weight-loss diet (6). Details can be found at **http://www.nhlbi.nih.gov/health/health-topics/topics/dash.**

Evaluating the Diet

Independent of your dietary plan, the question arises as to how well you are achieving the guidelines. How do you analyze your diet? The first thing to do is to determine what you are eating, without fooling yourself. The use of the **twenty-four-hour recall** method relies on your ability to remember, from a specific time in one day, what you ate during the previous 24 hours. You have to judge the size of the portion you have eaten and make a judgment of whether that day was representative of what you normally eat. Other people use **food records,** in which a person records what is eaten throughout the day. It is recommended that a person obtain food records for three or four days per week to have a better estimate of usual dietary intake. Because the simple act of recording food intake may change our eating habits, one has to try to eat as normally as possible when recording food intake. It is important to remember that the RDA standards are to be met over the long run, and variations from those standards will exist from day to day (161). The USDA developed an online resource, *MyPlate*, to promote healthy eating and physical activity to achieve one's body weight goal. We encourage you to log on to this website **(http://www.choosemyplate.gov/MyPlate)** to get a feel for its user-friendly nature.

> ### IN SUMMARY
>
> - The *Dietary Guidelines for Americans* is updated every five years, using the latest research, to inform the development of food, nutrition, and health policy and programs at the national level.
> - The *Guidelines* identified a variety of eating patterns (plans) to use in order to eat healthy and achieve a healthy body weight. They include the Healthy U.S.-Style Eating Patterns and its adaptations: the Healthy Mediterranean Style Eating Pattern and the Healthy Vegetarian Eating Pattern.
> - The Dietary Approaches to Stop Hypertension (DASH) food plan is an example of a healthy eating pattern.
> - The U.S. Department of Agriculture's *MyPlate* helps one track both healthy eating and physical activity.

BODY COMPOSITION

Obesity is a major problem in our society, being related to hypertension, elevated serum cholesterol, and adult-onset diabetes (99). In addition, there is growing concern that as the incidence of childhood obesity increases, so will the pool of obese adults. To deal with this problem, we must be able to assess the prevalence of overweight and obesity, as well as describe, in more specific terms, changes in body composition. This section presents a brief overview on how to do that. For those interested in a thorough discussion of body composition assessment issues, we refer you to Heyward and Wagner's *Applied Body Composition Assessment* and Heymsfield, Lohman, Wang, and Going's *Human Body Composition* in Suggested Readings, and Ratamess's chapter in the *ACSM's Resource Manual for Guidelines for Exercise Testing and Prescription* (115).

Methods of Assessing Overweight and Obesity

In the latter part of the twentieth century, one of the most common ways of making a judgment about whether a person was overweight was to use the Metropolitan Life Insurance height and weight tables (91). This has been replaced with a measure that has now been universally adopted—the Body Mass Index (BMI)—the ratio of body weight (in kilograms) to height (in meters) squared: BMI = wt [kg] ÷ ht [m²]. The BMI is easily calculated, and guidelines for classifying someone as overweight or obese have used percentile rankings or fixed BMI values. Current BMI standards that have been adopted worldwide include (99):

Underweight	<18.5
Normal	18.5-24.9
Overweight	25.0-29.9
Obesity–Class I	30.0-34.9
Obesity–Class II	35.0-39.9
Extreme Obesity–Class III	≥40

The BMI standards are for adults. Investigators and clinicians have relied on percentile cutoffs (e.g., 85th and 95th percentile) to classify the fatness of children without labeling them as overweight or obese. However, there is now agreement to use a BMI ≥95th percentile (for age and gender) for classifying obesity and a BMI ≥85th percentile but <95th percentile for classifying overweight in children (102, 103).

One of the major problems associated with height/weight tables and the BMI is that there is no way to know if the person is heavily muscled or simply overfat. One of the earliest uses of body composition analysis showed that with height/weight tables, "All-American" football players weighing 200 lbs would have been found unfit for military service and would not have received life insurance (7), even though they were lean. Clearly, there is a need to distinguish overweight from overfat, and that is the purpose of the next section of this chapter.

Methods of Measuring Body Composition

The most direct way to measure body composition is to do a chemical analysis of the whole body to determine the amount of water, fat, protein, and minerals.

This is a common method used in nutritional studies on rats, but it is useless in providing information for the average person—since the rats have to be "sacrificed" before analysis! Several methods of measuring body composition are found only in specialized laboratory or hospital settings because of cost, complexity, and the specialized personnel needed; they will only be described briefly with an appropriate reference for someone interested in more detail. The remainder of the methods are used in exercise physiology labs and fitness centers, and they will be addressed in more detail.

When using any of the body composition techniques, it is important to keep in mind that there is an inherent error involved in the estimations of percent body fat. The error is usually given as the standard error of estimate (SEE). If a technique estimates percent body fat as 20% and the SEE is ±2.5%, that means the actual percent body fat lies between 22.5% and 17.5% for 68% of subjects being measured as having 20% fat. Given that we don't know where in that range an individual is, caution is needed when interpreting percent body fat values. It is best to compare these estimates of percent body fat over time on the same subject, where the change in percent fat is indicative of changes in the fat mass or fat-free mass (115).

The following methods of measuring body composition are expensive and complex, and need specially trained personnel to carry them out.

Isotope Dilution Total body water (TBW) is determined by the isotope dilution method. In this method, a subject drinks an isotope of water (tritiated water–^3H_2O), deuterated water (^2H_2O), or ^{18}O-labeled water ($H_2^{18}O$) that is distributed throughout the body water (42, 124).

Photon Absorptiometry A beam of photons from iodine-125 is passed over a bone or bones, and the transmission of the photon beam through bone and soft tissue is used to determine mineral content and density (25, 83).

Potassium-40 Measures the amount of a naturally occurring radioactive isotope of potassium, ^{40}K, that is proportional to the mass of lean tissue (17).

Radiography An X-ray of a limb allows one to measure the widths of fat, muscle, and bone, and has been used extensively in tracing the growth of these tissues over time (49, 69, 72).

Ultrasound Sound waves are transmitted through tissues, and the echoes are received and analyzed. This technique has been used to measure the thickness of subcutaneous fat (18).

Nuclear Magnetic Resonance (NMR) Electromagnetic waves are transmitted through tissues, and the manner in which nuclei of specific tissues absorb and then release energy at a particular frequency (resonance) is used to determine body composition (18).

Total Body Electrical Conductivity (TOBEC) The subject lies in a large cylindrical coil while an electric current is injected into the coil. The electromagnetic field developed in the space enclosed by the cylindrical coil is affected by the subject's body composition (112, 130, 155).

Dual Energy X-Ray Absorptiometry (DEXA) In this technology, a single X-ray source is used to determine whole-body and regional estimates of lean tissue, bone, mineral, and fat with a high degree of accuracy (40, 83, 89, 115, 157). The SEE is approximately ±1.8%.

The following techniques are used more routinely in exercise physiology or fitness center settings: hydrostatic (underwater) weighing and air displacement plethysmography that assess body density; bioelectrical impedance analysis (BIA) that estimates total body water; and sum of skinfolds. They will be addressed in detail after we introduce you to the two-component model of body composition analysis.

IN SUMMARY

- The BMI uses a simple ratio of weight-to-height squared (kg/m²) to classify individuals as being normal weight, overweight, or obese. However, just like the old height-weight tables, the BMI does not consider the composition of the body weight (i.e., proportion of muscle tissue vs. fat tissue).
- Body composition can be measured in terms of total body water (isotope dilution, bioelectric impedance analysis), bone density (photon absorptiometry), lean tissue mass (potassium-40), density (underwater weighing, air displacement plethysmography), and thickness of various tissues (ultrasound, radiography, skinfolds).

Two-Component Model of Body Composition

In some of the conventional methods of determining body composition (e.g., underwater weighing and air displacement plethysmography) the investigator obtains an estimate of **whole-body density,** and from this calculates the percentage of the body that is fat and the percentage that is fat-free. This is the two-component body composition system described by Behnke that is commonly used to describe changes in body composition (7). The conversion of whole-body density values to fat and fat-free tissue components relies on "constants" used for each of those tissue components. Human fat tissue is believed to have a density of 0.900 g/ml, and fat-free tissue a density of 1.100 g/ml. Using these density values, Siri (137) derived an equation to calculate the percentage of body fat from whole-body density:

$$\% \text{ Body fat} = \frac{495}{\text{Density}} - 450$$

This equation is correct only if the density values for fat tissue and fat-free tissue are 0.900 and 1.100 g/ml, respectively. Investigators sensed that certain populations might have fat-free tissue densities different from that of 1.100 g/ml when they observed high values for body fatness for children and the elderly, and extremely low values (<0% body fat) in professional football players (51, 87, 166). Children have lower bone mineral contents, less potassium, and more water per unit fat-free mass, yielding a lower density for fat-free mass (87). Lohman (84) reports density values (g/ml) of 1.080 at age 6, 1.084 at age 10, and 1.097 for boys aged 15½. The lower values in the prepubescent child would overestimate percent body fat by 5%. In contrast to children, who have density values below 1.100 for the fat-free mass, African Americans were shown to have a density of 1.113 g/ml (125). The Siri equation would have to be modified as follows:

$$\% \text{ Body fat} = \frac{437}{\text{Density}} - 393$$

In order to determine the correct value for the fat-free mass, scientists use more sophisticated multi-component approaches in which the body is divided into three components (body water, protein + mineral, and fat) or four components (mineral, water, protein, and fat). These approaches are more complex, but they address many of the limitations found in the two-component model (59, 83, 86, 108). Heyward and Wagner's text (see Suggested Readings) provides guidance in choosing the most appropriate equation depending on age, race, gender, or other factors. The following sections will discuss how whole-body density values are determined by underwater weighing, air displacement plethysmography, BIA, and skinfold procedures.

Hydrostatic (Underwater) Weighing Density is equal to mass divided by volume (D = M/V). Because we already know body mass (body weight), we only have to determine body volume to calculate whole-body density (52). The **underwater weighing** method applies Archimedes' principle, which states that when an object is placed in water, it is buoyed up by a counterforce equal to the water it displaces. The volume of water displaced (spilled over) would equal the *loss of weight* while the object is completely submerged. Some investigators determine body volume by measuring the actual volume of water displaced; others measure weight while the subject is underwater and obtain body volume by subtracting the weight measured in water (M_W) from that measured in air (M_A), or ($M_A - M_W$). Both methods of determining volume are reproducible, but body fat percentage values are slightly but significantly (0.7%) lower with the volume displacement method (160). The weight of water displaced is converted to a volume by dividing by the density of the water (D_W) at the time of measurement:

$$D = \frac{M}{V} = \frac{M_A}{\dfrac{(M_A - M_W)}{D_W}}$$

This denominator must now be corrected for two other volumes: the volume of air in the lungs at the time of measurement [usually residual volume (V_R)] and the volume of gas in the gastrointestinal tract (V_{GI}). It is recommended that V_R be measured at the time that underwater weight is measured, but measurement on land with the subject in the same position is a suitable alternative (84). Residual volume can also be estimated with gender-specific regression equations or by taking 24% (males) or 28% (females) of vital capacity. However, the latter two procedures introduce measurement errors of 2% to 3% fat for a given individual (95). V_{GI} can be quite variable, and although some investigators ignore this measure, others assume a 100 ml volume for all subjects (22, 83).

The density equation can now be rewritten:

$$D = \frac{M}{V} = \frac{M_A}{\dfrac{(M_A - M_W)}{D_W} - V_R - V_{GI}}$$

Figure 18.2 shows the equipment used to measure underwater weight. Water temperature is measured to obtain the correct water density. The subject is weighed on land on a scale accurate to within 100 grams. The subject puts on a diver's belt with sufficient weight to prevent floating during the weighing procedure and sits on the chair suspended from the precision scale. The scale can be read to 10 grams and it has major divisions of 50 grams. The subject sits on the chair with the water at chin level and as a maximal exhalation is just about completed, the subject bends over and pulls the head under. When a maximal expiration is achieved, the subject holds that position for about five to ten seconds while the investigator reads the scale. This procedure is repeated six to ten times until the values stabilize. The weight of the diver's belt and chair (measured under water) are subtracted from this weight to obtain the true value for M_W.

If V_R were to be measured at the time underwater weight is measured, the subject would have to be breathing through a mouthpiece and valve assembly that could be activated at the correct time (111).

The following data were obtained on a white male, aged 36: $M_A = 75.20$ kg, $M_W = 3.52$ kg, $V_R = 1.43$ liters, $D_W = 0.9944$ at 34°C, $V_{GI} = 0.1$ liter.

$$D = \frac{M}{V} = \frac{75.20}{\dfrac{(75.20 - 3.52)}{0.9944} - 1.43 - 0.1} = \frac{75.20}{70.55} = 1.066$$

This density value is now used in Siri's equation to calculate the percentage of body fat:

$$\% \text{ Body fat} = \frac{495}{\text{Density}} - 450$$

$$14.3 = \frac{495}{1.066} - 450$$

The underwater weighing procedure in which V_R is measured (and not estimated) has been used as the "standard" against which other methods are compared. However, remember that due to the normal biological variability in the fat-free mass in a given population, the body fat percentage value is estimated to be within about ±2.0%–2.5% of the "true" value (83, 115).

Air Displacement Plethysmography Body density can also be calculated from body volume measurements obtained via air displacement plethysmography (in contrast to water displacement that is used in hydrostatic weighing). Small changes in pressure due to the change in the volume of air in a closed chamber are used to calculate the volume of the individual sitting in the chamber. The Bod Pod uses this technology to simplify the measurement of body volume and therefore the calculation of whole-body density (see Fig. 18.3). The information obtained is used in the same way as that collected in hydrostatic weighing (33). Although body fat percentage values derived from this method may not be the same as those from hydrostatic weighing, the differences are small (92). The SEE is approximately ±2.2–3.7% (115).

Bioelectrical Impedance Analysis (BIA) This is a simple, fast, and noninvasive method of obtaining information about body composition. Electrodes are placed on the end of two limbs, distant from each other (e.g., wrist to ankle, hand to hand, foot to foot) and a small electrical current, undetectable to the person being tested, is applied to one extremity (via source electrode) while the voltage drop (impedance) is measured at the other extremity (via sink or detector electrode) (83, 97). The current flows through all conducting material in the path between the electrodes, with lean tissue (mostly water and electrolytes) being a good conductor (low impedance) and fat tissue being a poor conductor (high impedance). The impedance value provides an estimate of total body water from which the fat-free mass and body fat can be calculated (115).

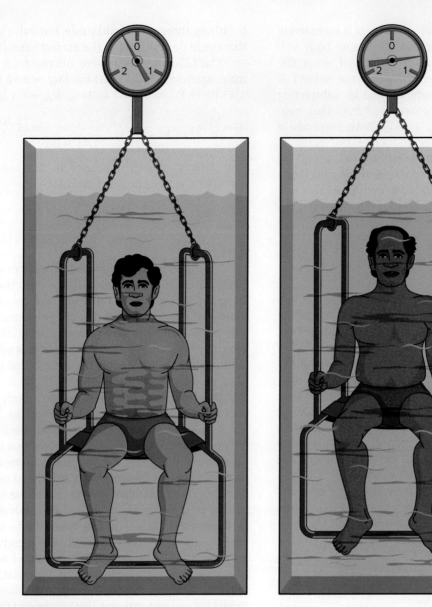

Figure 18.2 The underwater weighing technique illustrating two individuals with the same weight and height, but different body composition.

Early BIA models used a single frequency (50 kHz) and a low-level current (500 mA) that could not distinguish between intracellular and extracellular components of total body water. BIA devices developed to address these limitations use multiple frequencies within a range of 4 to 1000 kHz, and they may provide better estimates of the fat-free mass (83, 115, 128, 158). The SEE is about ±3.5%–5% (115).

However simple the BIA technique is, one must attend to a number of details in order to obtain reliable values (97, 115, 147):

■ Clean skin of oil, dirt, and lotions with alcohol prior to electrode placement.

■ Place electrodes exactly as described by the manufacturer. Incorrect or inconsistent placement of electrodes from test to test

will affect the accuracy and reliability of the measurement.

■ If needed for the calculation of body composition, careful measurements of height (to nearest 0.5 cm) and weight (to nearest 0.1 kg) should be obtained.

■ Exercise should be avoided for 12 hours prior to the measurement. Exercise affects BIA measurements because of increased blood flow to the skin, the warming of muscles, and sweating (dehydration).

■ Alcohol or diuretics (unless prescribed by a physician) should not be used for 48 hours prior to the test because hydration status is very important for an accurate BIA measurement.

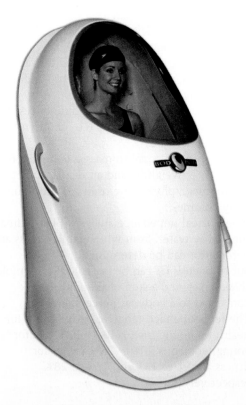

Figure 18.3 The Bod Pod system for measuring body volume using air displacement plethysmography.

Photo courtesy of www.cosmed.com

- Individuals should be instructed not to eat for four hours before the test and should drink only what is needed to maintain hydration.

- The phase of the menstrual cycle should be noted because of increased variability in the BIA measurement, between tests, in women,

Sum of Skinfolds Underwater weighing, although a good way to obtain a measurement of body density, is time consuming and requires special equipment and personnel. Paralleling the development of the advanced technologies used in body composition analysis, scientists developed equations that predicted body density from a collection of skinfold measurements. The skinfold method relies on the observation that within any population a certain fraction of the total body fat lies just under the skin (subcutaneous fat), and if one could obtain a representative sample of that fat, overall body fatness (density) could be predicted. Generally, these prediction equations were developed with the underwater weighing method used as the standard. For example, a group of college males and females would have body density measured by underwater weighing, and a variety of skinfold measures would also be obtained. The investigator would then determine what collection of skinfolds would most accurately predict the body density determined by underwater weighing.

Investigators found that subcutaneous fat represents a variable fraction of total fat (20%-70%), depending on age, sex, overall fatness, and the measurement technique used. At a specific body fatness, women have less subcutaneous fat than men, and older subjects of the same sex have less than younger subjects (86). Given that these variables could influence an estimate of body density, it is no surprise that of the more than 100 equations developed, most were found to be "population specific" and could not be used for groups of different ages or sex. This obviously creates problems for professionals in adult fitness programs or elementary or high school physical education teachers when they try to find the equation that works best for their particular group. Fortunately, a good deal of progress has been made to reduce these problems.

Jackson and Pollock (65) and Jackson, Pollock, and Ward (67) developed "generalized equations" for men and women—that is, equations that could be used across various age groups. In addition, these equations have been validated for athletic and nonathletic populations, including postpubescent athletes (84, 135, 136). In these equations, specific skinfold measurements are obtained and the values are used along with age to calculate body density. Jackson and Pollock (66) simplified this procedure by providing tabulated body fatness percentage values for different skinfold thicknesses across age. All that is needed is the sum of skinfolds to obtain a body fatness percentage value. Appendixes E and F show the percent body fat tables for men and women respectively, using the sum of three skinfolds. For example, a woman aged 25 with a sum of skinfolds equal to 50 mm has a body fat percentage equal to 22.9% (look to the right of the sum of skinfold column where 48-52 is shown, over to the second column—ages 23-27). Body fatness percentage derived from skinfold measures is estimated to have an error of about ±3.5% relative to the "true" value (85, 115).

The use of skinfold measurements was extended to children in the schools for early identification of obesity. Currently, the FITNESSGRAM uses the calf and triceps skinfolds to estimate percent body fat and to set criterion-referenced standards (see Chap. 15) for health. As an alternative, when skinfold measurements cannot be taken, the BMI is used with appropriate criterion-referenced cutoff values for health (164). For more on this, visit the FITNESSGRAM website **(http://www.fitnessgram.net).**

Body Fatness for Health and Fitness

We have already seen how the BMI is used to classify individuals relative to health and disease. How do we use information on body composition (e.g., percentage of body fat) to make judgments about one's status relative to health and fitness. Lohman, Houtkooper, and Going (82) recommend the following range of percent fat values for health and fitness for men and women:

Health Standards

	Men	Women
Young adults	8–22	20–35
Middle age	10–25	25–38
Elderly	10–23	25–35

Fitness Standards for Active Individuals

	Men	Women
Young adults	5–15	16–28
Middle age	7–18	20–33
Elderly	9–18	20–33

Now that we know how to obtain a percent body fatness measure and what the healthy and fitness percent body fat standards are, how can we determine the body weight associated with those values? In the following example, a female college student has 30% body fat and weighs 142 lbs. She wants to be at the low end of the healthy range, so her goal is 20% fat.

Step 1. Calculate fat-free weight:

100% − 30% fat = 70% fat-free
70% × 142 lb = 99.4 lb fat-free weight

Step 2. Goal weight $= \dfrac{\text{fat-free weight}}{(1 - \text{goal \% fat})}$, with goal % fat expressed as a fraction:

For 20% $= \dfrac{99.4 \text{ lb}}{(1 - .20)} = 124 \text{ lb}$

Her weight at her 20% goal is 124 lb.

Lohman (85) also provides values for body fat percentages that are below the optimal range: For boys, 6% to 10% is classified as low and <6% as very low. Comparable values for girls are 12% to 15% and <12%, respectively. There is great pressure in our society to be thin, and this can be carried to an extreme. A far-too-common problem in our high schools and colleges is an eating disorder known as **anorexia nervosa,** in which primarily young women have an exaggerated fear of getting fat. This fear leads to food restriction and increased exercise in an attempt to stay thin, when they are, in fact, already thin (48). **Bulimia nervosa** is an eating disorder in which large quantities of food are taken in (binging), only to be followed by self-induced vomiting or the use of laxatives to rid the body of the food that was eaten (purging). While anorexia nervosa is characterized by the cessation of the menstrual cycle in women and the development of an emaciated state, the majority of the bingers/purgers are in the normal weight range (161).

It is clear that to stay in the optimal body fat percentage range, one must balance the dietary consumption of calories with energy expenditure. We will now consider that topic.

IN SUMMARY

- In the two-component system of body composition analysis, the body is divided into fat-free and fat mass, with densities of 1.100 and 0.900, respectively. The estimate of the density of the fat-free mass must account for differences that exist in various populations (i.e., children and African Americans).
- Body density is equal to mass ÷ volume. Both underwater weighing and air displacement plethysmography can be used to determine body volume.
- Bioelectrical impedance analysis (BIA) estimates total body water, from which fat-free mass and percent fat can be determined.
- Subcutaneous fat can be "sampled" as skinfold thicknesses, and a sum of skinfolds can be converted to a body fat percentage.
- The recommended range of body fatness for health for young men is 8% to 22%, and for young women is 20% to 35%; values for fitness are 5% to 15% and 16% to 28%, respectively.

OBESITY AND WEIGHT CONTROL

In Chap. 14 we discussed the major risk factors associated with degenerative diseases. Although high blood pressure, cigarette smoking, elevated serum cholesterol, and inactivity have been accepted as major risk factors, more and more evidence points to obesity as being a separate and independent risk factor for coronary heart disease (CHD), and one directly tied to two of the major risk factors. A variety of diseases are linked to obesity: hypertension, type 2 diabetes, CHD, stroke, gallbladder disease, osteoarthritis, sleep apnea and respiratory problems, and some types of cancer (endometrial, breast, prostate, and colon). In addition, obesity is associated with complications of pregnancy, menstrual irregularities, hirsutism, stress incontinence, and psychological disorders (e.g., depression) (23, 99, 114, 117).

It should be no surprise that obesity is linked to an increased morbidity due to cardiovascular disease and some types of cancers. However, being overweight is not. Overweight was associated with a lower mortality from all causes, including cardiovascular disease (45). This information provides special urgency to promote strategies, including doing physical activity on a regular basis, to reduce the chance of a person moving from the overweight to the obese category. Let's take a more detailed look at obesity.

Obesity

If we use a BMI of ≥30 as a classification for obesity, the prevalence of obesity in U.S. adults increased from 15% in the 1976–1980 reporting period, to 23.3% in 1988–1994, to 30.9% in 1999–2000, to 32.2% in 2004, and to 35.9% for 2009–2010 (96, 104). When you include those who are classified as overweight (BMI 25.0–29.9), the prevalence of overweight and obesity was 69.2%. Consequently, more than two-thirds of the U.S. adult population is overweight, and one-third is obese. In addition, some ethnic groups were over-represented. More than half of non-Hispanic Black women were obese, and almost 80% were overweight. The good news is that the prevalence of obesity did not change between 2009 and 2010 and 2011 and 2012 (105).

All obesity is not the same. Studies suggest that not only is the relative body fatness related to an increased risk of CVD but the distribution of that fatness must also be considered. Individuals with a large waist circumference compared to hip circumference have a higher risk of CVD and sudden death (138, 139). These data suggest that in addition to skinfold or underwater weighing estimates of body density, measurements of waist and hip circumferences should be obtained (78, 79). Ratios of waist to hip circumference >0.95 for men and >0.8 for women are associated with the CVD risk factors of insulin resistance, high cholesterol, and hypertension, and such individuals are treated even if they are only borderline obese (9, 21, 26, 138). Given that the risk of these problems is associated with abdominal obesity, the BMI guidelines mentioned previously (99) use only waist circumference and recommend values of 102 cm (40 in) and 88 cm (35 in) to be used for men and women, respectively, when classifying those at high risk. Although various reviews support the continued use of circumference measurements to assess health risk (132), there is renewed interest in developing appropriate cutoff values for different racial groups since existing standards were derived primarily from Caucasian populations (60, 113, 142).

Unfortunately, obesity is not just a problem for adults. The prevalence of overweight and obesity in children and adolescents increased dramatically (from ~6% to ~15%) between the late 1970s and 2000; however, the rate of increase has slowed between 2000 and 2009–10 for both 6–11-year-olds (from 15.1% to 18.0%) and 12–19-year-olds (from 14.8% to 18.4%) (74, 96, 103, 106). Data for 2011–12 show no significant increase. However, a major concern is that the prevalence of those at the high end of the BMI scale (97th percentile for BMI) continues to increase at a fast rate (103). The increase in overweight and obesity in children over the past 35 years carries with it a disease burden (e.g., type 2 diabetes), formerly reserved for those over age 40 and overweight. What causes obesity?

Causes of Obesity

There is clearly no single cause of obesity. Obesity is related to a wide variety of genetic and environmental factors that can alter energy balance, which, in turn, leads to weight gain and obesity. Figure 18.4 provides a snapshot of some of the factors that can alter energy balance (98):

- Family history includes both the genetics involved as well as the lifestyle (physically active, planned meals vs. fast food, emotional environment, job security, etc.). Bouchard (13)

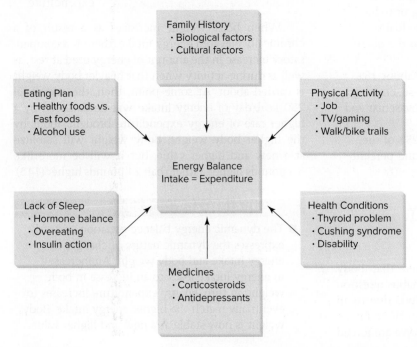

Figure 18.4 Factors related to energy balance and obesity.

and colleagues have determined, on the basis of an analysis of the relationships between and among nine types of relatives (spouses, parent-child, siblings, uncle-nephew, etc.), that 25% of body fat and fat mass is tied to genetic factors, and 30% is due to cultural transmission.

- Eating Plan–Is one of the healthy eating plans described earlier used in meal planning, or does fast food contribute substantial calories? Also, is alcohol consumption an issue?

- Physical activity–Is the person meeting the U.S. Physical Activity Guidelines (see Chap. 16)? Does the person have a sedentary job? How much time is spent watching TV or playing computer games?

- Health conditions such as having insufficient thyroid hormone (i.e., being hypothyroid) or having Cushing's syndrome (i.e., too much cortisol due to overproduction of ACTH)

- Medications like antidepressants and the corticosteroids (linked to Cushing's syndrome)

- Lack of sleep affects hormones involved in eating behavior (e.g., leptin) and provides more opportunities for eating.

Although there are many factors that can alter energy balance and cause obesity, the focus of attention is on two of them: diet and physical activity. The next section will address both relative to weight control.

IN SUMMARY

- Obesity is associated with an increased mortality from cardiovascular disease and some types of cancer, but being overweight is not. Emphasis should be on maintaining or reducing weight in the overweight individual to decrease the chance of migration to the obese category.
- About 36% of American adults and about 18% of children and adolescents are obese, creating a great health burden due to cardiovascular and metabolic disease.
- Genetic factors account for about 25% of the transmissible variance for fat mass and percentage of body fat; culture accounts for 30%.

DIET, PHYSICAL ACTIVITY, AND WEIGHT CONTROL

The Framingham Heart Study showed that body weight increases as we age. A reasonable question to ask is whether this gain in weight was due to an increase in caloric intake. Interestingly, caloric intake decreased over the same age span (15). We are forced to conclude that energy expenditure decreased faster than the decrease in caloric intake, and as a result, weight gain occurred (11). This weight gain problem can be corrected by understanding and dealing with one or both sides of the energy balance equation. We will deal with the energy balance equation first, and then discuss how modifications in energy intake can affect weight loss. Finally, we will explore the variables on the energy expenditure side of the equation.

Energy Balance

Weight gain occurs when there is a chronic increase in caloric intake compared to energy expenditure. A net gain of about 3500 kcal is needed to add 1 lb (454 grams) of adipose tissue. We are all familiar with the energy balance equation:

Change in energy stores = energy intake − energy expenditure

What is implied by this equation is that an excess energy intake of 250 kcal/day will cause body weight to increase 1 pound in 14 days (250 kcal/day × 14 day = 3500 kcal = 1 pound). At the end of one year, the person will have gained about 24 pounds. As reasonable as this equation may appear, we know that a weight gain of that magnitude will not occur. The equation is a "static" energy balance equation that does not consider the effect that the weight gain will have on energy expenditure (143).

The energy balance equation can be expressed in a manner to account for the dynamic nature of energy balance in biological systems:

Rate of change of energy stores = rate of change of energy intake − rate of change of energy expenditure

When body weight increases as a result of a chronically elevated energy intake, there is a compensatory increase in the amount of energy used at rest, as well as during activity when that heavier body weight is carried about. At some point, then, the additional 250 kcal/day of energy intake will be balanced by a higher rate of energy expenditure brought about by the higher body weight. Body weight will stabilize at a new and higher value, but it will be more like 3.5 pounds higher, rather than 24 pounds higher (143).

IN SUMMARY

- The dynamic energy balance equation correctly expresses the dynamic nature of changes in energy intake and body weight. An increase in energy intake leads to an increase in body weight; in turn, energy expenditure increases to eventually match the higher energy intake. Body weight is now stable at a new and higher value.

Diet and Weight Control

A good diet provides the necessary nutrients and calories to provide for tissue growth and regeneration and to meet the daily energy requirements of work and play. In our society, we are fortunate to have a variety of foods to meet these needs. However, we tend to consume more than the recommended amount of fat, which some believe is related to our country's obesity problem. The hypothesis that the fat content of the diet is an important aspect of weight control revolves around the factors driving energy intake. There is a mandatory need for carbohydrate oxidation by the nervous system, and we are driven to eat what is used (43, 57, 126). If we eat a high-fat diet, we will take in a considerable amount of fat while consuming the necessary carbohydrates to refill the carbohydrate stores. This fat is stored, and body weight will increase. As mentioned earlier, as body weight increases, daily energy expenditure increases until an energy balance is achieved at a new and higher body weight. In this sense, the elevation of body weight and fat mass due to a high-fat/high-calorie diet is a compensatory mechanism that results in weight maintenance.

However, while a great deal of attention is focused on the composition of the diet, we should not forget that calories count in any weight-loss or weight-maintenance program. For example, studies in which subjects were switched from a high-fat to a low-fat diet, *while maintaining a constant caloric intake,* showed no change in energy expenditure or body weight (57, 81, 121, 149). In addition, in conditions in which a negative caloric balance was imposed to achieve weight loss, the composition of the diet (high-fat vs. low-fat) did not matter (56). In this sense, one should not get carried away with a high-carbohydrate diet and consume calories in excess of what is needed (44). In fact, when a variety of popular diets (Atkins, Ornish, Weight Watchers, and Zone) were compared over the course of one year, each modestly reduced body weight, with no difference between diets. However, as Figure 18.5 shows the best predictor of weight loss was the degree to which individuals adhered to the diet—no matter which one (32, 47, 101, 122).

Consistent with these findings, in the newly released set of guidelines from the American Heart Association and the American College of Cardiology for the management of overweight and obesity, a wide variety of diets are recommended for weight loss (39, 68). The diets are to be prescribed within a framework of a comprehensive lifestyle intervention that includes exercise (see later section) and counseling. These diets include high-protein, low-fat, low or high glycemic load, vegetarian, and Mediterranean types with the primary focus on energy (calorie) restriction to achieve weight loss. The guidelines recommend using "trained interventionists" to deliver the program, which included a maintenance phase when weight-loss goals were achieved. The trained interventionists included a broad range of health professionals, including registered dietitians, psychologists, exercise specialists, health counselors, and professionals in training (68). In contrast to dietary strategies to achieve weight

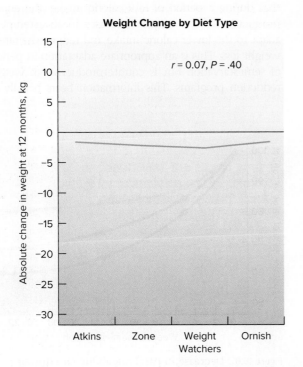

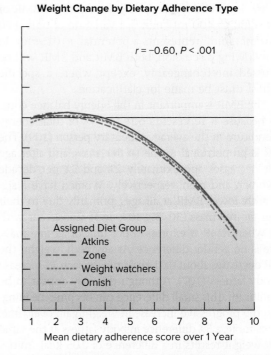

Figure 18.5 One-year changes in body weight as a function of diet group and dietary adherence level for all study participants.

loss in which the primary focus is on energy restriction, a parallel set of guidelines were provided to reduce the risk of cardiovascular and metabolic disease. Those guidelines focused on the health-related quality of the diet as described earlier in this chapter, including the use of the DASH and Mediterranean-style diets (39).

IN SUMMARY

- Calories do count and must be considered in any diet aimed at achieving or maintaining a weight-loss goal. However, the composition of the diet is important in terms of risk of cardiovascular and metabolic diseases, and good health.

Energy Expenditure and Weight Control

The other side of the energy balance equation involves the expenditure of energy and includes the basal metabolic rate, thermogenesis (shivering and nonshivering), and physical activity/exercise. We will examine each of these relative to its role in energy balance.

Basal Metabolic Rate   Basal metabolic rate (BMR) is the rate of energy expenditure measured under standardized conditions (i.e., immediately after rising, 12 to 18 hours after a meal, in a supine position in a thermoneutral environment). Because of the difficulty of achieving these conditions during routine measurements, investigators have measured **resting metabolic rate (RMR)** instead. In this latter procedure, the subject reports to the lab about four hours after eating a light meal and after a period of time (30 to 60 minutes), the metabolic rate is measured (94). Given the low level of oxygen uptake measured for BMR or RMR (200 to 400 ml $\cdot$ min^{-1}), a variation of only ± 20 to 40 ml $\cdot$ min^{-1} represents a potential $\pm 10\%$ error. In the following discussion, both BMR and RMR will be discussed interchangeably, except where a specific contrast must be made for clarification.

The BMR is important in the energy balance equation because it represents 60% to 75% of total energy expenditure in the average sedentary person (109). The BMR is proportional to the fat-free mass, and after age 20 it decreases approximately 2% and 3% per decade in women and men, respectively. Women have a significantly lower BMR at all ages, primarily due to their lower fat-free mass (30, 37, 107, 163). Consistent with this, when RMR is expressed per unit of fat-free mass, there is no gender difference. At any body weight, the RMR decreases about 0.01 kcal/min for each 1% increase in body fatness (107). Although this may appear to be insignificant, this small difference can become meaningful in the progressive increase in weight gain over time. For example, a 5% difference in body fatness at the same body weight results in a difference of 0.05 kcal $\cdot$ min^{-1}, or 3 kcal $\cdot$ hr^{-1}, which is equal to 72 kcal $\cdot$ d^{-1}. It must be emphasized that the percentage of body fat makes only a small contribution to the BMR. This was confirmed in a study examining the relationship of body composition to BMR; fat mass did not improve the prediction of BMR based on the fat-free mass alone (30).

Part of the variation in BMR between individuals is due to a genetic predisposition to be higher or lower (13). The range (± 3 SD) in normal BMR values is about $\pm 21\%$ from the average value, and such variation helps to explain the observation that some have an easier time maintaining body weight than others. If an average adult male has a BMR of 1500 kcal $\cdot$ d^{-1}, those at $+3$ SD can take in an additional 300 kcal $\cdot$ d^{-1} (21% of 1500 kcal) to maintain weight, whereas others at the low end of the range (-3 SD) would have to take in 300 fewer kcals (37, 50).

The fat-free mass is not the only factor influencing the BMR. In 1919, Benedict (8) showed that prolonged dieting (reduction from about 3100 kcal to 1950 kcal) was associated with a 20% decrease in the BMR expressed per kilogram of body weight. This observation was confirmed in the famous Minnesota Starvation Experiment (73) and is shown in Figure 18.6. In this figure the BMR is expressed as a percent of the value measured before the period of semi-starvation. The percent decrease in BMR is larger "per man" because of the loss of lean tissue (as well as fat tissue); however, when the value is expressed per kilogram of body weight or per unit of surface area (m²), the BMR is still shown to be reduced. A decrease in the concentration of one of the thyroid hormones (T_3) and a reduced level of sympathetic nervous system activity have been implicated in this lower BMR due to caloric restriction (14). What these data mean is that during a period of low caloric intake, the energy production of the tissues decreases in an attempt to adapt to the lower caloric intake and reduce the rate of weight loss. This is an appropriate adaptation in periods of semi-starvation but is counterproductive in weight-reduction programs. This information bears heavily on

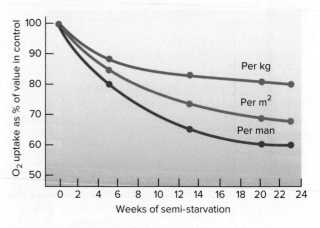

Figure 18.6   Decrease in basal metabolic rate during 24 weeks of semi-starvation.

the use of very-low-calorie diets as a primary means of weight reduction (36, 46, 110, 156, 159).

The BMR is also responsive to periods of overfeeding. In the dieting experiment of Benedict (8) mentioned earlier, when the subjects were allowed a day of free eating, the BMR was elevated on the following day. Further, in long-term (14 to 20 days) overfeeding to cause obesity, increases in resting and basal metabolic rates have been recorded. In essence, during the dynamic phase of weight gain (going from a lower to a higher weight), more calories are required per kilogram of body weight to maintain the weight gain than to simply maintain normal body weight (50, 134). This increased heat production due to an excess caloric intake, called **thermogenesis,** will be discussed in the next section. However, before leaving this discussion of the BMR, we need to mention the effect of exercise training. When careful measurements are made in which the RMR is expressed per kilogram of fat-free mass, the RMR is similar for trained and untrained individuals, and resistance and endurance training do not affect the value (19, 20).

IN SUMMARY

- The BMR represents the largest fraction of total energy expenditure in sedentary persons. The BMR decreases with age, and women have lower BMR values than men.
- The fat-free mass is related to both the gender difference and to the decline in BMR with age. A reduction in caloric intake by dieting or fasting can reduce the BMR.

Thermogenesis Core temperature is maintained at about 37°C by balancing heat production with heat loss. Under thermoneutral conditions, the BMR (RMR) provides the necessary heat, but under cold environmental conditions, the process of shivering is actuated, and 100% of the energy required for involuntary muscle contraction appears as heat to maintain core temperature. In addition, some animals (including newborn humans) produce heat by a process called nonshivering thermogenesis, involving brown adipose tissue (BAT). This type of adipose tissue is rich in mitochondria and increases heat production in response to norepinephrine (NE) and other hormones. Recently, BAT has been discovered in adult humans, and a variety of studies indicate that it may play a role in preventing weight gain with age. The interest has now shifted to the "browning" of white adipose tissue. Some white adipose tissue has brown-like (beige) adipocytes that are responsive to stimuli used to engage brown adipose tissue. Clearly, this is an area we will hear more about in the future (12, 80, 123).

Thermogenesis involves more than brown adipose tissue. The heat generated due to the food we consume accounts for about 10% to 15% of our total daily energy expenditure; this is called the *thermic effect of food* (15, 109). Generally, this is determined by having a subject ingest a test meal (700–1000 kcal), and the elevation in the metabolic rate is measured following the meal. This portion of our daily energy expenditure is influenced by genetic factors (13, 109), is lower in obese than in lean individuals (71, 129), and is influenced by the level of spontaneous activity and the degree of insulin resistance (144). However, because it represents such a small part of the overall daily energy expenditure, it is not a good predictor of subsequent obesity.

IN SUMMARY

- Thermogenesis (heat production) results from shivering, from the impact of norepinephrine on brown adipose tissue (nonshivering type), and from the ingestion of food.
- The thermic effect of food represents only 10% to 15% of total energy expenditure and is not predictive of obesity.

Physical Activity and Exercise Physical activity constitutes the most variable part of the energy expenditure side of the energy balance equation, being 5% to 40% of the daily energy expenditure (24, 109). There are those who have sedentary jobs and who do little physical activity during their leisure time. Others may have strenuous jobs or expend 300 to 1000 kcal during their leisure time every day or two. Just how important is physical activity in weight control? Epidemiological evidence suggests an inverse association between physical activity and body weight, with body fat being more favorably distributed in those who are physically active (34, 118). Consistent with these observations, various studies have shown an inverse relationship between the number of steps accumulated throughout the day and the BMI (see Fig. 18.7) (58, 148).

From a weight-loss perspective, one would think that a caloric deficit that results from an increase in energy expenditure through physical activity is equivalent to a caloric deficit due to a decrease in caloric intake. However, as Ross et al. (120) pointed out, leading authorities (99) have stated that the addition of exercise makes only a modest contribution to weight loss. How can this be the case, given the equivalency of the caloric deficit induced by either diet or exercise? Ross et al. (120) showed that in the majority of weight-loss studies in which a diet treatment was compared to an exercise treatment, the energy deficit caused by exercise was only a fraction of that caused by diet. In this situation, it is not surprising that weight loss due to diet was greater than that due to exercise; however, the weight loss due to exercise was as expected. The exercise-induced weight loss, 30% of that due to diet, was equivalent to the caloric deficit associated with the exercise (28%

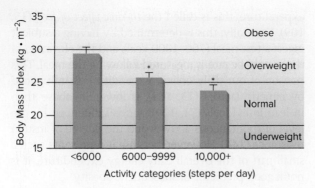

Figure 18.7 Body Mass Index varies with the number of steps taken per day.

of that due to diet). In a study to determine whether an exercise-calorie is the same as a diet-calorie, Ross et al. (119) did a controlled experiment designed to achieve a 700 kcal/day energy deficit due to either exercise alone or diet alone. Both dietary intake and the structured exercise programs were carefully monitored to ensure compliance. Both groups lost 7.5 kg over 12 weeks–exactly what was expected from the 58,800 kcal deficit (700 kcal/day times 84 days). However, the exercise group lost more total fat, thus preserving muscle. Another group in this study did the same amount of exercise (700 kcal/day) but were told to increase their caloric intake by 700 kcal/day to maintain weight! Not only did they increase their $\dot{V}O_2$ max like the other exercise group, they also decreased their abdominal and visceral fat in spite of no weight loss (119). This is additional evidence to support the proposition that persons who are overweight or obese gain health benefits from exercise, even when weight is not lost.

These results were supported in a more recent study that compared subjects who underwent a six-month 25% caloric restriction with those who had a 12.5% caloric restriction plus an exercise intervention equal to a 12.5% reduction in caloric intake (116). Both groups lost the same amount of weight, similar to what was mentioned earlier. There is little question that a calorie of aerobic exercise is really equal to a calorie of diet restriction as far as change in body weight is concerned; however, the exercise intervention yields results (e.g., increase in $\dot{V}O_2$ max) that cannot be realized by a diet-alone approach to weight loss (116, 119).

In both of these studies, caloric intake was carefully monitored, as demanded by the research design. What happens when an exercise intervention is used and the subjects are simply told to not change their dietary intake? In a recent study, overweight and obese men and women were randomly assigned to either a control group or one of the following exercise groups: those who did 400 kcal/session or 600 kcal/session. The participants

did five sessions a week for ten months. Although the exercise sessions were carefully monitored to make sure the subjects expended the necessary calories, they were simply told to not change their diet. Weight loss averaged 3.9 kg and 5.2 kg for the 400 and 600 kcal/session groups, respectively, while the control group gained 0.5 kg. The weight loss was due entirely to loss of body fat and represented a clinically significant weight loss in terms of risk of chronic diseases (35). These results were consistent with an earlier study that examined the effect of different amounts of exercise (energy expenditures equivalent to jogging 20 miles/wk vs. jogging 12 miles per week vs. walking 12 miles per week) on weight loss in subjects who were told to maintain a stable body weight. Weight loss over the nine-month study for the three groups was 2.9 kg vs. 0.6 kg vs. 0.9 kg, respectively, compared to a weight gain of 1.0 kg for the control group (140). More body fat than weight was lost, signifying an increase in fat-free mass. The emphasis in these studies was on vigorous exercise, except for the walking group in the last study.

Two well-controlled physical activity interventions focused on moderate-intensity physical activity, with half done in a structured setting and half done at home. Doing 180–370 minutes of physical activity per week (with no dietary restriction) resulted in a weight loss of about 1.5 kg over the 12-month studies (64, 90). Again, fat loss exceeded weight loss. Overall, weight loss follows a dose-response pattern, being greater with higher levels of energy expenditure.

IN SUMMARY

- There is an inverse relationship between physical activity and body weight.
- Exercise is as effective as diet in achieving weight loss when matched in terms of caloric deficit; however fitness effects occur only in those doing the exercise.
- When weight loss occurs with an exercise and diet program, less lean body mass is lost than when the same weight loss is achieved by diet alone.

Weight Loss vs. Weight Maintenance Strange as it may seem, given what has just been presented, exercise is not required to achieve weight loss. All that is necessary is a caloric deficit, the magnitude of which is easily controlled by diet (56). However, as mentioned previously, the use of exercise as a part of a weight-loss program might maintain a higher lean body mass and RMR and result in an optimal body fatness at a higher body weight.

Although exercise might not be an essential ingredient in a weight-loss program, it is in a weight-maintenance program (141). A major unresolved question

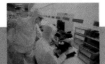

Successful Losers—How Much Exercise Is Needed to Keep the Weight Off?

There is general agreement that most U.S. adults need more physical activity. The question is, how much? The systematic increase in the prevalence of obesity over the past 25 years has provided a strong incentive to address this issue and, to some extent, we are making progress.

In Chap. 16 we presented the *U.S. Physical Activity Guidelines* recommendation that all adults should do at least 150 minutes of moderate-intensity or 75 minutes of vigorous-intensity physical activity per week (see Suggested Readings). There is clear evidence that this amount of physical activity results in significant health benefits. This is a minimal recommendation, with clear support that "more is better." So, doing 300 minutes per week of moderate-intensity or 150 minutes per week of vigorous-intensity physical activity results in additional benefits, including maintaining or losing weight. This is consistent with both the 2002 Institute of Medicine (IOM) report (63) and the most recent ACSM position stand on the issue of physical activity and weight (1), in which they recommend:

■ 150-250 min/wk of moderate-intensity physical activity to prevent weight gain

■ 250 min/wk of moderate-intensity physical activity to achieve significant weight loss

■ 250 minutes per week of moderate-intensity physical activity may be needed to prevent weight regain after weight lost

Regarding the last point, Dr. Rena Wing of the University of Pittsburgh and Dr. James Hill of the University of Colorado formed the National Weight Control Registry (NWCR) in 1993 to gain some insights into what made "successful losers"–individuals who lost weight and kept it off. To be included in the registry, individuals had to have lost substantial weight (≥13.6 kg [30 lb]) and kept it off for at least one year. Some of the findings follow (145):

■ The average weight loss of the registrants was 33.6 kg, and they kept the weight off for an average of 5.2 years, which placed most in the normal (57.9%) or overweight (29.9%) BMI range.

■ About 88% limit foods high in fat and sugar, 44% limit the amount of food consumed, and 44% count calories.

■ A total of 75% of registrants expend more than 1000 kcal/week, and 54% expend more than 2000 kcal/week (about 200 min/wk of moderate-intensity physical activity).

The NWCR has provided unique and helpful insights into what makes a successful loser. The seven key habits for long-term success at weight loss include (145):

1. High level of physical activity
2. Limit television watching–63% watch less than 10 hours a week
3. Low-calorie, low-fat diet–1380 kcal/day, with less than 30% fat
4. Consistent diet–eat the same foods regularly
5. Breakfast consumption–at least 78% eat breakfast daily
6. High dietary restraint (good control over eating)
7. Self-monitoring–more than 50% weigh weekly and track their daily food intake

Clearly, these messages from those who have been successful in maintaining weight loss have great value for both the professional and the client working toward that goal.

---

is, how much? However, some of the general exercise recommendations for health and fitness presented in Chap. 16 would be considered reasonable for weight-maintenance programs. The primary factor involved in energy expenditure is the total work accomplished, so low-intensity, long-duration exercise is as good as high-intensity, short-duration exercise in expending calories. For the sedentary, overweight person, moderate-intensity exercise is the proper choice because it can be done for longer periods of time in each exercise session and can be done each day. Recent well-controlled physical activity interventions showed that regular participation in moderate-intensity physical activity of 180 minutes or more per week (with no dietary restriction) was associated with a weight loss of about 1.5 kg over 8 to 12 months, indicating that the subjects were weight stable over that time (64, 90, 140). Although the magnitude of weight change was small, the message it conveys is important: Only 30 minutes or more of moderate-intensity physical activity per day is enough to prevent migration from one BMI level to the next–an important effect considering the prevalence of overweight and obesity in our society. However, as we saw in Chap. 16, "more is better" when it comes to physical activity and health, including maintaining a healthy body weight. It is clear that virtually any form of exercise contributes to fat loss and the maintenance of body weight. The important thing is to just do it. See Clinical Applications 18.2 for information on "successful losers."

IN SUMMARY

■ To prevent weight gain, 150–250 min/wk of moderate-intensity physical activity is recommended.

■ To achieve significant weight loss or to prevent weight regain after weight loss, >250 min/wk of moderate-intensity physical activity is recommended.

STUDY ACTIVITIES

1. What is the difference between an RDA standard and a Daily Value?
2. Which two minerals are believed to be inadequate in women's diets?
3. Relative to coronary heart disease, what fats should we limit in our diet?
4. Describe nutrient density in the context of the five food groups in the U.S. Style Healthy Eating Pattern.
5. Describe the two-component model of body composition assessment. Why should a different body density equation be used for children in contrast to adults?
6. What is the principle of underwater weighing?
7. Given a 20-year-old college male, 180 lb, 28% fat, what is his target body weight to achieve 17% fat?
8. Is obesity more related to genetics or the environment?
9. If a person consumes 120 kcal per day in excess of need, what weight gain does the static energy balance equation predict compared to the dynamic energy balance equation?
10. What happens to the BMR when a person goes on a prolonged low-calorie diet?
11. What are the differences in outcomes when someone uses diet alone, versus a combination of diet and exercise, to achieve a weight-loss goal?
12. What is the thermic effect of food?
13. In contrast to the general physical activity recommendation for achieving significant health benefits, how much physical activity may be needed to prevent weight gain or maintain weight once it has been lost?

SUGGESTED READINGS

Heyward, V. H., and D. R. Wagner. 2004. *Applied Body Composition Assessment*. 2nd ed. Champaign, IL: Human Kinetics.

Heymsfield S., T. Lohman, Z.M. Wang, and S. Going. 2005. *Human Body Composition*. 2nd ed. Champaign, IL: Human Kinetics.

U.S. Department of Health and Human Services. 2008. *2008 Physical Activity Guidelines for Americans*. Washington, D.C.: U.S. Department of Health and Human Services.

U.S. Department of Agriculture. 2016. *Dietary Guidelines for Americans 2015-2020* (http://health.gov/dietaryguidelines/2015/)

Wardlaw, G. M., A. M. Smith, and A. L. Collene. 2013. *Contemporary Nutrition, A Functional Approach*. New York, NY: McGraw-Hill Companies.

REFERENCES

1. **American College of Sports Medicine.** Appropriate physical activity intervention strategies for weight loss and prevention of weight regain for adults. *Medicine & Science in Sports & Exercise* 41: 459-471, 2009.
2. **American College of Sports Medicine.** Exercise and physical activity for the older adult. *Medicine & Science in Sports & Exercise* 41: 1510-1530, 2009.
3. **American College of Sports Medicine.** Physical activity and bone health. *Medicine & Science in Sports & Exercise* 36: 1985-1996, 2004.
4. **American College of Sports Medicine.** The female athlete triad. *Medicine & Science in Sports & Exercise* 39: 1867-1882, 2007.
5. **American Dietetic Association.** Position of the American Dietetic Association: health implications of dietary fiber. *Journal of the American Dietetic Association* 108: 993-1000, 2002.
6. **Azadbakht L, Mirmiran P, Esmaillzadeh A, Azizi T, and Azizi F.** Beneficial effects of dietary approaches to stop hypertension eating plan on features of the metabolic syndrome. *Diabetes Care* 28: 2823-2831, 2005.
7. **Behnke AR, Welham WC, and Feen BG.** The specific gravity of healthy men: body weight volume as an index of obesity. *Journal of the American Medical Association* 118: 495-498, 1942.
8. **Benedict F.** *Human Vitality and Efficiency Under Prolonged Restricted Diet.* The Carnegie Institution of Washington, 1919.
9. **Björntrop P.** Regional patterns of fat distribution. *Annals of Internal Medicine* 103: 994-995, 1985.
10. **Björntrop P.** The fat cell: a clinical view. In *Recent Advances in Obesity Research: II*, edited by Bray G. Westport: Technomic, 1978, pp. 153-168.
11. **Blair SN and Nichaman MZ.** The public health problem of increasing prevalence rates of obesity and what should be done about it. *Mayo Clinic Proceedings* 77: 109-113, 2002.
12. **Bonet ML, Oliver P, and Palou A.** Pharmacological and nutritional agents promoting browning of white adipose tissue. *Biochimica et Biophysica Acta* 1831: 969-985, 2013.
13. **Bouchard C.** Heredity and the path to overweight and obesity. *Medicine & Science in Sports & Exercise* 23: 285-291, 1991.
14. **Bray GA.** Effect of caloric restriction on energy expenditure in obese patients. *Lancet* 2: 397-398, 1969.
15. **Bray GA.** The energetics of obesity. *Medicine & Science in Sports & Exercise* 15: 32-40, 1983.
16. **Bray GA, Nielsen SJ, and Popkin BM.** Consumption of high fructose corn syrup in beverages may play a role in the epidemic of obesity. *American Journal of Clinical Nutrition* 79: 537-543, 2004.
17. **Brodie DA.** Techniques of measurement of body composition. Part I. *Sports Medicine* 5: 11-40, 1988.
18. **Brodie DA.** Techniques of measurement of body composition. Part II. *Sports Medicine* 5: 74-98, 1988.
19. **Broeder CE, Burrhus KA, Svanevik LS, and Wilmore JH.** The effects of aerobic fitness on resting metabolic rate. *American Journal of Clinical Nutrition* 55: 795-801, 1992.
20. **Broeder CE, Burrhus KA, Svanevik LS, and Wilmore JH.** The effects of either high-intensity resistance or endurance training on resting metabolic rate. *American Journal of Clinical Nutrition* 55: 802-810, 1992.
21. **Brozek J, Grande F, Anderson JT, and Keys A.** Densitometric analysis of body composition: revision

of some quantitative assumptions. *Annals of the New York Academy of Sciences* 110: 113–140, 1963.

22. **Buskirk ER.** Underwater weighing and body density: a review of procedures. In *Techniques for Measuring Body Composition*, edited by Brozek J, and Henschel A. National Research Council, 1961.

23. **Calle EE, Thun MJ, Petrelli JM, Rodriguez C, and Heath CW, Jr.** Body-mass index and mortality in a prospective cohort of U.S. adults. *New England Journal of Medicine* 341: 1097-1105, 1999.

24. **Calles-Escandon J and Horton ES.** The thermogenic role of exercise in the treatment of morbid obesity: a critical evaluation. *American Journal of Clinical Nutrition* 55: 533S-537S, 1992.

25. **Cameron JR and Sorenson J.** Measurement of bone mineral in vivo: an improved method. *Science* 142: 230-232, 1963.

26. **Campaigne BN.** Body fat distribution in females: metabolic consequences and implications for weight loss. *Medicine & Science in Sports & Exercise* 22: 291- 297, 1990.

27. **Centers for Disease Control and Prevention.** Trends in intake of energy and macronutrients–United States 1971-2000. *Morbidity & Mortality Weekly Report* 53: 80-82, 2004.

28. **Cha SH, Wolfgang M, Tokutake Y, Chohnan S, and Lane MD.** Differential effects of central fructose and glucose on hypothalamic malonyl-CoA and food intake. *Proceedings of the National Academy of Sciences* 105: 16871-16875, 2008.

29. **Coniglio JG.** Fat. In *Nutrition Reviews' Present Knowledge in Nutrition*. Washington, D.C.: The Nutrition Foundation, 1984, pp. 79-89.

30. **Cunningham JJ.** Body composition as a determinant of energy expenditure: a synthetic review and a proposed general prediction equation. *American Journal of Clinical Nutrition* 54: 963-969, 1991.

31. **Dahlquist A.** Carbohydrates. In *Nutrition Reviews' Present Knowledge in Nutrition*. Washington, D.C.: The Nutrition Foundation, 1984, pp. 116-130.

32. **Dansinger ML, Gleason JA, Griffith JL, Selker HP, and Schaefer EJ.** Comparison of the Atkins, Ornish, Weight Watchers, and Zone diets for weight loss and heart disease risk reduction: a randomized trial. *JAMA* 293: 43-53, 2005.

33. **Dempster P and Aitkens S.** A new air displacement method for the determination of human body composition. *Medicine & Science in Sports & Exercise* 27: 1692-1697, 1995.

34. **DiPietro L.** Physical activity, body weight, and adiposity: an epidemiologic perspective. *Exercise and Sport Sciences Reviews* 23: 275-303, 1995.

35. **Donnelly JE, Honas JJ, Smith BK, Mayo MS, Gibson CA, Sullivan DK, et al.** Aerobic exercise alone results in clinically significant weight loss for men and women: Midwest Exercise Trial-2. *Obesity* 21: E219- E228, 2013.

36. **Donnelly JE, Jakicic J, and Gunderson S.** Diet and body composition: effect of very low calorie diets and exercise. *Sports Medicine* 12: 237-249, 1991.

37. **DuBois EF.** Basal energy, metabolism at various ages: man. In *Metabolism: Clinical and Experimental*, edited by Altman PL, and Dittmer DS. Bethesda, MD: Federation of American Societies for Experimental Biology, 1968.

38. **Eastwood M.** Dietary fiber. In *Nutrition Reviews' Present Knowledge in Nutrition*. Washington, D.C.: The Nutrition Foundation, 1984, pp. 156-175.

39. **Eckel RH, Jakicic JM, Ard JD, Houston N, Hubbard VS, Nonas CA, et al.** 2013 AHA/ACC guidelines on lifestyle management to reduce cardiovascular risk. *Journal of the American College of Cardiology*. doi: 10.1016/j.jacc.2013.11.003.

40. **Ellis KJ, Shypailo RJ, Pratt JA, and Pond WG.** Accuracy of dual-energy x-ray absorptiometry for body-composition measurements in children. *American Journal of Clinical Nutrition* 60: 660-665, 1994.

41. **Fan JY, Song YQ, Wang YY, Hui RT, Zhang WL.** Dietary glycemic index, glycemic load, and risk coronary heart disease, stroke, and stroke mortality; a systematic review with meta-analysis. *PLOS ONE* 7: e52182, 2012.

42. **Finberg L.** Clinical assessment of total body water. In *Body-Composition Assessments in Youth and Adults*, edited by Roche AF. Columbus, OH: Ross Laboratories, 1985.

43. **Flatt JP.** Dietary fat, carbohydrate balance, and weight maintenance. *Annals of the New York Academy of Sciences* 683: 122-140, 1993.

44. **Flatt JP.** Use and storage of carbohydrate and fat. *American Journal of Clinical Nutrition* Suppl. 61: 952S-959S, 1995.

45. **Flegal KM, Graubard BI, Williamson DF, and Gail MH.** Cause-specific excess deaths associated with underweight, overweight, and obesity. *JAMA* 298: 2028-2037, 2007.

46. **Foster GD, Wadden TA, Feurer ID, Jennings AS, Stunkard AJ, Crosby LO, et al.** Controlled trial of the metabolic effects of a very-low-calorie diet: short- and long-term effects. *American Journal of Clinical Nutrition* 51: 167-172, 1990.

47. **Franz MJ, VanWormer JJ, Crain AL, Boucher JL, Histon T, Caplan W, et al.** Weight-loss outcomes: a systematic review and meta-analysis of weight-loss clinical trials with a minimum 1-year follow-up. *Journal of the American Dietetic Association* 107: 1755-1767, 2007.

48. **Garfinkle PE and Garner DM.** *Anorexia Nervosa*. New York, NY: Brunner/Mazel, 1982.

49. **Garn SM.** Radiographic analysis of body composition. In *Techniques for Measuring Body Composition*, edited by Brozek J and Henschel A. National Research Council, 1961.

50. **Garrow JS.** *Energy Balance and Obesity in Man*. New York NY: Elsevier North-Holland, 1978.

51. **Going S, Williams D, and Lohman T.** Aging and body composition: biological changes and methodological issues. *Exercise and Sport Sciences Reviews* 23: 411-458, 1995.

52. **Goldman RF and Buskirk ER.** Body volume measurement by underwater weighing: description of a method. In *Techniques for Measuring Body Composition*, edited by Brozek J, and Henschel A. National Research Council, 1961.

53. **Guthrie HA and Picciano MF.** *Human Nutrition*. St. Louis, MO: Mosby, 1995.

54. **Ha V, Jayalath VH, Cozma AI, Mirrahimi A, de Souza RJ, and Sievenpiper, JL.** Fructose-containing sugars, blood pressure and cardiometabolic risk: a critical review. *Current Hypertension Reports* 15: 281-297, 2013.

55. **Hallberg L.** Iron. In *Nutrition Reviews' Present Knowledge in Nutrition*. Washington, D.C.: The Nutrition Foundation, 1984, pp. 459-478.

56. **Hill J.** Obesity treatment: can diet composition play a role? *American College of Physicians* 119: 694-697, 1993.

57. **Hirsch J.** Role and benefits of carbohydrate in the diet: key issues for future dietary guidelines. *American Journal of Clinical Nutrition* Suppl. 61: 996S-1000S, 1995.

58. **Hornbuckle LM, Bassett DR, Jr., and Thompson DL.** Pedometer-determined walking and body composition variables in African-American women. *Medicine and Science in Sports and Exercise* 37: 1069-1074, 2005.

59. **Houtkooper LB and Going SB.** *Body Composition: How Should It Be Measured? Does It Affect Performance?* Barrington, IL: Gatorade Sports Science Institute, 1994.

60. **Huxley R, Mendis S, Zheleznyakov E, Reddy S, and Chan J.** Body mass index, waist circumference and waist : hip ratio as predictors of cardiovascular risk–a review of the literature. *European Journal of Clinical Nutrition* 64: 16-22, 2010.

61. **Institute of Medicine.** *Dietary Reference Intakes for Calcium and Vitamin D.* Washington, D.C.: National Academy of Sciences, 2010.

62. **Institute of Medicine.** *Dietary Reference Intakes for Water, Potassium, Sodium, Chloride, and Sulfate.* Washington, D.C.: National Academies Press, 2004.

63. **Institute of Medicine.** *Dietary Reference Intakes for Energy, Carbohydrate, Fiber, Fat, Fatty Acids, Cholesterol, Protein, and Amino Acids.* Washington, D.C.: National Academies Press, 2002.

64. **Irwin ML, Yasui Y, Ulrich CM, Bowen D, Rudolph RE, Schwartz RS, et al.** Effect of exercise on total and intra-abdominal body fat in postmenopausal women: a randomized controlled trial. *JAMA* 289: 323-330, 2003.

65. **Jackson AS and Pollock ML.** Generalized equations for predicting body density of men. *British Journal of Nutrition* 40: 497-504, 1978.

66. **Jackson AS and Pollock ML.** Practical assessment of body composition. *Physician and Sportsmedicine* 13: 76-90, 1985.

67. **Jackson AS, Pollock ML, and Ward A.** Generalized equations for predicting body density of women. *Medicine and Science in Sports and Exercise* 12: 175-181, 1980.

68. **Jensen MD, Ryan DH, Apovian CM, Ard JD, Comuzzie AG, Donato KA, et al.** 2013 AHA/ACC/TOS guideline for management of overweight and obesity in adults: a report of the American College of Cardiology/American Heart Association Task Force on Practice Guidelines and The Obesity Society. *Circulation.* Published online before print November 12, 2013, doi: 10.1161/ 01.cir.0000437739.71477.ee.

69. **Johnston FE and Malina RM.** Age changes in the composition of the upper arm in Philadelphia children. *Human Biology: An International Record of Research* 38: 1-21, 1966.

70. **Jones DW.** Dietary sodium and blood pressure. *Hypertension* 43: 932-935, 2004.

71. **Jung RT, Shetty PS, James WP, Barrand MA, and Callingham BA.** Reduced thermogenesis in obesity. *Nature* 279: 322-323, 1979.

72. **Katch FI.** Assessment of lean body tissues by radiography and bioelectrical impedance. In *Body-Composition Assessment in Youths and Adults,* edited by Roche AF. Columbus, OH: Ross Laboratories, 1985.

73. **Keys A.** *The Biology of Human Starvation.* Minneapolis, MN: The University of Minnesota Press, 1950.

74. **Knittle JL.** Obesity in childhood: a problem in adipose tissue cellular development. *Journal of Pediatrics* 81: 1048-1059, 1972.

75. **Kris-Etherton P, Daniels SR, Eckel RH, Engler M, Howard BV, Krauss RM, et al.** Summary of the scientific conference on dietary fatty acids and cardiovascular health: conference summary from the Nutrition Committee of the American Heart Association. *Circulation* 103: 1034-1039, 2001.

76. **Kristo AS, Matthan NR, and Lichtenstein AH.** Effects of diets differing in glycemic index and glycemic load on cardiovascular risk factors: review of randomized controlled feeding trials *Nutrients* 5: 1071-1080, 2013.

77. **Lane MD and Cha SH.** Effect of glucose and fructose on food intake via malonyl-CoA signaling in the brain. *Biochemical and Biophysical Research Communications* 382: 1-5, 2009.

78. **Lapidus L, Bengtsson C, Larsson B, Pennert K, Rybo E, and Sjostrom L.** Distribution of adipose tissue and risk of cardiovascular disease and death: a 12 year follow up of participants in the population study of women in Gothenburg, Sweden. *British Medical Journal (Clinical Research Ed)* 289: 1257-1261, 1984.

79. **Larsson B, Svardsudd K, Welin L, Wilhelmsen L, Bjorntorp P, and Tibblin G.** Abdominal adipose tissue distribution, obesity, and risk of cardiovascular disease and death: 13 year follow up of participants in the study of men born in 1913. *British Medical Journal (Clinical Research Ed)* 288: 1401-1404, 1984.

80. **Lee P, Swarbrick MM, and Ho KKY.** Brown adipose tissue in adult humans: a metabolic renaissance. *Endocrine Reviews* 34: 413-438, 2013.

81. **Leibel RL, Hirsch J, Appel BE, and Checani GC.** Energy intake required to maintain body weight is not affected by wide variation in diet composition. *American Journal of Clinical Nutrition* 55: 350-355, 1992.

82. **Lohman T, Houtkooper LB, and Going S.** Body fat measurement goes high-tech. *ACSM's Health & Fitness Journal* 1: 30-35, 1997.

83. **Lohman TG.** *Advances in Body Composition Assessment.* Champaign, IL: Human Kinetics, 1992.

84. **Lohman TG.** Applicability of body composition techniques and constants for children and youths. In *Exercise and Sport Sciences Reviews,* edited by Pandolf KB. New York, NY: Macmillan, 1986, pp. 325-357.

85. **Lohman TG.** Body composition methodology in sports medicine. *Physician and Sportsmedicine* 10: 47- 58, 1982.

86. **Lohman TG and Going SB.** Multicomponent models in body composition research: opportunities and pitfalls. In *Human Body Composition,* edited by Ellis KJ, and Eastman JD. New York, NY: Plenum Press, 1993, pp. 53-58.

87. **Lohman TG, Slaughter MH, Boileau RA, Bunt J, and Lussier L.** Bone mineral measurements and their relation to body density in children, youth and adults. *Human Biology: An International Record of Research* 56: 667-679, 1984.

88. **Ma XY, Liu JP, and Songf ZY.** Glycemic load, glycemic index and risk of cardiovascular diseases: a meta-analysis of prospective studies. *Atherosclerosis.* 223: 491-496, 2012.

89. **Mazess RB, Barden HS, Bisek JP, and Hanson J.** Dual-energy x-ray absorptiometry for total-body and regional bone-mineral and soft-tissue composition. *American Journal of Clinical Nutrition* 51: 1106-1112, 1990.

90. **McTiernan A, Sorensen B, Irwin ML, Morgan A, Yasui Y, Rudolph RE, et al.** Exercise effect on weight and body fat in men and women. *Obesity* 15: 1496-1512, 2007.

91. **Metropolitan Life Insurance Company.** New weight standards for men and women. *Statistical Bulletin Metropolitan Life Insurance Company* 40: 1-4, 1959.

92. **Millard-Stafford ML, Collins MA, Evans EM, Snow TK, Cureton KJ, and Rosskopf LB.** Use of air displacement plethysmography for estimating body fat in a four-component model. *Medicine and Science in Sports and Exercise* 33: 1311-1317, 2001.

93. **Mirrahimi A, de Souza RJ, Chiavaroli L, Sievenpiper JL, Beyene J, Hanley AJ, et al.** Associations of glycemic index and load with coronary heart disease events: a systematic review and meta-analysis of prospective cohorts. *Journal of the American Heart Association* 1: e000752, 2012.

94. **Mole PA.** Impact of energy intake and exercise on resting metabolic rate. *Sports Medicine* 10: 72-87, 1990.

95. **Morrow JR, Jr., Jackson AS, Bradley PW, and Hartung GH.** Accuracy of measured and predicted residual lung volume on body density measurement. *Medicine & Science in Sports & Exercise* 18: 647-652, 1986.

96. **National Center for Health Statistics.** *Health, United States, 2012: With Special Feature on Emergency Care.* Hyattsville, MD.: National Center for Health Statistics, 2013, 205.

97. **National Institutes of Health.** *Bioelectrical impedance analysis in body composition measurement: NIH Technology Assessment Conference statement.* Bethesda, MD: National Institutes of Health, 1994.

98. **National Institutes of Health: National Heart, Lung, and Blood Institute.** *What causes overweight and obesity?* http://www.nhlbi.nih.gov/health/health-topics/topics/obe/causes#.

99. **National Institutes of Health.** Clinical guidelines on the identification, evaluation, and treatment of overweight and obesity in adults. *Obesity Research* 6 (Suppl 2), 1998.

100. **National Research Council.** *Recommended Dietary Allowances.* Washington, D.C.: National Academy Press, 1989.

101. **Nordmann AJ, Nordmann A, Briel M, Keller U, Yancy WS, Jr., Brehm BJ, et al.** Effects of low-carbohydrate vs low-fat diets on weight loss and cardiovascular risk factors: a meta-analysis of randomized controlled trials. *Archives of Internal Medicine* 166: 285-293, 2006.

102. **Ogden CL and Flegal KM.** Changes in terminology for childhood overweight and obesity. *National Health Statistics Reports.* No. 25, June 25, 2010.

103. **Ogden CL, Carroll MD, Curtin LR, Lamb MM, and Flegal KM.** Prevalence of high body mass index in US children and adolescents, 2007-2008. *JAMA* 303: 242-249, 2010.

104. **Ogden CL, Carroll MD, Curtin LR, McDowell MA, Tabak CJ, and Flegal KM.** Prevalence of overweight and obesity in the United States, 1999-2004. *JAMA* 295: 1549-1555, 2006.

105. **Ogden CL, Carroll MD, Kit BK, and Flegal KM.** Prevalence of obesity among adults: United States, 2011-2012. *NCHS Data Brief.* Number 131, October 2013.

106. **Ogden CL, Flegal KM, Carroll MD, and Johnson CL.** Prevalence and trends in overweight among US children and adolescents, 1999-2000. *JAMA* 288: 1728-1732, 2002.

107. **Passmore R.** Energy metabolism at various weights: man. Part II. Resting: adults. In *Metabolism: Clinical and Experimental*, edited by Altman PL, and Dittmer DS. Bethesda, MD: Federation of American Societies for Experimental Biology, 1968, pp. 344-345.

108. **Pietrobelli A, Heymsfield SB, Wang ZM, and Gallagher D.** Multi-component body composition models: recent advances and future directions. *European Journal of Clinical Nutrition* 55: 69-75, 2001.

109. **Poehlman ET.** A review: exercise and its influence on resting energy metabolism in man. *Medicine and Science in Sports and Exercise* 21: 515-525, 1989.

110. **Poehlman ET, Melby CL, and Goran MI.** The impact of exercise and diet restriction on daily energy expenditure. *Sports Medicine* 11: 78-101, 1991.

111. **Pollock ML and Wilmore JH.** *Exercise in Health and Disease.* Philadelphia, PA: W. B. Saunders, 1990.

112. **Presta E, Casullo AM, Costa R, Slonim A, and Van Itallie TB.** Body composition in adolescents: estimation by total body electrical conductivity. *J Appl Physiol* 63: 937-941, 1987.

113. **Qiao Q and Nyamdorj R.** Is the association of type II diabetes with waist circumference or waist : hip ratio stronger than that with body mass index? *European Journal of Clinical Nutrition* 64: 3-34, 2010.

114. **Rabkin SW, Mathewson FA, and Hsu PH.** Relation of body weight to development of ischemic heart disease in a cohort of young North American men after a 26 year observation period: the Manitoba Study. *American Journal of Cardiology* 39: 452-458, 1977.

115. **Ratamess N.** Body composition status and assessment. In *ACSM's Resource Manual for Guidelines for Exercise Testing and Prescription*, edited by Swain DP. Baltimore, MD: Lippincott Williams & Wilkins, 2014, pp. 287-308.

116. **Redman LM, Heilbronn LK, Martin CK, Alfonso A, Smith SR, and Ravussin E.** Effect of calorie restriction with or without exercise on body composition and fat distribution. *Journal of Clinical Endocrinology and Metabolism* 92: 865-872, 2007.

117. **Rimm AA and White, PL.** Obesity: its risks and hazards. In *Obesity in America*, edited by U.S. Department of Health EaWNIH. Publication No. 79-359, 1979.

118. **Rising R, Harper IT, Fontvielle AM, Ferraro RT, Spraul M, and Ravussin E.** Determinants of total daily energy expenditure: variability in physical activity. *American Journal of Clinical Nutrition* 59: 800-804, 1994.

119. **Ross R, Dagnone D, Jones PJ, Smith H, Paddags A, Hudson R, et al.** Reduction in obesity and related comorbid conditions after diet-induced weight loss or exercise-induced weight loss in men: randomized, controlled trial. *Ann Intern Med* 133: 92-103, 2000.

120. **Ross R, Freeman JA, and Janssen I.** Exercise alone is an effective strategy for reducing obesity and related comorbidities. *Exercise and Sport Sciences Reviews* 28: 165-170, 2000.

121. **Roust LR, Hammel KD, and Jensen MD.** Effects of isoenergetic, low-fat diets on energy metabolism in lean and obese women. *American Journal of Clinical Nutrition* 60: 470-475, 1994.

122. **Sacks FM, Bray GA, Carey VJ, Smith SR, Ryan DH, Anton SD, et al.** Comparison of weight-loss diets with different compositions of fat, protein and carbohydrates. *New England Journal of Medicine* 360: 859-873, 2009.

123. **Saely CH, Geiger K, and Drexel H.** Brown versus white adipose tissue: a mini-review. *Gerontology* 58: 15-23, 2012.

124. **Schoeller D.** Measurement of total body water: isotope dilution techniques. In *Body-Composition Assessment in Youths and Adults*, edited by Roche AF. Columbus, OH: Ross Laboratories, 1985, pp. 24-29.

125. **Schutte JE, Townsend EJ, Hugg J, Shoup RF, Malina RM, and Blomqvist CG.** Density of lean body mass is greater in blacks than in whites. *J Appl Physiol* 56: 1647-1649, 1984.

126. **Schutz Y.** Concept of fat balance in human obesity revisited with particular reference to *de novo* lipogenesis. *International Journal of Obesity* 28: S3-S11, 2004.

127. **Schwingshackl L and Hoffmann G.** Long-term effects of low glycemic index/load vs. high glycemic index/load diets on parameters of obesity and obesity-associated risks: a systematic review and meta-analysis. *Nutrition Metabolism and Cardiovascular Diseases.* 23: 699-706, 2013.

128. **Segal KR, Burastero S, Chun A, Coronel P, Pierson RN, Jr., and Wang J.** Estimation of extra-cellular and total body water by multiple-frequency bioelectrical-impedance measurement. *American Journal of Clinical Nutrition* 54: 26-29, 1991.

129. **Segal KR, Edano A, Blando L, and Pi-Sunyer FX.** Comparison of thermic effects of constant and relative caloric loads in lean and obese men. *American Journal of Clinical Nutrition* 51: 14-21, 1990.

130. **Segal KR, Gutin B, Presta E, Wang J, and Van Itallie TB.** Estimation of human body composition by electrical impedance methods: a comparative study. *Journal of Applied Physiology* 58: 1565-1571, 1985.

131. **Segal MS, Gollub E, and Johnson RJ.** Is the fructose index more relevant with regards to cardiovascular disease than the glycemic index? *European Journal of Nutrition* 46: 406-417, 2007.

132. **Seidell JC.** Waist circumference and waist/hip ratio in relation to all-cause mortality, cancer and sleep apnea. *European Journal of Clinical Nutrition* 64: 35-41, 2010.

133. **Sheard NF, Clark NG, Brand-Miller JC, Franz MJ, Pi-Sunyer FX, Mayer-Davis E, et al.** Dietary carbohydrate (amount and type) in the prevention and management of diabetes: a statement by the American Diabetes Association. *Diabetes Care* 27: 2266-2271, 2004.

134. **Sims EA, Danforth E, Jr., Horton ES, Bray GA, Glennon JA, and Salans LB.** Endocrine and metabolic effects of experimental obesity in man. *Recent Progress in Hormone Research* 29: 457-496, 1973.

135. **Sinning WE, Dolny DG, Little KD, Cunningham LN, Racaniello A, Siconolfi SF, et al.** Validity of "generalized" equations for body composition analysis in male athletes. *Medicine & Science in Sports & Exercise* 17: 124-130, 1985.

136. **Sinning WE and Wilson JR.** Validity of "generalized" equations for body composition analysis in women athletes. *Research Quarterly for Exercise Sport* 55: 153-160, 1984.

137. **Siri WE.** Body composition from fluid spaces and density: analysis of methods. In *Techniques for Measuring Body Composition,* edited by Brozek J, and Henschel A. Washington, D.C.: National Academy of Sciences, 1961, pp. 223-244.

138. **Sjöström LV.** Morbidity of severely obese subjects. *American Journal of Clinical Nutrition* 55: 508S-515S, 1992.

139. **Sjöström LV.** Mortality of severely obese subjects. *American Journal of Clinical Nutrition* 55: 516S-523S, 1992.

140. **Slentz CA, Duscha BD, Johnson JL, Ketchum K, Aiken LB, Samsa GP, et al.** Effects of the amount of exercise on body weight, body composition, and measures of central obesity: STRRIDE–a randomized controlled study. *Archives of Internal Medicine* 164: 31-39, 2004.

141. **Stefanick ML.** Exercise and weight control. *Exercise and Sport Sciences Reviews* 21: 363-396, 1993.

142. **Stevens J, Katz EG, and Huxley RR.** Associations between gender, age and waist circumference. *European Journal of Clinical Nutrition* 64: 6-15, 2010.

143. **Swinburn B and Ravussin E.** Energy balance or fat balance? *American Journal of Clinical Nutrition* 57: 766S-770S; discussion 770S-771S, 1993.

144. **Tataranni PA, Larson DE, Snitker S, and Ravussin E.** Thermic effect of food in humans: methods and results from use of a respiratory chamber. *American Journal of Clinical Nutrition* 61: 1013-1019, 1995.

145. **Thomas JG, Bond DS, Hill JO, and Wing RR.** The national weight control registry. *ACSM's Health & Fitness Journal* 15: 8-12, 2011.

146. **Thompson CA and Thompson PA.** Healthy lifestyle and cancer prevention. *ACSM's Health & Fitness Journal* 12: 18-26, 2008.

147. **Thompson DL.** Body composition. In *Fitness Professional's Handbook.* Eds. Howley ET and Thompson, DL. Champaign, IL: Human Kinetics, 2017.

148. **Thompson DL, Rakow J, and Perdue SM.** Relationship between accumulated walking and body composition in middle-aged women. *Medicine and Science in Sports and Exercise* 36: 911-914, 2004.

149. **Tremblay A.** Dietary fat and body weight set point. *Nutrition Reviews* 62: S75-77, 2004.

150. **U.S. Department of Agriculture.** What we eat in America, NHANES 2009-2010. http://www.ars.usda.gov/services/docs.htm?docid=13793.

151. **U.S. Department of Agriculture.** *Dietary Guidelines for Americans.* Washington, D.C.: U.S. Department of Agriculture, 2010.

152. **U.S. Department of Agriculture.** *Dietary Guidelines for Americans.* Washington, D.C.: U.S. Department of Agriculture, 2015-20.

153. **U.S. Department of Health and Human Services.** 2008 *Physical Activity Guidelines for Americans.* Washington, D.C.: U.S. Department of Health and Human Services, 2008.

154. **U.S. Senate Select Committee on Nutrition and Human Needs.** *Eating in America: Dietary Goals for the U.S.* Washington, D.C.: U.S. Government Printing Office, 1977.

155. **Van Itallie T.** Clinical assessment of body fat content in adults: potential role of electrical impedance methods. In *Body-Composition Assessment in Youths and Adults,* edited by Roche AF. Columbus, OH: Ross Laboratories, 1985, pp. 5-8.

156. **Van Itallie TB.** Conservative approaches to treatment. In *Obesity in America,* edited by Bray G. Department of Health, Education, and Welfare. NIH Publication No. 79-359, 1979.

157. **Van Loan MD, Keim NL, Berg K, and Mayclin PL.** Evaluation of body composition by dual energy x-ray absorptiometry and two different software packages. *Medicine & Science in Sports & Exercise* 27: 587-591, 1995.

158. **Van Marken Lichtenbelt WD, Westerterp KR, Wouters L, Luijendijk SC.** Validation of bioelectrical-impedance measurements as a method to estimate body-water compartments. *American Journal of Clinical Nutrition* 60: 159-166, 1994.

159. **Vasselli JR, Cleary MP, and Van Itallie TB.** Obesity. In *Nutrition Reviews' Present Knowledge in Nutrition.* Washington, D.C.: The Nutrition Foundation, 1984, pp. 35-36.

160. **Ward A, Pollock ML, Jackson AS, Ayres JJ, and Pape G.** A comparison of body fat determined by underwater weighing and volume displacement. *American Journal of Physiology* 234: E94-96, 1978.

161. **Wardlaw GM, Smith AM, and Collene AL.** *Contemporary Nutrition–A Functional Approach.* New York, NY: McGraw-Hill, 2013.

162. **Weinberger MH.** Sodium and blood pressure 2003. *Current Opinion in Cardiology* 19: 353-356, 2004.

163. **Weinsier RL, Schutz Y, and Bracco D.** Reexamination of the relationship of resting metabolic rate to fat-free mass and to the metabolically active components of fat-free mass in humans. *American Journal of Clinical Nutrition* 55: 790-794, 1992.

164. **Welk GJ and Meredith MD (eds).** FITNESSGRAM®/ACTIVITYGRAM® *Reference Guide* (3rd ed). Dallas, TX: The Cooper Institute, 2008.

165. **Williams MH.** *Nutrition for Health, Fitness, & Sport.* New York, NY: McGraw-Hill, 2010.

166. **Wilmore JH.** Body composition in sport and exercise: directions for future research. *Medicine & Science in Sports & Exercise* 15: 21-31, 1983.

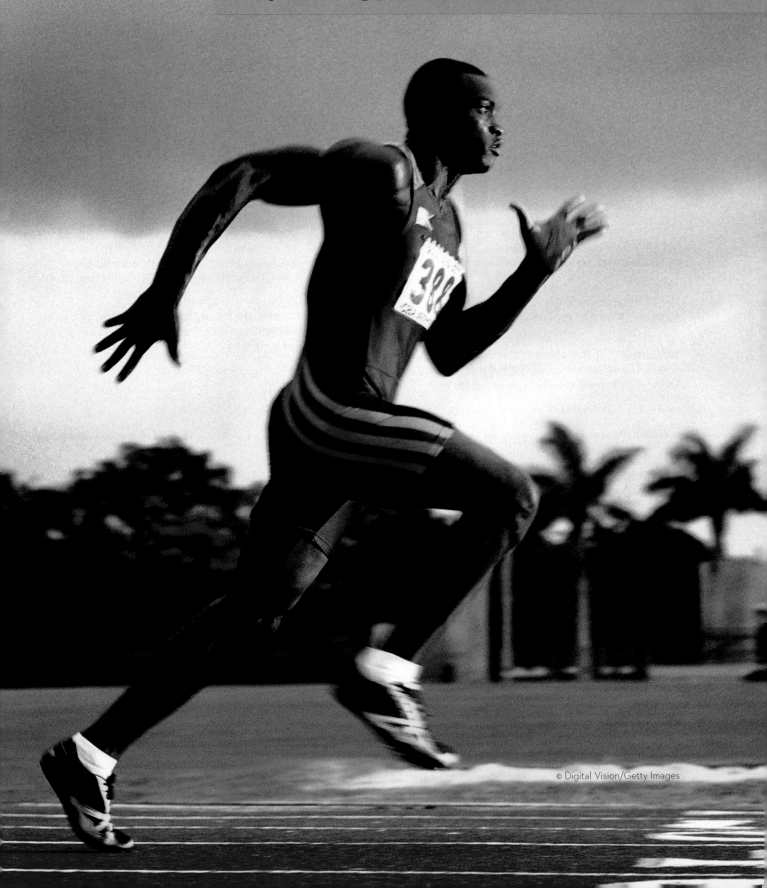

Physiology of Performance

© Digital Vision/Getty Images

Factors Affecting Performance

■ Objectives

By studying this chapter, you should be able to do the following:

1. Identify factors affecting maximal performance.
2. Provide evidence for and against the central nervous system being a site of fatigue.
3. Identify potential neural factors in the periphery that may be linked to fatigue.
4. Explain the role of cross-bridge cycling in fatigue.
5. Summarize the evidence on the order of recruitment of muscle fibers with increasing intensities of activity and the type of metabolism upon which each is dependent.

6. Describe the factors limiting performance in all-out activities lasting less than ten seconds.
7. Describe the factors limiting performance in all-out activities lasting 10–180 seconds.
8. Discuss the subtle changes in the factors affecting optimal performance as the duration of a maximal performance increases from three minutes to four hours.

■ Outline

■ Key Terms

central fatigue
peripheral fatigue
free radicals

In the last few chapters, we focused on proper exercise and nutrition for health and fitness. The emphasis was on *moderation* in both to reduce the risk factors associated with a variety of diseases. We must now change that focus to discuss the factors limiting physical performance.

Performance goals require much more time, effort, and risk of injury than fitness goals. What are the requirements for optimal performance? To answer this question, we must ask another: What kind of performance? It is clear that the requirements for the best performance in the 400-meter run are different from those associated with the marathon. Figure 19.1 shows a diagram of factors influencing performance (8). Every performance requires a certain amount of strength, as well as the "skill" to apply that strength in the best way. Further, energy must be supplied in the manner needed or performance will suffer. Different activities require differing amounts of energy from aerobic and anaerobic processes. Both the environment (altitude and heat) and diet (carbohydrate and water intake) play a role in endurance performance. In addition, best performances require a psychological commitment to "go for the gold." The purpose of this chapter is to expand on this diagram and discuss the factors limiting performance in a variety of activities, which will point the way to the remaining chapters. However, before we discuss these factors, we will summarize the potential sites of fatigue that would clearly affect performance.

SITES OF FATIGUE

Fatigue is simply defined as an inability to maintain a power output or force during repeated muscle contractions (28). As the two examples of the 400-meter run and the marathon suggest, the causes of fatigue vary and are usually specific to the type of physical activity. Figure 19.2 provides a summary of potential sites of fatigue (28). The discussion of mechanisms starts at the brain, where a variety of factors can influence the "will to win," and continues to the cross-bridges of the muscles themselves. There is evidence to support many of the sites listed in Fig. 19.2 as "weak links" in the development of the muscle tension needed for optimal performance. However, there is far from perfect agreement among scientists about the exact causes of fatigue. The reasons for this include (a) the fiber type and training state of the subject, (b) whether the muscle was stimulated voluntarily or electrically, (c) the use of both amphibian and mammalian muscle preparations, with some isolated from the body, and (d) the intensity and duration of the exercise and whether it was continuous or intermittent activity (61, 62). Table 19.1 provides a summary of the advantages and disadvantages of the various approaches scientists use to study fatigue (1). Clearly, depending on the nature of the exercise, the subject, and the experimental approach used to study fatigue, different results may be obtained. Within the scope of these limitations, we now provide a summary of the evidence about each weak link and apply the information to specific types of performances.

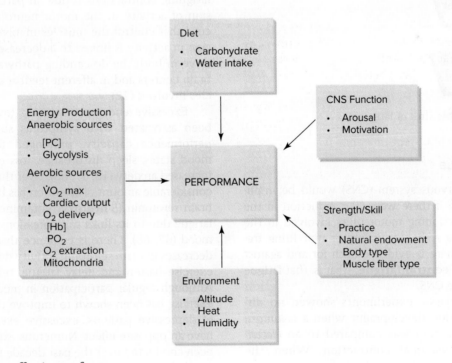

Figure 19.1 Factors affecting performance.

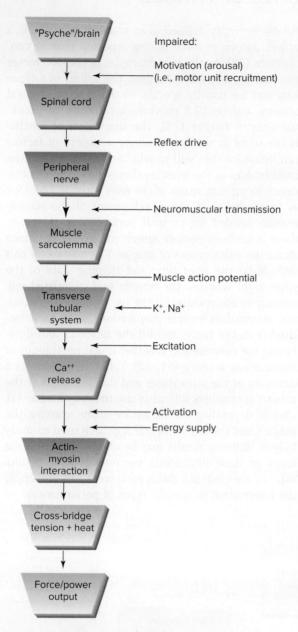

Possible Fatigue Mechanisms

"Psyche"/brain

Impaired:

Motivation (arousal)
(i.e., motor unit recruitment)

Spinal cord

Reflex drive

Peripheral nerve

Neuromuscular transmission

Muscle sarcolemma

Muscle action potential

Transverse tubular system

K^+, Na^+

Excitation

Ca^{++} release

Activation
Energy supply

Actin-myosin interaction

Cross-bridge tension + heat

Force/power output

Figure 19.2 Possible sites of fatigue.

Central Fatigue

The central nervous system (CNS) would be implicated in fatigue if there were (a) a reduction in the number of functioning motor units involved in the activity or (b) a reduction in motor unit firing frequency (20). There is evidence both for and against the concept of "**central fatigue**"–that is, that fatigue originates in the CNS.

Merton's classic experiments showed no difference in tension development when a *voluntary* maximal contraction was compared to an *electrically induced* maximal contraction. When the muscle was fatigued by voluntary contractions,

electrical stimulation could not restore tension (48). This suggested that the CNS was not limiting performance, and that the "periphery" was the site of fatigue.

In contrast, the early work of Ikai and Steinhaus (32) showed that a simple shout during exertion could increase what was formerly believed to be "maximal" strength. Later work showed that electrical stimulation of a muscle fatigued by voluntary contractions resulted in an increase in tension development (33). These studies suggest that the upper limit of voluntary strength is "psychologically" set, given that certain motivational or arousal factors are needed to achieve a physiological limit (33). In agreement with these results (that the CNS can limit performance) are two studies by Asmussen and Mazin (6, 7). Their subjects lifted weights 30 times a minute, causing fatigue in two to three minutes. Following a two-minute pause, the lifting continued. These investigators showed that when either a physical diversion, consisting of the contraction of nonfatigued muscles, or a mental diversion, consisting of doing mental arithmetic, was used between fatiguing bouts of exercise, work output was greater than when nothing was done during the pause. They also found that if a person did a series of muscle contractions to the point of fatigue with the eyes closed, simply opening the eyes restored tension (6). These studies suggest that alterations in central nervous system "arousal" can facilitate motor unit recruitment to increase strength and alter the state of fatigue. There is convincing evidence that impairment of the voluntary activation of muscle during fatiguing contractions is due, in part, to the depression of activity in the motor neurons of the spinal cord that control the muscles involved. The depression in activity is linked to a decrease in stimulatory drive in both the descending pathways from higher brain centers and in afferent feedback from the muscles involved (22).

Excessive endurance training (overtraining) has been associated with symptoms such as reduced performance capacity, prolonged fatigue, altered mood states, sleep disturbance, loss of appetite, and increased anxiety (18, 67, 68). Over the past decade, a considerable amount of attention has been directed at brain serotonin (5-hydroxytryptamine) as a factor in fatigue due to its links to depression, sleepiness, and mood (67, 68). There is evidence that increases and decreases in brain serotonin activity during prolonged exercise hasten and delay fatigue, respectively (17). Although regular participation in moderate-intensity exercise has been shown to improve the mood states of depressive patients, excessive exercise seems to have an opposite effect. Numerous experiments have been conducted over the past decade to try to understand the connection between serotonin and fatigue,

Muscle in vivo	Advantages	All physiological mechanisms present Fatigue can be central or peripheral All types of fatigue can be studied Stimulation patterns appropriate for fiber types and stage of fatigue
	Disadvantages	Mixture of fiber types Complex activation patterns Produces correlative data; hard to identify mechanisms Experimental interventions very limited
Isolated muscle	Advantages	Central fatigue eliminated Dissection simple
	Disadvantages	Mixture of fiber types Inevitable extracellular gradients of O_2, CO_2, K^+, lactic acid Mechanisms of fatigue biased by presence of extracellular gradients Drugs cannot be applied rapidly because of diffusion gradients
Isolated single fiber	Advantages	Only one fiber type present Force and other changes (ionic, metabolic) can be unequivocally correlated Fluorescent measurements of ions, metabolites, membrane potential, etc., possible Easy and rapid application of extracellular drugs, ions, metabolites, etc.
	Disadvantages	Environment different to in vivo K^+ accumulation and other in vivo changes absent Prone to damage at physiological temperatures Small size makes analysis of metabolites difficult
Skinned fiber	Advantages	Precise solutions can be applied Possible to study myofibrillar properties, SR release and uptake, AP/Ca^{2+} release coupling Metabolic and ionic changes associated with fatigue can be studied in isolation
	Disadvantages	Relevance to fatigue can be questionable May lose important intracellular constituents Relevant metabolites to study must be identified in other systems

but the answer remains elusive (67, 68). However, recent studies indicate that it is not the serotonin alone, but the ratio of serotonin to dopamine that contributes to tiredness on the one hand and arousal on the other, and that brain levels of norepinephrine also contribute to the picture (45, 46).

The CNS is intimately involved in exercise, including the psyching-up prior to exercise (70), the recruitment of motor units, and the continual feedback from a host of receptors sensing tension, temperature, blood gases, blood pressure, and other variables. The brain integrates these various signals and generates commands that automatically reduce power output to protect the organism. In this sense, exercise begins and ends in the brain (35). Noakes and others (37, 53–55, 65) have developed the "central governor" model of central fatigue that focuses primarily on the conscious and subconscious brain and does not involve the spinal cord or motor unit. This model has many novel aspects, but it has attracted some criticism (74). Let us now examine some of the events outside the CNS that are tied to the fatigue process.

Peripheral Fatigue

Although there is evidence that the CNS is linked to fatigue, its contribution is estimated to be about 10% (26). The vast majority of evidence points to the periphery (**peripheral fatigue**), where neural, mechanical, or energetic events can hamper tension development (23, 75).

Neural Factors If you are looking for potential sites of fatigue, you might track the movement of the action potential from the nerve to the muscle and, within the muscle, its progress along the sarcolemma and t-tubule to the sarcoplasmic reticulum (SR) where Ca^{++} is stored. When the Ca^{++} is released, it interacts with regulatory proteins (e.g., troponin) that cause movement of the cross-bridges to generate tension. Finally, the Ca^{++} must be pumped back into the SR to allow the muscle to relax before the next contraction. Let's take a look at the evidence to see if any of these sites is implicated in the fatigue process.

Neuromuscular Junction
The action potential appears to reach the neuromuscular junction even when fatigue occurs (48). In addition, evidence based on simultaneous measurements of electrical activity at the neuromuscular junction and in the individual muscle fibers suggests that the neuromuscular junction is not the site of fatigue (12, 26).

Sarcolemma and Transverse Tubules
It has been hypothesized that the sarcolemma might be the site of fatigue due to its inability to maintain Na^+ and K^+ concentrations during repeated stimulation. When the Na^+/K^+ pump cannot keep up, K^+ accumulates outside the membrane and decreases inside the cell. This results in a depolarization of the cell and a reduction in action potential amplitude (63). The gradual depolarization of the sarcolemma could result in altered t-tubule function, including a block of the t-tubule action potential. If the latter occurs, Ca^{++} release from the SR will be affected, as will muscle contraction (3). However, the evidence indicates that the typical reduction in the size of the action potential amplitude has little effect on force output by the muscle. In addition, the lower frequency of action potential firing with repeated stimulation of muscle seems to protect the muscle from further fatigue (rather than cause fatigue) by shifting the activation to a lower, more optimal, rate of firing (23). This does not mean that the t-tubule is not involved in the fatigue process. Under certain stimulation conditions an action potential block can occur in the t-tubule, leading to a reduction in Ca^{++} release from the SR (23, 26, 29). As a result, myosin cross-bridge activation would be adversely affected. One of the beneficial effects of training is an increase in the capacity of the Na^+/K^+ pump, which may contribute to the maintenance of the Na^+/K^+ gradient and reduce the potential for fatigue via this mechanism (26, 29).

IN SUMMARY

- Increases in CNS arousal facilitate motor unit recruitment to increase strength and alter the state of fatigue.
- Repeated stimulation of the sarcolemma can result in a reduction in the size and frequency of action potentials; however, shifts in the optimal frequency needed for muscle activation preserve force output.
- Under certain conditions, an action potential block can occur in the t-tubule to result in a reduction in Ca^{++} release from the SR.

Mechanical Factors
The primary mechanical factor that may be related to fatigue is cross-bridge "cycling." The action of the cross-bridge depends on (a) the functional arrangement of actin and myosin, (b) Ca^{++} being available to bind with troponin to allow the cross-bridge to bind with the active site on actin, and (c) ATP, which is needed for both the activation of the cross-bridge to cause movement and the dissociation of the cross-bridge from actin. Exercise, especially eccentric exercise, can cause a physical disruption of the sarcomere and reduce the capacity of the muscle to produce tension (5). However, a high H^+ concentration, which generally occurs with heavy exercise, may contribute to fatigue in a variety of ways (23, 24, 27, 61, 62):

- Reduce the force per cross-bridge
- Reduce the force generated at a given Ca^{++} concentration (related to H^+ ion interference with Ca^{++} binding to troponin)
- Inhibit SR Ca^{++} release

Consistent with this, data from skinned muscle fibers studied at room temperature (~20°C) showed that an increase in the H^+ concentration was linked to a decrease in force and the maximal velocity of shortening. However, when experiments in both skinned and intact muscle fibers were done at 30°C (a more physiological temperature), the acidosis decreased force by only 10% and did not accelerate the rate of fatigue. The latter results are consistent with data from exercising humans in which force recovered before the H^+ concentration did (57).

One sign of fatigue in isometric contractions is a longer "relaxation time"–the time from peak tension development to baseline tension. This appears to be an important aspect of fatigue in fast-twitch fibers. This longer relaxation time could be due to a slowing of the SR's ability to pump Ca^{++} and/or to slowing of cross-bridge cycling, but the latter appears to be most important (57). This longer relaxation time would result in a reduction in stride rate, a feature of fatigue in 400-m races (57). Although H^+ is implicated in this longer relaxation time, the accumulation of inorganic phosphate (P_i) from the breakdown of ATP is also involved (26). That is where we will now turn our attention.

IN SUMMARY

- The cross-bridge's ability to "cycle" is important in continued tension development. Fatigue may be related, in part, to the effect of a high H^+ concentration and the inability of the sarcoplasmic reticulum to rapidly take up Ca^{++}. The end result may be a longer relaxation time, which affects the rate of muscle contraction.

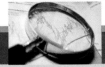

Radical Production During Exercise Contributes to Muscle Fatigue

Free radicals (radicals) are molecules that contain an unpaired electron in their outer orbital. This unpaired electron results in molecular instability; therefore, radicals are highly reactive and capable of damaging proteins, lipids, and DNA in the cell (30). Radical-mediated damage to cellular constituents is called oxidative stress, and high levels of oxidative stress can lead to cellular dysfunction.

Interestingly, although regular exercise provides many health benefits, exercise promotes the production of radicals in skeletal muscles, and prolonged and/or intense exercise can lead to oxidative stress in the exercising muscle. Importantly, this exercise-induced oxidative damage is a key contributor to muscle fatigue during prolonged exercise (i.e., >30 minutes' duration) (39, 40, 44).

The mechanism(s) to explain why radicals promote muscle fatigue remains an active topic of research. Cur-rent evidence indicates that radical production can contribute to muscle fatigue in two important ways. First, radicals can damage key contractile proteins including myosin and troponin (14). Damage to these muscle proteins reduces the calcium sensitivity of myofilaments and limits the number of myosin cross-bridges bound to actin (64). It follows that when fewer myosin cross-bridges are bound to actin, muscle force production is reduced (i.e., fatigue occurs). A second mechanism to explain how radicals can contribute to muscle fatigue is that high radical production can depress sodium/potassium pump activity in skeletal muscle (40). Impaired sodium/potassium pump function results in problems in achieving fiber excitation-contraction coupling, which impairs force production (40).

Because radicals contribute to muscle fatigue, it is feasible that antioxidant supplementation can re-tard exercise-induced muscle fatigue. Nonetheless, studies using antioxidant vitamins (e.g., vitamins E and C) do not support the concept that dietary antioxidants can improve human performance (59). In contrast, experiments using the powerful antioxidant N-acetyl-cysteine reveal that this unique antioxidant can delay fatigue during prolonged submaximal exercise (40, 43). Although optimal levels of this antioxidant can postpone fatigue, high doses of antioxidants (i.e., above the optimal dose) can impair muscle performance (15). Further, daily supplementation with high doses of antioxidants (e.g., vitamins C and E) has been reported to depress training-induced adaptations in skeletal muscles (47). Therefore, indiscriminant antioxidant supplementation could be detrimental to athletic performance. For more details about the role that free radicals play in muscle fatigue, see Cheng et al. in Suggested Readings.

Energetics of Contraction Fatigue can be viewed as the result of a simple imbalance between the ATP requirements of a muscle and its ATP-generating capacity (62). As described in Chap. 3, when exercise begins and the need for ATP accelerates, a series of ATP-generating reactions occur to replenish the ATP.

- As the cross-bridges use ATP and generate ADP, phosphocreatine provides for the immediate resynthesis of the ATP (PC + ADP → ATP + C).

- As the phosphocreatine becomes depleted, ADP begins to accumulate and the myokinase reaction occurs to generate ATP (ADP + ADP → ATP + AMP).

- The accumulation of all these products stimulates glycolysis to generate additional ATP, which may result in an H^+ accumulation (9).

However, as ATP demand continues to exceed supply, a variety of reactions occur in the cell that limit work and protect the cell from damage. Remember that ATP is needed to pump ions and maintain cell structure. In this sense, fatigue serves a protective function. What are the signals to the muscle cell that energy utilization must slow down? When ATP-generating mechanisms cannot keep up with ATP use, inorganic phosphate (P_i) begins to accumulate in the cell (P_i and ADP are not being converted to ATP). An increase in P_i in the muscle has been shown to inhibit maximal force, and the higher the P_i concentration, the lower the force measured during recovery from fatigue. The P_i seems to act directly on the cross-bridges to reduce its binding to actin (23, 24, 42, 57, 73) and also inhibits calcium release from the sarcoplasmic reticulum (2, 19, 26, 57). However, the accumulation of P_i reduces the total ATP cost per unit of force, suggesting an improvement in efficiency (42). What is interesting is that the cell does not run out of ATP, even in cases of extreme fatigue. Typically, the ATP concentration falls to only 70% of its pre-exercise level. The factors that cause fatigue reduce the rate of ATP utilization faster than ATP generation so that ATP concentration is maintained. This is believed to be a protective function aimed at minimizing changes in cellular homeostasis with continued stimulation. Other novel factors may be related to fatigue (see A Closer Look 19.1).

In Chap. 8, we linked the different methods of ATP production to the different muscle fiber types that are recruited during activity. We will briefly summarize this information as it relates to our discussion of fatigue. Figure 19.3 shows the pattern of recruitment of muscle fiber types with increasing intensities of exercise. Up to about 40% of $\dot{V}O_2$ max, the type I slow-twitch oxidative muscle fiber is recruited to provide tension development (62). This fiber type is dependent on a continuous supply of blood to provide the oxygen needed for the generation of ATP from carbohydrates and fats. Any factor limiting the oxygen supply to this fiber type (e.g., altitude, dehydration, blood loss, or anemia) would cause a reduction in tension development in these fibers and necessitate the recruitment of type IIa fibers to generate tension.

Between 40% and 75% $\dot{V}O_2$ max, type IIa fast-twitch, fatigue-resistant fibers are recruited in addition to the type I fibers (62). These fast-twitch fibers are rich in mitochondria, as are the type I fibers, making them dependent on oxygen delivery for tension development. They also have a great capacity to produce ATP via anaerobic glycolysis. The mitochondrial

content of type IIa fibers is sensitive to endurance training, so that with detraining, more of the ATP supply would be provided by glycolysis, leading to lactate production (see Chap. 13). If oxygen delivery to this fiber type is decreased, or if the ability of the fiber to use oxygen is decreased (due to low mitochondrial number), tension development will fall, requiring type IIx fiber recruitment to maintain tension.

Type IIx is the fast-twitch muscle fiber with a low mitochondrial content. This fiber can generate great tension via anaerobic sources of energy, but it fatigues quickly. It is recruited at about 75% $\dot{V}O_2$ max, adding to the tension from type I and type IIa fibers and making heavy exercise dependent upon its ability to develop tension (62).

Both Central and Peripheral Fatigue

In the preceding section a variety of metabolites generated by working muscles (e.g., H^+, Pi) were implicated in fatigue because of their effect on force development at the periphery (i.e., reduced force generated per cross bridge). However, these same metabolites may be implicated in central fatigue. As you may recall from Chaps. 9 and 10, skeletal muscle contains group III/IV afferent (sensory) nerve fibers, the ends of which can sense both mechanical (e.g., force) and chemical (e.g., H^+) stimuli. Consequently, information about contractile events at the periphery is sent back to the central nervous system (CNS), at both the spinal and supraspinal levels, where motor neuron activation can be modified. Under usual circumstances, the type III/IV fibers are crucial to having a normal cardiorespiratory and hemodynamic response to exercise—as described in Chaps. 9 and 10. However, when the concentration of the various metabolites associated with muscle contraction increases to very high levels, feedback from type III/IV fibers to the CNS can lead to the inhibition of motor unit recruitment—an example of central fatigue. This, of course, would lead to a reduction in muscle force production and performance (4).

Although the primary focus of this text has been on the fitness and performance of individuals stuck (by gravity) on the earth, we are all familiar with the weakness and instability of astronauts as they emerge from

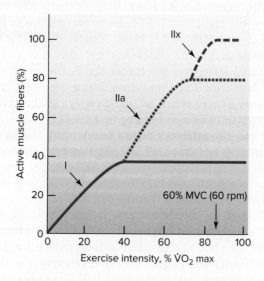

Figure 19.3 Order of muscle fiber type recruitment in exercise of increasing intensity.

McArdle, W., Katch, F., and Katch, V., *Exercise Physiology: Energy, Nutrition, and Human Performance.* Baltimore, MD: Lippincott Williams & Wilkins, 2001.

Muscle Adaptations to Space Travel: Questions and Answers with Dr. Robert H. Fitts

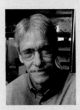

Courtesy of Robert H. Fitts

Dr. Fitts is Professor Emeritus in the Department of Biological Sciences at Marquette University. His primary research interests include excitation contraction coupling and muscle mechanics, and the mechanism of muscle adaptation to space flight and programs of regular exercise. His research also focuses on elucidating the cellular causes of muscle fatigue. He was awarded the American College of Sports Medicine's Citation Award in 1999 for his research accomplishments and received the Researcher of the Year Award from Marquette University in 2000.

QUESTION: What changes occur in skeletal muscle due to space travel?

ANSWER: The primary change in skeletal muscle with space travel is fiber atrophy due to a selective loss in the myofilaments. The antigravity muscles of the legs are more affected than arm muscles, and primarily slow muscles like the soleus are more affected than fast-twitch muscles such as the gastrocnemius. Due to the loss of myofilaments, muscle fibers generate less force and power. Following short-duration (≤3 weeks) space flight, slow type I fibers show an elevated maximal shortening velocity, which is not caused by an expression of fast-type myosin. It has been hypothesized that the increased velocity results from a selective loss of the thin filament actin, which increases the space between the filaments, causing the myosin cross-bridge to detach sooner at the end of the power stroke. Recent results from International Space Station (ISS) experiments have shown the elevated velocity to be a transient change, with slow fiber velocity showing a significant decline following long-duration flights. This change, plus additional fiber atrophy, contributes to the considerably greater loss in slow fiber power after long-duration flights, compared to short-duration flights. Space flight appears to increase the muscle's reliance on carbohydrates and reduce its ability to oxidize fats. This metabolic change is not caused by a reduced activity of any of the enzymes of the β-oxidative pathway or the Krebs cycle. The loss in fiber power and increased reliance on carbohydrates cause a reduced work capacity. In addition, post-flight crew members experience muscle soreness due to an increased susceptibility to eccentric contraction-induced fiber damage.

QUESTION: Do animal studies mimic the changes experienced by humans?

ANSWER: Many of the space flight-induced changes in skeletal muscle are observed in rodents, nonhuman primates, and humans. Fiber atrophy caused by the selective loss of myofilaments has been observed in all species. However, there are species differences in the time course of the adaptive process. For example, rats flown in space show a faster rate of fiber atrophy than do humans. Flights as short as two or three weeks have been shown to increase soleus muscle velocity in both rats, and humans, but in rats, the increase was in part due to a conversion of approximately 20% of the slow type I fibers to fast-twitch fibers containing fast myosin isozymes. In humans, short-duration space flight does not cause fiber type conversion. However, recent data suggest that such conversions (slow-twitch to fast-twitch) do occur in humans following long-duration (six months) space flight.

QUESTION: Are there any intervention (training) strategies being employed to reduce the impact of space flight on skeletal muscle?

ANSWER: The primary countermeasure used to protect skeletal muscle from microgravity-induced loss has employed endurance exercise on either a bicycle or treadmill. This type of modality has not been completely successful, as crew members still lose up to 20% of their leg muscle mass following six months in space. High-intensity exercise has been incorporated into the countermeasure program on the ISS, but the loads have been insufficient to adequately protect limb muscle size or power. Recently, a new high-resistance device has been installed on the ISS, but its effectiveness has not yet been established. (Readers are directed to two articles by Dr. Fitts on the effects of space flight on muscle structure and function in Suggested Readings.)

the Space Shuttle after returning from space. With the International Space Station (ISS) now in orbit and crews rotating on a regular basis, it should be no surprise that physiologists have been studying the impact of prolonged weightlessness on muscle function (25). Ask the Expert 19.1 provides some insights into why astronauts are weaker when they return to earth.

IN SUMMARY

- Metabolites such as H$^+$ and Pi, generated by muscle contraction, can reach levels that can reflexively reduce motor unit recruitment and cause fatigue through the action of type III/IV afferent nerve fibers.

FACTORS LIMITING ALL-OUT ANAEROBIC PERFORMANCES

As exercise intensity increases, muscle fiber recruitment progresses from type I → type IIa → type IIx. This means that the ATP supply needed for tension development becomes more and more dependent upon anaerobic metabolism (62). In this way, fatigue is specific to the type of task undertaken. If a task requires only type I fiber recruitment, then the factors limiting performance will be very different from those associated with tasks requiring type IIx fibers. With this review and summary in mind, let's now examine the factors limiting performance.

Ultra Short-Term Performances (Ten Seconds or Less)

The events that fit into this category include the shot put, high jump, long jump, and 50- and 100-meter sprints. These events require that tremendous amounts of energy be produced in a short period (high-power events), and type II muscle fibers must be recruited. Figure 19.4 shows that maximal performance is limited by the fiber type distribution (type I versus type II) and by the number of muscle fibers recruited, which is influenced by the level of motivation and arousal (32). Optimal performance is also affected by skill and technique, which are dependent on practice. It should be no surprise that the anaerobic sources of ATP–the ATP-PC system and glycolysis–provide the energy. However, in these ultra-short events, the energy release necessary for performance is determined primarily by the demand generated via neuromuscular drive, and is not limited by the intramuscular energy supply (13). Chapter 20 provides tests for anaerobic power, and Chap. 21 provides a detailed list of the activities dependent upon such

power. There is evidence that ingestion of creatine can influence performance in high-power exercise; see Chap. 25 for details.

IN SUMMARY

- In events lasting ten seconds or less, optimal performance is dependent on the recruitment of appropriate type II fibers to generate the great forces that are needed.
- Motivation and arousal are required, as well as the skill needed to direct the force.
- The primary energy sources are anaerobic, with the focus on phosphocreatine.

Short-Term Performances (10–180 Seconds)

Maximal performances in the 10- to 60-second range are still predominantly (>70%) anaerobic, using the high-force, fast-twitch fiber, but when a maximal performance is extended to three minutes, about 60% of the energy comes from the slower aerobic, ATP-generating processes. As a result of this transition from anaerobic to aerobic energy production, maximal running speed decreases as the duration of the race increases from 10 to 180 seconds. Given that the ATP-PC system can supply ATP for only several seconds, the vast majority of the ATP will be derived from anaerobic glycolysis (see Chap. 3). Figure 19.5 shows that this will cause an accumulation of H^+ in muscle as well as blood. The elevated H^+ concentration may actually interfere with the continued production of ATP via glycolysis, or the contractile machinery itself, by interfering with troponin's ability to bind with Ca^{++}. However, it must be added that following exhausting exercise, muscle tension recovers before the H^+ concentration does, indicating the complex nature of the fatigue process (27, 60, 61, 71). In an effort to slow H^+ accumulation, some athletes have attempted to ingest buffers prior to a

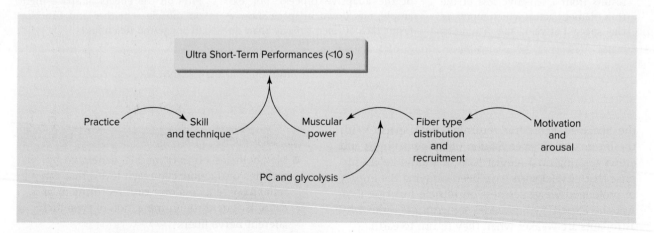

Figure 19.4 Factors affecting fatigue in ultra short-term events.

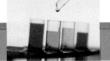
Brenda Bigland-Ritchie, Ph.D.

Brenda Bigland-Ritchie has had a major impact on our understanding of muscle, with a special focus on how it functions and what causes it to fatigue. Brenda Bigland completed her undergraduate degree at University College London, and was awarded a fellowship to work in the Physiology Department from which she had just graduated. As a graduate student she was encouraged by Nobel Prize winner A.V. Hill (see Chap. 0) to examine the oxygen cost of doing positive and negative work in humans, to parallel the experiments he had done in shortening and lengthening contractions in isolated muscle in which heat production was shown to be dramatically different for the two types of contractions. In a very clever design Brenda Bigland, Murdoch Ritchie (her future husband), and Bud Abbott arranged two bicycles back to back such that one rider pedaled forward and one pedaled backward; the same muscles were involved, but one muscle group was being lengthened while the other was being shortened. They showed, in a now classic study published in 1952, that positive work (shortening) required much more energy than negative work at the same power output, confirming Hill's observations in isolated muscle. She also published papers on the relationship between muscle force, velocity and integrated electromyographic (IEMG) activity measured with electrodes on the skin surface, and in other experiments, motor unit activity during voluntary contractions in human muscle. Bigland-Ritchie stepped away from doing her own research for about 20 years, after her first child was born in 1953. In 1956, her husband accepted a position at the Albert Einstein College of Medicine in the Bronx, N.Y., and the family immigrated to the United States. Later, when her children were of high school age, she was concerned that she could never return to science because she had been away from it for so long. Her husband encouraged her to work part-time in his lab and over the next few years they published three papers together. She then accepted a position at Hunter College to teach one section of a physiology course, and found that she not only enjoyed the teaching, but that she could learn as well as any of her much younger students. With the encouragement of her husband, she returned to England to write her Ph.D. thesis on the basis of her research done years earlier; she discovered that by examining her old data in the light of recent experimental findings, new ideas began to emerge. She was awarded her Ph.D. in 1969.

After her husband accepted a position at Yale University, she joined the faculty at nearby Quinnipiac College. It was there that she and her colleague Joe Woods wrote and submitted an NIH research grant that was funded, and she was able to continue her research in muscle physiology. Using the positive-negative work model from her earlier work they showed that both IEMG activity and oxygen uptake were much lower during lengthening contractions (negative work) compared to positive work.

Bigland-Ritchie's research raised serious questions about the use of surface IEMG activity as a means to investigate muscle function and fatigue. She devised techniques using fine-wire electrodes to monitor EMG activity within muscle itself, in order to study motor unit activity during exercise and fatigue. Her focus of attention was on the various sites of fatigue: was it in the CNS, neuromuscular junction, or in muscle itself? Much of what we know about fatigue (summarized at the beginning of this chapter) was due to her research and that of her students and her many colleagues. For more on this interesting scientist, we encourage you to read the two chapters by Bigland-Ritchie and by Thomas et al. in Suggested Readings.

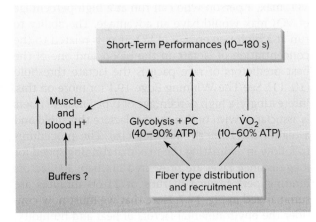

Figure 19.5 Factors affecting fatigue in short-term events.

race. This procedure is discussed in detail in Chap. 25, which deals with ergogenic aids and performance. See A Look Back, Important People in Science for information on someone who had a major impact on our understanding of fatigue.

IN SUMMARY

- In short-term performances lasting 10–180 seconds, there is a shift from 70% of the energy supplied anaerobically at 10 seconds to 60% being supplied aerobically at 180 seconds.
- Anaerobic glycolysis provides a substantial portion of the energy, resulting in elevated lactate levels.

FACTORS LIMITING ALL-OUT AEROBIC PERFORMANCES

As the duration of an all-out performance increases, more demand is placed on the aerobic sources of energy. In addition, environmental factors such as heat and humidity, and dietary factors such as water and carbohydrate ingestion, play a role in fatigue.

Moderate-Length Performances (3–20 Minutes)

Although 60% of ATP production is derived from aerobic processes in a 3-minute maximal effort, the value jumps to 90% in a 20-minute all-out performance. Given this dependence on oxidative energy production, the factors limiting performance include both the cardiovascular system, which delivers oxygen-rich blood to the muscles, and the mitochondrial content of the muscles involved in the activity. Because speed is a prerequisite in races lasting fewer than 20 minutes, type IIa fibers, which are rich in mitochondria, are involved in supplying the ATP aerobically (in addition to the already recruited type I fibers). Races lasting less than 20 minutes are run at 90%-100% of maximal aerobic power, so the athlete with the highest $\dot{V}O_2$ max has a distinct advantage. However, because type IIx fibers are also recruited, lactate and H^+ production are increased, and H^+ accumulation would affect tension development as previously described (27, 60, 61, 72). Figure 19.6 summarizes the factors affecting performances requiring a high maximal oxygen uptake. The maximal stroke volume is the crucial key to a high cardiac output (see Chap. 13) and is influenced by both genetics and training. The arterial oxygen content (CaO_2) is influenced by the arterial hemoglobin content [Hb], the fraction of inspired oxygen (FIO_2), and PO_2 of the inspired air. Chapter 24 discusses the effect of altitude (low PO_2) on $\dot{V}O_2$ max, and Chap. 25 discusses the use of blood doping (to raise the [Hb]) and oxygen breathing on aerobic performance. Training programs are discussed in Chap. 21.

IN SUMMARY

- In moderate-length performances lasting 3–20 minutes, aerobic metabolism provides 60%-90% of the ATP, respectively.
- These activities require an energy expenditure near $\dot{V}O_2$ max, with type II fibers being recruited in addition to the type I fibers.
- Any factor interfering with oxygen delivery (e.g., altitude or anemia) would decrease performance because it is so dependent on aerobic energy production. High levels of H^+ accompany these types of activities.

Intermediate-Length Performances (21–60 Minutes)

In all-out performances lasting 21-60 minutes, the athlete will generally work at <90% $\dot{V}O_2$ max. A high $\dot{V}O_2$ max is certainly a prerequisite for success, but now other factors come into play. For example, an individual who is an "economical" runner can move at a higher speed for the same amount of oxygen compared to a runner who is not economical. The importance of both $\dot{V}O_2$ max and running economy in predicting distance running performance was recently confirmed (41), and evidence exists that both are important in shorter (e.g., 1,500 m) races (34). Differences in running economy are due to biomechanical and/or bioenergetic factors. In this case, measurements of both $\dot{V}O_2$ max and running economy would be needed to predict performance (see Chap. 20). However, another variable must be considered. Because races of this duration are not run at $\dot{V}O_2$ max, a person who can run at a high percentage of $\dot{V}O_2$ max would have an advantage. The ability to run at a high percentage of $\dot{V}O_2$ max is related to the concentration of lactate in the blood, and one of the best predictors of race pace is the lactate threshold (10, 11). See The Winning Edge 19.1 for more on this. Interestingly, a high percentage of type I muscle fibers is associated with both a greater lactate threshold and a higher mechanical efficiency (16). The procedures to follow in estimating the maximal running speed for long-distance races are presented in Chap. 20. Factors limiting performance in runs of 21-60 minutes are summarized in Fig. 19.7. Note that we must now consider the environmental factors of heat and humidity, as well as the state of hydration of the runner. The heat load will require that a portion of the cardiac

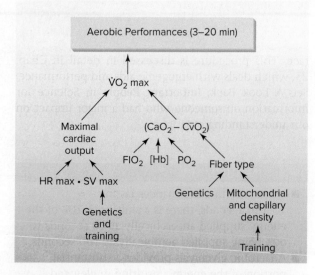

Figure 19.6 Factors affecting fatigue in aerobic performances lasting 3-20 minutes.

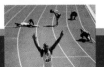

THE WINNING EDGE 19.1

Is Maximal Oxygen Uptake Important in Distance-Running Performance?

$\dot{V}O_2$ max is directly related to the rate of ATP generation that can be maintained during a distance race, even though it is not run at 100% $\dot{V}O_2$ max. The rate of ATP generation is dependent on the actual $\dot{V}O_2$ that can be maintained during the run (ml · kg^{-1} · min^{-1}), which is a function of the runner's $\dot{V}O_2$ max and the percent $\dot{V}O_2$ max at which the runner can perform. To run a 2:15 marathon, the runner would have to maintain a $\dot{V}O_2$ of about 60 ml · kg^{-1} · min^{-1} throughout the race. A runner working at 80% $\dot{V}O_2$ max would need a $\dot{V}O_2$ max of 75 ml · kg^{-1} · min^{-1}. In this way, the $\dot{V}O_2$ max sets the upper limit for energy production in endurance events, but does not determine the final performance. It is clear that both the percent of $\dot{V}O_2$ max that can be maintained over the course of the run (estimated by the lactate threshold) and running economy have a dramatic impact on the speed that can be maintained over distance (10, 11, 41). Interestingly, the progressive reduction in $\dot{V}O_2$ max with age appears to be the primary physiological mechanism associated with a reduction in the endurance performance of master athletes, along with the reduction in the velocity at the lactate threshold (69).

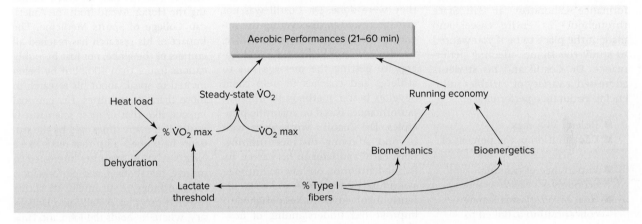

Figure 19.7   Factors affecting fatigue in aerobic performances lasting 21-60 minutes.

output be directed to the skin, pushing the cardiovascular system closer to maximum at any running speed. Chapters 23 and 24 deal with the effects of dehydration and environmental heat loads on performance. See A Look Back–Important People in Science for a physiologist who had a major role in discovering the factors linked to endurance performance.

IN SUMMARY

- Intermediate-length activities lasting 21–60 minutes are usually conducted at less than 90% $\dot{V}O_2$ max and are predominantly aerobic.
- Given the length of the activity, environmental factors such as heat, humidity, and the state of hydration of the subject play a role in the outcome.

Long-Term Performances (1–4 Hours)

Performances of 1-4 hours are clearly aerobic performances involving little anaerobic energy production. Using the shorter aerobic performances (60 minutes or less) as a lead-in, the longer the performance, the greater the chance that environmental factors will play a role in the outcome. In addition, for performances greater than one hour, the ability of the muscle and liver carbohydrate stores to supply glucose may be exceeded (see Chap. 23). Glucose supplementation during long-term performances provides the fuel needed not only for ATP generation for the cross-bridges, but also for the protection of muscle membrane excitability (66). As pointed out in Chap. 4, fatty acids can provide substantial fuel during prolonged muscular work at intensities <60% $\dot{V}O_2$ max. However, for the many endurance activities that are performed at higher exercise intensities (e.g., marathon running), muscle fibers must have carbohydrate to oxidize or performance will decline. Some have wondered if this same model could be used for predicting performance in "ultra" type performances (see A Closer Look 19.2). Chapter 23 provides information about the optimal dietary strategies for performance in long-term events, including the consumption of fluids and carbohydrates during the run. Figure 19.8 summarizes the factors limiting performance in long-distance running events. Almost

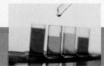
Dr. David L. Costill, Ph.D., Advanced the Study of Endurance Performance

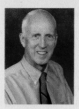

Courtesy of Ball State University Photo Service

Dr. David Costill has had a major impact on our understanding of the factors affecting endurance performance. Dr. Costill completed his Ph.D. at The Ohio State University and, after a two-year appointment at the State University of New York at Cortland, assumed a position at Ball State University. He directed the Human Performance Laboratory at Ball State throughout his entire career and made it the place to be if you wanted to study the factors affecting performance. Dr. Costill and his students addressed a variety of variables influencing endurance performance:

- Role of $\dot{V}O_2$ max
- Contribution of the percent of $\dot{V}O_2$ max
- Importance of running economy
- How blood/plasma lactate concentration is linked to performance

- Strategies for loading muscle glycogen (see Chap. 23)
- Fluid replacement–with emphasis on characteristics of sports drinks (see Chap. 23)
- Role of muscle fiber type (see Chap. 8)
- Whether ergogenic aids work (e.g., caffeine; L-carnitine–see Chap. 25)

Many of the studies dealing with these variables have become "classics" that investigators cite decades after they were done. Dr. Costill was not just interested in discovering the science behind endurance performance; he also committed his time and energy to getting the message out to athletes and coaches to help them develop better methods to improve performances based on scientific principles. Dr. Costill's work went well beyond studying distance running. Both early and later in his career, he focused attention on how to improve swimming performance, and he is currently involved in studies designed to improve our understanding of how to prevent deleterious changes in the

muscles of astronauts who spend long periods of time on the International Space Station. He has always practiced what he preached, being involved in distance running early in his career, and now Master's swimming–where he is swimming faster than he did when he was in college!

Dr. Costill provided exemplary service to the American College of Sports Medicine over his career, including serving as its president. His research has been recognized with numerous awards over the past 30 years, including the Honor Award from the American College of Sports Medicine. The impact of his research has reached all corners of the globe, not just by publications (more than 400), but by being invited to speak about his research in more than 30 countries. His personal impact, like that of most scientists, is multiplied many times over by the students he trained–a list that reads like a "who's who" of scientists interested in muscle, metabolism, and performance. He continues to maintain an active research program at Ball State University, where he holds the John and Janis Fisher Chair in Exercise Science.

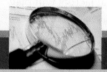

A CLOSER LOOK 19.2

Factors Affecting Performance in Ultra-Endurance Events

In contrast to the duration of endurance performances just mentioned, ultra-endurance events are in a class of their own. Examples include 166-km mountain runs (51), Triple Iron Triathlons (11.6-km swim, 540-km bike, 126.6-km run) (36), and a Paris to Beijing run (8500 km in 161 days) (50). In a recent study to evaluate the factors related to ultra-endurance performance, 14 subjects ran as many kilometers as possible in 24 hours on a treadmill. They covered an average of 149.2 km in 18 h 39 min of actual treadmill running in

the 24 hours. Two of the most important variables related to performance included $\dot{V}O_2$ max and the percentage of $\dot{V}O_2$ max that they could maintain over the 24 hours (49), two of the three variables linked to the regular endurance performances we just discussed.

Studies that have tracked metabolic responses before and after ultra-endurance events find that fat oxidation is markedly elevated after an ultra-endurance race, with plasma free fatty acids being 3.5 times higher (31). Given the low

% $\dot{V}O_2$ max maintained in many of these events (<60%), the metabolic response is not surprising (see Chap. 4). However, it doesn't mean that carbohydrate is not important, as some studies have shown a 50% reduction in muscle glycogen stores (31). Although ultra-endurance runs increase the potential for hyponatremia (a dangerous condition in which the body's sodium store is diluted because of the ingestion of too much water–see Chap. 23), only 4% of the runners experienced a mild form of the condition (56).

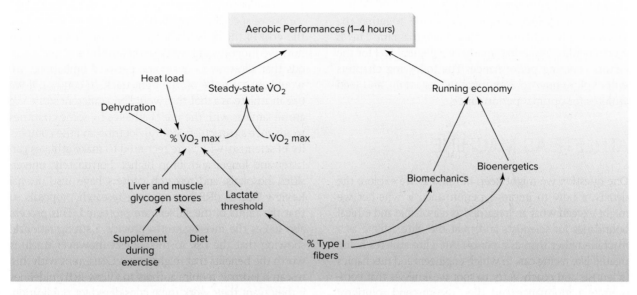

Figure 19.8 Factors affecting fatigue in aerobic performances lasting one to four hours.

all of the top 50 fastest times for men running a marathon are held by Kenyan or Ethiopian runners **http://www.iaaf.org/records/toplists/road-running/marathon/outdoor/men/senior/2015**

Investigators examined several of the variables in Figure 19.8 to help explain the incredible success of these runners. Compared to measurements made in elite European marathoners, Kenyan runners were found to be similar in $\dot{V}O_2$ max, the percent of $\dot{V}O_2$ max that could be maintained during the race, and oxidative enzyme activity in leg muscle involved in running. The evidence was contradictory regarding differences in the percent of type I muscle fibers. However, there was evidence that the Kenyan runners had lower blood lactate values at a given exercise intensity, and a better running economy. The running economy values were associated with the Kenyan's linear (ectomorphic) build and were comparable to the two best ever measured in Caucasian marathoners (38). Wilber and Pitsiladis (76) suggest that it may be more than physiology influencing the success of these Kenyan runners:

- Consistent running training from a young age as a method of getting to and from school and moderate-volume, high-intensity training at altitude (2000–3000 m)
- High motivation to succeed to improve socioeconomic status

The latter factor, *high motivation to succeed to improve economic status,* may also be driving some inappropriate behaviors–using performance-enhancing drugs (PEDs) like erythropoietin (see Chap. 25) to win the race and the prize money. Although more Kenyan runners who used PEDs are being identified, lax drug enforcement procedures in Kenya probably contributed to this problem in the first place (21). In May 2016, the World Anti-Doping Agency judged Kenya's Anti-Doping Agency "noncompliant," which can have a major impact on the ability of Kenya's athletes to compete internationally. We are sure to hear more about this in the near future. If we were to address long-distance cycling performance, a variety of other variables (e.g., minimizing air resistance and rolling resistance) would have to be considered (see Chap. 25 for more on this).

IN SUMMARY

- In long-term performances of one to four hours' duration, environmental factors play a more important role as the muscle and liver glycogen stores try to keep up with the rate at which carbohydrate is used.
- Diet, fluid ingestion, and the ability of the athlete to deal with heat and humidity all influence the final outcome.

In conclusion, the factors limiting performance are specific to the type of performance. Short-term explosive performances are dependent on type IIx fibers that can generate great power through anaerobic processes. In contrast, longer-duration aerobic events require a cardiovascular system that can deliver oxygen at a high rate to muscle fibers with many mitochondria. It is clear that the testing and training of athletes must focus on the factors limiting performance for the specific event. For example, dietary carbohydrate and fluid ingestion are more crucial for the long-distance runner than for the high jumper. A review article by Abbiss and Laursen in Suggested Readings pulls together the various models of fatigue into a single diagram. This is worth reading now that you have a general feel for the factors affecting performance. The following chapters will explore how to appropriately test, train, and feed athletes for optimal performance.

ATHLETE AS MACHINE

One question we might keep in mind as we explore the details of how to improve performance is whether we might exceed what are regarded as reasonable and ethical boundaries for scientists and treat the elite athlete as a machine rather than as a person. Are elite athletes being treated like racing cars in which engineers and mechanics (scientists and coaches) try to spot weaknesses that compromise performance and then recommend solutions? Some may say yes and indicate the worthiness of such an enterprise. Others may suggest that this has the potential to be dehumanizing if the athlete is reduced to no more than a collection of working parts that are evaluated by a variety of specialists. Much would appear to depend on the goal of the research. If we are trying to understand how we function and we develop healthy and safe methods that allow us to overcome personal limitations, we would appear to be on the right track. In contrast, if we use an athlete as a tool, that would be a different story. We are all familiar with the use of athletes by some countries to advance a particular political doctrine and the complicity of scientists who were recruited to make athletes run faster and longer and jump higher. Fortunately, universities, hospitals, and research centers have Institutional Review Boards (IRBs) to approve research proposals so that the rights of the subject are protected. This process also forces the investigator to provide a strong rationale showing that the risk to the subject (however small) is worth the benefits that might occur. Consistent with this, research journals require authors to follow IRB guidelines if they want their work to be considered for publication. In this way, we can move forward in our understanding of the physiological mechanisms underlying fatigue while protecting the rights of the subject.

STUDY ACTIVITIES

1. List the factors influencing performance.
2. Is the limiting factor for strength development located in the CNS or out in the periphery? Support your position.
3. Tracing the path the action potential takes from the time it leaves the motor end plate, where might the "weak link" be in the mechanisms coupling excitation to contraction?
4. When fatigue occurs, ATP is still present in the cell. What is the explanation for this?
5. Describe the pattern of recruitment of muscle fiber types during aerobic activities of progressively greater intensity.
6. As the duration of a maximal effort increases from 10 seconds or less to between 10 and 180 seconds, what factor becomes limiting in terms of energy production?
7. Draw a diagram of the factors limiting maximal running performances of 1500 m to 5 km.
8. Although a high $\dot{V}O_2$ max is essential to world-class performance, what role does running economy play in a winning performance?
9. Given that lactate accumulation will adversely affect endurance, what test might be an indicator of maximal sustained running (swimming, cycling) speed?
10. What is the role of environmental factors, such as altitude and heat, in very long-distance performances lasting one to four hours?

SUGGESTED READINGS

Abbiss, C. R., and P. B. Laursen. 2005. Models to explain fatigue during prolonged endurance cycling. *Sports Medicine* 35: 865-98.

Bigland-Ritchie, B. Looking Back. In *Fatigue*, Edited by Enoka RM, Gandevia SC, McComas AJ, Stuart DG, and Thomas CK. New York, NY: Plenum Press, 1995, pp. 1-9.

Cheng AJ, Yamada T, Rassier D, Andersson DC, Westerblad H, and Lanner JT. ROS/RNS and contractile function in skeletal muscle during fatigue and recovery. *Journal of Physiology*. 2016 Feb 9. doi: 10.1113/JP270650. [Epub ahead of print]

Daniels, J. T. 2005. *Daniels' Running Formula*, 2nd ed. Champaign, IL: Human Kinetics.

Fitts, R. H., S. W. Trappe, D. L. Costill, P. M. Gallagher, A. C. Creer, et al. 2010. Prolonged space flight-induced alterations in the structure and function of human skeletal muscle fibres. *Journal of Physiology* 588: 3567-92.

Fitts, R. H., P. A. Colloton, S. W. Trappe, D. L. Costill, J. L. W. Bain, and D. A. Riley. 2013. Effects of prolonged space flight on human skeletal muscle enzyme and substrate profiles. *Journal of Applied Physiology* 115: 667-79.

Thomas CK, Enoka RM, Gandevia SC, McComas AJ, and Stuart DG. The scientific contributions of Brenda Bigland-Ritchie. In *Fatigue*, Edited by Enoke RM, Gandevia SC, McComas AJ, Stuart DG, and Thomas CK. New York, NY: Plenum Press, 1995, pp. 11-26.

REFERENCES

1. **Allen DG, Lamb GD, and Westerblad H.** Skeletal muscle fatigue: cellular mechanisms. *Physiological Reviews* 88: 287-332, 2008.

2. **Allen DG and Westerblad H.** Role of phosphate and calcium stores in muscle fatigue. *Journal of Physiology* 536: 657-665, 2001.

3. **Allen DG, Westerblad H, Lee JA, and Lannergren J.** Role of excitation-contraction coupling in muscle fatigue. *Sports Medicine* 13: 116-126, 1992.

4. **Amann M, Sidhu SK, Weavil JC, Mangum TS, and Venturelli M.** Autonomic responses to exercise: group III/IV muscle afferents. *Autonomic Neuroscience: Basic and Clinical* 188: 19-23, 2015.

5. **Appell HJ, Soares JM, and Duarte JA.** Exercise, muscle damage and fatigue. *Sports Medicine* 13: 108-115, 1992.

6. **Asmussen E and Mazin B.** A central nervous component in local muscular fatigue. *European Journal of Applied Physiology and Occupational Physiology* 38: 9-15, 1978.

7. **Asmussen E and Mazin B.** Recuperation after muscular fatigue by "diverting activities." *European Journal of Applied Physiology and Occupational Physiology* 38: 1-7, 1978.

8. **Åstrand P-O and Rodahl K.** *Textbook of Work Physiology.* 2nd edition, New York: McGraw-Hill, 1977.

9. **Banister EW and Cameron BJ.** Exercise-induced hyperammonemia: peripheral and central effects. *International Journal of Sports Medicine* 11 (Suppl 2): S129-142, 1990.

10. **Bassett DR Jr. and Howley ET.** Limiting factors for maximum oxygen uptake and determinants of endurance performance. *Medicine & Science in Sports & Exercise* 32: 70-84, 2000.

11. **Bassett DR Jr. and Howley ET.** Maximal oxygen uptake: "classical" versus "contemporary" viewpoints. *Medicine & Science in Sports & Exercise* 29: 591-603, 1997.

12. **Bigland-Ritchie B.** EMG and fatigue of human voluntary and stimulated contractions. In *Human Muscle Fatigue: Physiological Mechanisms.* London: Pitman Medical, 1981, pp. 130-156.

13. **Bundle MW and Weyand PG.** Sprint exercise performance: does metabolic power matter? *Exercise and Sports Sciences Reviews* 40: 174-182, 2012.

14. **Coirault C, Guellich A, Barbry T, Samuel JL, Riou B, and Lecarpentier Y.** Oxidative stress of myosin contributes to skeletal muscle dysfunction in rats with chronic heart failure. *American Journal of Physiology* 292: H1009-1017, 2007.

15. **Coombes JS, Powers SK, Rowell B, Hamilton KL, Dodd SL, Shanely RA, et al.** Effects of vitamin E and alpha-lipoic acid on skeletal muscle contractile properties. *Journal of Applied Physiology* 90: 1424-1430, 2001.

16. **Coyle EF.** Integration of the physiological factors determining endurance performance ability. *Exercise and Sport Sciences Reviews* 23: 25-63, 1995.

17. **Davis JM, Alderson NL, and Welsh RS.** Serotonin and central nervous system fatigue: nutritional considerations. *American Journal of Clinical Nutrition* 72: 573S-578S, 2000.

18. **Davis JM and Bailey SP.** Possible mechanisms of central nervous system fatigue during exercise. *Medicine & Science in Sports & Exercise* 29: 45-57, 1997.

19. **Duke AM and Steele DS.** Mechanisms of reduced SR Ca^{12} release induced by inorganic phosphate in rat skeletal muscle fibers. *American Journal of Physiology - Cell Physiology* 281: C418-429, 2001.

20. **Edwards R.** Human muscle function and fatigue. In *Human Muscle Fatigue: Physiological Mechanisms.* London: Pitman Medical, 1981.

21. **Eichner ER.** Top marathon performance: interesting debate and troubling trends. *Current Sports Medicine Reports* 14: 2-3, 2015.

22. **Enoka RM, Baudry S, Rudroff T, Farina D, Klass M, and Duchateau J.** Unraveling the neurophysiology of muscle fatigue. *Journal of Electromyography and Kinesiology* 21: 208-219, 2011.

23. **Fitts RH.** Cellular mechanisms of muscle fatigue. *Physiological Reviews* 74: 49-94, 1994.

24. **Fitts RH.** The cross-bridge cycle and skeletal muscle fatigue. *Journal of Applied Physiology* 104: 551-558, 2008.

25. **Fitts RH, Riley DR, and Widrick JJ.** Functional and structural adaptations of skeletal muscle to microgravity. *Journal of Experimental Biology* 204: 3201-3208, 2001.

26. **Fitts RH.** The muscular system: fatigue processes. In *ACSM's Advanced Exercise Physiology*, edited by Tipton CM, Sawka MN, Tate CA, and Terjung RL. Baltimore, MD: Lippincott Williams & Wilkins, 2006, pp. 178-196.

27. **Fuchs F, Reddy Y, and Briggs FN.** The interaction of cations with the calcium-binding site of troponin. *Biochimica et Biophysica Acta* 221: 407-409, 1970.

28. **Gibson H and Edwards RH.** Muscular exercise and fatigue. *Sports Medicine* 2: 120-132, 1985.

29. **Green HJ.** Membrane excitability, weakness, and fatigue. *Canadian Journal of Applied Physiology 5 Revue Canadienne de Physiologie Appliquee* 29: 291-307, 2004.

30. **Halliwell B and Gutteridge J.** *Free Radicals in Biology and Medicine.* Oxford: Oxford Press, 2007.

31. **Helge JW, Rehrer NJ, Pilegaard H, Manning P, Lucas SJE, Gerrard DF, et al.** Increased fat oxidation and regulation of metabolic genes with ultraendurance exercise. *Acta Physiologica* 191: 77-86, 2007.

32. **Ikai M and Steinhaus AH.** Some factors modifying the expression of human strength. *Journal of Applied Physiology* 16: 157-163, 1961.

33. **Ikai M and Yabe K.** Training effect of muscular endurance by means by voluntary and electrical stimulation. *Internationale Zeitschrift Fur Angewandte Physiologie, Einschliesslich Arbeitsphysiologie* 28: 55-60, 1969.

34. **Ingham SA, Whyte GP, Pedlar C, Bailey DM, Dunman N, and Nevill AM.** Determinants of 800-m and 1500-m running performance using allometric models. *Medicine & Science in Sports & Exercise* 40: 345-350, 2008.

35. **Kayser B.** Exercise starts and ends in the brain. *European Journal of Applied Physiology* 90: 411-419, 2003.

36. **Knechtle B and Kohler G.** Running performance, not anthropometric factors, is associated with race success in a triple iron triathlon. *British Journal of Sports Medicine* 43: 437-441, 2009.

37. **Lambert EV, St Clair Gibson A, and Noakes TD.** Complex systems model of fatigue: integrative homeostatic control of peripheral physiological systems during exercise in humans. *British Journal of Sports Medicine* 39: 52-62, 2005.

38. **Larsen HB and Sheel AW.** The Kenyan runners. *Scandinavian Journal of Medicine and Science in Sports.* 25 (Suppl 4): 110-118, 2015.

39. **Matuszczak Y, Farid M, Jones J, Lansdowne S, Smith MA, Taylor AA, et al.** Effects of N-acetylcysteine on glutathione oxidation and fatigue during handgrip exercise. *Muscle & Nerve* 32: 633-638, 2005.

40. **McKenna MJ, Medved I, Goodman CA, Brown MJ, Bjorksten AR, Murphy KT, et al.** N-acetylcysteine attenuates the decline in muscle Na^+, K^+-pump activity and delays fatigue during prolonged exercise in humans. *Journal of Physiology* 576: 279-288, 2006.

41. **McLaughlin JE, Howley ET, Bassett DR, Jr., Thompson DL, and Fitzhugh EC.** Test of the classic model for predicting endurance running performance. *Medicine & Science in Sports & Exercise* 42: 991-997, 2010.

42. **McLester JR, Jr.** Muscle contraction and fatigue. The role of adenosine 5'-diphosphate and inorganic phosphate. *Sports Medicine* 23: 287-305, 1997.

43. **Medved I, Brown MJ, Bjorksten AR, and McKenna MJ.** Effects of intravenous N-acetylcysteine infusion on time to fatigue and potassium regulation during prolonged cycling exercise. *Journal of Applied Physiology* 96: 211-217, 2004.

44. **Medved I, Brown MJ, Bjorksten AR, Murphy KT, Petersen AC, Sostaric S, et al.** N-acetylcysteine enhances muscle cysteine and glutathione availability and attenuates fatigue during prolonged exercise in endurance-trained individuals. *Journal of Applied Physiology* 97: 1477-1485, 2004.

45. **Meeusen R and Watson P.** Amino acids and the brain: do they play a role in "central fatigue"? *International Journal of Sport Nutrition and Exercise Metabolism* 17: S37-S46, 2007.

46. **Meeusen R, Watson P, Hasegawa H, Roelands B, and Piacentini MF.** Central fatigue: the serotonin hypothesis and beyond. *Sports Medicine* 36: 881-909, 2006.

47. **Merry TL and Ristow M.** Do antioxidant supplements interfere with skeletal muscle adaptations to exercise training? *Journal of Physiology.* 2015 Dec 7. doi: 10.1113/JP270654 [Epub ahead of print]

48. **Merton PA.** Voluntary strength and fatigue. *Journal of Physiology* 123: 553-564, 1954.

49. **Millet GY, Banfi JC, Kerherve H, Morin JB, Vincent L, Estrade C, et al.** Physiological and biological factors associated with a 24 h treadmill ultra-marathon performance. *Scandinavian Journal of Medicine & Science in Sports* 21: 54-61, 2011.

50. **Millet GY, Morin JB, Degache F, Edouard P, Feasson L, Verney J, et al.** Running from Paris to Neijing: biomechanical and physiological consequences. *European Journal of Applied Physiology* 107: 731-738, 2009.

51. **Millet GY, Tomazin K, Verges S, Vincent C, Bonnefoy R, Boisson RC, Gergele L, Feasson L, and Martin V.** Neuromuscular consequences of an extreme mountain ultra-marathon. *PLOS ONE* 6: No. e17059, 2011.

52. **Nielsen B and Nybo L.** Cerebral changes during exercise in the heat. *Sports Medicine* 33: 1-11, 2003.

53. **Noakes TD and St Clair Gibson A.** Logical limitations to the "catastrophe" models of fatigue during exercise in humans. *British Journal of Sports Medicine* 38: 648-649, 2004.

54. **Noakes TD, St Clair Gibson A, and Lambert EV.** From catastrophe to complexity: a novel model of integrative central neural regulation of effort and fatigue during exercise in humans. *British Journal of Sports Medicine* 38: 511-514, 2004.

55. **Noakes TD, St Clair Gibson A, and Lambert EV.** From catastrophe to complexity: a novel model of integrative central neural regulation of effort and fatigue during exercise in humans: summary and conclusions. *British Journal of Sports Medicine* 39: 120-124, 2005.

56. **Page AJ, Reid SA, Speedy DB, Mulligan GP, and Thompson J.** Exercise-associated hyponatremia, renal function, and nonsteroidal antiinflammatory drug use in an ultraendurance mountain run. *Clinical Journal of Sport Medicine* 17: 43-48, 2007.

57. **Place N, Yamada T, Bruton JD, and Westerblad H.** Muscle fatigue: from observations in humans to underlying mechanisms studies in intact single muscle fibers. *European Journal of Applied Physiology* 110: 1-15, 2010.

58. **Powers S and Jackson M.** Exercise-induced oxidative stress: cellular mechanisms and impact on skeletal muscle force production. *Physiological Reviews* 88: 1243-1276, 2008.

59. **Powers SK, DeRuisseau KC, Quindry J, and Hamilton KL.** Dietary antioxidants and exercise. *Journal of Sports Sciences* 22: 81-94, 2004.

60. **Roberts D and Smith DJ.** Biochemical aspects of peripheral muscle fatigue. A review. *Sports Medicine* 7: 125-138, 1989.

61. **Sahlin K.** Metabolic factors in fatigue. *Sports Medicine* 13: 99-107, 1992.

62. **Sale DG.** Influence of exercise and training on motor unit activation. In *Exercise and Sport Sciences Reviews*, edited by Pandolf K. New York, NY: Macmillan, 1987, vol. 15, pp. 95-151.

63. **Sejersted OM and Sjogaard G.** Dynamics and consequences of potassium shifts in skeletal muscle and heart during exercise. *Physiological Reviews* 80: 1411-1481, 2000.

64. **Smith MA and Reid MB.** Redox modulation of contractile function in respiratory and limb skeletal muscle. *Respiratory Physiology & Neurobiology* 151: 229-241, 2006.

65. **St Clair Gibson A and Noakes TD.** Evidence for complex system integration and dynamic neural regulation of skeletal muscle recruitment during exercise in humans. *British Journal of Sports Medicine* 38: 797-806, 2004.

66. **Stewart RD, Duhamel TA, Foley KP, Ouyang J, Smith IC, and Green HJ.** Protection of muscle membrane excitability during prolonged cycle exercise with glucose supplementation. *Journal of Applied Physiology* 103: 331-339, 2007.

67. **Struder HK and Weicker H.** Physiology and pathophysiology of the serotonergic system and its implications on mental and physical performance. Part I. *International Journal of Sports Medicine* 22: 467-481, 2001.

68. **Struder HK and Weicker H.** Physiology and pathophysiology of the serotonergic system and its implications on mental and physical performance. Part II. *International Journal of Sports Medicine* 22: 482-497, 2001.

69. **Tanaka H and Seals DR.** Dynamic exercise performance in Masters athletes: insight into the effects of primary human aging on physiological functional capacity. *Journal of Applied Physiology* 95: 2152-2162, 2003.

70. **Tod D, Iredale F, and Gill N.** 'Psyching-up' and muscular force production. *Sports Medicine* 33: 47-58, 2003.

71. **Trivedi B and Danforth WH.** Effect of pH on the kinetics of frog muscle phosphofructokinase. *Journal of Biological Chemistry* 241: 4110-4112, 1966.

72. **Tupling AR.** The sarcoplasmic reticulum in muscle fatigue and disease: role of the sarco(endo)plasmic reticulum Ca^{21}-ATPase. *Canadian Journal of Applied Physiology 5 Revue Canadienne de Physiologie Appliquee* 29: 308-329, 2004.

73. **Vandenboom R.** The myofibrillar complex and fatigue: a review. *Canadian Journal of Applied Physiology 5 Revue Canadienne de Physiologie Appliquee* 29: 330-356, 2004.

74. **Weir JP, Beck TW, Cramer JT, and Housh TJ.** Is fatigue all in your head? A critical review of the central governor model. *British Journal of Sports Medicine* 40: 573-586; discussion 586, 2006.

75. **Westerblad H, Lee JA, Lannergren J, and Allen DG.** Cellular mechanisms of fatigue in skeletal muscle. *American Journal of Physiology* 261: C195-209, 1991.

76. **Wilber RL and Pitsiladis YP.** Kenyan and Ethiopian distance runners: what makes them so good? *International Journal of Sports Physiology and Performance* 7: 92-102, 2012.

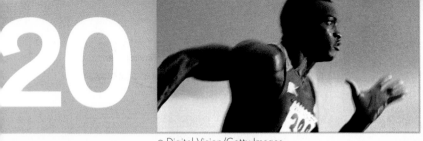

© Digital Vision/Getty Images

20

Laboratory Assessment of Human Performance

■ Objectives

By studying this chapter, you should be able to do the following:

1. Discuss the factors that determine the effectiveness of a physiological test of athletic performance.
2. Define "specificity of $\dot{V}O_2$ max."
3. Explain the difference between $\dot{V}O_2$ max and $\dot{V}O_2$ peak.
4. Discuss the physiological rationale for the assessment of the lactate threshold in the endurance athlete.
5. Describe methods for the assessment of anaerobic power.
6. Discuss the techniques used to evaluate muscular strength.

■ Outline

■ Key Terms

critical power
dynamic
dynamometer

isokinetic
power test

Quebec 10-second test
Wingate test

In general, there have been two principal approaches to the assessment of physical performance: (1) field tests of physical fitness and performance, which include a variety of measurements requiring basic performance demands, and (2) laboratory assessments of physiological capacities such as maximal aerobic power ($\dot{V}O_2$ max), anaerobic power, and exercise economy. It can be argued that physical fitness testing is important for an overall assessment of general conditioning, particularly in terms of evaluating student progress in a conditioning class (1, 68). However, the use of these test batteries does not provide the detailed physiological information needed to assess an athlete's level of conditioning or potential weaknesses. Therefore, more specific laboratory tests are required to provide detailed physiological information about performance in specific athletic events. This chapter will discuss tests designed to measure physical work capacity and performance in athletes. Specifically, much of this chapter will focus on both laboratory and field tests to evaluate the maximum energy transfer capacities discussed in Chaps. 3 and 4. The performance tests described in this chapter differ from the exercise tests described in Chap. 15 in several ways. Recall that the exercise tests described in Chap. 15 were targeted toward assessing cardiorespiratory fitness in healthy adults entering or actively engaged in a "health-related" exercise program. In contrast, the exercise tests described in this chapter are targeted toward measurement of performance in athletes actively engaged in competitive sports. Let's begin with a discussion of the theory and ethics of laboratory assessment of performance.

LABORATORY ASSESSMENT OF PHYSICAL PERFORMANCE: THEORY AND ETHICS

Designing laboratory tests to assess physical performance requires an understanding of those factors that contribute to success in a particular sport or athletic event. In general, physical performance is determined by the individual's capacity for maximal energy output (i.e., maximal aerobic and anaerobic processes), muscular strength, coordination/economy of movement, psychological factors (e.g., motivation and tactics), and the environment (32, 79). Figure 20.1 illustrates the components that interact to determine the quality of physical performance. Many athletic events require a combination of several factors for an outstanding performance to occur. However, often, one or more of these factors plays a dominant role in determining athletic success. In golf, there is little need for a high-energy output, but proper coordination is essential. Sprinting 100 meters

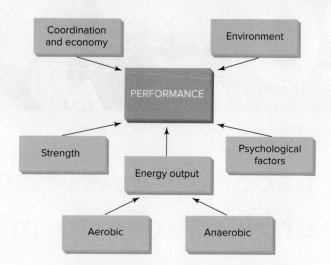

Figure 20.1 Factors that contribute to physical performance. See text for details.

requires not only good technique but a high anaerobic power output. In distance running, cycling, or swimming, a high capacity for aerobic production of ATP is essential for success. Again, laboratory evaluation of performance requires an understanding of those factors that are important for optimal performance in a particular athletic event. Thus, a test that stresses the same energy production systems required by a particular sport or athletic event is required to provide a valid assessment of physical performance.

A key concern in the performance of "athletic" laboratory testing is maintaining respect for the athlete's human rights. Therefore, laboratory testing should be performed only on athletes who are volunteers and have given written consent prior to testing. Further, prior to testing, the exercise scientist has the responsibility of informing the athlete about the purpose of the tests and the potential risks or discomfort associated with laboratory testing.

WHAT THE ATHLETE GAINS BY PHYSIOLOGICAL TESTING

Laboratory measurement of physical performance can be expensive and time consuming. An obvious question arises: What does the athlete gain by laboratory testing? A testing program can benefit the athlete and coach in at least three major ways:

1. Physiological testing can provide information regarding an athlete's strengths and weaknesses in his/her sport; this information can be used as baseline data to plan individual exercise training programs. As discussed earlier, athletic success in most sports involves the interaction

of several physiological components (Fig. 20.1). In the laboratory, the exercise scientist can often measure these physiological components separately and provide the athlete with information about which physiological components require improvement in order for the athlete to raise his/her level of athletic performance. This information provides the rationale for an individual exercise prescription that concentrates on the identified areas of weakness (53).

2. Laboratory testing provides feedback to the athlete about the effectiveness of a training program (53). For example, comparing the results of physiological tests performed before and after a period of training provides a basis for evaluating the success of the training program (5).

3. Laboratory testing educates the athlete about the physiology of exercise (53). By participating in laboratory testing, the athlete learns more about those physiological parameters that are important to success in his/her sport. This is important because athletes with a basic understanding of exercise physiology will likely make better personal decisions regarding the design of both exercise training and nutritional programs.

WHAT PHYSIOLOGICAL TESTING WILL NOT DO

Laboratory testing of the athlete is not a magical aid for the identification of future Olympic gold medalists (53). Although laboratory testing can provide valuable information concerning an athlete's strengths and weaknesses, this type of testing has limitations in that it is difficult to simulate in the laboratory the physiological and psychological demands of many sports. Therefore, it is challenging to predict athletic performance from any single battery of laboratory measurements. Performance in the field is the ultimate test of athletic success, and laboratory testing should be considered primarily a training aid for the coach and athlete (53).

COMPONENTS OF EFFECTIVE PHYSIOLOGICAL TESTING

For laboratory testing to be effective, several key factors need consideration (53):

1. The physiological variables to be tested should be relevant to the sport. For example, measurement of maximal handgrip strength in a distance runner is not relevant to the athlete's event. Therefore, only those physiological components that are important for a particular sport should be measured.

2. Physiological tests should be valid and reliable. Valid tests are tests that measure what they are supposed to measure. Reliable tests are tests that are reproducible. Based on these definitions, the need for tests that are both valid and reproducible is clear (20). (See A Closer Look 20.1.)

3. Tests should be as sport specific as possible. For instance, the distance runner should be tested while running (i.e., treadmill), and the cyclist should be tested while cycling.

4. Tests should be repeated at regular intervals. One of the main purposes of laboratory testing is to provide the athlete with systematic feedback concerning training effectiveness. Therefore, to meet this objective, tests should be performed on a regular basis.

5. Testing procedures should be carefully controlled. The need to rigidly administer the laboratory test relates to the reliability of tests. For tests to be reliable, the testing protocol should be standardized. Factors to be controlled include the instructions given to the athletes prior to testing, the testing protocol itself, the calibration of instruments involved in testing, environmental conditions (i.e., temperature and humidity), the time of the day for testing, prior exercise, diet standardization, and other factors such as sleep, illness, hydration status, or injury.

6. Test results should be clearly explained to the coach and athlete. This final step is a key goal of effective laboratory testing.

IN SUMMARY

- Designing laboratory tests to assess physical performance requires an understanding of those factors that contribute to success in a particular sport. Physical performance is determined by the interaction of the following factors: (a) maximal energy output, (b) muscular strength, (c) coordination/economy of movement, (d) psychological factors such as motivation and tactics, and (e) environmental conditions (e.g., heat/humidity, altitude, etc.).

- To be effective, physiological tests should be (a) relevant to the sport, (b) valid and reliable, (c) sport specific, (d) repeated at regular intervals, (e) standardized, and (f) interpreted to the coach and athlete.

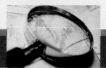

A CLOSER LOOK 20.1

Reliability of Physiological Performance Tests

For a physiological test of human performance to be useful, the test must be reliable. That is, the test results must be reproducible. Several factors influence the reliability of physiological performance tests. These include the caliber of athletes tested, the type of ergometer (instrument for measuring work output) used during the test, and the specificity of the test.

Physiological tests of performance are more reliable when highly trained and experienced athletes are tested (38). The explanation for this observation appears to be that these

athletes are highly motivated to perform and they are better able to pace themselves in a reproducible manner during a performance test. That is, high-caliber athletes may have a better "feel" for pace, and their perceptions of fatigue are less variable than those of less experienced athletes (38).

It is clear that some ergometers are more unvarying than others in providing a constant resistance. For instance, an ergometer that maintains its calibration and delivers a constant power output during a test would

result in a more reproducible test of human performance than an ergometer that provides variable power outputs during the test.

Exercise tests with a movement pattern and intensity that mimics the actual sporting event are more reliable than tests that do not imitate the event (38, 39). For example, testing racing cyclists on a cycle ergometer at an exercise intensity close to the intensity of competition should be a more reliable performance test than testing these athletes on other types of ergometers, such as treadmills.

DIRECT TESTING OF MAXIMAL AEROBIC POWER

Let's begin our discussion of the laboratory assessment of human performance by describing tests to measure the maximal oxygen uptake ($\dot{V}O_2$ max) of athletes. Exercise testing to determine $\dot{V}O_2$ max dates back to studies conducted more than 90 years ago by the British scientist A.V. Hill. Indeed, A.V. Hill coined the term $\dot{V}O_2$ *max* in the early 1920s (3). *Maximal oxygen uptake* was first mentioned in Chap. 4 and is defined as the highest oxygen uptake that an individual can obtain during exercise using large muscle groups (i.e., legs) (1). Although several tests to estimate $\dot{V}O_2$ max exist (12, 89), the most accurate means of determination is by direct laboratory measurement. Direct measurement of $\dot{V}O_2$ max is generally performed using a motorized treadmill or cycle ergometer, and open-circuit spirometry is used to measure pulmonary gas exchange as discussed in Chap. 1. However, $\dot{V}O_2$ max has also been measured during swimming, cross-country skiing, bench stepping, ice skating, and rowing (8, 12, 54, 57, 64, 95).

Historically, the measurement of $\dot{V}O_2$ max has been considered the test of choice for predicting success in endurance events such as distance running (11, 16, 27, 28, 34, 45, 53, 63, 101). For example, relative $\dot{V}O_2$ max (i.e., $\dot{V}O_2$ max expressed in $ml \cdot kg^{-1} \cdot min^{-1}$) has been shown to be the single most important factor in predicting distance running success in a heterogeneous (i.e., different $\dot{V}O_2$ max) group of athletes (17, 18, 28). The logical explanation for this finding is that because distance

running is largely an aerobic event (see Chaps. 4 and 19), those individuals with a high $\dot{V}O_2$ max will have an advantage over individuals with lower aerobic capacities. However, as one would expect, the correlation between $\dot{V}O_2$ max and distance running performance is low in a homogeneous (i.e., similar $\dot{V}O_2$ max) group of runners (15, 75). This finding indicates that although a high $\dot{V}O_2$ max is important in determining distance running success, other variables are also important. Therefore, measurement of $\dot{V}O_2$ max is only one in a battery of tests that should be used in evaluating the performance capacity of endurance athletes.

Specificity of Testing

Clearly, a valid test to determine $\dot{V}O_2$ max should involve the specific movement used by the athlete in his or her event (7, 8, 69). For example, if the athlete is a distance runner, it is important that $\dot{V}O_2$ max be assessed during running. Likewise, if the athlete being evaluated is a trained cyclist, the exercise test should be performed on the cycle ergometer. Further, specific testing procedures have been established for cross-country skiers and swimmers as well (54, 57, 64).

Exercise Test Protocol

Although the first exercise tests to determine $\dot{V}O_2$ max were performed in the 1920s, rigorous studies to optimize laboratory exercise tests were not performed until the 1940s and 1950s. An early leader in the development of graded exercise tests was Dr. Robert

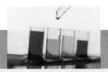

Robert Bruce Was a Pioneer in the Development of the Graded Exercise Test

Robert Arthur Bruce (1916–2004) completed his medical school training in 1943 at the University of Rochester. After finishing his medical residency in 1946, he joined the faculty at the University of Rochester. Dr. Bruce later (1950) became the chief of cardiology at the University of Washington Medical School, where he remained until his retirement from academic medicine in 1987.

Early in his career, Dr. Bruce recognized that an exercise test could play an important role in the clinical evaluation of cardiac patients. He published his first paper on exercise testing in 1949 and

concluded that a standardized exercise test provides key diagnostic information about cardiac patients. Dr. Bruce continued to explore exercise testing protocols for patient testing, and in 1963, he conceived and validated a multistage exercise protocol that was designed to evaluate the patient's exercise performance and provide important diagnostic information from the measurement of heart rate, blood pressure, and ECG changes during exercise. Subsequently, the standard Bruce Exercise Test evolved into its present form with seven 3-minute stages. This test became known as

the "Bruce Protocol" and remains a widely used treadmill protocol to evaluate cardiac patients.

Dr. Bruce developed his exercise test for patient populations in the clinical laboratory. Nonetheless, the Bruce graded exercise test was the conceptual model behind many of the current graded exercise tests that are used in the exercise physiology laboratory to evaluate both $\dot{V}O_2$ max and the lactate threshold in athletes. Because of his early research accomplishments in the area of clinical exercise testing, Dr. Bruce is considered to be a pioneer of the graded exercise test.

Bruce, a cardiologist at the University of Washington (see A Look Back–Important People in Science).

A test to determine $\dot{V}O_2$ max generally begins with a submaximal "warm-up" exercise period that may last three to five minutes. After the warm-up, the exercise intensity can be increased in several ways: (1) the work rate can be increased to a load that in preliminary experiments has been shown to represent a load near the predicted maximal load for the subject, (2) the load can be increased stepwise each minute until the subject reaches a point at which the power output cannot be maintained, or (3) the load may be increased stepwise every two to four minutes until the subject cannot maintain the desired work rate. When any one of these procedures is carefully followed, it yields approximately the same $\dot{V}O_2$ max as the others (1, 49, 73, 104), although an exercise protocol that does not exceed 10 to 12 minutes seems preferable (10, 49).

The criteria to determine if $\dot{V}O_2$ max was introduced in Chap. 15. Because of the importance of this measure, some important issues will be reviewed here. The primary criterion to determine if $\dot{V}O_2$ max has been reached during an incremental exercise test is a plateau in oxygen uptake with a further increase in work rate (94). This concept is illustrated in Figure 20.2. Unfortunately, when testing untrained subjects, a plateau in $\dot{V}O_2$ is rarely observed during an incremental exercise test. Does this mean that the subject did not reach his or her $\dot{V}O_2$ max? This possibility exists, but it is also possible that the subject

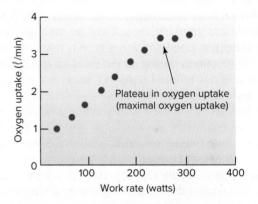

Figure 20.2 Changes in oxygen uptake during an incremental cycle ergometer test designed to determine $\dot{V}O_2$ max. The observed plateau in $\dot{V}O_2$ with an increase in work rate is considered to be the "gold standard" for validation of $\dot{V}O_2$ max.

reached his or her $\dot{V}O_2$ max at the last work rate but could not complete another exercise stage; therefore, a plateau in $\dot{V}O_2$ was not observed. In light of this possibility, several investigators have suggested that the validity of a $\dot{V}O_2$ max test be determined from not one but several criteria. In Chap. 15, it was discussed that a blood lactate concentration of >8 mmoles $\cdot$ liter^{-1} during the last stage of exercise could be used as one of the criteria to determine if $\dot{V}O_2$ max has been reached. However, to avoid the difficulty of taking blood samples and subsequent analysis for lactate levels, investigators have proposed additional criteria that do not involve blood sampling. For example, Williams et al. (100) and McMiken and Daniels (58) have proposed that a $\dot{V}O_2$ max test be judged as valid if any two of the following criteria are met: (1) a respiratory exchange ratio of ≥1.15, (2) a heart rate during the last exercise stage that is ±10 beats per minute within the subject's predicted maximum heart rate, or (3) a plateau in $\dot{V}O_2$ with an increase in work rate.

Note that the criteria for reaching $\dot{V}O_2$ max discussed above is appropriate for both men and women between the ages 20-49. However, recent evidence suggests that the end criteria for reaching $\dot{V}O_2$ max should be adjusted for both sex and age for individuals >50 years old (24). For more details on this topic, see Edvardsen et al. (2014) in the Suggested Readings.

Determination of Peak $\dot{V}O_2$ in Paraplegic Athletes

Again, by definition, $\dot{V}O_2$ max is the highest $\dot{V}O_2$ that can be attained during exercise using large muscle groups (1). However, subjects with injuries to or paralysis of their lower limbs can have their aerobic fitness evaluated through arm ergometry, which substitutes arm cranking for cycling or running. Given the aforementioned definition of $\dot{V}O_2$ max, the highest $\dot{V}O_2$ obtained during an incremental arm ergometry test is not referred to as $\dot{V}O_2$ max, but is termed the *peak $\dot{V}O_2$* for arm exercise.

The protocols used to determine peak $\dot{V}O_2$ during arm ergometry are similar in design to the previously mentioned treadmill and cycle ergometer protocols (84, 86). Research indicates that in subjects who are not specifically arm trained, a higher peak $\dot{V}O_2$ is obtained during arm ergometry if the test begins at some predetermined load that represents approximately 50% to 60% of peak $\dot{V}O_2$ during arm work (97). A logical explanation for these findings is that an "accelerated" incremental arm testing protocol that rapidly reaches a high power output might limit muscular fatigue early in the test, allowing the subject to reach a higher power output and therefore obtain a higher peak $\dot{V}O_2$.

In an effort to provide a more specific form of testing for paraplegics who are wheelchair racing athletes, some laboratories have modified a wheelchair by connecting the wheels to a cycle ergometer in such a way that the resistance to turn the wheels can be adjusted in the same manner as the load is altered on the cycle ergometer (81). This allows wheelchair athletes to be tested using the exact movement that they use during a race; therefore, it is superior to using arm ergometry to evaluate peak $\dot{V}O_2$ in this population.

IN SUMMARY

- The measurement of $\dot{V}O_2$ max requires the use of large muscle groups and should be specific to the movement required by the athlete in his or her event or sport.
- A $\dot{V}O_2$ max test for men and women aged 20-49 years can be judged to be valid if two of the following criteria are met: (a) respiratory exchange ratio ≥1:15, (b) HR during the last test stage that is ±10 beats per minute within the predicted HR max, and/or (c) plateau in $\dot{V}O_2$ with an increase in work rate.
- Arm crank ergometry and wheelchair ergometry are commonly used to determine the peak $\dot{V}O_2$ in paraplegic athletes.

LABORATORY TESTS TO PREDICT ENDURANCE PERFORMANCE

Exercise physiologists, coaches, and athletes have long searched for a single laboratory test that can predict success in endurance events. Numerous tests have been developed in an effort to predict athletic performance. In this section, we describe two well-developed laboratory tests—lactate threshold and critical power—that are useful in predicting endurance performance. Also, another laboratory test to predict performance, called "peak running velocity," is introduced in Research Focus 20.1. Let's begin with a discussion of the lactate threshold.

Use of the Lactate Threshold to Evaluate Performance

Studies reveal that a laboratory measurement that predicts the maximal steady-state running speed is useful in predicting success in distance running events from two miles to the marathon (19, 25, 26, 48-50, 51, 74, 91, 92). A common measurement to estimate this maximal steady-state speed is the determination of the lactate threshold. Recall that the lactate threshold represents an exercise intensity wherein blood lactate levels begin to systematically increase. Because fatigue is associated with high levels of blood and muscle lactate, it is logical that the lactate threshold is related to endurance performance in events lasting longer than 12 to 15 minutes (52). Although much of the research examining the role of the lactate threshold in predicting endurance performance has centered around distance running, the same principles apply to predicting performance in endurance cycling, swimming, and cross-country skiing.

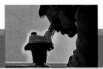
Measurement of Peak Running Velocity to Predict Performance in Distance Running

The lactate threshold and critical power measurements have generally been used to predict performance in endurance events lasting longer than 20 minutes (e.g., 10-kilometer run). In an effort to develop a laboratory or field test to predict performance in endurance events lasting fewer than 20 minutes (e.g., 5-kilometer run), researchers have developed a test called "peak running velocity" (66, 67, 85). The test is easy to administer and can be performed on a treadmill or track. For example, the measurement of peak running velocity on a treadmill involves a short test of progressively increasing the treadmill speed every 30 seconds (0% grade) until volitional fatigue. Peak running velocity (meters · second⁻¹) is defined as the highest speed that can be maintained for more than five seconds' duration (85).

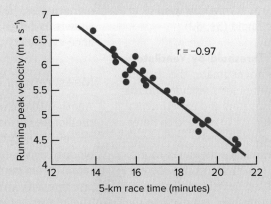

Figure 20.3 Relationship between running peak velocity and finish time of a 5-kilometer (km) race.

Data from Scott, B.K., and Houmard, J. A., "Peak Running Velocity is Highly Related to Distance Running Performance," *International Journal of Sports Medicine* 15: 504–507, 1994.

Studies confirm that peak running velocity is an excellent predictor of success in endurance events such as a 5-kilometer run. This point is illustrated by the strong correlation between peak running velocity and 5-kilometer race time (see Fig. 20.3). Surprisingly, similar findings have been reported for longer running events (e.g., 10–90 kilometers) as well (67). Therefore, peak running velocity is a useful laboratory or field test to predict endurance performance.

Direct Determination of Lactate Threshold Similar to the assessment of $\dot{V}O_2$ max, the determination of the lactate threshold requires athletes to be tested in a manner that simulates their competitive movements (i.e., specificity of testing). Testing protocols to determine the lactate threshold generally begin with a two- to five-minute warm-up at a low work rate followed by a stepwise increase in the power output every one to three minutes (76, 92, 95, 98, 99, 104). In general, the stepwise increases in work rate are small in order to provide better resolution in the determination of the lactate threshold (104).

To determine the blood concentration of lactate, blood samples are obtained at each work rate from a catheter (an indwelling tube) placed in an artery or vein in the subject's arm or from a small puncture of the fingertip. After the test, these blood samples are chemically analyzed for lactate, and the concentration at each exercise stage is then graphed against the oxygen consumption at the time the sample is removed. This concept is illustrated in Figure 20.4. How is the lactate threshold determined? Recall that the definition of the lactate threshold is the exercise intensity before there is a systematic and continuous rise in blood lactate concentration. Although several techniques are available, a simple and common procedure is to allow two independent investigators to

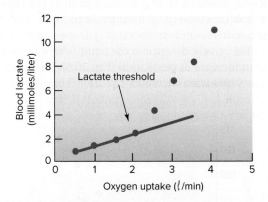

Figure 20.4 Typical graph of the changes in blood lactate concentrations during an incremental exercise test. The sudden rise in blood lactate is called the "lactate threshold."

subjectively pick the lactate "breakpoint" by visual inspection of the lactate/$\dot{V}O_2$ plot (76, 98). If the two investigators disagree as to where the threshold occurs, a third investigator is used to arbitrate.

In practice, the lactate "break point" can often be chosen by using a ruler and drawing a straight line through the lactate concentrations at the first several work rates. The last point on the line is considered the lactate threshold (Fig. 20.4). The obvious advantage of this technique is its simplicity. The disadvantage is that not all investigators agree that this procedure yields valid and reliable results (76). In light of this concern, several researchers have proposed that complex computer programs be used to more accurately predict the lactate threshold or that an arbitrary lactate value (e.g., 4 mM) be used as an indication of the lactate threshold (31, 52).

Prediction of the Lactate Threshold by Ventilatory Alterations A technique to estimate the lactate threshold that does not require blood withdrawal has obvious appeal to both investigators and experimental subjects. This need for a noninvasive method to determine the lactate threshold has led to the widespread use of ventilatory and gas exchange measures to estimate the lactate threshold. Recall from Chap. 10 that the rationale for the use of the ventilatory threshold as a "marker" of the lactate threshold is linked to the belief that the increase in blood lactate concentration at the lactate threshold stimulates ventilation via hydrogen ion influence on the carotid bodies. Although there are several noninvasive techniques in use today (4, 13, 87), the least complex procedure to estimate the lactate threshold by gas exchange is to perform an incremental exercise test similar to the previously discussed test used to determine the lactate threshold. Upon completion of the test, the minute ventilation at each work rate during the test is graphed as a function of the oxygen uptake. Figure 20.5 illustrates this procedure. Similar to the determination of the lactate threshold, a common procedure is to allow two independent researchers to visually inspect the graph and subjectively determine the point where there is a sudden increase in ventilation (Fig. 20.5). The point at which ventilation increases rapidly is considered the

ventilatory threshold and is used as an estimate of the lactate threshold. The error in predicting the lactate threshold from the ventilator threshold is estimated to range from 12% to 17% (36). Therefore, this technique has been criticized for a lack of precision (36, 76). Nonetheless, the ventilatory threshold has been shown to be useful in predicting success in endurance events (29, 75).

Measurement of Critical Power

Another laboratory measurement that can be used to predict performance in endurance events is critical power. Note that critical power and the lactate threshold are highly correlated. However, from an exercise intensity viewpoint, critical power represents an exercise intensity that is above the lactate threshold (52). The concept of **critical power** is based upon the notion that athletes can maintain a specific submaximal power output (i.e., exercise intensity) without fatigue (35, 46). Figure 20.6 illustrates the critical power concept for running performance. In this illustration, running speed is plotted on the y-axis, and the time that the athlete can run at this speed prior to exhaustion is plotted on the x-axis. Critical power is defined as the running speed (i.e., power output) at which the running speed/time curve reaches a plateau. Therefore, in theory, the critical power is considered the highest power output that can be maintained indefinitely (44). In practice, however, this is not the case. In fact, most athletes fatigue within 30 to 60 minutes when exercising at their critical power (35).

Critical power can be determined in the laboratory by having subjects perform a series of five to seven timed exercise trials to exhaustion. This is generally accomplished over several days of testing. The results are graphed, and critical power is determined by subjective assessment of the point where the power/time curve begins to plateau or by using a mathematical technique (see references

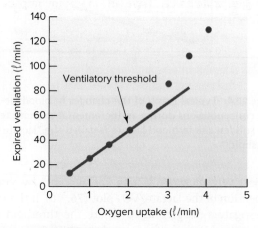

Figure 20.5 Example of the ventilatory threshold determination. Note the linear rise in ventilation up to an oxygen uptake of 2.0 l/min–above which ventilation begins to increase in an alinear fashion. This break in linearity of ventilation is termed the *ventilatory threshold* and can be used as an estimate of the lactate threshold.

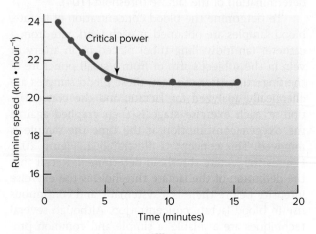

Figure 20.6 Concept of critical power.

35, 41, and 46 for details). Although Figure 20.6 illustrates the critical power measurement for running, the same principle of measurement can be applied to other endurance sports (e.g., cycling and rowing) (35, 40).

How well does critical power predict performance? Several studies have reported that critical power is significantly correlated with performance in endurance events lasting 3–100 minutes (e.g., r = 0.67 − 0.85) (35, 40, 46). Therefore, critical power is a useful laboratory predictor of success in endurance sports.

Is critical power a better predictor of success in endurance events than other laboratory measures such as the lactate threshold or $\dot{V}O_2$ max? The answer remains controversial because many investigators argue that $\dot{V}O_2$ max is the best single predictor of endurance performance success (17, 18, 28). However, in events lasting approximately 30 minutes, the lactate threshold, $\dot{V}O_2$ max, and critical power appear to be similar in their abilities to predict performance (46). This is not surprising, considering that critical power is dependent upon both $\dot{V}O_2$ max and the lactate threshold. Indeed, critical power is highly correlated to both $\dot{V}O_2$ max and the lactate threshold (46, 62). In other words, a subject with a high $\dot{V}O_2$ max and lactate threshold will also possess a high critical power. See Lundby and Roback (2015) and Vanhatalo et al. (2011) in Suggested Readings for more details on the critical power concept.

IN SUMMARY

- Common laboratory tests to predict endurance performance include measurement of the lactate threshold, critical power, and peak running velocity. All these measurements have proven useful in predicting performance in endurance events.
- The lactate threshold can be determined during an incremental exercise test using any one of several exercise modalities (e.g., treadmill, cycle ergometer, etc.). The lactate threshold represents an exercise intensity at which blood lactate levels begin to systematically increase.
- Success in distance running performance can be estimated by using both the lactate threshold and measurements of running economy.
- Critical power is defined as the running speed (i.e., power output) at which the running speed/time curve reaches a plateau.
- Peak running velocity (meters · second^{-1}) can be determined on a treadmill or track and is defined as the highest speed that can be maintained for more than five seconds.

TESTS TO DETERMINE EXERCISE ECONOMY

The topic of exercise economy was first introduced in Chap. 1. The economy of a particular sport movement (e.g., running or cycling) has a major influence on the energy cost of the sport and consequently interacts with $\dot{V}O_2$ max in determining endurance performance (15, 21, 61). For example, a runner who is uneconomical will expend a greater amount of energy to run at a given speed than will an economical runner. With all other variables being equal, the more economical runner would likely defeat the less economical runner in head-to-head competition. Therefore, the measurement of exercise economy is useful when performing a battery of laboratory tests to evaluate an athlete's performance potential.

How is exercise economy evaluated? Conceptually, exercise economy is assessed by graphing energy expenditure during a particular activity (e.g., running, cycling) at several speeds. In general, the energy costs of running, cycling, or swimming can be determined using similar methods. Let's use running as an example to illustrate this procedure. The economy of running is quantified by measuring the steady-state oxygen cost of running on a horizontal treadmill at several speeds. The oxygen requirement of running is then graphed as a function of running speed (9, 37). Figure 20.7 illustrates the change in $\dot{V}O_2$ in two runners at a variety of running speeds. Notice that at any given speed, runner B requires less oxygen and therefore expends less energy than runner A (i.e., runner B is more economical than runner A). A marked difference in running economy between athletes can have an important impact on performance.

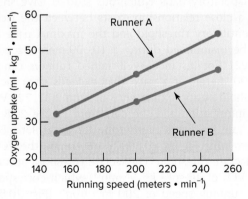

Figure 20.7   An oxygen cost-of-running curve for two subjects. Note the higher $\dot{V}O_2$ cost of running at any given running speed for subject A when compared to subject B. See text for details.

ESTIMATING SUCCESS IN DISTANCE RUNNING USING THE LACTATE THRESHOLD AND RUNNING ECONOMY

Over the past 30 years, many investigators used laboratory tests to predict performance in a variety of sports (see reference 71 for examples). The sport that has received the most attention is distance running. Theoretically, the prediction of potential performance in any endurance sport involves the use of similar laboratory measurements ($\dot{V}O_2$ max, economy of movement, etc.). We will use distance running as an example of how an exercise scientist can use laboratory measurements to estimate an athlete's performance in a particular event. Let's begin our discussion with a brief overview of the physiological factors that contribute to distance running success. As previously mentioned, an excellent test for determining an endurance runner's potential is $\dot{V}O_2$ max. However, other factors can also influence the pace that can be maintained for races of different lengths. For example, energy produced via anaerobic pathways (e.g., glycolysis) contributes to the ability to maintain a specified pace during shorter distance runs (e.g., 1500 meters) (11). In longer runs (5,000 to 10,000 meters), running economy and the lactate threshold also play important roles in determining success (25, 75, 92). To predict endurance performance, we must determine the athlete's maximal race pace that can be maintained for a particular racing distance.

To illustrate how performance in distance running might be estimated, consider an example of predicting performance in a 10,000-meter race. We begin with an assessment of the athlete's running economy and then perform an incremental treadmill test to determine $\dot{V}O_2$ max and the lactate threshold. The test results for our runner are graphed in Figure 20.8. How do we determine the maximal race pace from the laboratory data? Numerous studies have shown that a close relationship exists between the lactate or ventilatory threshold and the maximal pace that can be maintained during a 10,000-meter race (25, 75, 92). For instance, well-trained runners can run 10,000 meters at a pace that exceeds their lactate threshold by approximately 5 m · min⁻¹ (37, 72). With this information and the data from Figure 20.8, we can now predict a finish time for an athlete. First, we examine Figure 20.8(*b*) to determine the $\dot{V}O_2$ at the lactate threshold. The lactate threshold occurred at a $\dot{V}O_2$ of 40 ml · kg⁻¹ · min⁻¹, which corresponds to a running speed of 200 m · min⁻¹ (Fig. 20.8(*a*)). Assuming that the athlete can exceed this speed by 5 m · min⁻¹, the projected average race pace for a 10,000-meter run would be 205 m · min⁻¹. Therefore,

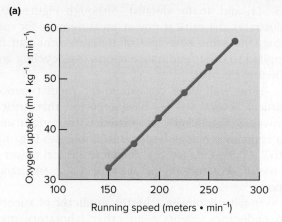

(a)

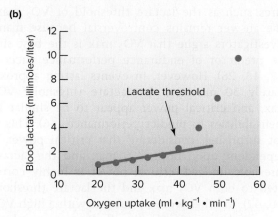

(b)

Figure 20.8 Incremental exercise test results for a hypothetical runner. These test results can be used to predict performance in an endurance race. See text for details.

an estimate of the athlete's finish time could be obtained by dividing 10,000 meters by his predicted running speed (m · min⁻¹):

Estimated finish time = 10,000 m ÷ 205 m · min⁻¹

= 48.78 min

Although theoretical predictions of performance, such as the example presented here, can generally estimate performance with a reasonable degree of precision, a number of outside factors can influence racing performance. For example, motivation and race tactics play an important role in distance running success. Environmental conditions (heat/humidity, altitude, etc.) also influence an athlete's ultimate performance (see Chaps. 19 and 24). For information on the ability of laboratory testing to predict future champions, see The Winning Edge 20.1.

IN SUMMARY

- Success in an endurance event can be predicted by a laboratory assessment of the athlete's movement economy and lactate threshold. These parameters can be used to determine the maximal race pace that an athlete can maintain for a given racing distance.

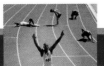

THE WINNING EDGE 20.1

Exercise Physiology Applied to Sports—Can Laboratory Testing of Young Athletes Predict Future Champions?

Many magazine articles have proclaimed the ability of laboratory testing in children to predict future athletic champions. For example, it has been argued that determination of skeletal muscle fiber type (via a muscle biopsy) in youth athletes and/or a genetic analysis can be used to predict the future athletic success of these individuals. The truth is that there are no laboratory measurements that accurately predict the "ultimate" athletic ability of anyone. Indeed, athletic success depends on numerous physiological and psychological factors, many of which are difficult, if not impossible, to measure in the laboratory. As mentioned earlier, the primary benefits of laboratory testing of athletes are to provide the individual with information about his or her strengths and weaknesses in a sport, to offer feedback about the effectiveness of the conditioning program, and to educate the athlete about the physiology of exercise (2).

Barker, A. R., and Armstrong, N., "Exercise Testing Elite Young Athletes," *Medicine and Sport Science* 56: 106–125, 2011.

DETERMINATION OF ANAEROBIC POWER

To assess maximal anaerobic power, it is essential that the test employed use the muscle groups involved in the sport (i.e., specificity) and utilize the energy pathways used in the performance of the event. Tests to assess maximal anaerobic power are generally classified into (1) ultra short-term tests designed to test the maximal capacity of the "ATP-PC system" and (2) short-term tests to evaluate the overall anaerobic capacity, which measures the maximal capacity for ATP production by both the ATP-PC system and anaerobic glycolysis (6, 33). Remember that events lasting fewer than 10 seconds primarily use the ATP-PC system to produce ATP, while events lasting 30–60 seconds utilize anaerobic glycolysis as the major bioenergetic pathway to synthesize ATP. This principle is illustrated in Figure 20.9 and should be remembered when designing tests to evaluate an athlete's anaerobic power for a specific sport.

Tests of Ultra Short-Term Maximal Anaerobic Power

Several practical "field tests" have been developed to assess the maximal capacity of the ATP-PC system to produce ATP over a very short time period (e.g., one–ten seconds) (55). These tests are generally referred to as **power tests.** Recall from Chap. 1 that power is defined as:

$$Power = (F \times D) \div T$$

where F is the force generated, D is the distance over which the force is applied, and T is the time required to perform the work.

Jumping Power Tests For many years, tests such as the standing long jump (formerly called the broad jump) and vertical jump have been used as field tests to evaluate an individual's explosive anaerobic power. The standing long jump is the distance covered in a horizontal leap from a crouched position, whereas the vertical jump is the distance between the standing reach height and the maximum jump-and-touch height. Both tests probably fail to adequately assess an individual's maximal ATP-PC system capacity because of their brief duration. Moreover, neither test is considered a good predictor of running success in a short dash (e.g., 40–100 yards) (42, 80, 88). Nonetheless, the vertical jump test is considered valuable in predicting vertical leaping ability of athletes and is widely used by coaches in professional football, soccer, and basketball as one of the many performance tests used to evaluate athletic potential.

Running Power Tests for American Football The 40-yard dash remains a popular test to evaluate power output in football players. The athlete generally

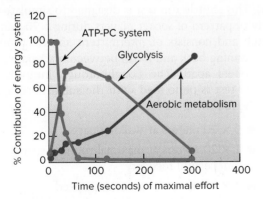

Figure 20.9 The percent contribution of the ATP-PC system, anaerobic glycolysis, and aerobic metabolism as a function of time during a maximal effort.

performs two to three timed 40-yard dashes with full recovery between efforts. The fastest time recorded is considered an indication of the individual's power output. Although a 40-yard dash is a rather specific test of power output for football players, there is little evidence that a 40-yard run in a straight line is a reliable predictor of an athlete's success at a particular position. Perhaps a shorter run (e.g., 10–20 yards), with several changes in direction, might provide a more specific test of power output in football players (57).

Stuart and colleagues (90) developed an anaerobic fitness test for football players that is designed to evaluate the athlete's ability to perform repeated short bursts of power. The test is conducted in the following way. After a brief warm-up, the athlete performs a series of ten timed 40-yard dashes (maximum effort), with a 25-second recovery between dashes. The 25-second recovery period is designed to simulate the elapsed time between plays in a football game. The athletes' time for each 40-yard dash is converted to running speeds (i.e., yards per second) and is graphed as a function of trial number. Specifically, running speed is graphed on the y-axis and the trial number is graphed on the x-axis. This procedure is illustrated in Figure 20.10 where line A represents data from a well-conditioned athlete and line B is data from a less fit athlete. Notice that both lines A and B have negative slopes (fatigue slope). This demonstrates that each of the two athletes is slowing down with each succeeding 40-yard trial. Athletes who are highly conditioned will be able to maintain faster 40-yard dash times over the ten trials when compared to less conditioned athletes, and therefore will have a less negative fatigue slope. In an effort to establish a set of standards for this test, Stuart and co-workers proposed that athletes be classified into one of four

TABLE 20.1 Classification of Fitness Levels for Football Players on the Basis of a Series of 40-Yard Dash Times

Level	Category	Percentage of Maximal Velocity Maintained*
1	Superior	≥90%
2	Good	85%–89%
3	Sub-par	80%–84%
4	Poor	≤79%

*The "percentage of the maximal velocity maintained" is calculated by averaging the velocity of the last three trials and dividing by the average velocity over the first three trials. This ratio is then expressed as a percentage. See text for further details.

fitness levels on the basis of the maximal running velocity percentage that can be maintained over the final three 40-yard dash trials (see Table 20.1). For example, a fitness level of 1-2 is labeled as a good to superior fitness level for players of any position. In contrast, fitness levels of 3 or below are considered to be subpar to poor fitness levels for a football player.

Running Tests for Soccer Soccer (called football outside of North America) remains the most popular sport in many countries around the world. Therefore, it is not surprising that numerous performance tests have been developed for soccer players (14, 60, 77, 78). Included in these performance tests are both tests of motor skills required for soccer and fitness tests. The design of a fitness test for soccer is complicated by the fact that soccer is a complex game requiring intermittent bursts of maximal running followed by periods of walking and/or slow running. Therefore, soccer is a sport that utilizes both anaerobic and aerobic bioenergetic pathways to produce the required ATP. A popular field test to determine both performance and metabolic responses of soccer athletes is the Loughborough Intermittent Shuttle Test developed at Loughborough University in England (65). This shuttle run test is designed to simulate the activity pattern of soccer players during a 90-minute match and consists of intermittent shuttle running (i.e., running back and forth) between markers placed 20 meters apart. The Loughborough intermittent shuttle test is performed with the subjects completing the following runs:

- 3 × 20 meters at walking pace
- 1 × 20 meters at maximal running speed with four-second recovery
- 3 × 20 meters at a running speed corresponding to 55% of individual $\dot{V}O_2$ max
- 3 × 20 meters at a running speed corresponding to 95% of individual $\dot{V}O_2$ max

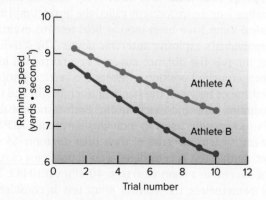

Figure 20.10 Illustration of the use of a series of timed 40-yard dashes to determine the anaerobic fitness of football players. In this illustration, athlete A shows a small but constant decline in running speed with each additional dash. In contrast, athlete B shows a large systematic decline in speed across dash trials. Therefore, athlete A is considered to be in better condition than athlete B. See text for details.

This block of exercise is repeated continuously for 90 minutes. In practice, the 20-meter distance is marked on the ground (or floor), and walking and running speeds are dictated by audio signals produced from a computer. Sprint times for the maximal 20-meter runs are recorded throughout the test by infrared photoelectric cells and represent one of the measured performance variables. That is, soccer players with the highest fitness levels will be able to maintain a higher percentage of their maximal sprint speed throughout the shuttle test. Further, the total distance covered during the test is also measured as a performance variable. During this shuttle test, it is estimated that 22% of the total exercise time is spent at or above 95% $\dot{V}O_2$ max, whereas the activity level for the remainder of the test is 55% $\dot{V}O_2$ max or below (65). Complete details of the numerous tests used to evaluate soccer performance are beyond the scope of this chapter, and the reader is referred to O'Reilly and Wong (2012) in Suggested Readings for more details about performance testing of soccer players.

Cycling Power Tests   The **Quebec 10-second test** was developed to assess ultra short-term anaerobic power in cyclists (88). The technical error of this test is small, and the procedure is highly reliable (6). The test is performed on a friction-braked cycle ergometer that contains a photocell capable of measuring flywheel revolutions; the number of flywheel revolutions and resistance against the flywheel are electrically relayed to a computer for analysis. The design of the test is simple. After a brief warm-up, the subject performs two all-out 10-second cycling trials separated by a rest period. The initial resistance on the cycle flywheel is determined by the subject's weight (about 0.09 kg per kg of body weight). Upon a verbal start command by the investigator, the subject begins pedaling at 80 rpm, and the load is rapidly adjusted within two to three seconds of the desired load. The subject then pedals as fast as possible for 10 seconds. Strong verbal encouragement is provided throughout the test. After a 10-minute rest period, a second test is performed and the results of the two tests averaged. The test results are reported in peak joules per kg of body weight and total joules per kg of body weight.

In addition to the evaluation of cyclists, the Quebec 10-second test has been used to test ultra short-term anaerobic power in nonathletes, runners, speed skaters, biathletes, and body builders. For complete details of these results, see reference 6.

Tests of Short-Term Anaerobic Power

As illustrated in Figure 20.9, the ATP-PC system for production of ATP during intense exercise is important for short bursts of exercise (1–10 seconds),

whereas glycolysis becomes an important metabolic pathway for energy production in events lasting longer than 15 seconds. In an effort to evaluate the maximal capacity for anaerobic glycolysis to produce ATP during exercise, several short-term anaerobic power tests have been developed. Like other performance tests, anaerobic power tests should involve the specific muscles used in a particular sport.

Cycling Anaerobic Power Tests   Researchers at the Wingate Institute in Israel have developed a maximal effort cycling test **(Wingate test)** designed to determine both peak anaerobic power and mean power output over the 30-second test. This test has been shown to be highly reproducible and offers an excellent means of evaluating anaerobic power output in cyclists (43). The test is administered in the following manner. The subject performs a short, two- to four-minute warm-up on the cycle ergometer at an exercise intensity sufficient to elevate heart rate to 150 to 160 beats · min^{-1}. After a three- to five-minute rest interval, the test begins with the subject pedaling the cycle ergometer as fast as possible without resistance on the flywheel. After the subject reaches full pedaling speed (e.g., two to three seconds), the test administrator quickly increases the flywheel resistance to a predetermined load. This predetermined load is an estimate (based on body weight) of a workload that would exceed the subject's predicted $\dot{V}O_2$ max by 20% to 60% (see Table 20.2). The subject continues to pedal as rapidly as possible, and the pedal rate is recorded every five seconds during the test. The

TABLE 20.2	The Resistance Setting for the Wingate Test Is Based on the Subject's Body Weight	
Subject's Body Weight (kg)	**Resistance Setting on the Flywheel (kg)**
20–24.9	1.75
25–29.9	2.0
30–34.9	2.5
35–39.9	3.0
40–44.9	3.25
45–49.9	3.5
50–54.9	4.0
55–59.9	4.25
60–64.9	4.75
65–69.9	5.0
70–74.9	5.5
75–79.9	5.75
80–84.9	6.25
≥85	6.5

Noble, B., *Physiology of Exercise and Sport.* St. Louis, MO: C. V. Mosby, 1986.

highest power output over the first few seconds is considered the peak power output and is indicative of the maximum rate of the ATP-PC system to produce ATP during this type of exercise. The decline in power output during the test is used as an index of anaerobic endurance and presumably represents the maximal capacity to produce ATP via a combination of the ATP-PC system and glycolysis. The decrease in power output is expressed as the percentage of peak power decline. The peak power output obtained during a Wingate test occurs near the beginning of the test, and the lowest power output is recorded during the last five seconds of the test. The difference in these two power outputs (i.e., highest power output minus lowest power output) is then divided by the peak power output and expressed as a percentage. For instance, if the peak power output was 600 watts and the lowest power output during the test was 200 watts, then the decline in power output would be computed as:

$$(600 - 200) \div 600 = .666 \times 100\% = 67\%$$

The 67% decline in power output means that the athlete decreases his or her peak power output by 67% over the 30-second exercise period.

Since the introduction of the Wingate test, a number of modifications to the original protocol have been proposed (23, 30, 43, 70, 82). For example, sport scientists have also developed a test for the measurement of anaerobic power on a cycle ergometer that involves 60 seconds of maximal exercise and uses variable resistance loading (30). The test design permits the measurement of both peak anaerobic power (i.e., peak ATP-PC system power) and mean (glycolytic) power output over the 60-second maximal exercise bout. The test is designed as follows. The subject performs a five-minute warm-up at a low work rate (e.g., 120 watts). After a two-minute recovery, the subject begins pedaling as fast as possible with no load against the cycle flywheel. When peak pedaling speed is obtained (i.e., three seconds), the investigator quickly increases the load on the flywheel to 0.095 kg resistance per kg of body weight. The subject continues to pedal as fast as possible at this load for 30 seconds; at the 30-second point, the load on the flywheel is reduced to 0.075 kg resistance per kg of body weight for the remainder of the test. The subject's power output during the test is continuously monitored electronically, and work output is recorded as peak power output (joules per kg per second) and mean power output (joules per kg per second) during the entire test.

The rationale for the variable load is that although a high resistance is required to elicit maximal anaerobic power, such a resistance is too great for a supra-maximal test of 60 seconds' duration (30). By reducing the resistance midway through the test, the workload becomes more manageable, which enables the subject to complete a maximal effort test for the entire 60-second period. The major difference between this test and the Wingate test is that the variable resistance design permits the measurement of peak anaerobic power and maximal anaerobic power over 60 seconds' duration. This type of test is useful for athletes who compete in events lasting between 45 and 60 seconds. Note that while this test maximally taxes both the ATP-PC system and glycolysis, because of the test duration, the aerobic system is also activated (see Chaps. 3 and 4). Therefore, although the energy required to perform 60 seconds of maximal exercise comes primarily (e.g., 70%) from anaerobic pathways, the aerobic energy contribution may reach 30%.

Running Anaerobic Power Tests   Maximal distance runs from 35 to 800 meters have been used to evaluate anaerobic power output in runners (83, 93, 103). This type of test can be used to determine improvement within individuals as a result of a training regimen. One example of a valid and reliable running anaerobic test is the "running anaerobic sprint test" (RAST) (102). This running anaerobic sprint test is easy to administer and is a reliable predictor of success in sprint races (103). In this test, subjects perform a series of six 35-meter maximal sprints with a 10-second recovery between runs. Each sprint is timed, and peak power is calculated (power = (body mass × distance^2)/time^3) for each of the individual sprints. Mean power is then calculated as the average of the peak power of the six runs. The mean power output from this test has been shown to be a reasonable predictor of running performance at 100, 200, and 400 meters (103).

Sport-Specific Tests   Ultra short-term and short-term sport-specific anaerobic tests can be developed to meet the needs of team sports or individual athletic events *not previously discussed here*. The tests can be designed to measure the peak power output in a few seconds or measure mean power output during a period of 10 to 60 seconds, depending upon the energy demands of the sport.

For example, tests can be developed for tennis, basketball, ice skating, swimming, and so on. In some cases, time or distance covered would be the dependent variable measured rather than a direct measurement of power output (6). This type of sport-specific test provides the coach and athlete with direct feedback about the athlete's present level of fitness and subsequent periodic testing can be used to evaluate the success of training programs.

To evaluate maximal anaerobic power in team sports such as basketball, handball, and soccer the "maximal anaerobic shuttle running test" (MASRT) was developed (22). This test is designed to evaluate anaerobic fitness of athletes involved in team sports that require a high anaerobic power output to be successful. Importantly, this test is both valid and reliable (22). The MASRT involves an intermittent shuttle run between two parallel lines and is easy to administer by a single assessor. It has been argued that this test is sensitive enough to identify even small changes in anaerobic performance in team sport players (22). This type of anaerobic fitness test is useful for evaluating team sport athlete's response to a training program.

IN SUMMARY

- Anaerobic power tests are classified as (a) ultra short-term tests to determine the maximal capacity of the ATP-PC system and (b) short-term tests to evaluate the maximal capacity for anaerobic glycolysis.
- Ultra short-term and short-term power tests should be sport specific in order to provide the athlete and coach with feedback about the athlete's current fitness level.

EVALUATION OF MUSCULAR STRENGTH

Muscular strength is defined as the maximum force that can be generated by a muscle or muscle group (1). The measurement of muscular strength is a common practice in the evaluation of training programs for American football players, shot-putters, weight lifters, and other power athletes. Strength testing can monitor both training progress and the rehabilitation of injuries (56). Muscular strength can be assessed by using one of four methods: (1) isometric testing, (2) free-weight testing, (3) isokinetic testing, and (4) variable resistance testing. Before we discuss these methods of strength measurement, let's consider some general guidelines for the selection of a strength-testing method.

Criteria for Selection of a Strength-Testing Method

The criteria for selecting a method of strength testing include the following factors (80): specificity, ease of data acquisition and analysis, cost, and safety. Given the importance of proper strength-test selection, a brief discussion of each of these factors is warranted.

Specificity of strength testing considers the muscles involved in the sport movement, the movement pattern and contraction type, and the velocity of the contraction. For example, the measurement of sport-specific strength should use the muscle groups involved in the activity. Further, the testing mode should simulate the type of contraction used in the sport (isometric vs. dynamic). If the contraction used in the sport is dynamic, further consideration should be given to whether the contraction is concentric or eccentric. A final level of specificity is the velocity of shortening. There is a degree of velocity specificity in strength training; speed and power athletes perform better on high-velocity power tests than on low (96). Therefore, there is a justification for trying to make the velocity of test contractions similar to those used in the sport.

Factors such as convenience and time required for strength measurements are important considerations when measurements are made on a large number of athletes (47). Currently, a number of companies market strength measurement devices that are interfaced with computer analysis packages. These devices greatly reduce the time required for strength measurement and analysis.

Much of the commercially available computerized equipment for strength measurement is expensive. The high cost of this equipment may prevent its purchase by physical therapy, exercise science, or athletic programs with small budgets. In these cases, the physical therapist, exercise scientist, or coach must choose the best available option within his/her budget.

A final concern for the selection of a strength-testing method is the safety of the technique. Safety should be a key concern for any measurement of strength. Clearly, strength-measurement techniques that put the athlete at high risk of injury should be avoided.

Isometric Measurement of Strength

Measurement of isometric strength requires a device that permits testing of the sport-specific muscle groups. These devices are commercially available from numerous sources. Most of the isometric testing devices available today are computerized instruments that are capable of measuring both isometric and dynamic force in a variety of muscle groups. Figure 20.11 illustrates one of these devices being used to measure leg strength during a knee extension. As the subject generates maximal isometric force, the computerized tensiometer (tension-measuring device) measures the force produced, and this information is recorded and displayed on an electronic panel on the instrument.

The measurement of isometric strength is typically performed at several joint angles. Isometric testing at each joint angle usually consists of two or more trials of maximal contractions (contraction duration of approximately five seconds), and the best of these trials is considered to be the measure of strength.

Advantages of isometric testing using computerized equipment include the fact that these tests are generally simple and safe to administer. For example,

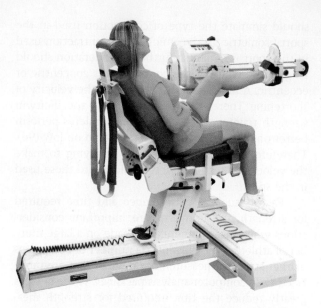

Figure 20.11 Use of a commercially available dynamometer to measure force during a knee extension.

Photo courtesy of Biodex Medical Systems, Inc.

computerized measurement of isometric strength has been used in physical therapy to evaluate training progress in injured limbs. It has been argued that since the isometric tensiometer can be used to measure static strength at many different joint angles with a low risk of injury, this technique might be more effective in evaluating strength gains during therapeutic training than conventional weight-lifting tests (57). Disadvantages of isometric testing include the high cost of some commercial devices and the fact that many sport activities involve dynamic movements. Further, because strength differs over the full range of joint movement, isometric measurements must be made at numerous joint angles; this increases the amount of time required to perform a test.

Free-Weight Testing of Strength

The term *isotonic* means constant tension. This term is often applied to conventional weight-lifting exercise because the weight of the barbell or dumbbell remains constant as the weight is lifted over the range of movement. In a strict sense, application of the term *isotonic* to weight lifting is not appropriate because the actual force or torque applied to the weight does not remain constant over the full range of movement. Acceleration and deceleration of the limbs during a weight-lifting movement often cause variation in the force applied. Therefore, in place of the term isotonic, the term **dynamic** is now commonly used to describe this type of muscle activity when exercising with a constant external resistance, such as free weights or weight stacks on machines where the resistance remains constant throughout the range of motion. The most common measure of dynamic strength is the one-repetition maximum, but tests involving three to six repetitions have been employed.

The one-repetition maximum (1-RM) method of evaluating muscular strength involves the performance of a single, maximal lift. This refers to the maximal amount of weight that can be lifted during one complete dynamic repetition of a particular movement (e.g., bench press). To test the 1-RM for any given muscle group, the subject selects a beginning weight that is close to the anticipated 1-RM weight. If one repetition is completed, the weight is increased by a small increment and the trial repeated. This process is continued until the maximum lifting capacity is obtained. The highest weight moved during one repetition is considered the 1-RM. The 1-RM test can be performed using free weights (barbells) or an adjustable resistance exercise machine. For more details of the 1-RM test, see Powers et al. (2017) in Suggested Readings.

Because of safety concerns, some physical therapists and exercise scientists have recommended that a dynamic test consisting of three or six repetitions be substituted for the 1-RM test. The rationale is that the incidence of injury may be less with a weight that can be lifted a maximum of three or six times compared to the heavier weight that can be lifted during a 1-RM contraction.

In addition to the use of free weights or machines, maximal strength can be measured using dynamometers. A **dynamometer** is a device capable of measuring mechanical force. Hand-grip dynamometers have been used to evaluate grip strength for many years. Dynamometers operate in the following way. When force is applied to the dynamometer, a steel spring is compressed and moves a pointer along a scale. By calibrating the dynamometer with known weights, one can determine how much force is required to move the pointer a specified distance on the scale. Figure 20.12 illustrates the use of a hand-grip dynamometer to assess grip strength.

The advantages of dynamic strength testing include low cost of equipment and the fact that force is dynamically applied, which may simulate sport-specific movements. The disadvantages of free-weight testing using a 1-RM technique include the possibility of subject injury and the fact that it does not provide information concerning the force application over the full range of motion. This point will be discussed again in the next section.

Isokinetic Assessment of Strength

Over the past several years, many commercial computer-assisted devices to assess dynamic muscular force (i.e., dynamometer) have been developed. The most common type of computerized strength measurement device on the market is an isokinetic

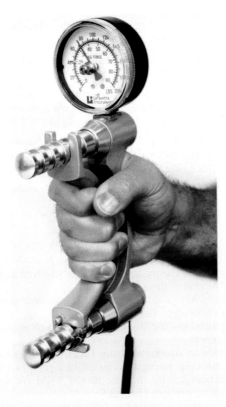

Figure 20.12 Use of the typical hand-grip dynamometer.

Photo Courtesy of Lafayette Instrument Company

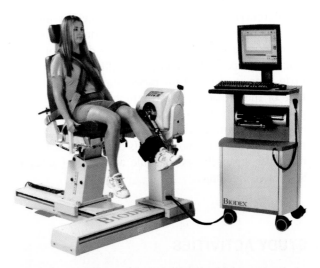

Figure 20.13 Use of a commercially available computer-assisted isokinetic dynamometer to measure strength during a knee extension.

Photo courtesy of Biodex Medical Systems, Inc.

dynamometer, which provides variable resistance. The term **isokinetic** means moving at a constant rate of speed. A variable-resistance isokinetic dynamometer is an electronic-mechanical instrument that maintains a constant speed of movement while varying the resistance during a particular movement. The resistance offered by the instrument is an accommodating resistance, which is designed to match the force generated by the muscle. A force transducer inside the instrument constantly monitors the muscular force generated at a constant speed and relays this information to a computer, which calculates the average force generated over each time period and joint angle during the movement. An example of this type of instrument is pictured in Figure 20.13.

A typical computer printout of data obtained during a maximum-effort leg extension on a computerized isokinetic dynamometer is illustrated in Figure 20.14. This type of strength assessment provides significantly more information than that supplied by a 1-RM test. The force curve pictured in Figure 20.14 illustrates that the subject generates the smallest amount of force early in the movement pattern and the greatest amount of force during the middle portion of the movement. The 1-RM test provides only the final outcome, which is the maximum amount of weight lifted during this particular movement. That is, a 1-RM test does not provide information about the differences in force generation

over the full range of movement. Therefore, a computer-assisted isokinetic dynamometer offers several advantages over the more traditional 1-RM test. Importantly, isokinetic strength testing has been shown to be highly reliable (59).

Variable-Resistance Measurement of Strength

Several commercial companies market weight machines that vary the resistance (weight) during dynamic muscular contractions. The measurement of strength using a variable-resistance device is similar in principle to isotonic tests using 1-RM or three to six repetitions, with the exception that the variable-resistance machine creates a variable resistance over the range of movement. This variable resistance is typically achieved via a "cam," which in theory is designed to vary the resistance according to physiological and mechanical factors that determine force generation by muscles over the normal range of movement.

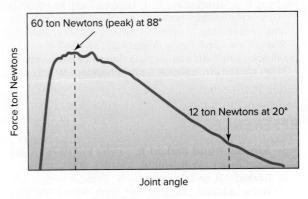

Figure 20.14 Example of a computer printout from a computer-assisted isokinetic dynamometer during a maximal-effort knee extension.

Potential advantages of these devices include the fact that most sport movement patterns are performed using variable forces, and the design of these machines makes adjustment of weight easy; therefore, little time is required for measurement. A disadvantage of these machines is the high cost; this is compounded by the fact that several individual machines are often required to measure strength in different muscle groups. For more details on the evaluation of muscular strength, see Baechle and Earle (2012) in Suggested Readings.

IN SUMMARY

- Muscular strength is defined as the maximum force that can be generated by a muscle or muscle group.
- Evaluation of muscular strength is useful in assessing training programs for athletes involved in power sports or events.
- Muscular strength can be evaluated using any one of the following techniques: (a) isometric, (b) free-weight testing, (c) isokinetic, or (d) variable-resistance devices.

STUDY ACTIVITIES

1. Discuss the rationale behind laboratory tests designed to assess physical performance in athletes. How do these tests differ from general physical fitness tests?
2. Define maximal oxygen uptake. Why might relative $\dot{V}O_2$ max be the single most important factor in predicting distance running success in a heterogeneous group of runners?
3. Discuss the concept of "specificity of testing" for the determination of $\dot{V}O_2$ max. Give a brief overview of the design of an incremental test to determine $\dot{V}O_2$ max. What criteria can be used to determine the validity of a $\dot{V}O_2$ max test?
4. Briefly explain the technique employed to determine the lactate threshold and the ventilatory threshold.
5. Describe how the economy of running might be evaluated in the laboratory.
6. Discuss the theory and procedures involved in predicting success in distance running.
7. Explain how short-term maximal anaerobic power can be evaluated by field tests.
8. Describe how the Wingate test is used to assess anaerobic power.
9. Provide an overview of the 1-RM technique to evaluate muscular strength. Why might a computer-assisted dynamometer be superior to the 1-RM technique in assessing strength changes?
10. Discuss the advantages and disadvantages of each of the following types of strength measurement: (1) dynamic, (2) free weights, (3) isokinetic, and (4) variable resistance.

SUGGESTED READINGS

Baechle, T. R., and R. W. Earle. 2012. *Essentials of Strength Training and Conditioning.* Champaign, IL: Human Kinetics.

Castagna, C., V. Manzi, F. Impellizzeri, M. Weston, and J. C. Barbero Alvarez. 2010. Relationship between endurance field tests and match performance in young soccer players. *Journal of Strength and Conditioning Research* 24: 3227-33.

Edvardsen, E., E. Hem, and S.A. Anderssen. 2014. End criteria for reaching maximal oxygen uptake must be strict and adjusted to sex and age: A cross-sectional study. *PLOS ONE.* 9: e85276.

Hudgins, B., J. Scharfenberg, N. T. Triplett, and J. M. McBride. 2013. Relationship between jumping ability and running performance in events of varying distance. *Journal of Strength and Conditioning Research* 27: 563-567.

Lundby, C., and P. Robach. 2015. Performance enhancement: What are the physiological limits? *Physiology* 30: 282-292.

Machado, F. et al. 2013. Incremental test design, peak aerobic running speed, and endurance performance in runners. *Journal of Science and Medicine in Sport* 16: 577-582.

Miller, T. (Editor). *NSCA's Guide to Tests and Assessments.* 2012. Champaign, IL: Human Kinetics.

Noordhof, D. A., P. F. Skiba, and J. J. de Koning. 2013. Determining anaerobic capacity in sporting activities. *International Journal of Sports Physiology and Performance* 8: 475-482.

O'Reilly, J., and S. Wong. 2012. The development of aerobic and skill assessment in soccer *Sports Medicine* 42: 1029-1040.

Powers, S., and S. Dodd. 2017. *Total Fitness and Wellness.* San Francisco: CA Pearson.

Vanhatalo, A., A. M. Jones, and M. Burnley. 2011. Application of critical power in sport. *International Journal of Sports Physiology and Performance* 6: 128-136.

REFERENCES

1. **Åstrand P and Rodahl K.** *Textbook of Work Physiology.* Champaign, IL: Human Kinetics, 2003.
2. **Barker AR and Armstrong N.** Exercise testing elite young athletes. *Medicine and Sport Science* 56: 106-125, 2011.
3. **Bassett DR Jr. and Howley ET.** Limiting factors for maximum oxygen uptake and determinants of endurance performance. *Medicine & Science in Sports & Exercise* 32: 70-84, 2000.
4. **Beaver WL, Wasserman K, and Whipp BJ.** A new method for detecting anaerobic threshold by gas exchange. *Journal of Applied Physiology* 60: 2020-2027, 1986.
5. **Bentley DJ, Newell J, and Bishop D.** Incremental exercise test design and analysis: implications for

performance diagnostics in endurance athletes. *Sports Medicine* 37: 575-586, 2007.

6. **Bouchard C.** Testing anaerobic power and capacity. In *Physiological Testing of the High Performance Athlete*, edited by MacDougall J, Wenger H, and Green H. Champaign, IL: Human Kinetics, 1991, pp. 175-222.

7. **Bouckaert J and Pannier J.** Specificity of $\dot{V}O_{2\,max}$ and blood lactate determinations in runners and cyclists. *International Archives of Physiology and Biochemistry* 93: 30-31, 1984.

8. **Bouckaert J, Pannier JL, and Vrijens J.** Cardiorespiratory response to bicycle and rowing ergometer exercise in oarsmen. *European Journal of Applied Physiology and Occupational Physiology* 51: 51-59, 1983.

9. **Bransford DR and Howley ET.** Oxygen cost of running in trained and untrained men and women. *Medicine and Sport Science* 9: 41-44, 1977.

10. **Buchfuhrer MJ, Hansen JE, Robinson TE, Sue DY, Wasserman K, and Whipp BJ.** Optimizing the exercise protocol for cardiopulmonary assessment. *Journal of Applied Physiology* 55: 1558-1564, 1983.

11. **Bulbulian R, Wilcox AR, and Darabos BL.** Anaerobic contribution to distance running performance of trained cross-country athletes. *Medicine & Science in Sports & Exercise* 18: 107-113, 1986.

12. **Burke EJ.** Validity of selected laboratory and field tests of physical working capacity. *Research Quarterly* 47: 95-104, 1976.

13. **Caiozzo VJ, Davis JA, Ellis JF, Azus JL, Vandagriff R, Prietto CA, et al.** A comparison of gas exchange indices used to detect the anaerobic threshold. *Journal of Applied Physiology* 53: 1184-1189, 1982.

14. **Castagna C, Manzi V, Impellizzeri F, Weston M, and Barbero Alvarez JC.** Relationship between endurance field tests and match performance in young soccer players. *Journal of Strength and Conditioning Research* 24: 3227-3233, 2010.

15. **Conley DL and Krahenbuhl GS.** Running economy and distance running performance of highly trained athletes. *Medicine & Science in Sports & Exercise* 12: 357-360, 1980.

16. **Costill DL.** A scientific approach to distance running. *Los Altos: Track and Field News Press* 14: 12-40, 1979.

17. **Costill DL.** Metabolic responses during distance running. *Journal of Applied Physiology* 28: 251-255, 1970.

18. **Costill DL.** The relationship between selected physiological variables and distance running performance. *Journal of Sports Medicine and Physical Fitness* 7: 61-66, 1967.

19. **Costill DL, Thomason H, and Roberts E.** Fractional utilization of the aerobic capacity during distance running. *Medicine & Science in Sports & Exercise* 5: 248-252, 1973.

20. **Currell K and Jeukendrup AE.** Validity, reliability and sensitivity of measures of sporting performance. *Sports Medicine* 38: 297-316, 2008.

21. **Daniels J and Daniels N.** Running economy of elite male and elite female runners. *Medicine & Science in Sports & Exercise* 24: 483-489, 1992.

22. **Dardouri W, Gharbi Z, Selmi MA, Sassi RH, Moalla W, and Souissi N.** Reliability and validity of a new maximal anaerobic shuttle running test. *International Journal of Sports Medicine* 35: 310-315, 2013.

23. **Dotan R and Bar-Or O.** Load optimization for the Wingate anaerobic test. *European Journal of Applied Physiology and Occupational Physiology* 51: 409-417, 1983.

24. **Edvardsen E, Hem E, and Anderssen SA.** End criteria for reaching maximal oxygen uptake must be strict and adjusted to sex and age: a cross-sectional study. *PLOS One.* 9: e85276, 2014.

25. **Farrell PA, Wilmore JH, Coyle EF, Billing JE, and Costill DL.** Plasma lactate accumulation and distance running performance. *Medicine and Sport Science* 11: 338-344, 1979.

26. **Foster C.** Blood lactate and respiratory measurement of the capacity for sustained exercise. In *Physiological Assessment of Human Fitness*, edited by Maud P, and Foster C. Champaign, IL: Human Kinetics, 1995, pp. 57-72.

27. **Foster C.** $\dot{V}O_{2\,max}$ and training indices as determinants of competitive running performance. *Journal of Sports Sciences* 1: 13-27, 1983.

28. **Foster C, Daniels J, and Yarbough R.** Physiological correlates of marathon running and performance. *Australian Journal of Sports Medicine* 9: 58-61, 1977.

29. **Gaskill SE, Ruby BC, Walker AJ, Sanchez OA, Serfass RC, and Leon AS.** Validity and reliability of combining three methods to determine ventilatory threshold. *Medicine & Science in Sports & Exercise* 33: 1841-1848, 2001.

30. **Gastin P, Lawson D, Hargreaves M, Carey M, and Fairweather I.** Variable resistance loadings in anaerobic power testing. *International Journal of Sports Medicine* 12: 513-518, 1991.

31. **Grant S, McMillan K, Newell J, Wood L, Keatley S, Simpson D, et al.** Reproducibility of the blood lactate threshold, 4 mmol.l(-1) marker, heart rate and ratings of perceived exertion during incremental treadmill exercise in humans. *European Journal of Applied Physiology* 87: 159-166, 2002.

32. **Green H.** What do tests measure? In *Physiological Testing of the High Performance Athlete*, edited by MacDougall J, Wenger H, and Green H. Champaign, IL: Human Kinetics, 1991.

33. **Green S.** Measurement of anaerobic work capacities in humans. *Sports Medicine* 19: 32-42, 1995.

34. **Hagan RD, Smith MG, and Gettman LR.** Marathon performance in relation to maximal aerobic power and training indices. *Medicine & Science in Sports & Exercise* 13: 185-189, 1981.

35. **Hill DW.** The critical power concept: a review. *Sports Medicine* 16: 237-254, 1993.

36. **Hopker JG, Jobson SA, and Pandit JJ.** Controversies in the physiological basis of the 'anaerobic threshold' and their implications for clinical cardiopulmonary exercise testing. *Anaesthesia* 66: 111-123, 2011.

37. **Hopkins P and Powers SK.** Oxygen uptake during submaximal running in highly trained men and women. *American Corrective Therapy Journal* 36: 130-132, 1982.

38. **Hopkins WG, Hawley JA, and Burke LM.** Design and analysis of research on sport performance enhancement. *Medicine & Science in Sports & Exercise* 31: 472-485, 1999.

39. **Hopkins WG, Schabort EJ, and Hawley JA.** Reliability of power in physical performance tests. *Sports Medicine* 31: 211-234, 2001.

40. **Housh DJ, Housh TJ, and Bauge SM.** The accuracy of the critical power test for predicting time to exhaustion during cycle ergometry. *Ergonomics* 32: 997-1004, 1989.

41. **Housh TJ, Cramer JT, Bull AJ, Johnson GO, and Housh DJ.** The effect of mathematical modeling on critical velocity. *European Journal of Applied Physiology* 84: 469-475, 2001.

42. **Hudgins B, Scharfenberg J, Triplett NT, and McBride JM.** Relationship between jumping ability

and running performance in events of varying distance. *Journal of Strength and Conditioning Research* 27:563-567, 2013.

43. **Jacobs I.** The effects of thermal dehydration on performance of the Wingate anaerobic test. *International Journal of Sports Medicine* 1: 21-24, 1980.

44. **Jones AM, Vanhatalo A, Burnley M, Morton RH, and Poole DC.** Critical power: implications for determination of $\dot{V}O_2$ max and exercise tolerance. *Medicine & Science in Sports & Exercise* 42: 1876-1890, 2010.

45. **Kenney WL and Hodgson JL.** Variables predictive of performance in elite middle-distance runners. *British Journal of Sports Medicine* 19: 207-209, 1985.

46. **Kolbe T, Dennis SC, Selley E, Noakes TD, and Lambert MI.** The relationship between critical power and running performance. *Journal of Sports Science* 13: 265-269, 1995.

47. **Kraemer W and Fry A.** *Physiological Assessment of Human Fitness,* edited by Maud P, and Foster C. Champaign, IL: Human Kinetics, 1995, pp. 115-138.

48. **LaFontaine TP, Londeree BR, and Spath WK.** The maximal steady state versus selected running events. *Medicine & Science in Sports & Exercise* 13: 190-193, 1981.

49. **Lawler J, Powers SK, and Dodd S.** A time-saving incremental cycle ergometer protocol to determine peak oxygen consumption. *British Journal of Sports Medicine* 21: 171-173, 1987.

50. **Lehmann M.** Correlations between laboratory testing and distance running performance in marathoners of similar ability. *International Journal of Sports Medicine* 4: 226-230, 1983.

51. **Lorenzo S, Minson CT, Babb TG, and Halliwill JR.** Lactate threshold predicting time trial performance: impact of heat and acclimation. *Journal of Applied Physiology* 111: 221-227, 2011.

52. **Lundby, C and Robach, P.** Performance enhancement: what are the physiological limits? *Physiology* 30: 282-292, 2015.

53. **MacDougall J and Wenger H.** The purpose of physiological testing. In *Physiological Testing of the High Performance Athlete,* edited by MacDougall J, Wenger H, and Green H. Champaign, IL: Human Kinetics, 1991.

54. **Magel JR and Faulkner JA.** Maximum oxygen uptakes of college swimmers. *Journal of Applied Physiology* 22: 929-933, 1967.

55. **Margaria R, Aghemo P, and Rovelli E.** Measurement of muscular power (anaerobic) in man. *Journal of Applied Physiology* 21: 1662-1664, 1966.

56. **Mayhew T and Rothstein J.** Measurement of muscle performance with instruments. In *Measurement of Muscle Performance with Instruments,* edited by Rothstein J. New York, NY: Churchill Livingstone, 1985, pp. 57-102.

57. **McArdle W, Katch F, and Katch V.** *Exercise Physiology: Energy, Nutrition, and Human Performance.* Baltimore, MD: Lippincott Williams & Wilkins, 2001.

58. **McMiken DF and Daniels JT.** Aerobic requirements and maximum aerobic power in treadmill and track running. *Medicine & Science in Sports & Exercise* 8: 14-17, 1976.

59. **Meeteren J, Roebroeck ME, and Stam HJ.** Test-retest reliability in isokinetic muscle strength measurements of the shoulder. *Journal of Rehabilitation Medicine* 34: 91-95, 2002.

60. **Mirkov D, Nedeljkovic A, Kukolj M, Ugarkovic D, and Jaric S.** Evaluation of the reliability of soccer-specific field tests. *Journal of Strength and Conditioning Research* 22: 1046-1050, 2008.

61. **Morgan DW and Craib M.** Physiological aspects of running economy. *Medicine & Science in Sports & Exercise* 24: 456-461, 1992.

62. **Moritani T, Nagata A, deVries HA, and Muro M.** Critical power as a measure of physical work capacity and anaerobic threshold. *Ergonomics* 24: 339-350, 1981.

63. **Murase Y, Kobayashi K, Kamei S, and Matsui H.** Longitudinal study of aerobic power in superior junior athletes. *Medicine & Science in Sports & Exercise* 13: 180-184, 1981.

64. **Mygind E, Larsson B, and Klausen T.** Evaluation of a specific test in cross-country skiing. *Journal of Sports Sciences* 9: 249-257, 1991.

65. **Nicholas CW, Nuttall FE, and Williams C.** The Loughborough intermittent shuttle test: a field test that simulates the activity pattern of soccer. *Journal of Sports Sciences* 18: 97-104, 2000.

66. **Noakes TD.** Implications of exercise testing for prediction of athletic performance: a contemporary perspective. *Medicine & Science in Sports & Exercise* 20: 319-330, 1988.

67. **Noakes TD, Myburgh KH, and Schall R.** Peak treadmill running velocity during the $\dot{V}O_2$ max test predicts running performance. *Journal of Sports Sciences* 8: 35-45, 1990.

68. **Noble B.** *Physiology of Exercise and Sport.* St. Louis, MO: C. V. Mosby, 1986.

69. **Pannier JL, Vrijens J, and Van Cauter C.** Cardiorespiratory response to treadmill and bicycle exercise in runners. *European Journal of Applied Physiology and Occupational Physiology* 43: 243-251, 1980.

70. **Parry-Billings M.** The measurement of anaerobic power and capacity: studies on the Wingate anaerobic test. *Snipes J* 9: 48-58, 1986.

71. **Peronnet F and Thibault G.** Mathematical analysis of running performance and world running records. *Journal of Applied Physiology* 67: 453-465, 1989.

72. **Pollock ML.** Submaximal and maximal working capacity of elite distance runners. Part I: cardiorespiratory aspects. *Annals of the New York Academy of Sciences* 301: 310-322, 1977.

73. **Pollock ML, Bohannon RL, Cooper KH, Ayres JJ, Ward A, White SR, et al.** A comparative analysis of four protocols for maximal treadmill stress testing. *American Heart Journal* 92: 39-46, 1976.

74. **Pollock ML, Jackson AS, and Pate RR.** Discriminant analysis of physiological differences between good and elite distance runners. *Research Quarterly for Exercise and Sport* 51: 521-532, 1980.

75. **Powers S.** Ventilatory threshold, running economy, and distance running performance of trained athletes. *Research Quarterly for Exercise and Sport* 54: 179-182, 1983.

76. **Powers SK, Dodd S, and Garner R.** Precision of ventilatory and gas exchange alterations as a predictor of the anaerobic threshold. *European Journal of Applied Physiology and Occupational Physiology* 52: 173-177, 1984.

77. **Psotta R, Bunc V, Hendl J, Tenney D, and Heller J.** Is repeated-sprint ability of soccer players predictable from field-based or laboratory physiological tests? *Journal of Sports Medicine and Physical Fitness* 51: 18-25, 2011.

78. **Rampinini E, Bishop D, Marcora SM, Ferrari Bravo D, Sassi R, and Impellizzeri FM.** Validity of simple field tests as indicators of match-related physical performance in top-level professional soccer players. *International Journal of Sports Medicine* 28: 228-235, 2007.

79. **Reiman M and Manske R.** *Functional Testing in Human Performance.* Champaign, IL: Human Kinetics, 2009.

80. **Sale D.** Testing strength and power. In *Physiological Testing of the High Performance Athlete*, edited by MacDougall J, Wenger H, and Green H. Champaign, IL: Human Kinetics, 1991, pp. 21-106.

81. **Sawka MN, Foley ME, Pimental NA, Toner MM, and Pandolf KB.** Determination of maximal aerobic power during upper-body exercise. *Journal of Applied Physiology* 54: 113-117, 1983.

82. **Schenau G.** Can cycle power output predict sprint running performance? *European Journal of Applied Physiology* 63: 255-260, 1991.

83. **Schnabel A and Kindermann W.** Assessment of anaerobic capacity in runners. *European Journal of Applied Physiology and Occupational Physiology* 52: 42-46, 1983.

84. **Schwade J, Blomqvist CG, and Shapiro W.** A comparison of the response to arm and leg work in patients with ischemic heart disease. *American Heart Journal* 94: 203-208, 1977.

85. **Scott BK and Houmard JA.** Peak running velocity is highly related to distance running performance. *International Journal of Sports Medicine* 15: 504-507, 1994.

86. **Shaw DJ, Crawford MH, Karliner JS, DiDonna G, Carleton RM, Ross J, Jr., et al.** Arm-crank ergometry: a new method for the evaluation of coronary artery disease. *American Journal of Cardiology* 33: 801-805, 1974.

87. **Sherrill DL, Anderson SJ, and Swanson G.** Using smoothing splines for detecting ventilatory thresholds. *Medicine & Science in Sports & Exercise* 22: 684-689, 1990.

88. **Simoneau JA, Lortie G, Boulay MR, and Bouchard C.** Tests of anaerobic alactacid and lactacid capacities: description and reliability. *Canadian Journal of Applied Sport Sciences* 8: 266-270, 1983.

89. **Storer TW, Davis JA, and Caiozzo VJ.** Accurate prediction of $\dot{V}O_2$ max in cycle ergometry. *Medicine & Science in Sports & Exercise* 22: 704-712, 1990.

90. **Stuart M, Powers S, and Nelson J.** Development of an anaerobic fitness test for football players. (Unpublished observations).

91. **Tanaka K and Matsuura Y.** Marathon performance, anaerobic threshold, and onset of blood lactate accumulation. *Journal of Applied Physiology* 57: 640-643, 1984.

92. **Tanaka K, Matsuura Y, Kumagai S, Matsuzaka A, Hirakoba K, and Asano K.** Relationships of anaerobic threshold and onset of blood lactate accumulation with endurance performance. *European Journal of Applied Physiology and Occupational Physiology* 52: 51-56, 1983.

93. **Taunton JE, Maron H, and Wilkinson JG.** Anaerobic performance in middle and long distance runners. *Canadian Journal of Applied Sport Sciences* 6: 109-113, 1981.

94. **Taylor HL, Buskirk E, and Henschel A.** Maximal oxygen intake as an objective measure of cardio-respiratory performance. *Journal of Applied Physiology* 8: 73-80, 1955.

95. **Thoden J.** Testing aerobic power. In *Physiological Testing of the High Performance Athlete*, edited by MacDougall J, Wenger H, and Green H. Champaign, IL: Human Kinetics, 1991, pp. 107-174.

96. **Thorland WG, Johnson GO, Cisar CJ, Housh TJ, and Tharp GD.** Strength and anaerobic responses of elite young female sprint and distance runners. *Medicine & Science in Sports & Exercise* 19: 56-61, 1987.

97. **Walker R, Powers S, and Stuart MK.** Peak oxygen uptake in arm ergometry: effects of testing protocol. *British Journal of Sports Medicine* 20: 25-26, 1986.

98. **Wasserman K, Whipp BJ, Koyl SN, and Beaver WL.** Anaerobic threshold and respiratory gas exchange during exercise. *Journal of Applied Physiology* 35: 236-243, 1973.

99. **Weltman A, Snead D, Stein P, Seip R, Schurrer R, Rutt R, and Weltman J.** Reliability and validity of a continuous incremental treadmill protocol for the determination of lactate threshold, fixed blood lactate concentrations, and $\dot{V}O_{2max}$. *International Journal of Sports Medicine* 11: 26-32, 1990.

100. **Williams JH, Powers SK, and Stuart MK.** Hemoglobin desaturation in highly trained athletes during heavy exercise. *Medicine & Science in Sports & Exercise* 18: 168-173, 1986.

101. **Wyndham CH, Strydom NB, van Rensburg AJ, and Benade AJ.** Physiological requirements for world-class performances in endurance running. *South African Medical Journal* 43: 996-1002, 1969.

102. **Zacharogiannis E, Pardisis G, and Tziortzis S.** An evaluation of tests of anaerobic power and capacity. *Medicine & Science in Sports & Exercise* 36: S116, 2004.

103. **Zagatto AM, Beck WR, and Gobatto CA.** Validity of the running anaerobic sprint test for assessing anaerobic power and predicting short-distance performances. *Journal of Strength and Conditioning Research* 23: 1820-1827, 2009.

104. **Zhang YY, Johnson MC, II, Chow N, and Wasserman K.** Effect of exercise testing protocol on parameters of aerobic function. *Medicine & Science in Sports & Exercise* 23: 625-630, 1991.

21

© Digital Vision/Getty Images

Training for Performance

■ Objectives

By studying this chapter, you should be able to do the following:

1. Design a sport-specific training program based on an analysis of the energy systems utilized by the activity.
2. Define the terms *overload, specificity,* and *reversibility.*
3. Compare and contrast the use of interval training and continuous training to improve the maximal aerobic power in athletes.
4. Discuss the differences between training for anaerobic power and training for the improvement of strength.
5. List the advantages and disadvantages of different equipment types in weight training.
6. Define delayed-onset muscle soreness (DOMS). Outline the factors that contribute to its development.
7. Discuss the use of static and ballistic stretching to improve flexibility.
8. Discuss the differences between conditioning goals during (1) the off-season, (2) the preseason, and (3) in-season.
9. List and discuss several common training errors.

■ Outline

delayed-onset muscle soreness
   (DOMS)
dynamic stretching
hypertrophy
overtraining

progressive resistance exercise (PRE)
proprioceptive neuromuscular
   facilitation (PNF)
repetition
rest interval

set
static stretching
tapering
variable-resistance exercise
work interval

Traditionally, coaches and trainers have planned conditioning programs for their teams by following regimens used by teams that have successful win-loss records. This type of reasoning is not sound because win-loss records alone do not scientifically validate the conditioning programs used by the successful teams. In fact, the successful team might be victorious by virtue of its superior athletes and not its outstanding conditioning program. Clearly, the planning of an effective athletic conditioning program is best achieved by the application of proven physiological training principles. Optimizing training programs for athletes is important because failure to properly condition an athletic team results in a poor performance and often defeat. This chapter presents an overview of how to apply scientific principles to the development of an athletic conditioning program.

TRAINING PRINCIPLES

The overall objective of a sport conditioning program is to improve performance. Depending upon the specific sport, this can be achieved by increasing the muscle's ability to generate force and power, improving muscular efficiency, and/or increasing muscular endurance (8, 9, 70). Recall that throughout this book (e.g., Chaps. 3, 4, 13, 19, and 20), emphasis has been placed on the fact that dissimilar sport activities use different metabolic pathways or "energy systems" to produce the ATP needed for movement. An understanding of exercise metabolism is important to the coach or trainer because the design of a conditioning program to optimize athletic performance requires knowledge of the principal energy systems utilized by the sport. Let's consider a few examples. The performance of a 60-meter dash uses the ATP-PC system almost exclusively to produce the needed ATP. In contrast, a marathon runner depends on aerobic metabolism to provide the energy needed to complete the race. However, most sport activities use multiple energy pathways. For instance, soccer uses a combination of metabolic pathways to provide the needed ATP. Knowledge of the relative anaerobic-aerobic contributions to ATP production during an activity is the cornerstone of planning a

conditioning program. A well-designed conditioning program allocates the appropriate amount of aerobic and anaerobic conditioning time to match the energy demand of the sport. For instance, if an activity derives 40% of its ATP from anaerobic pathways and 60% from aerobic pathways (e.g., 1500-meter run), the training program should be divided 40%/60% between anaerobic/aerobic training (8). Table 21.1 contains a list of various sports and an estimation of their predominant energy systems. The coach and athlete can use this information to allocate the appropriate amount of time to training each energy system.

This discussion does not necessarily imply that power athletes (e.g., sprinters) should not perform aerobic training. On the contrary, aerobic exercise during the preseason to strengthen tendons and ligaments is generally recommended for all athletes. Note, however, that performing concurrent training (i.e., resistance training and endurance [aerobic] exercise) can possibly reduce strength gains compared to strength training alone (92). Therefore, designing the appropriate training program to optimize the benefit to the athlete requires careful planning. More will be said about concurrent training later in the chapter.

Overload, Specificity, and Reversibility

The terms *overload*, *specificity*, and *reversibility* were introduced in Chap. 13 and are repeated here only briefly. Recall that an organ system (e.g., cardiovascular, skeletal muscle, etc.) increases its capacity in response to a training overload. That is, the training program must stress the system above the level to which it is accustomed. While a training overload is required to achieve improvements in performance, too much overload without sufficient time for recovery can result in overtraining. **Overtraining** is defined as an accumulation of training stress that impairs an athlete's ability to perform training sessions and results in long-term decrements of performance (95). Overtraining is commonly associated with both physiological and psychological symptoms (e.g., chronic fatigue, mood disturbance, etc.). Recovery from overtraining can restore performance capacity, but may require several weeks or months of reduced exercise training.

TABLE 21.1	The Predominant Energy Systems for Selected Sports		
	% ATP CONTRIBUTION BY ENERGY SYSTEM		
Sport/Activity	ATP-PC	Glycolysis	Aerobic
Baseball	80	15	5
Basketball	80	10	10
Field hockey	60	20	20
Football	90	10	—
Golf (swing)	100	—	—
Gymnastics	90	10	—
Ice hockey:			
Forwards/ defense	80	20	—
Goalie	95	5	—
Rowing	20	30	50
Soccer:			
Goalie/wings/ strikers	80	20	—
Halfbacks	60	20	20
Swimming:			
Diving	98	2	—
50 meters	95	5	—
100 meters	80	15	—
200 meters	30	65	5
400 meters	20	40	40
1500 meters	10	20	70
Tennis	70	20	10
Track and field:			
100/200 meters	98	2	—
Field events	90	10	—
400 meters	40	55	5
800 meters	10	60	30
1500 meters	5	35	60
5000 meters	2	28	70
Marathon	—	2	98
Volleyball	90	10	—
Wrestling	45	55	—

Fox, E., and Mathews, D., *Interval Training: Conditioning for Sports and General Fitness.* Philadelphia, PA: W.B. Saunders, 1974.

A related term, *overreaching*, is also commonly used in the exercise training literature. Overreaching is commonly defined as excessive training that leads to a short-term decrement in performance; with adequate rest intervals between training sessions, this type of training can lead to improved performance (95). As you can see, overtraining and overreaching are similar terms and it is often difficult to distinguish between the two (95). To avoid confusion this chapter will refer to an extreme accumulation of training stress as overtraining, and the term overreaching will not be used.

The concept of specificity refers not only to the specific muscles involved in a particular movement, but also to the energy systems that provide the ATP required to complete the movement under competitive conditions. Therefore, training programs should use not only those muscle groups engaged during competition, but also the energy systems that will be providing the ATP. For instance, specific training for a sprinter would involve running high-intensity dashes. Similarly, specific training for a marathoner would involve long distance runs in which virtually all the ATP needed by the working muscles would be derived from aerobic metabolism.

When an athlete stops training, the training effect is quickly lost, and this is referred to as the reversibility of training. For example, studies have demonstrated that within two weeks after the cessation of training, significant reductions in $\dot{V}O_2$ max can occur (23, 24). Specifically, a classic study demonstrated that after 20 days of bed rest, a group of subjects showed a 25% reduction in $\dot{V}O_2$ max and maximal cardiac output (86). This large detraining-induced decrement in $\dot{V}O_2$ max clearly demonstrates the rapid reversibility of training.

Influence of Gender and Initial Fitness Level

At one time, it was believed that conditioning programs for women had special requirements that differed from those used to train men. However, it is now clear that men and women respond to training programs in a similar fashion (7, 12, 89). Therefore, the same general approach to physiological conditioning can be used in planning programs for men and women. This does not mean that men and women should perform identical exercise training sessions (e.g., same volume and intensity). Indeed, individual training programs should be designed appropriately to match the level of fitness and maturation of the athlete, regardless of gender. Individual "exercise prescriptions" is an important concern in the design of training programs and is discussed in further detail in later sections of this chapter.

It is a common observation that individuals differ greatly in the degree to which their performance benefits from training programs. Many factors contribute to the observed individual variations in the training response. One of the most important influences is the athlete's beginning level of fitness. In general, the amount of training improvement is always greater in those who are less conditioned at the beginning of the training program. It has been demonstrated that sedentary, middle-aged men with heart disease may improve their $\dot{V}O_2$ max by as much as 50%, whereas the same training program in normal, active adults improves $\dot{V}O_2$ max by only 10%–20%. Similarly, conditioned athletes may improve their level of conditioning by only 3%–5% following an increase in training intensity. However, this 3%–5% improvement in the trained athlete may be the difference between winning an Olympic gold medal and failing to place in the event.

Influence of Genetics

As discussed in Chap. 13, it is clear that genetics play an important role in how an individual responds to a training program (4, 10, 83). For instance, a person with a high genetic endowment for endurance sports responds differently to endurance training than does someone with a markedly different genetic profile. Indeed, recent research has provided genetic clues as to why some individuals are "high responders" to training and improve their fitness levels quickly to a greater extent than do "low responders" (10). For this reason, and the fact that athletes begin conditioning programs at different levels of fitness, training programs should be individualized. It is unrealistic to expect each athlete on the team to perform the same amount of work or to exercise at the same work rate during training sessions.

Note that while training can greatly improve performance, there is no substitute for genetically inherited athletic talent if the individual is to compete at a world-class level. Indeed, there is a limit to how much training can improve aerobic power. Therefore, those individuals with a low genetic endowment for aerobic power cannot, under any training program, increase their $\dot{V}O_2$ max to world-class levels. Åstrand and Rodahl (8) have commented that if you want to become a world-class athlete, you must choose your parents wisely. Although this comment was made in jest, genetics does play a key role in determining athletic potential. A Closer Look 21.1 examines this issue in more detail and explores the physiological limits for performance enhancement.

Similar to aerobic exercise, genetics also play a key role in determining the performance level that can be achieved in anaerobic sports (e.g., sprinting in track and field) (13, 67). Indeed, it is well known that training can only improve anaerobic performance to a small degree. The primary reason is that the type of skeletal muscle fiber that is best suited for anaerobic performance (i.e., fast fibers, type IIx) is determined early in development, and the relative percentage of muscle fiber types does not vary widely over the lifetime. Therefore, anaerobic capacity appears to be largely genetically determined because the percentage of fast/anaerobic fibers is a primary determinant of anaerobic capacity.

IN SUMMARY

- The general objective of sport conditioning is to improve performance by increasing muscle force/power output, improving muscular efficiency, and/or improving muscle endurance.
- A conditioning program should allocate the appropriate amount of training time to match the aerobic and anaerobic energy demands of the sport.
- Muscles respond to training as a result of a progressive overload. When an athlete stops training, a rapid decline in fitness occurs due to detraining (reversibility).
- In general, men and women respond to conditioning in a similar fashion. The amount of training improvement is always greater in those individuals who are less conditioned at the onset of the training program.
- Genetics play an important role in performance in both endurance (aerobic) exercise and anaerobic exercise.

COMPONENTS OF A TRAINING SESSION: WARM-UP, WORKOUT, AND COOL DOWN

Every training session should consist of three components: (1) warm-up, (2) workout, and (3) cool down. This idea was first introduced in Chap. 16 and is mentioned only briefly here. The warm-up prior to a training workout has two primary objectives. First, warm-up exercises increase cardiac output and blood flow to the skeletal muscles to be used during the training session. Second, the warm-up activity results in an increase in muscle temperature, which elevates muscle enzyme activity. The duration of the warm-up is generally from 10 to 20 minutes, depending on environmental conditions and the nature of the training activity. Although limited data exist, a recent review concludes that a proper warm-up may reduce the possibility of muscle injury due to pulls or strains (33, 94) and may also improve physical performance (34). Nonetheless, additional research is needed to definitively demonstrate whether a warm-up can deter exercise-induced injuries.

Immediately following the training session, a period of low-intensity "cool-down" exercises should be performed. The objective of a cool down is to return "pooled" blood from the exercised skeletal muscles back to the central circulation. Similar to the warm-up, the length of the cool down may vary from 10 to 20 minutes, depending on environmental conditions and the nature of the training session.

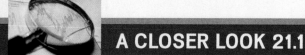
Enhancement in Endurance Performance: What Are the Physiological Limits?

Elite endurance performance relies on many factors including appropriate training, proper nutrition, motivation, and several key physiological determinants. Although many physiological factors contribute to endurance performance, three key elements of success include: (1) a high $\dot{V}O_2$ max; (2) superior exercise economy/efficiency; and (3) a high lactate threshold and critical power. Let's discuss how much training can improve each of these important physiological determinants of endurance performance success.

How much can training improve $\dot{V}O_2$ max?

The genetic makeup of an individual is referred to as a "genotype." Fig. 21.1 illustrates the fact that genetics plays an important role in determining $\dot{V}O_2$ max. For example, individuals labeled as "genotype A" (bottom line) possess a relatively low $\dot{V}O_2$ max

$(35 \text{ ml} \cdot \text{kg}^{-1} \cdot \text{min}^{-1})$ in the untrained state and often, these individuals are also "low responders" to exercise as training results in only small improvements in their $\dot{V}O_2$ max (e.g., 5% or less). Clearly, the genetic makeup of these individuals will not permit them to achieve the $\dot{V}O_2$ max that is required to become a champion endurance athlete (i.e., approximately 80 ml $\cdot$ kg^{-1} $\cdot$ min^{-1}). In contrast, individuals labeled as "genotype E" enjoy the ideal genetic makeup required for champion endurance athletes. Indeed, these individuals possess an elevated $\dot{V}O_2$ max (e.g., 53 ml $\cdot$ kg^{-1} $\cdot$ min^{-1}) in the untrained state and are commonly "high responders" to exercise training as training can often increase their $\dot{V}O_2$ max by 50% (i.e., training-induced improvement of $\dot{V}O_2$ max from 53 to 80 ml $\cdot$ kg^{-1} $\cdot$ min^{-1}).

The genotypes labeled as B–D in Fig. 21.1 further illustrate the range of genetic differences that exist across

the population. Specifically, the $\dot{V}O_2$ max (untrained state) of these individual's spans from 40 to 48 ml $\cdot$ kg^{-1} $\cdot$ min^{-1} and their training-induced improvement in maximal aerobic power can range from 15% to 35%. From the examples illustrated in Fig. 21.1, it is clear that in order to achieve a $\dot{V}O_2$ max of 80 ml $\cdot$ kg^{-1} $\cdot$ min^{-1}, it is essential that athletes begin with a baseline $\dot{V}O_2$ max between 53 and 60 ml $\cdot$ kg^{-1} $\cdot$ min^{-1} because training can only increase $\dot{V}O_2$ max by approximately 50%. Further, note that Fig. 21.1 also illustrates that regardless of the genetic makeup of the individual, the training-induced increase in $\dot{V}O_2$ max typically reaches a plateau within the first 24–30 months of training. Therefore, following the first 24–30 months of training, further advances in endurance performance must come from improvements in exercise economy and/or increases in the lactate threshold or critical power.

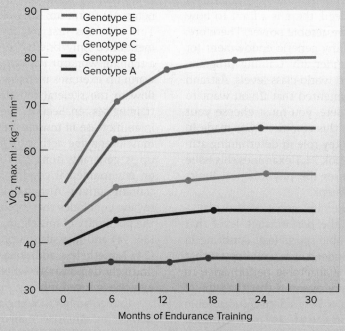

Figure 21.1 Illustration of the impact of genetics (i.e., genotype) on $\dot{V}O_2$ max in both the untrained state and following 30 months of endurance training (each group performed similar training protocols). Genotype E (top line) illustrates the individual with the genetic makeup of a champion endurance athlete. Genotype A (bottom line) exemplifies the genetic makeup of an individual that has very limited genetic potential to become a champion endurance athlete. Notice that training-induced increases in $\dot{V}O_2$ max often reach a plateau at around 24-30 months of training. See text for more details.

How much can training improve exercise economy/efficiency?

Although training improvements in $\dot{V}O_2$ max often reach a plateau within the first 24–30 months of training, exercise economy/efficiency can increase throughout the career of championship endurance athletes. For example, Paula Radcliffe (current world record holder in the marathon) improved her running economy by 15% during 9 years of training (56). This enhancement in exercise economy was achieved by exercise training alone without any specific attempts to alter running style. Similarly, muscular efficiency has been shown to improve by 8% in an elite cyclist during 7 years of training (23). It is not clear if training-induced improvements in exercise economy/efficiency are dependent upon the genetic makeup of the individual (65). Also, the mechanism(s) responsible for exercise-induced improvement in exercise economy/efficiency remain a topic of debate.

How much can training improve the lactate threshold or critical power?

Both the lactate threshold and critical power can be improved in elite athletes during several years of training. For instance, the elite marathon runner Paula Radcliffe improved both her lactate threshold and critical power output during 10 years of training (56). In particular, this champion athlete improved her lactate threshold and critical power by approximately 30% over a decade of training. Similar to running economy, it is unknown if training-induced improvements in the lactate threshold and critical power are impacted significantly by genetics.

Summary–what are the physiological limits to performance enhancement?

- Training-induced improvements in $\dot{V}O_2$ max are greatly influenced by the genetic makeup (i.e., genotype) of the individual. Training improvements in $\dot{V}O_2$ max ranges from 5% to 50% (depending upon genotype) and often reach a plateau during the first 24–30 months of training.

- Exercise training can improve exercise economy by as much as 15% during several years of training.

- Training-induced improvements in both the lactate threshold and critical power can reach approximately 30% during 10 years of exercise training.

See Lundby and Robach (2015) and Joyner and Coyle (2008) in the Suggested Readings for more details on the physiological limitations to performance enhancement.

IN SUMMARY

- Every training session should consist of a warm-up period, a workout session, and a cool-down period.
- Although limited data exist, it is feasible that a warm-up reduces the risk of muscle and/or tendon injury during exercise.

TRAINING TO IMPROVE AEROBIC POWER

Recall from Chap. 13 that endurance training improves $\dot{V}O_2$ max by increasing both maximal cardiac output and the a-$\bar{v}$ O_2 difference (i.e., increasing the muscle's ability to extract O_2). Therefore, a training program designed to improve maximal aerobic power must overload the circulatory system and stress the oxidative capacities of skeletal muscles as well. As in all training regimens, specificity is critical. The athlete should stress the specific muscles to be used in his or her sport. Therefore, runners should train by running, cyclists should train on the bicycle, swimmers should swim, and so forth.

There are three principal aerobic training methods used by athletes: (1) interval training, (2) long, slow distance (low-intensity), and (3) high-intensity, continuous exercise. Controversy exists as to which of these training methods results in the greatest improvement in $\dot{V}O_2$ max. Indeed, there does not appear to be a magic training formula for all athletes to follow. However, evidence suggests that training intensity is a key factor in improving $\dot{V}O_2$ max (50, 76, 77). Nonetheless, from a psychological standpoint, it would appear that a mixing of all three methods provides the needed variety to prevent the athlete from becoming bored with a single and rather monotonous training program.

Note that improvement of $\dot{V}O_2$ max is only one variable related to endurance. Recall from Chap. 20 that although a high $\dot{V}O_2$ max is important for success in endurance events, both movement economy and the lactate threshold are also important variables that contribute to endurance performance. Therefore, training to improve endurance performance should not only be geared toward the improvement of $\dot{V}O_2$ max, but should also increase the lactate threshold and improve running economy (see Closer Look 21.1 for more details on the physiological limits for improving the lactate threshold and exercise economy). A brief discussion of various training methods used to improve endurance performance follows.

Interval Training

Interval training involves the performance of repeated exercise bouts, with brief recovery periods in between. The length and intensity of the **work interval** depends on what the athlete is trying to accomplish.

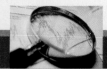
High-Intensity Interval Training—New Interest in an Old Training Method

The use of interval training as a method of conditioning endurance athletes first gained world-wide attention over 60 years ago when Roger Banister ran the first sub-4 minute mile. Here's the story. When Banister broke the 4-minute mile barrier in 1954, he was a medical student with limited time for training. His solution to his time management problem was to avoid time-consuming long distance runs and instead he performed short daily training sessions using high-intensity interval training (HIIT). For example, his typical daily workout was to run 6-10 × 400 meter intervals at near maximal effort resulting in 55-60 seconds of intense exercise. The fact that this training program allowed Bannister to break the world record for the mile run provided the first practical evidence that this form of training was a highly effective conditioning technique for endurance athletes.

Recently, a renewed interest in HIIT has emerged in both the scientific and popular literature because HIIT has been demonstrated to be a highly effective and time-saving method of training for endurance athletes and individuals interested in health-related fitness. For example, research reveals that as few as 30 seconds of high-intensity exercise promotes rapid and significant physiological adaptations. Specifically, even low-volume HIIT results in an increase in mitochondrial volume in the trained skeletal muscles. The exercise-induced signaling pathways that trigger this adaptation in skeletal muscles were discussed in Chap. 13 and involve the activation of PGC-1α which promotes mitochondrial biogenesis. For a summary of the physiological adaptations associated with HIIT see Gibala et al. (2012) in Suggested Readings.

For instance, a longer work interval requires a greater involvement of aerobic energy production, whereas a shorter, more intense interval provides greater participation of anaerobic metabolism. Therefore, interval training that is designed to improve $\dot{V}O_2$ max typically involves intervals longer than 50-60 seconds to increase the involvement of aerobic ATP production. Further, it is believed that high-intensity intervals are more effective in improving aerobic power, and perhaps the lactate threshold, than low-intensity intervals (29, 31, 59). These improvements are likely due to the recruitment of fast-twitch (types IIa and IIx) fibers during this type of high-intensity exercise (26).

Recently, the term high-intensity interval training (HIIT) has been coined to describe high-intensity intervals lasting 30-120 seconds. A relatively short high-intensity exercise bout lasting 30 seconds would be expected to involve a significant amount of energy production from anaerobic energy sources. Nonetheless, abundant evidence indicates that HIIT promotes significant improvements in the aerobic capacity (i.e., increased mitochondrial volume) in the trained skeletal muscles (40). For more details and a brief history of HIIT, see A Closer Look 21.2.

One obvious advantage of interval training over continuous running at slower speeds is that this method of training provides a means of performing large amounts of high-intensity exercise in a short time. Further, this training method offers two ways of providing a training overload. For example, the interval training prescription can be modified to provide "overload" in terms of increasing either the total number of exercise intervals performed or the intensity of the work interval. Adjustments to either of these factors allow the coach or athlete to alter the workout plan to accomplish specific training goals. How does one design an interval workout? A complete discussion of the theory and rationale of designing an interval training program to improve athletic performance is beyond the scope of this chapter; therefore, only an overview of interval training will be provided here. In planning an interval training session, the following variables need to be considered: (1) length of the work interval, (2) intensity of the effort, (3) duration of the rest interval, (4) number of interval sets, and (5) the number of work repetitions. The length of the work interval refers to the distance to be covered during the work effort. The intensity of the work effort during interval training can be monitored from a 10-second HR count upon completion of the interval (i.e., 10-second HR count × 6 = HR per min). In general, exercise HRs should reach 85%-100% of the maximal HR during interval training. The time between work efforts is termed the **rest interval** and consists of light activity such as walking. The length of the rest interval is generally expressed as a ratio of the duration of the work interval. For example, if the work interval for running 400 meters was 75 seconds, a rest interval of 75 seconds would result in a 1:1 ratio of work to rest. Generally, the rest interval should be at least as long as the work interval (8). In planning an interval training program for athletes who are not already highly trained, a work:rest ratio of 1:3 or 1:2 may be preferable. As a general rule in young adult athletes, the HR should drop to approximately 120-130 beats · min⁻¹ near the end of the recovery interval (8).

A **set** is a specified number of work efforts performed as a unit. For instance, a set may consist of

8 × 400-meter runs with a prescribed rest interval between each run. The term **repetition** is the number of work efforts within one set. In the example just provided, 8 × 400-meter runs constituted one set of 8 repetitions. The number of repetitions and sets performed per workout depends on the purpose of the particular training session and the fitness levels of the athletes involved. For more details on interval training, see reference 62.

Long, Slow-Distance Exercise

The use of long, slow-distance runs (or cycle rides, long swims, etc.) became a popular means of training for endurance events in the 1970s. In general, this method of training involves performing exercise at a low intensity (i.e., 50%–65% $\dot{V}O_2$ max or approximately 60%–70% of max HR) for durations that are generally greater in length than the normal competition distance. Although it seems reasonable that this type of training is a useful means of preparing an athlete to compete in long endurance competitions (marathon running), evidence suggests that short-term, high-intensity exercise is superior to long-term, low-intensity exercise in improving $\dot{V}O_2$ max (50).

One of the historical reasons that athletes have used training sessions of long duration is the common belief that improvements in endurance are proportional to the volume of training performed. Indeed, many coaches and athletes believe that improvements in athletic performance are directly related to how much work was performed during training, and that athletes can reach their potential only by doing long-duration exercise bouts. However, evidence by Costill et al. contradicts this belief (22). Indeed, a classic study demonstrated that athletes training 1.5 hours per day performed as well as athletes training 3 hours per day (22). In fact, the athletes who trained 3 hours per day performed more poorly in some events than the group training 1.5 hours per day. This study illustrates the point that "more" is not always better in endurance training. Therefore, coaches and athletes should carefully consider the volume of training required to reach maximal benefits from long, slow-distance exercise.

High-Intensity, Continuous Exercise

Again, research suggests that continuous, high-intensity exercise is an outstanding means of improving $\dot{V}O_2$ max and the lactate threshold in athletes (25, 27, 30, 50). Although the exercise intensity that promotes the greatest improvement in $\dot{V}O_2$ max may vary from athlete to athlete, it appears that exercise intensities between 80% and 100% $\dot{V}O_2$ max are optimal (see Fig. 21.2) (76). Further, evidence also indicates that a work rate that is equal to or slightly above the lactate threshold provides improvement in maximum aerobic power (76, 88).

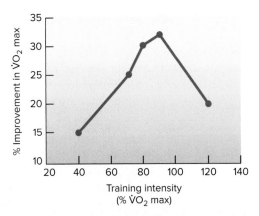

Figure 21.2 Relationship between training intensity and percent improvement in $\dot{V}O_2$ max.

Data from Knuttgen, H. G., Nordesjo, L.O., Ollander, B., and Saltin, B., "Physical Conditioning Through Interval Training with Young Male Adults," *Medicine and Science in Sports* 5: 220–226, 1973.

How does the athlete monitor their exercise intensity during a training session? A precise quantification of training intensity during exercise is complicated, but the measurement of exercise heart rate can be used as an estimate of an athlete's relative training intensity. An example of a heart rate-based training intensity scale to prescribe and monitor training of endurance athletes is presented in Table 21.2. Obviously, standardizing exercise intensity based on heart rate alone has limitations and fails to account for individual variation among athletes in the relationship between heart rate and blood lactate concentration. Nonetheless, the advantage of this type of intensity scale is the simplicity because athletes can easily measure their heart rates during exercise using electronic heart rate monitors. For more details on using heart rate to monitor training intensity, see Seiler (2010) in Suggested Readings.

Altitude Training Improves Exercise Performance at Sea Level

Whether or not exercise training at high altitude improves endurance performance at sea level remains a controversial topic, as altitude training is not consistently reported to be advantageous in improving $\dot{V}O_2$ max and performance at sea level (90). Nonetheless, for many years, endurance athletes believed that living and training at high altitude (e.g., <6000 feet above sea level) enhances performance compared to living and training at sea level (69, 91). However, this may not always be true because athletes cannot perform as much high-intensity exercise training at altitude compared to sea level. Therefore, by performing less training, a form of detraining could actually occur while living and training at altitude. So, how can athletes design a training program to optimize the physiological benefits of living at altitude without the potentially negative detraining effects?

Training in Athletes
A practical variable to monitor exercise intensity is heart rate expressed as a percent of heart rate max. Note that the exercise intensity zones presented in this table are arbitrary, beginning with a relatively low-intensity zone (zone 1) and ending with a high-intensity zone (zone 5).

Intensity Zone	% Heart Rate Max	%$\dot{V}O_2$ Max	Blood Lactate Levels (mmol · L^{-1})	Typical Training Duration in Zone
1	60–71	50–65	0.8–1.5	1–3 hours
2	72–82	66–80	1.5–2.5	1–2 hours
3	83–87	81–87	2.6–4.0	30–90 minutes
4	88–92	88–93	4.1–6.0	10–40 minutes
5	93–100	94–100	>6.1	5–10 minutes

This altitude-training riddle appeared to be solved when researchers developed the altitude training modality known as "Live-High, Train-Low" (63). This training program requires the athlete to spend most of the day resting and sleeping at altitude, but the athlete performs exercise training sessions at a much lower altitude. This approach affords the athlete the benefit of altitude acclimatization, and by training at a low altitude, the athlete's ability to perform intense training sessions is not hampered by high altitude. This type of altitude training program has been argued to provide significant performance gains compared to training and living at sea level (63). Nonetheless, debate on this topic continues and some authors suggest that altitude training is not beneficial for elite athletes. See Lundby and Robach (2016) in the Suggested Readings for more details on the impact of altitude training on exercise performance at sea level. Note that the issue of altitude training is discussed again in Chap. 24.

IN SUMMARY

- Historically, training to improve maximal aerobic power has used three methods: (1) interval training, (2) long, slow-distance exercise, and (3) high-intensity, continuous exercise.
- Although controversy exists as to which of the training methods results in the greatest improvement in $\dot{V}O_2$ max, growing evidence suggests that it is intensity and not duration that is the most important factor in improving $\dot{V}O_2$ max.
- The concept that "Live-High, Train-Low" altitude training program provides significant endurance performance gains compared to training and living at sea level remains controversial and additional research is required to confirm that this practice will improve performance at sea level in elite athletes.

INJURIES AND ENDURANCE TRAINING

An important question associated with any type of endurance training is what type of training program presents the lowest risk of injury to the athlete. At present, a clear answer to this question is not available. However, a review of exercise-training-induced injuries suggests that the majority of training injuries are a result of overtraining (e.g., overuse injuries) and occur in the knee (57, 75). The overuse injury can come from either short-term, high-intensity exercise or long-term, low-intensity exercise (75). A commonsense guideline to avoid overuse injuries is to avoid large increases in training volume or intensity. Perhaps the most useful general rule for increasing the training load is the "ten percent rule" (75). In short, the ten percent rule suggests that training intensity or duration should not be increased more than ten percent per week to avoid an overtraining injury. For example, a runner running 50 miles per week could increase his/her weekly distance to 55 miles (10% of 50 = 5) the following week.

In addition to overtraining, several other exercise-induced injury risk factors have been identified (75). Among these factors are musculotendonous imbalance of strength and/or flexibility, footwear problems (i.e., excessive wear), anatomical malalignment, poor running surface, and disease (e.g., arthritis and old fracture) (14).

Note that gender is not an injury risk factor for endurance training (75). Similar to male athletes, it appears that most of the leg injuries in female runners are the result of overtraining (75). This may be especially true for poorly conditioned women beginning training programs.

- The majority of training injuries are a result of overtraining (e.g., overuse injuries) and can come from either short-term, high-intensity exercise or prolonged, low-intensity exercise.
- A useful rule for increasing the training load is the "ten percent rule." The ten percent rule states that training intensity or duration should not be increased more than ten percent per week to avoid an overtraining injury.

TRAINING TO IMPROVE ANAEROBIC POWER

Athletic events lasting fewer than 60 seconds depend largely on anaerobic production of the necessary energy. In general, training to improve anaerobic power centers around the need to enhance either the ATP-PC system or anaerobic glycolysis (lactate system) (74). However, some activities require major contributions of both of these anaerobic metabolic pathways to provide the necessary ATP for competition (see Table 21.1). Moreover, many activities require ATP production from both aerobic and anaerobic sources. For example, running an 800-meter race is typically performed at a power output that exceeds $\dot{V}O_2$ max by ~30%. Exercise at work rates that exceed $\dot{V}O_2$ max is possible because the ATP used to perform at these high work rates comes from the combination of both aerobic sources and anaerobic sources. Therefore, energy to perform this type of sporting event requires the "pooled" ATP production from both aerobic and anaerobic sources (i.e., oxidative phosphorylation, anaerobic glycolysis, and the ATP-PC system).

Anaerobic training is commonly defined as exercise that is performed at intensities above $\dot{V}O_2$ max where the primary aim is to stimulate anaerobic energy production (55). High-intensity anaerobic training lasting two to ten seconds is often termed *speed or sprint training*, whereas the term *speed endurance training* is commonly used to describe all forms of anaerobic training lasting longer than ten seconds (55). Identical to aerobic endurance training, it is critical that the anaerobic training program use the specific muscle groups that are required by the athlete during competition.

Training to Improve the ATP-PC System

Sports such as football, weight lifting, and short dashes in track (100 meters) depend on the ATP-PC system to provide the bulk of the energy needed for competition. Therefore, optimal performance requires a training program that will maximize ATP production via the ATP-PC pathway.

Training to improve the ATP-PC system involves a special type of interval training. To maximally stress the ATP-PC metabolic pathway, short, high-intensity intervals (five to ten seconds' duration) using the muscles utilized in competition are ideal. Because of the short durations of this type of interval, limited lactate is produced and recovery is rapid. The rest interval may range between 30 and 60 seconds, depending on the fitness levels of the athletes. For example, a training program for football players might involve repeated 30- to 40-yard dashes with several directional changes with a 30-second rest period between efforts. The number of repetitions per set would be determined by the athletes' fitness levels, environmental factors, and perhaps other considerations.

Training to Improve the Glycolytic System

After approximately ten seconds of a maximal effort, there is a growing dependence on energy production from anaerobic glycolysis (32). To improve the capacity of this energy pathway, the athlete must overload the "system" via short-term, high-intensity efforts. In general, high-intensity intervals of 20–60 seconds' duration are useful in overloading this metabolic pathway.

This type of anaerobic training is both physically and psychologically demanding and thus requires a high commitment on the part of the athlete. Further, this type of training may drastically reduce muscle glycogen stores. For these reasons, athletes often alternate hard-interval training days and light training sessions. For more details on training for improved anaerobic performance, see Ask the Expert 21.1 and Iaia and Bangsbo (2010) in Suggested Readings.

- Training to improve anaerobic power involves a special type of interval training. In general, the intervals are of short duration and consist of high-intensity exercise.

TRAINING TO IMPROVE MUSCULAR STRENGTH

The goal of a strength-training program is to increase the maximum amount of force and power that can be generated by a particular muscle group. In general, any muscle that is regularly exercised at a high intensity (i.e., intensity near its maximum force-generating capacity) will become stronger. Strength-training exercises can be classified into three categories: (1) isometric or static, (2) dynamic or isotonic (includes variable-resistance exercise), and (3) isokinetic. Recall that isometric exercise is the

Training to Improve Anaerobic Performance: Questions and Answers with Dr. Michael Hogan

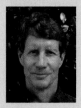

Courtesy of Michael Hogan

Michael Hogan, Ph.D., Professor in the Department of Medicine at the University of California–San Diego, is an internationally known exercise physiologist whose research focuses on delivery and utilization of oxygen in skeletal muscle. Dr. Hogan has published more than 160 research articles, and his work is widely cited in the scientific literature. Further, he has been a leader in numerous scientific organizations, including the American College of Sports Medicine and the American Physiological Society. In addition to being an internationally known scientist, Dr. Hogan continues to be an active competitor and coach in the pole vault. As a collegiate athlete, Dr. Hogan was a four-year letterman in track and field and a school record holder in the pole vault at the University of Notre Dame. In the years following his graduation from college, Dr. Hogan has continued to train and compete in the pole vault and has excelled in both national and international age-group championships in this event. In this box feature, Dr. Hogan answers questions related to training to improve anaerobic power.

QUESTION: In designing a training program to improve anaerobic power, should weekly training sessions be planned on a "hard-easy" cycle?

ANSWER: Absolutely! This is possibly even more critical in anaerobic power training versus aerobic training. The reason for this is that to improve anaerobic capacity, extremely high-intensity exercise needs to be conducted to totally activate the type IIx fibers within the muscle. Recall from Chap. 7 that due to the size principle, type IIx muscle fibers are the last fibers recruited during the muscle activation process. An important component of anaerobic training is to work during the "hard" cycle at an extremely high intensity that subsequently results in increasing muscle fiber size (thereby increasing the total amount of PC and ATP available) so that muscle power is increased. A key concern is the duration of the "hard-easy" cycles, as each individual athlete will be different in how much high-intensity exercise can be endured before the athlete "breaks down" and injury ensues. Knowing the proper balance of "hard-easy" is the difference between an Olympic gold medal and an injured athlete.

QUESTION: In sports or athletic events (e.g., 200-meter dash) that require energy from both the ATP-PC system and glycolysis, is it possible to design a training program to improve energy production from each of these bioenergetic systems?

ANSWER: Yes, these bioenergetic systems can be improved, although not to the degree that adaptation to endurance training (i.e., cardiovascular and oxidative enzyme changes) can be accomplished with aerobic training. The key to anaerobic performance that requires high ATP turnover rates for a short period (~30 seconds) is to have as much capacity in the glycolytic and ATP-PC systems and to minimize the factors that lead to fatigue in these short, high-intensity exercise bouts. Studies have demonstrated that glycolytic enzymes can be increased in all fiber types by high-intensity training so that more ATP can be generated anaerobically when necessary. Anaerobic training will also improve aerobic capacity (mitochondrial content) of the muscle, which can be important in that: (1) increased aerobic production of ATP will result in "sparing" of the ATP-PC and a lower rate of lactate production; and (2) increased mitochondria will also result in a more rapid resynthesis of PC during recovery from exercise and thereby, permit a subsequent high-intensity exercise bout to begin with a higher basal level of PC (important in sports with rapid start-stops like soccer or basketball). Anaerobic training will also improve the speed at which phosphocreatine (PC) can be degraded so that a faster ATP turnover is possible. It appears that PC levels are minimally affected by training; however, creatine supplementation increases resting levels of PC, thereby potentially improving anaerobic performance.

QUESTION: Recently, much interest has focused upon high-intensity training as a means of improving both anaerobic and aerobic power. Please define high-intensity training and discuss the evidence that this type of training can improve both anaerobic and aerobic bioenergetic systems.

ANSWER: Abundant evidence indicates that high-intensity interval training (HIIT), which is characterized by brief repeated bursts of intense exercise (e.g., 30–60 seconds of exercise at 100%–120% $\dot{V}O_2$ max), can significantly improve not only anaerobic bioenergetic pathways but maximal aerobic power as well. This has surprised some scientists because, historically, it has been believed that HIIT would improve only anaerobic power. Nonetheless, it is now clear that HIIT can induce many adaptations in muscle normally associated with traditional endurance exercise training, including increased mitochondrial volume and improved endurance performance. In fact, there is growing evidence that HIIT may provide fitness and health benefits above and beyond what can be derived from exclusive low-intensity aerobic training, likely due to a greater activation of adaptive responses resulting from the intense cellular stress of HIIT that is not generated by low-intensity aerobic activity.

application of force without joint movement, and that dynamic exercise involves force application with joint movement (see Chaps. 8 and 20). **Variable-resistance exercise** is the term used to describe exercise performed on machines such as Nautilus equipment, which provide a variable amount of resistance during the course of a dynamic contraction. Isokinetic exercise is the exertion of force at a constant speed. Although isometric exercise has been shown to improve strength, isotonic and isokinetic strength training are generally preferred in the preparation of athletes because isometric training does not increase strength over the full range of motion—only at the specific joint angle maintained during training.

What physiological adaptations occur as a result of strength training? This issue was discussed in Chap. 13 and will be addressed only briefly here. One of the obvious and perhaps most important physiological changes that occurs following a strength-training program is the increase in muscle mass. Recall from Chap. 8 that the amount of force that can be generated by a muscle group is proportional to the cross-sectional area of the muscle. Therefore, larger muscles exert greater force than smaller muscles. Recall that almost all of the increase in muscle size via resistance training is due to **hypertrophy** (an increase in muscle fiber diameter due to an increase in myofibrils) (2, 3, 42–44, 58, 87, 89).

Progressive Resistance Exercise

The most common form of strength training is weight lifting using free weights or various types of weight machines (i.e., dynamic or isokinetic training). To improve strength, weight training must employ the overload principle by periodically increasing the amount of weight (resistance) used in a particular exercise. This method of strength training was first described in 1940s by Delorme and Watkins and is called **progressive resistance exercise (PRE).** Since this early work, numerous other systems of training to improve muscular strength have been proposed, but the concept of PRE is the basis for most weight-training programs.

Resistance training workouts are prescribed around the exercise intensity and the volume of exercise performed. The exercise intensity of resistance training is expressed in terms of the repetitions maximum (RM), where 1-RM is the greatest weight that can be lifted one time. The volume of resistance training is established by the number of repetitions (reps) and sets that are performed. Sets are the number of times a specific exercise is performed, and reps are the number of times a movement is repeated within a set.

General Strength-Training Principles

Muscles increase in strength when they are overloaded by contracting at relatively high tensions. If muscles are not overloaded, no improvement in strength occurs. The first application of the overload principle was used by the famous Olympic wrestler, *Milo of Crotona* (500 B.C.). Milo incorporated overload in his training routine by carrying a bull calf on his back each day until the animal reached maturity. Since the days of Milo, athletes have applied the principle of overload to training by lifting heavy objects.

The optimal training regimen for optimal improvement of strength remains controversial. Indeed, there does not appear to be a simple formula for strength training that meets the needs of everyone (1). Therefore, the exercise prescription for strength training should be tailored to the individual. However, a general guideline for a strength-training prescription is as follows: In general, the recommended intensity of training is 8–12 maximal repetitions (RM) and practiced in multiple sets (1). Rest days between workouts seem critical for optimal strength improvement (1). Therefore, a training schedule of two to four days per week is recommended for novice or immediate individuals (1). For advanced weight training, a frequency of four to six days per week is recommended when using split routines (i.e., training one to three different muscle groups per training session) (1).

A common belief among coaches and athletes is that strength increases in direct proportion to the volume of training (i.e., number of sets performed). Although a physiological link exists between training volume and strength gains, the optimal number of sets to improve strength continues to be debated. Nonetheless, two recent reviews conclude that multiple sets (i.e., two or more sets) of resistance exercise result in greater hypertrophy and strength gains compared to one set alone (60, 61). It appears likely that the optimal number of sets for maximal improvement of muscular strength may vary among subjects of different ages and fitness levels (1). Further, it is clear that weight-training programs incorporating extremely high training volumes (e.g., >10 sets) are not required for optimal strength gains (38, 80).

Similar to other training methods, strength training should involve those muscles used in competition. Indeed, strength-training exercises should stress the muscles in the same movement pattern used during the athletic competition. For instance, a shot-putter should perform exercises that strengthen the specific muscles of the arm, chest, back, and legs that are involved in "putting the shot."

A final concern in the design of strength-training programs for sport performance is that the speed of muscle shortening during training should be similar to those speeds used during the event. For example, many sports require a high velocity of movement. Studies have shown that strength-training programs using high-velocity movements in a sport-specific movement pattern produce superior gains in strength/power-oriented sports. Table 21.3 provides an overview of resistance training guidelines for training programs to emphasize gains in maximal strength or muscular endurance. For a complete overview of progression models of strength training, see the ACSM position stand (2009) in Suggested Readings. Further, see The Winning Edge 21.1 for information on periodization of strength training to improve strength gains.

Free Weights Versus Machines

Over the years, controversy has centered around the question of whether training with free weights (barbells) or various types of weight machines (Nautilus, Life Fitness, etc.) produces greater strength gains in athletes. It is clear that both free weights and machines are effective at improving strength. Research shows that free-weight training leads to greater strength improvements in free-weight tests, whereas machine training results in greater strength performance on machine tests (1). When a neutral testing device is used to measure strength, strength improvement from free weights and machines are similar (1, 66). A recent review published by the American College of

TABLE 21.3	Resistance Training Guidelines for Training Programs That Emphasize Maximal Strength or Muscular Endurance				

Frequency per Week	Number of Sets per Exercise	Number of Repetitions per Set	Intensity (Percentage of 1-RM)	Rest Interval Between Sets
Resistance Training Programs to Maximize Strength Gains				
Novice Trainer				
2–3 total body sessions	1–3	8–12	60%–70%	2–3 minutes
Intermediate Trainer				
3 total body sessions, 4 split routines	Multiple (>2 sets)	8–12	60%–70%	2–3 minutes
Advanced Trainer				
4–6 split routines	Multiple (>2 sets)	1–12	80%–100% in a periodized program	2–3 minutes

Frequency per Week	Number of Sets per Exercise	Number of Repetitions per Set	Intensity (Percentage of 1-RM)	Rest Interval Between Sets
Resistance Training Programs to Emphasize Muscular Endurance				
Novice Trainer				
2–3 total body sessions	Multiple (>2 sets)	10–15	Low (e.g. 30%–50%)	1 minute
Intermediate Trainer				
3 total body sessions, 4 split routines	Multiple (>2 sets)	10–15	Low (e.g., 30%–50%)	1 minute
Advanced Trainer				
4–6 split routines	Multiple (>2 sets)	10–25	Range 30%–60%	1 minute for 10–15 reps, 1–2 minutes for 15–25 reps

Note the following definitions: Novice trainer—less than 1 year of experience with resistance training; intermediate trainer—2–3 years of experience with resistance training; advanced trainer— ≥3 years of experience with resistance training; split routine—body is divided into different areas with each trained in a separate training session.

Data from "American College of Sports Medicine Position Stand. Progression Models in Resistance Training for Healthy Adults. *Medicine & Science in Sports & Exercise* 41: 687-708, 2009.

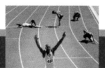
Periodization of Strength Training

Resistance training workouts are structured around the exercise intensity and the number of "sets" and "reps." Further, when working with athletic populations interested in maximal performance, a strength coach may also specify the rest periods between exercises and sets, the type of muscle action (eccentric or concentric), the number of training sessions per week, and the training volume (the total number of reps done in a workout). Periodized strength training uses these variables to develop workouts to achieve optimal gains in strength, power, motor performance, and/or hypertrophy over the course of the year leading up to the competitive season (1). Periodization describes a systematic process in which the volume and intensity of training are varied over time. For example, in "linear periodization," the individual is progressed from high volume/low intensity to low volume/high intensity over a specified time period (e.g., months). Are periodized resistance training programs better than nonperiodized programs?

A recent literature review concluded that periodized programs are more effective in promoting maximal strength than are nonperiodized programs for men and women of all age groups and individuals with varying backgrounds in resistance training (i.e., novice or athletes) (84). Consistent with the overload principle, periodization-induced additions to volume, intensity, and frequency resulted in improved strength gains. Several types of periodization have been formulated and are discussed in both Harries et al. (2015) and the American College of Sports Medicine Position Stand on Progression Models in Resistance Training for Healthy Adults located in Suggested Readings.

Sports Medicine concludes that each training mode has some advantages. For example, weight machines are regarded as safer to use, easy to learn, and they allow performance of some exercises that are difficult to achieve with free weights (e.g., knee extension) (1). Advantages of training with free weights include the fact that lifting free weights forces the athlete to control both balance and stabilizing factors. This type of training could be useful because most sports require the athlete to maintain balance and body stability during competition. Table 21.4 summarizes some of the advantages and disadvantages of strength training

TABLE 21.4	Summary of Potential Advantages and Disadvantages of Weight-Training Programs Using Various Types of Equipment		
Program	Equipment	Advantages	Disadvantages
Isometric	Variety of home-designed devices	Minimal cost; less time required	Not directly applicable to most sport activities; may become boring; progress is difficult to monitor
Dynamic	Free weights	Low cost; specialized exercises may be designed to simulate a particular sport movement; progress easy to monitor	Injury potential due to dropping weights; increase in workout time due to time required to change weights
Dynamic	Commercial weight machines (i.e., Life Fitness®)	Generally safe; progress easy to monitor; small amount of time required to change weight	Does not permit specialized exercise; high cost
Variable resistance	Commercial devices (e.g., Nautilus®)	Has a cam system that provides a variable resistance that changes to match the joint's ability to produce force over the range of motion; progress easy to monitor; safety	High cost; limited specialized exercises
Isokinetic	Commercial isokinetic devices (e.g., Cybex®)	Allows development of maximal resistance over full range of motion; exercises can be performed at a variety of speeds	High cost; limited specialized exercises

Modified from Åstrand, P., and Rodahl, K., *Textbook of Work Physiology*. Champaign, IL: Human Kinetics, 2003.

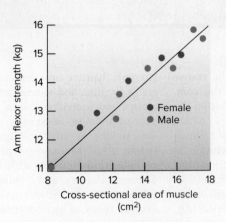

Figure 21.3   Arm flexor strength of men and women graphed as a function of muscle cross-sectional area.

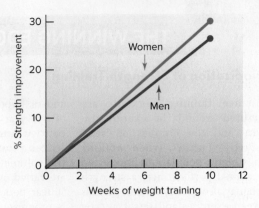

Figure 21.4   Strength changes in men and women as a result of a 10-week strength-training program.

using isometric, dynamic (free weights, Nautilus, etc.), and isokinetic machines.

Gender Differences in Response to Strength Training

It is well established that when absolute strength (i.e., total amount of force applied) is compared in untrained men and women, men are typically stronger. This difference is greatest in the upper body, where men are approximately 50% stronger than women, whereas men are only 30% stronger than women in the lower body (78). However, this sex difference in strength is eliminated when force production in men and women is compared on the basis of the cross-sectional area of muscle. Figure 21.3 illustrates this point. Notice that as the cross-sectional area of muscle increases (x-axis), the arm flexor strength (y-axis) increases in a linear fashion and is independent of sex. That is, human muscle can generate 3-4 kg of force per cm² of muscle cross-section, regardless of whether the muscle belongs to a male or a female.

An often-asked question is "Do women gain strength as rapidly as men when training with weights?" A classic study answered this question and compared the strength change between a group of untrained men and women before and after 10 weeks of resistance training (93). The results revealed that no differences existed between sexes in the percentage of strength gained during the training period (see Fig. 21.4). Similar findings have been reported in other studies, and they demonstrate that untrained men and women respond similarly to weight training (52). However, the aforementioned studies are considered short-term training periods and may not reflect what occurs over long-term training. For instance, it is generally believed that men exhibit a greater degree

of muscular hypertrophy than women as a result of long-term weight training. This gender difference in muscular hypertrophy appears to be related to the fact that men have 20-30 times higher blood levels of testosterone (52).

IN SUMMARY

- Improvement in muscular strength can be achieved via progressive overload by using either isometric, isotonic, or isokinetic exercise.
- Isotonic or isokinetic training seems preferable to isometric exercise in developing strength gains in athletes, because isometric strength gains occur only at the specific joint angles that are held during isometric training.
- Men are generally larger than women and exhibit greater absolute strength than females. However, when muscle force production is normalized to muscle cross-sectional area, no differences exist in the force production of skeletal muscle between men and women.

CONCURRENT STRENGTH AND ENDURANCE TRAINING PROGRAMS

Strength and endurance training are often performed concurrently by athletes and fitness enthusiasts. As discussed in Chap. 13, the performance of combined strength- and endurance-training programs does not impair aerobic training-induced increases in endurance capacity but concurrent training can antagonize the strength gains achieved by resistance training alone (28, 47, 49, 85, 92).

Note that these interference effects are muscle group specific whereby decrements in strength gains are found in the legs and not in upper-body muscles (92). Moreover, whether or not the combination of resistance and endurance training impedes strength gains depends on several factors, including the endurance training modality, the volume and frequency of endurance training, and the way the two training methods are integrated (71, 85, 92). For example, although the mechanism remains unknown, resistance training performed concurrently with running exercise training has a greater decrement on strength gains than cycling exercise (92). Further, the volume of endurance training completed plays an important role in determining whether concurrent training has a negative impact on strength gains (92). Specifically, endurance exercise training performed more than three days per week and ≥30-40 minutes per day appears to represent a threshold where concurrent training interferes with strength gains. Finally, the scheduling of strength and endurance training on the same day can impact strength gains. For instance, performing an endurance training workout immediately prior to engaging in a resistance training session could have a negative impact on the athlete's training effort during the resistance training session (85).

What are the practical implications for athletes regarding the question of whether to engage in concurrent training? Clearly, research suggests that concurrent training can impair the development of both maximal strength and power compared to resistance training alone (92). Therefore, athletes whose sport requires maximal strength and power output (i.e., 100 meter sprinters, etc.) should limit concurrent training. However, if an athlete's sport is not dependent upon maximal power output, concurrent training will not have a negative impact on performance unless the combination of resistance and endurance exercise training results in overtraining. Moreover, careful planning of concurrent training by engaging in cycling exercise and/or avoiding high-volume endurance training (i.e., ≥3 days/week and ≥30 minutes/day) can prevent concurrent training-induced decrements in strength gains (92).

IN SUMMARY

- The performance of combined strength- and endurance-training does not impair training-induced increases in endurance but this concurrent training can impair the strength gains achieved by resistance training alone.

- Concurrent training-induced impairment of muscular strength gains is muscle group specific whereby a decrease in strength gains occurs in the legs but not in upper-body muscles.
- Whether or not the combination of resistance and endurance training impedes strength gains depends on several factors, including the endurance training modality, the volume of endurance training, and the way the two training methods are integrated.
- Athletes whose sport requires maximal strength and power output should limit concurrent training. However, if an athlete's sport is not dependent upon maximal power output, concurrent training will not have a negative impact on performance unless the concurrent training results in overtraining.

NUTRITIONAL INFLUENCE ON TRAINING-INDUCED SKELETAL MUSCLE ADAPTATIONS

As discussed in Chaps. 8 and 13, skeletal muscle is a highly adaptable tissue with the capacity to change its functional capacity in response to exercise training. These functional consequences of exercise-induced muscle adaptations are primarily determined by the mode of training (e.g. endurance exercise vs. resistance exercise). However, emerging evidence suggests that exercise training-induced muscle adaptations are also influenced by nutrition and nutrient availability (48). Recall that an introduction to nutrition and exercise was provided in Chap. 18 and the impact of nutrition on exercise performance is addressed in Chap. 23. In the following sections, we highlight the influence of nutrition and nutrient supply on skeletal muscle adaptation to exercise training. Specifically, we will discuss the impact of carbohydrate and protein availability on muscle adaptation to exercise training and will review the evidence that supplementation with mega doses of antioxidants has the potential to diminish the normal training responses to endurance exercise.

Carbohydrate Availability in Skeletal Muscle Influences Endurance Training Adaptation

During exercise, skeletal muscle obtains carbohydrate as a fuel source primarily from glycogen stores in the muscle. In this regard, evidence shows that low muscle glycogen levels can have a positive influence on endurance training-induced skeletal muscle adaptation (18). Indeed, beginning an exercise training session with low muscle glycogen levels promotes a greater muscle adaptation compared to the same training performed with normal or high muscle glycogen concentrations (48). Specifically, starting a workout with low muscle glycogen levels results in increased protein synthesis of a number of proteins involved in training adaptation. The mechanism to explain this response is that exercise during conditions of low muscle glycogen increases the activation of PGC-1α (i.e., master regulator of mitochondrial biogenesis) in skeletal muscle due to greater stimulation of both AMP kinase and p38 which serve as upstream promoters of PGC-1α activation (48). This higher activation of PGC-1α during exercise will result in increased mitochondrial biogenesis which is an important muscle adaptation to endurance exercise.

How can an endurance athlete design a training program to effectively use the knowledge that training with low glycogen levels accelerates training adaptation? One approach could be to limit dietary carbohydrate intake and therefore deplete muscle glycogen levels by the failure to resynthesis glycogen following training sessions. However, this approach has been shown to result in chronic fatigue and impair the athlete's ability to train. The second and perhaps best approach would be to engage in training twice a day every second day. By training twice a day, the endurance athlete would begin the second training session of the day with lower muscle glycogen levels compared to the first training session which should be advantageous for training adaptation. Indeed, research shows that this method is effective and suggests that this training pattern is superior to training once a day (45).

Protein Availability in Skeletal Muscle Influences Muscle Protein Synthesis Following Exercise

Research shows that providing high-quality (e.g., milk or whey) protein (e.g., milk or whey) to athletes immediately before or following a training session increases the rate of muscle protein synthesis following exercise (81). This is true for both endurance exercise training and resistance exercise training (81). Moreover, protein supplementation may also accelerate gains in anaerobic power (79). Therefore, both endurance and power athletes should carefully plan their protein intake around workouts to optimize training adaptations. For more details on the timing and amount of protein required for optimal exercise-induced protein synthesis, see Chap. 23 and Pasiakos et al. (2015) in Suggested Readings.

Supplementation with Mega Doses of Antioxidants

Both endurance and resistance exercises result in increased free radical production in active skeletal muscles. In this regard, studies indicate that exercise-induced free radical production can promote oxidative damage to cells and contributes to muscular fatigue during prolonged exercise. The fact that contracting muscles produce radicals has motivated some athletes to use antioxidant supplements in an effort to prevent exercise-induced free radical damage and muscle fatigue. However, whether or not antioxidant supplements are helpful or harmful to the athlete remains debatable and emerging evidence indicates that supplementation with mega doses of antioxidants can block training adaptations. For example, supplementation with mega doses of the antioxidants, vitamins E and C (i.e., 400 i.u. vitamin E and 1000 mg vitamin, C), can diminish important exercise-induced adaptations in skeletal muscle. Indeed, recall from Chap. 13 that exercise-induced production of free radicals is a required signal to stimulate the expression of numerous skeletal muscle proteins including antioxidant enzymes and mitochondrial proteins. Therefore, it is not surprising that blocking radical stimulated signaling pathways in skeletal muscle by consuming mega doses of antioxidants can blunt exercise-induced muscle adaptations.

IN SUMMARY

- Exercise-induced muscle adaptations are influenced by nutrition and nutrient availability.
- Beginning an endurance training session with low muscle glycogen levels has a positive influence on muscle adaptation to training.
- Consumption of high-quality protein before or after an exercise training session can increase the rate of muscle protein synthesis.
- Consuming mega doses of the antioxidants, vitamins E and C, can blunt important exercise-induced adaptations in skeletal muscle.

MUSCLE SORENESS

It is a common experience for novice exercisers and sometimes even veteran athletes to notice a **delayed-onset muscle soreness (DOMS)** that appears 24–48 hours after strenuous or unaccustomed exercise. The search for an answer to the question of "What causes DOMS?" has extended over many years. A number of possible explanations have been proposed, including a buildup of lactate in muscle, muscle spasms, and torn muscle and connective tissue. It is clear that lactate does not cause this type of soreness. Based on present evidence, it appears that DOMS is due to tissue injury caused by excessive mechanical force exerted upon muscle and connective tissue resulting in microtrauma to these tissues (6, 16, 18, 35, 64). Evidence to support this viewpoint comes from electron microscopy studies in which electron micrographs taken of muscles suffering from DOMS reveal microscopic tears in these muscle fibers (36).

How does DOMS occur, and what is the physiological explanation for it? Complete answers to these questions are not currently available (for reviews, see references 6, 17, and 82). However, current evidence suggests that DOMS occurs in the following manner (6, 82): (1) strenuous muscular contractions (especially eccentric contractions) result in structural damage in muscle (i.e., disruption of sarcomeres); (2) membrane damage occurs, including damage to the membranes of the sarcoplasmic reticulum; (3) calcium leaks out of the sarcoplasmic reticulum and collects in the mitochondria, which inhibits ATP production; (4) the buildup of calcium also activates enzymes (proteases), which degrade cellular proteins, including contractile proteins (41); (5) membrane damage combines with a breakdown of muscle proteins and results in an inflammatory process, which includes an increase in prostaglandins/histamine production and production of free radicals (19); and finally (6) the accumulation of histamines and edema surrounding muscle fibers stimulates free nerve endings (pain receptors), which results in the sensation of pain in the muscle (64) (see Fig. 21.5).

How does one avoid being a victim of DOMS following exercise? It appears that DOMS occurs most frequently following intense exercise using muscles that are unaccustomed to being worked (17, 21). Further, eccentric exercise (i.e., lengthening contractions) increases the risk for the development of DOMS compared to concentric exercise. Therefore, a general recommendation for the avoidance of DOMS is to slowly begin a specific exercise during the first five to ten training sessions. This pattern of slow progression allows the exercised muscles to "adapt" to the exercise stress and therefore reduces the incidence or severity of DOMS (see Research

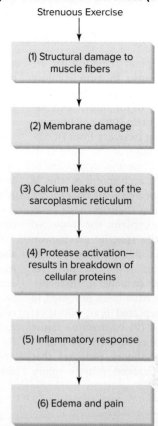

Proposed Steps Leading to Delayed-Onset Muscle Soreness (DOMS)

Strenuous Exercise

(1) Structural damage to muscle fibers

(2) Membrane damage

(3) Calcium leaks out of the sarcoplasmic reticulum

(4) Protease activation—results in breakdown of cellular proteins

(5) Inflammatory response

(6) Edema and pain

Figure 21.5 Proposed model to explain the occurrence of delayed-onset muscle soreness (DOMS) resulting from strenuous muscular exercise.

Focus 21.1). For more information on DOMS, see Lewis et al. (2012) in Suggested Readings and Clinical Applications 21.1. Also, many manufacturers produce compression garments for use during training and sports competition. A common manufacturer claim about the benefits compression clothing is that they improve recovery from exercise-induced muscle soreness. Further, manufacturers also claim that compression clothing improves endurance exercise performance–see a Winning Edge 21.2 for information on the impact of compression clothing on DOMS and sports performance.

IN SUMMARY

- Delayed-onset muscle soreness (DOMS) occurs due to microscopic tears in muscle fibers or connective tissue. This results in activation of proteases, inflammation, and muscle edema (i.e., swelling), which results in pain within 24–48 hours after strenuous exercise.

Protection Against Exercise-Induced Muscle Soreness: The Repeated Bout Effect

Performing a bout of unfamiliar exercise often results in muscle injury and DOMS. This is particularly true when the bout of unfamiliar exercise involves eccentric actions. Interestingly, following recovery from DOMS, a subsequent bout of the same exercise results in minimal symptoms of muscle injury and soreness; this is called the "repeated bout effect" (72). Although many theories have been proposed to explain the repeated bout effect, the specific mechanism responsible for this exercise-induced protection is unknown and continues to be debated. In general, three primary theories have been proposed to explain the repeated bout effect: (1) neural theory, (2) connective tissue theory, and (3) cellular theory (72).

The neural theory proposes that the exercise-induced muscle injury occurs in a relatively small number of active type II (fast) fibers. In the subsequent exercise bout, a change occurs in the pattern of recruitment of muscle fibers to increase motor unit activation to recruit a larger number of muscle fibers. This results in the contractile stress being distributed over a larger number of fibers. Hence, there is a reduction in stress within individual fibers, and no muscle injury occurs during subsequent exercise bouts.

The connective tissue theory argues that muscle damage due to the initial exercise bout results in an increase in connective tissue to provide more protection to the muscle during the stress of exercise. This increased connective tissue is postulated to be responsible for the repeated bout effect.

Finally, the cellular theory predicts that exercise-induced muscle damage results in the synthesis of new proteins (e.g., stress proteins and cytoskeletal proteins) that improve the integrity of the muscle fiber. The synthesis of these "protective proteins" reduces the strain on the muscle fiber and protects the muscle from exercise-induced injury.

Which of these theories best explains the repeated bout effect is unknown. It seems unlikely that one theory can explain all the various observations associated with the repeated bout effect. Thus, it is possible that the repeated bout effect occurs through the interaction of various neural, connective tissue, and cellular factors that respond to the specific type of exercise-induced muscle injury (72). This idea is summarized in Fig. 21.6.

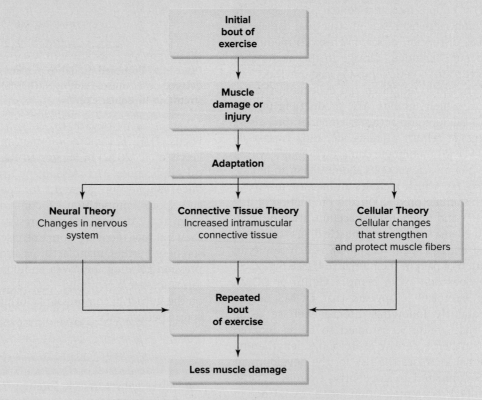

Figure 21.6 Proposed theories to explain the "repeated bout effect." Briefly, an initial bout of exercise results in muscle injury. This muscular injury results in a physiological adaptation, which occurs via changes in the nervous system, muscle connective tissue, and/or cellular changes within muscle fibers. One or all of these adaptations serve to protect the muscle from injury during a subsequent bout of exercise.

Figure redrawn from McHugh, M. P., Connolly, D. A., Eston, R. G., and Gleim, G. W., "Exercise-Induced Muscle Damage and Potential Mechanisms for the Repeated Bout Effect," *Sports Medicine* 27: 157–170, 1999.

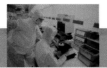
Treatment of Delayed Onset Muscle Soreness

Delayed onset muscle soreness (DOMS) often appears within 24–48 hours following a strenuous and/or unaccustomed exercise bout. In many cases, the muscle pain associated with DOMS is significant and can result in a loss of training time. Therefore, many studies have explored treatment strategies to alleviate the pain and discomfort associated with DOMS. The most common and well-documented treatments for DOMS are: (1) rest, ice, compression, and elevation and (2) the use of nonsteroidal anti-inflammatory drugs (e.g., aspirin, ibuprofen, or naproxen).

The most recommended initial treatment for minor soft tissue (e.g., skeletal muscle) injuries is rest, ice, compression, and elevation (often abbreviated as RICE). The strategy of RICE is to reduce swelling and inflammation of the injured muscle to lessen pain and accelerate healing. Specifically, rest of the injured muscles lowers the risk of further tissue damage and the application of ice to the injured muscle reduces both blood flow and swelling. Continuous compression (wearing compression garments or elastic bandages) around the injured muscle is an effective means to reduce swelling and lessen pain associated with DOMS. In addition to compression, elevation of the injured muscle is another means of decreasing swelling. Collectively, the RICE treatment of soft tissue injury is widely considered to be an effective treatment for DOMS.

While the use of nonsteroidal anti-inflammatory drugs such as aspirin and ibuprofen is a common treatment to relieve pain associated with DOMS, a review of the scientific literature reveals that many discrepancies exist on the efficacy of these drugs. Nonetheless, many well-controlled studies suggest that anti-inflammatory drug treatment can reduce the pain associated with severe DOMS. Unfortunately, the specific type of nonsteroidal anti-inflammatory drug, dosage, and treatment pattern that is most effective in lessening the pain associated with DOMS remains in question. Further, athletes and active individuals should be warned that high doses and prolonged use of nonsteroidal anti-inflammatory drugs is often associated with adverse gastrointestinal effects (e.g., stomach irritation).

Many other treatments for DOMS have also been explored; however, the effectiveness of these therapies remains unclear. In general, there is limited support for the concept that stretching or massage is effective in reducing the pain associated with DOMS. Moreover, other treatments such as acupuncture, ultrasound, herbal remedies, and antioxidants do not consistently relieve the pain associated with DOMS.

In summary, the most documented effective treatments to relieve pain from DOMS are RICE and treatment with nonsteroidal anti-inflammatory drugs. Clearly, treatment using the RICE approach is effective in reducing both pain and swelling associated with DOMS. While over the counter medications are frequently used to treat DOMS, controversy remains regarding the type, dosage, and treatment pattern with nonsteroidal anti-inflammatory drugs that is most effective in reducing the pain associated with DOMS. Clearly, additional research on this topic is warranted. See Jones et al. (2015) and Connolly et al. (2003) in the Suggested Readings for more details on the treatment of DOMS.

TRAINING TO IMPROVE FLEXIBILITY

Historically, it has been believed that improvement of flexibility via stretching reduces the risk of exercise-induced injury. Nonetheless, at present, limited evidence exists to support the concept that stretching prevents injuries during exercise and participation in many sports (5, 46, 73). Further, a general consensus is that stretching in addition to warm-up does not reduce the risk of overuse injuries (73). See McHugh and Cosgrave (2010) in Suggested Readings for more information regarding the role of stretching in preventing or reducing muscle soreness after exercise.

Although improved flexibility may not reduce the risk of exercise-induced injury, the ability to move joints through a full range of motion is important in many sports. Indeed, loss of flexibility can result in a reduction of movement efficiency. Therefore, many athletic trainers and coaches recommend regular stretching exercises to improve flexibility and perhaps optimize the efficiency of movement.

Two general stretching techniques are in use today: (1) **static stretching** (continuously holding a stretch position) and (2) **dynamic stretching** (sometimes referred to as ballistic stretching if movements are not controlled). Although both techniques result in an improvement in flexibility, static stretching is considered to be superior to dynamic stretching because (1) there is less chance of injury, (2) static stretching causes less muscle spindle activity when compared to dynamic stretching, and (3) there is less chance of inducing muscle injury. Stimulation of muscle spindles during dynamic stretching can produce a stretch reflex and therefore result in muscular contraction. This type of muscular contraction counteracts the desired lengthening of the muscle and may increase the chance of injury.

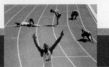
Do Compression Garments Benefit Athletes During Competition and Recovery from Training?

Elastic compression clothing can be worn to compress both the lower and upper limbs via the pressure applied to the skin and musculature. Historically, lower body compression garments have been used in medicine to treat a variety of circulatory disorders (e.g., postural hypotension, varicose veins, or deep vein thrombosis). For these patients, wearing compression clothing improves venous return and reduces tissue swelling. Based on the evidence that compression garments increase venous return, many athletic apparel companies promote compression clothing for use during exercise, creating a new category of sports clothing. Manufacturers claim that wearing compression clothing enhances recovery from exercise by accelerating lactate removal from the blood and improving recovery following damaging exercise. Some manufacturers also assert that compression clothing improves endurance performance. However, to date, limited scientific evidence exists to support most of these claims. Let's examine the evidence for and against the benefits of wearing compression garments during exercise.

Do compression garments improve recovery from exercise?

Several companies claim that a key benefit of using compression garments is the increased removal of the metabolic byproduct lactate from skeletal muscles, which could aid in recovery from exercise. However, studies investigating the effects of compression clothing on lactate removal following exercise are inconsistent. In fact, most studies conclude that compression clothing does not speed up lactate removal from the blood following exercise (68). Further, even if compression clothing increased lactate elimination, blood lactate concentration alone is not an established biomarker of the quality of recovery from exercise.

Several studies support the concept that wearing compression clothing can aid in the recovery from exercise-induced muscle damage (i.e., DOMS). Specifically, wearing compression clothing for 3-4 days following the exercise-induced muscle damage reduces muscle swelling and lowers the pain associated with DOMS (30, 51, 68). These findings are not surprising given that treatment of DOMS using compression is an established treatment approach to reduce the pain and swelling associated with soft tissue injuries.

Do compression garments improve exercise performance?

In addition to wearing compression garments during recovery, many athletes also wear compression clothing in their event in hopes of improving performance. However, a recent review concluded that wearing compression garments does not improve running performance in events ranging from 400 meters to the half-marathon (i.e., 13.1 miles) (30). Nonetheless, compression garments do appear to have a small positive effect on running economy (30); yet, the mechanism(s) to explain this compression-induced benefit on running economy is unclear.

Interestingly, some studies also suggest that compression clothing results in small improvements in time-to-exhaustion during laboratory exercise tests (reviewed in 30). The mechanism(s) to explain this finding is unclear but could be linked to a placebo effect of wearing compression garments. That is, wearing compression clothing during exercise could exert a positive psychological influence that leads to a lower perceived exertion during exercise (reviewed in 30). The explanation for a lower perceived exertion could be that test subjects have positive perceptions about the outcome of the exercise test when wearing compression clothing.

Exercise benefits of compression clothing—conclusions

Athletes and coaches are continuously searching for training aids that enhance both performance and recovery from training. Many advertisements claim that compression garments improve both performance and recovery; however, scientific evidence to support these claims is limited. In this regard, although the number of studies investigating the effects of wearing compression clothing is growing, there is a need for additional well-designed experiments to determine the impact on compression garments on both exercise performance and recovery. Indeed, the current research is highly inconsistent with some studies reporting exercise benefits of compression clothing, whereas other reports find no benefits. Several factors can account for the inconsistency in the literature including differences in study design, training status of subjects, small sample size in many studies, and differences in types of compression clothing. In regard to the types of compression clothing, a major problem in studying the physiological effects of compression clothing is most investigations do not measure the amount of external pressure applied to the body by the compression garment. This is important because differing levels of compression could have diverse physiological effects during both exercise and recovery.

Despite the fact that the current literature suggests that compression clothing provides few benefits for training or competition, the use of compression garments remains popular among athletes. Clearly, further investigation into the effects of wearing compression garments is required to identify the physiological influence of these garments and to better understand whether compression clothing can aid performance or recovery.

Thirty minutes of static stretching exercises performed twice per week will improve flexibility within five weeks. It is recommended that the stretch position be held for 10 seconds at the beginning of a flexibility program and increased to 60 seconds after several training sessions. Each stretch position should be repeated three to five times, with the number increased up to ten repetitions. Overload is applied by increasing the range of motion during the stretch position and increasing the amount of time the stretch position is held.

Preceding a static stretch with an isometric contraction of the muscle group to be stretched is an effective means of improving muscle relaxation and may enhance the development of flexibility. This stretching technique is called **proprioceptive neuromuscular facilitation (PNF).** The procedure generally requires two people and is performed as follows: A training partner moves the target limb passively through its range of motion; after reaching the end point of the range of motion, the target muscle is isometrically contracted (against the partner) for six to ten seconds. The target muscle is then relaxed and is again stretched by the partner to a greater range of motion. The physiological rationale for the use of PNF stretching is that muscular relaxation follows an isometric contraction because the contraction stimulates the Golgi tendon organs, which inhibit contraction during the subsequent stretching exercise.

IN SUMMARY

- Limited evidence exists to support the notion that improved joint mobility (flexibility) reduces the incidence of exercise-induced injury.
- Stretching exercises are often recommended to improve flexibility and optimize the efficiency of movement.
- Improvement in flexibility can be achieved via static or dynamic stretching, with static stretching being the preferred technique.

YEAR-ROUND CONDITIONING FOR ATHLETES

It is common for today's athletes to engage in year-round conditioning exercises. This is necessary to prevent gain of excessive body fat and to prevent extreme physical detraining between competitive seasons. The training periods of athletes can be divided into three phases: (1) off-season training, (2) preseason training, and (3) in-season training, and can incorporate the periodization techniques discussed earlier in this chapter (see The Winning Edge 21.1). A brief description of each training period follows.

Off-Season Conditioning

In general, the objectives of off-season conditioning programs are to (1) prevent excessive fat weight gain, (2) maintain muscular strength or endurance, (3) sustain ligament and bone integrity, and (4) retain a reasonable skill level in the athlete's specific sport. Obviously, the exact nature of the off-season conditioning program will vary from sport to sport. For example, a football player would spend considerably more time performing strength-training exercises than would a distance runner. Conversely, the runner would incorporate more running into an off-season conditioning program than would the football player. Hence, specific exercises should be selected on the basis of the sport's demands.

No matter what the sport, it is critical that an off-season conditioning program provide variety for the athlete. Further, off-season conditioning programs generally use a training regimen that is composed of low-intensity, high-volume work. This combination of low-intensity training and variety may prevent the occurrence of "overtraining syndromes" and the development of psychological staleness. Figure 21.7 contains a list of some recommended training activities for off-season conditioning.

Off-season conditioning allows athletes to concentrate on fitness areas where they may be weak. Therefore, it is important that off-season programs be designed for the individual. For instance, a basketball player may lack leg strength and power and therefore have a limited vertical jump. Therefore, this athlete should engage in an off-season conditioning program that improves leg strength and power production to enhance vertical jumping capacity.

Preseason Conditioning

The principal objective of preseason conditioning (e.g., 8–12 weeks prior to competition) is to increase to a maximum the capacities of the predominant energy systems used in a particular sport. In the transition from off-season conditioning to preseason conditioning,

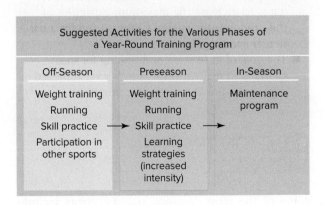

Suggested Activities for the Various Phases of a Year-Round Training Program		
Off-Season	Preseason	In-Season
Weight training	Weight training	Maintenance program
Running	Running	
Skill practice →	Skill practice →	
Participation in other sports	Learning strategies (increased intensity)	

Figure 21.7 Recommended activities for the various phases of year-round training.

there is a gradual shift from low-intensity, high-volume exercise to high-intensity, low-volume exercise. As in all phases of a training cycle, the program should be sport specific.

In general, the types of exercise performed during preseason conditioning are similar to those used during off-season conditioning (Fig. 21.7). The principal difference between off-season and preseason conditioning is the intensity of the conditioning effort. During preseason conditioning, the athlete applies a progressive overload by increasing the intensity of workouts, whereas off-season conditioning involves high-volume, low-intensity workouts.

In-Season Conditioning

The goal of in-season conditioning for most sports is to maintain the fitness level achieved during the preseason training program. For instance, in a sport such as football, in which there is a relatively long competitive season, the athlete must be able to maintain strength and endurance during the entire season. A complicating factor in planning an in-season conditioning program for many team sports is that the season may not have a clear-cut ending. That is, at the end of the regular season, playoff games may extend the season an additional several weeks. Therefore, it is difficult in these types of sports to plan a climax in the conditioning program, and so there is the need for a maintenance training program.

IN SUMMARY

- Year-round conditioning programs for athletes include an off-season program, a preseason program, and an in-season program.
- The general objectives of an off-season conditioning program are to prevent excessive fat weight gain, maintain muscular strength and endurance, maintain bone and ligament strength, and preserve a reasonable skill level in the athlete's specific sport.
- The primary objective of preseason conditioning is to increase the maximum capacities of the predominant energy systems used for a particular sport.
- The goal of in-season conditioning for most sports is to maintain the fitness level achieved during the preseason training program.

COMMON TRAINING MISTAKES

Some of the most common training errors include (1) overtraining, (2) undertraining, (3) using exercises and work-rate intensities that are not sport specific,

(4) failure to plan long-term training schedules to achieve specific goals, and (5) failure to taper training prior to a competition. Let's discuss each of these training errors briefly.

Overtraining may be a more significant problem than undertraining for several reasons. First, overtraining (workouts that are too long or too strenuous) may result in injury or reduce the athlete's resistance to disease (see Chap. 6). Further, overtraining may result in a psychological staleness, which can be identified by a general lack of enthusiasm on the part of the athlete. The general symptoms of overtraining include (1) elevated heart rate and blood lactate levels at a fixed submaximal work rate, (2) loss in body weight due to a reduction in appetite, (3) chronic fatigue, (4) psychological staleness, (5) multiple colds or sore throats, and/or (6) a decrease in performance (see Fig. 21.8). An overtrained athlete may exhibit one or all of these symptoms (11, 37, 53). Therefore, it is critical that coaches and trainers recognize the classic symptoms of overtraining and be prepared to reduce their athletes' workloads when overtraining symptoms appear. Recall that specific training programs should be planned for athletes when possible to compensate for individual differences in genetic potential and fitness levels. This is an important point to remember when planning training programs for athletic conditioning.

For more details on overtraining, see Halson and Jeukendrup (2004) in Suggested Readings and reference 95.

Another common mistake in the training of athletes is the failure to plan sport-specific training exercises. Often, coaches or trainers fail to understand the importance of the law of specificity, and they develop training exercises that do not enhance the energy

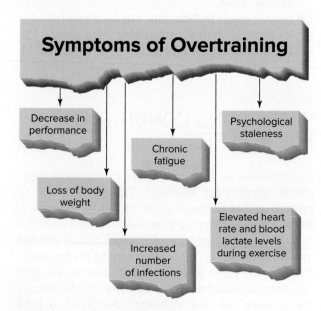

Figure 21.8 Common symptoms of overtraining.

capacities of the skeletal muscles used in competition. This error can be avoided by achieving a broad understanding of the training principles discussed earlier in this chapter.

Further, coaches, trainers, and athletes should plan and record training schedules designed to achieve specific fitness objectives at various times during the year. Failure to plan a training strategy may result in the misuse of training time and ultimately result in inferior performance.

Finally, failure to reduce the intensity and volume of training prior to competition is also a common training error. Achieving a peak athletic performance requires a healthy blend of proper nutrition, training, and rest. Failure to reduce the training volume and/or intensity prior to competition results in inadequate rest and compromises performance. Therefore, in an effort to achieve peak performance, athletes should reduce their training load for several days prior to competition; this practice is called **tapering.** The goal of tapering is to provide time for muscles to resynthesize glycogen to maximal levels and to allow muscles to heal from training-induced damage. Although the optimum length of a taper period continues to be debated, a reduced training load of 3–21 days has been used successfully in both strength and

endurance sports (54). Indeed, runners and swimmers can reduce their training load by approximately 60% for up to 21 days without a reduction in performance (20, 39, 54).

IN SUMMARY

- Common mistakes in training include undertraining, (1) overtraining, (2) performing nonspecific exercises during training sessions, (3) failing to carefully schedule a long-term training plan, and (4) failing to taper training prior to a competition.
- Symptoms of overtraining include (1) elevated heart rate and blood lactate levels at a fixed submaximal work rate, (2) loss in body weight due to a reduction in appetite, (3) chronic fatigue, (4) psychological staleness, (5) increased number of infections, and/or (6) a decrease in performance.
- Tapering is the term applied to short-term reduction in training load prior to competition. Research has shown that tapering prior to a competition is useful in improving performance in both strength and endurance events.

STUDY ACTIVITIES

1. Explain how knowledge of the energy systems used in a particular activity or sport might be useful in designing a sport-specific training program.
2. Provide an outline of the general principles of designing a training program for the following sports: (1) football, (2) soccer, (3) basketball, (4) volleyball, (5) distance running (5000 meters), and (6) 200-meter dash (track).
3. Define the following terms as they relate to interval training: (1) work interval, (2) rest interval, (3) work-to-rest ratio, and (4) set.
4. How can interval training be used to improve both aerobic and anaerobic power?
5. List and discuss the three most common types of training programs used to improve $\dot{V}O_2$ max.
6. Discuss the practical and theoretical differences between an interval training program used to improve

the ATP-PC system and a program designed to improve the ATP production via glycolysis.
7. List the general principles of strength development.
8. Define the terms *isometric, isotonic, dynamic,* and *isokinetic.*
9. Outline the model to explain delayed-onset muscle soreness.
10. Discuss the use of static and dynamic stretching to improve flexibility. Why is a high degree of flexibility not desired in all sports?
11. List and discuss the objectives of (1) off-season conditioning, (2) preseason conditioning, and (3) in-season conditioning.
12. What are some of the more common errors made in the training of athletes?

SUGGESTED READINGS

ACSM. 2009. American College of Sports Medicine position stand. Progression models in resistance training for healthy adults. *Medicine & Science in Sports & Exercise* 41: 687–708.

Fradkin, A. J., T. R. Zazryn, and J. M. Smoglia. 2010. Effects of warming-up on physical performance: a systematic review with meta-analysis. *Journal of Strength and Conditioning Research* 24: 140–48.

Gibala, M., J. Little, M. MacDonald, and J. Hawley. 2012. Physiological adaptations to low-volume, high intensity interval training in health and disease. *Journal of Physiology* 590(5): 1077–1084.

Haff, G. and N. T. Triplett. 2016. Essentials of strength and conditioning. Champaign, IL. Human Kinetics.

Harries, S., D. Lubans, and R. Callister. 2015. Systematic review and meta-analysis of linear and undulating periodized resistance training programs on muscular strength. 29: 1113–1125.

Hawley, J. A. 2009. Molecular responses to strength and endurance training: are they incompatible? *Applied Physiology Nutrition and Metabolism* 34: 355–61.

Iaia, F. M., and J. Bangsbo. 2010. Speed endurance training is a powerful stimulus for physiological adaptations and performance improvements of athletes. *Scandinavian Journal of Medicine and Sciences in Sports* 20 (Suppl 2): 11-23.

Joyner, M.J. and E.F. Coyle. 2008. Endurance exercise performance: the physiology of champions. *Journal of Physiology* 586:35-44

Krieger, J. W. 2010. Single vs. multiple sets of resistance exercise for muscle hypertrophy: A meta-analysis. *Journal of Strength and Conditioning Research* 24: 1150-59.

Lewis, P., D. Ruby, and C. Bush-Joseph. 2012. Muscle soreness and delayed onset muscle soreness. *Clinics in Sports Medicine* 31: 255-262.

Lundby, C. and P. Robach. 2015. Performance enhancement: what are the physiological limits? *Physiology.* 30: 282-292.

Lundby, C. and P. Robach. 2016. Does altitude training increase exercise performance in elite athletes? *Experimental Physiology* 101:783-788.

McHugh, M. P., and C. H. Cosgrave. 2010. To stretch or not to stretch: the role of stretching in injury prevention and performance. *Scandinavian Journal of Medicine and Sciences in Sports* 20: 169-81.

Pasiakos, S., T. McLellan, and H. Lieberman. 2015. The effects of protein supplements on muscle mass, strength, and aerobic and anaerobic power in health adults: A systematic review. *Sports Medicine* 45:111-131.

Seiler, S. 2010. What is best practice for training intensity and duration distribution in endurance athletes? *International Journal of Sports Physiology and Performance* 5: 276-91.

Wilson, J. M., P. J. Marin, M. R. Rhea, S. M. Wilson, J. P. Loenneke, and J. C. Anderson. 2012. Concurrent training: a meta-analysis examining interference of aerobic and resistance exercises. *Journal of Strength and Conditioning Research* 26: 2293-2307.

Wyatt, F., A. Donaldson, and E. Brown. 2013. The overtraining syndrome: a meta-analytic review. *Journal of Exercise Physiology* 16: 12-23.

REFERENCES

1. **ACSM.** American College of Sports Medicine position stand. Progression models in resistance training for healthy adults. *Medicine & Science in Sports & Exercise* 41: 687-708, 2009.

2. **Alway SE, Sale DG, and MacDougall JD.** Twitch contractile adaptations are not dependent on the intensity of isometric exercise in the human triceps surae. *European Journal of Applied Physiology and Occupational Physiology* 60: 346-352, 1990.

3. **Alway SE, Stray-Gundersen J, Grumbt WH, and Gonyea WJ.** Muscle cross-sectional area and torque in resistance-trained subjects. *European Journal of Applied Physiology and Occupational Physiology* 60: 86-90, 1990.

4. **Amir O, Amir R, Yamin C, Attias E, Eynon N, Sagiv M, et al.** The ACE deletion allele is associated with Israeli elite endurance athletes. *Experimental Physiology* 92: 881-886, 2007.

5. **Andersen J.** Stretching before and after exercise: effect on muscle soreness and injury risk. *Journal of Athletic Training* 40: 218-220, 2005.

6. **Armstrong RB.** Mechanisms of exercise-induced delayed onset muscular soreness: a brief review. *Medicine & Science in Sports & Exercise* 16: 529-538, 1984.

7. **Astorino TA, Allen RP, Roberson DW, Jurancich M, Lewis R, McCarthy K, et al.** Adaptations to high-intensity training are independent of gender. *European Journal of Applied Physiology* 2010.

8. **Åstrand P and Rodahl K.** *Textbook of Work Physiology.* Champaign, IL: Human Kinetics, 2003.

9. **Berger R.** *Applied Exercise Physiology.* Philadelphia, PA: Lea & Febiger, 1982.

10. **Bouchard C, Sarzynski MA, Rice TK, Kraus WE, Church TS, Sung YJ, et al.** Genomic predictors of maximal oxygen uptake response to standardized exercise training programs. *Journal of Applied Physiology* 110:1160-1170, 2011.

11. **Bowers R and Fox E.** *Sports Physiology.* New York, NY: McGraw-Hill, 1992.

12. **Burke E.** Physiological similar effects of similar training programs in males and females. *Research Quarterly* 48: 510-517, 1977.

13. **Calvo M, Rodas G, Vallejo M, Estruch A, Arcas A, Javierre C, et al.** Heritability of explosive power and anaerobic capacity in humans. *European Journal of Applied Physiology* 86: 218-225, 2002.

14. **Carvalho AC, Junior LC, Costa LO, and Lopes AD.** The association between runners' lower limb alignment with running-related injuries: a systematic review. *British Journal of Sports Medicine* 45: 339, 2011.

15. **Chapman R, Karlsen T, Resaland G, Ge R, Harber M, Witkowski S, et al.** Defining the dose of altitude training: how high to live for optimal sea level performance. *Journal of Applied Physiology* 116: 595-603, 2014.

16. **Clarkson PM, Byrnes WC, McCormick KM, Turcotte LP, and White JS.** Muscle soreness and serum creatine kinase activity following isometric, eccentric, and concentric exercise. *International Journal of Sports Medicine* 7: 152-155, 1986.

17. **Clarkson PM, Nosaka K, and Braun B.** Muscle function after exercise-induced muscle damage and rapid adaptation. *Medicine & Science in Sports & Exercise* 24: 512-520, 1992.

18. **Clarkson PM and Sayers SP.** Etiology of exercise-induced muscle damage. *Canadian Journal of Applied Physiology* 24: 234-248, 1999.

19. **Close GL, Ashton T, McArdle A, and Maclaren DP.** The emerging role of free radicals in delayed onset muscle soreness and contraction-induced muscle injury. *Comparative Biochemistry and Physiology Part A: Molecular & Integrative Physiologyl* 142: 257-266, 2005.

20. **Costill D.** Effects of reduced training on muscular power in swimmers. *Physician and Sports Medicine* 13: 94-101, 1985.

21. **Costill DL, Coyle EF, Fink WF, Lesmes GR, and Witzmann FA.** Adaptations in skeletal muscle following strength training. *Journal of Applied Physiology* 46: 96-99, 1979.

22. **Costill DL, Thomas R, Robergs RA, Pascoe D, Lambert C, Barr S, et al.** Adaptations to swimming training: influence of training volume. *Medicine & Science in Sports & Exercise* 23: 371-377, 1991.

23. **Coyle, EF.** Improved muscular efficiency displayed as Tour de France champion matures. *Journal of Applied Physiology* 98:2191-2196, 2007.

24. **Coyle EF, Martin WH, III, Sinacore DR, Joyner MJ, Hagberg JM, and Holloszy JO.** Time course of loss of adaptations after stopping prolonged intense endurance training. *Journal of Applied Physiology* 57: 1857-1864, 1984.

25. **Davies CT, and Knibbs AV.** The training stimulus: the effects of intensity, duration and frequency of effort on maximum aerobic power output. *Internationale Zeitschrift für angewandte Physiologie, einschliesslich Arbeitsphysiologie* 29: 299-305, 1971.

26. **Deschenes M.** Short review: motor coding and motor unit recruitment pattern. *Journal of Applied Sport Science Research* 3: 33-39, 1989.

27. **Dudley GA, Abraham WM, and Terjung RL.** Influence of exercise intensity and duration on biochemical adaptations in skeletal muscle. *Journal of Applied Physiology* 53: 844-850, 1982.

28. **Dudley GA, and Djamil R.** Incompatibility of endurance- and strength-training modes of exercise. *Journal of Applied Physiology* 59: 1446-1451, 1985.

29. **Fox E, and Mathews D.** *Interval Training: Conditioning for Sports and General Fitness*. Philadelphia, PA: W. B. Saunders, 1974.

30. **Engel F, Holmberg H, and Sperlich B.** Is there evidence that runners can benefit from wearing compression clothing? *Sports Medicine* DOI.1007/s40279-016-0546-5, 2016.

31. **Fox EL, Bartels RL, Billings CE, O'Brien R, Bason R, and Mathews DK.** Frequency and duration of interval training programs and changes in aerobic power. *Journal of Applied Physiology* 38: 481-484, 1975.

32. **Fox EL, Robinson S, and Wiegman DL.** Metabolic energy sources during continuous and interval running. *Journal of Applied Physiology* 27: 174-178, 1969.

33. **Fradkin AJ, Gabbe BJ, and Cameron PA.** Does warming up prevent injury in sport? The evidence from randomised controlled trials? *Journal of Science and Medicine in Sport* 9: 214-220, 2006.

34. **Fradkin AJ, Zazryn TR, and Smoliga JM.** Effects of warming-up on physical performance: a systematic review with meta-analysis. *Journal of Strength and Conditioning Research* 24: 140-148, 2010.

35. **Friden J, and Lieber RL.** Structural and mechanical basis of exercise-induced muscle injury. *Medicine & Science in Sports & Exercise* 24: 521-530, 1992.

36. **Friden J, Sjöström M, and Ekblom B.** Myofibrillar damage following intense eccentric exercise in man. *International Journal of Sports Medicine* 4: 170-176, 1983.

37. **Fry RW, Grove JR, Morton AR, Zeroni PM, Gaudieri S, and Keast D.** Psychological and immunological correlates of acute overtraining. *British Journal of Sports Medicine* 28: 241-246, 1994.

38. **Galvao D, and Taafee D.** Single- vs. multiple-set resistance training: recent developments in the controversy. *Journal of Strength and Conditioning Research* 18: 660-667, 2004.

39. **Gibala MJ, MacDougall JD, and Sale DG.** The effects of tapering on strength performance in trained athletes. *International Journal of Sports Medicine* 15: 492-497, 1994.

40. **Gibala M, Little J, MacDonald M, and Hawley J.** Physiological adaptations to low-volume, high intensity interval training in health and disease. *Journal of Physiology* 590(5): 1077-1084, 2012.

41. **Gissel H, and Clausen T.** Excitation-induced Ca^{2+} influx and skeletal muscle cell damage. *Acta Physiologica Scandinavica* 171: 327-334, 2001.

42. **Gonyea W, Ericson GC, and Bonde-Petersen F.** Skeletal muscle fiber splitting induced by weight-lifting exercise in cats. *Acta Physiologica Scandinavica* 99: 105-109, 1977.

43. **Gonyea WJ.** Role of exercise in inducing increases in skeletal muscle fiber number. *Journal of Applied Physiology* 48: 421-426, 1980.

44. **Gonyea WJ, Sale DG, Gonyea FB, and Mikesky A.** Exercise induced increases in muscle fiber number. *European Journal of Applied Physiology and Occupational Physiology* 55: 137-141, 1986.

45. **Hansen A, Fischer C, Plomgaard P, Andersen J, Saltin B, and Pedersen B.** Skeletal muscle adaptation: training twice every second day vs. training once daily. *Journal of Applied Physiology* 98: 93-99, 2005.

46. **Hart L.** Effect of stretching on sport injury risk: a review. *Clinical Journal of Sport Medicine* 15: 113, 2005.

47. **Hawley JA.** Molecular responses to strength and endurance training: are they incompatible? *Applied Physiology Nutrition and Metabolism* 34: 355-361, 2009.

48. **Hawley J, Burke L, Phillips S, and Spriet L.** Nutritional modulation of training-induced skeletal muscle adaptations. *Journal of Applied Physiology* 110: 834-845, 2011.

49. **Hickson RC.** Interference of strength development by simultaneously training for strength and endurance. *European Journal of Applied Physiology and Occupational Physiology* 45: 255-263, 1980.

50. **Hickson RC, Bomze HA, and Holloszy JO.** Linear increase in aerobic power induced by a strenuous program of endurance exercise. *Journal of Applied Physiology* 42: 372-376, 1977.

51. **Hill J, Howatson G, van Someren K, Leeder J, and Pedlar C.** Compression garments and recovery from exercise-induced muscle damage: a meta-analysis. *British Journal of Sports Medicine* 48:1340-1346, 2014.

52. **Holloway JB, and Baechle TR.** Strength training for female athletes: a review of selected aspects. *Sports Medicine* 9: 216-228, 1990.

53. **Hooper SL, Mackinnon LT, Howard A, Gordon RD, and Bachmann AW.** Markers for monitoring overtraining and recovery. *Medicine & Science in Sports & Exercise* 27: 106-112, 1995.

54. **Houmard JA, Costill DL, Mitchell JB, Park SH, Hickner RC, and Roemmich JN.** Reduced training maintains performance in distance runners. *International Journal of Sports Medicine* 11: 46-52, 1990.

55. **Iaia FM, and Bangsbo J.** Speed endurance training is a powerful stimulus for physiological adaptations and performance improvements of athletes. *Scandinavian Journal of Medicine and Sciences in Sports* 20 (Suppl 2): 11-23, 2010.

56. **Jones, AM.** The physiology of the world record holder for the women's marathon. *International Journal of Sports Science & Coaching*. 1:101-115, 2006.

57. **Junior LC, Carvalho AC, Costa LO, and Lopes AD.** The prevalence of musculoskeletal injuries in runners: a systematic review. *British Journal of Sports Medicine* 45: 351-352, 2011.

58. **Kelley G.** Mechanical overload and skeletal muscle fiber hyperplasia: a meta-analysis. *Journal of Applied Physiology* 81: 1584-1588, 1996.

59. **Knuttgen HG, Nordesjo LO, Ollander B, and Saltin B.** Physical conditioning through interval training with young male adults. *Medicine & Science in Sports* 5: 220-226, 1973.

60. **Krieger JW.** Single versus multiple sets of resistance exercise: a meta-regression. *Journal of Strength and Conditioning Research* 23: 1890-1901, 2009.

61. **Krieger JW.** Single vs. multiple sets of resistance exercise for muscle hypertrophy: a meta-analysis. *Journal of Strength and Conditioning Research* 24: 1150-1159, 2010.

62. **Laursen PB, and Jenkins DG.** The scientific basis for high-intensity interval training: optimising training programmes and maximising performance in highly trained endurance athletes. *Sports Medicine* 32: 53-73, 2002.

63. **Levine BD, and Stray-Gundersen J.** Living high-training low: effect of moderate-altitude acclimatization with low-altitude training on performance. *Journal of Applied Physiology* 83: 102-112, 1997.

64. **Lewis P, Ruby D, and Bush-Joseph C.** Muscle soreness and delayed onset muscle soreness. *Clinics in Sports Medicine* 31: 255-262, 2012.

65. **Lunby, C and Robach P.** Performance enhancement: what are the physiological limits? Physiology. 30:282-292, 2015.

66. **Manning RJ, Graves JE, Carpenter DM, Leggett SH, and Pollock ML.** Constant vs variable resistance knee extension training. *Medicine & Science in Sports & Exercise* 22: 397-401, 1990.

67. **Maridaki M.** Heritability of neuromuscular performance and anaerobic power in preadolescent and adolescent girls. *Journal of Sports Medicine and Physical Fitness* 46: 540-547, 2006.

68. **Marques-Jimenez, D, Calleja-Gonzalez J, Arratibel I, Delextrat A, and Terrados N.** Are compression garments effective for recovery of exercise-induced muscle damage? A systematic meta-analysis. *Physiology & Behavior* 153:133-148, 2016.

69. **Mazzeo RS.** Physiological responses to exercise at altitude: an update. *Sports Medicine* 38: 1-8, 2008.

70. **McArdle W, Katch F, and Katch V.** *Exercise Physiology: Energy, Nutrition, and Human Performance.* Baltimore, MD: Lippincott Williams & Wilkins, 1996.

71. **McCarthy JP, Pozniak MA, and Agre JC.** Neuromuscular adaptations to concurrent strength and endurance training. *Medicine & Science in Sports & Exercise* 34: 511-519, 2002.

72. **McHugh MP, Connolly DA, Eston RG, and Gleim GW.** Exercise-induced muscle damage and potential mechanisms for the repeated bout effect. *Sports Medicine* 27: 157-170, 1999.

73. **McHugh MP, and Cosgrave CH.** To stretch or not to stretch: the role of stretching in injury prevention and performance. *Scandinavian Journal of Medicine and Sciences in Sports* 20: 169-181, 2010.

74. **Medbo JI, and Burgers S.** Effect of training on the anaerobic capacity. *Medicine & Science in Sports & Exercise* 22: 501-507, 1990.

75. **Micheli L.** Injuries and prolonged exercise. In *Prolonged Exercise*, edited by Lamb D, and Murray R. Indianapolis, IN: Benchmark Press, 1988, pp. 393-407.

76. **Midgley AW, McNaughton LR, and Jones AM.** Training to enhance the physiological determinants of long-distance running performance: can valid recommendations be given to runners and coaches based on current scientific knowledge? *Sports Medicine* 37: 857-880, 2007.

77. **Midgley AW, McNaughton LR, and Wilkinson M.** Is there an optimal training intensity for enhancing the maximal oxygen uptake of distance runners?: empirical research findings, current opinions, physiological rationale and practical recommendations. *Sports Medicine* 36: 117-132, 2006.

78. **Morrow JR, Jr., and Hosler WW.** Strength comparisons in untrained men and trained women athletes. *Medicine & Science in Sports & Exercise* 13: 194-197, 1981.

79. **Passiakos, SM, McLellan TM, and Lieberman HR.** The effects of protein supplements on muscle mass, strength, and aerobic and anaerobic power in healthy adults: A systematic review. 45: 111-131, 2015.

80. **Peterson MD, Rhea MR, and Alvar BA.** Applications of the dose-response for muscular strength development: a review of meta-analytic efficacy and reliability for designing training prescription. *Journal of Strength and Conditioning Research* 19: 950-958, 2005.

81. **Phillips S.** Dietary protein requirements and adaptive advantages in athletes. *British Journal of Nutrition* 108: S158-S167, 2012.

82. **Proske U, and Allen TJ.** Damage to skeletal muscle from eccentric exercise. *Exercise and Sport Sciences Reviews* 33: 98-104, 2005.

83. **Rankinen T, Bray MS, Hagberg JM, Perusse L, Roth SM, Wolfarth B, et al.** The human gene map for performance and health-related fitness phenotypes: the 2005 update. *Medicine & Science in Sports & Exercise* 38: 1863-1888, 2006.

84. **Rhea MR, and Alderman BL.** A meta-analysis of periodized versus nonperiodized strength and power training programs. *Research Quarterly for Exercise & Sport* 75: 413-422, 2004.

85. **Sale DG, Jacobs I, MacDougall JD, and Garner S.** Comparison of two regimens of concurrent strength and endurance training. *Medicine & Science in Sports & Exercise* 22: 348-356, 1990.

86. **Saltin B, Blomqvist G, Mitchell JH, Johnson RL, Jr., Wildenthal K, and Chapman CB.** Response to exercise after bed rest and after training. *Circulation* 38: VII 1-78, 1968.

87. **Schoenfeld B.** Potential mechanisms for a role of metabolic stress in hypertrophic adaptations to resistance training. *Sports Medicine* 43: 179-194, 2013.

88. **Seiler S.** What is best practice for training intensity and duration distribution in endurance athletes? *International Journal of Sports Physiology and Performance* 5: 276-291, 2010.

89. **Staron RS, Malicky ES, Leonardi MJ, Falkel JE, Hagerman FC, and Dudley GA.** Muscle hypertrophy and fast fiber type conversions in heavy resistance-trained women. *European Journal of Applied Physiology and Occupational Physiology* 60: 71-79, 1990.

90. **Vogt M, and Hoppeler H.** Is hypoxia training good for muscles and exercise performance? *Progress in Cardiovascular Diseases* 52: 525-533, 2010.

91. **Wehrlin JP, Zuest P, Hallen J, and Marti B.** Live high-train low for 24 days increases hemoglobin mass and red cell volume in elite endurance athletes. *Journal of Applied Physiology* 100: 1938-1945, 2006.

92. **Wilson JM, Marin PJ, Rhea MR, Wilson SM, Loenneke JP, and Anderson JC.** Concurrent training: a meta-analysis examining interference of aerobic and resistance exercises. *Journal of Strength and Conditioning Research* 26: 2293-2307, 2012.

93. **Wilmore JH.** Alterations in strength, body composition and anthropometric measurements consequent to a 10-week weight training program. *Medicine & Science in Sports* 6: 133-138, 1974.

94. **Woods K, Bishop P, and Jones E.** Warm-up and stretching in the prevention of muscular injury. *Sports Medicine* 37: 1089-1099, 2007.

95. **Wyatt F, Donaldson A, and Brown E.** The overtraining syndrome: A meta-analytic review. *Journal of Exercise Physiology* 16:12-23, 2013.

© Digital Vision/Getty Images

Training for the Female Athlete, Children, Special Populations, and the Masters Athlete

■ Objectives

By studying this chapter, you should be able to do the following:

1. Describe the incidence of amenorrhea in female athletes versus the general population.

2. List those factors thought to contribute to "athletic" amenorrhea.

3. Discuss the general recommendations for training during menstruation.

4. List the general guidelines for exercise during pregnancy.

5. Define the term *female athlete triad*.

6. Discuss the possibility that chronic exercise presents a danger to (1) the cardiopulmonary system or (2) the musculoskeletal system of children.

7. List those conditions in individuals with type 1 diabetes that might limit their participation in a vigorous training program.

8. Explain the rationale for the selection of an insulin injection site for people with type 1 diabetes prior to a training session.

9. List the precautions that people with asthma should take during a training session.

10. Discuss the question "does exercise promote seizures in people with epilepsy?"

11. Graph the change in muscle mass and muscular strength that occur with age.

12. Discuss the factors that contribute to the age-related changes in muscle mass and muscular strength.

13. Discuss the impact of aging on $\dot{V}O_2$ max in both men and women.

14. Outline the factor(s) that are responsible for the age-related decline in endurance performance.

■ Outline

amenorrhea	bulimia	female athlete triad
anorexia nervosa	dysmenorrhea	growth plate (epiphyseal plate)
articular cartilage	epilepsy	sarcopenia

The general physiological principles of exercise training to improve performance apply to anyone interested in improving athletic performance (see Chap. 21). However, when planning competitive training programs for special populations, several specific issues require individual consideration. For example, special training concerns exist for both the female athlete and children. Also, there are specific guidelines for the training of people with diabetes, asthma, or epilepsy. Finally, a growing number of masters athletes are competing in endurance events. How does aging affect their physiological capability and ability to train? This chapter addresses each of these issues. Let's begin our discussion with the topic of exercise training for the female athlete.

FACTORS IMPORTANT TO WOMEN INVOLVED IN VIGOROUS TRAINING

The involvement of women in competitive athletics has increased markedly over the past several decades. Previously, many of the decisions regarding the participation of women in sports and exercise programs was made on the basis of limited, or absent, physiological information. Research concerning women and exercise was scarce until recent years. Although many questions concerning the female athlete remain to be answered, research reveals that there is no reason to limit the healthy female athlete from active participation in endurance or power sports (13, 68). In fact, the general responses of females to exercise and training are essentially the same as those described for males (68), with the exception that exercise thermoregulation is moderately impaired in female athletes during the luteal phase of the menstrual cycle (76). The fact that men and women respond to exercise training in a similar manner is logical because the cellular mechanisms that regulate most physiological and biochemical responses to exercise are generally the same for both sexes. However, there are several specific concerns related to female participation in vigorous training. In this section, we will discuss four key issues related to the female athlete: (1) exercise and the menstrual cycle, (2) eating disorders, (3) bone mineral disorders, and (4) exercise during pregnancy.

Exercise and Menstrual Disorders

Over the past several years, there have been increasing reports concerning the influence of intense exercise training on the length of the menstrual cycle (23). Indeed, there are numerous reports in the literature of female athletes who experience "athletic" amenorrhea. The term **amenorrhea** is defined an absence or cessation of menses.

The incidence of athletic amenorrhea varies markedly across different sports. For example, the incidence of amenorrhea in the general population is approximately 3%, whereas the rate of amenorrhea ranges from 12% to 69% in female athletes (2, 27, 56). The highest incidence of amenorrhea (e.g., 50%-69%) occurs in sports that require a low percentage of body fatness to achieve competitive success' such as distance running or ballet (85).

What causes menstrual cycle dysfunction in athletes? In general, amenorrhea is caused by disruptions in the normal signaling processes between the hypothalamus and the pituitary gland. The specific cause(s) of these disrupted signaling processes in female athletes may vary across individuals, but can be due to several factors, including overtraining, psychological stress, and low energy availability (48, 74, 85). Although some studies linked a low percentage of body fat with athletic amenorrhea, evidence does not fully support the notion that low body fat alone is the principal cause of amenorrhea (85). Whatever the cause of amenorrhea in athletes, the risk of developing it increases as a function of the total amount of training (21, 45). Figure 22.1 illustrates this point. As the weekly training distance increases, the incidence of athletic amenorrhea increases in proportion to the increase in training stress. This finding can be interpreted to mean that too much training either directly or indirectly influences the incidence of amenorrhea. There are at least three ways in which training might influence normal reproductive function. First, exercise alters blood concentrations of numerous hormones (4, 36, 37), which may result in a modification of feedback to the hypothalamus (see Chap. 5). This, in turn, may influence the release of female reproductive hormones and therefore modify the menstrual cycle. A second possibility is that high training mileage may result in increased psychological stress. Psychological stress may disrupt the menstrual cycle by increasing blood levels of catecholamines or endogenous opiates,

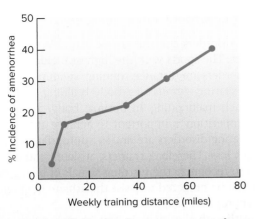

Figure 22.1 The relationship between training distance and the incidence of amenorrhea. Notice that as the training distance increases, there is a direct increase in the incidence of amenorrhea.

which play a role in regulating the reproductive system. Finally, prolonged and intense exercise training can result in low energy availability, which is a major risk factor for the development of athletic amenorrhea (74). Energy availability is defined as dietary energy intake minus exercise energy expenditure. It follows that high levels of exercise energy expenditure without adequate dietary energy intake would result in low energy availability in cells, which can impair the normal reproductive signaling processes and result in amenorrhea (74). For a review of the reproductive system and exercise in women, see Orio et al. (2013) in Suggested Readings. For a discussion about menstrual dysfunction associated with the female athlete triad, see A Closer Look 22.1.

Training and Menstruation

The consensus opinion among physicians is that there is little reason for the healthy female athlete to avoid training or competition during menses (50). Indeed, evidence exists that outstanding performances and world records have been established during all phases of the menstrual cycle (30). Therefore, it is not recommended that the female athlete alter her training or competitive schedule because of menses.

Dysmenorrhea (painful menstruation) can be problematic for females because the incidence of dysmenorrhea is higher in athletic populations than in nonathletic groups. The explanation for this observation is unknown. However, it is possible that prostaglandins (a type of naturally occurring fatty acid) are responsible for dysmenorrhea in both athletes and nonathletes. The release of prostaglandins begins just prior to the onset of menstrual flow and may last for two to three days after menses begin. These prostaglandins cause the smooth muscle in the uterus to contract, which in turn causes ischemia (reduced blood flow) and pain (50).

Although athletes who experience dysmenorrhea can continue to train, this is often difficult because physical activity may increase the discomfort. Athletes who experience severe dysmenorrhea should see a physician for treatment (50). Often, dysmenorrhea pain can be treated with over-the-counter medications, which can be taken without interrupting training schedules.

The Female Athlete and Eating Disorders

Eating disorders are illnesses that cause severe disturbances in eating behaviors. In the United States, it is estimated that over 10 million women and 1 million men will suffer from a clinically significant eating disorder in their lifetime (57). Indeed, the perceived low social acceptance for individuals with a high percentage of body fat and an emphasis on having the "perfect" body have increased the incidence of eating disorders (64). Two of the more common eating disorders that affect both female and male athletes are anorexia nervosa and bulimia (87). Because of the relatively high occurrence of these eating disorders in female athletes, we discuss both the symptoms and health consequences of these abnormal eating behaviors.

Anorexia Nervosa   **Anorexia nervosa** is an eating disorder that is unrelated to any specific physical disease. The end result of extreme anorexia nervosa is a state of starvation in which the individual becomes emaciated due to a refusal to eat. The psychological cause is unclear, but it seems to be linked to an unfounded fear of fatness that may be related to family or societal pressures to be thin (28). It appears that individuals with the highest probability of developing anorexia nervosa are upper-middle-class, young females who are extremely self-critical. The incidence of anorexia nervosa in the United States is estimated to be approximately 1 out of every 100 adolescent girls (46, 81).

The person with anorexia may use a variety of techniques to remain thin, including starvation, exercise, and laxatives (46, 87). The effects of anorexia include excessive weight loss, cessation of menstruation, and, in extreme cases, death. Because this is a serious mental and physical disorder, medical treatment by a team of professionals (physician, psychologist, nutritionist) is necessary to correct the problem. Treatment may require years of psychological counseling and nutritional guidance. The first step in seeking professional treatment for anorexia nervosa is the recognition that a problem exists. Figure 22.2 illustrates common symptoms. See Joy et al. (2016) in the Suggested Readings for more details on the diagnosis and treatment of eating disorders in athletes.

Bulimia   **Bulimia** (also referred to as bulimia nervosa) is overeating (called binge eating) followed by vomiting (called purging) (69). The person with

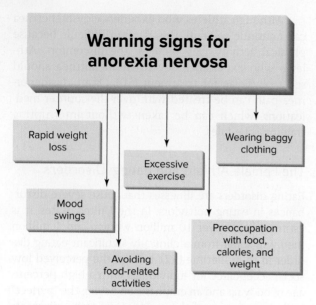

Figure 22.2 Warning signs for anorexia nervosa.

bulimia repeatedly ingests large quantities of food and then forces himself or herself to vomit to prevent weight gain. Bulimia may result in damage to the teeth and the esophagus due to vomiting of stomach acids. Like anorexia nervosa, bulimia is most common in female athletes, has a psychological origin, and requires professional treatment when diagnosed. The incidence of bulimia has been estimated as between 1% and 3% among U.S. females aged 13-20 (81).

Most people with bulimia look normal and are of normal weight. Even when their bodies are slender, their abdomens may protrude due to being stretched by frequent eating binges. Common symptoms are illustrated in Fig. 22.3.

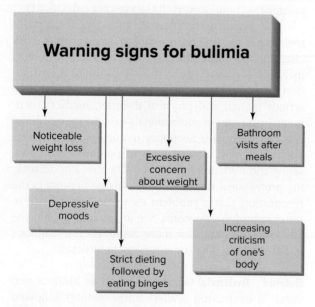

Figure 22.3 Warning signs for bulimia.

Eating Disorders: Final Comments

Eating disorders continue to be a problem in female athletes. The sports with the highest incidence of eating disorders are distance running, swimming, diving, figure skating, gymnastics, body building, and ballet. Although maintaining an optimal body composition for competition is important to achieve athletic success, eating disorders are not an appropriate means of weight loss. Therefore, trainers, athletes, and coaches need to recognize the warning signals of eating disorders and be prepared to assist the athlete in obtaining the appropriate help.

Although the focus in this chapter is on eating disorders in female athletes, it is important to note that eating disorders also occur in female nonathletes. Interestingly, in the nonathletes, exercise has been suggested as a useful intervention to treat eating disorders (51). Indeed, studies indicate that regular exercise can improve the biological and social outcomes in many patients with eating disorders (51).

Bone Mineral Disorders and the Female Athlete

A growing concern for the female athlete is the loss of bone mineral content (osteoporosis). In general, there are two major causes of bone loss in the female athlete (1, 32):

1. Estrogen deficiency due to amenorrhea
2. Inadequate calcium intake due to eating disorders

Unfortunately, many female athletes suffer bone loss due to both amenorrhea and the inadequate calcium intake associated with an eating disorder (1, 32, 33). Although exercise training has been shown to reduce the rate of bone loss due to estrogen deficiency and low calcium intake, exercise cannot completely reverse this process (1). Therefore, the only solution to the problem of bone mineral loss in the female athlete is to correct the estrogen deficiency and/or increase the calcium intake to normal levels. In both cases, a physician should be involved in prescribing the correct treatment for the individual athlete (see A Closer Look 22.1).

Exercise During Pregnancy

Chapter 17 provided an overview of the current exercise guidelines for fitness during pregnancy. As discussed in that chapter, it is generally agreed that women who are physically fit prior to pregnancy can continue to perform regular exercise during pregnancy (3, 12, 73). Indeed, guidelines by the American College of Obstetricians and Gynecologists state that pregnancy should not be a state of confinement, and women with uncomplicated pregnancies should be encouraged to engage in regular physical activity (8). Importantly, exercise training during pregnancy has

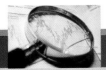

The Female Athlete Triad and beyond

Female athlete triad–origin and definition The **female athlete triad** was first described in 1992 as a common medical problem in female athletes. Specifically, the female athlete triad is defined as a medical condition that is commonly observed in physically active young girls and women and involves three components: (1) low energy availability with or without disordered eating; (2) menstrual dysfunction; and (3) low bone mineral density (56). Research indicates that these problems are interrelated as illustrated in Fig. 22.4. It is widely believed that the required factor underpinning the triad is low energy availability. Indeed, low energy availability is a major risk factor for the development of both menstrual dysfunction and low bone mineral density. Let's discuss the physiological connection between low energy availability and the development of menstrual dysfunction and low bone mineral density.

Low energy availability is defined as an energy deficiency that exists due to an imbalance between dietary energy intake and daily energy expenditure (71). This imbalance results in inadequate energy available to support the cellular activities to maintain homeostasis and provide the energy required for skeletal muscles engaged in both activities of daily living and sports activities. The cause of low energy availability is inadequate energy (i.e., food) intake that may or may not be linked to eating disorders. As discussed earlier, eating disorders are illnesses that cause severe disturbances in eating behaviors. However, athletes that expend large amounts of energy (i.e., calories) during training can reach a state of low energy balance without suffering from an eating disorder. Under these circumstances, the athlete simply does not consume sufficient calories to meet their daily energy requirement.

Regardless of the cause of the depleted energy availability, low energy availability plays a casual role in both menstrual disturbances and low bone density (10, 17, 56, 63, 71, 79). Menstrual dysfunction can be caused by several factors including abnormal levels of hormones, inadequate fat stores, and exercise-related stress. In this regard, low energy availability can alter the levels of hormones involved in the regulation of the menstrual cycle by altering the normal pattern of release of luteinizing hormone; this is important because luteinizing hormone plays a key role in control of the menstrual cycle (71). If energy availability remains low for prolonged periods, the menstrual cycle is temporarily "switched off" due to disruptions in the normal endocrine signaling that regulates the cycle (17, 85). This resulting menstrual dysfunction leads to a reduced production of estrogen by the ovaries and subsequently, low blood levels of estrogen. This is important because a low blood estrogen level promotes the loss of bone minerals due to increased bone resorption (17, 85). Further, low energy availability has a negative impact on bone density independent of the estrogen effects (56).

Female athlete triad model

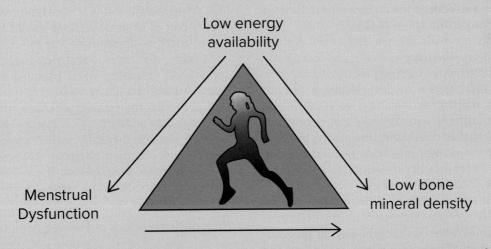

Figure 22.4 Interrelationships between the three components that compose the female athlete triad. It is believed that an energy imbalance resulting in low available energy promotes menstrual problems such as amenorrhea. Amenorrhea is associated with lowered blood levels of estrogen, which increases the risk of bone mineral loss. Further, decreased energy intake may lead to deficiencies in both calcium and vitamin D consumption and may also contribute to a loss of bone minerals.

(Continued)

Incidence of the female athlete triad Estimates of the prevalence of the female athlete triad vary widely in the literature. For example, the prevalence of all three components of the female athlete triad (i.e., low energy availability, low bone density, and menstrual dysfunction) ranges from 0% to 16% across various populations of female athletes (48). Not surprisingly, the incidence of all three components are higher in athletes in sports require a low percent of body fat and involve high daily energy expenditures (e.g., endurance athletes and ballet). Studies reveal that 3%-27% of all female athletes exhibit at least two of the triad conditions whereas as many as 78% of female athletes can exhibit one component (48, 53).

Negative health consequences associated with the female athlete triad For athletes presenting to a physician with low available energy, early intervention is required to prevent the progression to serious clinical problems that include amenorrhea and osteoporosis (low bone mineral content) (56). Indeed, evidence indicates that the health problems associated with the female athlete triad progress from optimal bone health and normal menstrual function along a spectrum toward subclinical (undetectable) health problems to a more severe and detectable health problem (i.e., osteoporosis and menstrual dysfunction) (56). The key to prevention of the severe health problems associated with the female athlete triad is early diagnosis and treatment. For details on diagnosis and treatment of the female athlete triad, see Joy et al. (2014, 2016).

Recent proposal to replace the term female athlete triad with new terminology known as "Relative energy deficiency in sport" Growing evidence indicates that the cause of the female athlete triad is low energy intake (resulting in low energy availability), which leads to health problems because of the energy required for maintaining cellular homeostasis is not available. Therefore, in a consensus statement published by the scientists working with the International Olympic Committee (IOC), the authors reasoned that the medical condition known as the female athlete triad is not composed of three entities but rather is a syndrome (i.e., combination of symptoms associated with a morbid process) that results from low energy availability. They contend that low energy availability affects many physiological functions including metabolic rate, menstrual function, bone health, immunity, cellular protein synthesis, cardiovascular, and psychological health (71). These authors also argue that low energy available is not limited to female athletes but also impacts male athletes. Therefore, the scientists working with the IOC conclude that new terminology is required to more accurately describe the clinical syndrome originally known as the female athlete triad (71). This new recommendation is that the female athlete triad terminology be abandoned and in the future, we refer to the problems associated with the female athlete triad as "relative energy deficiency in sports." These authors propose that the term "relative energy deficiency syndrome" be defined as impaired physiological function including metabolic rate, menstrual function, bone health, immunity, protein synthesis, cardiovascular health caused by relative energy deficiency (71). This proposal to replace the term "female athlete triad" is relatively new and therefore, it is too early to know if this new term becomes widely accepted by exercise scientists and sport medicine physicians.

many benefits for mothers such as reduction in excessive weight gain, reduced risk for gestational diabetes, and better postpartum recovery (18).

Although pregnant women can safely perform low- to moderate-intensity exercise, can female athletes maintain an active training program during pregnancy? The short answer to this question is yes, but some qualifications exist. First, both recreational and competitive athletes with uncomplicated pregnancies can continue to train during pregnancy, but they should carefully monitor their body temperature during exercise to prevent hyperthermia (8). Specifically, pregnant athletes should avoid high-intensity and/or long training sessions that raise body core temperature above 1.5°C (8). In this regard, aquatic exercise is considered an excellent form of training for pregnant athletes because it allows cardiovascular conditioning in a medium that facilitates accelerated heat loss.

It is also important that pregnant athletes maintain adequate hydration during training by consuming fluid at regular intervals (e.g., every 15 minutes) during exercise. Fluid balance can be monitored by weighing before and after the exercise session. Any loss of body weight is fluid loss and should be replaced by drinking the appropriate amount of fluid (e.g., 0.5-kg weight loss = 500 ml fluid). Moreover, the energy cost of exercise sessions should be estimated and balanced by appropriate energy intake.

Finally, it is also critical that pregnant athletes apply good judgment when planning exercise programs. Athletes should be aware that it may be necessary to reduce the training intensity and volume as the pregnancy advances (8). Importantly, it is recommended that all physically active women be examined regularly by their physician to assess the effects of their exercise programs on the developing fetus, and adjustments should be made if appropriate (8).

Risk of Knee Injury in Female Athletes

Knee injuries are common in many sports. Although the risk of knee injuries varies across sports, studies reveal that compared to males, post-pubescent female athletes are at 3.5 times higher risk for a noncontact anterior cruciate ligament (ACL) injury (16, 34, 84). A noncontact ACL injury is a sports injury where the athlete tears the ACL during an awkward movement that does not involve direct contact with another athlete.

These types of noncontact ACL injuries comprise ~70% of all sports-related ACL injuries and are commonly observed in sports such as soccer, basketball, team handball, and volleyball (84). Further, knee injuries such as ACL injuries occur at a higher rate in female athletes compared to male athletes at a similar level of competition (34, 88). For example, in a study of male and female professional basketball players, female athletes suffered 60% more ACL injuries than males (88). This increased risk of knee injury in female athletes is not limited to professional athletes and affects both collegiate and high school athletes as well (34, 89). For example, National Collegiate Athletic Association statistics reveal that women sustain ACL injuries at a rate that is almost 4 times higher than men in basketball and 2.4 times higher than men in soccer (34).

Why are females at a greater risk for ACL injuries? Unfortunately, a definitive answer to this question is not available. However, it has been speculated that several factors may play a role in placing women at higher risk for knee injuries; these include fluctuation in sex hormones during the menstrual cycle, gender differences in knee anatomy, and dynamic neuromuscular imbalances (34, 84). A discussion of the evidence to support each of these potential risk factors follows.

In reference to sex hormones and knee injuries, studies reveal that the risk of ACL injury is increased in female athletes during the follicular and ovulatory phase of the menstrual cycle (34). However, the direct link between sex hormones and the increased risk of tear of the ACL remains unclear. In this regard, some investigators propose that sex hormones influence the structure of the ACL, perhaps compromising both the strength of the ligament and/or proprioceptive feedback (34). Nonetheless, direct evidence to support this concept is limited.

Studies investigating gender differences in knee anatomy as a determinant of the risk of knee injuries have failed to provide definitive evidence that anatomical explanations are responsible for gender differences in the rate of knee injuries. For example, although women are more likely to have knee joint laxity (loose joint) than men, this fact has not been correlated to the higher rate of knee injury in women (34). Therefore, it does not appear that gender differences in knee anatomy can explain why females are at higher risk for ACL injuries.

Dynamic neuromuscular imbalance in the knee is an area of research related to ACL tears in women that continues to grow. Dynamic neuromuscular imbalance refers to a combination of imbalanced factors, including muscular strength, proprioception, and landing biomechanics. In regard to muscle strength, women have less quadriceps and hamstring strength than men, even when normalizing for body weight. This is significant because exercises that strengthen both the quadriceps and hamstring muscles provide protection against knee injury (19, 52). Evidence also

suggests that the higher incidence of knee injury in women may be linked to an imbalance in knee proprioceptive and neuromuscular control in female athletes (34). Nonetheless, more detailed studies are required before a firm conclusion can be reached on the role that proprioception plays in gender differences in knee injury. Finally, emerging evidence reveals that compared to men, women run, jump, and land differently when playing sports (34). This is important because the usual mechanism for noncontact ACL injury involves a deceleration in limb speed before changing directions or landing with the knee between full extension and 20 degrees of flexion (34). In this regard, compared to males, female athletes tend to land with knee angles that pose a greater risk of ACL injury (34). Therefore, a neuromuscular difference between males and females that affects landing or other movement strategies may partly explain why female athletes are at greater risk for knee injuries in sports compared to male athletes.

In summary, compared to males, female athletes are at high risk for certain types of knee injuries (e.g., ACL injury). Current evidence suggests that male/female differences in dynamic neuromuscular imbalance (e.g., leg muscle strength, jumping and landing strategies) may contribute to gender differences in the risk of knee injuries. Although several studies have explored the effectiveness of neuromuscular training programs in reducing the incidence of ACL injuries in female athletes, convincing evidence does not exist that these training programs significantly reduce the risk of injury. For a detailed discussion of programs aimed at reducing ACL injury in women, see Voskanian (2013) in Suggested Readings.

IN SUMMARY

- The incidence of amenorrhea in female athletes appears to be highest in distance runners and ballet dancers when compared to other sports. Although the cause of amenorrhea in female athletes is not clear, it appears likely that multiple factors (e.g., the amount of training and psychological stress) are involved.
- There appears to be little reason for female athletes to avoid training during menstruation unless they experience severe discomfort due to dysmenorrhea. Athletes who experience severe dysmenorrhea should see a physician for treatment.
- Two of the more common eating disorders are anorexia nervosa and bulimia.
- The female athlete triad is a medical condition that is commonly observed in physically active young girls and women and involves three components: (1) low energy availability with or without disordered eating; (2) menstrual dysfunction; and (3) low bone mineral density.

- Short-term, low-intensity exercise does not appear to have negative consequences during pregnancy. However, data suggest that long-duration or high-intensity training should be carefully monitored during pregnancy.
- Female athletes are at greater risk for knee injuries compared to males. Evidence suggests that male/female differences in dynamic neuromuscular imbalance (e.g., differences in leg muscle strength and/or jumping and landing strategies) may contribute to gender differences in the risk of knee injuries.

SPORTS CONDITIONING FOR CHILDREN

There are many unanswered questions about the physiologic responses of the healthy child to various types of exercise. This is due to the limited number of investigators studying children and exercise, and because of ethical considerations in studying children. For instance, few investigators would puncture a child's artery, take a muscle biopsy, or expose a child to harsh environments (e.g., heat, cold, high altitudes) to satisfy scientific curiosity. Because of these ethical constraints, current knowledge concerning training for children is limited primarily to the impact of training on the cardiovascular and musculoskeletal system. The following discussion addresses some of the important issues concerning child participation in vigorous conditioning programs.

Training and the Cardiopulmonary System

As youth sports teams increase in popularity, one of the first questions asked is, "Are the hearts of children strong enough for intensive sports conditioning?" In other words, is there a possibility of "overtraining" young athletes, with the end result being permanent damage to the cardiovascular system? The answer to this question is no. Children involved in endurance sports such as running or swimming improve their maximal aerobic power comparable to adults and show no indices of damage to the cardiopulmonary system (7, 54, 65, 75). Moreover, identical to adults, children significantly improve their cardiopulmonary fitness in response to high-intensity interval training without evidence of physical complications (26). Over the past several years, children have safely trained for and completed marathon runs in less than four hours. If proper techniques of physical training are employed, with a progressive increase in cardiopulmonary stress, children appear to adapt to endurance

training in a fashion similar to adults (6). Further, the risk of cardiac sudden death in young endurance athletes is small (See Clinical Applications 22.1).

Training and the Musculoskeletal System

Evidence indicates that organized training in a variety of team sports (e.g., swimming, basketball, volleyball, track and field) does not adversely affect growth and development in children (67). This is true for both boys (38) and girls (9). In fact, moderate physical training has been shown to augment or optimize growth in children and reduce the risk of obesity and type 2 diabetes (35, 38). Therefore, many investigators have concluded that regular physical activity is necessary for normal growth and development. However, is there danger of overtraining and injury to bones and cartilage (11, 39, 42)?

One of the long-standing concerns with intense endurance or resistance training in children is that the growing bones of a child are more susceptible to certain types of mechanical injury than those of the adult, primarily because of the presence of growth cartilage (67). Growth cartilage is found in children at three major anatomical locations (67): (1) **growth plate** (also called the **epiphyseal plate**); (2) **articular cartilage** (i.e., cartilage at joints); and (3) muscle-tendon insertions. The location of the growth plate for the knee joint is illustrated in Fig. 22.5. The growth plate is the site of bone growth in long bones. The time at which

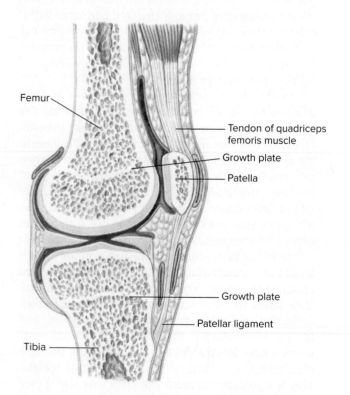

Figure 22.5 Location of the growth plate (epiphyseal plate) associated with the long bones in the leg.

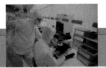
Risk of Sudden Cardiac Death in Young Athletes

Cardiovascular-related sudden death is the leading cause of mortality in athletes less than 18 years of age (62). However, in healthy young athletes, the risk of sudden cardiac injury or death during participation in sports or exercise is relatively small. For example, the incidence of sudden death in young athletes is estimated to range from 1–3 deaths per 100,000 athletes (31, 60, 62). Importantly, almost all of these deaths resulted from congenital heart defects and did not result from exercise per se (31).

Four cardiovascular abnormalities account for the majority of sudden cardiac deaths in young athletes: (1) hypertrophic cardiomyopathy (pathologically enlarged heart); (2) congenital (inherited) abnormalities of the coronary arteries; (3) aortic aneurysms; and (4) congenital stenosis (narrowing) of the aortic valve (31).

Can a medical exam identify athletes at risk for sudden death? In many cases, yes. A medical history and a physical exam from a qualified physician are good tools for detecting heart disease that could pose a risk for the young athlete participating in sports (25). However, some cardiac abnormalities that can cause death during sports participation are difficult to detect during routine medical examination (31). Nonetheless, a medical exam along with a cardiac evaluation (cardiac imaging and stress testing) can potentially reduce the risk of sudden cardiac death by identifying those young athletes who are predisposed to cardiac injury (31, 60). See Lithwick et al. (2016) in the Suggested Readings for more information on cardiac screening of young athletes.

---

bone growth ceases varies from bone to bone, but growth is generally complete by 18–20 years of age (67). Upon completion of growth, growth plates ossify (harden with calcium) and disappear, and growth cartilage is replaced by a permanent "adult" cartilage.

Can children perform heavy endurance training or strength training without long-term musculoskeletal problems? Currently, there are no published reports or case studies indicating that endurance exercise has adverse effects on bone growth in children and adolescents. In fact, growing evidence indicates that, compared to sedentary children, regular endurance exercise training results in increased bone mineral content (80). Further, studies have investigated the effects of resistance exercise training on children (6–12 years of age) and have concluded that supervised resistance exercise does not damage bone, muscle, or the epiphyseal plate (41, 86). Moreover, recent reviews on the effects of resistance exercise on children have concluded that under proper supervision, resistance training can be performed safely in youth athletes without bone or cartilage injury (11, 39, 42, 61). In fact, it is well established that resistance training has numerous health benefits in children. For example, weight training has been shown to promote bone health by increasing bone mineral density to prepubertal boys and girls (11). It is also clear that resistance training is effective in promoting muscular strength in prepubertal boys and girls (40, 43). Interestingly, this training-induced muscular strength is achieved with limited hypertrophy in prepubertal children (11). Therefore, the resistance training-induced increase in muscular strength in children appears to be achieved primarily by changes in the nervous system alone (e.g., improved motor unit recruitment, etc.). For more details on resistance training in children and adolescents, see Faigenbaum et al. (2015).

Progress in Pediatric Exercise Science

As discussed earlier, our knowledge about pediatric exercise science has developed slowly because of ethical concerns of using children in research. Nonetheless, knowledge in this field has expanded during the past several years. One of the pioneers promoting research in pediatric exercise science was Dr. Oded Bar-Or (see A Look Back–Important People in Science). Moreover, the creation of the scientific journal *Pediatric Exercise Science* has stimulated additional research in exercise during childhood. Therefore, it is anticipated that scientific knowledge of pediatric exercise science will grow rapidly during the coming years.

> **IN SUMMARY**
>
> - Current evidence indicates that endurance training is not detrimental to the growth and development of the cardiovascular system in children. Further, there is no evidence that endurance exercise training has a negative impact on bone and cartilage health.
> - The risk of sudden cardiac death in youth athletes is extremely low (1–3 deaths per 100,000 athletes).
> - The consensus of current scientific evidence indicates that under proper supervision, resistance training can be performed safely in youth athletes without bone or cartilage injury.
> - Resistance training in prepubertal children has been shown to increase both bone density and muscular strength with limited muscle hypertrophy.

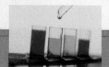
Oded Bar-Or Was a Pioneer in Pediatric Exercise Physiology

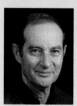

Courtesy of
Marilyn Bar-Or

Oded Bar-Or (1937–2005) was born and raised in Jerusalem, Israel. He was trained as a medical doctor at Hadassah Medical School (Israel), and following graduation, he traveled to the United States to begin postdoctoral research training in exercise physiology in the laboratory of Dr. Elsworth Buskirk at Pennsylvania State University. After completing his postdoctoral studies in 1969, Dr. Bar-Or returned to Israel and established the Department of Sports Medicine at the Wingate Institute. During his tenure at the Wingate Institute, Dr. Bar-Or and his colleagues earned international acclaim in sports science research, and his research group developed the Wingate Anaerobic Power Test that remains in use today (Chap. 20).

In 1981, Professor Bar-Or left the Wingate Institute to join the faculty at McMaster University in Hamilton, Ontario (Canada). Upon arrival at McMaster, he established the Children's Exercise and Nutrition Center and began a lifelong quest to increase our knowledge about pediatric exercise science. During his tenure at McMaster, his research focused on understanding the physiological differences between adults and children in their response to exercise. A major portion of this work was dedicated to resolving how children differ from adults in their cardiorespiratory and thermoregulatory responses to exercise in hot environments. Indeed, Dr. Bar-Or was one of the first investigators to study children's thermoregulatory responses and acclimatization to exercise. Dr. Bar-Or's legacy in pediatric exercise physiology includes 158 research publications, and he also authored or coauthored ten books on a variety of topics in pediatric sports medicine and exercise physiology.

COMPETITIVE TRAINING FOR PEOPLE WITH DIABETES

As discussed in Chap. 17, there is a beneficial effect of exercise on diabetes, and physicians often recommend regular exercise for people with this condition as a part of their therapeutic regimen (i.e., to help maintain control of blood glucose levels). We will focus our discussion on people with type 1 diabetes, because people with type 2 diabetes are less likely on engage in training for performance purposes. Can people with type 1 diabetes train vigorously and take part in competitive athletics? The answer to this question is a qualified yes. In people with long-term diabetes that have microvascular complications (damage to small blood vessels) or neuropathy (nerve damage), exercise should be limited and extensive training is not generally recommended (15, 67). However, in individuals who maintain good blood glucose control and are free from other medical complications, diabetes in itself should not limit the type of exercise or sporting event.

What precautions should the athlete with diabetes take to allow safe participation in training programs? An overview of exercise training for fitness in diabetic populations was presented in Chap. 17 and will be reviewed here only briefly. The key to safe participation in sport conditioning for the athlete with diabetes is to learn to avoid hypoglycemic episodes during training (78). Because people with diabetes vary in their response to insulin, each athlete, in cooperation with his or her personal physician, must determine the appropriate combination of exercise, diet, and insulin for optimal control of blood glucose concentrations. In general, exercise should take place after a meal and should be part of a regular routine. It is often recommended that a reduction in the amount of insulin injected be considered on days in which the athlete is engaged in strenuous training (15, 77). A major concern for the athlete with diabetes is the site of the insulin injection prior to exercise. Insulin injected subcutaneously in the leg prior to running (or other forms of leg exercise) results in an increased rate of insulin uptake due to elevated leg blood flow. This could result in exercise-induced hypoglycemia and may be avoided by using an insulin injection site in the abdomen or the arm. Conversely, if the training regimen requires arm exercise (e.g., rowing), the site of insulin injection should be away from the working muscle (e.g., abdomen). Having a glucose solution or carbohydrate snack available during training sessions may help avoid hypoglycemic incidents during workouts.

Can people with diabetes obtain the same benefits from training as those without the condition? The consensus answer to this question is yes. Although untrained children with diabetes tend to be less fit than normal children (58), young children with diabetes respond to a conditioning program in a manner similar to that of healthy children (67). Empirical observations suggest that when the blood glucose of the athlete with diabetes is carefully regulated, he or she can compete and excel in a variety of competitive sports.

TRAINING FOR PEOPLE WITH ASTHMA

It is generally agreed that most children, adolescents, and adults with asthma can safely participate in all sports, with the exception of SCUBA diving, provided they are able to control exercise-induced bronchospasms via medication or careful monitoring of activity levels (70). In fact, evidence suggests that aerobic training can reduce airway inflammation and improve asthmatic symptoms in some asthma patients (66). A prerequisite for planning training programs for people with this condition is that the proper therapeutic regimen for managing the athlete's particular type of asthma be worked out prior to commencement of a vigorous training program (see Chap. 17). When the asthma is under control, planning the training schedule for asthmatic athletes is identical to planning for athletes without asthma (see Chap. 21). However, as mentioned in Chap. 17, it is often recommended that the asthmatic athlete keep an inhaler (containing a bronchodilator) handy during training sessions, and that workouts be conducted with other athletes in case a major attack occurs.

The issue of the safety of a person with asthma participating in SCUBA diving continues to be debated. A recent review concludes that despite the risks of SCUBA diving, many asthmatic individuals can safely dive if they are at low risk for an asthma attack during diving (24). The following guidelines are recommended. To determine if the asthmatic is a good candidate to dive, the patient should have a thorough medical exam that includes a review of patient history, spirometry, allergy testing, and bronchial challenges (24). Further, for pulmonary patients that plan to dive, their asthma should be well controlled on the day of the dive (24). Finally, asthmatic patients that want to dive should not exhibit exercise-, emotion-, or cold-induced asthma (24). However, a recent review on the subject suggests that people with asthma with normal airway function at rest who do not exhibit exercise-induced asthma have a risk of barotrauma during diving similar to that of healthy individuals.

EPILEPSY AND PHYSICAL TRAINING

The term **epilepsy** refers to a transient disturbance of brain function, which may be characterized by a loss of consciousness, muscle tremor, and sensory disturbances. Because the occurrence of epileptic seizures is not easily predicted, should people with epilepsy engage in vigorous training programs? Unfortunately, there is little information available to answer this question. Before a clear-cut recommendation for the participation of people with epilepsy in athletics can be made, two fundamental questions must be answered. First, does intense physical activity increase the risk of an epileptic seizure? Second, does the occurrence of a seizure during a particular sports activity expose the athlete to unnecessary risk? Let's examine the available evidence concerning each of these questions.

Does Exercise Promote Seizures?

There is one rare type of epileptic seizure that has been shown to be induced by exercise per se (22). These are tonic (continuous motor activity) seizures, which have been reported to occur during a variety of sports activities. Fortunately, this type of seizure can be controlled in most instances by anticonvulsant drugs.

However, stress is among the most commonly reported causes of seizures in people with epilepsy (5). For example, patients report that the frequency of their seizures increases if they are exposed to an increase in excitement, tension, sadness, or other strong emotions (5). Given that exercise is physical stress, does exercise per se promote seizures?

As for other types of seizure disorders, physicians remain divided in their opinions as to whether exercise increases the risk of seizure occurrence. A report by Gotze et al. (49) suggests that exercise does not increase the risk of seizures in children or adolescents with epilepsy. In fact, Gotze (49) argues that exercise appears to reduce the incidence of seizures by increasing the threshold. In support of these claims, reviews on epilepsy and sports have concluded that there is a reduction in the number of seizures during exercise (3, 5). In contrast, Kuijer (59) has suggested that the person with epilepsy is at an increased risk of experiencing a seizure during exercise and during recovery from exercise. In this regard, several factors related to exercise have been hypothesized to increase the risk of seizures: (1) physical fatigue, (2) hyperventilation, (3) hypoxia, (4) hyperthermia, (5) hypoglycemia, (6) electrolyte imbalance, and (7) emotional stress associated with competitive sports. In conclusion, division exists in the medical community concerning the risk of exercise and seizures. Clearly, generalizations about exercise and the epileptic patient cannot be made. Each patient is unique concerning the type, frequency, and severity of epileptic seizures (5). Therefore, physicians, parents, and coaches must make case-by-case decisions on the wisdom of competitive sports for individual patients. However, people with epilepsy who are judged to be healthy enough to engage in rigorous physical activity should be encouraged to exercise (5). Indeed, a recent review on exercise and epilepsy concludes that people with epilepsy should include exercise as a complementary therapy, not only for seizure control, but also to promote good physical and mental health (5).

Another specific concern for the participation of people with epilepsy in contact sports is whether a blow to the head might mediate a seizure. Again, physicians remain divided in their opinions but at present, no studies exist to prove that repeated head trauma in people with epilepsy causes a recurrence of seizures (47). See Pimentel et al. (2015) in Suggested Readings for more details.

Risk of Injury Due to Seizures

Clearly, there are many competitive sports activities (e.g., football, boxing) during which the occurrence of a seizure would expose the athlete to a risk of harm. However, the occurrence of a seizure during many types of daily routine activities (e.g., climbing stairs) or recreational sports (e.g., SCUBA diving, sky diving, mountain climbing) could also pose a threat to the person with epilepsy (47). Whether the person with epilepsy should participate in physical training or sports must be determined on an individual basis by the use of common sense and advice from a physician. The benefit-risk ratio of sports participation may vary greatly from case to case and is dependent on the exact nature of the patient's epilepsy and the sport being considered. A child with only a minor seizure problem may, with the aid of medication, experience only a rare seizure with

little visible alteration in behavior or consciousness due to the seizure. This type of person could likely participate in most training activities without harm (5, 14, 49). In contrast, a person who experiences frequent and major seizures would not be a candidate for many types of sports. For a detailed discussion of epilepsy and exercise, see Pimental et al. (2015) in Suggested Readings.

> **IN SUMMARY**
>
> - Questions about safe participation for people with epilepsy in training programs must be answered on an individual basis.
> - The benefit-risk ratio of sports participation may vary greatly from case to case and depends on the type of epilepsy involved and the sport being considered.

EXERCISE PERFORMANCE AND TRAINING FOR MASTERS ATHLETES

There are a growing number of people over the age of 50 that compete in competitive athletic events. These "masters athletes" represent an interesting subgroup of older adults because they possess unique physiological characteristics that could be termed as "exceptionally successful aging" (82). The masters athlete often trains on a daily basis and strives to maintain athletic performances that he/she achieved at earlier ages. However, a decline in athletic performance at advancing ages is inevitable. In the following segments, we describe the age-related changes in muscular strength and endurance performance and discuss the physiological reasons for the decline in physical capabilities with age.

Age-Related Changes in Muscular Strength

Aging results in a progressive decrease in muscular strength. Although changes in the nervous system do occur during aging, much of the loss in strength with aging is due to a decline in muscle mass. The age-related loss of muscle mass is termed **sarcopenia,** and the rate of muscle loss with age is illustrated in Fig. 22.6. Age-related sarcopenia occurs due to both a decrease in fiber size and a decrease in the number of fibers present in the muscle (44). However, much of the age-related loss in muscle mass is due to a loss of muscle fibers (44, 72). The mechanisms responsible for this age-related loss of muscle remain unclear. Nonetheless, it appears that a number of factors contribute to sarcopenia, including inactivity, free radical-mediated damage (oxidative

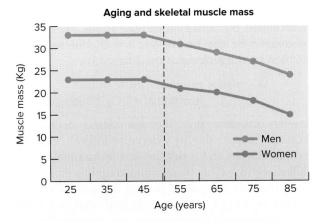

Aging and skeletal muscle mass

Figure 22.6 Aging results in a loss of muscle mass with aging in both men and women.

Data from Buford, T. W., Anton, S. D., Judge, A. R., Marzetti, E., Wohlgemuth, S. E., Carter, C. S., et al., "Models of Accelerated Sarcopenia: Critical Pieces for Solving the Puzzle of Age-Related Muscle Atrophy," Ageing Research Reviews 9: 369-383, 2010; Faulkner, J. A., Larkin, L. M., Claflin, D. R., Brooks, S. V., "Age-Related Changes in the Structure and Function of Skeletal Muscles," *Clinical and Experimental Pharmacology and Physiology* 34: 1091-1096, 2007.

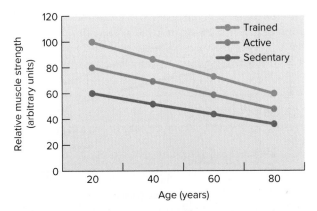

Figure 22.7 Aging is associated with a significant loss of muscular strength. Notice, however, that regular strength training can greatly delay this age-related loss in muscle force production.

Modifed from Buford, T. W., Anton, S. D., Judge, A. R., Marzetti, E., Wohlgemuth, S. E., Carter, C. S., et al., "Models of Accelerated Sarcopenia: Critical Pieces for Solving the Puzzle of Age-Related Muscle Atrophy," Ageing Research Reviews 9: 369-383, 2010; Faulkner, J. A., Larkin, L. M., Claflin, D. R., Brooks, S. V., "Age-Related Changes in the Structure and Function of Skeletal Muscles," *Clinical and Experimental Pharmacology and Physiology* 34: 1091-1096, 2007.

stress) to muscle fibers, inflammation, and decreases in anabolic hormones such as testosterone (20).

Note in Fig. 22.6 that there is little loss of muscle mass before the age of 50. However, after age 50, there is a progressive loss of skeletal muscle mass in both men and women. The rate of muscle loss with aging is variable across individuals, but both men and women tend to lose muscle mass at a rate of 1%-2% per year after the age of 50 (20). Therefore, men and women can lose 40%-60% of their total muscle mass from age 50 to age 80.

Although aging results in a loss of muscle mass and strength in all people, a lifelong program of strength training can maintain a relatively high level of muscle strength across the life span. For example, Fig. 22.7 illustrates the age-related change in leg muscle strength in three individuals that differ in exercise habits. In this illustration, the trained individual has maintained a lifetime of resistance training (2-3 days/ week). The active individual is engaged in routine walking exercise (~5000 steps/3-5 days week) but does not engage in resistance training. The sedentary individual does not participate in regular exercise and is the classic "couch potato." Note that the rate of muscle strength loss with aging does not differ between these individuals. Nonetheless, the resistance-trained individual maintains a higher level of leg muscle strength across the life span compared to both the active and sedentary individual. Therefore, while strength training cannot prevent age-related muscle loss, an individual who engages in regular resistance training can maintain a much higher level of muscular strength throughout the life span compared to less active individuals.

Aging and Endurance Performance

Similar to the age-related loss of muscular strength, aging also results in a decline in endurance performance and $\dot{V}O_2$ max. For example, Fig. 22.8 illustrates the changes in men's and women's 10,000 (10K)-meter running times with advancing age. Note that 10K-performance times increase (i.e., decreased performance) with age in a curvilinear fashion, with the most rapid changes in performance occurring after approximately age 60. Similarly, $\dot{V}O_2$ max also declines with age in trained men and women (Fig. 22.9). Notice that limited change occurs in $\dot{V}O_2$ max until age 40 (55). However, the age-related decline in $\dot{V}O_2$ max in both men and women is approximately a 1% loss per

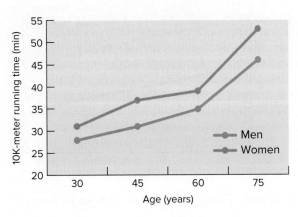

Figure 22.8 Changes in men's and women's 10,000 (10K)-meter running times with advancing age.

Data from World Masters Athletics.

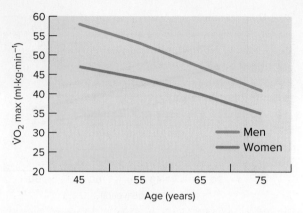

Figure 22.9 The age-related decline in $\dot{V}O_2$ max in both endurance trained men and women.

Data from Jackson, A. S., Sui, X., Hebert, J. R., Church, T. S., and Blair, S. N., "Role of Lifestyle and Aging on the Longitudinal Change in Cardiorespiratory Fitness," *Archives of Internal Medicine* 169: 1781–1787, 2009.

year after age 40. Although endurance training can increase the $\dot{V}O_2$ max of people of all ages, endurance exercise cannot prevent the age-related decline in $\dot{V}O_2$ max. However, individuals that maintain an active program of endurance training throughout the life span can sustain a higher $\dot{V}O_2$ max compared to sedentary individuals (Fig. 22.10).

What factors contribute to the age-related decline in endurance performance and $\dot{V}O_2$ max? Recall from Chap. 20 that the primary determinants of endurance performance are $\dot{V}O_2$ max, exercise economy, and the maximal exercise intensity that can be sustained during endurance exercise (i.e., lactate threshold). Let's discuss the impact of aging on each of these factors.

Maximal aerobic capacity ($\dot{V}O_2$ max) is the upper limit of maximal energy production via oxidative phosphorylation and is a major determinant of

endurance exercise performance. Recall that $\dot{V}O_2$ is determined by both cardiac output and the uptake of oxygen by the tissues (i.e., a-v̄ O_2 difference) as defined by the Fick equation (Chap. 13):

$$\dot{V}O_2 \text{ max} = \text{maximal cardiac output} \times \text{maximal a-v̄ } O_2 \text{ difference}$$

Studies indicate that the age-related decline in $\dot{V}O_2$ max occurs due to a decrease in both maximal cardiac output and a decline in the maximal a-v̄ O_2 difference (82). This point is illustrated in Fig. 22.11. Note that the age-related decline in maximal cardiac output is due to a decrease in both maximal heart rate and the maximal stroke volume. Clearly, the age-related decline in maximal heart rate plays an important role in the decrease in maximal cardiac output. For example, the maximal heart rate can decline by approximately 60 beats per minute from age 20 to 60. The age-related decay in the maximal oxygen extraction (a-v̄ O_2 difference) is likely due to a combination of factors, including a decreased capillary density and mitochondrial volume (82).

Exercise economy is measured as the steady-state oxygen consumption during exercising at a submaximal exercise intensity below the lactate threshold. Exercise economy is important for endurance performance, because, compared to inefficient athletes, efficient athletes use less energy to perform a given exercise task. Several studies indicate that exercise economy does not change with age; therefore, changes in economy are not a major factor in explaining the age-related decline in endurance performance (Fig. 22.11).

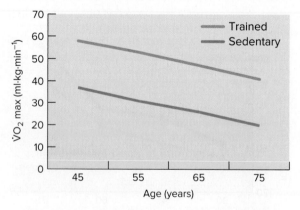

Figure 22.10 Changes in $\dot{V}O_2$ max with age for men.

Data from Jackson, A. S., Sui, X., Hebert, J. R., Church, T. S., and Blair, S. N., "Role of Lifestyle and Aging on the Longitudinal Change in Cardiorespiratory Fitness," *Archives of Internal Medicine* 169: 1781–1787, 2009.

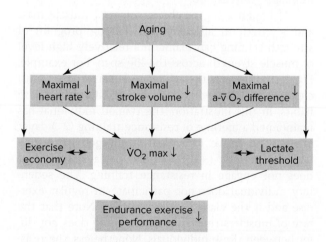

Figure 22.11 Factors and physiological mechanisms responsible for the age-related decline in endurance exercise performance in healthy adults. Down arrows indicate decreases, whereas horizontal arrows indicate no change.

Figure has been modified from Tanaka, H., and Seals, D.R., "Endurance Exercise Performance in Masters Athletes: Age-Associated Changes and Underlying Physiological Mechanisms," *Journal of Physiology* 586: 55–63, 2008.

The ability to work at a high percentage of one's maximal oxygen uptake during submaximal exercise is an important determinant of endurance performance and is often evaluated in the laboratory by measurement of the lactate threshold (Chap. 20). The lactate threshold does not change with age when expressed relative to the $\dot{V}O_2$ max (82). Therefore, age-related changes in the lactate threshold are not a key factor in determining the decline in endurance performance with age (82).

To summarize, success in endurance events is dependent upon $\dot{V}O_2$ max, exercise economy, and the lactate threshold. Aging does not appear to have a negative impact on the lactate threshold or exercise economy. In contrast, aging results in a progressive decline in $\dot{V}O_2$ max, which is the primary factor that contributes to the age-related decline in endurance performance.

IN SUMMARY

- Aging results in a decline in both muscle mass and muscular strength.
- Most of the age-related decline in both skeletal muscle mass and strength occur following age 50.
- Regular bouts of resistance exercise training can assist in maintaining muscle mass and muscular strength throughout the life span.
- Aging is associated with a progressive decline in endurance performance.
- The major factor contributing to the age-related decline in endurance performance is a decrease in $\dot{V}O_2$ max, which occurs due to a decline in both maximal cardiac output and maximal a-$\bar{v}$ O_2 difference.
- Endurance exercise training can protect against age-related decreases in $\dot{V}O_2$ max, but cannot completely halt this decline.

Training Guidelines for Masters Athletes

A detailed discussion of exercise training for the masters athlete is beyond the scope of this chapter.

Nonetheless, an overview of some of the key considerations for training of masters athletes are presented. First, it is important for any masters athlete to gain medical clearance prior to beginning a rigorous exercise training program. A complete medical exam should include a physical exam along with an exercise stress test to ensure that rigorous exercise does not pose a health risk for the older athlete.

The basic principles of exercise training to improve performance were presented in Chap. 21, and these apply to both young and masters athletes. Identical to younger athletes, the masters athlete should avoid overtraining and be aware of the key signs of overtraining, such as an excessive feeling of fatigue at rest, reduced ability to perform a workout, higher resting heart rate, and disrupted sleep.

Training programs for masters athletes must be customized for each individual because differences in genetic capacities for adaptation vary from individual to individual. Add to this fact differences in age, training status, and competitive schedule, and the importance of planning individual training programs for masters athletes becomes obvious. A critical consideration in planning training programs for all masters athletes is to avoid overuse injuries by scheduling adequate recovery periods between rigorous workouts. Indeed, scheduling rest days between challenging workouts becomes more important as athletes increase in age. For more details on the impact of lifelong endurance exercise on cardiovascular fitness, see Trappe et al. (2013) in Suggested Readings.

IN SUMMARY

- All masters athletes should gain medical clearance prior to beginning a rigorous exercise training program.
- The fundamental principles of exercise training apply to people of all ages.
- Training programs for masters athletes must be customized to meet the needs of the individual and consider such factors as age and current training status.

STUDY ACTIVITIES

1. Outline several possible causes of "athletic" amenorrhea.
2. What is the current recommendation for training and competition during menstruation?
3. Discuss the role of prostaglandins in mediating dysmenorrhea.
4. Based on present information, what are reasonable guidelines for advising the pregnant athlete concerning the intensity and duration of training?
5. Define the *female athlete triad*.
6. What factors contribute to bone mineral loss in the female athlete?
7. Discuss the notion that intense exercise might result in permanent damage to (a) the cardiovascular system or (b) the musculoskeletal system in children.
8. What is the recommendation for people with type 1 diabetes with no physical complications for entering a competitive training program?
9. What factors should be considered when advising the diabetic athlete concerning safe participation in athletic conditioning? Include in your discussion suggestions concerning meal timing, injection sites for insulin, and the availability of glucose drinks during training sessions.

10. What is the current opinion concerning the safe participation of people with asthma in competitive athletics?
11. Define the term *epilepsy*.
12. Discuss the possibility that exercise increases the risk of seizures for people with epilepsy.
13. What factors should be considered in assessing the risk-to-benefit ratio of sports participation for people with epilepsy?

14. Graph the change in both muscle mass and muscular strength with age.
15. What factors contribute to the age-related changes in muscle mass and muscular strength?
16. Discuss the impact of aging on $\dot{V}O_2$ max in both men and women.
17. What factor(s) are responsible for the age-related decline in endurance performance?

SUGGESTED READINGS

Armstrong, N., and A. R. Barker. 2011. Endurance training and elite young athletes. *Medicine and Sport Science* 56: 59-83.

Armstrong, N., and A. M. McManus. 2011. Physiology of elite young male athletes. *Medicine and Sport Science* 56: 1-22.

Blaize, A., K. Pearson, and S. Newcomer. 2015. Impact of material exercise during pregnancy on offspring chronic disease susceptibility. *Exercise and Sport Sciences Reviews* 43:198-203.

Faigenbaum, A., R. Loyd, J. MacDonald, and G. Myer. 2015. Citius, altius, Fortius: beneficial effects of resistance training for young athletes. *British Journal of Sports Medicine* doi:10.1136/bjsports-2015-094621.

Joy E. et al. 2014 Female athlete triad coalition consensus statement on treatment and return to play of the female athlete triad. *Current Sports Medicine Reports* 13:219-231.

Joy E., A. Kussman, and A. Nattiv. 2016 Update on eating disorders in athletes: A comprehensive narrative review with a focus on clinical assessment and management. *British Journal of Sports Medicine* 50:154-162.

Lithwick D, et al. 2016 Pre-participation screening in the young competitive athlete: International recommendations and a Canadian perspective. *British Columbia Medical Journal* 58: 145-151.

Lloyd, R. S., A. D. Faigenbaum, M. H. Stone, J. L. Oliver, I. Jeffreys, J. A. Moody, et al. 2013. Position statement on youth resistance training: the 2014 international consensus. *British Journal of Sports Medicine*, September 20, 2013, doi: 10.1136/bjsports-2013-092952.

Morton, A. R., and K. D. Fitch. 2011. Australian Association for Exercise and Sports Science position statement on exercise and asthma. *Journal of Science and Medicine in Sport* 14: 312-316.

Nascimento, S. L., F. G. Surita, and J. G. Cecatti. 2012. Physical exercise during pregnancy: a systematic review. *Current Opinion in Obstetrics and Gynecology* 24: 387-394.

Orio, F., G. Muscogiuri, A. Ascione, F. Marciano, A. Volpe, G. La Sala, et al. 2013. Effects of physical exercise on the female reproductive system. *Minerva Endocrinologica* 38: 305-319.

Pimentel J., R. Tojal, and J. Morgado. 2015. Epilepsy and physical exercise. Seizure. 25: 87-94.

Trappe, S., E. Hayes, A. Galpin, L. Kaminsky, B. Jemiolo, W. Fink, et al. 2013. New records in aerobic power among octogenarian lifelong endurance athletes. *Journal of Applied Physiology* 114: 3-10.

Voskanian, N. 2013. ACL injury prevention in female athletes: review of the literature and practical considerations in implementing an ACL prevention program. *Current Reviews in Musculoskeletal Medicine* 6: 158-163.

REFERENCES

1. **Ackerman KE, and Misra M.** Bone health and the female athlete triad in adolescent athletes. *Physician and Sports Medicine* 39: 131-141, 2011.
2. **Andersen AE.** Anorexia nervosa and bulimia: a spectrum of eating disorders. *Journal of Adolescent Health Care* 4: 15-21, 1983.
3. **Arida RM, Cavalheiro EA, de Albuquerque M, da Silva AC, and Scorza FA.** Physical exercise in epilepsy: the case in favor. *Epilepsy and Behavior* 11: 478-479, 2007.
4. **Arida RM, Scorza FA, Terra VC, Cysneiros RM, and Cavalheiro EA.** Physical exercise in rats with epilepsy is protective against seizures: evidence of animal studies. *Arquivos de Neuro-psiquiatria* 67: 1013-1016, 2009.
5. **Arida R, Guimaraes de Almeda AC, Cavalheiro EA, and Scorza F.** Experimental and clinical findings from physical exercise as complementary therapy for epilepsy. *Epilepsy and Behavior* 26: 273-278, 2013.
6. **Armstrong N, and Barker AR.** Endurance training and elite young athletes. *Medicine and Sport Science* 56: 59-83, 2011.
7. **Armstrong N, and McManus AM.** Physiology of elite young male athletes. *Medicine and Sport Science* 56: 1-22, 2011.

8. **Artal R, and O'Toole M.** Guidelines of the American College of Obstetricians and Gynecologists for exercise during pregnancy and the postpartum period. *British Journal of Sports Medicine* 37: 6-12; discussion 12, 2003.
9. **Åstrand P.** Girl swimmers. *Acta Paediatric Scandinavica* 147(Suppl): 1-75, 1963.
10. **Barrack MT, Ackerman KE, and Gibbs JC.** Update on the female athlete triad. *Current Reviews in Musculoskeletal Medicine* 6: 195-204, 2013.
11. **Behm DG, Faigenbaum AD, Falk B, and Klentrou P.** Canadian Society for Exercise Physiology position paper: resistance training in children and adolescents. *Applied Physiology Nutrition and Metabolism* 33: 547-561, 2008.
12. **Beilock SL, Feltz DL, and Pivarnik JM.** Training patterns of athletes during pregnancy and postpartum. *Research Quarterly for Exercise & Sport* 72: 39-46, 2001.
13. **Benjamin HJ.** The female adolescent athlete: specific concerns. *Pediatric Annals* 36: 719-726, 2007.
14. **Bennett D.** Sports and epilepsy: to play or not to play. *Seminars in Neurology* 1: 345-357, 1981.
15. **Bhaskarabhatla KV, and Birrer R.** Physical activity and diabetes mellitus. *Comprehensive Therapy* 31: 291-298, 2005.

16. **Bien DP.** Rationale and implementation of anterior cruciate ligament injury prevention warm-up programs in female athletes. *Journal of Strength and Conditioning Research* 25: 271-285, 2011.

17. **Birch K.** Female athlete triad. *British Medical Journal* 330: 244-246, 2005.

18. **Blaize, A, Pearson K, and Newcomer S.** Impact of maternal exercise during pregnancy on offspring chronic disease susceptibility. *Exercise and Sport Sciences Reviews* 43:198-203, 2015.

19. **Brophy RH, Silvers HJ, and Mandelbaum BR.** Anterior cruciate ligament injuries: etiology and prevention. *Sports Medicine and Arthroscopy Review* 18: 2-11, 2010.

20. **Buford TW, Anton SD, Judge AR, Marzetti E, Wohlgemuth SE, Carter CS, et al.** Models of accelerated sarcopenia: critical pieces for solving the puzzle of age-related muscle atrophy. *Ageing Research Reviews* 9: 369-383, 2010.

21. **Bullen BA, Skrinar GS, Beitins IZ, von Mering G, Turnbull BA, and McArthur JW.** Induction of menstrual disorders by strenuous exercise in untrained women. *New England Journal of Medicine* 312: 1349-1353, 1985.

22. **Burger LJ, Lopez RI, and Elliott FA.** Tonic seizures induced by movement. *Neurology* 22: 656-659, 1972.

23. **Castelo-Branco C, Reina F, Montivero AD, Colodron M, and Vanrell JA.** Influence of high-intensity training and of dietetic and anthropometric factors on menstrual cycle disorders in ballet dancers. *Gynecological Endocrinology* 22: 31-35, 2006.

24. **Coop CA, Adams KE, and Webb CN.** SCUBA diving and asthma: Clinical recommendations and safety. *Clinical Reviews in Allergy & Immunology* 50:18-22, 2016.

25. **Corrado D, Basso C, Pavei A, Michieli P, Schiavon M, and Thiene G.** Trends in sudden cardiovascular death in young competitive athletes after implementation of a preparticipation screening program. *JAMA* 296: 1593-1601, 2006.

26. **Costigan S, Eather, N, Plotnikoff R, Taaffe D, and Lubans D.** High-intensity interval training for improving health-related fitness in adolescents: a systematic review and meta-analysis. *British Journal of Sports Medicine* 49:1253-1261, 2015.

27. **Dale E, Gerlach DH, and Wilhite AL.** Menstrual dysfunction in distance runners. *Obstetrics & Gynecology* 54: 47-53, 1979.

28. **Dalle Grave R.** Eating disorders: progress and challenges. *European Journal of Internal Medicine* 22: 153-160, 2011.

29. **De Souza MJ.** Menstrual disturbances in athletes: a focus on luteal phase defects. *Medicine & Science in Sports & Exercise* 35: 1553-1563, 2003.

30. **De Souza MJ, and Metzger DA.** Reproductive dysfunction in amenorrheic athletes and anorexic patients: a review. *Medicine & Science in Sports & Exercise* 23: 995-1007, 1991.

31. **Drezner J, and Corrado D.** Is there evidence for recommending electrocardiogram as part of the pre-participation examination? *Clinical Journal of Sport Medicine* 21: 18-24, 2011.

32. **Drinkwater BL, Bruemner B, and Chesnut CH, III.** Menstrual history as a determinant of current bone density in young athletes. *JAMA* 263: 545-548, 1990.

33. **Drinkwater BL, Nilson K, Chesnut CH, III, Bremner WJ, Shainholtz S, and Southworth MB.** Bone mineral content of amenorrheic and eumenorrheic athletes. *New England Journal of Medicine* 311: 277-281, 1984.

34. **Dugan SA.** Sports-related knee injuries in female athletes: what gives? *American Journal of Physical Medicine & Rehabilitation* 84: 122-130, 2005.

35. **Ekblom B.** Effect of physical training in adolescent boys. *Journal of Applied Physiology* 27: 350-355, 1969.

36. **Enea C, Boisseau N, Fargeas-Gluck MA, Diaz V, and Dugue B.** Circulating androgens in women: exercise-induced changes. *Sports Medicine* 41: 1-15, 2011.

37. **Enea C, Boisseau N, Ottavy M, Mulliez J, Millet C, Ingrand I, et al.** Effects of menstrual cycle, oral contraception, and training on exercise-induced changes in circulating DHEA-sulphate and testosterone in young women. *European Journal of Applied Physiology* 106: 365-373, 2009.

38. **Eriksson BO.** Physical training, oxygen supply and muscle metabolism in 11-13-year old boys. *Acta Physiologica Scandinavica. Supplementum* 384: 1-48, 1972.

39. **Faigenbaum AD, Kraemer WJ, Blimkie CJ, Jeffreys I, Micheli LJ, Nitka M, et al.** Youth resistance training: updated position statement paper from the National Strength and Conditioning Association. *Journal of Strength and Conditioning Research* 23: S60-79, 2009.

40. **Faigenbaum AD, Loud RL, O'Connell J, Glover S, and Westcott WL.** Effects of different resistance training protocols on upper-body strength and endurance development in children. *Journal of Strength and Conditioning Research* 15: 459-465, 2001.

41. **Faigenbaum AD, Milliken LA, and Westcott WL.** Maximal strength testing in healthy children. *Journal of Strength and Conditioning Research* 17: 162-166, 2003.

42. **Faigenbaum AD, and Myer GD.** Resistance training among young athletes: safety, efficacy and injury prevention effects. *British Journal of Sports Medicine* 44: 56-63, 2010.

43. **Faigenbaum AD, Loyd RS, and Myer GD.** Youth resistance training: past practices, new perspectives, and future directions. *Pediatric Exercise Science* 25: 591-604, 2013.

44. **Faulkner JA, Larkin LM, Claflin DR, and Brooks SV.** Age-related changes in the structure and function of skeletal muscles. *Clinical and Experimental Pharmacology and Physiology* 34: 1091-1096, 2007.

45. **Feicht CB, Johnson TS, Martin BJ, Sparkes KE, and Wagner WW, Jr.** Secondary amenorrhoea in athletes. *Lancet* 2: 1145-1146, 1978.

46. **Fitzpatrick KK, and Lock J.** Anorexia nervosa. *BMJ Clinical Evidence (Online)* 2011: 2011.

47. **Fountain NB, and May AC.** Epilepsy and athletics. *Clinics in Sports Medicine* 22: 605-616, x-xi, 2003.

48. **Gibbs JC, Williams NI, and De Souza MJ.** Prevalence of individual and combined components of the female athlete triad. *Medicine & Science in Sports & Exercise* 45: 985-996, 2013.

49. **Gotze W, Kubicki S, Munter M, and Teichmann J.** Effect of physical exercise on seizure threshold (investigated by electroencephalographic telemetry). *Diseases of the Nervous System* 28: 664-667, 1967.

50. **Hale R.** Factors important to women engaged in vigorous physical activity. In *Sports Medicine*, edited by Strauss R. Philadelphia, PA: W. B. Saunders, 1984.

51. **Hausenblas HA, Cook BJ, and Chittester NI.** Can exercise treat eating disorders? *Exercise and Sport Sciences Reviews* 36: 43-47, 2008.

52. **Hewett TE, Lindenfeld TN, Riccobene JV, and Noyes FR.** The effect of neuromuscular training on the incidence of knee injury in female athletes: a prospective study. *American Journal of Sports Medicine* 27: 699-706, 1999.

53. **Hoch AZ, et al.** Prevalence of the female athlete triad in high school athletes and sedentary students. *Clinical Journal of Sport Medicine* 19:421-428, 2009.

54. **Ingjer F.** Development of maximal oxygen uptake in young elite male cross-country skiers: a longitudinal study. *Journal of Sports Sciences* 10: 49-63, 1992.

55. **Jackson AS, Sui X, Hebert JR, Church TS, and Blair SN.** Role of lifestyle and aging on the longitudinal change in cardiorespiratory fitness. *Archives of Internal Medicine* 169: 1781-1787, 2009.

56. **Joy E et al.** Female athlete triad coalition consensus statement on treatment and return to play of the female athlete triad. *Current Sports Medicine Reports* 13:219-231, 2014.

57. **Joy E, Kussman A, and Nattiv A.** 2016 Update on eating disorders in athletes: A comprehensive narrative review with a focus on clinical assessment and management. *British Journal of Sports Medicine* 50:154-162, 2016.

58. **Komatsu WR, Gabbay MA, Castro ML, Saraiva GL, Chacra AR, de Barros Neto TL, and Dib SA.** Aerobic exercise capacity in normal adolescents and those with type 1 diabetes mellitus. *Pediatric Diabetes* 6: 145-149, 2005.

59. **Kuijer A.** Epilepsy and exercise, electroencephalographical and biochemical studies. In *Advances in Epileptology: The X Epilepsy International Symposium,* edited by Wada J, and Penry J. New York, NY: Raven Press, 1980.

60. **La Gerche A, Baggish AL, Knuuti J, Prior DL, Sharma S, Heidbuchel H, et al.** Cardiac imaging and stress testing asymptomatic athletes to identify those at risk of sudden cardiac death. *JACC Cardiovascular Imaging* 6: 993-1007, 2013.

61. **Lloyd RS, Faigenbaum AD, Stone MH, J. L. Oliver, I. Jeffreys, J. A. Moody, et al.** Position statement on youth resistance training: the 2014 international consensus. *British Journal of Sports Medicine,* September 20, 2013, doi: 10.1136/bjsports-2013-092952.

62. **Luong, MW, Morrison B, Lithwick D, Isserow SH, Heibron B, and Krahn A.** Sudden cardiac death in young competitive athletes. *British Columbia Medical Journal* 58:138-144, 2016.

63. **Manore MM, Kam LC, and Loucks AB.** The female athlete triad: components, nutrition issues, and health consequences. *Journal of Sports Sciences* 25 Suppl 1: S61-71, 2007.

64. **Martinsen M, Bratland-Sanda S, Eriksson AK, and Sundgot-Borgen J.** Dieting to win or to be thin? A study of dieting and disordered eating among adolescent elite athletes and non-athlete controls. *British Journal of Sports Medicine* 44: 70-76, 2010.

65. **McManus AM, and Armstrong N.** Physiology of elite young female athletes. *Medicine and Sport Science* 56: 23-46, 2011.

66. **Mendes FA, Almeida FM, Cukier A, Stelmach R, Jacob-Filho W, Martins MA, et al.** Effects of aerobic training on airway inflammation in asthmatic patients. *Medicine & Science in Sports & Exercise* 43: 197-203, 2011.

67. **Micheli L.** *Pediatric and Adolescent Sports Medicine.* Philadelphia, PA: W. B. Saunders, 1984.

68. **Micheli LJ, Smith A, Biosca F, and Sangenis P.** Position statement on girls and women in sport. IOC, 2002.

69. **Miller CA, and Golden NH.** An introduction to eating disorders: clinical presentation, epidemiology, and prognosis. *Nutrition in Clinical Practice* 25: 110-115, 2010.

70. **Morton AR, and Fitch KD.** Australian Association for Exercise and Sports Science position statement on exercise and asthma. *Journal of Science and Medicine in Sport* 14: 312-316, 2011.

71. **Mountjoy M et al.** The IOC consensus statement: beyond the female athlete triad-relative energy deficiency in sport. *British Journal of Sports Medicine* 48:491-497, 2014.

72. **Narici MV, and Maffulli N.** Sarcopenia: characteristics, mechanisms and functional significance. *British Medical Bulletin* 95: 139-159, 2010.

73. **Nascimento SL, Surita FG, and Cecatti JG.** Physical exercise during pregnancy: a systematic review. *Current Opinion in Obstetrics and Gynecology* 24:387-394, 2012.

74. **Nattiv A, Loucks AB, Manore MM, Sanborn CF, Sundgot-Borgen J, and Warren MP.** American College of Sports Medicine position stand. The female athlete triad. *Medicine & Science in Sports & Exercise* 39: 1867-1882, 2007.

75. **Nottin S, Vinet A, Stecken F, N'Guyen LD, Ounissi F, Lecoq AM, et al.** Central and peripheral cardiovascular adaptations to exercise in endurance-trained children. *Acta Physiologica Scandinavica* 175: 85-92, 2002.

76. **Pivarnik JM, Marichal CJ, Spillman T, and Morrow JR, Jr.** Menstrual cycle phase affects temperature regulation during endurance exercise. *Journal of Applied Physiology* 72: 543-548, 1992.

77. **Pruett E.** Insulin and exercise in the non-diabetic man. In *Exercise Physiology,* edited by Fotherly K, and Pal S. New York, NY: Walter de Gruyter, 1985.

78. **Roberts A, et al.** Do youth with type 1 diabetes exercise safely? A focus on patient practices with glycemic outcomes. *Pediatric Diabetes* doi: 10.1111/pedi.12402, 2016.

79. **Scheid JL, and De Souza MJ.** Menstrual irregularities and energy deficiency in physically active women: the role of ghrelin, PYY and adipocytokines. *Medicine and Sport Science* 55: 82-102, 2010.

80. **Specker B, Thiex N, and Sudhagoni R.** Does exercise influence pediatric bone? A systematic review. *Clinical Orthopaedics and Related Research* 473:3658-3672, 2015.

81. **Stice E, Marti CN, and Rohde P.** Prevalence, incidence, impairment, and course of the proposed DSM-5 eating disorder diagnoses in an 8-year prospective community study of young women. *Journal of Abnormal Psychology* 122: 445-457, 2013.

82. **Tanaka H, and Seals DR.** Endurance exercise performance in masters athletes: age-associated changes and underlying physiological mechanisms. *Journal of Physiology* 586: 55-63, 2008.

83. **Torstveit MK, and Sundgot-Borgen J.** The female athlete triad exists in both elite athletes and controls. *Medicine & Science in Sports & Exercise* 37: 1449-1459, 2005.

84. **Voskanian N.** ACL injury prevention in female athletes: review of the literature and practical considerations in implementing an ACL prevention program. *Current Reviews in Musculoskeletal Medicine* 6: 158-163, 2013.

85. **Warren MP, and Chua A.** Exercise-induced amenorrhea and bone health in the adolescent athlete. *Annals of the New York Academy of Sciences* 1135: 244-252, 2008.

86. **Weltman A, Janney C, Rians CB, Strand K, Berg B, Tippitt S, et al.** The effects of hydraulic resistance strength training in pre-pubertal males. *Medicine & Science in Sports & Exercise* 18: 629-638, 1986.

87. **Yager J, and Andersen AE.** Clinical practice: anorexia nervosa. *New England Journal of Medicine* 353: 1481-1488, 2005.

88. **Zelisko JA, Noble HB, and Porter M.** A comparison of men's and women's professional basketball injuries. *American Journal of Sports Medicine* 10: 297-299, 1982.

89. **Zilmer D.** Gender specific injury patterns in high school varsity basketball. *Journal of Women's Health* 1: 69-76, 1992.

23

© Digital Vision/Getty Images

Nutrition, Body Composition, and Performance

■ Objectives

By studying this chapter, you should be able to do the following:

1. Describe the effect of various carbohydrate diets on muscle glycogen and on endurance performance during heavy exercise.

2. Contrast the "classic" method of achieving a supercompensation of the muscle glycogen stores with the "modified" method.

3. Describe some potential problems when glucose is ingested immediately prior to exercise and how these problems can be avoided.

4. Describe the importance of blood glucose as a fuel in prolonged exercise and the role of carbohydrate supplementation during the performance.

5. Explain why multiple carbohydrates have to be consumed during prolonged exercise when blood glucose is used at a very high rate.

6. Describe the need for protein during the adaptation to a new, more strenuous exercise level with the protein need when the adaptation is complete.

7. Describe the recommended range of protein intake for athletes, and indicate dietary factors that would demand using the top end of the range.

8. Describe the recommended fluid replacement strategies to use before exercise, during exercise of different durations, and following exercise.

9. Describe the salt requirement of the athlete compared to that of the sedentary individual and the recommended means of maintaining sodium balance.

10. Provide a brief summary of the effects of vitamin supplementation on performance.

11. Characterize the role of the precompetition meal on performance and the rationale for limiting fats and proteins.

12. Explain why one must be careful in recommending specific body fatness values for individual athletes.

■ Outline

This chapter on nutrition, body composition, and performance is an extension of Chap. 18 because the primary emphasis must be on achieving health-related goals before performance-related goals are examined. In fact, the information presented here must be examined in light of what the average person needs. Does an athlete need additional protein? What percentage of body fat is a reasonable goal for an athlete? We will address these questions in that order. For a more detailed look at these issues, see Suggested Readings for *Clinical Sports Nutrition* by Burke and Deakin, *Nutrition for Health, Fitness and Sport* by Williams, Anderson, and Rawson, and the 2016 ACSM position stand on *Nutrition and Athletic Performance*.

In Chap. 18, we indicated the recommended range of nutrient intakes:

■ Adults should get 45%–65% of their calories from carbohydrates, 20%–35% from fat, and 10%–35% from protein.

This simple statement is important because it sets the stage for a discussion of what athletes should and do eat to support vigorous training programs and provide the fuel for the diverse performances that make up competitive athletics.

CARBOHYDRATE

The recommended range for carbohydrate intake is quite broad to meet the needs of the whole population and allow one to address special needs linked to a reduced capacity for using carbohydrates (e.g., people with type 2 diabetes). Because carbohydrate oxidation makes up a larger percentage of total energy production as exercise intensity increases, it should be no surprise that most athletes need more carbohydrate than the average person. This section considers the use of carbohydrates in the days prior to a performance, during the performance itself, and post-performance. However, the information is also applicable for planning training sessions where the demand for carbohydrate is great.

Carbohydrate Diets and Performance

In 1967, three studies were published from the same Swedish laboratory that set the stage for our understanding of the role of muscle glycogen in performance (1, 10, 69). Hermansen et al. (72) showed muscle glycogen to be systematically depleted during

heavy (77% $\dot{V}O_2$ max) exercise, and when exhaustion occurred, glycogen content was near zero. Ahlborg et al. (1) found that work time to exhaustion was directly related to the initial glycogen store in the working muscles. Bergström et al. (10) confirmed and extended this by showing that by manipulating the quantity of carbohydrate in the diet, the concentration of glycogen in muscle could be altered and, along with it, the time to exhaustion. In their study, subjects consumed 2800 kcal/day using either a low-CHO (fat and protein) diet, a mixed diet, or a high-carbohydrate diet in which 2300 kcal came from carbohydrate. Glycogen contents of the quadriceps femoris muscle were, respectively, 0.63 (low), 1.75 (average), and 3.31 (high) g/100 g muscle, and performance time for exercise at 75% $\dot{V}O_2$ max averaged 57, 114, and 167 minutes. Figure 23.1 shows these results. In brief, the muscle glycogen content and performance time could be varied with diet. These laboratory findings were confirmed by Karlsson and Saltin (82), who had trained subjects run a 30-km race twice, once following a high-carbohydrate diet and the other time after a mixed diet. The initial muscle glycogen level was 3.5 g/100 g muscle following the CHO diet and 1.7 g/100 g muscle following the mixed diet. The best performance of all subjects occurred during the high-CHO diet. Interestingly, the pace at the start of the race was not faster; instead, the additional CHO allowed subjects to maintain the pace for a longer

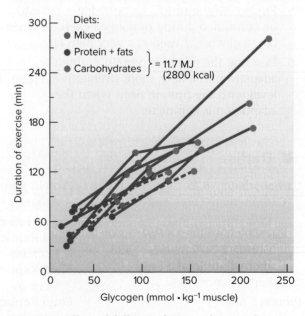

Figure 23.1 Effect of different diets on the muscle glycogen concentration and work time to exhaustion.

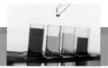

Jonas Bergström, M.D., Ph.D.—From the Needle Biopsy Technique and Muscle Glycogen to Much, Much More

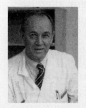

Courtesy of
Dr. Bengt Lindholm

Dr. Jonas Bergström had a major impact on the field of exercise physiology, even though most of his research work focused on renal function, in which he had an international reputation. A multitalented man, he pursued medicine only after deciding to give up a career as a recognized jazz musician. He studied medicine at the Karolinska Institute in Stockholm, Sweden, and graduated in 1956. He did subsequent training in renal physiology and biochemistry, and his thesis work, *Muscle Electrolytes in Man*, resulted in the development of the percutaneous (needle) muscle biopsy technique. The introduction of that technique allowed numerous investigators around the world to study muscle function and metabolism at rest and during exercise—studies that revolutionized our understanding of exercise physiology, be it in muscle fiber typing, substrate use during exercise, or adaptation to spaceflight. The classic studies on muscle glycogen use during exercise that were just described were made possible because of this technique, and Dr. Bergström was a lead scientist in those studies.

When he started his career as a physician, there was little that could be done for those in renal failure. He was the leading force in securing the funds, space, and support to develop a chronic dialysis program in Sweden. However, his extensive background in biochemistry and metabolism allowed him to have a major impact on nutritional factors related to renal function. His research led to the development of special low-protein diets that could reduce the buildup of urea in the blood, and its associated symptoms, which postponed the need for dialysis for months and years. His research also addressed issues related to blood pressure and blood volume during dialysis, the make-up of the fluids used in dialysis (to reduce protein breakdown), and the importance of preventing inflammation in renal disease patients through proper diet. His work impacted the care of renal disease patients around the world, and he was recognized with numerous awards throughout his career for his outstanding contributions. Dr. Bergström died in 2001.

Source: "Obituary of Jonas Bergström (1929–2001)," *Nephrology Dialysis Transplantation* 17: 936–938, 2002.

period. An important finding in this study was that compared to those on the high-CHO diet, pace did not fall off for those on the mixed diet until about halfway through the race (about one hour or so). This suggests that the normal mixed diet used in the study would be suitable for run or cycle races lasting less than one hour. See A Look Back–Important People in Science for an individual who had a major impact on our understanding of this aspect of exercise physiology, even though it was not his primary research focus.

Given the importance of muscle glycogen in prolonged endurance performance, it is no surprise that investigators have tried to determine what conditions will yield the highest muscle glycogen content. In 1966, Bergström and Hultman (11) had subjects do one-legged exercise to exhaust the glycogen store in the exercised leg while not affecting the resting leg's glycogen store. When this procedure was followed with a high-carbohydrate diet, the glycogen content was more than twice as high in the previously exercised leg, compared to the control leg. Further, they found that in subjects who had the high-carbohydrate diet following the protein/fat diet (plus doing exhausting exercise), the muscle glycogen stores were higher than when the mixed diet preceded the high-carbohydrate treatment (11). This combination of information led to the following *classical method* of achieving a muscle glycogen **supercompensation:**

- Prolonged, strenuous exercise to exhaust muscle glycogen store
- A fat/protein diet for three days while continuing to train
- A high-carbohydrate diet (90% CHO) for three days, with inactivity

There were some practical problems with this approach to achieving a high muscle glycogen content, given that it required seven days to prepare for a race. Further, some subjects could not tolerate either the extremely low- (high fat and protein) or high- (90%) carbohydrate diets. Sherman (114, 115) proposed a *modified plan* that causes supercompensation. The plan requires a tapering of the workout from 90 minutes to 40 minutes while eating a 50% CHO diet (350 g/day). This is followed by two days of 20-minute workouts while eating a 70% CHO diet (500–600 g/day) and, finally, a day of rest prior to the competition with the 70% CHO diet (or 500–600 g/day). This regimen was shown to be effective in increasing the glycogen stores to *high values* consistent with good performance (see Fig. 23.2). Studies have shown that when carbohydrate intake is about 10 g/kg body weight using foods with

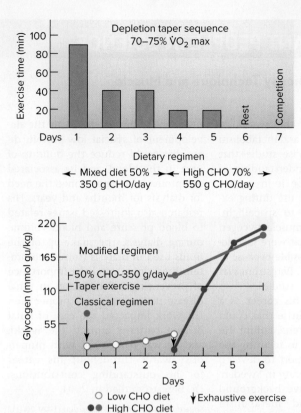

Figure 23.2 Modification of the classic glycogen loading technique to achieve high muscle glycogen levels with minimal changes in a training or diet routine. Glycogen levels are in glucose units (gu) per kilogram (kg).

a high glycemic index (see Chap. 18), only one day was needed to achieve very high muscle glycogen levels in all muscle fiber types (18, 50). The elevated muscle glycogen levels can last as long as five days, depending on the level of activity and the amount of carbohydrate ingested during that time (6). What is needed for the day-to-day replenishment of muscle glycogen?

It takes about 24 hours to replenish muscle glycogen following prolonged, strenuous exercise, provided that about 500-700 g of carbohydrate are ingested (36, 50, 55, 77). The point that must be emphasized is that a person who is eating 55%-60% of calories from carbohydrate is already consuming what is needed to replace muscle glycogen on a day-to-day basis. If an athlete requires 4000 kcal per day for caloric balance and 55%-60% is derived from carbohydrates, then 2200-2400 kcal (55%-60% of 4000 kcal) or 550-600 g of carbohydrate will be consumed. This quantity is consistent with what is needed to restore muscle glycogen to normal levels 24 hours after strenuous exercise (3). This is important for training considerations, and this "regular" diet would require little or no change to meet the carbohydrate load (500-600 g/day) described by Sherman to achieve supercompensation (114, 115). Consistent with this, the 2016 ACSM position stand on Nutrition and Athletic Performance (3) makes the

following recommendations for providing high levels of carbohydrate for training sessions and competitions:

- General fueling for events lasting less than 90 min: 7-12 g · kg^{-1} · d^{-1} for daily fuel needs.
- Carbohydrate loading for events greater than 90 min of sustained or intermittent exercise: 10-12 g · kg^{-1} · d^{-1} for 36-48 hours before competitions.

However, concerns have been raised because most of these guidelines have been based on male subjects, who have high or very high caloric intakes. When applied to women, results are not as consistent. Given that glycogen is stored with water (~3 grams water per gram of carbohydrate), athletes need to be aware of a potential feeling of fullness and heaviness, especially for those doing weight-bearing exercise (113).

Before leaving this section we want to address one more question: is there any advantage to doing endurance training when muscle glycogen stores are low? There is some support for this notion of "training low" in that cell signaling responses that drive muscle adaptations are activated to a greater degree compared to when muscle glycogen levels are high. However, this is countered by evidence showing that under those circumstances ("training low"), the quality of the workout (e.g., intensity, number of repetitions) that can be maintained is reduced, and with it, the adaptations to training. Consequently, although there is sound theory for "training low," any benefits to performance are unclear (3, 16, 17).

IN SUMMARY

- Performance in endurance events is improved by a diet high in carbohydrates due primarily to the increase in muscle glycogen.
- When workouts are tapered over several days while additional CHO (70% of dietary intake) is consumed, a "supercompensation" of the glycogen store can be achieved.

Carbohydrate Intake Prior to or During a Performance

The focus on muscle glycogen as the primary carbohydrate source in heavy exercise has always diminished the role that blood glucose plays in maintaining carbohydrate oxidation in muscle. In Coggan and Coyle's review (31), they correct this perception for exercises that last three to four hours, in which blood glucose and muscle glycogen share equally in contributing to carbohydrate oxidation. In fact, as muscle glycogen decreases, the role that blood glucose plays increases until, at the end of three to four hours of exercise, it may be the sole source of carbohydrate. This is what makes blood glucose an important fuel in prolonged work, and why so much attention has been directed at trying to maintain the blood glucose concentration.

Unfortunately, the liver glycogen supply also decreases with time during prolonged exercise, and because gluconeogenesis can supply glucose at a rate of only 0.2–0.4 g/min when the muscles may be consuming it at a rate of 1–2 g/min, hypoglycemia is a real possibility. Hypoglycemia (blood glucose concentration <2.5 mmoles/liter) results when the rate of blood glucose uptake is not matched by release from the liver and/or small intestine. Hypoglycemia has been shown to occur during exercise at 58% $\dot{V}O_2$ max for 3.5 hours and at 74% $\dot{V}O_2$ max for 2.5 hours (39). However, the number of subjects who demonstrate central nervous system dysfunction varied from none (51) to only 25% of the subjects (39). Although no absolutely clear association exists between hypoglycemia and fatigue, the availability of blood glucose as an energy source is, without question, linked to the performance of prolonged (three to four hours) strenuous exercise (31). How should carbohydrate be taken in before and during exercise to maintain the high rate of carbohydrate oxidation needed for performance?

Carbohydrate Intake Prior to a Performance The timing and the type of carbohydrate are important to top off the body's carbohydrate stores prior to a performance. One of the earliest studies showed that when 75 g of glucose were ingested 30–45 minutes before exercise requiring 70%–75% $\dot{V}O_2$ max, plasma glucose and insulin were elevated at the start of exercise, and muscle glycogen was used at a *faster rate* during the exercise (34). This is counter to the goal of sparing muscle glycogen, and performance was shown to decrease 19% with such a treatment (53). In contrast to this early study, various reviews of this topic indicate that the blood glucose and plasma insulin responses to pre-exercise glucose feedings are quite variable (some will experience a lowering of blood glucose; most will not), and that, in general, performance in prolonged exercise is either improved or not affected (3, 81, 114). The pre-exercise carbohydrate feeding is viewed as a means of topping off both muscle and liver glycogen stores. Generally, such procedures result in carbohydrates being used at a higher rate, but because of the large amount of carbohydrate ingested, the plasma glucose concentration is maintained for a longer period. Jeukendrup provides the following observations and recommendations relative to pre-exercise feedings (81):

■ The fall in blood glucose during submaximal exercise (62%–72% $\dot{V}O_2$ max) following ingestion of 75 g of carbohydrate an hour before the exercise cannot be prevented by ingesting a smaller (~22 g) or larger (>155 g) amount of carbohydrate.

■ High glycemic index carbohydrates taken in an hour before exercise lead to higher blood glucose and insulin responses, compared to moderate or low glycemic index carbohydrates.

■ The hypoglycemic response is quite variable, with some athletes being much more susceptible than others. Interestingly, this responsiveness is not linked to insulin sensitivity.

■ To minimize the risk of hypoglycemia, carbohydrates can be ingested just prior to the exercise (in last five minutes) or during the warm-up.

■ The form in which the carbohydrate is ingested does not matter. One can use a solid, gel, or liquid carbohydrate product. Clearly, the type should be left to the athlete.

Athletes who are more responsive to pre-exercise carbohydrate feedings (i.e., experience symptoms of hypoglycemia) should test different types of carbohydrate (low, moderate, high glycemic index), ingest carbohydrates just before the performance or during the warm-up, or if that doesn't work, avoid carbohydrates in the 90 minutes before exercise (81). Consistent with this, the 2016 ACSM position stand's recommendation (3) for pre-event fueling for carbohydrate is to consume 1–4 g · kg^{-1}, 1–4 hours before exercise, but with the following caveats.

■ Timing, amount, and type of carbohydrate should be chosen to suit the individual's needs and preferences.

■ Low-glycemic choices may provide a more sustained source of carbohydrate when it cannot be consumed during exercise.

Carbohydrate Intake During a Performance In contrast to the pre-exercise feeding studies in which there was some variability in the outcome, there is a great deal of consensus that feeding carbohydrate during exercise delays fatigue and improves performance. Interestingly, the improved performance appears to have nothing to do with sparing the muscle glycogen store. Muscle glycogen is depleted at the same rate during prolonged vigorous (70%–75% $\dot{V}O_2$ max) exercise, with or without carbohydrate ingestion; however, liver glycogen is not (28, 31). The ingestion of carbohydrate appears to spare the liver glycogen store by directly contributing carbohydrate for oxidation. If additional carbohydrate is not ingested during prolonged exercise, the blood glucose concentration decreases as the liver stores are depleted, resulting in an inadequate rate of carbohydrate oxidation by muscle. Central nervous system activation of muscle is diminished by hypoglycemia, resulting in a reduced

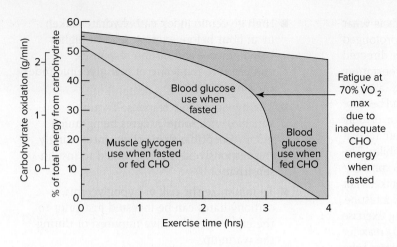

Figure 23.3 Blood glucose and muscle glycogen use when subjects fasted or were fed carbohydrates (CHO) during prolonged exercise.

power output (101). Consistent with that, the rating of perceived exertion (RPE) is lower with carbohydrate supplementation during prolonged exercise (24, 121). Figure 23.3 shows Coggan and Coyle's model of how carbohydrate is supplied to muscle during prolonged exercise under fasted and fed conditions. The rate of muscle glycogen depletion is not different; however, when fed carbohydrates, the subjects last longer due to the increased availability of blood glucose. This effect varies with the dose, with a greater rate of ingestion (i.e., 60 g/hr vs. 15 g/hr) leading to better performances (117). When is the best time to consume carbohydrates during exercise?

Coggan and Coyle indicate that carbohydrates either can be ingested throughout exercise or can be taken 30 minutes before the anticipated time of fatigue, with no difference in the outcome (31). This is consistent with their contention that it is the increased availability of glucose late in exercise that delays fatigue. In exercise tests at 75% $\dot{V}O_2$ max, the time to fatigue was extended by about 45 minutes with carbohydrate ingestion. Because muscles use blood glucose at the rate of about 1–1.3 g/min late in exercise, sufficient carbohydrate should be ingested to provide an additional 45–60 g (45 min × 1 to 1.3 g/min) of carbohydrate. There is general agreement that this can be achieved when carbohydrates are taken in at the rate of about 30–60 g/hr during exercise (24). The 120–240 g of glucose consumed (4 hrs × 30 to 60 g/hr) provides for the 45–60 g needed at the end of exercise, but also supports the elevated carbohydrate metabolism throughout exercise. Glucose, sucrose, or **glucose polymer** solutions are all successful in maintaining the blood glucose concentration during exercise, but the palatability of the solution is improved if glucose polymer solutions are used for concentrations above 10%. There is evidence that carbohydrate ingestion during exercise also improves performance in shorter (45–60 min) and more intense (>75% $\dot{V}O_2$ max) endurance activities and during intermittent team sports (26). The 2016 ACSM position stand recommends the following for carbohydrate intake during performance (3):

- During endurance exercise of 1–2.5 hours, including "stop and start" sports like soccer, 30–60 g · hr⁻¹ should be consumed in either liquid, solid or gel forms, and the athlete should practice using these products during training sessions.

- During ultra-endurance exercise of 2.5–3 hours, up to 90 g · hr⁻¹ should be consumed, but products providing a mix of transportable carbohydrates (e.g., glucose:fructose mixture) are needed to meet this high rate of carbohydrate oxidation. The fructose is transported, independent of glucose, from the GI tract to the blood, allowing more carbohydrate to be transported compared to glucose alone.

Is there anything that can be added to these drinks to have a larger impact on performance? For an update on carbohydrate drinks and performance, see "Ask the Expert 23.1."

A new question regarding carbohydrate drinks has arisen: Does simply rinsing the mouth with the drink at regular intervals during the performance result in an improved performance? The answer appears to be yes when applied to time-trial performances in both cyclists (27) and runners (111). In one of the studies, brain centers (as observed using MRI) associated with reward were activated with the carbohydrate mouth rinse whether it was sweet (glucose) or not (maltodextrin) (27). In contrast, Beelen et al. (7) found no improvement in time-trial performance with this procedure when performed with well-fed subjects (versus those who fasted overnight). The 2016 ACSM position stand recommends the following for sustained high-intensity exercise lasting 45–75 minutes (3):

- Use small amounts of a range of drinks and sport products that contain easily digested carbohydrates. This can also be used as a mouth rinse to activate reward centers in the CNS and enhance perceptions of well-being and increase self-selected exercise intensity.

Carbohydrate Drinks and Performance:
Questions and Answers with Dr. Ronald J. Maughan

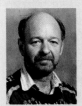

Courtesy of Ronald J. Maughan

Ron Maughan obtained his B.Sc. (Physiology) and Ph.D. from the University of Aberdeen, and held a lecturing position in Liverpool before returning to Aberdeen where he stayed for more than 20 years. He then moved to the School of Sport, Exercise and Health Sciences at Loughborough University, England. He now has a visiting post at St Andrews University, Scotland. He chairs the Nutrition Working Group of the International Olympic Committee. His research interests are in the physiology, biochemistry, and nutrition of exercise performance, with an interest in both the basic science of exercise and the applied aspects that relate to health and performance in sport.

QUESTION: Athletes use carbohydrate drinks to improve performance. What type of athlete would benefit most from this strategy?

ANSWER: All athletes will find these drinks useful in some training and competition situations. During exercise, they are especially important when the exercise time exceeds about 30–40 minutes, but some benefits may be apparent sooner than that. They provide carbohydrate as an energy source, and this is especially important if there has not been an opportunity for complete recovery of the body's carbohydrate stores since the last training session or competition. Carbohydrate is a more efficient fuel than fat–it requires less oxygen for a given energy demand–so ensuring an adequate supply is crucial to performance. These drinks also promote water absorption and supply some electrolytes, so they are particularly important when sweat losses are high. Athletes should get into the habit of using these drinks in training as well as in competition. Training sessions feel easier, the risk of heat illness

is greatly reduced, and the quality of training may be better maintained: this is important for those who take exercise for fun as well as for the elite athlete. The reduction in the perception of effort is especially important for those who exercise for health. If the exercise feels easier, they are more likely to stick to an exercise program, and these effects may be felt in exercise of less than 30 minutes duration. Strength and power athletes may train for long periods, but often do not have the awareness of the need for rehydration that exists in endurance sports. Of course, the calories in these drinks need to be taken into account, and those on an energy-restricted diet may limit their use of sport drinks for this reason.

QUESTION: Given the existing research support for this strategy, what are the most important questions remaining to be answered?

ANSWER: Many questions remain to be answered, but these relate mostly to the application of the basic science in practical situations. The main ingredients of carbohydrate-electrolyte sports drinks (water, sugar, and salt) have not changed substantially, but we need to have a better understanding of the optimum formulation for use in different situations. We now know that a mixture of different carbohydrates, including both glucose and fructose, can increase the availability and oxidation of ingested carbohydrates and can enhance performance compared to drinks that contain only glucose. There are situations in which a higher or a lower carbohydrate content would be better, and athletes have to recognize that different drinks may be better suited to different exercise and environmental conditions. They also need to recognize

how to assess their own individual fuel and hydration needs and how these change in different situations. There is some debate about the need for electrolyte replacement in different situations, and we need to learn how to identify those at risk of over- or underhydration. We also need to learn how to communicate current knowledge more effectively to athletes and coaches, and this is perhaps the biggest challenge we face at present.

QUESTION: Are there any differences between these traditional carbohydrate drinks and the new "energy drinks" being advertised to improve performance?

ANSWER: The new energy drinks are mostly very high in sugar, and thus, energy, and they also usually contain caffeine to give a feeling of more energy. These drinks can have disadvantages in some situations. Because of the high carbohydrate content, the osmolality of these drinks is very high, and the body actually secretes water into the small intestine after they have been ingested. Although this is a transient effect, it exacerbates any existing dehydration and can cause gastrointestinal discomfort. Some of the newer energy drinks do not contain energy at all: they contain only caffeine (plus a few flavorings, etc.) or other purported stimulants to give a feeling of more energy. Although moderate doses of caffeine can help performance, the very high doses in some of these products can increase the risk of dehydration due to increased urine loss and can lead to over-arousal that results in poorer performance in some skilled tasks. Some athletes also report that they find it difficult to sleep at night when they have used high doses of caffeine in competitions held in late afternoon or evening.

In summary, consuming carbohydrate during exercise helps maintain the necessary rate of carbohydrate oxidation associated with good performance:

- For performances less than 75 minutes, only small amounts of carbohydrate are needed, including its use as a mouth rinse.

- For performances of 1–2.5 hours, 30–60 g of carbohydrate should be consumed per hour.

- For performance of 2.5–3 hours, up to 90 g of carbohydrate should be consumed per hour.

Either a single (e.g., glucose) or a multiple transportable (e.g., glucose:fructose) form of carbohydrate can be used for the first two conditions, but only a multiple transportable mixture should be used for the last condition to achieve the needed high rate of delivery of carbohydrate (3, 79, 80). One final point: Even when the blood glucose concentration is maintained by either glucose infusion or ingestion during exercise, the subject will eventually stop; this indicates that fatigue is related to more than the delivery of fuel to muscles (31).

Carbohydrate Intake Post-Performance

The degree of muscle glycogen depletion varies with the duration and intensity of the exercise. The limiting factor in muscle glycogen synthesis is glucose transport across the cell membrane. Following a bout of heavy exercise, there is an increase in the muscle cell's permeability to glucose, an increase in glycogen synthase activity, and an increase in the muscle's sensitivity to insulin (77). To take advantage of these factors, carbohydrates (1.0–1.5 g $\cdot$ kg^{-1}) need to be consumed within 30 minutes after exercise and at 2-hour intervals for up to 6 hours if one wants to replace glycogen stores quickly. High glycemic foods are better in this regard. Further, the combined ingestion of a smaller amount of carbohydrate (0.8 g $\cdot$ kg^{-1} $\cdot$ hr^{-1}) with a small amount of protein (0.2 – 0.4 g $\cdot$ kg^{-1} $\cdot$ hr^{-1}) has been shown to be as effective as the ingestion of 1.2 g $\cdot$ kg^{-1} $\cdot$ hr^{-1} of carbohydrate (3, 8, 17). However, if time is not crucial, eating a balance of carbohydrates, fats, and protein will achieve both carbohydrate replacement and the promotion of an optimal rate of muscle protein synthesis needed for tissue repair and hypertrophy. Consistent with this, the 2016 ACSM position stand recommends the following (3):

- For speed refueling, when there is less than 8 hours between two carbohydrate-demanding exercise sessions, 1–1.2 g $\cdot$ kg^{-1} $\cdot$ h^{-1} of carbohydrate should be consumed for the first 4 hours.

IN SUMMARY

- From 1 to 4 g $\cdot$ kg^{-1} of carbohydrate should be consumed 1–4 hours before exercise, but, timing, amount, and type of carbohydrate should be chosen to suit the individual's needs and preferences.
- The ingestion of glucose solutions during exercise extends performance by providing carbohydrate to the muscle at a time when muscle glycogen is being depleted.
- Depending on the duration of the endurance performance, from 30 to 90 g $\cdot$ hr^{-1} of carbohydrate should be consumed during exercise to maintain the high rate of carbohydrate oxidation.
- To restore glycogen stores quickly after exercise, carbohydrates should be consumed at the rate of 1 to 1.2 g $\cdot$ kg^{-1} $\cdot$ h^{-1} for the first 4 hours.

PROTEIN

The adult RDA for protein is 0.8 gm $\cdot$ kg^{-1} $\cdot$ d^{-1} and is easily met by a diet having 12% of its energy (kcal) as protein. For example, if the daily energy requirement for an adult male weighing 72 kg is 2900 kcal/day, then about 348 kcal are taken in as protein (12% of 2900 kcal). At 4 kcal/g, this person would consume approximately 87 g protein per day, representing 1.2 g $\cdot$ kg^{-1} $\cdot$ d^{-1} (87 g/70 kg), or 50% more than the RDA standard. Does an athlete have to take in more protein than specified in the RDA, or is the normal diet adequate? Confusing as it may seem, the answer to both questions appears to be yes.

Protein Requirements and Exercise

Adequacy of protein intake has been based primarily on nitrogen (N)-balance studies. Protein is about 16% N by weight, and when N-intake (dietary protein) equals N-excretion, the person is in N-balance. Excretion of less N than one consumes is called positive N-balance, and the excretion of more N than one consumes is called negative N-balance. This latter condition, if maintained, is inconsistent with good health due to the potential loss of lean body mass. Based on these N-balance studies, it was generally believed that the 0.8 g $\cdot$ kg^{-1} $\cdot$ d^{-1} RDA standard was adequate for those engaged in prolonged exercise. In these studies, urinary N excretion was usually used as an index of N-excretion, because about 85% of N is excreted this way (89). However, some experiments suggest this method of measurement may underestimate amino acid utilization in exercise. Lemon and Mullin (90) found that although there was no difference in urinary N excretion compared to rest, the loss of N in sweat increased 60- to 150-fold during exercise, suggesting that as much as 10% of the energy requirement of the exercise was met by the oxidation of amino acids.

Other studies, using different techniques, supported these observations. Muscle has been shown to release the amino acid alanine in proportion to exercise intensity (52), and the alanine is used in gluconeogenesis in the liver to generate new plasma glucose. Several investigators have infused a stable isotope (^{13}C-label) of the amino acid leucine to study the rate at which amino acids are mobilized and oxidized during exercise. In general, the rate of oxidation (measured by the appearance of $^{13}CO_2$) is higher during exercise than at rest in rats and humans (41, 73, 127). Taken as a group, these studies suggest that amino acids are used as a fuel during exercise to a greater extent than previously believed. They also suggest that the protein requirement for those involved in prolonged exercise is higher than the RDA (89). However, there is more to the story.

Whole-Body Nitrogen Balance Studies   The ability to maintain N-balance during exercise appears to be dependent on the following (19, 21, 88–90):

- The training state of the subject
- The quality and quantity of protein consumed
- Total calories consumed
- The body's carbohydrate store
- The intensity, duration, and type (resistance versus endurance) of exercise

If measurements of protein utilization are made during the first few days of an exercise program, formerly sedentary subjects show a negative N-balance (Fig. 23.4). However, after about 12–14 days of training, this condition disappears and the person can maintain N-balance (61). So, depending on the point into the training program where the measurements are made, one could conclude either that more protein is needed during the adaptation to exercise or that protein needs can be met by the RDA after the adaptation is complete (21). Butterfield indicates that in N-balance studies, the length of time needed to achieve a new steady state depends on the magnitude of the change in the level of N-intake and the absolute amount of N consumed, and that the recommended minimum of a ten-day adaptation period may be inadequate when N-intake is very large (19).

Another factor influencing the conclusion one would reach about protein needs during exercise is whether the person is in caloric balance–that is, taking in enough kcal to cover the cost of the added exercise. For example, it has been shown that by increasing the energy intake 15% more than that needed to maintain weight, an increase in N-retention occurred during exercise when these subjects consumed only 0.57 g · kg^{-1} · d^{-1} of egg white protein (21). In a parallel study by the same group (120), a 15% deficit in energy intake was created while subjects consumed either 0.57 or 0.8 g · kg^{-1} · d^{-1} egg white protein. When taking in 15% fewer calories than needed, the 0.8 g · kg^{-1} · d^{-1} protein intake was associated with a negative N-balance of 1 g · d^{-1}. However, when the subjects did one or two hours of exercise, the negative N-balance improved to a loss of only 0.51, or 0.27 g · d^{-1}, respectively. During the treatment in which the subjects were in caloric balance, the RDA of 0.8 g · kg^{-1} · d^{-1} was sufficient to achieve a positive N-balance for both durations of exercise. It is clear, then, that to make proper judgments about the adequacy of the protein intake, the person must be in energy balance.

A final nutritional factor that can influence the rate of amino-acid metabolism during exercise is the availability of carbohydrate. Lemon and Mullin (91) showed that the quantity of urea found in sweat was cut in half when subjects were carbohydrate loaded as opposed to carbohydrate depleted (see Fig. 23.5). Further,

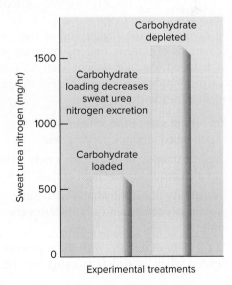

Figure 23.5   Effect of initial muscle glycogen levels on sweat urea nitrogen excretion during exercise. A high muscle glycogen level decreases the excretion of urea nitrogen in sweat during exercise.

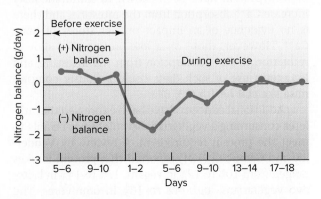

Figure 23.4   Effect of exercise on nitrogen balance.

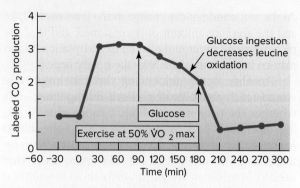

Figure 23.6 Effect of glucose ingestion on the rate of metabolism of the amino acid leucine. Glucose ingestion decreases the rate of amino acid oxidation.

as Fig. 23.6 shows, the ingestion of glucose during the latter half of a three hour exercise test at 50% $\dot{V}O_2$ max reduces the rate of oxidation of the amino acid leucine (41). So, not only is caloric balance important in protein metabolism, but the ability of the diet to provide adequate carbohydrate must also be considered.

Protein Requirements for Athletes

How much protein does an athlete need? To answer that question, one needs to consider the fact that the RDA for protein varies from country to country ($0.8\text{-}1.2\text{ g}\cdot\text{kg}^{-1}\cdot\text{d}^{-1}$), and that most of these standards do not consider vigorous exercise done by athletes. The Dutch did, and offered $1.5\text{ g}\cdot\text{kg}^{-1}\cdot\text{d}^{-1}$ as the standard for athletes (87). So, again, how much protein is needed? Previous guidelines recommended different protein intakes for elite endurance athletes (e.g., $1.2\text{-}1.4\text{ g}\cdot\text{kg}^{-1}\cdot\text{d}^{-1}$) and elite strength training athletes (e.g., $1.2\text{-}1.7\text{ g}\cdot\text{kg}^{-1}\cdot\text{d}^{-1}$). The 2016 ACSM position stand (3) recommends a single range of $1.2\text{-}2.0\text{ g}\cdot\text{kg}^{-1}\cdot\text{d}^{-1}$ with the caveat that the higher end of the range is for short periods of intense training or when energy intake is reduced (e.g., for weight loss). In fact, the position stand emphasizes the point that the protein requirement varies with:

- Training status of the athlete, with experienced athletes needing less.
- Current training regime, with a new training stimulus requiring the high end of the range.
- Availability of carbohydrate, with more protein needed when carbohydrates are limited.
- Availability of energy, with more protein needed when an athlete is losing weight.

Current questions revolve around the timing of protein intake for optimal gains in muscle mass, and whether some types of protein are better than others (see The Winning Edge 23.1).

Another way to approach this question is to consider the protein requirement of a human from childhood to adulthood. The RDA for protein is $1.5\text{ g}\cdot\text{kg}^{-1}\cdot\text{d}^{-1}$ during the second six months of life, decreasing to $0.95\text{ g}\cdot\text{kg}^{-1}\cdot\text{d}^{-1}$ by ages 4–8, and reaching the adult value of $0.8\text{ g}\cdot\text{kg}^{-1}\cdot\text{d}^{-1}$ by age 18. During this period, an individual may increase body weight by a factor of ten (15 lb to 150 lb). This is not unlike what was previously mentioned about the adaptation to exercise. During the initial days of an exercise training program when the muscles are adapting to the new exercise, the protein requirement might be higher than the RDA, and data of Gontzea (61, 62) support this proposition. However, after the person has adapted to the exercise, the requirement would revert to the RDA.

At the beginning of this section on the protein requirements for athletes, a question was raised: Does an athlete have to take in more protein than the RDA, or is the normal diet adequate? During intense endurance training or strength training, the requirement of protein may be higher than the RDA. So the answer is yes to that part of the question. It is also yes to the second part, in that the average person typically takes in 50% more than the RDA for protein. Brotherhood reports that an average athlete's diet is about 16% protein, exceeding $1.5\text{ g}\cdot\text{kg}^{-1}\cdot\text{d}^{-1}$ (88% more than RDA!). These values exceed the RDA of young children who are in a chronic state of positive nitrogen balance, and approach the upper limit of the recommendations (3, 19, 86, 87, 88). In support of dietary protein intake being sufficient, two studies found that protein supplements provided no advantage in terms of strength gains in a resistance training program in both young experienced trained athletes (72) and in older individuals experiencing sarcopenia (22).

Some concern has been raised about consuming too much dietary protein, especially with regard to amenorrheic athletes (20). High-protein diets lead to an increase in Ca^{++} excretion, and for many years, it was believed that the Ca^{++} was of bone origin and of real concern for the amenorrheic athlete (48, 68). Recent studies suggest otherwise. Short-term diets high in protein have been shown to simultaneously increase Ca^{++} absorption from the intestine, and there is no evidence of an impact on net stores of bone Ca^{++}. However, those on a low-protein diet show a reduction in Ca^{++} absorption from the intestine, and long-term use of such diets could seriously compromise skeletal health (83, 84).

Additional concerns have been expressed that athletes consuming a vegetarian diet might not be able to meet the protein requirement. A review by Venderley and Campbell (124) reported that protein intakes ranged from 10% to 12% in vegans, 12% to 14% in lacto-ovo vegetarians, and 14% to 18% in omnivores. The lacto-ovo vegetarians have easy access to high-quality

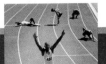
Timing of Protein Intake for Maximum Effect

There is no question that following a resistance training workout, muscle protein synthesis (MPS) is increased. But it is increased even more when amino acids are either ingested or infused, compared to a fasted state. For obvious practical reasons, the focus has been on ingestion rather than infusion, and the following observations have been made about how to obtain optimal results (71, 78, 106):

- MPS is activated most strongly when amino acids are available in the first hour following the workout.
  - This approach to timing of protein intake is even more important for older adults.
- Whey protein (20% of milk protein) is digested more rapidly than casein protein (80% of milk protein) or soy protein and yields a higher level of essential amino acids (EAA) in the blood, with the EAA being a driving force for MPS.
  - Casein protein provides a longer and more sustained EAA response, making milk a good post-exercise drink because it contains both proteins naturally.
- There is only limited information on the impact of these post-exercise protein feedings over the course of a full resistance-training program, but the available evidence supports the recommendation.
- The amount of high-quality protein needed post-exercise to optimally stimulate MPS is modest (~25 g), containing 8-10 g of EAA (3,106). Though others (78) recommend >35 g, this amount has not been shown to further enhance MPS (3).

A recent review raised some questions about this idea of a post-exercise "anabolic window" relative to protein synthesis. The authors note that many studies used both pre- and post-exercise protein supplementation, making it difficult to evaluate the timing issue. Further, the majority of studies failed to match total protein intake between conditions, and the supplement usually contained overly conservative amounts (10-20 g) of protein. Finally, since the studies used primarily untrained subjects, it was not clear how the results applied to trained subjects (4). Related to the issue of the amount of protein used, an analysis of studies in which a positive effect on muscle and strength was observed, protein supplements were about 60% greater than the habitual protein intake of the subjects (13). This is clearly an exciting area of research, and we are sure to see a more complete picture in the near future.

---

and easily accessed protein in eggs and milk products. On the other hand, athletes who are vegans do not, and they may benefit from careful dietary planning with a sports-related registered dietician to realize performance goals (3, 124). See Suggested Readings for a review by Fuhrman and Ferreri, and a position stand by Borrione, Grasso, Quaranta, and Parisi that address this issue.

> ### IN SUMMARY
>
> - The range of protein requirements for athletes is 1.2-2.0 g · kg^{-1} · d^{-1} with the top part of the range needed for those engaged in new training programs, or consuming inadequate amounts of calories or carbohydrates.

WATER AND ELECTROLYTES

Chapter 12 described in some detail the need to dissipate heat during exercise to minimize the increase in core temperature. The primary mechanism for heat loss at high work rates in a comfortable environment, and at all work rates in a hot environment, is the evaporation of sweat. Sweat rates increase linearly with exercise intensity, and in hot weather, sweat rates can reach 2.8 liters per hour (33). In spite of attempts to replace water during marathon races, some runners lose 8% of their body weight (33). Given that water losses in excess of 2% adversely affect endurance performance, especially in hot weather, there is a clear need to maintain water balance (2, 3). Of course, more than water is lost in sweat. An increased sweat rate means that a wide variety of electrolytes, such as Na^+, K^+, Cl^-, and Mg^{++}, are lost as well (33). These electrolytes are needed for normal functioning of excitable tissues, enzymes, and hormones. It should be no surprise then that investigators have been concerned about the optimal way to replace water and electrolytes to reduce the chance of health-related problems and increase the chance of optimal performance (93).

Fluid Replacement—Before Exercise

The goal of prehydrating is to be euhydrated (have a normal body water content) before the exercise or competition begins. In general, with sufficient time (8-24 hours) between the end of one exercise (competition) and the next, foods and beverages consumed at meals will be sufficient. If the time frame is too short, the following steps can be taken (2, 3):

- Slowly drink beverages (e.g., ~5-10 ml · kg^{-1}) 2-4 hours before exercise to achieve urine that is pale yellow in color, and to allow sufficient time for excess fluid to be voided.

- Using beverages with sodium in them or salted snacks would help retain the fluid.

Some investigators have used large volumes of water or have taken glycerol (94) to create a hyperhydrated state (body water content greater than normal) prior to exercise; in fact, some studies provide guidelines for an optimal dose of glycerol to accomplish this goal (63, 123). However, there is no clear evidence that better performances will result compared to euhydration (2), and the practice of using glycerol has been banned by the World Anti-Doping Agency (http://list.wada-ama.org/list/s5-diuretics-and-other-masking-agents/).

Fluid Replacement—During Exercise

The goal of drinking beverages during exercise is to reduce the chance of becoming excessively dehydrated (2% body weight loss from water deficit) (2). Fortunately, for some sports in which play is intermittent (football, tennis, golf), water replacement during the activity is possible, but some athletes may need reminders to drink fluids during breaks in the action (58). However, in athletic events such as marathon running, there are no formal breaks in the activity to allow for replacement. In these latter activities, in which a high rate of heat production is coupled with the potential problems of environmental heat and humidity, the athlete is at great risk. Studies confirm the need to replace fluids as they are lost during exercise in order to maintain moderate heart rate and body temperature responses (65, 107). Figure 23.7 shows changes in esophageal temperature, heart rate, and rating of perceived exertion during two hours of exercise at 62%-67% $\dot{V}O_2$ max under four conditions of fluid replacement: (a) no fluid, (b) small fluid (300 ml/hr), (c) moderate fluid (700 ml/hr), and (d) large fluid (1200 ml/hr). The fluid was a "sport drink" containing 6% carbohydrate and electrolytes (40). As you can see, there were marked differences in the responses over time. The lowest heart rate, body temperature, and rating of perceived exertion were associated with the highest rates of fluid replacement (37, 40). It must be added that although most of the attention on fluid replacement is directed at those who participate in prolonged endurance exercise, it is clear that the same message must reach those who participate in intermittent exercise (116). Given that fluid replacement during exercise is clearly beneficial, how much fluid should be taken at one time? Should it be warm or cold? Should it contain electrolytes and glucose?

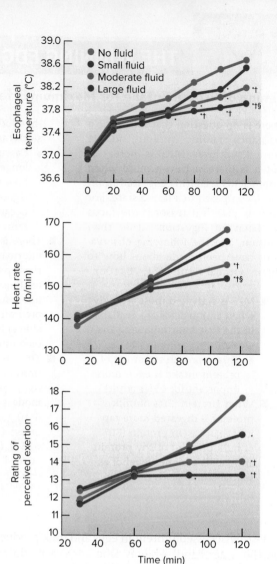

Figure 23.7 Core temperature (esophageal temperature), heart rate, and perceived exertion during 120 min of exercise when subjects ingested no fluid, or small (300 ml/hr), moderate (700 ml/hr), or large (1,200 ml/hr) volumes of fluid. A rating of 17 for perceived exertion corresponds to "Very Hard," 15 is "Hard," and 13 is "Somewhat Hard." Values are means ±SE.

°Significantly lower than no fluid, P < 0.05.
†Significantly lower than small fluid, P < 0.05.
§Significantly lower than moderate fluid, P < 0.05.

Costill and colleagues (35, 38) provided some of the original answers to these questions. One study examined the effects of fluid volume, temperature, glucose concentration, and the intensity of exercise on the rate at which fluid leaves the stomach to the small intestine. They determined this by giving the subject the fluid in question and then, 15 minutes later, aspirating the contents of the stomach. Figure 23.8 summarizes the results of that study. A glucose concentration above 139 mM (2.5%) slowed gastric emptying (i.e., increased residue; Fig. 23.8(a)). The optimal volume to ingest was 600 ml (Fig. 23.8(b)), and colder drinks appeared to be

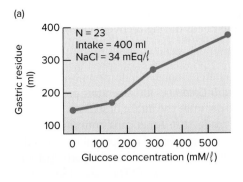

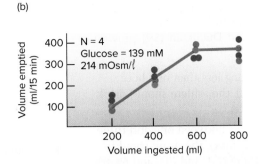

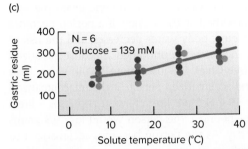

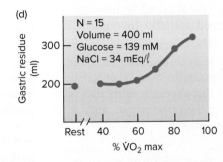

Figure 23.8 Effect of fluid volume, glucose concentration, solute temperature, and the intensity of exercise on the rate of fluid absorption from the gastrointestinal tract.

emptied faster (i.e., decreased residue; Fig. 23.8(c)). Finally, exercise had no effect on gastric emptying until the intensity exceeded 65%–70% $\dot{V}O_2$ max (Fig. 23.8(d)). Using the same technique, which has been shown to be valid (54), studies have confirmed that intensities below 75% $\dot{V}O_2$ max do not affect the rate of gastric emptying (95), and that there is no difference between running and cycling in the rate of gastric emptying for exercise intensities of 70% to 75% $\dot{V}O_2$ max (74, 99, 110). However, dehydration and/or high body temperature have been shown to delay gastric emptying (96, 109). While most of the later work supports the findings shown in Fig. 23.8, the one exception is with regard to the carbohydrate content of the drink.

In the original study (35), the effectiveness of a drink was evaluated 15 minutes after ingestion by aspirating the contents of the stomach. Davis and colleagues (44, 45) questioned the use of the aspiration technique, because it simply measures how much fluid leaves the stomach, not how much is actually absorbed into the blood from the small intestine. They used heavy water (D_2O) as a tracer of fluid absorption from the gastrointestinal tract to the blood and found that a 6% glucose-electrolyte solution was absorbed as fast as or faster than water at rest (45) or during exercise (44). Two additional studies that used the aspiration technique (92, 103) found that when either a 10% glucose solution or glucose polymer solutions containing 5%–10% carbohydrate were ingested at 15- to 20-minute intervals during prolonged exercise at 65%–70% $\dot{V}O_2$ max, there was no difference in the gastric emptying rate of either solution compared to water. The improved performance of the carbohydrate drinks in the most recent studies may be related to the experimental procedures, which included the

ingestion of small volumes (~200 ml) at regular intervals (15–20 minutes) during prolonged exercise, with the aspiration occurring at the end of the entire exercise session (not 15 minutes after ingestion). An additional benefit of these glucose solutions is that the extra carbohydrate helps to maintain the blood glucose during exercise (see earlier discussion). It must be added, however, that drinks containing more than 8% glucose remain in the stomach longer, with subjects complaining of gastrointestinal distress (2, 3). If fluid intake is most important and carbohydrate is secondary, a drink should be fashioned accordingly.

Because sweat rates vary so much among individuals, it is recommended that individuals estimate their sweat rates (measure weight pre- and post-exercise [competition], and account for the volume of fluid ingested) to determine how much to drink. Also, they should "practice" drinking the beverage in routine workouts to determine if it works for them. The following should be considered for a sport beverage (2):

- A temperature between 15 and 21°C has been a classic recommendation, however, new information suggests a temperature of 0.5°C (3) or making the solution in the form of an ice slurry (119) to help lower core temperature.
- ~20–30 mEq · L^{-1} sodium and 2–5 mEq · L^{-1} potassium
- 5%–10% carbohydrate

The greatest rates of carbohydrate delivery occur when a mixture of sugars is used (e.g., glucose and fructose) as described earlier (2, 3). Interestingly, and in contrast to popular beliefs, caffeine consumption does *not* create a water-electrolyte imbalance or hyperthermia, or reduce exercise-heat tolerance (3, 5).

A range of values are given for the electrolyte and carbohydrates to allow drinks to better meet expected demands. Gisolfi and Duchman (59) provide the following guidelines:

- During exercise lasting less than one hour (80%–130% $\dot{V}O_2$ max), the athlete should drink 500–1000 ml of water.

- For exercise durations between one and three hours (60%–90% $\dot{V}O_2$ max), the drink should contain 10–20 mEq of Na^+, and Cl^-, and 6%–8% carbohydrate, with 500–1000 ml/hr meeting the carbohydrate need, and 800–1600 ml/hr meeting the fluid need.

- For events of more than three hours' duration, the drink should contain 20–30 mEq of Na^+ and Cl^-, and 6%–8% carbohydrate, with 500–1000 ml/hr meeting the carbohydrate and fluid needs of most athletes.

Gisolfi, C. V., and Duchman, S. M., "Guidelines for Optimal Replacement Beverages for Different Athletic Events," *Medicine and Science in Sports and Exercise* 24: 679-687, 1992.

Allowances must be made for individual differences in the frequency and volume of ingestion (58). The addition of salt to the drink enhances its palatability, maintains plasma osmolality to stimulate thirst (118), promotes fluid and carbohydrate absorption, and replenishes some of the electrolytes lost during the activity. An additional reason sodium has been added to the drinks is related to concerns that have been raised about the potential for hyponatremia, a dangerously low Na^+ concentration that can occur when a person hydrates only with water or hypotonic drinks during extremely long (>4 hours), ultra-endurance athletic events (2, 3, 99, 125). (See The Winning Edge 23.2.)

Fluid Replacement—After Exercise

Gisolfi and Duchman (59) also provided a drink for recovery that is consistent with the need to replenish electrolytes and muscle glycogen: The drink should contain 30–40 mEq of Na^+ and Cl^- and deliver 50 g of carbohydrate per hour. If an individual has to rehydrate quickly, it is recommended that ~1.5 liters of fluid be ingested for every kilogram of weight lost to compensate for the increased urine output (2, 3). One can use a sport drink or other beverages to rehydrate following exercise, and cold (e.g., 10°C) drinks appear to be more effective (104). One study compared a carbohydrate-electrolyte (CE) drink to skim milk. The subjects consumed 150% of the body weight lost as a result of doing an exercise bout in the heat. Three hours after they ingested the beverages, the subjects achieved euhydration with the CE drink and were slightly hyperhydrated with the skim milk. The milk provided 113 gm of carbohydrate vs. 137 for the CE drink, but the milk also provided 75 gm of protein–allowing the milk to address multiple needs during recovery (126).

Salt (NaCl)

One of the *Dietary Guidelines for Americans* presented in Chap. 18 was to decrease the intake of sodium. Although the point was made that Americans consume two to three times the amount needed for optimal health, is the dietary intake sufficient for an athlete who participates in regular vigorous physical activity? The mass of sodium in the body determines the water content, given the way water is reabsorbed at the kidney. If a person becomes sodium depleted, body water decreases, and the risk of heat injury increases. An untrained and unacclimatized individual (see Chap. 24) loses more Na^+ in sweat than a trained and acclimatized person. If the unacclimatized person has 1.9 g Na^+ per liter of sweat and loses 5 liters of sweat (11 pounds), the person would lose 9.5 grams of Na^+ per day. As the person becomes acclimatized to heat, the sodium content in sweat decreases to about half that, and Na^+ loss is about 5 g/day. Given that Na^+ is 40% of NaCl by weight, a person would have to consume 12.5 g of salt per day to meet that demand. It is generally believed that an individual with a high Na^+ loss can stay in sodium/water balance by simply adding salt to food at mealtime, rather than by consuming salt tablets (129). The best single practical test of the success of salt/water replacement procedures is to obtain a nude body weight measure in the morning, after voiding. Additional information about adequate hydration can be obtained by measuring urine specific gravity of the morning urine (2). The general dietary routine followed by athletes must be successful, because early-morning body weight remains relatively constant despite large daily sweat losses. Given what has just been presented, you might think there is no disagreement about whether dehydration impairs exercise performance–but you would be wrong. See the "point-counterpoint" of Noakes and Sawka in Suggested Readings.

IN SUMMARY

- Fluid replacement during exercise reduces the heart rate, body temperature, and perceived exertion responses to exercise, and the greater the rate of fluid intake, the lower the responses.
- Cold drinks are absorbed faster than warm drinks, and when exercise intensity exceeds 65%–70% $\dot{V}O_2$ max, gastric emptying decreases.
- For exercise lasting less than one hour, the focus is on water replacement only. When exercise duration exceeds one hour, drinks should contain Na^+, Cl^-, and carbohydrate.
- Salt needs are easily met at mealtime, and salt tablets are not needed. In fact, most Americans take in more salt than is required (see Chap. 18).

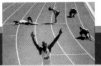
Hyponatremia

A primary driving force shaping fluid replacement recommendations over the past 60 years was the potential for dehydration during athletic events due to inadequate consumption of fluids. Over the past decade, a different problem, hyponatremia, has surfaced–that associated with drinking too much fluid during long-term athletic events and diluting the body's sodium level (3, 98, 99). The normal range of the serum sodium concentration is 135-145 mEq $\cdot$ L^{-1}. The risks associated with hyponatremia vary with the sodium concentration (112):

- *Mild* (Na$^+$ = 131-134 mEq $\cdot$ L^{-1})– generally causes no symptoms
- *Moderate* (Na$^+$ = 126-130 mEq $\cdot$ L^{-1})–can result in bloating, malaise, headache, nausea, vomiting, fatigue, confusion, and persistent and involuntary leg movements
- *Severe* (Na$^+$ <126 mEq $\cdot$ L^{-1})– can cause altered mental status, coma, seizures, and even death

The most recent consensus statement (70) classifies individuals into only two categories based on the following signs and symptoms, rather than serum Na$^+$ levels (which may not be readily available at a competition site):

- *Mild*–lightheadedness, dizziness, nausea, puffiness, and body weight gain.
- *Moderate*–vomiting, headache, phantom running, seizure, coma, signs of impending brain herniation, dyspnea, and frothy sputum.

The risk factors associated with hyponatremia include the following (23):

- Individual factors
  - Genetic predisposition for high sodium sweat rates (49)
  - Variation in symptoms at the same sodium concentration (112)

- Overdrinking–drinking too much relative to need
- Exercise duration >4 hr of continuous physical activity
- Low body weight <20 BMI
- Women–smaller stature; slower speeds
- Pre-exercise overhydration
- Insufficient sodium in foods consumed
- Weight gain–fluid retention during race

Given these risk factors, it is no surprise that in marathons, symptomatic hyponatremia is more likely to occur in smaller individuals who run slowly, sweat less, and drink relatively large volumes of water and other hypotonic fluids before, during, and after the race (2). In response to this problem, the ACSM released recommendations from their Roundtable Series on the topic: hydration and physical activity (25):

- Work to minimize risk of both hyponatremia and dehydration. Athletes are encouraged to neither underhydrate nor overhydrate, because each has significant consequences. Dehydration, especially during warm/hot weather conditions, occurs more frequently and is also life threatening. The message is to drink intelligently, not maximally.
- Athletes should determine their typical sweat rate during a practice run (e.g., 60 min).
  - Measure weight lost, e.g., 1.9 kg (1.9 L)
  - Add volume of fluid consumed, e.g., +0.5 L
  - Subtract volume of urine excreted, if any, e.g., 0.0 L
  - Sweat rate = 1.9 L + 0.5 L – 0.0 L = 2.4 L/60 min = 0.04 L/min or 40 ml/min
- Drink to match fluid loss and on a schedule. The fluid should

be consumed over a set period of time, rather than rapidly in a "catch-up" fashion. If athletes are not sweating much and are not thirsty, fluid replacement should be modest.
- Consume salty foods and beverages. Foods and beverages with sodium help promote fluid retention and stimulate thirst. Those performing long-duration exercise should consume snacks and fluids containing sodium to help prevent hyponatremia.

The consensus statement (70) recommends the following treatments, which vary with the severity of the hyponatremia. Remember, this is a life-threatening situation.

For mild hyponatremia:

- Observation (restrict hypotonic and isotonic fluids until urinating freely)
- Administration of intravenous hypertonic saline solution (HTS)
- Administration of oral HTS
  - Concentrated bouillon.
  - 3% NaCl (100 ml), preferably flavored.
  - Equivalent volumes of other high sodium drinks (e.g., 3%-9%).

For moderate hyponatremia:

- Administration of intravenous HTS:
  - 100 ml bolus of 3% NaCl, repeated twice if there is no clinical improvement.
  - Comparable amounts of more concentrated Na$^+$ containing solutions (e.g., 10 ml of 20% NaCl).
  - In some situations (e.g., more severe signs and symptoms), it may be appropriate to administer larger boluses initially, rather than waiting to assess improvement.

MINERALS

Iron

A vast majority of the body's iron is found in hemo-globin in the red blood cells (erythrocytes) that are involved in oxygen transport to tissues (see Chap. 10). Other iron-containing molecules include myoglobin and the cytochromes in the electron transport chains of mitochondria. The remainder of the body's iron is stored in various tissues, primarily tied to the protein ferritin, with the serum ferritin (SF) levels being a good index of the body's iron store (128).

As mentioned in Chap. 18, iron deficiency is the most common nutritional deficiency. The groups of athletes with the highest risk of iron depletion and deficiency include female athletes, distance runners, and vegetarians (and those who eat little red meat) (46). Iron depletion may be as high as 20%–35% in women runners, in contrast to 3.5%–8% in male runners; however, because some use different cut-off values for SF, it is difficult to make comparisons across studies. Anemia is much less common, being about 5%–7% in female athletes (66). As iron stores are depleted, the iron containing compounds ferritin, hemoglobin, transferrin, myoglobin, and cytochromes become depleted. Given that hemoglobin is a necessary part of the oxygen-transport process, it is not surprising that in individuals with iron-deficiency anemia, endurance and work performance are decreased (57, 60, 66). Interestingly, when the low-hemoglobin condition is corrected in iron-deficient animals by transfusion, $\dot{V}O_2$ max is brought back to normal, but not endurance time. This suggests that while hemoglobin levels may be high enough to achieve a normal $\dot{V}O_2$ max, iron deficiency affects the iron-containing cytochromes (electron transport chain) that are involved in oxidative phosphorylation, and endurance performance is adversely affected (42). In a similar study (43), iron supplementation brought the $\dot{V}O_2$ max back to normal values faster than that of mito-chondrial activity (measured by pyruvate oxidase activity) and endurance performance (see Fig. 23.9).

What causes iron deficiency in athletes? A com-bination of factors are linked to iron deficiency in athletes (46, 66):

- High iron requirement due to
  - Blood loss in GI tract
  - Greater red blood cell damage due to simple "pounding" on hard surfaces
  - Hemoglobin loss in urine and sweat
  - Variable blood loss in menses
- Low iron intake linked to
  - Low energy intake, including dieting for weight loss
  - Vegetarian diets
  - Diets low in red meat

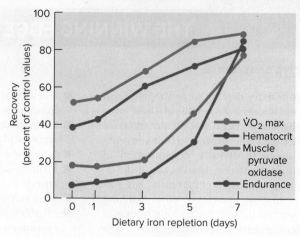

Figure 23.9 Recovery of various physiological capacities with iron repletion. Note that recovery of endurance lagged behind $\dot{V}O_2$ max.

Consistent with this, Diehl et al. (47) have shown decreases in serum ferritin over the course of a field hockey season and from one hockey season to the next in female athletes. The average value at the end of the season in third-year players was $10.5\ \mu g \cdot L^{-1}$ (below the $12\ \mu g \cdot L^{-1}$ standard), indicating iron deple-tion (67). A recent study indicated that even though female athletes may have some iron-status variables in the normal range, they may still be in a state of non-anemic iron depletion. This argues for better tracking of female athletes over their careers (64). Iron defi-ciency and anemia are also concerns for the military. Two studies from Israel indicate that 24% of female recruits were anemic (32), and 4.5% of males had he-moglobin levels below $12\ g \cdot dl^{-1}$ (100).

Generally, when a person has a deficiency in iron stores, there is an increased uptake of dietary iron. Unfortunately, athletes do not appear to follow that pattern. Factors that can affect the absorption of iron include (46):

- Facilitators
  - Amount of heme iron in food. Heme iron (found in meat) is more readily absorbed than non-heme iron (found in vegetables), but less than 15% of dietary iron is heme iron
  - Vitamins A and C
  - Peptides from partial digestion of meat protein
- Inhibitors
  - Cereal grains, legumes, nuts, peanut butter, bran, soy products
  - Tea, coffee, red wine, some spices
  - Peptides from partial digestion of plant proteins

Given the impact of so many variables on iron sta-tus, especially in women, it should be no surprise that supplementation may be needed (46, 66). This is especially the case for those on vegetarian diets (3, 12, 56). Some may choose to take an iron supplement each day as an ounce of prevention, but such a practice is not without problems (e.g., intolerance, overdose, drug interactions) and should not be done indiscriminately (3, 46, 66, 129). Consistent with that, 15% of male recreational marathon runners showed signs of iron overload due to iron supplementation (91).

VITAMINS

Chapter 18 provided the details about the RDA for each vitamin. Many of these vitamins are directly involved in energy production, acting as coenzymes in mitochondrial reactions associated with aerobic metabolism. Unfortunately, the old adage that "if a little is good, more will be better" has been applied to the question of whether the RDA for athletes is higher than that for sedentary people, rather than a factual research base. The major reviews of this issue over the past 30 years have systematically concluded that, in general:

- Vitamin supplementation is unnecessary for the athlete on a well-balanced diet.

- People who are *clearly deficient* in certain vitamins have improved performance when values return to normal.

- Individuals taking large doses of fat-soluble vitamins or vitamin C should be concerned about toxicity (9, 29, 122, 129).

The central concern raised by these reviewers is for the small athlete on a low-energy diet who may not make wise food selections, a point reinforced in a recent set of recommendations. In these situations, a single RDA multivitamin/mineral pill might be appropriate (3). The existence of a vitamin D deficiency in the general population and vitamin D's role in muscle function has generated renewed interest in vitamin D supplementation; however, the research is controversial about its ability to enhance performance (102, 108). That said, it is recommended that those athletes at a high risk of vitamin D deficiency (indoor athletes and those living in northerly latitudes) should have vitamin D levels checked annually (3, 30, 85, 102). Finally, some vitamins (e.g., C and E) aimed at countering the reactive oxygen species (free radicals) generated by exercise may actually interfere with the muscle's adaptation to training (14, 97, 105). See A Closer Look 19.1 for more on this. Additional information on the use of nutritional supplements to improve athletic performance is presented in Chap. 25, where ergogenic aids are discussed.

IN SUMMARY

- Iron deficiency in athletes may be related to an inadequate intake of dietary iron as well as a potentially greater loss in sweat and feces. In spite of this deficiency, athletes may absorb less than what a sedentary group of anemic individuals absorbs. Iron supplementation may be recommended for female athletes as a result of an annual clinical assessment of iron status.

- Vitamin supplementation is unnecessary for an athlete on a well-balanced diet. However, for those with a clear deficiency, supplementation is warranted.

PRECOMPETITION MEAL

The two most important nutritional practices associated with optimal performance in endurance exercise are (a) to eat a high-carbohydrate diet in the days preceding competition when the intensity and duration of workouts are reduced, and (b) to drink liquids at regular intervals during the competition. Consistent with our previous discussion, the purposes of the precompetition meal are the following (3, 130):

- To provide adequate hydration

- To provide carbohydrate to "top off" already high carbohydrate stores in the liver

- To avoid the sensation of hunger on a relatively empty stomach

- To minimize GI tract problems (gas, diarrhea)

- To allow the stomach to be relatively empty at the start of competition

Unfortunately, the type of precompetition meal served at various universities throughout this country may rely more on tradition than nutrition. The standard rare steak before a boxing match or football game to bring out the animal instinct, or careful planning to make sure that the color of the Jell-O° is the same as it was when the team won last year's championship, are less than rational, but may be useful in pulling the team together to get ready for competition. Problems arise when the precompetition meal is responsible for poor performance because of its own characteristics (high fat and protein) or the inability of the athlete to tolerate the meal without vomiting or experiencing diarrhea due to the emotion associated with competition. These latter events would cause dehydration, a condition inconsistent with optimal performance. It is clear that beyond what is recommended in the nutrient makeup of a precompetition meal, the ability of the athlete to tolerate it must be considered (3, 129).

°Jell-O is a registered trademark of General Foods, Inc.

Nutrients in Precompetition Meal

To achieve the purposes of the precompetition meal, the following general guidelines are provided (3):

- Sufficient fluid should be consumed to maintain hydration.
- Carbohydrates should make up the majority of the meal, but large amounts of simple sugars, especially fructose, should be avoided because of the potential for gastrointestinal problems such as diarrhea.
- The meal should be low in fats and fiber to facilitate gastric emptying.
- Protein should make up a small part of the meal because the metabolism of protein increases the acid load that must be buffered and finally excreted by the kidneys.
- The foods should be familiar to and well liked by the athlete.

Table 23.1 presents two precompetition meals that meet these considerations. These meals should be eaten about three hours prior to competition (129). Some coaches and athletes prefer one of the commercially available liquid meals as the precompetition meal because of convenience. These liquid meals can also be consumed throughout the day (along with additional water) when events or games are scheduled over long periods. Given that some people may not react favorably to any new "food," these liquid meals should be tried on practice days rather than on game day to make sure they are suitable.

IN SUMMARY

- The precompetition meal should provide for hydration and adequate carbohydrate to "top off" stores while minimizing hunger symptoms, gas, and diarrhea.
- Varieties of commercially available liquid meals are consistent with these goals.

TABLE 23.1 Two Examples of Precompetition Meals Containing 500–600 Kilocalories

Meal A	Meal B
Glass of orange juice	One cup low-fat yogurt
One bowl of oatmeal	One banana
Two pieces of toast with jelly	One toasted bagel
Sliced peaches with skim milk	One ounce of turkey breast
	One-half cup raisins

Williams MH, Anderson DE, and Rawson ES. *Nutrition for Health, Fitness and Sport.* New York, NY: McGraw-Hill, 2013.

BODY COMPOSITION AND PERFORMANCE

In Chap. 18, we discussed body composition from a health perspective, with the range of body fatness values, using the two-component system, associated with health and fitness being:

Health	Fitness
Males: 8%–22% fat	5%–15% fat
Females: 20%–35% fat	16%–28% fat

The question is, are these values optimal for athletic performance?

Table 23.2 lists a summary of body fatness values by sport (131). Many are average values and do not represent the range that might be observed in a study. For example, a study might find an average value of 12% body fat for a group of football players, but the range might be 5%–19%. In a sport or activity in which body weight must be carried along (e.g., running or jumping), there is a negative correlation between body fatness and performance (130, 131).

There is little question that regular measurements of body composition are useful for athletes to monitor changes during the season as well as over the off-season. In this way, the athlete will know whether changes in body weight represent gains or losses of body fatness. What is more difficult is providing a fixed absolute recommendation about what body fatness should be for optimal performance for each individual.

One of the main reasons one must be careful in making absolute recommendations, such as "This athlete should reduce her percent body fat from 15.6% to 14.0%," is that the athlete may already be 14% body fat. Each *individual estimate* of body fatness, even done by the most accurate technique, has an error in measurement that cannot be ignored. With some methods such as underwater weighing and with careful measurement, percent fat can be estimated with an error of about 2.5% fat. So when an athlete is measured as being 15.0% body fat, the true value may be as high as 17.5% and as low as 12.5% (75). Other techniques have larger errors, which would only complicate one's ability to make a specific absolute body fatness recommendation to an athlete (see discussion in Chap. 18).

Another reason caution must be used in making an absolute recommendation for each athlete is that it ignores the normal variation in body fatness found in elite athletes in any particular sport. An elite group of volleyball players may have an average value of 12%, but the range among the team members might be 6%–16%. No one would think of telling the athlete with

TABLE 23.2 Percent Body Fat Values for Male and Female Athletes

Athletic Group or Sport	Male	Female
Baseball	11.8–14.2	—
Basketball	7.1–10.6	20.8–26.9
Canoeing	12.4	—
Football		
Backs	9.4–12.4	—
Linebackers	13.7	—
Linemen	15.5–19.1	—
Quarterbacks, kickers	14.1	—
Gymnastics	4.6	9.6–23.8
Ice hockey	13–15.1	—
Jockeys	14.1	—
Orienteering	16.3	18.7
Pentathlon	—	11.0
Racquetball	8.3	14.0
Skiing		
Alpine	7.4–14.1	20.6
Cross-country	7.9–12.5	15.7–21.8
Nordic combined	8.9–11.2	—
Ski jumping	14.3	—
Soccer	9.6	—
Speed skating	11.4	—
Swimming	5.0–8.5	20.3
Tennis	15.2–16.3	20.3
Track and field		
Distance runners	3.7–18.0	15.2–19.2
Middle distance runners	12.4	—
Sprinters	16.5	19.3
Discus	16.3	25.0
Jumpers/hurdlers	—	20.7
Shot put	16.5–19.6	28.0
Volleyball	—	21.3–25.3
Wrestling	4.0–14.4	

Wilmore, J. H., "Body Composition in Sport and Exercise: Directions for Future Research," *Medicine and Science in Sports and Exercise* 15: 21–31, 1983.

6% body fat to increase body fatness to reach the team average, and the same advice holds true for the one at 16% body fatness who is playing with world-class skill. A recommendation to alter body composition to achieve better performance must be made against the background of present performance and general health status as seen in sleeping patterns, adequate diet, mental outlook, and so on. The implementation of longer workouts or a reduction in caloric intake might change the percent body fat in the appropriate direction, but either one could adversely affect the athlete's ability to tolerate a workout or to study for exams. Wilmore's (130) observation of one of the best female distance runners who held most of the American middle distance records should be remembered when making such recommendations: The champion was 17% body fat when most of the elite female runners were <12%.

Monitoring body fatness in athletes by one of the body composition techniques described in Chap. 18 is a reasonable procedure to follow because it allows a coach or trainer to observe *changes* in body fatness over the course of a season and from one year to the next. The information is also useful to the athletes who, when they finish their competitive careers, must attend to what is a reasonable body weight in order to be within the optimal body fatness range for health and fitness.

IN SUMMARY

- The body fat percentage consistent with excellence in performance is different for men and women and varies within gender from sport to sport. Average values for a team should not be applied to any single individual without regard to overall health status as seen in diet, sleep, and mental outlook. Further, it is "natural" for some athletes to have a higher body fatness than others in order to perform optimally.

STUDY ACTIVITIES

1. What procedures would you follow to cause a supercompensation of muscle glycogen?
2. How could glucose ingestion prior to exercise actually increase the rate of glycogen depletion? What could be done to minimize this effect?
3. Does carbohydrate ingestion during exercise slow down muscle glycogen depletion? Does it improve performance?
4. As the need for carbohydrate increases during prolonged exercise, explain why multiple forms of carbohydrate have to be consumed, and not just glucose.
5. What is the recommended range of protein intake for athletes, and what dietary factors supports use of the high end of the range?
6. What would you recommend to an athlete to reduce the chance of dehydration during exercise?
7. What causes hyponatremia, and who is most susceptible?
8. What factors contribute to iron deficiency in female athletes? What can be done to address these factors?
9. Does an athlete need additional vitamins for optimal performance? Explain.
10. What are the primary considerations for a precompetition meal?
11. Given a champion female distance runner with 17% body fat, what should you consider before recommending that she decrease her percent fat to 15%?

SUGGESTED READINGS

American College of Sports Medicine. 2016. Nutrition and athletic performance. *Medicine and Science in Sports and Exercise* 48:543-568.

Borrione, P., L. Grasso, F. Quaranta, and A. Parisi. 2009. FIMS position statement 2009: vegetarian diet and athletes. *International SportMed Journal* 10: 53-60.

Burke, L. M., and V. Deakin. 2015. *Clinical Sports Nutrition.* New York, NY: McGraw-Hill.

Fuhrman, J., and D. M. Ferreri. 2010. Fueling the vegetarian (vegan) athlete. *Current Sports Medicine Reports* 9: 233-41.

Noakes, T. D., and M. N. Sawka. 2007. Point-counterpoint: does dehydration impair exercise performance? *Medicine and Science in Sports and Exercise* 39: 1209-17.

Williams, M. H., D. E. Anderson, and E. S. Rawson. 2017. *Nutrition for Health, Fitness and Sport.* New York, NY: McGraw-Hill.

REFERENCES

1. **Ahlborg B.** Muscle glycogen and muscle electrolytes during prolonged physical exercise. *Acta Physiologica Scandinavica* 70: 129-142, 1967.

2. **American College of Sports Medicine.** Exercise and fluid replacement. *Medicine and Science in Sports and Exercise* 39: 2007.

3. **American College of Sports Medicine.** Nutrition and athletic performance. *Medicine and Science in Sports and Exercise* 48: 543-568, 2016.

4. **Aragon AA and Schoenfeld BJ.** Nutrient timing revisited: is there a post-exercise anabolic window. *Journal of the International Society of Sports Nutrition.* 10: 5-16, 2013.

5. **Armstrong LE, Casa DJ, Maresh CM, and Ganio MS.** Caffeine, fluid-electrolyte balance, temperature regulation, and exercise-heat tolerance. *Exercise and Sport Sciences Reviews* 35: 135-140, 2007.

6. **Arnall DA, Nelson AG, Quigley J, Lex S, Dehart T, and Fortune P.** Supercompensated glycogen loads persist 5 days in resting trained cyclists. *European Journal of Applied Physiology* 99: 251-256, 2007.

7. **Beelen M, Berghuis J, Bonoparte B, Ballak SB, Jeukendrup AE, and van Loon LJC.** Carbohydrate mouth rinsing in the fed state: lack of enhancement of time-trial performance. *International Journal of Sport Nutrition and Exercise Metabolism* 19: 2009.

8. **Beelen M, Burke LM, Gibala MJ, and van Loon, LJC.** Nutritional strategies to promote post-exercise recovery. *International Journal of Sports Nutrition and Exercise Metabolism.* 20: 515-532, 2010.

9. **Belko AZ.** Vitamins and exercise: an update. *Medicine and Science in Sports and Exercise* 19: S191-196, 1987.

10. **Bergström J, Hermansen L, Hultman E, and Saltin B.** Diet, muscle glycogen and physical performance. *Acta Physiol Scand* 71: 140-150, 1967.

11. **Bergström J and Hultman E.** Muscle glycogen synthesis after exercise: an enhancing factor localized to the muscle cells in man. *Nature* 210: 309-310, 1966.

12. **Borrione P, Grasso L, Quaranta F, and Parisi A.** FIMS position statement 2009: vegetarian diet and athletes. *International SportMed Journal* 10: 53-60, 2009.

13. **Bosse JD and Dixon BM.** Dietary protein to maximize resistance training: a review and examination of protein spread and change theories. *Journal of the International Society of Sports Nutrition* 9: 42-53, 2012.

14. **Braakhuis AJ.** Effect of vitamin C on physical performance. *Current Sports Medicine Reports* 11: 180-184, 2012.

15. **Brotherhood JR.** Nutrition and Sports Performance. *Sports Medicine.* 1: 350-389, 1984.

16. **Burke LM.** Fueling strategies to optimize performance: training high or training low? *Scandinavian Journal of Medicine and Science in Sports.* 20(Suppl 2): 48-58, 2010.

17. **Burke LM, Hawley JA, Wong SHS, and Jeukendrup AE.** Carbohydrates for training and competition. *Journal of Sports Sciences.* 29(S1): S17-S27, 2011.

18. **Bussau VA, Fairchild TJ, Rao A, Steele P, and Fournier PA.** Carbohydrate loading in human muscle: an improved 1 day protocol. *European Journal of Applied Physiology* 87: 290-295, 2002.

19. **Butterfield G.** Amino acids and high protein diets. In *Ergogenics: Enhancement of Performance in Exercise and Sport,* edited by Lamb D, and Williams M. Carmel, CA: Brown & Benchmark, 1991, pp. 87-117.

20. **Butterfield GE.** Whole-body protein utilization in humans. *Medicine and Science in Sports and Exercise* 19: S157-165, 1987.

21. **Butterfield GE and Calloway DH.** Physical activity improves protein utilization in young men. *British Journal of Nutrition* 51: 171-184, 1984.

22. **Campbell WW.** Synergistic use of higher-protein diets or nutritional supplements with resistance training to counter sarcopenia. *Nutrition Reviews* 65: 416-422, 2007.

23. **Carter III R.** Exertional heat illness and hyponatremia: an epidemiological prospective. *Current Sports Medicine Reports* 7: S20-S27, 2008.

24. **Carter J, Jeukendrup AE, Mundel T, and Jones DA.** Carbohydrate supplementation improves moderate and high-intensity exercise in the heat. *Pflugers Arch* 446: 211-219, 2003.

25. **Casa DJ, Clarkson PM, and Roberts WO.** American College of Sports Medicine roundtable on hydration and physical activity: consensus statements. *Current Sports Medicine Reports* 4: 115-127, 2005.

26. **Cermak NM and van Loon L.** The use of carbohydrate during exercise as an ergogenic aid. *Sports Medicine* 43: 1139-1155, 2013.

27. **Chambers ES, Bridge MW, and Jones DA.** Carbohydrate sensing in the human mouth: effects on exercise performance and brain activity. *Journal of Applied Physiology-London* 587: 1779-1794, 2009.

28. **Chryssanthopoulos C, Williams C, and Nowitz A.** Influence of a carbohydrate-electrolyte solution ingested during running on muscle glycogen utilisation in fed humans. *International Journal of Sports Medicine* 23: 279-284, 2002.

29. **Clarkson P.** Vitamins and trace minerals. In *Ergogenics: Enhancement of Performance in Exercise and Sport,* edited by Lamb D, and Williams M. Carmel, CA: Brown & Benchmark, 1991, pp. 123-182.

30. **Close GL, Russell J, Cobley JN, Owens DJ, Wilson G, Gregson W, et al.** Assessment of vitamin D concentration in non-supplemented professional athletes and health adults during the winter months in the UK: implications for skeletal muscle function. *Journal of Sport Sciences* 31: 344-353, 2013.

31. **Coggan AR, and Coyle EF.** Carbohydrate ingestion during prolonged exercise: effects on metabolism and performance. *Exercise and Sport Sciences Reviews* 19: 1-40, 1991.

32. **Constantini N, Dubnov G, Foldes AJ, Mann G, Magazanik A, and Siderer M.** High prevalence of iron deficiency and anemia in female military recruits. *Military Medicine* 171: 866-869, 2006.

33. **Costill DL.** Sweating: its composition and effects on body fluids. *Annals of the New York Academy of Sciences* 301: 160-174, 1977.

34. **Costill DL, Coyle E, Dalsky G, Evans W, Fink W, and Hoopes D.** Effects of elevated plasma FFA and insulin on muscle glycogen usage during exercise. *Journal of Applied Physiology* 43: 695-699, 1977.

35. **Costill DL and Saltin B.** Factors limiting gastric emptying during rest and exercise. *Journal of Applied Physiology* 37: 679-683, 1974.

36. **Costill DL, Sherman WM, Fink WJ, Maresh C, Witten M, and Miller JM.** The role of dietary carbohydrates in muscle glycogen resynthesis after strenuous running. *American Journal of Clinical Nutrition* 34: 1831-1836, 1981.

37. **Coyle E.** Fluid and carbohydrate replacement during exercise: how much and why? Barrington, IL: Gatorade Sports Science Institute, 1994.

38. **Coyle EF, Costill DL, Fink WJ, and Hoopes DG.** Gastric emptying rates for selected athletic drinks. *Research Quarterly* 49: 119-124, 1978.

39. **Coyle EF, Hagberg JM, Hurley BF, Martin WH, Ehsani AA, and Holloszy JO.** Carbohydrate feeding during prolonged strenuous exercise can delay fatigue. *Journal of Applied Physiology* 55: 230-235, 1983.

40. **Coyle EF and Montain SJ.** Benefits of fluid replacement with carbohydrate during exercise. *Medicine and Science in Sports and Exercise* 24: S324-330, 1992.

41. **Davies C.** Glucose inhibits CO_2 production from leucine during whole body exercise in man. *Journal of Physiology* 332: 40-41, 1982.

42. **Davies KJ, Donovan CM, Refino CJ, Brooks GA, Packer L, and Dallman PR.** Distinguishing effects of anemia and muscle iron deficiency on exercise bioenergetics in the rat. *American Journal of Physiology* 246: E535-543, 1984.

43. **Davies KJ, Maguire JJ, Brooks GA, Dallman PR, and Packer L.** Muscle mitochondrial bioenergetics, oxygen supply, and work capacity during dietary iron deficiency and repletion. *American Journal of Physiology* 242: E418-427, 1982.

44. **Davis JM, Burgess WA, Slentz CA, Bartoli WP, and Pate RR.** Effects of ingesting 6% and 12% glucose/electrolyte beverages during prolonged intermittent cycling in the heat. *European Journal of Applied Physiology and Occupational Physiology* 57: 563-569, 1988.

45. **Davis JM, Lamb DR, Burgess WA, and Bartoli WP.** Accumulation of deuterium oxide in body fluids after ingestion of D2O-labeled beverages. *Journal of Applied Physiology* 63: 2060-2066, 1987.

46. **Deakin V.** Prevention, detection and treatment of iron depletion and deficiency in athletes. In *Clinical Sports Nutrition*, edited by Burke LM, and Deakin V. New York, NY: McGraw-Hill, 2010, pp. 222-267.

47. **Diehl DM, Lohman TG, Smith SC, and Kertzer R.** Effects of physical training and competition on the iron status of female field hockey players. *International Journal of Sports Medicine* 7: 264-270, 1986.

48. **Drinkwater BL, Nilson K, Chesnut CH, III, Bremner WJ, Shainholtz S, and Southworth MB.** Bone mineral content of amenorrheic and eumenorrheic athletes. *New England Journal of Medicine* 311: 277-281, 1984.

49. **Eichner ER.** Genetic and other determinants of sweat rate. *Current Sports Medicine Reports* 7: S36-S40, 2008.

50. **Fairchild TJ, Fletcher S, Steele P, Goodman C, Dawson B, and Fournier PA.** Rapid carbohydrate loading after a short bout of near maximal-intensity exercise. *Medicine and Science in Sports and Exercise* 34: 980-986, 2002.

51. **Felig P, Cherif A, Minagawa A, and Wahren J.** Hypoglycemia during prolonged exercise in normal men. *New England Journal of Medicine* 306: 895-900, 1982.

52. **Felig P and Wahren J.** Amino acid metabolism in exercising man. *Journal of Clinical Investigation* 50: 2703-2714, 1971.

53. **Foster C, Costill DL, and Fink WJ.** Effects of pre-exercise feedings on endurance performance. *Medicine and Science in Sports* 11: 1-5, 1979.

54. **Foster C and Thompson NN.** Serial gastric emptying studies: effect of preceding drinks. *Medicine and Science in Sports and Exercise* 22: 484-487, 1990.

55. **Friedman JE, Neufer PD, and Dohm GL.** Regulation of glycogen resynthesis following exercise. Dietary considerations. *Sports Medicine* 11: 232-243, 1991.

56. **Fuhrman J and Ferreri DM.** Fueling the vegetarian (vegan) athlete. *Current Sports Medicine Reports* 9: 233-241, 2010.

57. **Gardner GW, Edgerton VR, Senewiratne B, Barnard RJ, and Ohira Y.** Physical work capacity and metabolic stress in subjects with iron deficiency anemia. *American Journal of Clinical Nutrition* 30: 910-917, 1977.

58. **Garth AK and Burke LM.** What do athletes drink during competitive sporting activities? *Sports Medicine.* 43: 539-564, 2013.

59. **Gisolfi CV and Duchman SM.** Guidelines for optimal replacement beverages for different athletic events. *Medicine and Science in Sports and Exercise* 24: 679-687, 1992.

60. **Gledhill N.** The influence of altered blood volume and oxygen transport capacity on aerobic performance. *Exercise and Sport Sciences Reviews* 13: 75-93, 1985.

61. **Gontzea I, Sutzescu P, and Dumitrache S.** The influence of adaptation of physical effort on nitrogen balance in man. *Nutrition Reports International* 11: 231-236, 1975.

62. **Gontzea I, Sutzescu P, and Dumitrache S.** The influence of muscular activity on nitrogen balance, and on the need of man for protein. *Nutrition Reports International* 10: 35-43, 1974.

63. **Goulet EDB.** Glycerol-induced hyperhydration: a method for estimating the optimal load of fluid to be ingested before exercise to maximize endurance performance. *Journal of Strength and Conditioning Research* 24: 74-78, 2010.

64. **Gropper SS, Blessing D, Dunham K, and Barksdale JM.** Iron status of female collegiate athletes involved in different sports. *Biological Trace Element Research* 109: 1-14, 2006.

65. **Hamilton MT, Gonzalez-Alonso J, Montain SJ, and Coyle EF.** Fluid replacement and glucose infusion during exercise prevent cardiovascular drift. *Journal of Applied Physiology* 71: 871-877, 1991.

66. **Haymes EM.** Iron. In *Sports Nutrition,* edited by Driskell JA, and Wolinsky I. Boca Raton, FL: CRC Taylor & Francis, 2006, pp. 203–216.

67. **Haymes EM.** Nutritional concerns: need for iron. *Medicine and Science in Sports and Exercise* 19: S197–200, 1987.

68. **Hegsted M, Schuette SA, Zemel MB, and Linkswiler HM.** Urinary calcium and calcium balance in young men as affected by level of protein and phosphorus intake. *Journal of Nutrition* 111: 553–562, 1981.

69. **Hermansen L, Hultman E, and Saltin B.** Muscle glycogen during prolonged severe exercise. *Acta Physiol Scand* 71: 129–139, 1967.

70. **Hew-Butler T, Rosner MH, Fowkes-Godek S, Dugas JP, Hoffman MD, Lewis DP, Maughan RJ, Miller KC, Montain SJ, Rehrer NJ, Roberts WO, Rogers IR, Siegel AJ, Stuempfle KJ, Winger JM, and Vernalis JG.** Statement of the Third International Exercise-Associated Hyponatremia Consensus Development Conference, Carlsbad, California 2015. *Clinical Journal of Sports Medicine.* 25: 303–320, 2015.

71. **Hoffman J.** Protein intake: effect of timing. *Strength and Conditioning Journal* 29: 26–34, 2007.

72. **Hoffman J, Ratamess N, and Kang J.** Effects of protein supplementation on muscular performance and resting hormonal changes in college football players. *Journal of Sports Science and Medicine* 6: pp. 85–92 2007.

73. **Hood DA and Terjung RL.** Amino acid metabolism during exercise and following endurance training. *Sports Medicine* 9: 23–35, 1990.

74. **Houmard JA, Egan PC, Johns RA, Neufer PD, Chenier TC, and Israel RG.** Gastric emptying during 1 h of cycling and running at 75% $\dot{V}O_2$ max. *Medicine and Science in Sports and Exercise* 23: 320–325, 1991.

75. **Houtkooper L and Going S.** Body composition: how should it be measured? Does it affect performance? Barrington, IL: Gatorade Sports Science Institute, 1994.

76. **Institute of Medicine.** Water. In *Dietary Reference Intakes for Energy, Carbohydrate, Fiber, Fat, Protein and Amino Acids (Macronutrients).* Washington, D.C.: National Academy Press, 2002, pp. 73–185.

77. **Ivy JL.** Muscle glycogen synthesis before and after exercise. *Sports Medicine* 11: 6–19, 1991.

78. **Ivy JL and Ferguson LM.** Optimizing resistance exercise adaptations through the timing of post-exercise carbohydrate-protein supplementation. *Strength and Conditioning Journal* 32: 30–36, 2010.

79. **Jeukendrup A.** A step towards personalized sports nutrition: carbohydrate intake during exercise. *Sports Medicine.* 44: S25–S33, 2014.

80. **Jeukendrup AE.** Nutrition for endurance sports: marathon, triathlon, and road cycling. *Journal of Sport Sciences.* 29: S91–S99, 2011.

81. **Jeukendrup A and Killer SC.** The myths surrounding pre-exercise carbohydrate feeding. *Ann Nutri Metab* 57: 18–25, 2010.

82. **Karlsson J and Saltin B.** Diet, muscle glycogen, and endurance performance. *Journal of Applied Physiology* 31: 203–206, 1971.

83. **Kerstetter JE, O'Brien KO, Caseria DM, Wall DE, and Insogna KL.** The impact of dietary protein on calcium absorption and kinetic measures of bone turnover in women. *Journal of Clinical Endocrinology and Metabolism* 90: 26–31, 2005.

84. **Kerstetter JE, O'Brien KO, and Insogna KL.** Dietary protein, calcium metabolism, and skeletal

85. **Lanteri P, Lombardi G, Colombini A, and Banfi G.** Vitamin D in exercise: physiologic and analytical concerns. *Clinica Chimica Acta* 415: 45–53, 2013.

86. **Lemon PW.** Do athletes need more dietary protein and amino acids? *International Journal of Sport Nutrition* 5 (Suppl): S39–61, 1995.

87. **Lemon PW.** Effect of exercise on protein requirements. *Journal of Sports Sciences* 9 Spec No: 53–70, 1991.

88. **Lemon PW.** Protein and amino acid needs of the strength athlete. *International Journal of Sport Nutrition* 1: 127–145, 1991.

89. **Lemon PW.** Protein and exercise: update 1987. *Medicine and Science in Sports and Exercise* 19: S179–190, 1987.

90. **Lemon PW and Mullin JP.** Effect of initial muscle glycogen levels on protein catabolism during exercise. *Journal of Applied Physiology* 48: 624–629, 1980.

91. **Mettler S and Zimmermann MB.** Iron excess in recreational marathon runners. *European Journal of Clinical Nutrition* 64: 490–494, 2010.

92. **Mitchell JB, Costill DL, Houmard JA, Flynn MG, Fink WJ, and Beltz JD.** Effects of carbohydrate ingestion on gastric emptying and exercise performance. *Medicine and Science in Sports and Exercise* 20: 110–115, 1988.

93. **Murray R.** Fluid needs in hot and cold environments. *International Journal of Sport Nutrition* 5 (Suppl): S62–73, 1995.

94. **Nelson JL and Roberts RA.** Exploring the potential ergogenic effects of glycerol hyperhydration. *Sports Medicine* 37: 981–1000, 2007.

95. **Neufer PD, Young AJ, and Sawka MN.** Gastric emptying during exercise: effects of heat stress and hypohydration. *European Journal of Applied Physiology and Occupational Physiology* 58: 433–439, 1989.

96. **Neufer PD, Young AJ, and Sawka MN.** Gastric emptying during walking and running: effects of varied exercise intensity. *European Journal of Applied Physiology and Occupational Physiology* 58: 440–445, 1989.

97. **Nikolaidis MG, Kerksick CM, Lamprecht M, and McAnulty.** Does vitamin C and E supplementation impair the favorable adaptations of regular exercise? *Oxidative Medicine and Cellular Longevity.* Article number 707941, 2012.

98. **Noakes T.** Hyponatremia in distance runners: fluid and sodium balance during exercise. *Current Sports Medicine Reports* 1: 197–207, 2002.

99. **Noakes TD, Norman RJ, Buck RH, Godlonton J, Stevenson K, and Pittaway D.** The incidence of hyponatremia during prolonged ultraendurance exercise. *Medicine and Science in Sports and Exercise* 22: 165–170, 1990.

100. **Novack V, Finestone AS, Constantini N, Shpilberg O, Weitzman S, and Merkel D.** The prevalence of low hemoglobin values among new infantry recruits and nonlinear relationship between hemoglobin concentration and physical fitness. *American Journal of Hematology* 82: 128–133, 2007.

101. **Nybo L.** CNS fatigue and prolonged exercise: effect of glucose supplementation. *Medicine and Science in Sports and Exercise* 35: 589–594, 2003.

102. **Ogan D and Pritchett K.** Vitamin D and the athlete: risks, recommendations and benefits. *Nutrients* 5: 1856–1868, 2013.

103. **Owen MD, Kregel KC, Wall PT, and Gisolfi CV.** Effects of ingesting carbohydrate beverages during exercise in the heat. *Medicine and Science in Sports and Exercise* 18: 568-575, 1986.

104. **Park SG, Bae YJ, Lee YS, and Kim BJ.** Effects of rehydration fluid temperature and composition on body weight retention upon voluntary drinking following exercise-induced dehydration. *Nutrition Research and Practice* 6: 126-131, 2012.

105. **Peternelj TT and Coombes JS.** Antioxidant supplementation during exercise training: beneficial or detrimental? *Sports Medicine* 41: 1043-1069, 2011.

106. **Phillips SM.** The science of muscle hypertrophy: making dietary protein count. *Proceedings of the Nutrition Society* 70: 100-103, 2011.

107. **Pitts G, Johnson R, and Consolazio F.** Work in the heat as affected by intake of water, salt and glucose. *American Journal of Physiology* 142: 353-359, 1944.

108. **Powers S, Nelson WB, and Larson-Meyer E.** Antioxidant and vitamin D supplements for athletes: sense or nonsense? *Journal of Sport Sciences.* 29: S47-S55, 2011.

109. **Rehrer NJ, Beckers EJ, Brouns F, ten Hoor F, and Saris WH.** Effects of dehydration on gastric emptying and gastrointestinal distress while running. *Medicine and Science in Sports and Exercise* 22: 790-795, 1990.

110. **Rehrer NJ, Brouns F, Beckers EJ, ten Hoor F, and Saris WH.** Gastric emptying with repeated drinking during running and bicycling. *International Journal of Sports Medicine* 11: 238-243, 1990.

111. **Rollo I, Cole M, Miller R, and Williams C.** Influence of mouth rinsing a carbohydrate solution on 1-hr running performance. *Medicine and Science in Sports and Exercise* 42: 798-804, 2010.

112. **Sallis RE.** Fluid balance and dysnatremias in athletes. *Current Sports Medicine Reports* 7: S14-S19, 2008.

113. **Sedlock DA.** The latest on carbohydrate loading: a practical approach. *Current Sports Medicine Reports* 7: 209-213, 2008.

114. **Sherman W.** Carbohydrate feedings before and after exercise. In *Perspectives in Exercise Science and Sports Medicine*, edited by Lamb R, and Williams M. New York, NY: McGraw-Hill, 1991.

115. **Sherman W.** Carbohydrates, muscle glycogen, and muscle glycogen supercompensation. In *Ergogenic Aids in Sports*, edited by Williams M. Champaign, IL: Human Kinetics, 1983, pp. 3-26.

116. **Shi X and Gisolfi CV.** Fluid and carbohydrate replacement during intermittent exercise. *Sports Medicine* 25: 157-172, 1998.

117. **Smith JW, Zachwieja JJ, Peronnet F, Passe DH, Massicote D, Lavoie C, et al.** Fuel selection and cycling endurance performance with ingestion of [13C] glucose: evidence for a carbohydrate dose response. *Journal of Applied Physiology* 108: 1520-1529, 2010.

118. **Stachenfeld NS.** Sodium ingestion, thirst, and drinking during endurance exercise. *Sports Science Exchange.* 27(122): 1-5, 2014.

119. **Tan PMS and Lee JKW.** The role of fluid temperature and form on endurance performance in the heat. *Scandinavian Journal of Medicine and Science in Sports and Exercise.* 25 (Suppl 1): 39-51, 2015.

120. **Todd K, Butterfield G, and Calloway D.** Nitrogen balance in men with adequate and deficit energy intake at 3 levels of work. *Journal of Nutrition* 114: 2107-2118, 1984.

121. **Utter AC, Kang J, Nieman DC, Dumke CL, McAnulty SR, Vinci DM, et al.** Carbohydrate supplementation and perceived exertion during prolonged running. *Medicine and Science in Sports and Exercise* 36: 1036-1041, 2004.

122. **Van der Beek EJ.** Vitamins and endurance training: food for running or faddish claims? *Sports Medicine* 2: 175-197, 1985.

123. **Van Rosendal SP, Osborne MA, Fassett RG, and Coombes JS.** Guidelines for glycerol use in hyperhydration and rehydration associated with exercise. *Sports Medicine* 40: 113-139, 2010.

124. **Venderley AM and Campbell WW.** Vegetarian diets : nutritional considerations for athletes. *Sports Medicine* 36: 293-305, 2006.

125. **Vrijens DM and Rehrer NJ.** Sodium-free fluid ingestion decreases plasma sodium during exercise in the heat. *Journal of Applied Physiology* 86: 1847-1851, 1999.

126. **Watson P, Love TD, Maughan RJ, and Shirreffs SM.** A comparison of the effects of milk and a carbohydrate-electrolyte drink on the restoration of fluide capacity in a hot, humid environment. *European Journal of Applied Physiology* 104: 633-642, 2008.

127. **White TP and Brooks GA.** [U-14C]glucose, alanine, and leucine oxidation in rats at rest and two intensities of running. *American Journal of Physiology* 240: E155-165, 1981.

128. **Widmaier EP, Raff H, and Strang KT.** *Vander's Human Physiology.* New York, NY: McGraw-Hill, 2008.

129. **Williams MH, Anderson DE, and Rawson ES.** *Nutrition for Health, Fitness and Sport.* New York, NY: McGraw-Hill, 2013.

130. **Wilmore J.** Body composition and sports medicine: research considerations. In *Report of the Sixth Ross Conference on Medical Research.* Columbus, OH: Ross Laboratories, 1984, pp. 78-82.

131. **Wilmore JH.** Body composition in sport and exercise: directions for future research. *Medicine and Science in Sports and Exercise* 15: 21-31, 1983.

24

© Digital Vision/Getty Images

Exercise and the Environment

■ Objectives

By studying this chapter, you should be able to do the following:

1. Describe the changes in atmospheric pressure, air temperature, and air density with increasing altitude.

2. Describe how altitude affects sprint performances and explain why that is the case.

3. Explain why distance running performance decreases at altitude.

4. Draw a graph to show the effect of altitude on $\dot{V}O_2$ max and list the reasons for this response.

5. Graphically describe the effect of altitude on the heart rate and ventilation responses to submaximal work, and explain why these changes are appropriate.

6. Describe the process of adaptation to altitude and the degree to which this adaptation can be complete.

7. Explain why such variability exists among athletes in the decrease in $\dot{V}O_2$ max upon exposure to altitude, the degree of improvement in $\dot{V}O_2$ max at altitude, and the gains made upon return to sea level.

8. Describe the potential problems associated with training at high altitude and how one might deal with them.

9. Explain the circumstances that caused physiologists to reevaluate their conclusions that humans could not climb Mount Everest without oxygen.

10. Explain the role that hyperventilation plays in helping to maintain a high oxygen-hemoglobin saturation at extreme altitudes.

11. List and describe the factors influencing the risk of heat injury.

12. Provide suggestions for the fitness participant to follow to minimize the likelihood of heat injury.

13. Describe in general terms the guidelines suggested for running road races in the heat.

14. Describe the three elements in the heat stress index, and explain why one is more important than the other two.

15. List the factors influencing hypothermia.

16. Explain what the wind chill index is relative to heat loss.

17. Explain why exposure to cold water is more dangerous than exposure to air of the same temperature.

18. Describe what the "clo" unit is and how recommendations for insulation change when one does exercise.

19. Describe the role of subcutaneous fat and heat production in the development of hypothermia.

20. List the steps to follow to deal with hypothermia.

21. Explain how carbon monoxide can influence performance, and list the steps that should be taken to reduce the impact of pollution on performance.

By now it should be clear that performance is dependent on more than simply having a high $\dot{V}O_2$ max. In Chap. 23, we saw the role of diet and body composition on performance, and in Chap. 25, we will formally consider "ergogenic" or work-enhancing aids and performance. Sandwiched between these chapters is a discussion of how the environmental factors of altitude, heat, cold, and pollution can influence performance.

ALTITUDE

In the late 1960s, when the Olympic Games were scheduled to be held in Mexico City, our attention was directed at the question of how altitude (2300 meters at Mexico City) would affect performance. Previous experience at altitude suggested that many performances would not equal former Olympic standards or, for that matter, the athlete's own personal record (PR) at sea level. On the other hand, some performances were actually expected to be better because they were conducted at altitude. Why? What happens to $\dot{V}O_2$ max with altitude? Can a sea-level resident ever completely adapt to altitude? We will address these and other questions after a brief review of the environmental factors that change with increasing altitude.

Atmospheric Pressure

The **atmospheric pressure** at any spot on earth is a measure of the weight of a column of air directly over that spot. At sea level, the weight (and height) of that column of air is greatest. As one climbs to higher and higher altitudes, the height and, of course, the weight of the column are reduced. Consequently, atmospheric pressure decreases with increasing altitude, the air is less dense, and each liter of air contains fewer molecules of gas. Since the *percentages* of O_2, CO_2, and N_2 are the same at altitude as at sea level, any change in the partial pressure of each gas is due solely to the change in the atmospheric or barometric pressure (see Chap. 10). The decrease in the partial pressure of O_2 (PO_2) with increasing altitude has a direct effect on the saturation of hemoglobin with oxygen (HbO_2) and, consequently, oxygen transport. For example, at 2000 m altitude the HbO_2 is 93%, at 3000 m it is 86%, and at 4000 m it is 73%. This lower PO_2 is called **hypoxia,** with **normoxia** being the term to describe the PO_2 under sea-level conditions. The term **hyperoxia** describes a condition in which the inspired PO_2 is greater than that at sea level (see Chap. 25). In addition to the hypoxic condition at altitude, the air temperature and humidity are lower, adding potential temperature regulation problems to the hypoxic stress of altitude. How do these changes affect performance? To answer that question, we will divide performances into short-term anaerobic performances and long-term aerobic performances.

Short-Term Anaerobic Performance

In Chaps. 3 and 19, we described the importance of the anaerobic sources of ATP in maximal performances lasting two minutes or less. If this information is correct, and we think it is, then the short-term anaerobic races shouldn't be affected by the low PO_2 at altitude because O_2 transport to the muscles is not limiting performance. Table 24.1 shows this to be the

Olympic Games	Short Races: Men				Short Races: Women			
	100 m	200 m	400 m	800 m	100 m	200 m	400 m	800 m
1964 (Tokyo)	10.0 s	20.3 s	45.1 s	1 m 45.1 s	11.4 s	23.0 s	52.0 s	2 m 1.1 s
1968 (Mexico City)	9.9 s	19.8 s	43.8 s	1 m 44.3 s	11.0 s	22.5 s	52.0 s	2 m 0.9 s
% change*	+1.0	+2.5	+2.9	+0.8	+3.5	+2.2	0	+0.2

*+ sign indicates improvement over 1964 performance.

From Howley, E. T., "Effect of Altitude on Physical Performance," Stull, G. A., Cureton, T. K., *Encyclopedia of Physical Education, Fitness and Sports: Training, Environment, Nutrition, and Fitness*. Reston, VA: American Alliance for Health, Physical Education, Recreation and Dance.

case when the sprint performances of the 1968 Mexico City Olympic Games (~2300 m) were compared to those in the 1964 Tokyo Olympic Games (sea level) (61). The performances improved in all but one case, in which the time for the 400-meter run for the women was the same. The reasons for the improvements in performance include the "normal" gains made over time from one Olympic Games to the next and the fact that the density of the air at altitude offers less resistance to movements at high speeds. Improvements in the 100-meter and 400-meter races for each increase of 1000 meters in altitude have been estimated to be about 0.08 seconds and 0.06 seconds, respectively (6, 92). Consistent with this, in the following Olympics (Munich 1972; altitude 1860 ft [567 m]) the sprint times for the men were all slower compared to Mexico City, however, this was not the case for the women, who turned in faster times in three of the races. It must be added that some of the performances were tainted by the systematic use of performance enhancing drugs by the East German team. The issue of lower air resistance sparked controversy over Bob Beamon's fantastic performance in the long jump in the Mexico City Games (see A Closer Look 24.1).

IN SUMMARY

- The atmospheric pressure, PO_2, air temperature, and air density decrease with altitude.
- The lower air density at altitude offers less resistance to high-speed movement, and sprint performances are either not affected or are improved.

Long-Term Aerobic Performance

Maximal performances in excess of two minutes are primarily dependent on oxygen delivery, and, in contrast to the short-term performances, are clearly affected by the lower PO_2 at altitude. Table 24.2 shows the results of the distance running events from 1500 meters up through the marathon and the 50,000-meter walk, and as you can see, performance was diminished at all

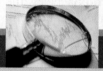

A CLOSER LOOK 24.1

Jumping Through Thin Air

In the 1968 Olympic Games in Mexico City, Bob Beamon shattered the world record in the long jump with a leap of 29 feet 2.5 inches (8.90 m), 21.75 inches (55 cm) longer than the existing world record. Because the record was achieved at altitude where air density is less than that at sea level, some questions were raised about the true magnitude of the achievement. A variety of analyses have been made to determine just how much would have been gained by doing the long jump at altitude (117). The calculations had to

consider the mass of the jumper, a drag coefficient based on the frontal area exposed to the air while jumping, and the difference in the air density between sea level and Mexico City. The result indicated that approximately 2.4 cm (less than an inch) would have been gained by doing the jump at altitude where the air density is less. Subsequent calculations addressed the effect of the favorable wind speed (~2 ms⁻¹) that existed at the time of the jump, as well as the effect of altitude. The authors considered the effect of the wind

speed on both the run phase leading to take off and the jump itself, and concluded that the combination of altitude and wind speed could account for as much as 31 cm. This does not diminish Beamon's incredible achievement—the second-place jumper was 68 cm behind (118)! Scientists have tried to predict the effect of altitude on running performances by considering the opposing factors of lower air density and the reduced availability of oxygen (86). The latter factor is discussed relative to long-distance races.

Olympic Games	Long Races: Men					
	1500 m	3000 m	5000 m	10,000 m	Marathon	50,000 m Walk
1964 (Tokyo)	3 m 38.1 s	8 m 30.8 s	13 m 48.8 s	28 m 24.4 s	2 h 12 m 11.2 s	4 h 11 m 11.2 s
1968 (Mexico City)	3 m 34.9 s	8 m 51.0 s	14 m 05.0 s	29 m 27.4 s	2 h 20 m 24.6 s	4 h 20 m 13.6 s
% change*	+1.5	−3.9	−1.9	−3.7	−6.2	−3.6

*+ sign indicates improvement over 1964 performance.

From Howley, E. T., "Effect of Altitude on Physical Performance," Stull, G. A., Cureton, T. K., *Encyclopedia of Physical Education, Fitness and Sports: Training, Environment, Nutrition, and Fitness.* Reston, VA: American Alliance for Health, Physical Education, Recreation and Dance.

distances but the 1500-meter run (61). This performance is worthy of special note, given that it was expected to be affected, as were the others. It is more than just of passing interest that the record setter was Kipchoge Keino, who was born and raised in Kenya at an altitude similar to that of Mexico City. Did he possess a special adaptation due to his birthplace? We will come back to this question in a later section. We would like to continue our discussion of the effect of altitude on performance by asking, "Why did the performance fall off by as much as 6.2% in the long-distance races?"

Maximal Aerobic Power and Altitude

The decrease in distance running performance at altitude is similar to what occurs when a trained runner becomes untrained–it would clearly take longer to run a marathon! The similarity in the effect is related to a decrease in maximal aerobic power that occurs with detraining and with increasing altitude.

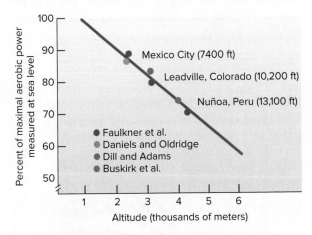

Figure 24.1 Changes in maximal aerobic power with increasing altitude. The sea-level value for maximal aerobic power is set to 100%.

Howley, E. T., "Effect of Altitude on Physical Performance," Stull, G. A., Cureton, T. K., *Encyclopedia of Physical Education, Fitness and Sports: Training, Environment, Nutrition, and Fitness.* Reston, VA: American Alliance for Health, Physical Education, Recreation and Dance.

Figure 24.1 shows that $\dot{V}O_2$ max decreases in a linear fashion, being about 12% lower at 2400 meters (7400 feet), 20% lower at 3100 meters (10,200 feet), and 27% lower at about 4000 meters (13,100 feet) (16, 27, 32, 39). Although it should be no surprise that endurance performance decreases with such changes in $\dot{V}O_2$ max, why does $\dot{V}O_2$ max decrease?

Cardiovascular Function at Altitude Maximal oxygen uptake is equal to the product of the maximal cardiac output and the maximal arteriovenous oxygen difference, $\dot{V}O_2 = CO \times (CaO_2 - C\bar{v}O_2)$. Given this relationship, the decrease in $\dot{V}O_2$ max with increasing altitude could be due to a decrease in cardiac output and/or a decrease in oxygen extraction. It will become clear in the following paragraphs that oxygen extraction is a major factor causing a decrease in $\dot{V}O_2$ max at all altitudes, with decreases in maximal cardiac output contributing primarily at higher altitudes.

Maximal cardiac output is equal to the product of maximal heart rate and maximal stroke volume. In several studies, the maximal heart rate was unchanged at altitudes of 2300 meters (37, 88), 3100 meters (47), and 4000 meters (16), while changes in maximal stroke volume were somewhat inconsistent (66). If these two variables, maximal stroke volume and maximal heart rate, do not change much at these altitudes, then the decrease in $\dot{V}O_2$ max must be due to a difference in oxygen extraction.

Although oxygen extraction ($CaO_2 - C\bar{v}O_2$) could decrease due to a decrease in the arterial oxygen content (CaO_2) or an increase in the mixed venous oxygen content ($C\bar{v}O_2$), the primary cause is the desaturation of the arterial blood due to the low PO_2 at altitude. The lower atmospheric PO_2 causes the alveolar PO_2 to be lower. This reduces the pressure gradient for oxygen diffusion between the alveolus and the pulmonary capillary blood, thus lowering the arterial PO_2. As you recall from Chap. 10, as the arterial PO_2 falls, there is a reduction in the volume of oxygen bound to hemoglobin. At sea level, hemoglobin is about 96%–98% saturated with oxygen. However, at 2300 meters and 4000 meters, saturation falls to 88% and 71%, respectively. These decreases in the oxygen saturation of hemoglobin are similar to the reductions in $\dot{V}O_2$ max at these altitudes described earlier. Because maximal oxygen transport is the product of the maximal cardiac output and the arterial oxygen content, the capacity to transport oxygen to the working muscles at altitude is reduced due to desaturation, even though maximal cardiac output may be unchanged during acute exposures up to altitudes of 4000 meters (66). However, it must be added that a variety of studies have shown a decrease in maximal heart rate at altitude. Although some of these decreases have been observed at altitudes of 3100 meters (32) and 4300 meters (37), it is more common to find lower maximal heart rates above altitudes of 4300 meters. For example, compared to maximal HR at sea level, maximal HR was observed to be 24–33 beats/minute lower at 4650 meters (15,300 feet) and 47 beats/minute lower at about 6100 meters (20,000 feet) (51, 91). This depression in maximal heart rate is reversed by acute restoration of normoxia, or the use of atropine (51). This altitude-induced bradycardia suggests that myocardial hypoxia may trigger the slower heart rate to decrease the work and, therefore, the oxygen demand of the heart muscle.

As mentioned earlier, during an acute exposure to altitude, stroke volume during exercise is only slightly reduced, if at all. However, prolonged exposures to altitude result in a reduction in plasma volume that leads to a lower end diastolic volume and stroke volume (80). This means that $\dot{V}O_2$ max decreases at a faster rate at the higher altitudes due to the combined effects of the desaturation of hemoglobin and the decrease in maximal cardiac output.

This desaturation of arterial blood at altitude affects more than $\dot{V}O_2$ max. The cardiovascular responses to submaximal work are also influenced. Due to the fact that each liter of blood is carrying less oxygen, more liters of blood must be pumped per minute in order to compensate. This is accomplished through an increase in the HR response, since the stroke volume response is at its highest point already, or it is actually lower at altitude due to the hypoxia (2). This elevated HR response is shown in Fig. 24.2 (47). This has implications for more than the performance-based athlete. The average person who participates in an exercise program will have to decrease the intensity of exercise at altitude in order to stay in the target heart rate zone. Remember, the exercise prescription needed for a cardiovascular training effect includes a proper duration of exercise to achieve an appropriate total caloric expenditure (see Chap. 16). If the intensity is too high, the person will have more difficulty achieving that goal.

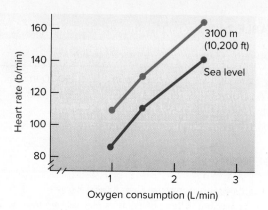

Figure 24.2 The effect of altitude on the heart rate response to submaximal exercise.

Respiratory Function at Altitude In the introduction to this section, we mentioned that the air is less dense at altitude. This means that there are fewer O_2 molecules per liter of air, and if a person wanted to consume the same number of liters of O_2, pulmonary ventilation would have to increase. At 5600 meters (18,400 feet), the atmospheric pressure is one-half that at sea level, and the number of molecules of O_2 per liter of air is reduced by one-half; therefore, a person would have to breathe twice as much air to take in the same amount of O_2. The consequences of this are shown in Fig. 24.3, which presents the ventilation responses of a subject who exercised at work rates demanding a $\dot{V}O_2$ of about 1–2 L · min^{-1} at sea level and at three altitudes exceeding 4000 meters. The pulmonary ventilation is elevated at all altitudes, reaching values of almost 180 L · min^{-1} at 6400 meters (21,000 feet) (91). This extreme ventilatory response requires the respiratory muscles, primarily the diaphragm, to work so hard that fatigue may occur. We will see more on this in a later section dealing with the assault on Mount Everest.

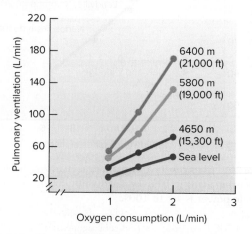

Figure 24.3 The effect of altitude on the ventilation response to submaximal exercise.

- Distance-running performances are adversely affected at altitude due to the reduction in the PO_2, which causes a decrease in hemoglobin saturation and $\dot{V}O_2$ max.
- Up to moderate altitudes (~4000 meters), the decrease in $\dot{V}O_2$ max is due primarily to the decrease in the arterial oxygen content brought about by the decrease in atmospheric PO_2. At higher altitudes, the rate at which $\dot{V}O_2$ max falls is increased due to a reduction in maximal cardiac output.
- Submaximal performances conducted at altitude require higher heart rate and ventilation responses due to the lower oxygen content of arterial blood and the reduction in the number of oxygen molecules per liter of air, respectively.

Acclimatization to High Altitude

The low PO_2 at altitude triggers an increase in the hypoxia inducible factor-1 (HIF-1) that is present in most cells of the body. HIF-1 activates genes associated with erythropoietin (EPO) production that is involved in red blood cell production, vascular endothelial growth factors that are involved in the generation of new blood vessels, and nitric oxide synthase that promotes the synthesis of nitric oxide that is involved in vasodilation (102, 106). In the high-altitude populations of the Andes in South America, the acclimatization response to the low PO_2 at altitude is to produce additional red blood cells to compensate for the desaturation of hemoglobin. In the mining community of Morococha, Peru, where people reside at altitudes above 4540 meters, hemoglobin levels of $211 \text{ g} \cdot \text{L}^{-1}$ have been measured, in contrast to the normal $156 \text{ g} \cdot \text{L}^{-1}$ of the sea-level residents in Lima, Peru. This higher hemoglobin compensates rather completely for the low PO_2 at those altitudes (64):

> Sea level: $156 \text{ g} \cdot \text{L}^{-1}$ times $1.34 \text{ ml } O_2 \cdot \text{g}^{-1}$ at 98% saturation $= 206 \text{ ml} \cdot \text{L}^{-1}$
>
> 4,540 m: $211 \text{ g} \cdot \text{L}^{-1}$ times $1.34 \text{ ml } O_2 \cdot \text{g}^{-1}$ at 81% saturation $= 224 \text{ ml} \cdot \text{L}^{-1}$

One of the best tests of the degree to which these high-altitude residents have adapted is found in the $\dot{V}O_2$ max values measured at altitude. Average values of 46–$50 \text{ ml} \cdot \text{kg}^{-1} \cdot \text{min}^{-1}$ were measured on the altitude natives (67, 77–79), which compares favorably with sea-level natives in that country and in ours.

There is no question that any sea-level resident who makes a journey to altitude and stays a while will experience an acclimatization process that includes an increase in red blood cell number. However, the adaptation will probably never be as complete as seen in the permanent residents. This conclusion is drawn from a study that compared $\dot{V}O_2$ max values of several different groups: (a) Peruvian lowlanders and Peace Corps volunteers who came to altitude as adults, (b) lowlanders who came to altitude as children and spent their growing years at altitude, and (c) permanent altitude residents (39). The $\dot{V}O_2$ max values were $46 \text{ ml} \cdot \text{kg}^{-1} \cdot \text{min}^{-1}$ for the altitude residents and those who arrived there as children. In contrast, the lowlanders who arrived as adults and spent only one to four years at altitude had values of $38 \text{ ml} \cdot \text{kg}^{-1} \cdot \text{min}^{-1}$. This indicates that to have complete acclimatization, one must spend the developmental years at high altitude. This may help explain the surprisingly good performance of Kipchoge Keino's performance in the 1500-meter run at the Mexico City Olympic Games mentioned earlier, because he spent his childhood at an altitude similar to that of Mexico City.

The elevated hemoglobin concentration of the Peruvian permanent-altitude residents was believed to be the primary means by which humans adapted in order to live at high altitudes. That is no longer the case. It has become clear that those who live at high altitudes in Tibet have achieved that level of acclimatization by a different means compared to those who live in the Andes (73, 100, 111, 126). Tibetan residents adapt by increasing the oxygen saturation of hemoglobin, rather than the concentration of hemoglobin, which may be 30 g/L lower than Andeans living at comparable altitudes. Tibetan Sherpas' superior performance at extreme altitudes is linked, not to an exceptional $\dot{V}O_2$ max at altitude, but to better lung function, capillary density, forearm blood flow, maximal cardiac output, and level of oxygen saturation of hemoglobin (42, 102). The different types of adaptations observed in these populations is related to the natural selection of those with unique genes that promote either an increase in red blood cell production (e.g., Andean) or an increase in oxygen saturation (Tibetan) that is a result of an increase in nitric oxide in the lungs that promotes an increase in blood flow (107, 111, 126).

- Andeans adapt to high altitude by producing more red blood cells to counter the desaturation caused by the lower PO_2. Andean altitude residents who spent their growing years at altitude show a rather complete adaptation as seen in their arterial oxygen content and $\dot{V}O_2$ max values. Lowlanders who arrive as adults show only a modest adaptation.
- In contrast, Tibetan high-altitude residents adapt by increasing the oxygen saturation of the existing hemoglobin, a result of increased blood flow to the lungs due to high nitric oxide levels.

Training for Competition at Altitude

It was clear to many of the middle- and long-distance runners who competed in the Olympic Trials or Games in 1968 that the altitude was going to have a detrimental effect on performance. Using $\dot{V}O_2$ max as an indicator of the impact on performance, scientists studied the effect of immediate exposure to altitude, the rate of recovery in $\dot{V}O_2$ max as the individual stayed at altitude, and whether $\dot{V}O_2$ max was higher than the prealtitude value upon return to sea level. The results were interesting, not due to the general trends that were expected, but to the extreme variability in response among the athletes. For example, the decrease in $\dot{V}O_2$ max upon ascent to a 2300-meter altitude ranged from 8.8% to 22.3% (99); at 3090 meters, it ranged from 13.9% to 24.4% (34); and at 4000 meters the decrease ranged from 24.8% to 34.3% (17). One of the major conclusions that could be drawn from these data is that the best runner at sea level might not be the best at altitude if that person had the largest drop in $\dot{V}O_2$ max. Why such variability? Studies of this phenomenon suggest that the variability in the decrease in $\dot{V}O_2$ max across individuals relates to the degree to which athletes experience desaturation of arterial blood during maximal work (68, 74, 87). Chapter 10 described the effect that arterial desaturation has on $\dot{V}O_2$ max of superior athletes at sea level. If such desaturation can occur under sea-level conditions, then the altitude condition should have an additional impact, with the magnitude of the impact being greater on those who suffer some desaturation at sea level. Consistent with that, exposure to a simulated altitude of 3000 meters resulted in a 20.8% decrease in $\dot{V}O_2$ max for trained subjects and only a 9.8% decrease for untrained subjects (68).

The decrease in $\dot{V}O_2$ max upon exposure to altitude was not the only physiological response that varied among the athletes. There also was a variable response in the size of the increase in $\dot{V}O_2$ max as the subjects stayed at altitude and continued to train. One study, lasting 28 days at 2300 meters, found the $\dot{V}O_2$ max to increase from 1% to 8% over that time (99). Some found the $\dot{V}O_2$ max to gradually improve over a period of 10–28 days (28, 32, 88), while others (37, 47) did not. In addition, when the subjects returned to sea level and were retested, some found the $\dot{V}O_2$ max to be higher than before they left (28, 32), whereas others found no improvements (16, 39, 46). Why was there such variability in response?

There are several possibilities. If an athlete was not in peak condition before ascending to altitude, the combined stress of the exercise and altitude could increase the $\dot{V}O_2$ max over time while at altitude and show an additional gain upon return to sea level. Evidence exists both for (99) and against

(1, 36, 115) the idea that the combination of altitude and exercise stress leads to greater changes in $\dot{V}O_2$ max than exercise stress alone. Another reason for the variability is related to the altitude at which the training was conducted. When runners trained at high (4000 meters) altitude, the intensity of the runs (relative to sustained sea-level speeds) had to be reduced to complete a workout due to the reduction in $\dot{V}O_2$ max that occurs at altitude. As a result, the runner might actually "detrain" while at altitude, and subsequent performance at sea level might not be as good as it was before going to altitude (16). Daniels and Oldridge (28) provided a way around this problem by having runners alternate training at altitude (7–14 days) and at sea level (5–11 days). Using an altitude of only 2300 meters, the runners were still able to train at "race pace," and detraining did not occur. In fact, 13 personal records were achieved by the athletes when they raced at sea level. The focus on gaining the benefits of acclimation to altitude has resulted in a strategy in which the athlete lives at high altitude but trains at low altitude–in some cases, without ever leaving low altitude. See The Winning Edge 24.1.

IN SUMMARY

- When athletes train at altitude, some experience a greater decline in $\dot{V}O_2$ max than others. This may be due to differences in the degree to which each athlete experiences a desaturation of hemoglobin. Remember, some athletes experience desaturation during maximal work at sea level.
- Some athletes show an increase in $\dot{V}O_2$ max while training at altitude, whereas others do not. This may be due to the degree to which the athlete was trained before going to altitude.
- In addition, some athletes show an improved $\dot{V}O_2$ max upon return to sea level, whereas others do not. Part of the reason may be the altitude at which they train. Those who train at high altitudes may actually "detrain" due to the fact that the quality of their workouts suffers at the high altitudes. To get around this problem, athletes can alternate low-altitude and sea-level exposures, or follow a "live high, train low" program.

The Quest for Everest

The most obvious tie between exercise and altitude is mountain climbing. The climber faces the stress of altitude, cold, solar radiation, and, of course, the work of climbing up steep slopes or sheer rock walls. A goal of some mountaineers has been to climb Mount Everest, at 8848 meters, the highest mountain on earth.

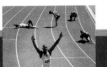
Live High, Train Low, or the Reverse!

There is great interest in the "live high, train low" strategy as a way of improving endurance performance. The "live high" refers to being exposed to a low PO_2 to obtain an increase in the amount of hemoglobin, and "train low" refers to doing exercise at sea level (or a very low altitude) to not affect the intensity and/or duration of the workouts. There is clear evidence that some athletes perform better after doing a LHTL program, but many do not (24). A wide variety of factors are thought to affect the outcome: type of subjects (elite vs. trained), length of the study, intensity and volume of training, the altitude (be it real or simulated), and the length of stay at altitude (129). Lundby et al. (70, 71) attempted to explain the discrepancies by examining some of these factors.

Subjects: there is a big difference between *elite* subjects and *trained*

subjects, in the sense that elite subjects might not be as responsive to altitude or, for that matter, any other kind of training due to the training they are currently doing.

Baseline values: If an athlete has a low level of some physiological measure (e.g., $\dot{V}O_2$ max), there is a greater potential for it to increase due to an intervention, compared to someone with an already high baseline $\dot{V}O_2$ max. For example, although there was a linear relationship between the increase in hemoglobin mass (Hb_{mass}) and the increase in $\dot{V}O_2$ max after LHTL, there was an inverse relationship between the baseline level of Hb_{mass} and the increase in Hb_{mass} that occurred due to LHTL. In essence, the ones who improved the most had the lowest levels of hemoglobin mass at baseline (71).

Research design: Few of the more than 100 altitude training studies included a control group, which opens the door for misinterpretation of results, when it might be a placebo effect rather than an altitude effect causing a change in performance. In this regard, Lundby et al. (70, 71) encourage all future studies, especially those using normobaric hypoxia (sleeping/living in a low percent oxygen environment at sea level to simulate the altitude experience) to include a placebo-controlled, double-blind design (see Chap. 25).

In summary, LHTL may increase performance in some athletes, but certainly not all, and the potential response seems to be lower for those with high baseline levels of Hb_{mass} (70, 71). We are sure to hear more about this exciting topic in the years ahead.

Figure 24.4 shows various early attempts to climb Everest during the twentieth century (125). Special note should be made of Hillary and Tensing, who were the first to do it in 1963, and Messner and Habeler, who, to the amazement of all, did it without supplemental oxygen in 1978. See Messner in Suggested Readings for complete details on how they accomplished this feat. This achievement brought scientists

back to Everest in 1981 asking how this was possible. This section provides some background to this fascinating story.

In 1924, Norton's climbing team attempted to scale Everest without O_2 and almost succeeded–they stopped only 300 meters from the summit (83). This 1924 expedition was noteworthy because data were collected on the climbers and porters by physicians

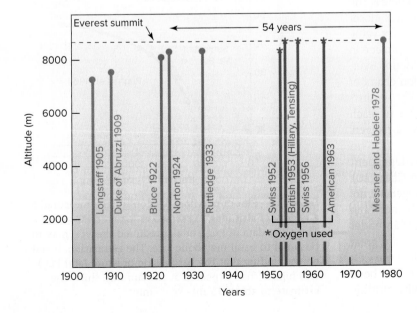

Figure 24.4 The highest altitudes attained by climbers in the twentieth century. In 1924, the climbers ascended within 300 meters of the summit without supplemental oxygen. It took another 54 years to climb those last 300 meters.

and scientists associated with the attempt. The story of this assault is good reading for those interested in mountain climbing and provides evidence of the keen powers of observation of the scientists. Major Hingston noted the respiratory distress associated with climbing to such heights, stating that at 5800 meters (19,000 feet) "the very slightest exertion, such as the tying of a bootlace, the opening of a ration box, the getting into a sleeping bag, was associated with marked respiratory distress." At 8200 meters (27,000 feet), one climber "had to take seven, eight, or ten complete respirations for every single step forward. And even at that slow rate of progress he had to rest for a minute or two every twenty or thirty yards" (83). Pugh, who made observations during a 1960-1961 expedition to Everest, believed that fatigue of the respiratory muscles may be the primary factor limiting such endeavors at extreme altitudes (91). Further, Pugh's observations of the decreases in $\dot{V}O_2$ max at the extreme altitudes suggested that $\dot{V}O_2$ max would be just above basal metabolism at the summit, making the task an unlikely one at best. How then did Messner and Habeler climb Everest without supplemental O_2?

This was one of the primary questions addressed by the 1981 expedition to Everest. As mentioned earlier, $\dot{V}O_2$ max decreases with altitude due to the lower barometric pressure, which causes a lower PO_2 and a desaturation of hemoglobin. In effect, the $\dot{V}O_2$ max at the summit of Everest was predicated on the observed rate of decrease in $\dot{V}O_2$ max at lower altitudes and then extrapolated to the barometric pressure at the top of the mountain. One of the first major findings of the 1981 expedition was that the barometric pressure at the summit was 17 mm Hg higher than previously believed (121, 124). This higher barometric pressure increased the estimated inspired PO_2 and made a big difference in the predicted $\dot{V}O_2$ max. Figure 24.5 shows that the $\dot{V}O_2$ max predicted from the 1960-1961 expedition was near the basal metabolic rate, whereas the value predicted from the 1981 expedition was closer to 15 ml · kg^{-1} · min^{-1} (121, 124). This $\dot{V}O_2$ max value was confirmed in the Operation Everest II project in which subjects did a simulated ascent of Mount Everest over a 40-day period in a decompression chamber (27, 112). This $\dot{V}O_2$ max value of 15 ml · kg^{-1} · min^{-1} helps to explain how the climbers were able to reach the summit without the aid of supplemental oxygen. However, it was not the only reason.

The arterial saturation of hemoglobin is dependent upon the arterial PO_2, PCO_2, and pH (see Chap. 10). A low PCO_2 and a high pH cause the oxygen hemoglobin curve to shift to the left so that hemoglobin is more saturated under these conditions than under normal conditions. A person who can ventilate great volumes in response to hypoxia can exhale more CO_2 and cause the pH to become elevated. It has been shown that those who successfully deal with altitude

have strong hypoxic ventilatory drives, allowing them to have a higher arterial PO_2 and oxygen saturation (105). In fact, when alveolar PCO_2 values were obtained at the top of Mount Everest in the 1981 expedition, the climbers had values much lower than expected (122). This ability to hyperventilate, coupled with the barometric pressure being higher than expected, resulted in higher arterial PO_2, and, of course, $\dot{V}O_2$ max values. How high must your $\dot{V}O_2$ max be to climb Mount Everest?

Figure 24.5 shows that the climbers in the 1981 expedition had $\dot{V}O_2$ max values at sea level that were higher than those of the 1960-1961 expedition. In fact, several of the climbers had been competitive marathon runners (121), and, given the need to transport oxygen at these high altitudes to do work, having such a high $\dot{V}O_2$ max would appear to be a prerequisite to success in climbing without oxygen. Subsequent measurements on other mountaineers who had scaled 8500 meters or more without oxygen confirmed this by showing them to possess primarily type I muscle fibers and to have an average $\dot{V}O_2$ max of 60 ± 6 ml · kg^{-1} · min^{-1} (84). However, there was one notable exception: One of the subjects in this study was Messner, who had climbed Mount Everest without oxygen; his $\dot{V}O_2$ max was 48.8 ml · kg^{-1} · min^{-1} (84). West et al. (123) provide food for thought in this regard: "It remains for someone to elucidate the evolutionary processes responsible for man being just able to reach the highest point on Earth while breathing ambient air." However, there is more to consider in climbing Mount Everest than a person's $\dot{V}O_2$ max.

It has been a common experience in mountain climbing, especially with prolonged exposure to high altitudes, for climbers to lose weight secondary to a loss

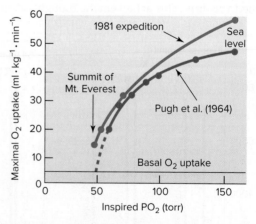

Figure 24.5 Plot of maximal oxygen uptake measured at a variety of altitudes, expressed as inspired PO_2 values. The 1964 data of Pugh et al. predicted the $\dot{V}O_2$ max to be equal to basal metabolic rate. The estimation, based on the finding that the barometric pressure (and PO_2) was higher than expected at the summit, shifts the estimate to about 15 ml · kg^{-1} · min^{-1}.

of appetite (65). Clearly, if a large portion of this weight loss were muscle, it would have a negative impact on the climber's ability to scale the mountain. Some research work from both simulated and real ascents of Mount Everest provides some insight into what changes are taking place in muscle and what may be responsible for those changes. In the Operation Everest II 40-day simulation of an ascent to Mount Everest, the subjects experienced a 25% reduction in the cross-sectional area of type I and type II muscle fibers, and a 14% reduction in muscle area (46, 72). These and other observations (e.g., shifts in myosin from fast to slow isoforms) were supported by data from real high-altitude ascents that combined exercise with severe hypoxia (33, 56, 60). What could have caused these changes? The Operation Everest II data on nutrition and body composition showed that caloric intake decreased 43% from 3136 to 1789 kcal/day over the course of the 40-day exposure to hypoxia. The subjects lost an average of 7.4 kg, with most of the weight from lean body mass, despite the availability of palatable food (98). This and other studies (119) showed that hypoxia itself suppresses both hunger and food intake, resulting in weight loss and changes in body composition. Whether such changes in muscle mass are linked directly to changes in $\dot{V}O_2$ max, they would clearly affect performance.

IN SUMMARY

- Climbers reached the summit of Mount Everest without oxygen in 1978. This surprised scientists who thought $\dot{V}O_2$ max would be just above resting $\dot{V}O_2$ at that altitude. They later found that the barometric pressure was higher than they previously had thought and that the estimated $\dot{V}O_2$ max was about 15 ml·kg^{-1}·min^{-1} at this altitude.
- Those who are successful at these high altitudes have a great capacity to hyperventilate. This drives down the PCO_2 and the [H$^+$] in blood and allows more oxygen to bind with hemoglobin at the same arterial PO_2.
- Finally, those who are successful at climbing to extreme altitudes must contend with the loss of appetite that results in a reduction in body weight and in the cross-sectional area of type I and type II muscle fibers.

HEAT

Chapter 12 described the changes in body temperature with exercise, how heat loss mechanisms are activated, and the benefits of acclimation to heat. This section extends that discussion by considering the prevention of thermal injuries during exercise.

Hyperthermia

Our core temperature (37°C) is within a few degrees of a value (45°C) that could lead to death (see Chap. 12). Given that, and the fact that distance running races, triathlons, fitness programs, and football games occur during the warmer part of the year, the potential for heat injury, **hyperthermia,** is increased (14, 49, 63). Heat injury is not an all-or-none affair, but includes a series of stages that need to be recognized and attended to in order to prevent a progression from the least to the most serious (62). These stages include **exercise-induced muscle cramps, heat syncope, heat exhaustion,** and **heat stroke.** Table 24.3 summarizes each stage, identifying signs, symptoms, and the immediate care that should be provided (21). Special attention is directed at heatstroke, a medical emergency that can lead to death. There is an urgency to lower core temperature as soon and as fast as possible, and cold-water and ice-water immersion are the recommended approaches to accomplish that goal (5, 20, 22). Although it is important to recognize and deal with these problems, it is better to prevent them from happening.

Figure 24.6 shows the major factors related to heat injury. Each one independently influences susceptibility to heat injury:

Fitness A high level of fitness is related to a lower risk of heat injury (45). Fit subjects can tolerate more work in the heat (34), acclimate faster (14), and sweat more (12). However, very fit individuals can still develop exercise-related heatstroke (5).

Acclimation Exercise in the heat for 10–14 days, either at low intensity (<50% $\dot{V}O_2$ max) and long duration (60–100 min) or at moderate intensity (75% $\dot{V}O_2$ max) and short duration (30–35 min), accomplish the following (5, 14, 48, 59, 69, 94):

- Increases plasma volume, skin blood flow, and sweating
- Increases $\dot{V}O_2$ max, maximal cardiac output, and power output at the LT
- Lowers body temperature and heart rate responses to submaximal exercise
- Reduces salt loss in sweat and the chance of sodium depletion
- Increases aerobic exercise performance

This acclimation process is the best protection against exertional heatstroke and heat exhaustion (5). The National Athletic Trainers' Association provides a plan for football that phases in the intensity and duration of activity, as well as the equipment that is worn. This is important because the first 2–3 weeks of preseason presents the greatest risk of heat illness (21).

TABLE 24.3　Exertional Heat Illnesses

Heat Illness	Signs and Symptoms	Immediate Care
Exercise-induced muscle cramps: sudden involuntary muscle contractions during or after exercise	Visible cramping May involve multiple muscle groups	Rest, passive stretching, icing, massage Rehydrate
Heat syncope: orthostatic dizziness attributed to dehydration, hypotension, venous pooling	Brief episode of fainting associated with dizziness, tunnel vision	Move to shaded area Elevate legs above level of heart Cool skin Rehydrate
Heat exhaustion: inability to effectively exercise in the heat due to cardiovascular insufficiency, hypotension, or central fatigue	Excessive fatigue Fainting Confusion, disorientation	Move to shared area Remove excess clothing/equipment Elevate legs above level of heart Cool with ice towels and fans Rehydrate Refer to physician
Exertional heat stroke: characterized by neuropsychiatric impairment and a high body temperature; medical emergency	Disorientation, confusion, dizziness, hysteria Rectal temperature >40.5°C Hot sweaty skin	Remove excess clothing/equipment Lower core temperature to <38.9°C (<102°F) within 30 minutes Use pool/tub of cold (15°C/60°F) water; vigorously circulate the water If medical personnel are available, place intravenous fluid line Transfer to medical facility

Table is based on "National Athletic Trainers' Association Position Statement: Exertional Heat Illness," *Journal of Athletic Training* 50: 986–1000, 2015.

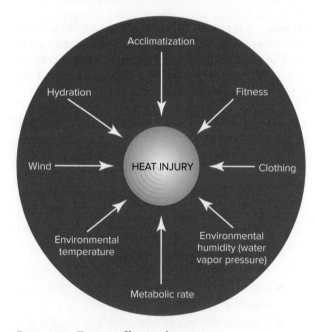

Figure 24.6　Factors affecting heat injury.

Hydration　Inadequate hydration reduces sweat rate and increases the chance of heat injury (101, 103, 104). Chapter 23 discussed the procedures for fluid replacement. Generally, there are no differences among water, electrolyte drinks, or carbohydrate-electrolyte drinks in replacing body water during exercise (19, 25, 131). However, drinks with sodium seem to stimulate thirst, which can increase voluntary drinking (110).

Environmental Temperature　Convection and radiation heat-loss mechanisms are dependent on a temperature gradient from skin to environment. Exercising in temperatures greater than skin temperatures results in a heat gain. Evaporation of sweat must then compensate if body temperature is to remain at a safe value. See the later discussion on the use of the Wet Bulb Globe Temperature as a guide to reducing the risk of heat injury.

Clothing　Expose as much skin surface as possible to encourage evaporation. Choose materials, such as cotton, that will "wick" sweat to the surface for evaporation. In that regard, cotton and synthetic (e.g., polyester) fabrics performed similarly in terms of thermoregulation and subjective sensations during exercise (11, 30, 109). However, fabrics impermeable to water will increase the risk of heat injury. Figure 24.7 shows the influence of different military uniforms on the body temperature response to treadmill running (75). Because many exercise-related heat injuries occur during the first four days of American football practice, attention to limiting clothing, as well as attending to acclimation and hydration are advised (5).

Humidity (Water Vapor Pressure)　Evaporation of sweat is dependent on the water vapor pressure gradient between skin and environment. In warm/hot environments, the relative humidity is a good index of the water vapor pressure, with a lower relative

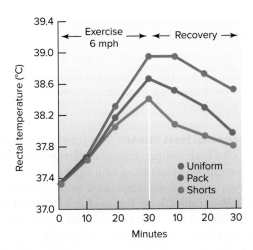

Figure 24.7 The effect of different types of uniforms on the body temperature response to treadmill running.

humidity facilitating evaporation. In a recent study, time to exhaustion at 70% $\dot{V}O_2$ max decreased linearly when relative humidity was increased from 24% to 40%, 60%, and 80% on four separate days. Interestingly, there was no difference in heart rate or core temperature between trials (76). See the later discussion on the use of the Wet Bulb Globe Temperature as a guide to reducing the risk of heat injury.

Metabolic Rate Given that core temperature is proportional to work rate, metabolic heat production plays an important role in the overall heat load the body experiences during exercise. As one begins to overheat, decreasing the pace lowers the metabolic rate and the physiological strain. However, if the pace cannot be voluntarily decreased (e.g., coach directing the drills) heat-related problems can increase (20).

Wind Wind places more air molecules into contact with the skin and can influence heat loss in two ways. If a temperature gradient for heat loss exists between the skin and the air, wind will increase the rate of heat loss by convection. In a similar manner, wind increases the rate of evaporation, assuming the air can accept moisture. During self-paced exercise in the heat, wind reduces physiological strain and improves performance (113).

Even the time of day is a consideration when it comes to exercise performance during heat exposure. With its typical diurnal variation, core temperature is lower and the body's heat storage capacity is higher in the morning, compared to the afternoon, when resting core temperature is elevated (94). When male cyclists rode to exhaustion at 65% $\dot{V}O_2$ max in a warm environment (35°C, 60% RH), time to exhaustion was longer in the morning trial (45.8 min) compared to the afternoon trial (40.5 min). Core temperature was lower in the morning trial for the first 25 minutes,

but was no different at exhaustion (54). The results suggested that the greater heat storage capacity contributed to the difference.

For a practical guide on the prevention and treatment of heat-related illness, see Howe and Boden in Suggested Readings.

IMPLICATIONS FOR FITNESS

The person exercising for fitness needs to be educated about all of the previously listed factors. Suggestions might include:

- Providing information on heat illness symptoms: cramps, lightheadedness, and so on
- Exercising in the cooler part of the day to avoid heat gain from the sun or structures heated by the sun
- Gradually increasing exposure to high heat/humidity to safely acclimatize
- Drinking water before, during, and after exercise and weighing in each day to monitor hydration
- Wearing only shorts and a tank top to expose as much skin as possible
- Taking heart rate measurements several times during the activity and reducing exercise intensity to stay in the target heart rate (THR) zone

The latter recommendation is most important. The heart rate is a sensitive indicator of dehydration, environmental heat load, and acclimation. Variation in any of these factors will modify the heart rate response to any fixed, submaximal exercise. Furthermore, the relationship between % $\dot{V}O_2$ max and % HRR is maintained during exercise in the heat (127, 128). It is therefore important for fitness participants to monitor heart rate on a regular basis and to slow down to stay within the THR zone. Age is sometimes raised as a predisposing factor related to heat injury, but that may not be the case after you account for the factors mentioned previously. We would like to direct the interested reader to a brief and clearly written review of this topic by Kenney and Munce in Suggested Readings.

IMPLICATIONS FOR PERFORMANCE

Heat injury has been a concern in athletics for decades. Initially, the vast majority of attention was focused on football because of the large number of heat-related deaths associated with that sport (15). Emphasis on preseason conditioning to improve fitness and promote acclimation, drinking water during practice and games, and weighing in each day to monitor hydration resulted in a steady reduction of heat-related deaths throughout the early 1990s. However, since that time, there has been an increase in the number of heat-related deaths in football, especially at the high school level. In fact, among U.S. high school athletes, heat illness is the leading cause of death and disability (44).

There is a need to return to the vigilance and practices that resulted in the low death rates of the early 1990s. It might be added that during the time that the number of heat-related deaths in football players was decreasing, there was an increase in the number of deaths in another athletic activity—long-distance road races (49, 63). In response to this problem, and on the basis of sound research, the American College of Sports Medicine developed a Position Stand on the Prevention of Thermal Injuries During Distance Running (3), parts of which have been updated (5). The elements recommended in this position statement are consistent with what we previously presented:

Medical Director

- A sports medicine physician should work with the race director to enhance safety and coordinate first-aid measures.

Race Organization

- Minimize environmental heat load by planning races for the cooler months and at a time of day (before 8:00 A.M. or after 6:00 P.M.) to reduce solar heat gain.

- Use an environmental heat stress index (see the next section, "Environmental Heat Stress") to help make decisions about whether to run a race. See Roberts in Suggested Readings for more on this.

- Have a water station every 2–3 km; encourage runners to drink 150–300 milliliters of water every 15 minutes.

- Clearly identify the race monitors and have them look for those who might be in trouble due to heat injury.

- Have traffic control for safety.

- Use radio communication throughout the race course.

Medical Support

- Medical director coordinates ambulance service with local hospitals and has the authority to evaluate or stop runners who appear to be in trouble.

- Medical director coordinates medical facilities at race site to provide first aid.

Competitor Education

- Provide information about factors related to heat illness that were discussed previously.

- Encourage the "buddy system" (see Chap. 17). The primary focus in these recommendations is on safety.

Environmental Heat Stress   The previous discussion mentioned high temperature and relative humidity as factors increasing the risk of heat injuries. To quantify the overall heat stress associated with any environment, a Wet Bulb Globe Temperature (**WBGT**) guide was developed (3). This overall heat stress index is composed of the following measurements:

Dry Bulb Temperature (T_{db})

- Ordinary measure of air temperature taken in the shade

Black Globe Temperature (T_g)

- Measure of the radiant heat load taken in direct sunlight

Wet Bulb Temperature (T_{wb})

- Measurement of air temperature with a thermometer whose mercury bulb is covered with a wet cotton wick. This measure is sensitive to the relative humidity (water vapor pressure) and provides an index of the ability to evaporate sweat.

The formula used to calculate the WBGT index shows the importance of this latter wet bulb temperature in determining heat stress (3):

$$WBGT = 0.7\ T_{wb} + 0.2\ T_g + 0.1\ T_{db}$$

The risk of exertional heatstroke (EHS) is classified as follows (5, 97):

■ WBGT ≤50.0°F (≤10.0°C)	Risk of hypothermia; EHS can occur
■ WBGT 50–65°F (10–18.3°C)	Low risk of both hypothermia and hyperthermia; EHS can occur
■ WBGT 65.1–72.0°F (18.4–22.2°C)	Caution: risk of heat illness increases; high-risk persons monitored or do not compete
■ WBGT 72.1–78.0°F (22.3–25.6°C)	Extreme caution; risk of hyperthermia increased for all
■ WBGT 78.1–82.0°F (25.7–27.8°C)	Extreme caution; high risk for unfit, non-acclimatized
■ WBGT ≥82.1°F (≥27.9°C)	Extreme risk of hyperthermia; cancel or postpone

In spite of the wide acceptance of the WBGT index, it has been criticized because it is an environmental heat stress index and not a representation of human heat strain (93). Specific attention was directed at the WBGT index's tendency to underestimate heat-stress risk when evaporation of sweat is restricted (e.g., high humidity and/or low air movement). Further, since it is a climatic index, it does not account for metabolic heat production or clothing. The consensus panel concluded that it is therefore difficult to establish absolute cut-off values across sports and across the broad range of participants who might differ in terms of fitness and acclimatization. They suggest that the WBGT index be used as a guideline to implement preventive counter measures to offset the potential risk of heat illness (93). The most recent position statement of the National Athletic Trainers' Association does just that with an example that includes recommended rest breaks, length of practice, and so forth to prevent heat injury (21). We are sure that this new approach will influence the development of future guidelines for athletic competitions conducted in the heat.

In addition to environmental factors contributing to the risk of heat injury, there is no question about their impact on performance. For example, the fastest marathons are run at environmental temperatures of 10.6–12.8°C for men and 11.6–13.6°C for women; times are systematically slower with higher environmental temperatures (35). Not surprisingly, precooling the body prior to exercise in the heat has the potential to improve performance. A recent review on practical approaches to accomplish this concluded that cold drinks were most effective, followed by cooling packs and a cooled room (120). These various methods should be tested and individualized during training to minimize disruption to the athlete (93).

IN SUMMARY

- Heat injury is influenced by environmental factors such as temperature, water vapor pressure, acclimation, hydration, clothing, and metabolic rate. The fitness participant should be educated about the signs and symptoms of heat injury; the importance of drinking water before, during, and after the activity; gradually becoming acclimated to the heat; exercising in the cooler part of the day; dressing appropriately; and checking the HR on a regular basis.
- Road races conducted in times of elevated heat and humidity need to reflect the coordinated wisdom of the race director and medical director to minimize heat and other injuries. Concerns include running the race at the correct time of the day and season of the year; frequent water stops; traffic control; race monitors to identify and stop those in trouble; and communication between race monitors, medical director, ambulance services, and hospitals.

- The heat stress index includes dry bulb, wet bulb, and globe temperatures. The wet bulb temperature, which is a good indicator of the water vapor pressure, is more important than the other two in determining overall heat stress.

COLD

Altitude and heat stress are not the only environmental factors having an impact on performance. A WBGT of 10°C or less is associated with hypothermia. **Hypothermia** results when heat loss from the body exceeds heat production and is defined clinically as a core temperature below 35°C (95°F), which is a drop of about 2°C (3.5°F) below normal body temperature (4). Cold air facilitates this process in more ways than are readily apparent. First, and most obvious, when air temperature is less than skin temperature, a gradient for heat loss exists for convection, and physiological mechanisms involving peripheral vasoconstriction and shivering come into play to counter this gradient. Second, and less obvious, cold air has a low water vapor pressure, which encourages the evaporation of moisture from the skin to further cool the body. The combined effects can be deadly, as witnessed in Pugh's report of three deaths during a "walking" competition over a 45-mile distance (89).

Hypothermia, based on core temperature, can range in severity from mild to severe (4):

- Mild hypothermia
  - 35°C (95°F)—maximal shivering
  - 34°C (93.2°F)—amnesia, poor judgment
- Moderate hypothermia
  - 33°C (91.4°F)—ataxia, apathy
  - 31°C (87.8°F)—shivering ceases, pupils dilate
  - 29°C (85.2°F)—unconscious
- Severe hypothermia
  - 28°C (82.4°F)—ventricular fibrillation
  - 26°C (78.8°F)—no response to pain
  - 24°C (75.2°F)—hypotension, bradycardia
  - 19°C (66.2°F)—EEG silence
  - 13.7°C (56.7°F)—lowest temperature for adult survival

Figure 24.8 shows the factors related to hypothermia. These include environmental factors such as temperature, water vapor pressure, wind, and whether air or water is involved; insulating factors such as clothing and subcutaneous fat; the characteristics of the individuals involved (e.g., age and gender); and the capacity for sustained heat production, including fuels available (23). We will now comment on each of these relative to hypothermia. For a thorough presentation on this topic, see the American

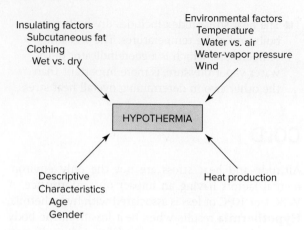

Figure 24.8 Factors affecting hypothermia.

College of Sports Medicine's Position Stand (4) and the National Athletic Trainers' Association position statement (18).

Environmental Factors

Heat loss mechanisms introduced in Chap. 12 included conduction, convection, radiation, and evaporation. Given that hypothermia is the result of higher heat loss than heat production, understanding how these mechanisms are involved will facilitate a discussion of how to deal with this problem.

Conduction, convection, and radiation are dependent on a temperature gradient between skin and environment; the larger the gradient, the greater the rate of heat loss. What is surprising is that the environmental temperature does not have to be below freezing to cause hypothermia. In effect, other environmental factors interact with temperature to create the dangerous condition by facilitating heat loss—namely, wind and water.

Wind Chill Index The rate of heat loss at any given temperature is directly influenced by the wind speed. Wind increases the number of cold air molecules coming into contact with the skin so that heat loss is accelerated. The **wind chill index** indicates what the "effective" temperature is for any combination of temperature and wind speed. Siple and Passel (108) developed a formula for predicting how fast heat would be lost at different wind speeds and temperatures:

Wind chill (kcal · m^{-2} · h^{-1}) =

$$[\sqrt{WV \times 100} + 10.45 - XV] \times (33 - T_A)$$

where WV = wind velocity (m · s^{-1}); 10.45 is a constant; 33 is 33°C, which is taken as the skin temperature; and T_A = ambient dry bulb temperature in °C. Siple and Passel estimated how long it would take for exposed flesh to freeze and tabulated the levels of "danger" associated with combinations of wind speed and temperature.

This formula (41), which had been used for many years, was thought to overestimate the effect of increasing wind speed on tissue freezing and underestimate the effect of decreasing temperature (29). The following wind chill formula has been adopted by the National Weather Service (**http://www.crh.noaa.gov/dtx/New_Wind_Chill.php**):

Wind chill (°F) = 35.74 + 0.6215 (T) − 35.75 (V$^{0.16}$) + 0.4275T (V$^{0.16}$)

where wind speed (V) is in mph and temperature (T) is in °F.

Table 24.4 provides the calculated wind chill temperatures for a variety of wind speeds and temperatures, along with estimates of the time it would take for frostbite to occur. Keep in mind that if you are running, riding, or cross-country skiing into the wind, you must add your speed to the wind speed to evaluate the full impact of the wind chill. For example, cycling at 20 mph into calm air at 0°F is equivalent to a wind chill temperature of −22° (23). When wind is coupled with rain, heat loss is dramatically increased compared to wind alone (130), and that leads us to the next section.

Water The thermal conductivity of water is about 25 times greater than that of air, so you can lose heat 25 times faster in water compared to air of the same temperature (57). Figure 24.9 shows death can occur in only a few hours when a person is shipwrecked in cold water. Unlike air, water offers little or no insulation at the skin-water interface, so heat is rapidly lost from the body. Given that movement in such cold water would increase heat loss from the arms and legs, the recommendation is to stay as still as possible in long-term immersions (4, 57). The impact that insulation, both body fat and clothing, has on the rate of heat loss will be considered next.

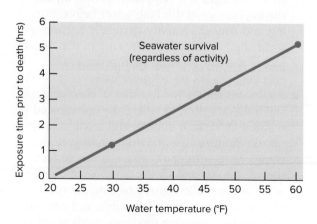

Figure 24.9 The effect of different water temperatures on survival of shipwrecked individuals.

TABLE 24.4 Wind Chill Chart

WIND (MPH)	TEMPERATURE (°F)																	
Calm	40	35	30	25	20	15	10	5	0	−5	−10	−15	−20	−25	−30	−35	−40	−45
5	36	31	25	19	13	7	1	−5	−11	−16	−22	−28	−34	−40	−46	−52	−57	−63
10	34	27	21	15	9	3	−4	−10	−16	−22	−28	−35	−41	−47	−53	−59	−66	−72
15	32	25	19	13	6	0	−7	−13	−19	−26	−32	−39	−45	−51	−58	−64	−71	−77
20	30	24	17	11	4	−2	−9	−15	−22	−29	−35	−42	−48	−55	−61	−68	−74	−81
25	29	23	16	9	3	−4	−11	−17	−24	−31	−37	−44	−51	−58	−64	−71	−78	−84
30	28	22	15	8	1	−5	−12	−19	−26	−33	−39	−46	−53	−60	−67	−73	−80	−87
35	28	21	14	7	0	−7	−14	−21	−27	−34	−41	−48	−55	−62	−69	−76	−82	−89
40	27	20	13	6	−1	−8	−15	−22	−29	−36	−43	−50	−57	−64	−71	−78	−84	−91
45	26	19	12	5	−2	−9	−16	−23	−30	−37	−44	−51	−58	−65	−72	−79	−86	−93
50	26	19	12	4	−3	−10	−17	−24	−31	−38	−45	−52	−60	−67	−74	−81	−88	−95
55	25	18	11	4	−3	−11	−18	−25	−32	−39	−46	−54	−61	−68	−75	−82	−89	−97
60	25	17	10	3	−4	−11	−19	−26	−33	−40	−48	−55	−62	−69	−76	−84	−91	−98

Frostbite Times   ■ 30 minutes   ■ 10 minutes   ■ 5 minutes

Wind Chill (°F) = 35.74 + 0.6215T − 35.75 (V$^{0.16}$) + 0.4275 (V$^{0.16}$)

Where T = Air Temperature (°F)   V = Wind Speed (mph)

(Effective 11/01/01)

■ Hypothermia is influenced by natural and added insulation, environmental temperature, vapor pressure, wind, water immersion, and heat production.

■ The wind chill index describes how wind lowers the effective temperature at the skin such that convective heat loss is greater than what it would be in calm air at that same temperature.

■ Water causes heat to be lost by convection 25 times faster than it would be by exposure to air of the same temperature.

Insulating Factors

The rate at which heat is lost from the body is inversely related to the insulation between the body and the environment. The insulating quality is related to the thickness of subcutaneous fat, the ability of clothing to trap air, and whether the clothing is wet or dry.

Subcutaneous Fat An excellent indicator of total body insulation per unit surface area (through which heat is lost) is the average subcutaneous fat thickness (52). Pugh and Edholm's (90) observation that a "fat" man was able to swim for seven hours in 16°C water with no change in body temperature, whereas a "thin" man had to leave the water in 30 minutes with a core temperature of 34.5°C, supports this statement. Long-distance swimmers tend to be fatter than short-course swimmers. The higher body fatness does more than help maintain body temperature; fatter swimmers are more buoyant, requiring less energy to swim at any set speed (55). In addition, body fatness plays a role in the onset and magnitude of the shivering response to cold exposure (see later discussion in the "Heat Production" section).

Clothing Clothing can extend our natural subcutaneous fat insulation to allow us to sustain very cold environments. The insulation quality of clothing is given in **clo** units, where 1 clo is the insulation needed at rest (1 MET) to maintain core temperature when the environment is 21°C, the RH = 50%, and the air movement is 6 m · min⁻¹ (13). Still air next to the body has a clo rating of 0.8. As the air temperature falls, clothing with a higher clo value must be worn to maintain core temperature, because the gradient between skin and environment increases (85). Figure 24.10 shows the insulation needed at different energy expenditures across a broad range of temperatures from −50 to +30°C (−60 to +80°F) (13). It is clear that as heat production increases, insulation must decrease to maintain core temperature. By

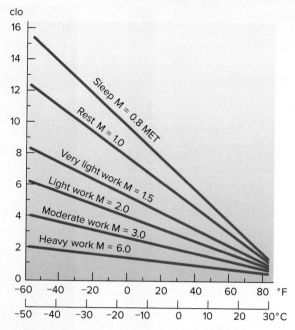

Figure 24.10 Changes in the insulation requirement of clothing (plus air) with increasing rates of energy expenditure over environmental temperatures of −50 to +30°C.

wearing clothing in layers, insulation can be removed piece by piece because less insulation is needed to maintain core temperature. By following these steps, sweating, which can rob the clothing of its insulating value, will be minimized. A practical example of how clothing helps maintain body temperature (and comfort) can be seen in the following study. Heat loss from the head increases linearly from +32°C to −21°C, with about half of the entire heat production being lost through the head when the temperature is −4°C. Wearing a simple "helmet" with a clo rating of 3.5 allows an individual to stay out indefinitely at 0°C (40).

Clothing offers insulation by trapping air, which is a poor conductor of heat. If the clothing becomes wet, the insulating quality decreases because the water can now conduct heat away from the body at a faster rate (57). A primary goal, then, is to avoid wetness due either to sweat or to weather. This problem is exacerbated by the cold environment's very low water vapor pressure. Recall from Chap. 12 that the water vapor pressure in the environment is the primary factor influencing evaporation and that at low environmental temperatures, the water vapor pressure is low even when the relative humidity is high. Think of a time when you finished playing a game indoors and stepped outside into cold, damp weather to cool off. You noticed "steam" coming off your body; how is this possible when the RH is near 100%? The water vapor pressure is high at the skin surface, since the skin temperature is elevated, so a gradient for water vapor pressure exists. You will cool off very fast under these circumstances. This is why cold, wet, windy environments carry an extra risk of hypothermia. The wind not only provides for greater convective heat loss as described in the wind chill chart, but it also accelerates evaporation (50).

Heat Production

Figure 24.10 shows that the amount of insulation needed to maintain core temperature decreases as energy expenditure increases. This is also true for our "natural" insulation, subcutaneous fat. McArdle et al. (81) showed that when fat men (27.6% fat) were immersed for one hour in 20°C, 24°C, and 28°C water, the resting $\dot{V}O_2$ and core temperature did not change compared to values measured in air. In thinner men (<16.8% fat), the $\dot{V}O_2$ increased to counter the rapid loss of heat; however, the core temperature still decreased. When these same subjects did exercise in the cold water, requiring a $\dot{V}O_2$ of 1.7 L·min^{-1}, the fall in body temperature was either prevented or retarded (82), showing the importance of high rates of heat production in preventing hypothermia. Other studies support these observations, showing an earlier onset and greater magnitude of shivering in lean subjects when exposed to cold air (114). Similar findings have been reported for fit subjects (8).

Fuel Use Shivering can increase oxygen consumption to 1000 ml/min during resting immersion in cold water, and like moderate exercise of the same intensity, fat is a primary fuel to support shivering in well-fed individuals (4). However, it is clear that inadequate carbohydrate stores may lead to hypoglycemia, which can affect one's ability to shiver. Further, bursts of shivering lead to greater muscle glycogen depletion. Consequently, having adequate carbohydrate stores is important to reduce the risk for hypothermia (4). Given the importance of body fatness and body type in the metabolic response to cold exposure, are there differences due to gender and age?

Descriptive Characteristics

Subject characteristics, such as gender and age, influence the metabolic and body temperature responses to cold exposure.

Gender Sex differences in response to cold water exposure are linked to a woman's higher body fatness, thicker subcutaneous layer, less lean mass, and higher surface area-to-mass ratio, compared to men of the same weight and age. At rest, women show a faster reduction in body temperature than do men, even when subcutaneous fat thickness is the same. In contrast, when exercise is done in cold water, women and men of the same body fatness have similar decreases in body temperature. Consequently, any gender differences in core temperature responses to cold exposure can be explained primarily on the basis of differences in body composition and anthropometry (23). It must be added that amenorrheic women cannot maintain core temperature during exercise in the cold as well as eumenorrheic women can (4).

Age In general, individuals over 60 years may be less tolerant to cold exposures than younger individuals because the ability of older individuals to vasoconstrict skin blood vessels and conserve heat is reduced. They also have less thermal sensitivity. That is, their response to a decrease in temperature is reduced, allowing time for greater heat loss. In contrast to adults, children have a larger surface area-to-mass ratio and less subcutaneous fat. This results in a faster fall in core temperature with cold water exposure and a greater risk of hypothermia. Similar to the gender differences (or lack thereof) mentioned earlier, 11- to 12-year-old boys with the same subcutaneous fat as men had the same core temperature response when doing exercise in cold air (4). See A Look Back–Important People in Science for an individual who had a major impact on our understanding of the physiology of how humans adapt to extreme environments.

IN SUMMARY

- Subcutaneous fat is the primary "natural" insulation and is effective in preventing rapid heat loss when a person is exposed to cold water.
- Clothing extends this insulation, and the insulation value of clothing is described in clo units, where a value of 1 describes what is needed to maintain core temperature while sitting in a room set at 21°C and 50% RH with an air movement of 6 m·s^{-1}.
- The amount of insulation needed to maintain core temperature is less when one exercises because the metabolic heat production helps maintain the core temperature. Clothing should be worn in layers when exercising so one can shed one insulating layer at a time as body temperature increases.
- Heat production increases with exposure to cold, with an inverse relationship between the increase in $\dot{V}O_2$ and body fatness. Women cool faster than men when exposed to cold water, exhibiting a longer delay in the onset of shivering and a lower $\dot{V}O_2$, despite a greater stimulus to shiver.

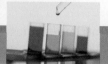
L. G. C. E. Pugh Furthered Our Understanding of How to Survive and Function Well in Extreme Environments

In this chapter that deals with the effect of cold, heat, and altitude on performance, we thought it would be appropriate to highlight an individual who had a major impact on our understanding of the physiology involved in adapting to adverse environments: **Lewis Griffith Cresswell Evans (L.G.C.E.) Pugh, M.D.**

L.G.C.E. Pugh was born in 1909 in England. He attended New College, Oxford, and completed his B.A. in 1931. He then studied natural sciences during 1931–1933 and medicine until 1938, at which time he received his B.M. and M.A. degrees. He was a competitive downhill and cross-country skier and qualified for England's 1936 Winter Olympics. In 1939, he entered the army as a medical officer and served in Europe and the Middle East. In 1943, he was sent to the Mountain Warfare Training Centre in Lebanon to select, train, and evaluate troops for mountain warfare. There he became involved in the systematic study of the interaction of altitude, environmental temperature, nutrition, clothing, and fitness on human performance, and he developed training manuals based on his work. Following the war he was involved in British navy research expeditions to the Arctic, and in 1950, he accepted a position in the Medical Research Council's Division in Human Physiology to study the effects of extreme environments.

Dr. Pugh was a major participant in several high-altitude expeditions during the 1950s and 1960s. The first, in 1952, gave him insight into what kinds of clothing, nutrition, hydration, and oxygen were required for humans to function at extreme altitudes. His work was recognized as being crucial to the success of the 1953 British expedition to Mt. Everest in which Edmund Hillary and Tenzing Norgay were the first to reach the summit. In the late 1950s, he joined Edmund Hillary for an Antarctic expedition in which he studied human tolerance to extreme cold; it was also during this time that the two planned to return to Everest. Dr. Pugh was the principal scientist in the 1960–1961 Scientific and Mountaineering Expedition to Everest that provided ground-breaking, and yet fundamental, information about how humans adapt to chronic exposure to high altitude. In addition, in the late 1960s, he was involved in helping athletes prepare for the Olympic Games that were to take place in Mexico City at an altitude of ~2300 m. His life's work revolved around understanding how humans adapt to exercise in extreme environments, and his findings are as relevant today as they were 60 years ago. He died in 1994.

Sources: Hansen, Peter H.; "Pugh, (Lewis) Griffith Cresswell Evans (1909–1994), physiologist and mountaineer," *Oxford Dictionary of National Biography*; The Register of L. G. C. E. Pugh Papers 1940–1986. San Diego, CA: Mandeville Special Collections Library, Geisel Library, University of California.

Dealing with Hypothermia

As body temperature falls, the person's ability to carry out coordinated movements is reduced, speech is slurred, and judgment is impaired. As mentioned earlier, people can die from hypothermia, and the condition must be dealt with when it occurs. The following steps on how to do this are taken from the National Athletic Trainers' Association position statement on cold injuries (18):

- **Mild hypothermia**
  - Remove wet or damp clothing.
  - Insulate the person with warm dry clothing or blankets, covering the head.
  - Move person to warm environment with shelter from wind and rain.
  - When rewarming, apply heat only to the trunk and other areas of heat transfer (axilla, chest wall, groin).
  - Provide warm, nonalcoholic fluids and food containing 6%–8% carbohydrate.

- **Moderate/severe hypothermia**
  - Determine if CPR is necessary and activate emergency medical system.
  - Remove wet or damp clothing.
  - Insulate the person with warm, dry clothing or blankets, covering the head.
  - Move person to warm environment with shelter from wind and rain.
  - When rewarming, apply heat only to the trunk and other areas of heat transfer (axilla, chest wall, groin).
  - If physician is not present, initiate rewarming strategies immediately and continue during transport.
  - During treatment/transit, continue to monitor vital signs and be prepared for airway management.

IN SUMMARY

- For mild hypothermia, get the person out of the wind, rain, and cold; remove wet clothing and put on dry clothing; for rewarming, apply heat only to the trunk and other areas of heat transfer; and provide warm drinks and food.
- For moderate/severe hypothermia do as noted earlier, check vital signs, activate emergency medical system, and transport.

AIR POLLUTION

Air pollution includes a variety of gases and particulates that are products of the combustion of fossil fuels. The "smog" that results when these pollutants are in high concentration can have a detrimental effect on health and performance. The gases can affect performance by decreasing the capacity to transport oxygen, increasing airway resistance, and altering the perception of effort required when the eyes "burn" and the chest "hurts." A study on traffic policemen, who are routinely exposed to a full range of pollutants throughout their workday, makes the point. Although their physiological responses were normal at rest, during an exercise test, about one-third of the policemen experienced ECG changes and elevated blood pressure responses, with the vast majority of those individuals also experiencing a desaturation of hemoglobin (116). In addition, children living in an air-polluted environment had significantly lower $\dot{V}O_2$ max values compared to those living in areas with better air quality (132).

The physiological responses to these pollutants are related to the amount, or "dose," received. The major factors determining the dose are the concentration of the pollutant, the duration of the exposure to the pollutant, and the volume of air inhaled (concentration $\times$ time $\times$ V_E). This last factor increases during exercise and is one reason why physical activity should be curtailed during times of peak pollution levels (38). The following discussion focuses on the major air pollutants: particulate matter, ozone, sulfur dioxide, and carbon monoxide.

Particulate Matter

The air is full of microscopic and submicroscopic particles, many of which can be tied to motor vehicles (especially diesels) and industrial sources. Over the past five years, more attention has been focused on the very small particles because of their potential to promote pulmonary infection and actually cross the epithelium to enter the circulation (26, 43). Fine (<2.5 μm diameter), and especially ultrafine (<0.1 μm diameter), particles interact with environmental factors to promote local inflammation and oxidative stress that can lead to impaired pulmonary, cardiovascular, and immune function (26, 43). For example, when an endurance-training program was conducted in an urban versus a rural setting, there were no differences in gains in $\dot{V}O_2$ max; however, in the urban setting (with its high level of ultrafine particulate pollution), there was an increase in inflammatory biomarkers (9, 10). Consequently, athletes, especially those susceptible to pulmonary diseases (e.g., asthma), should minimize exposure whenever possible (see section on carbon monoxide). A case in point is that exposure to particulate matter prior to

exercise was associated with ECG abnormalities during exercise (43).

Ozone

The ozone we breathe is generated by the reaction of UV light and emissions from internal combustion engines. While a single two-hour exposure to a high ozone concentration, 0.75 part per million (ppm), decreases $\dot{V}O_2$ max, others studies show that a two-hour exposure to less than half that concentration, 0.3 ppm, increases inflammatory biomarkers and decreases lung function (31). The impact on $\dot{V}O_2$ max follows a does response pattern: for every 0.017 ppm increase in ozone, aerobic fitness decreases 1.5% (43). Finally, prolonged exposure (6-12 hours) to only 0.12 ppm (the U.S. air quality standard) decreases lung function and increases respiratory symptoms. Interestingly, an adaptation to ozone exposure can occur, with subjects showing a diminished response to subsequent exposures during the "ozone season." However, concern about long-term lung health suggests that it would be prudent to avoid heavy exercise during the time of day when ozone and other pollutants are elevated (38).

Sulfur Dioxide

Sulfur dioxide (SO_2) is produced by smelters, refineries, and electrical utilities that use fossil fuel for energy generation. SO_2 does not affect lung function in normal subjects, but it causes bronchoconstriction in people with asthma. These latter responses are influenced by the temperature and humidity of the inspired air, as mentioned in Chap. 17. Nose breathing is encouraged to "scrub" the SO_2, and drugs like cromolyn sodium and β_2-agonists can partially block the response to SO_2 in someone with asthma (38).

Carbon Monoxide

Carbon monoxide (CO) is derived from the burning of fossil fuel, coal, oil, gasoline, and wood, as well as from cigarette smoke. Carbon monoxide can bind to hemoglobin to form carboxyhemoglobin (HbCO) and decrease the capacity for oxygen transport. This has the potential to affect the physiological responses to submaximal exercise (53) and $\dot{V}O_2$ max, as does altitude. The carbon monoxide concentration [HbCO] in blood is generally less than 1% in nonsmokers, but may be as high as 10% in smokers (95). Horvath et al. (58) found that the critical concentration of HbCO needed to decrease $\dot{V}O_2$ max was 4.3%. Figure 24.11 shows the relationship between the blood HbCO concentration and the decrease in $\dot{V}O_2$ max; beyond 4.3% HbCO, $\dot{V}O_2$ max decreases 1% for each 1% increase in HbCO (96).

In contrast, when one performs light work, at about 40% $\dot{V}O_2$ max, the [HbCO] can be as high as 15% before endurance is affected. The cardiovascular system has the capacity to compensate with a larger

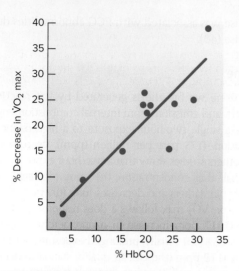

Figure 24.11 The effect of the concentration of carbon monoxide in the blood on the change in $\dot{V}O_2$ max.

cardiac output when the HbO_2 concentration is reduced during submaximal work (58, 95, 96). Because it takes two to four hours to remove half the CO from the blood after the exposure has been removed, CO can have a lasting effect on performances (38).

Unfortunately, it is difficult to predict what the actual [HbCO] will be in any given environment. One must consider the previous exposure to the pollutant, as well as the length of time and rate of ventilation associated with the current exposure. As a result, Raven (95) provides the following guidelines for exercising in an area with air pollution:

- Reduce exposure to the pollutant prior to exercise because the physiological effects are time- and dose-dependent.

- Stay away from areas where you might receive a "bolus" dose of CO: smoking areas, high-traffic areas, urban environments.

- Do not schedule activities around the times when pollutants are at their highest levels (7–10 A.M. and 4–7 P.M.) due to traffic.

The **Air Quality Index (AQI)** is a measure of the quality of the air for five major air pollutants regulated by the Clean Air Act: ground-level ozone, particulate matter, carbon monoxide, sulfur dioxide, and nitrogen dioxide. Figure 24.12 shows a color-coded chart of the AIQ, with the interpretation of what the numerical values mean. Information on the AIQ is generally provided in a local community's weather forecast and should be suited to the individual–some will experience symptoms at lower levels of pollution than others (17).

IN SUMMARY

- Air pollution can affect performance. Exposure to ozone decreases $\dot{V}O_2$ max and respiratory function, and sulfur dioxide causes bronchoconstriction in people with asthma.
- Carbon monoxide binds to hemoglobin and reduces oxygen transport.
- To prevent problems associated with pollution of any type, reduce exposure time, stay away from "bolus" amounts of the pollutant, and schedule activity at the least polluted part of the day.
- The Air Quality Index should be monitored to determine if conditions are safe for exercising outdoors.

Air Quality Index Levels of Health Concern	Numerical Value	Meaning
Good	0 to 50	Air quality is considered satisfactory, and air pollution poses little or no risk.
Moderate	51 to 100	Air quality is acceptable; however, for some pollutants there may be a moderate health concern for a very small number of people who are unusually sensitive to air pollution.
Unhealthy for Sensitive Groups	101 to 150	Members of sensitive groups may experience health effects. The general public is not likely to be affected.
Unhealthy	151 to 200	Everyone may begin to experience health effects; members of sensitive groups may experience more serious health effects.
Very Unhealthy	201 to 300	Health warnings of emergency conditions. The entire population is more likely to be affected.
Hazardous	301 to 500	Health alert: everyone may experience more serious health effects.

Figure 24.12 The Air Quality Index (AQI)–A Guide to Air Quality and Your Health. AIRNow website.
Available at: https://airnow.gov/index.cfm?action=aqibasics.aqi.

STUDY ACTIVITIES

1. Describe the changes in barometric pressure, PO_2, and air density with increasing altitude.
2. Why is sprint performance not affected by altitude?
3. Explain why maximal aerobic power decreases at altitude and what effect this has on performance in long-distance races.
4. Graphically describe the effect of altitude on the HR and ventilation responses to submaximal work and provide recommendations for fitness participants who occasionally exercise at altitude.
5. Describe the physiological processes by which high-altitude residents in the Andes adapt to altitude compared to those who live in Tibet.
6. While training at altitude can be beneficial, how could someone "detrain"? How can you work around this problem?
7. It was formerly believed that a person could not climb Mount Everest without oxygen because the estimated $\dot{V}O_2$ max at altitude was close to basal metabolic rate. When two climbers accomplished the feat in 1978, scientists had to determine how this was possible. What were the primary reasons allowing the climb to take place without oxygen?
8. List and describe the factors related to heat injury.
9. What is the heat stress index, and why is the wet bulb temperature weighed so heavily in the formula?
10. List the factors related to hypothermia.
11. Explain what the wind chill index is relative to convective heat loss.
12. What is a clo unit, and why is the insulation requirement less when you exercise?
13. What would you do if a person had hypothermia?
14. Explain how carbon monoxide can influence $\dot{V}O_2$ max and endurance performance.
15. What steps would you follow to minimize the effect of pollution on performance?

SUGGESTED READINGS

Howe, A. S., and B. P. Boden. 2007. Heat-related illness in athletes. *American Journal of Sports Medicine* 35: 1384–95.

Kenney, W. L., and T. A. Munce. 2003. Invited review: aging and human temperature regulation. *Journal of Applied Physiology* 95: 598–603.

Messner, R. 1999. *Everest: Expedition to the Ultimate.* Seattle, WA: Mountaineers Books. (A story of the first trip to the summit by Messner and Habeler without oxygen.)

Roberts, W. O. Determining a "do not start" temperature for a marathon on the basis of adverse outcomes. *Medicine and Science in Sports and Exercise* 2: 226–232, 2010.

REFERENCES

1. **Adams WC, Bernauer EM, Dill DB, and Bomar JB, Jr.** Effects of equivalent sea-level and altitude training on $\dot{V}O_2$ max and running performance. *Journal of Applied Physiology* 39: 262–266, 1975.
2. **Alexander JK, Hartley LH, Modelski M, and Grover RF.** Reduction of stroke volume during exercise in man–following ascent to 3,100 m altitude. *Journal of Applied Physiology* 23: 849–858, 1967.
3. **American College of Sports Medicine.** Position stand: heat and cold illnesses during distance running. *Medicine and Science in Sports and Exercise* 28: i–x, 1996.
4. **American College of Sports Medicine.** Position stand: prevention of cold injuries during exercise. *Medicine and Science in Sports and Exercise* 38: 2012–2029, 2006.
5. **American College of Sports Medicine.** Position stand. Exertional heat illness during training and competition. *Medicine and Science in Sports and Exercise* 39: 556–572, 2007.
6. **Arsac LM.** Effect of altitude on the energetics of human best performances in 100 m running: a theoretical analysis. *European Journal of Applied Physiology.* 87: 78–84, 2002.
7. **Balke B, Nagle FJ, and Daniels J.** Altitude and maximum performance in work and sports activity. *JAMA* 194: 646–649, 1965.
8. **Bittel JH, Nonotte-Varly C, Livecchi-Gonnot GH, Savourey GL, and Hanniquet AM.** Physical fitness and thermoregulatory reactions in a cold environment in men. *Journal of Applied Physiology* 65: 1984–1989, 1988.
9. **Bos I, De Boever P, Vanparijs J, Pattyn N, Panis LI, and Meeusen R.** Subclinical effects of aerobic training in urban environment. *Medicine and Science in Sports and Exercise.* 45: 439–447, 2013.
10. **Brauner EV, Forchhammer L, Moller P, Simonsen J, Glasius M, Wahlin P, et al.** Exposure to ultrafine particles from ambient air and oxidative stress-induced DNA damage. *Environmental Health Perspectives* 115: 1177–1182, 2007.
11. **Brazaitis M, Kamandulis S, Skurvydas A, and Daniuseviciute L.** The effect of two kinds of t-shirts on physiological and psychological thermal responses during exercise and recovery. *Applied Ergonomics* 42: 46–51, 2010.
12. **Buono MJ and Sjoholm NT.** Effect of physical training on peripheral sweat production. *Journal of Applied Physiology* 65: 811–814, 1988.
13. **Burton A and Edholm O.** *Man in a Cold Environment .* London: Edward Arnold, 1955.
14. **Buskirk E and Bass D.** Climate and exercise. In *Science and Medicine of Exercise and Sport*, edited by Johnson W, and Buskirk E. New York, NY: Harper & Row, 1974, pp. 190–205.
15. **Buskirk E and Grasley W.** Heat injury and conduct of athletics. In *Science and Medicine of Exercise and Sport*, edited by Johnson W, and Buskirk E. New York, NY: Harper & Row, 1974, pp. 206–210.
16. **Buskirk ER, Kollias J, Akers RF, Prokop EK, and Reategui EP.** Maximal performance at altitude and on return from altitude in conditioned runners. *Journal of Applied Physiology* 23: 259–266, 1967.
17. **Campbell ME, Li Q, Gingrich SE, Macfarlane RG, and Cheng S.** Should people be physically active outdoors on smog alert days? *Canadian Journal of Public Health* 96: 24–28, 2005.
18. **Cappaert TA, Stone JA, Castellani JW, Krause BA, Smith D, and Stephens BA.** National Athletic Trainers'

Association postion statement: environmental cold injuries. *Journal of Athletic Training* 43: 640-658, 2008.

19. **Carter JE and Gisolfi CV.** Fluid replacement during and after exercise in the heat. *Medicine and Science in Sports and Exercise* 21: 532-539, 1989.

20. **Casa DJ, Armstrong LE, Kenny GP, O'Conner FG, and Huggins RA.** Exertional heat stroke: new concepts regarding cause and care. *Current Sports Medicine Reports* 11: 115-123, 2012.

21. **Casa DJ, DeMartini JK, Bergeron MF, Csillan D, Eichner ER, Lopez RM, Ferrara MS, Miller KC, O'Connor F, Sawka MN, and Yeargin SW.** National Athletic Trainers' Association Position Statement: exertional heat illnesses. *Journal of Athletic Training.* 50: 986-1000, 2015.

22. **Casa DJ, McDermott BP, Lee EC, Yeargin SW, Armstrong LE, and Maresh CM.** Cold water immersion: the gold standard for exertional heatstroke treatment. *Exercise and Sport Sciences Reviews* 35: 141-149, 2007.

23. **Castellani JW and Young AJ.** Health and performance challenges during sports training and competition in cold weather. *British Journal of Sports Medicine.* 46: 788-791, 2012.

24. **Chapman RF, Stray-Gundersen J, and Levine BD.** Individual variation in response to altitude training. *Journal of Applied Physiology* 85: 1448-1456, 1998.

25. **Costill DL, Cote R, Miller E, Miller T, and Wynder S.** Water and electrolyte replacement during repeated days of work in the heat. *Aviation, Space, and Environmental Medicine* 46: 795-800, 1975.

26. **Cutrufello PT, Smoliga JM, and Rundell KW.** Small things make a big difference: particulate matter and exercise. *Sports Medicine* 42: 1041-1068, 2012.

27. **Cymerman A, Reeves JT, Sutton JR, Rock PB, Groves BM, Malconian MK, et al.** Operation Everest II: maximal oxygen uptake at extreme altitude. *Journal of Applied Physiology* 66: 2446-2453, 1989.

28. **Daniels J and Oldridge N.** The effects of alternate exposure to altitude and sea level on world-class middle-distance runners. *Medicine and Science in Sports* 2: 107-112, 1970.

29. **Danielsson U.** Windchill and the risk of tissue freezing. *Journal of Applied Physiology* 81: 2666-2673, 1996.

30. **Davis JK, and Bishop PA.** Impact of clothing on exercise in the heat. *Sports Medicine* 43:695-706, 2013.

31. **Devlin RB, Duncan KE, Jardim M, Schmitt MT, Rappold AG, and Diaz-Sanchez D.** Controlled exposure of healthy young volunteers to ozone causes cardiovascular effects. *Circulation* 126: 104-111, 2012.

32. **Dill DB and Adams WC.** Maximal oxygen uptake at sea level and at 3,090-m altitude in high school champion runners. *Journal of Applied Physiology* 30: 854-859, 1971.

33. **Doria C, Toniolo L, Verratti V, Cancellara P, Pietrangelo T, Marconi V, et al.** Improved V̇O₂ uptake kinetics and shift in muscle fiber type in high-altitude trekkers. *Journal of Applied Physiology* 111:1597-1605, 2011.

34. **Drinkwater BL, Denton JE, Kupprat IC, Talag TS, and Horvath SM.** Aerobic power as a factor in women's response to work in hot environments. *Journal of Applied Physiology* 41: 815-821, 1976.

35. **Ely MR, Cheuvront SN, and Montain SJ.** Neither cloud cover nor low solar loads are associated with fast marathon performance. *Medicine and Science in Sports and Exercise* 39: 2029-2035, 2007.

36. **Engfred K, Kjaer M, Secher NH, Friedman DB, Hanel B, Nielsen OJ, et al.** Hypoxia and training-induced adaptation of hormonal responses to exercise in humans. *European Journal of Applied Physiology and Occupational Physiology* 68: 303-309, 1994.

37. **Faulkner JA, Kollias J, Favour CB, Buskirk ER, and Balke B.** Maximum aerobic capacity and running

performance at altitude. *Journal of Applied Physiology* 24: 685-691, 1968.

38. **Folinsbee L.** Discussion: exercise and the environment. In *Exercise, Fitness, and Health,* edited by Bouchard C, Shephard R, Stevens T, Sutton J, and McPherson B. Champaign, IL: Human Kinetics, 1990, pp. 179-183.

39. **Frisancho AR, Martinez C, Velasquez T, Sanchez J, and Montoye H.** Influence of developmental adaptation on aerobic capacity at high altitude. *Journal of Applied Physiology* 34: 176-180, 1973.

40. **Froese G and Burton AC.** Heat losses from the human head. *Journal of Applied Physiology* 10: 235-241, 1957.

41. **Gates D.** *Man and His Environment: Climate.* New York, NY: Harper & Row, 1972.

42. **Gilbert-Kawai ET, Milledge JS, Grocott MPW, and Martin DS.** King of the mountains: Tibetan and Sherpa physiological adaptations for life at high altitude. *Physiology.* 29: 388-402, 2014.

43. **Giles LV and Koehle MS.** The health effects of exercising in air pollution. *Sports Medicine.* 44: 223-249, 2014.

44. **Gilchrist J, Murphy M, Comstock RD, Collins C, McIlvain N, and Yard E.** Heat illness among high school athletes-United States, 2005-2009. *Morbidity and Mortality Weekly Report* 59: 1009-1013, 2010.

45. **Gisolfi CV and Cohen JS.** Relationships among training, heat acclimation, and heat tolerance in men and women: the controversy revisited. *Medicine and Science in Sports* 11: 56-59, 1979.

46. **Green HJ, Sutton JR, Cymerman A, Young PM, and Houston CS.** Operation Everest II: adaptations in human skeletal muscle. *Journal of Applied Physiology* 66: 2454-2461, 1989.

47. **Grover RF, Reeves JT, Grover EB, and Leathers JE.** Muscular exercise in young men native to 3,100 m altitude. *Journal of Applied Physiology* 22: 555-564, 1967.

48. **Guy JH, Deakin GB, Edwards AM, Miller CM, and Pyne DB.** Adaptation to hot environmental conditions: an exploration of the performance basis, procedures and future directions to optimize opportunities for elite athletes. *Sports Medicine.* 45: 303-311, 2015.

49. **Hanson PG and Zimmerman SW.** Exertional heatstroke in novice runners. *JAMA* 242: 154-157, 1979.

50. **Hardy J and Bard P.** Body temperature regulation. In *Medical Physiology,* edited by Mount-Castle V. St. Louis, MO: C. V. Mosby, 1974, pp. 1305-1342.

51. **Hartley LH, Vogel JA, and Cruz JC.** Reduction of maximal exercise heart rate at altitude and its reversal with atropine. *Journal of Applied Physiology* 36: 362-365, 1974.

52. **Hayward MG, and Keatinge WR.** Roles of subcutaneous fat and thermoregulatory reflexes in determining ability to stabilize body temperature in water. *Journal of Physiology* 320: 229-251, 1981.

53. **Hirsch GL, Sue DY, Wasserman K, Robinson TE, and Hansen JE.** Immediate effects of cigarette smoking on cardiorespiratory responses to exercise. *Journal of Applied Physiology* 58: 1975-1981, 1985.

54. **Hobson RM, Clapp EL, Watson P, and Maughan RJ.** Exercise capacity in the heat is greater in the morning than in the evening in man. *Medicine and Science in Sports and Exercise* 41: 174-180, 2009.

55. **Holmer I.** Physiology of swimming man. In *Exercise and Sport Sciences Reviews,* edited by Hutton R, and Miller D. Salt Lake City, UT: Franklin Institute, 1979.

56. **Hoppeler H, Kleinert E, Schlegel C, Claassen H, Howald H, Kayar SR, et al.** Morphological adaptations of human skeletal muscle to chronic hypoxia. *International Journal of Sports Medicine* 11 (Suppl 1): S3-9, 1990.

57. **Horvath SM.** Exercise in a cold environment. In *Exercise and Sport Sciences Reviews*, edited by Miller D. Salt Lake City, UT: Franklin Institute, 1981, pp. 221-263.

58. **Horvath SM, Raven PB, Dahms TE, and Gray DJ.** Maximal aerobic capacity at different levels of carboxyhemoglobin. *Journal of Applied Physiology* 38: 300-303, 1975.

59. **Houmard JA, Costill DL, Davis JA, Mitchell JB, Pascoe DD, and Robergs RA.** The influence of exercise intensity on heat acclimation in trained subjects. *Medicine and Science in Sports and Exercise* 22: 615-620, 1990.

60. **Howald H, Pette D, Simoneau JA, Uber A, Hoppeler H, and Cerretelli P.** Effect of chronic hypoxia on muscle enzyme activities. *International Journal of Sports Medicine* 11 (Suppl 1): S10-14, 1990.

61. **Howley E.** Effect of altitude on physical performance. In *Encyclopedia of Physical Education, Fitness, and Sports: Training, Environment, Nutrition, and Fitness*, edited by Stull G, and Cureton T. Salt Lake City, UT: Brighton, 1980, pp. 177-187.

62. **Hubbard R, and Armstrong LE.** Hyperthermia: new thoughts on an old problem. *Physician and Sportsmedicine* 17: 97-113, 1989.

63. **Hughson RL, Green HJ, Houston ME, Thomson JA, MacLean DR, and Sutton JR.** Heat injuries in Canadian mass participation runs. *Canadian Medical Association Journal* 122: 1141-1144, 1980.

64. **Hurtado A.** Animals in high altitudes: resident man. In *Handbook of Physiology: Section 4–Adaptation to the Environment*, edited by Dill D. Washington, D.C.: American Physiological Society, 1964.

65. **Kayser B.** Nutrition and energetics of exercise at altitude. Theory and possible practical implications. *Sports Medicine* 17: 309-323, 1994.

66. **Kollias J and Buskirk E.** Exercise and altitude. In *Science and Medicine of Exercise and Sport*, edited by Johnson W, and Buskirk E. New York, NY: Harper & Row, 1974.

67. **Kollias J, Buskirk ER, Akers RF, Prokop EK, Baker PT, and Picon-Reategui E.** Work capacity of long-time residents and newcomers to altitude. *Journal of Applied Physiology* 24: 792-799, 1968.

68. **Lawler J, Powers SK, and Thompson D.** Linear relationship between $\dot{V}O_{2\,max}$ and $\dot{V}O_{2\,max}$ decrement during exposure to acute hypoxia. *Journal of Applied Physiology* 64: 1486-1492, 1988.

69. **Lorenzo S, Halliwill JR, Sawka MN, and Minson CT.** Heat acclimation improves exercise performance. *Journal of Applied Physiology* 109: 1140-1147, 2010.

70. **Lundby C, and Robach P.** Does 'altitude training' increase exercise performance in elite athletes? *Experimental Physiology.* 101.7: 783-788, 2016.

71. **Lundby C, Millet GP, Calbet JA, Bärtsch P, and Subudhi AW.** Does 'altitude training' increase exercise performance in elite athletes? *British Journal of Sports Medicine.* 46: 792-795, 2012.

72. **MacDougall JD, Green HJ, Sutton JR, Coates G, Cymerman A, Young P, et al.** Operation Everest II: structural adaptations in skeletal muscle in response to extreme simulated altitude. *Acta Physiologica Scandinavica* 142: 421-427, 1991.

73. **Marconi C, Marzorati M, Grassi B, Basnyat B, Colombini A, Kayser B, et al.** Second generation Tibetan lowlanders acclimatize to high altitude more quickly than Caucasians. *Journal of Physiology* 556: 661-671, 2004.

74. **Martin D and O'Kroy J.** Effects of acute hypoxia on the $\dot{V}O_{2\,max}$ of trained and untrained subjects. *Journal of Sports Sciences* 11: 37-42, 1993.

75. **Mathews DK, Fox EL, and Tanzi D.** Physiological responses during exercise and recovery in a football uniform. *Journal of Applied Physiology* 26: 611-615, 1969.

76. **Maughan RJ, Otani H, and Watson P.** Influence of relative humidity on prolonged exercise capacity in a warm environment. *European Journal of Applied Physiology* 112: 2313-2321, 2012.

77. **Mazess RB.** Cardiorespiratory characteristics and adaptation to high altitudes. *American Journal of Physical Anthropology* 32: 267-278, 1970.

78. **Mazess RB.** Exercise performance at high altitude in Peru. *Federation Proceedings* 28: 1301-1306, 1969.

79. **Mazess RB.** Exercise performance of Indian and white high altitude residents. *Human Biology: An International Record of Research* 41: 494-518, 1969.

80. **Mazzeo RS.** Physiological responses to exercise at altitude–an update. *Sports Medicine* 38: 1-8, 2008.

81. **McArdle WD, Magel JR, Gergley TJ, Spina RJ, and Toner MM.** Thermal adjustment to cold-water exposure in resting men and women. *Journal of Applied Physiology* 56: 1565-1571, 1984.

82. **McArdle WD, Magel JR, Spina RJ, Gergley TJ, and Toner MM.** Thermal adjustment to cold-water exposure in exercising men and women. *Journal of Applied Physiology* 56: 1572-1577, 1984.

83. **Norton E.** *The Fight for Everest: 1924.* New York, NY: Longmans, Green, 1925.

84. **Oelz O, Howald H, Di Prampero PE, Hoppeler H, Claassen H, Jenni R, et al.** Physiological profile of world-class high-altitude climbers. *Journal of Applied Physiology* 60: 1734-1742, 1986.

85. **Pascoe DD, Shanley LA, and Smith EW.** Clothing and exercise. I: biophysics of heat transfer between the individual, clothing and environment. *Sports Medicine* 18: 38-54, 1994.

86. **Peronnet F, Thibault G, and Cousineau DL.** A theoretical analysis of the effect of altitude on running performance. *Journal of Applied Physiology* 70: 399-404, 1991.

87. **Powers SK, Martin D, and Dodd S.** Exercise-induced hypoxaemia in elite endurance athletes. Incidence, causes and impact on $\dot{V}O_2$ max. *Sports Medicine* 16: 14-22, 1993.

88. **Pugh L.** Athletes at altitude. *Journal of Physiology* 192: 619-646, 1967.

89. **Pugh LG.** Deaths from exposure on Four Inns Walking Competition, March 14-15, 1964. *Lancet* 1: 1210-1212, 1964.

90. **Pugh LG and Edholm OG.** The physiology of channel swimmers. *Lancet* 269: 761-768, 1955.

91. **Pugh LG, Gill MB, Lahiri S, Milledge JS, Ward MP, and West JB.** Muscular exercise at great altitudes. *Journal of Applied Physiology* 19: 431-440, 1964.

92. **Quinn MD.** The effects of wind and altitude in the 400-m sprint. *Journal of Sports Sciences* 22: 1073-1081, 2004.

93. **Racinais S, Alonso J-M, Coutts AJ, Flouris AD, Girard O, González-Alonso J, Hausswirth C, Jay O, Lee JKW, Mitchell N, Nassis GP, Nybo L, Pluim BM, Roelands B, Sawka MN, Wingo J, and Périad JD.** Consensus recommendations on training and competing in the heat. *Sports Medicine.* 45:925-938, 2015.

94. **Racinais S.** Different effects of heat exposure upon exercise performance in the morning and afternoon. *Scandinavian Journal of Medicine & Science in Sports* 20 Suppl. 3: 80-89, 2010.

95. **Raven P.** Effects of air pollution on physical performance. In *Encyclopedia of Physical Education, Fitness, and Sports: Training, Environment, Nutrition, and Fitness*, edited by Stull G, and Cureton T. Salt Lake City, UT: Brighton, 1980, pp. 201-216.

96. **Raven PB, Drinkwater BL, Ruhling RO, Bolduan N, Taguchi S, Gliner J, et al.** Effect of carbon monoxide and peroxyacetyl nitrate on man's maximal aerobic capacity. *Journal of Applied Physiology* 36: 288-293, 1974.

97. **Roberts WO.** Heat and cold: what does the environment do to marathon injury? *Sports Medicine* 37: 400-403, 2007.

98. **Rose MS, Houston CS, Fulco CS, Coates G, Sutton JR, and Cymerman A.** Operation Everest. II: Nutrition and body composition. *Journal of Applied Physiology* 65: 2545-2551, 1988.

99. **Roskamm H, Landry F, Samek L, Schlager M, Weidemann H, and Reindell H.** Effects of a standardized ergometer training program at three different altitudes. *Journal of Applied Physiology* 27: 840-847, 1969.

100. **Rupert JL and Hochachka PW.** Genetic approaches to understanding human adaptation to altitude in the Andes. *Journal of Experimental Biology* 204: 3151-3160, 2001.

101. **Saltin B.** Circulatory response to submaximal and maximal exercise after thermal dehydration. *Journal of Applied Physiology* 19: 1125-1132, 1964.

102. **Saunders PU, Pyne DB, and Gore CJ.** Endurance training at altitude. *High Altitude Medicine & Biology* 10: 135-148, 2009.

103. **Sawka MN, Francesconi RP, Young AJ, and Pandolf KB.** Influence of hydration level and body fluids on exercise performance in the heat. *JAMA* 252: 1165-1169, 1984.

104. **Sawka MN, Young AJ, Francesconi RP, Muza SR, and Pandolf KB.** Thermoregulatory and blood responses during exercise at graded hypohydration levels. *Journal of Applied Physiology* 59: 1394-1401, 1985.

105. **Schoene RB, Lahiri S, Hackett PH, Peters RM, Jr., Milledge JS, Pizzo CJ, et al.** Relationship of hypoxic ventilatory response to exercise performance on Mount Everest. *Journal of Applied Physiology* 56: 1478-1483, 1984.

106. **Semenza GL.** Hypoxia-inducible factors in physiology and medicine. *Cell* 148: 399-408, 2012.

107. **Simonson TS, McClain DA, Jorde LB, and Prchal JT.** Genetic determinants of Tibetan high-altitude adaptation. *Human Genetics* 131: 527-533, 2012.

108. **Siple P and Passel C.** Measurements of dry atmospheric cooling in subfreezing temperatures. *Proceedings of the American Philosophical Society* 89: 177-199, 1945.

109. **Sperlich B, Born DP, Lefter MD, and Holmberg HC.** Exercising in a hot environment: which t-shirt to wear? *Wilderness & Environmental Medicine* 24: 211-220, 2013.

110. **Stachenfeld NS.** Sodium ingestion, thirst, and drinking during endurance exercise. *Sports Science Exchange* 27(122): 1-5, 2014.

111. **Strohl KP.** Lessons in hypoxic adaptations from high-altitude populations. *Sleep Breath* 12: 115-121, 2008.

112. **Sutton JR, Reeves JT, Wagner PD, Groves BM, Cymerman A, Malconian MK, et al.** Operation Everest II: oxygen transport during exercise at extreme simulated altitude. *Journal of Applied Physiology* 64: 1309-1321, 1988.

113. **Teunissen LPJ, de Haan A, de Koning JJ, and Daanen HAM.** Effects of wind application on thermal perception and self-paced performance. *European Journal of Applied Physiology* 113: 1705-1717, 2013.

114. **Tikuisis P, Bell DG, and Jacobs I.** Shivering onset, metabolic response, and convective heat transfer during cold air exposure. *Journal of Applied Physiology* 70: 1996-2002, 1991.

115. **Vogt M and Hoppeler H.** Is hypoxia training good for muscles and exercise performance? *Progress in Cardiovascular Diseases* 52: 525-533, 2010.

116. **Volpino P, Tomei F, La Valle C, Tomao E, Rosati MV, Ciarrocca M, et al.** Respiratory and cardiovascular function at rest and during exercise testing in a healthy working population: effects of outdoor traffic air pollution. *Occupational Medicine* 54: 475-482, 2004.

117. **Ward-Smith AJ.** The influence of aerodynamic and biomechanical factors on long jump performance. *Journal of Biomechanics* 16: 655-658, 1983.

118. **Ward-Smith AJ.** Altitude and wind effects on long jump performance with particular reference to the world record by Bob Beamon. *Journal of Sport Sciences* 4: 89-99, 1986.

119. **Wasse LK, Sunderland C, King JA, Batterham RL, and Stensel DJ.** Influence of rest and exercise at a simulated altitude of 4,000 m on appetite, energy intake, and plasma concentrations of acylated ghrelin and peptide YY. *Journal of Applied Physiology* 112: 552-559, 2012.

120. **Wegmann M, Faude O, Poppendieck W, Hecksteden A, Frohlich M, and Meyer T.** Precooling and sports performance: a meta-analytical review. *Sports Medicine Volume* 42: 545-564, 2012.

121. **West JB, Boyer SJ, Graber DJ, Hackett PH, Maret KH, Milledge JS, et al.** Maximal exercise at extreme altitudes on Mount Everest. *Journal of Applied Physiology* 55: 688-698, 1983.

122. **West JB, Hackett PH, Maret KH, Milledge JS, Peters RM, Jr., Pizzo CJ, et al.** Pulmonary gas exchange on the summit of Mount Everest. *Journal of Applied Physiology* 55: 678-687, 1983.

123. **West JB, Lahiri S, Gill MB, Milledge JS, Pugh LG, and Ward MP.** Arterial oxygen saturation during exercise at high altitude. *Journal of Applied Physiology* 17: 617-621, 1962.

124. **West JB, Lahiri S, Maret KH, Peters RM, Jr., and Pizzo CJ.** Barometric pressures at extreme altitudes on Mt. Everest: physiological significance. *Journal of Applied Physiology* 54: 1188-1194, 1983.

125. **West JB and Wagner PD.** Predicted gas exchange on the summit of Mt. Everest. *Respiration Physiology* 42: 1-16, 1980.

126. **Wilson MJ, Julian CG, and Roach RC.** Genomic analysis of high-altitude adapatation: innovations and implications. *Current Sports Medicine Reports* 10: 59-61, 2011.

127. **Wingo JE.** Exercise intensity prescription during heat stress: a brief review. *Scandinavian Journal of Medicine and Science in Sports and Exercise* 25(Suppl 1): 90-95, 2015.

128. **Wingo JE, Ganio MS, and Cureton KJ.** Cardiovascular drift during heat stress: implications for exercise prescription. *Exercise and Sport Sciences Reviews.* 40: 88-94, 2012.

129. **Wolski LA, McKenzie DC, and Wenger HA.** Altitude training for improvements in sea level performance. Is the scientific evidence of benefit? *Sports Medicine* 22: 251-263, 1996.

130. **Yamane M, Oida Y, Ohnishi N, Matsumoto T, and Kitagawa K.** Effects of wind and rain on thermal responses of humans in a mildly cold environment. *European Journal of Applied Physiology* 109: 117-123, 2010.

131. **Yaspelkis BB, III, and Ivy JL.** Effect of carbohydrate supplements and water on exercise metabolism in the heat. *Journal of Applied Physiology* 71: 680-687, 1991.

132. **Yu IT, Wong TW, and Liu HJ.** Impact of air pollution on cardiopulmonary fitness in schoolchildren. *Journal of Occupational and Environmental Medicine* 46: 946-952, 2004.

© Digital Vision/Getty Images

Ergogenic Aids

The preceding chapters have described exercise and dietary plans related to performance. However, no presentation of factors affecting performance would be complete without a discussion of ergogenic aids. **Ergogenic aids** are defined as work-producing substances or phenomena believed to increase performance (98). For this reason they are also called *performance enhancing substances* (PES).

Ergogenic aids include, for example, nutrients, drugs, warm-up exercises, blood doping, oxygen breathing, music, and extrinsic biomechanical aids. Although we discussed nutritional issues related to performance in Chap. 23, we will provide additional detail about the role of dietary supplements as ergogenic aids in this chapter. In addition, we will discuss ergogenic aids related to aerobic performance (oxygen inhalation and blood doping) and anaerobic performance (blood buffers), as well as various drugs (amphetamines and caffeine), high-tech equipment, and physical warm-up. Note that anabolic steroids and growth hormone were discussed in Chap. 5.

Performance enhancing substances are used broadly at all levels of competition. The prevalence of elite athletes intentionally using doping is estimated to be about 14% to 39%, but the actual percent varies greatly among sports (33). Not surprisingly, a greater percentage of athletes use some types of PES (e.g., dietary supplements) more than others (e.g., drugs). Reasons elite athletes initially get into using PES include greater athletic success through better performance, financial gain, faster recovery, preventing nutritional deficiencies, and because they think others are using them (97). Among college athletes, those who use PES are much more likely to drink alcohol and use drugs, whether or not the latter improves or impedes performance (20). Although athletes criticize the way testing is carried out, they feel that the severity of the punishment is appropriate or not severe enough. Interestingly, coaches are still the main influence and source of information about PES for athletes (97); this problem may be compounded by the lack of knowledge physicians have about PES (96). Finally, given the limited resources available to deal with this problem, there is concern that the majority of the money is spent on anti-drug testing and not on educational programs to prevent the problem (97).

Although the attention of the reader will be focused on athletic performance, where an improvement of less than 1% would alter world records, it must be noted that industrial physiologists have long been concerned about the relationship of lighting, environmental temperature, and background noise (music) to performance in the workplace (98). Research work in this area must be done carefully, with special attention to the research design due to the number of factors that can influence the outcome of the study.

RESEARCH DESIGN CONCERNS

It is sometimes difficult to compare the results of one research study on ergogenic aids with another. The reason for this is that the effect of an ergogenic aid depends on a number of variables (98):

- Amount—too little or too much may show no effect
- Subject—the ergogenic aid may be effective in "untrained" subjects but not "trained" subjects, or vice versa
    - —the "value" of an ergogenic aid is determined by the subject
- Task—may work in short-term, power-related tasks, but not in endurance tasks, or vice versa
    - —may work for gross-motor, large-muscle activities and not with fine-motor activities, or vice versa
- Use—an ergogenic aid used on an acute (short-term) basis may show a positive effect, but in the long run may compromise performance, or vice versa

Given these variables, scientists are careful in designing experiments in order not to be "fooled" by the result. For example, an athlete may improve performance because he or she believes the substance improves performance, so the "belief" is more important than the substance in determining the outcome. Further, an investigator may "believe" in the ergogenic aid and inadvertently offer different levels of encouragement during the testing of athletes under the influence of the ergogenic aid. These problems are controlled for by using a **placebo** as a treatment condition and using a **double-blind research design,** respectively.

A placebo is a "look-alike" substance relative to the ergogenic aid under consideration, but it contains nothing that will influence performance. The need for such a control is seen in Figure 25.1, which describes the gain in strength by a group that was taking a placebo but was told it was an anabolic steroid. It is contrasted with the group's performance prior to taking the placebo. The rate and amount of strength gained was higher with the placebo, indicating the need for such a control if one is to isolate the true effect of a substance (4).

A double-blind research design is one in which neither the subject nor the investigator knows who is receiving the placebo or the substance under investigation. The subjects are randomly assigned to receive pill x or pill y. After all data are collected, the "code" is broken to find out which pill (x or y)

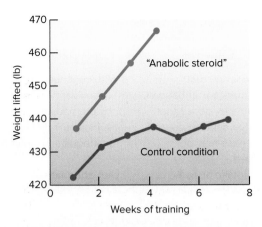

Figure 25.1 Changes in performance when subjects were told they were taking an anabolic steroid but were really taking a placebo.

was the placebo and which was the substance under investigation. These designs are complex and difficult to carry out, but they reduce the chance of subject or investigator bias (98).

The scientist must also be careful in the selection of subjects. If a substance is tested as a potential aid to sprinters, it would be reasonable to select subjects from that population so the results can be generalized to that group. Further, the tests used by the investigator should be as close as, or actually be, the performance task (e.g., 100-meter dash). In short, results obtained on a proper subject population but under controlled laboratory conditions using conventional physiological tests may not be useful when taken to the "field" (98).

IN SUMMARY

- Ergogenic aids are defined as substances or phenomena that are work producing and are believed to increase performance.
- Because an athlete's belief in a substance may influence performance, scientists use a placebo or look-alike substance to control for this effect. In addition, scientists use a double-blind research design in which the investigator and subject are both unaware of the treatment.

DIETARY SUPPLEMENTS

We discussed issues related to basic nutrition in Chap. 18 and provided additional detail about the role of nutrition in performance in Chap. 23. In this section, we go a step further and discuss the role that dietary supplements may play in athletic performance—a point of interest to many athletes. A survey of athletes indicated that more than 80% of U.S. Division I athletes and national or international elite athletes use dietary supplements (3, 91, 105). For more detail on dietary supplements and performance, see texts by Burke and Deakin in Suggested Readings and Williams, Anderson, and Rawson (155). We also encourage you to examine the website of the Australian Institute of Sport (http://www.ausport.gov.au/ais/nutrition), which systematically updates information on a wide variety of dietary supplements.

One has only to open a strength-training magazine to become aware of the incredible number of dietary supplements promoted as improving the effects of a workout, be it size or strength. Table 25.1 provides a summary of a number of dietary supplements used by strength-training athletes to increase strength, muscle mass, and athletic performance. The columns provide information about the claim made for each substance and the evidence for or against that claim. A quick reading of Table 25.1 indicates that little or no support exists for most of the supplements, with the exception of creatine and, perhaps, beta-alanine. We all know of the role of phosphocreatine (PC) in high-power events or at the onset of endurance exercise (see Chaps. 3 and 4). Numerous studies show that creatine supplementation can increase the muscle's creatine concentration. Does it affect performance? (See The Winning Edge 25.1 for more on this developing story.)

Some dietary supplements are aimed at improving endurance performance. Inorganic nitrate is found in green leafy vegetables and beetroot. Once ingested it is converted to nitrite, which, in turn, can be converted to nitric oxide, an important molecule in circulatory and metabolic function. Nitrate supplementation has been shown to have health benefits (e.g., lowering blood pressure) (27), and there is some evidence that it can lower the oxygen cost of submaximal exercise. However, its efficacy in high caliber athletes is unclear and additional research is needed (3, 27, 73). Another supplement, sodium phosphate, has been shown to increase $\dot{V}O_2$ max in both average and elite cyclists; however, its impact on endurance performance is not as clear cut (19). We are sure to see more on these dietary supplements in the years ahead.

The use of supplements of any kind needs to be approached with a "buyer beware" attitude. When the U.S. Congress passed the Dietary Supplements Health and Education Act in 1994, it opened the door for the manufacture and sale of dietary supplements, including some (e.g., prohormones) that were not originally envisioned (8, 145). The lack of regulation of these products means that between 10%-15% of supplements may contain contaminants which may elicit a positive drug test (105). A case in point is a recent study by Baume et al. (9). They examined 103 dietary supplements and found 3 that had an anabolic steroid in very large amounts that would

TABLE 25.1 Dietary Supplements for Strength Trainers

Supplement	Description	Claim	Evidence	Comment
Antioxidants (e.g., vitamins A, C, and E)	Chemicals that protect cells from oxidative damage caused by free radicals	Reduce muscle damage resulting from severe or eccentric exercise	Little evidence that performance is enhanced, but some evidence that oxidative damage caused by exercise may be lessened	With continued training, antioxidants produced by the body may be sufficient; if diet is inadequate, supplement
Proteins or branched-chain amino acids	High-protein diets or unique amino acid supplements	Meet greater protein needs associated with training	Dietary intake already exceeds upper limit of known protein requirements	Diet adequate
Lysine, arginine, and ornithine	Amino acids	Increase growth hormone secretion; promote muscle growth	May increase growth hormone, but of limited magnitude; no effect on muscle mass	Costly and ineffective
β-Alanine	Amino acid used in synthesis of carnosine	More carnosine will buffer acids better in muscle	No support for high-intensity exercise lasting <60s; some for >60s and <240s	Paraesthesia (tingling sensation on skin) can occur; more research needed
Creatine	Amino acid	Increases anaerobic power	Improves performance in selected tasks (e.g., repeated sprint bouts)	See The Winning Edge 25.1
Dehydroepi-androsterone (DHEA)	Precursor to testosterone	Enhances testosterone concentration and muscle mass	No effect on testosterone, strength, or muscle mass; banned by WADA and IOC	Increases estrogen levels and decreases HDL cholesterol; could result in a positive drug test for testosterone
Androstenedione (andro)	Precursor to testosterone	Enhances testosterone concentration and muscle mass	No effect on testosterone, strength, or muscle mass; banned by WADA and IOC	Increases estrogen levels and decreases HDL cholesterol; could result in a positive drug test for testosterone
Carnitine	Used in fat metabolism	Enhances fat use, decreases bodyfat	No deficiency in athletes; no effect on metabolic response to exercise	Diet adequate

From References 2, 3, 11, 23, 62, 65, 67, 72, 75, 88, 131, 140, 155, 160, 165 and Australian Institute of Sport. http://www.ausport.gov.au/ais/nutrition.

have generated a positive drug test. One creatine product revealed the presence of two anabolic steroids when urine samples were examined. To prevent the problems associated with using contaminated supplements, extensive testing of products by an independent lab may be warranted—or the athlete should only take those nutritional supplements recommended by a nutritionist/registered dietician (34). Some of the dietary supplements are banned by the World Anti-Doping Agency (WADA) and the International Olympic Committee (IOC).

For a summary of the effect of herbs on athletic performance, see a review by Williams in Suggested Readings.

IN SUMMARY

- For the most part, little evidence exists that dietary supplements provide a performance advantage to athletes, with the possible exception of creatine.

AEROBIC PERFORMANCE

Chapter 20 detailed the various tests used to evaluate the physiological factors related to endurance performance. Clearly, an increased ability to transport O_2 to the muscles and a delay in the onset of lactate production

Creatine Monohydrate

We are all familiar with the importance of phosphocreatine (PC) as an energy source during short-term, explosive exercise, and as the energy source that helps us to make the transition to the steady state of oxygen uptake during submaximal aerobic exercise (see Chaps. 3 and 4). Because of PC's importance in explosive exercise, there has been a great deal of interest in the potential of the dietary supplement creatine monohydrate to increase the muscle's concentration of PC and, hopefully, performance.

The total creatine concentration in muscle is about 120 mmol · kg^{-1}, and 2 grams are excreted per day. These 2 grams are replaced by diet (1 gram) and by synthesis (1 gram) from amino acids (35, 146). The first step in a typical creatine monohydrate "loading" plan consists of adding 20 to 25 grams to the diet per day for five to seven days (79). This results in ~20% increase in muscle creatine, which approaches what is thought to be the upper limit of the muscle's capacity to store creatine. There is evidence that this elevated level can be achieved with doses as low as 2 to 3 grams per day–given time (119). Independent of the means used to achieve the higher levels of creatine in muscle, there is great variability among subjects (35, 146):

■ Individuals with lower initial values (e.g., vegetarians) have greater increases, and some individuals with high presupplement values may not respond to the increased creatine. This has led to the terms *responders* and *nonresponders*.

■ The ingestion of glucose with the creatine reduces this variation and enhances uptake. In general, the short-term loading scheme appears to improve the ability to maintain muscular force and power output during various exhaustive bouts of exercise, including in older individuals (59, 123), but not without exception (146, 154). Studies that controlled for protein and energy intake show convincingly that it is the creatine itself that brings about these effects (32). In addition, creatine does not affect muscle glycogen, either at rest or following exhaustive exercise.

In contrast to scientists using a five- to seven-day loading regimen to determine the effect of an elevated muscle creatine concentration, athletes take the creatine supplement for long periods to improve performance. The elevated level of creatine in muscle achieved in the loading phase can be maintained by consuming 2 to 5 grams of creatine monohydrate per day. Interestingly, the "mechanism" for any increase in performance may be only indirectly related to the creatine. For example, greater gains in strength achieved in a weight-training program may be mediated by the athlete's ability to increase the intensity of training, which would, in turn, allow for a greater physiological adaptation (i.e., strength gain) to the training (118, 146). However, it must be noted that creatine supplementation does not reduce muscle damage resulting from severe exercise (117). What about the down side of creatine supplementation? Creatine supplementation appears to increase body mass, but this is probably due more to water retention than protein synthesis. Consequently, athletes who must "carry" their own body weight (e.g., runners) might have to be careful not to negatively affect performance (3, 35, 154). Use of a low-dose of creatine monohydrate (~2.3 g/day) (119) or of polyethylene glycosylated creatine (1.25-2.5 g/day) (63) avoided the weight gain, but resulted in improved performance. There are reports of gastrointestinal distress, nausea, and muscle cramping associated with the use of creatine; however, recent reports suggest that at least out to 21 months, there are no long-term adverse effects (8, 116). Since an Upper Level of Intake (UL) standard is not yet available for creatine (see Chap. 18 for a description of UL), the use of the Observed Safe Level (OSL) has been suggested as a first step. Based on existing research, an amount of 5 g per day appears to be a safe level for chronic consumption (126). Should it be banned? Volek (146) provides an interesting analogy: Creatine supplementation is linked to enhanced performance of high-intensity, repetitive bouts of exercise in the same way that carbohydrate supplementation is linked to improvements in endurance performance (see Chap. 23).

Recently, investigators have systematically evaluated the role that creatine might play in individuals with myopathies (disorders of muscle that can be acquired or genetic in nature). In those with muscular dystrophies, those taking creatine had greater gains in strength compared to those in a placebo group. In contrast, those with metabolic myopathies who took creatine experienced a deterioration in being able to do activities of daily living, with McArdle's disease patients experiencing an increase in muscle pain (76).

---

are related to improved performance. Two ergogenic aids have been used to try to influence O$_2$ delivery: the breathing of O$_2$-enriched mixtures and blood doping.

Oxygen

Given the importance of aerobic metabolism in the production of ATP for muscular work, it is not surprising that scientists have been interested in the effect of additional oxygen (hyperoxia) on performance. But to discuss this issue, we must ask the following question: How and when was the O$_2$ administered to achieve a higher PO$_2$ in the blood? In his insightful review of this topic, Welch (149) stressed the difficulty of comparing results from studies in which hyperoxia is achieved by increasing the percent of O$_2$ in the inspired air with

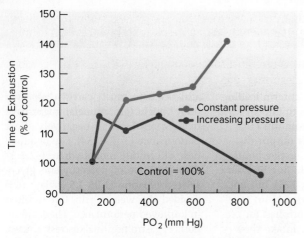

Figure 25.2 The effect of PO_2 on performance. Constant pressure experiments used oxygen-enriched gas mixtures at sea-level pressure, while the increasing pressure experiments used a hyperbaric chamber to increase the PO_2.

From Reference 130, New York: McGraw-Hill, Inc., 1987.

those that use a **hyperbaric** (high-pressure) **chamber** with 21% or higher O_2 mixtures. Figure 25.2 shows that performance (e.g., longer time to exhaustion) improves throughout the range of inspired oxygen pressures when O_2-enriched mixtures are used at a normal pressure of 1 atmosphere ("constant pressure"), compared to the use of a hyperbaric chamber ("increasing pressure"). A study using both weight-lifting tasks and an endurance treadmill run confirmed the lack of effect of hyperbaric hyperoxia on performance (125). The second part of the question is related to the time of administration of the supplemental O_2. Results vary depending on whether the O_2 is administered prior to, during, or following exercise. For that latter reason, this section on oxygen is organized by those conditions.

Prior to Exercise The rationale for the use of supplemental oxygen prior to exercise is to try to "store" additional oxygen in the blood so that more will be available at the onset of exercise. It has been estimated that the hemoglobin in arterial blood is about 97% saturated with O_2 at rest (200 ml O_2/L blood). Breathing 100% O_2 would increase the O_2 bound to hemoglobin by only 3%, or 6 milliliters. However, the amount of oxygen physically dissolved in solution is proportional to the arterial PO_2, and when the PO_2 increases from about 100 mm Hg (breathing 21% O_2 at sea level) to about 700 mm Hg (breathing 100% O_2), the dissolved oxygen increases from 3 ml/L to 21 ml/L. If a person has a total blood volume of 5 liters, approximately 100 milliliters of additional O_2 can be "stored" prior to exercise. However, if the person takes a few breaths between the time the O_2 breathing stops and the event begins, the O_2 store will return to that associated with air breathing (157).

The focus of attention on the use of oxygen prior to exercise has been on short-term exercise. In general, in runs of 880 yards or less, weight lifting, stair climbing, and swims of 200 yards or less, the O_2 breathing seemed to be beneficial (100, 157). In addition, evidence suggested that the O_2 breathing needed to take place within two minutes of the task (157). Some concern has been expressed about these findings due to the fact that in some cases the subjects knew they were breathing O_2, a factor that could have affected the results (157). Overall, considering the fact that O_2 cannot be breathed up to the start of a sprint event in swimming or track, any effect would be lost before the starter's gun is fired. Therefore, unless one participates in a breath-holding event, oxygen breathing prior to exercise will have little effect on performance.

During Exercise The rationale for the use of oxygen during exercise to improve performance is based on the proposition that muscle is hypoxic during exercise and additional O_2 delivery will alleviate the problem (150). If this is the case, then the additional O_2 in the blood during O_2 breathing should increase the delivery of O_2 to the muscle and improve performance. However, Welch et al. (150) showed that when one breathes hyperoxic gas mixtures, the increase in the O_2 content of arterial blood (CaO_2) is balanced by a decrease in blood flow to the working muscles such that O_2 delivery ($CaO_2 \times$ flow) is not different from normoxic (21% O_2) conditions. $\dot{V}O_2$ max is increased by only 2% to 5% with hyperoxia, which is about what would be expected, since maximal cardiac output doesn't change and the a-$\bar{v}O_2$ difference does not increase more than 5% to 6% ($\dot{V}O_2$ max $= \dot{Q}$ max $\times [CaO_2 - C\bar{v}O_2]$).

In spite of similarities in O_2 delivery during hyperoxia and normoxia, performance has been shown to increase dramatically as a result of an increase in inspired O_2. Figure 25.2 shows time to exhaustion to be improved by 40% while breathing 100% O_2 ($PO_2 = 700$ mm Hg). How could this be if O_2 delivery to muscles is not substantially different? The increased availability of O_2 has been shown to decrease pulmonary ventilation and reduce the work of breathing, a change that should lead to an increase in performance (149, 158, 159). In addition, those athletes who experience "desaturation" of hemoglobin during maximal work (see Chaps. 10 and 24) while breathing 21% O_2 could benefit by breathing oxygen-enriched gas mixtures (112). One study found that when sprinters did three repeat 300-meter sprints at different speeds on a treadmill while breathing 40% oxygen (compared to 21%), hemoglobin saturation was maintained and the fall in blood pH was less (103). Finally, the high PO_2 slows glycolysis during heavy exercise, resulting in a slower accumulation of lactate and H^+ in the plasma and extending the time to exhaustion (68, 149). The reduction in lactate formation in hyperoxia appears to be due to a reduction in the rate of glycogen breakdown so that it is better matched with its subsequent oxidation in the Krebs cycle (134). Given the impracticality of trying to provide O_2 mixtures to athletes during performance, this research on hyperoxia is more useful as a tool to answer questions related to the age-old question of what factor, O_2 delivery or the muscle's capacity to consume O_2, limits aerobic performance (149). However, some have used hyperoxia during training in an attempt to improve performance. A recent study had subjects breathe 60% O_2 (versus 21% O_2) during training to see if it would result in larger gains in $\dot{V}O_2$ max and performance. Subjects were able to exercise at an 8% higher work rate using 60% O_2, but changes in $\dot{V}O_2$ max and time to exhaustion were not different between treatments (106).

After Exercise The rationale for the use of supplemental oxygen after exercise is that the subject might recover more quickly following exercise and be ready to go again. Some of the early work showed just that, but because the subjects knew what gas they were breathing, the results have to be interpreted with caution (100, 157). Wilmore (157) summarized the effects of several studies and concluded that there was no benefit of O_2 breathing during recovery on heart rate, ventilation, and post-exercise oxygen uptake. This conclusion was supported by studies showing no effect of O_2 breathing on subsequent performance in all-out exercise (121).

IN SUMMARY

- Oxygen breathing before or after exercise seems to have little or no effect on performance, whereas oxygen breathing during exercise improves endurance performance.

Blood Doping

In Chap. 19, we described how $\dot{V}O_2$ max is directly linked to cardiac output and that a high $\dot{V}O_2$ max is very important to achieving excellence in endurance performances. Because maximal O_2 transport is equal to the product of maximal cardiac output ($\dot{Q}$ max) and the O_2 content of arterial blood (CaO_2), one way to improve O_2 delivery to tissue when $\dot{Q}$ max cannot change is to increase the quantity of hemoglobin in each liter of blood. **Blood doping** refers to the infusion of red blood cells (RBCs) in an attempt to increase the hemoglobin concentration ([Hb]) and, consequently, O_2 transport (CaO_2 is equal to the [Hb] × 1.34 ml O_2/gm Hb). Other terms to describe this are **blood boosting** and **blood packing,** with **induced erythrocythemia** being the proper medical term.

However, before we get into this topic, it must be remembered that an increase in blood volume (independent of an increase in the hemoglobin concentration) would also favorably affect $\dot{V}O_2$ max and aerobic performance (57).

In blood doping, a subject receives a transfusion of blood, which may be his or her own (**autologous transfusion**) or blood from a matched donor (**homologous transfusion**). The latter procedure is acceptable in times of medical emergencies but carries the risk of infection and blood-type incompatibility (56); it is therefore not recommended in blood-doping procedures. The need to use your own blood to achieve the goal of a higher [Hb] creates some interesting problems that led to confusion in the early days of research in this area. The primary problem was related to the mismatch between the maximum time blood could be refrigerated and the time period needed for the subject to produce new RBCs and bring the [Hb] back to normal before the reinfusion. Maximum storage time with refrigeration is three weeks, during which time about 1% of the RBCs are lost per day. In addition, some RBCs adhere to the storage containers or become so fragile that they will not function upon reinfusion. Because of these problems, only about 60% of the removed RBCs could be reinfused (56). The normal time period for replacement of the RBCs following a 400-milliliter donation is three to four weeks, and following a 900-milliliter donation, five to six weeks or more are required. If the blood were reinfused at the end of the three-week maximal storage time, the investigator might not have been able to achieve the condition of an increased [Hb] due to RBC loss (decreased 40%) and the below-normal (anemic) values in the subjects. Gledhill (56) makes a strong case for this as a primary reason why studies prior to 1978 showed inconsistent changes in $\dot{V}O_2$ max and performance with blood doping. Another major problem encountered in these early studies was the lack of an adequate research design. There was a need to have a group undergoing a **"sham" withdrawal** (needle placed in the arm but no blood is removed) and a **"sham" reinfusion** (needle placed in the arm but blood is not returned) to act as placebo controls.

The central factor allowing a more careful study of blood doping was the introduction of the freezer preservation technique, which allows the blood to be stored frozen for years with only a 15% RBC loss. This allows plenty of time for the subject to become **normocythemic** (achieve normal [Hb]), so that any effect of the reinfusion can be correctly evaluated (56).

The general findings were that reinfusions of single units (~450 milliliters) of blood showed small but insignificant increases in [Hb], $\dot{V}O_2$ max, and performance, whereas the infusion of two units (900 milliliters) significantly increased the [Hb] (8%–9%), $\dot{V}O_2$ max (4%–5%),

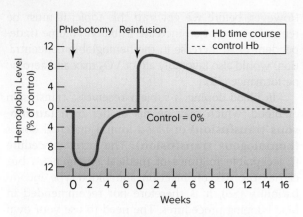

Figure 25.3 Changes in hemoglobin levels in blood following removal (phlebotomy) and reinfusion.

and performance (3%–34%). The infusion of three units (1350 milliliters) of blood caused slightly greater increases in [Hb] (10.8%) and $\dot{V}O_2$ max (6.6%). This large reinfusion caused borderline **erythrocythemia** to be approached, so a 1350-milliliter infusion probably represents the upper limit that can be used. Figure 25.3 shows a gradual reduction in [Hb] toward the normal value following reinfusion, indicating that increased O_2 transport is maintained for 10 to 12 weeks. This is an important point as far as performance gains are concerned (55). That said, there is no question that elite cyclists have used blood doping on a regular day-to-day routine to assist in training sessions as well as during competitions (142).

The classic study by Ekblom et al. in 1972 showed the impact of blood doping on $\dot{V}O_2$ max and performance (43). The improvements in performance (3%–34%) were much more variable than the changes in [Hb] or $\dot{V}O_2$ max. Part of the reason for this variation was the type of performance test used. The greatest change was observed in a running test to exhaustion that lasted less than ten minutes, and the smallest change was observed in a five-mile time trial, with the improvement being 51 seconds compared to a preinfusion run time of 30:17 (156). Early questions (41) about whether this procedure would "work in the field" were answered in a study on cross-country skiers (14), and judging by the number of cyclists that withdrew from the Tour de France when records of blood doping were uncovered suggests that there is little question of the advantage it provides. See A Look Back–Important People in Science for an individual who got this started.

Although the blood doping issue will always raise a question of ethics, Gledhill presents what amounts to a moral dilemma in the use of blood doping in getting athletes ready for performance at altitude. In Chap. 24, we discussed the changes in $\dot{V}O_2$ max and performance at altitude. Those athletes who stay at altitude experience a natural increase in RBC production to deal with the hypoxia. As Gledhill (56)

points out, those athletes who can afford to train at altitude accomplish what blood doping does in a manner that is acceptable to the International Olympic Committee. The availability of a recombinant DNA analog of **erythropoietin (EPO),** the hormone that stimulates red blood cell production, has complicated the picture.

Erythropoietin is used as a part of therapy for those who undergo chemotherapy or dialysis (due to kidney disease). The hormone stimulates red blood cell production to reduce the chance of anemia. This is crucial for a variety of patients, and investigators are trying to optimize the use of EPO (86). Although normal cross-country training does not seem to increase plasma levels of naturally occurring erythropoietin (12), acute exposure to 3000 and 4000 meters of simulated altitude has been shown to increase the concentration 1.8- and 3.0-fold, respectively (40). The real concern, of course, is the potential abuse of the DNA-derived analog of this hormone (recombinant human EPO [rhEPO]) to generate the effects of blood doping without having to undergo the blood withdrawals and reinfusions. Such abuse is not without its risks, in that RBC production can get out of hand, as seen in some studies where the increase in the hemoglobin concentration varied from 4% to 19% (83). This could lead to extremely high RBC levels in some athletes, which could impair blood flow to the heart and brain, resulting in a myocardial infarction or a stroke.

In fact, within four years of its introduction, about 20 top European cyclists died, unexpectedly. The EPO causes an increase in the hemoglobin concentration by a simultaneous increase in the red blood cell volume and a decrease in plasma volume, such that blood volume is relatively unchanged (83, 85). Like the blood-doping procedure, the hemoglobin concentration remains elevated for several weeks while the EPO concentration decreases, making detection difficult (83). It should be no surprise that finding those athletes who use blood doping or EPO to gain an advantage is crucial to the "fairness" principle in sport.

In 2002, an organization composed of scientists, pharmaceutical companies, and hematologists was formed to work systematically to prevent abuse of these products and unethical practices by athletes (5). Some progress has been made. For those using a homologous blood transfusion, tests can discriminate between the donor and the recipient by focusing on minor blood group factors (81, 147). For those reinfusing their own packed red blood cells, that same testing procedure will not work because the blood groups are obviously the same. However, systematic progress has been made with an approach that tracks an athlete's blood over years and notes changes in a variety of factors during that time (81). The term "hematological passport" has been applied to this approach, but concerns have been raised about its

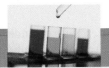

A LOOK BACK—IMPORTANT PEOPLE IN SCIENCE

Dr. Björn Ekblom, M.D., Ph.D., Studied Factors Affecting Oxygen Transport, Leading Others to "Blood Doping"

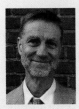

Courtesy of Arthur Forsberg

Björn Ekblom received his Ph.D. in 1969 and his M.D. in 1970 from the Karolinska Institutute in Stockholm, Sweden, and was appointed Professor of Physiology at the Karolinska Institute in 1977. The focus of his research early in his career was on maximal oxygen uptake ($\dot{V}O_2$ max), the physiological factors linked to $\dot{V}O_2$ max, and the effect of training on $\dot{V}O_2$ max in young and old subjects. Consistent with his interest in the factors affecting $\dot{V}O_2$ max, he examined the role of hemoglobin concentration on oxygen transport and $\dot{V}O_2$ max. In 1972, he published

"Responses to Exercise After Blood Loss and Reinfusion," which showed that as you lower or raise the hemoglobin concentration, you can alter $\dot{V}O_2$ max in a systematic manner. This paper set in motion the interest in the use of blood doping to alter oxygen transport, $\dot{V}O_2$ max, and endurance performance, which is currently a major problem in sports (see discussion in this chapter). Dr. Ekblom's studies also investigated the effect of EPO on $\dot{V}O_2$ max and, later, how to detect the presence of EPO in those who might use it in an unethical manner.

Dr. Ekblom made major contributions over the past 45 years in our understanding of $\dot{V}O_2$ max and the various factors that affect it. However, his research interests went well

beyond that. He studied temperature regulation during exercise, hemodynamic (i.e., blood pressure, cardiac output) responses to exercise, effects of training on patients with rheumatoid arthritis, and nutritional factors related to performance. In addition to making these important contributions to our understanding of the physiology related to physical training, he published a number of books and pamphlets related to conditioning and training for different sports. He has published more than 150 peer-reviewed articles, numerous books, eight major review articles, and more than 30 chapters in books. He is currently Professor Emeritus at the Karolinska Institute, where he continues his productive career.

---

ability to track subjects over time who are using EPO (13, 84). In addition, a promising technique involving the measurement of hemoglobin mass to catch those using autologous blood transfusions (83, 99, 110) has now been called into question. Limitations in the procedure exist, including inherent measurement error and the fact that the athlete would be exposed to carbon monoxide during the test (which could negatively affect performance) (84, 109). To demonstrate the difficulties involved in catching a cheat while new techniques are being developed to allow a scientist to distinguish rhEPO from natural EPO, drugs are being developed that will stimulate natural EPO production (84).

IN SUMMARY

- Blood doping refers to the reinfusion of red blood cells to increase the hemoglobin concentration and oxygen-carrying capacity of the blood.
- Due to improvements in blood storage techniques, blood doping has been shown to be effective in improving $\dot{V}O_2$ max and endurance performance.
- Erythropoietin (EPO) is a hormone that stimulates red blood cell production and is one of the most abused PES.

ANAEROBIC PERFORMANCE

Improvements in endurance performance focus on the supply of carbohydrate and oxygen to muscle (see previous sections on oxygen and blood doping in this chapter and on carbohydrate in Chap. 23). However, in short-term, all-out performances in which anaerobic energy sources provide the vast majority of energy for muscle contraction, the focus of attention shifts to the buffering of the H^+ released from muscle. This section considers a means by which investigators have tried to buffer the H^+ and improve performance.

Blood Buffers

Elevations in the $[H^+]$ in muscle can decrease the activity of phosphofructokinase (PFK) (141), which may slow glycolysis, interfere with excitation-contraction coupling events by reducing Ca^{++} efflux from the terminal cisternae of the sarcoplasmic reticulum (51), and reduce the binding of Ca^{++} to troponin (101). Decreases in muscle force development have been shown to be linked to increases in muscle $[H^+]$ in both frog muscle (47) and human muscle (138). Finally, when Adams and Welch (1) showed that performance times in heavy exercise (90% $\dot{V}O_2$ max) could be altered by breathing 60% O_2 compared to 21% or 17% O_2, the point of exhaustion was associated with the same arterial [H+]. The mechanisms involved in the regulation of the plasma [H+] were described in detail in Chap. 11. Briefly, the primary means by which H+ is buffered during exercise is through its reaction with the plasma bicarbonate reserve to form carbonic acid, which subsequently yields CO_2 that is exhaled (respiratory compensation). As the bicarbonate buffer store decreases, the ability to buffer H+ is reduced and the plasma [H+] will increase. Knowing this, scientists have explored ways of increasing the plasma buffer store to slow down the rate of H+ increase during strenuous exercise.

As early as 1932 (36), induced alkalosis (means unknown) was shown to extend run time to exhaustion from (min:sec) 5:22 to 6:04. Since that time, a variety of studies have supported these findings. On the basis of several reviews (18, 21, 69, 80, 104, 113, 120, 152), there appears to be agreement that:

- The optimal dose of bicarbonate used to improve performance was 0.3 g per kilogram of body weight (although 0.2 g/kg may be as effective (129))

- Tasks of a minute or less in duration, even at extremes of intensity, did not seem to benefit from the induced alkalosis

- Performance gains were shown for tasks of high intensity that lasted about one to ten minutes or that involved repeated bouts of high-intensity exercise with short recovery periods

However, when bicarbonate is taken over several days (in contrast to just before the test), there appears to be a dose-response effect, with $0.5 \text{ g} \cdot \text{kg}^{-1} \cdot \text{d}^{-1}$ being better than $0.3 \text{ g} \cdot \text{kg}^{-1} \cdot \text{d}^{-1}$ (39). Given the potential for blood buffers to have a positive impact on performance, one must be careful to not be fooled by an inadequately designed study, as mentioned at the beginning of this chapter. In the case of blood buffers, McClung and Collins (89) used a research design to help separate out the effect of being told you are getting the buffer (drug) from actually getting the drug. They had four treatments in which subjects were:

1. Told they were going to get the drug/Got the drug
2. Told they were going to get the drug/Did not get the drug
3. Told they were not going to get the drug/Got the drug
4. Told they were not going to get the drug/Did not get the drug

There were several important findings in this study that we need to keep in mind when we deal with ergogenic aids. The "Told drug/Did not get drug treatment (#2)" resulted in a better performance than the "Told they were not going to get the drug/ Got the drug treatment (#3)"–in effect, the pure pharmacological effect of the bicarbonate was not as good as the expectation that they were receiving the drug.

The positive impact of the buffers may be related to maintaining the oxygen saturation of hemoglobin during maximal exercise, as well as any improvements at the level of the muscle (102). The variability in the effectiveness of the sodium bicarbonate treatment points to inter-individual variation in the response to sodium bicarbonate, and that some short-term anaerobic activities are more dependent on the muscle or plasma [H+] as a primary cause of fatigue than others (114). Welch (149) indicates that while subjects may stop at the same [H+] within any exercise protocol, the differences that exist among studies in the "terminal" [H+] suggest the other factors are more limiting as far as performance is concerned. The use of these agents to cause an alkalosis is not without risks. Large doses of sodium bicarbonate can cause diarrhea and vomiting, both of which are sure to affect performance (3, 54, 80, 152). It appears that taking the sodium bicarbonate at least 120 minutes before exercise reduces the chance of these problems (22, 128). Research is needed to help determine what causes the variability between individuals (e.g., caliber of athlete, training history, gut tolerance); whether it can be used across several performance bouts in a short period of time (heats in a track and field competition); and how it interacts with other supplements (e.g., caffeine, nitrate, creatine) (21).

IN SUMMARY

- The ingestion of sodium bicarbonate improves the performance of high-intensity exercise of one to ten minutes' duration or repeated bouts of high-intensity exercise.

DRUGS

A variety of drugs have been used to aid performance. Some drugs are as common and "legal" as caffeine whereas others, like amphetamines, are banned from use. We will briefly examine each of these drugs, exploring how they might work to improve performance, as well as the evidence about whether or not they do. There is a widespread misconception that performance enhancing drugs (PED) are safe or that adverse effects are manageable. However, the majority of PED users are recreational weight lifters, not elite athletes, and the adverse health effects are greatly underappreciated (108).

Amphetamines

Amphetamines are stimulants that have been used primarily to recover from fatigue and improve endurance. In 1972, Golding (58) indicated that it was the most abused group of drugs at that time. Amphetamines are readily absorbed in the small intestine, and although the effects reach a peak 2 to 3 hours after ingestion, they persist for 12 to 24 hours (70, 82). Amphetamines are both a **sympathomimetic** drug (simulates catecholamine effects) and a central nervous system stimulant. The drug produces its effects by altering either the metabolism and synthesis of catecholamines or receptor affinity for catecholamines (70, 82).

The most consistent effect of amphetamines is to increase one's arousal or wakefulness, leading to a perception of increased energy and self-confidence (70). The drug affects the redistribution of blood flow, driving it away from the skin and splanchnic areas and delivering more to muscle or brain. This could lead to problems related to a decrease in lactic acid removal (see Chap. 3) and an increase in body temperature (see Chap. 12). Animal studies show that amphetamines can increase endurance-type performances. However, the dose of the drug was shown to be important, in that smaller doses (1–2 mg/kg) did not have an effect different from control, and large doses (16 mg/kg) appeared to reduce the ability of the rat to swim. Data collected using run tests on rats indicate the same detrimental effect of high doses (7.5–10 mg/kg) of amphetamines (70).

Ivy (70) concluded from an analysis of studies on human subjects that amphetamines extend endurance and hasten recovery from fatigue. Time to exhaustion was increased in spite of no effect on submaximal or maximal $\dot{V}O_2$ (24, 70). Two explanations have been offered. Ivy (70) believes that the endurance aspect of performance can be improved due to amphetamines' catecholamine-like effect in mobilizing free fatty acid (FFA) and sparing muscle glycogen, similar to that of caffeine (see the caffeine section next). Chandler and Blair (24) believe that the amphetamines may simply mask fatigue and interfere with the perception of the normal biological signals that fatigue has occurred. It is this latter conclusion that has raised the most concern about the safety of the athlete, in that during prolonged submaximal work, especially in a hot and/or humid environment, the decreased blood flow to the skin could cause hyperthermia, leading to death (26, 70, 82). Increased attention has been directed at this latter concern for athletes with attention deficit hyperactivity disorder (ADHD) who are prescribed stimulant medications (e.g., Ritalin) to control the condition (115). In addition, because these kinds of stimulant medications may have an ergogenic effect, a Therapeutic Use Exemption is needed (see the World Anti-Doping Agency at https://wada-main-prod.s3.amazonaws.com/resources/files/WADA-MI-ADHD-5.0.pdf).

As mentioned at the beginning of this section, amphetamines' major effect is in increasing wakefulness and producing a state of arousal. However, although amphetamines have restored reaction time in fatigued subjects, the drug does not affect reaction time in alert, motivated, and nonfatigued subjects (29). Given that athletes are usually alert and motivated prior to competition, Golding (58) suggests that amphetamines would be counterproductive, making users hyperirritable and interfering with their sleep. Finally, it is risky to extrapolate from data collected under tightly controlled laboratory conditions using discrete measures related to performance ($\dot{V}O_2$ max, endurance time, reaction time) to the actual performance in a skilled sport in front of a hostile audience for a national championship. That might be excitement enough. Sometimes, a drug used for one purpose finds its way into the sporting world because of its unique impact on muscle. See A Closer Look 25.1 for such an example.

IN SUMMARY

- Amphetamines have a catecholamine-like effect that leads to an increased arousal and a perception of increased energy and self-confidence.
- Although amphetamines improve the performance of fatigued subjects, they do not have this effect on alert, motivated, and nonfatigued subjects.

Caffeine

Caffeine is a stimulant that is found in a variety of common foods, drinks, and over-the-counter drugs (see Table 25.2). Caffeine has been viewed as an on-again, off-again ergogenic aid. Caffeine was banned by the International Olympic Committee (IOC) in 1962, then removed from the list of banned drugs in 1972. In 1984, the IOC again banned "high levels" in the urine that might have been the result of caffeine injections or suppositories; the standard was set at 12 µg/ml (143, 153). Caffeine is again off the list of banned substances. Part of the reason is the availability of caffeine in food and drinks, which makes it a difficult thing to track and control in an athlete's diet. Since the ban was lifted, analysis of caffeine levels in urine samples from athletes of many different sports show power lifters to have the highest concentration, followed by cyclists and body builders (144). Caffeine is absorbed rapidly from the GI tract and is significantly elevated in the blood at 15 minutes, with the peak concentration achieved at 60 minutes. Caffeine is diluted by body water, and the physiological response is proportional to the concentration in the body water. There is a natural variability in how people respond to caffeine, with evidence that chronic users are less responsive than abstainers (10, 143).

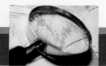
β_2-Agonists: Clenbuterol and Salbutamol

Clenbuterol is a drug that was developed to treat airway diseases such as asthma. Its chemical action in the body is to activate beta-2 receptors (β_2-agonists) in tissue (see Chaps. 5 and 17). Although the drug is useful in the treatment of airway diseases, in the early 1980s, it was discovered that clenbuterol is a powerful anabolic agent in skeletal muscles. Early studies showed that, in animals, a 14-day treatment with clenbuterol (2 mg/kg/day) resulted in a 10% to 20% increase in muscle mass, converted type I muscle fibers to type II fibers, and caused a selective hypertrophy of type II fibers (33, 163). Further, the time course of clenbuterol-induced muscular hypertrophy was rapid, with muscle growth beginning within two days after commencement of treatment.

With the discovery that clenbuterol is a powerful anabolic agent in skeletal muscle, scientific interest in the clinical use of this drug has grown. For example, this compound is potentially useful in the treatment of conditions that result in muscle wasting (i.e., aging, spinal cord injury, etc.) (87). Unfortunately, some athletes now use clenbuterol in an effort to increase muscle size and improve performance in power events (e.g., sprinting, football, etc.). What does the research say?

In two recent reviews of this issue, the authors were consistent in finding that inhaled β_2-agonists had no effect on either aerobic or anaerobic performances (28, 107). However, when the β_2-agonists were either ingested or infused, performance was favorably altered, but the two reviews differed in terms of how much:

- Collomp et al. (28) found that in almost all trials, following an acute or short-term administration of the drug at a therapeutic dosage, subjects showed improved performances, whatever the intensity.

- In a meta-analysis of the randomized controlled trials on this issue, Pluim et al. (107) showed that while some performances improved (e.g., endurance time at 80%-85% $\dot{V}O_2$ max), others did not (endurance time at 70% $\dot{V}O_2$ max), even though they were similar in nature. They concluded that while the overall effect of the β_2-agonists on performance was positive, the evidence was weak.

Clearly, this is an area in which additional research is needed to help clarify issues related to the dosage and duration of administration, type of athlete who benefits, and magnitude of change expected in standardized performance tests.

Salbutamol and salmeterol are β_2-agonists used to treat asthma: The former is short acting (4-6 hours) and the latter is long acting (~12 hours). The World Anti-Doping Agency (WADA) allows these drugs to be used without the athlete seeking a Therapeutic Use Exemption, a change from previous standards (162). However, if the level of salbutamol in the urine exceeds 1000 ng/ml, it is presumed not to be due to an intended therapeutic use. Unfortunately, the work of governing bodies like WADA will increase over time as novel designer drugs based on old formulations of β_2-agonists hit the market—they may be very difficult to detect (48).

Although caffeine can affect a wide variety of tissues, Figure 25.4 shows that its role as an ergogenic aid is based on its effects on skeletal muscle and the central nervous system, and in the mobilization of fuels for muscular work. The evidence for the enhanced function of skeletal muscle is based primarily on *in vitro* and *in situ* muscle preparations and shows that caffeine can directly potentiate skeletal muscle force, work, and power (111, 135, 143). This was shown most clearly in fatigued muscle and was believed to be due to increased Ca^{++} release from the ryanodine receptor that mediates the release of Ca^{++} from the sarcoplasmic reticulum (136). In a recent meta-analysis, caffeine ingestion was shown to have a small but positive impact (+7%) on knee extensor maximal strength, with little or no impact on other muscle groups; this is surprising, given that the drug obviously reached all muscles. In contrast, muscular endurance was improved by ~14% across muscle groups (148).

Caffeine has long been recognized as a stimulator of the central nervous system (CNS). Caffeine can pass the blood-brain barrier and affect a variety of brain centers, which usually leads to an increased alertness and decreased drowsiness (113, 143). The best evidence supporting caffeine as a CNS stimulant is in the decreased perception of fatigue during prolonged exercise in subjects who took it (31). Two reviews support this proposition, with findings that the rating of perceived exertion (RPE) is lower during exercise with caffeine ingestion, accounting for some of the improvement in performance (38, 136).

The role of caffeine in the mobilization of fuel has received considerable attention as the primary means by which it exerts its ergogenic effect. Caffeine has been shown to cause an elevation of glucose and an increase in fatty acid utilization. The elevated glucose could be due to the stimulation of the sympathetic nervous system and the resulting increase in catecholamines, which would increase the mobilization of glucose from the liver. On the other hand, the glucose concentration could be elevated due to a decreased rate of removal related to the suppression of insulin release by catecholamines (see Chap. 5) (143). However, some of these metabolic effects are not dependent on catecholamines; instead, they may be related to the

TABLE 25.2	Caffeine Content of Popular Drinks and Drugs	
Popular Beverages (8 oz)		**Caffeine (mg)**
Coffee, drip		115–175
Coffee, brewed		80–135
Coffee, instant		65–100
Tea, iced		47
Tea, brewed (import)		60
Tea, brewed (domestic)		40
Tea, green		15
Soft Drinks (12 oz)		
Low (e.g., root beer)		23
Most (e.g., colas)		⁓45
High (e.g., Mountain Dew)		⁓55
Jolt		71
Red Bull		80
Non-Prescription Drugs		
NoDoz		200
Vivarin		200
Midol		64
Pain Relievers		
Anacin analgesic		64 mg
Excedrin		130
Tylenol		0

From http://www.holymtn.com/tea/caffeine_content.htm and http://wilstar.com/caffeine.htm.

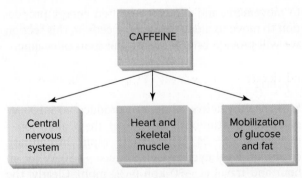

Figure 25.4 Factors influenced by caffeine that might cause an improvement in performance.

products of caffeine breakdown (e.g., theophylline), which are metabolic stimuli in their own right (60). Interestingly, when caffeine is coingested with glucose, the ingested glucose is oxidized at a higher rate than when the glucose is taken without caffeine (164).

Lipid mobilization has been shown to be increased as a result of caffeine ingestion. Figure 25.5 shows that the mechanism of action could be related either to the elevated catecholamines increasing the level of cyclic AMP in the adipose cell or to caffeine's blocking of phosphodiesterase activity, which is responsible for breaking down cyclic AMP. Van Handel

(143) believes that the latter mechanism is less likely, given the dose of caffeine needed. Plasma FFA increase quickly at rest after ingestion of caffeine (15 minutes) and continue to increase over the next several hours (143). However, during exercise, plasma FFA may (37, 137) or may not (31, 37, 44, 61, 71) be significantly elevated as a result of caffeine ingestion. In addition, while the respiratory exchange ratio may (44, 71) or may not (61, 137) be reduced, both glucose kinetics (124) and the lactate threshold (15, 37, 53) have been shown not to be affected by caffeine ingestion. In addition, there is variability in the effect of caffeine on improvements in work output or total work time, making it an ergogenic aid for some and not for others (37, 38, 44, 53, 61, 71, 133, 156). A recent review confirmed the variability in improvement in endurance performance (range 20.3% to 17.3%, with an average of 3.2%) (52). What causes such variability?

The ergogenic effect appears to be dose dependent and may vary with the type of subject (29); however, gender and menstrual cycle status do not appear to affect the pharmacokinetics of how caffeine is handled (93). Although some studies show physiological changes with doses as low as 5 to 7 mg/kg (31, 44), others find a 10 mg/kg dose to be inadequate (71). In fact, in other studies, a dose of 15 mg/kg was needed to see an increase in fat metabolism (94, 95). However, when restricted to improvements in sport-specific endurance performance, a dose of 3–6 mg/kg taken prior to or during the performance appears to be sufficient (52). There is now evidence that lower doses (e.g., <3 mg/kg) are ergogenic in some exercise and sport situations. These lower doses have been shown to improve vigilance, alertness, and mood, and have fewer side effects–suggesting that the effects are mediated through the CNS (132).

In contrast to earlier work, the manner in which the caffeine was ingested (e.g., regular coffee vs. anhydrous caffeine dissolved in water) had no impact on performance improvements (66). There is also evidence that patterns of caffeine use affect the response to exercise. For example, habitual caffeine users who abstain from caffeine for at least seven days will optimize the ergogenic effect (52). Further, heavy caffeine users (>300 mg/day) respond differently than those consuming little caffeine (37). Van Handel (143) makes the point that what an investigator observes in a controlled laboratory setting may be masked by a normal sympathetic nervous system response to competition. Given the potential side effects such as insomnia, diarrhea, anxiety, tremulousness, and irritability (143), and the variability among subjects in response to caffeine, one might not see much of an improvement in performance (42, 61, 133). Although caffeine has a diuretic effect, recent studies indicated that rehydration with caffeine-containing beverages during nonexercise periods of two-a-day practices did not hinder hydration status (46, 167).

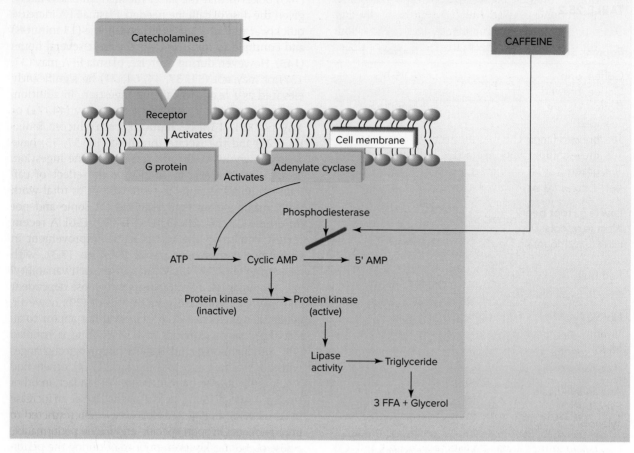

Figure 25.5 **Mechanisms by which caffeine might increase free fatty acid mobilization.**

IN SUMMARY

- Caffeine can potentially improve performance through changes in muscle or the central nervous system, or in the delivery of fuel for muscular work. Caffeine can elevate blood glucose and simultaneously increase the utilization of fat.
- Caffeine's ergogenic effect on performance is variable; it appears to be dose related and less pronounced in subjects who are daily users of caffeine.

MECHANICAL ERGOGENIC AIDS

Each of us is limited in the rate at which we can produce energy, both anaerobically and aerobically. In fact, many of the ergogenic aids discussed thus far focus on trying to stretch those limits (e.g., blood doping for aerobic performances and bicarbonate ingestion for anaerobic performances). In contrast to altering physiological processes like oxygen delivery to muscle or the buffering capacity of muscle, some sports have dealt with these limitations by designing equipment and techniques that lower the resistance to movement, and allow our limited energy production to move us along at higher speeds. In this section we will provide brief look into the sport of cycling.

Cycling

Most healthy active adults can produce ᴗ75-100 W of power continuously to propel them along on a bicycle at ᴗ16-24 kph (ᴗ10-15 mph). In contrast, champion level cyclists can produce ᴗ450 W for an hour and travel at ᴗ50 kph (ᴗ30 mph). Clearly, the champion rider can generate much more power, but why did it take ᴗ4-6 times as much power to go only 2-3 times faster? Much of it has to do with the forces acting against the rider as speed increases (77).

There are a variety of factors that contribute the drag or resistance to movement in cycling. The major retarding force acting on the cyclist at high riding speeds is air resistance. Aerodynamic drag increases as the square of the velocity. In effect, you are moving against more molecules of air the faster you go and you are hitting them at a faster rate. Power is the product of the drag and the velocity, so the power requirement of cycling increases as the cube of the velocity—which explains why it required so much additional energy to double the speed (77). How can aerodynamic drag be reduced to allow higher speeds to be reached at the same power output? Much attention is directed to the bicycle and its components, the cyclist's body position, clothing, and race strategies to reduce drag.

The Bicycle and its Components   Great advances have been made in the design of bicycles over the years to reduce resistance to movement. These include (77, 78):

- Frame. Round tubes on a bicycle frame cause the airstream to separate from the surface of the tube on impact, resulting in a lower pressure on the back of the tube that causes drag (pressure drag). Simply changing bicycle tubes from a round to a teardrop shape reduces drag. The frame should be "fitted" to the rider and smaller frames weigh less and cause less drag. Modern bicycle frames are made from carbon fiber, which increases stiffness in the crankset area, allowing for optimal power transfer from the rider to the wheels.

- Wheels. Wheels with round, steel spokes cause more drag than wheels with aero-shaped spokes; further, drag is proportional to the number of spokes. However, wheels with aero-shaped spokes have more drag than either flat-disc wheels or carbon fiber wheels having 3-4 spokes. In time trials (events in which individual cyclists race against a clock) a flat-disc wheel is typically used in the rear, while a tri-spoke wheel is used in the front to prevent crosswinds from affecting steering.

- Tires and rolling resistance. Rolling resistance due to tires is a small part of overall drag and rolling resistance actually decreases, as a proportion of overall drag, at higher speeds (because air resistance increases so dramatically with speed). Rolling resistance is related to the area of tire in contact with the ground and the degree to which it is deformed (flattened). Light-weight tires with thin side-walls that are inflated to high pressures (<120 psi [8 atm]) are characteristics associated with lower rolling resistance, and tubular type tires are better in this regard than clincher type.

- Components. Low-drag versions of some components such as cranks, handlebars, brakes, and seatposts are also available to lower air resistance.

A bicycle with all of these variables optimized to minimize air resistance enhances performance in those who ride at high speeds. It must be added that the total weight of the bike and rider is an important consideration when riding hills, and it should be no surprise that high-end bikes are light. However, the

Union Cycliste Internationale (UCI–the world governing body for the sport of cycling) mandates that road racing bikes must weight at least 6.8 kg because lighter bikes could compromise safety.

Body Position   When riding in an upright position with straight arms on the handlebars a large cross section of the body is presented to the air, offering great resistance to movement. To put this in perspective, at ⁓40 kph (⁓25 mph) the aerodynamic drag of the bicycle is only 20% to 25% of total aerodynamic drag, with the cyclist's body being the remainder. Consequently, body position is the most important factor in achieving low aerodynamic drag (78). Simply moving from the upright to the crouched or traditional racing position, with the hands on the lower part of the drop handlebars, decreases aerodynamic drag by 20%. Adopting a fully aerodynamic (aero) position in which the forearms rest on pads on the handlebars and the elbows are moved inward, lowers drag by 30% to 35% (7, 45). See Figure 25.6 for examples of such aerodynamic positions. It should be noted that the Obree and "superman" positions have been outlawed by the UCI.

Clothing and Other Gear   There is no question that loose-fitting clothing offers more resistance to airflow than tight-fitting clothing. Thus, bicycle racers choose skin-tight jerseys, shorts, and socks to reduce drag. Further, some materials (e.g. Lycra) are better at letting air flow by than others (e.g., wool or polypropylene), while still providing excellent breathability. Choosing an appropriate aero helmet and covering the shoes with a smooth material results in additional reductions in drag (78). It must be added that using clip-in pedals and hard carbon-fiber soles in cycling shoes helps power transfer to the pedals, and allows the cyclist to pull up on the pedals as well as push down.

Drafting   If a cyclist rides behind and in close proximity to another cyclist, the lead cyclist reduces the air resistance for the one that follows. This can lead to a reduction in the energy cost of cycling by ⁓30%. If the cyclist is behind a pack of riders, the reduction in the energy cost approaches 40%, and if riding behind a vehicle, 60% (Fig. 25.7) (90). In many road races the best rider is "sheltered" by team members who do most of the work; this allows their best rider to sprint to the finish at the end of the race (45).

It is clear that one can do a great number of things to lower air resistance and improve performance in cycle races. If you watch the Tour de France you will see a stage in which the cyclist rides alone (a time trial) and drafting, of course, is not a possibility. In these races the cyclist makes use of all of the equipment and clothing technologies mentioned above to be able to complete the race distance in the shortest time possible. In contrast,

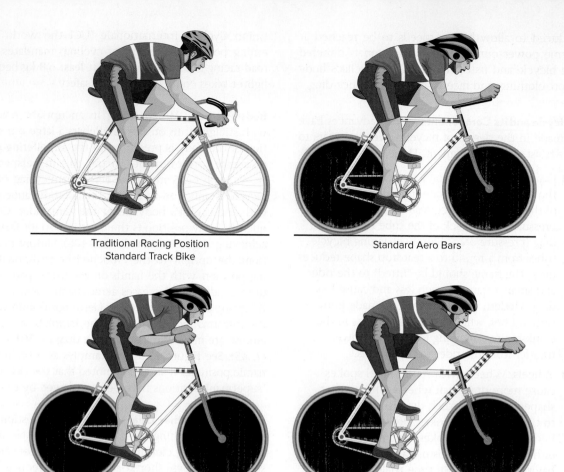

Traditional Racing Position
Standard Track Bike

Standard Aero Bars

The Obree Position

The Superman Position

Figure 25.6 Bicycle racing positions. From the 1890s until 1986, cyclists used the same traditional crouched racing position. Starting in 1986, aero bars (invented by Peter Pensayres and used in the Race Across America in 1986) allowed cyclists to rest on their elbows while maintaining a low aerodynamic riding posture. Graham Obree of Scotland pioneered two unique riding positions, which he used to set hour records in 1993 and 1994 (the Obree position and the Superman position).

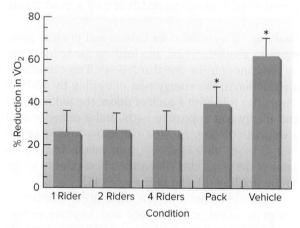

Figure 25.7 Reduction in $\dot{V}O_2$ resulting from drafting different numbers of riders and a vehicle at 40 km/hr.

in regular stages of the tour in which all riders are involved at the same time, you see more conventional, but still high-tech, bicycles, however drafting and other strategies are now used to win the stage.

An individual who makes a "breakaway" and tries to do it on his own is usually caught by the pack of cyclists before the stage is completed. The cyclist has to deal with the air resistance by himself, which demands a higher percent of maximal power output, and he has nothing left at the end.

PHYSICAL WARM-UP

Warming up prior to moderate or strenuous activity is a general recommendation made for those involved in fitness programs or athletes involved in various types of performance. Most of us accept this as a reasonable recommendation, but is there good scientific support for it? In Franks's original 1972 review (50), he found that 53% of the studies supported the proposition that warm-up was better than no warm-up, 7% the opposite, and 40% found no difference between the two. Concerns were raised about the wide variety of tasks and the methods used to evaluate the effectiveness of warm-up. In his 1983 review, Franks (49) analyzed the role of the participant (trained or untrained), the duration and intensity of the warm-up, and the type of performance as the variables involved in a determination of the effectiveness of warm-up. Before we summarize these findings, a few definitions must be presented.

Warm-up refers to exercise conducted prior to a performance, whether or not muscle or body temperature is elevated. Warm-up activities can be identical to the performance (baseball pitcher throwing with normal form and high speed to a catcher prior to the batter stepping up), directly related to the performance (shot-putter practicing at 75% of normal effort prior to a competition), or indirectly related to a performance (general activities to increase body temperature or arousal) (49). Generally, all three are used in a typical warm-up prior to performance, in the reverse order of the aforementioned descriptions.

The theoretical benefits of warm-up are physiological, psychological, and safety related. Physiological benefits would include less muscle resistance and faster enzymatic reactions at high body temperatures. This might lower the oxygen deficit at the onset of work (74, 122), decrease the RER during the subsequent activity (64), or cause a favorable shift in the lactate threshold (25). One review supported most of these effects, but questioned the impact of the warm-up on speeding up rate-limiting enzyme reactions (16). Increases in body temperature as a result of warm-up have been linked to improved performance (49). Skilled performances benefit from identical and direct warm-up, with indirect warm-up sometimes acting in a facilitatory manner. As an example, warm-up swings with a standard weight baseball bat were most effective for enhancing bat speed (92). The warm-up procedures can increase arousal, which is good up to a point, and provide the optimal "mental set" for improved performance (16, 49).

Stretching, as a part of warming up, has been recommended as a way to improve performance and reduce the risk of soft tissue injury. A recent study suggests that static stretching, especially longer than 45 seconds, be avoided before competition because of its negative impact on maximal muscle strength and explosive muscular performance (130). There is no question that stretching improves joint flexibility, but reviews on this topic provide little support that injury risk is reduced. Weldon and Hill (151) found that most of the available studies were of poor quality, and it was not possible to draw a definitive conclusion regarding stretching and exercise-related injuries. A group of researchers at the Centers for Disease Control and Prevention drew the same conclusion from their review of the literature, and indicated that there was not enough evidence to either endorse or discontinue routine stretching before or after exercise to prevent injuries (139). Witvrouw and colleagues (161) agreed with these general conclusions when applied to most sports. However, for those sports demanding high-intensity stretch-shortening cycles (e.g., soccer, basketball), stretching was viewed as important to keep the muscle-tendon unit compliant enough to store and release energy during explosive movements. Finally, Shrier's comment on the CDC article indicated that there was a need to separate out the effects of stretching outside of periods of exercise from the stretching that precedes exercise. There is evidence that the former approach is associated with injury prevention. Clearly, more research is needed (127). From a safety standpoint, apart from the potential for soft tissue injuries, some evidence suggests that warm-up reduces the "stress" experienced when doing strenuous work. In Barnard et al.'s (6) classic study, six of ten firefighters who did not warm up experienced an ischemic response (reduced myocardial blood flow) as shown by abnormalities on the ECG during strenuous exercise (see Chap. 17). All had normal ECG responses when a gradual warm-up preceded the strenuous exercise.

Warming up obviously affects a variety of factors, but is there evidence that it favorably affects performance? The answer is "yes," but with some caveats (17).

- In short-term performances (max effort of ≤10 s), a three- to five-minute warm-up improves performance. However, an intense warm-up may result in a decrement in performance due, in part, to a reduction in high-energy phosphates.
- Warm-up improves intermediate-term performances (>10 s, but ≤5 min), but not if the intensity is too low (≤40% $\dot{V}O_2$ max) or the recovery time is too long (5–10 minutes). The goal is to begin the performance with a slightly elevated baseline $\dot{V}O_2$, and be sufficiently recovered.
- For long-term performances (fatiguing effort for ≥5 minutes), an elevated baseline $\dot{V}O_2$ also improves performance. However, if the warm-up depletes muscle glycogen or increases thermal strain (by elevating body temperature too much), performance may suffer.

So, what is the recommended warm-up? For short-term performances, a warm-up at 40% to 60% $\dot{V}O_2$ max for five to ten minutes, followed by a five-minute recovery, is recommended. For intermediate- or long-term performances, the warm-up at 60% to 70% $\dot{V}O_2$ max for 5 to 10 minutes, with a ≤5 minute recovery, is recommended (17). This is similar to what Franks reported some 25 years ago (49). For a recent review on this topic applied to military fitness testing, see reference 166.

> **IN SUMMARY**
>
> ■ Warm-up activities can be identical to performance, directly related to performance, or indirectly related to performance (general warm-up). Warm-up causes both physiological and psychological changes that are beneficial to performance.

STUDY ACTIVITIES

1. What is an ergogenic aid?
2. Why must an investigator use a "placebo" treatment to evaluate the effectiveness of an ergogenic aid?
3. Provide a brief summary of the role that dietary supplements play in improving performance.
4. What is a double-blind research design?
5. Does breathing 100% O_2 improve performance? Recovery?
6. Breathing hyperoxic gas mixtures improves performance without changing O_2 delivery to tissue. How is this possible?
7. What is blood doping and why does it appear to improve performance now when it did not in the earliest investigations?
8. How might ingested buffers improve short-term performances?
9. Although amphetamines improve performance in fatigued individuals, they might not have this effect on motivated subjects. Why?
10. How might caffeine improve long-term performances? Can the results be extrapolated to "real" performances in the field?
11. Describe how high-speed cycling performance can be improved with equipment changes and riding techniques.
12. Describe the different types of warm-up activities and the mechanisms by which they may improve performance.

SUGGESTED READINGS

Burke, L. M., and V. Deakin. 2015. *Clinical Sports Nutrition.* New York: McGraw-Hill.

Williams, M. Dietary supplements and sports performance. *Journal of the International Society of Sports Nutrition* 3: 1–6, 2006.

REFERENCES

1. **Adams RP and Welch HG.** Oxygen uptake, acid-base status, and performance with varied inspired oxygen fractions. *Journal of Applied Physiology: Respiratory, Environmental and Exercise Physiology* 49: 863–868, 1980.
2. **Alvares TS, Meirelles CM, Bhambhani YN, Paschoalin VMF, and Gomes PSC.** L-arginine as a potential ergogenic aid in healthy subjects. *Sports Medicine* 41: 233–248, 2011.
3. **American College of Sports Medicine.** Nutrition and athletic performance. *Medicine and Science in Sports and Exercise.* 48: 543–568, 2016.
4. **Ariel G and Saville W.** Anabolic steroids: the physiological effects of placebos. *Medicine and Science in Sports* 4: 124–126, 1972.
5. **Ashenden MJ.** A strategy to deter blood doping in sport. *Haematologica* 87: 225–232, 2002.
6. **Barnard RJ, Gardner GW, Diaco NV, MacAlpin RN, and Kattus AA.** Cardiovascular responses to sudden strenuous exercise—heart rate, blood pressure, and ECG. *Journal of Applied Physiology: Respiratory, Environmental and Exercise Physiology* 34: 833–837, 1973.
7. **Bassett D, Kyle C, Passfield L, Broker J, and Burke E.** Comparing cycling world hour records, 1967–1996: modeling with empirical data. *Medicine & Science in Sports and Exercise* 31: 1665–1676, 1999.
8. **Baume N, Hellemans I, and Saugy M.** Guide to over-the-counter sports supplements for athletes. *Int Sport Med J* 8: 2–10, 2007.
9. **Baume N, Mahler N, Kamber M, Mangin P, and Saugy M.** Research of stimulants and anabolic steroids in dietary supplements. *Scandinavian Journal of Medicine & Science in Sports* 16: 41–48, 2006.
10. **Bell DG and McLellan TM.** Exercise endurance 1, 3, and 6 h after caffeine ingestion in caffeine users and nonusers. *Journal of Applied Physiology: Respiratory, Environmental and Exercise Physiology* 93: 1227–1234, 2002.
11. **Bellinger PM.** Beta-alanine supplementation for athletic performance: an update. *Journal of Strength and Conditioning Research.* 28: 1751–1770, 2014.
12. **Berglund B, Birgegard G, and Hemmingsson P.** Serum erythropoietin in cross-country skiers. *Medicine and Science in Sports and Exercise* 20: 208–209, 1988.
13. **Berglund B, Ekblom B, Ekblom E, Berglund L, Kallner A, Reinebo P, et al.** The Swedish Blood Pass project. *Scandinavian Journal of Medicine & Science in Sports* 17: 292–297, 2007.
14. **Berglund B and Hemmingson P.** Effect of reinfusion of autologous blood on exercise performance in cross-country skiers. *International Journal of Sports Medicine* 8: 231–233, 1987.
15. **Berry MJ, Stoneman JV, Weyrich AS, and Burney B.** Dissociation of the ventilatory and lactate thresholds following caffeine ingestion. *Medicine and Science in Sports and Exercise* 23: 463–469, 1991.
16. **Bishop D.** Warm up I: potential mechanisms and the effects of passive warm up on exercise performance. *Sports Medicine* 33: 439–454, 2003.
17. **Bishop D.** Warm up II: performance changes following active warm up and how to structure the warm up. *Sports Medicine* 33: 483–498, 2003.
18. **Bishop D, Edge J, Davis C, and Goodman C.** Induced metabolic alkalosis affects muscle metabolism and repeated-sprint ability. *Medicine and Science in Sports and Exercise* 36: 807–813, 2004.

19. **Buck CL, Wallman KE, Dawson B, and Guelfi KJ.** Sodium phosphate as an ergogenic aid. *Sports Medicine.* 43: 425-435, 2013.

20. **Buckman JF, Farris SG, and Yusko DA.** A national study of substance use behaviors among NCAA male athletes who use banned performance enhancing substances. *Drug and Alcohol Dependence.* 131: 50-55, 2013.

21. **Burke LM.** Practical considerations for bicarbonate loading and sports performance. In, *Nutritional Coaching Strategy to Modulate Training Efficiency. Nestlé Nutrition Institute Workshop Series.* 75: 15-26, 2013.

22. **Carr AJ, Slater GJ, Gore CJ, Dawson B, and Burke LM.** Effect of sodium bicarbonate on [HCO_3^-], pH, and gastrointestinal symptoms. *International Journal of Sport Nutrition and Exercise Metabolism.* 21: 189-194, 2011.

23. **Caruso J, Charles J, Unruh K, Giebel R, Learmonth L, and Potter W.** Ergogenic effects of β-alanine and carnosine: proposed future research to quantify their efficacy. *Nutrients* 4: 585-601, 2012.

24. **Chandler JV and Blair SN.** The effect of amphetamines on selected physiological components related to athletic success. *Medicine and Science in Sports and Exercise* 12: 65-69, 1980.

25. **Chwalbinska-Moneta J, and Hanninen O.** Effect of active warming-up on thermoregulatory, circulatory, and metabolic responses to incremental exercise in endurance-trained athletes. *International Journal of Sports Medicine* 10: 25-29, 1989.

26. **Clarkson PM and Thompson HS.** Drugs and sport. Research findings and limitations. *Sports Medicine* 24: 366-384, 1997.

27. **Clements WT, Lee SR, and Bloomer RJ.** Nitrate ingestion: a review of the health and performance effects. *Nutrients.* 6: 5224-5264, 2014.

28. **Collomp K, Le Panse B, Candau R, Lecoq AM, and De Ceaurriz J.** Beta-2 agonists and exercise performance in humans. *Science & Sport* 25: 281-290, 2010.

29. **Conlee R.** Amphetamine, caffeine, and cocaine. In *Perspectives in Exercise Science and Sports Medicine, Vol 4: Ergogenics-Enhancement of Performance in Exercise and Sports,* edited by Lamb D, and Williams M. New York, NY: McGraw-Hill, 1991, pp. 285-330.

30. **Costill DL, Dalsky GP, and Fink WJ.** Effects of caffeine ingestion on metabolism and exercise performance. *Medicine and Science in Sports* 10: 155-158, 1978.

31. **Cribb PJ, Williams AD, and Hayes A.** A creatine-protein-carbohydrate supplement enhances responses to resistance training. *Medicine and Science in Sports and Exercise* 39: 1960-1968, 2007.

32. **Criswell DS, Powers SK, and Herb RA.** Clenbuterol-induced fiber type transition in the soleus of adult rats. *European Journal of Applied Physiology and Occupational Physiology* 74: 391-396, 1996.

33. **De Hon O, Kuipers H, and van Bottenburg M.** Prevalence of doping use in elite sports: a review of numbers and methods. *Sports Medicine.* 45: 57-69, 2015.

34. **De Hon O and Coumans B.** The continuing story of nutritional supplements and doping infractions. *British Journal of Sports Medicine* 41: 800-805; discussion 805, 2007.

35. **Demant TW and Rhodes EC.** Effects of creatine supplementation on exercise performance. *Sports Medicine* 28: 49-60, 1999.

36. **Dill D, Edwards H, and Talbot J.** Alkalosis and the capacity for work. *Journal of Biological Chemistry* 97: LVII-LIX, 1932.

37. **Dodd SL, Brooks E, Powers SK, and Tulley R.** The effects of caffeine on graded exercise performance in caffeine naive versus habituated subjects. *European Journal of Applied Physiology and Occupational Physiology* 62: 424-429, 1991.

38. **Doherty M and Smith PM.** Effects of caffeine ingestion on rating of perceived exertion during and after exercise: a meta-analysis. *Scandinavian Journal of Medicine & Science in Sports* 15: 69-78, 2005.

39. **Douroudos II, Fatouros IG, Gourgoulis V, Jamurtas AZ, Tsitsios T, Hatzinikolaou A, et al.** Dose-related effects of prolonged $NaHCO_3$ ingestion during high-intensity exercise. *Medicine and Science in Sports and Exercise* 38: 1746-1753, 2006.

40. **Eckardt KU, Boutellier U, Kurtz A, Schopen M, Koller EA, and Bauer C.** Rate of erythropoietin formation in humans in response to acute hypobaric hypoxia. *Journal of Applied Physiology: Respiratory, Environmental and Exercise Physiology* 66: 1785-1788, 1989.

41. **Eichner E.** Blood doping results and consequences from the laboratory and the field. *Physician and Sportsmedicine* 15: 121-129, 1987.

42. **Eichner E.** The caffeine controversy: effects on endurance and cholesterol. *Physician and Sportsmedicine* 14: 124-132, 1986.

43. **Ekblom B, Goldbarg AN, and Gullbring B.** Response to exercise after blood loss and reinfusion. *Journal of Applied Physiology: Respiratory, Environmental and Exercise Physiology* 33: 175-180, 1972.

44. **Essig D, Costill D, and Van Handel P.** Effect of caffeine ingestion on utilization of muscle glycogen and lipid during leg ergometer cycling. *International Journal of Sports Medicine* 1: 86-90, 1980.

45. **Faria EW, Parker DL, and Faria IE.** The science of cycling: factors affecting performance - part 2. *Sports Medicine* 35: 313-337, 2005.

46. **Fiala KA, Casa DJ, and Roti MW.** Rehydration with a caffeinated beverage during the nonexercise periods of 3 consecutive days of 2-a-day practices. *International Journal of Sport Nutrition and Exercise Metabolism* 14: 419-429, 2004.

47. **Fitts RH and Holloszy JO.** Lactate and contractile force in frog muscle during development of fatigue and recovery. *American Journal of Physiology* 231: 430-433, 1976.

48. **Fragkaki AG, Georgakopoulos C, Sterk S, and Nielen MWF.** Spots doping: emerging designer and therapeutic β_2 agonists. *Clinica Chimica Acta.* 427: 242-258, 2013.

49. **Franks B.** Physical warm-up. In *Ergogenic Aids in Sport,* edited by Williams M. Champaign, IL: Human Kinetics, 1983, pp. 340-375.

50. **Franks B.** Physical warm-up. In *Ergogenic Aids and Muscular Performance,* edited by Morgan W. New York, NY: Academic Press, 1972, pp. 160-191.

51. **Fuchs F, Reddy Y, and Briggs FN.** The interaction of cations with the calcium-binding site of troponin. *Biochimica et Biophysica Acta* 221: 407-409, 1970.

52. **Ganio MS, Klau JF, Casa DJ, Armstrong LE, and Maresh CM.** Effect of caffeine on sport-specific endurance-performance: a systematic review. *Journal of Strength and Conditioning Research* 23: 315-324, 2009.

53. **Gastin P, Misner J, Boileau R, and Slaughter M.** Failure of caffeine to enhance exercise performance in incremental treadmill running. *Australian Journal of Science and Medicine in Sport* 22: 23-27, 1990.

54. **Gledhill N.** Bicarbonate ingestion and anaerobic performance. *Sports Medicine* 1: 177-180, 1984.

55. **Gledhill N.** Blood doping and related issues: a brief review. *Medicine and Science in Sports and Exercise* 14: 183-189, 1982.

56. **Gledhill N.** The influence of altered blood volume and oxygen transport capacity on aerobic performance. *Exercise and Sport Sciences Reviews* 13: 75-93, 1985.

57. **Gledhill N, Warburton D, and Jamnik V.** Haemoglobin, blood volume, cardiac function, and aerobic power. *Canadian Journal of Applied Physiology = Revue Canadienne de Physiologie Appliquee* 24: 54-65, 1999.

58. **Golding L.** Drugs and hormones. In *Ergogenic Aids and Muscular Performance*, edited by Morgan W. New York, NY: Academic Press, 1972.

59. **Gotshalk LA, Volek JS, Staron RS, Denegar CR, Hagerman FC, and Kraemer WJ.** Creatine supplementation improves muscular performance in older men. *Medicine and Science in Sports and Exercise* 34: 537-543, 2002.

60. **Graham T and Spriet L.** *Caffeine and Exercise Performance. Sports Science Exchange #60,* Vol. 9, Number 1, The Gatorade Sports Science Institute is located in Barrington, Il.

61. **Graham TE and Spriet LL.** Performance and metabolic responses to a high caffeine dose during prolonged exercise. *Journal of Applied Physiology: Respiratory, Environmental and Exercise Physiology* 71: 2292-2298, 1991.

62. **Heinonen OJ.** Carnitine and physical exercise. *Sports Medicine* 22: 109-132, 1996.

63. **Herda TJ, Beck TW, Ryan ED, Smith AE, Walter AA, Hartman MJ, et al.** Effects of creatine monohydrate and polyethylene glycosylated creatine supplementation on muscular strength, endurance, and power output. *Journal of Strength and Conditioning Research* 23: 818-826, 2009.

64. **Hetzler R.** Effect of warm-up on plasma free fatty acid responses and substrate utilization during submaximal exercise. *Research Quarterly for Exercise and Sport* 57: 223-228, 1986.

65. **Hobson RM, Saunders B, Ball G, Harris RC, and Sale C.** Effects of β-alanine supplementation on exercise performance: a meta-analysis. *Amino Acids* 43: 25-37, 2012.

66. **Hodgson AB, Randell RK, and Jeukendrup AE.** The metabolic and performance effects of caffeine compared to coffee during endurance exercise. *PLOS ONE.* 8: e59561, 2013.

67. **Hoffman JR, Emerson NS, and Stout JR.** β-alanine supplementation. *Current Sports Medicine Reports* 11: 189-195, 2012.

68. **Hogan MC, Cox RH, and Welch HG.** Lactate accumulation during incremental exercise with varied inspired oxygen fractions. *Journal of Applied Physiology: Respiratory, Environmental and Exercise Physiology* 55: 1134-1140, 1983.

69. **Horswill CA.** Effects of bicarbonate, citrate, and phosphate loading on performance. *International Journal of Sport Nutrition* 5 (Suppl): S111-119, 1995.

70. **Ivy J.** Amphetamines. In *Ergogenic Aids in Sport.* Champaign, IL: Human Kinetics, 1983.

71. **Ivy JL, Costill DL, Fink WJ, and Lower RW.** Influence of caffeine and carbohydrate feedings on endurance performance. *Medicine and Science in Sports* 11: 6-11, 1979.

72. **Jagim AR, Wright GA, Brice AG, and Doberstein ST.** Effects of beta-alanine supplementation on sprint endurance. *Journal of Strength and Conditioning Research.* 27: 526-532, 2013.

73. **Jones AM.** Dietary nitrate supplementation and exercise performance. *Sports Medicine.* 44: S35-S45, 2014.

74. **Jones AM, Koppo K, and Burnley M.** Effects of prior exercise on metabolic and gas exchange responses to exercise. *Sports Medicine* 33: 949-971, 2003.

75. **Juhn M.** Popular sports supplements and ergogenic aids. *Sports Medicine* 33: 921-939, 2003.

76. **Kley RA, Tarnopolsky MA, Vorgerd M.** Creatine for treating muscle disorders. Cochrane Database of Systematic Reviews 2013, No.: CD004760. DOI: 10.1002/14651858.CD004760.pub4.

77. **Kyle C.** Mechanical factors affecting the speed of a cycle. In *Science of Cycling,* edited by Burke ER. Champaign, IL: Human Kinetics, 1986 pp. 123-136.

78. **Kyle C.** Selecting cycling equipment. In *High-Tech Cycling,* edited by Burke ER. Champaign, IL: Human Kinetics, 2003, pp. 1-48.

79. **Law YLL, Ong WS, GillianYap TL, Lim SCJ, and Von Chia E.** Effects of two and five days of creatine loading on muscular strength and anaerobic power in trained athletes. *Journal of Strength and Conditioning Research* 23: 906-914, 2009.

80. **Linderman J and Fahey TD.** Sodium bicarbonate ingestion and exercise performance: an update. *Sports Medicine* 11: 71-77, 1991.

81. **Lippi G and Banfi G.** Blood transfusions in athletes: old dogmas, new tricks. *Clinical Chemistry and Laboratory Medicine* 44: 1395-1402, 2006.

82. **Lombardo J.** Stimulants and athletic performance (part 1 of 2): amphetamines and caffeine. *Physician and Sportsmedicine* 14: 128-142, 1986.

83. **Lundby C and Robach P.** Assessment of total haemoglobin mass: can it detect erythropoietin-induced blood manipulations? *European Journal of Applied Physiology* 108: 197-200, 2010.

84. **Lundby C, Robach P, and Saltin B.** The evolving science of detection of 'blood doping.' *British Journal of Pharmacology* 165: 1306-1315, 2012.

85. **Lundby C, Thomsen JJ, Boushel R, Koskolou M, Warberg J, Calbet JA, et al.** Erythropoietin treatment elevates haemoglobin concentration by increasing red cell volume and depressing plasma volume. *Journal of Physiology* 578: 309-314, 2007.

86. **Macdougall IC.** Meeting the challenges of a new millennium: optimizing the use of recombinant human erythropoietin. *Nephrol Dial Transplant* 13 (Suppl 2): 23-27, 1998.

87. **Maltin CA, and Delday MI.** Satellite cells in innervated and denervated muscles treated with clenbuterol. *Muscle & Nerve* 15: 919-925, 1992.

88. **Maughan RJ, King DS, and Lea T.** Dietary supplements. *Journal of Sports Sciences* 22: 95-113, 2004.

89. **McClung M and Collins D.** "Because I know it will!": placebo effects of an ergogenic aid on athletic performance. *Journal of Sport & Exercise Psychology* 29: 382-394, 2007.

90. **McCole SD, Claney K, Conte J-C, Anderson R, and Hagberg, JM.** Energy expenditure during bicycling. *Journal of Applied Physiology* 68: 748-753, 1990.

91. **McDowall JA.** Supplement use by young athletes. *Journal of Sport Science & Medicine* 6: 337-342, 2007.

92. **McCrary JM, Ackermann BJ, and Halaki M.** A systematic review of the effects of upper body warm-up on performance. *British Journal of Sports Medicine.* 49: 935-942, 2015.

93. **McLean C and Graham TE.** Effects of exercise and thermal stress on caffeine pharmacokinetics in men and eumenorrheic women. *Journal of Applied Physiology: Respiratory, Environmental and Exercise Physiology* 93: 1471-1478, 2002.

94. **McNaughton L.** Two levels of caffeine ingestion on blood lactate and free fatty acid responses during incremental exercise. *Research Quarterly for Exercise and Sport* 58: 255-259, 1987.

95. **McNaughton LR.** The influence of caffeine ingestion on incremental treadmill running. *British Journal of Sports Medicine* 20: 109-112, 1986.

96. **Momaya A, Fawal M, and Estes R.** Performance-enhancing substances in sports: a review of the literature. *Sports Medicine.* 45: 517-531, 2015.

97. **Morente-Sánchez J and Zabala M.** Doping in sport: a review of elite athletes' attitudes, beliefs, and knowledge. *Sports Medicine.* 43: 395-411, 2013.

98. **Morgan W.** Basic considerations. In *Ergogenic Aids and Muscular Performance*, edited by Morgan W. New York, NY: Academic Press, 1972.

99. **Morkeberg J, Sharpe K, Belhage B, Damsgaard R, Schmidt W, Prommer N, et al.** Detecting autologous blood transfusions: a comparison of three passport approaches and four blood markers. *Scandinavian Journal of Medicine & Science in Sports* 21: 235-243, 2011.

100. **Morris A.** Oxygen. In *Ergogenic Aids in Sports.* Champaign, IL: Human Kinetics, 1983.

101. **Nakamaru Y and Schwartz A.** The influence of hydrogen ion concentration on calcium binding and release by skeletal muscle sarcoplasmic reticulum. *Journal of General Physiology* 59: 22-32, 1972.

102. **Nielsen HB, Bredmose PP, Stromstad M, Volianitis S, Quistorff B, and Secher NH.** Bicarbonate attenuates arterial desaturation during maximal exercise in humans. *Journal of Applied Physiology: Respiratory, Environmental and Exercise Physiology* 93: 724-731, 2002.

103. **Nummela A, Hamalainen I, and Rusko H.** Effect of hyperoxia on metabolic responses and recovery in intermittent exercise. *Scandinavian Journal of Medicine & Science in Sports* 12: 309-315, 2002.

104. **Oopik V, Saaremets I, Medijainen L, Karelson K, Janson T, and Timpmann S.** Effects of sodium citrate ingestion before exercise on endurance performance in well trained college runners. *British Journal of Sports Medicine* 37: 485-489, 2003.

105. **Outram S and Stewart B.** Doping through supplement use: a review of the available evidence. *International Journal of Sport Nutrition and Exercise Metabolism.* 25: 54-59, 2015.

106. **Perry CG, Talanian JL, Heigenhauser GJ, and Spriet LL.** The effects of training in hyperoxia vs. normoxia on skeletal muscle enzyme activities and exercise performance. *Journal of Applied Physiology: Respiratory, Environmental and Exercise Physiology* 102: 1022-1027, 2007.

107. **Pluim BM, de Hon O, Staal JB, Limpens J, Kuipers H, Overbeek SE, et al.** β_2-agonists and physcial performance: a systematic review and meta analysis of randomized controlled studies. *Sports Medicine* 41: 39-57, 2011.

108. **Pope HG, Wood RI, Rogol A, Nyberg F, Bowers L, and Bhasin S.** Adverse health consequences of performance-enhancing drugs: an Endocrine Society Scientific Statement. *Endocrine Reviews.* 35: 341-375, 2014.

109. **Pottgiesser T, Echteler T, Sottas P-E, Umhau M, and Schumacher YO.** Hemoglobin mass and biological passport for detection of autologous blood doping. *Medicine and Science in Sports and Exercise* 44: 835-843, 2012.

110. **Pottgiesser T, Umhau M, Ahlgrim C, Ruthardt S, Roecker K, and Schumacher YO.** Hb mass measurement suitable to screen for illicit autologous blood transfusions. *Medicine and Science in Sports and Exercise* 39: 1748-1756, 2007.

111. **Powers SK and Dodd S.** Caffeine and endurance performance. *Sports Medicine* 2: 165-174, 1985.

112. **Powers SK, Lawler J, Dempsey JA, Dodd S, and Landry G.** Effects of incomplete pulmonary gas exchange on $\dot{V}O_2$ max. *Journal of Applied Physiology: Respiratory, Environmental and Exercise Physiology* 66: 2491-2495, 1989.

113. **Price M, Moss P, and Rance S.** Effects of sodium bicarbonate ingestion on prolonged intermittent exercise. *Medicine and Science in Sports and Exercise* 35: 1303-1308, 2003.

114. **Price MJ and Simons C.** The effect of sodium bicarbonate ingestion on high-intensity intermittent running and subsequent performance. *Journal of Strength and Conditioning Research* 24: 1834-1842, 2010.

115. **Putukian M, Kreher JB, Coppel DB, Glazer JL, McKeag DB, and White RD.** Attention deficit hyperactivity disorder and the athlete: an American Medical Society for Sports Medicine position statement. *Clinical Journal of Sports Medicine.* 21: 392-401, 2011.

116. **Rawson E and Clarkson P.** Scientifically debatable: is creatine worth its weight? *Sports Science Exchange #91*, Volume 16, Number 4, 2003 Gatorade Sports Science Institute, Barrington, Il.

117. **Rawson E, Coni M, and Miles M.** Creatine supplementation does not reduce muscle damage or enhance recovery from resistance exercise. *Journal of Strength and Conditioning Research* 21: 1208-1213, 2007.

118. **Rawson E and Persky A.** Mechanisms of muscular adaptations to creatine supplementation. *Int Sport Med J* 8: 43-53, 2007.

119. **Rawson ES, Stec MJ, Frederickson SJ, and Miles MP.** Low-dose creatine supplementation enhances fatigue resistance in the absense of weight gain. *Nutrition* 27: 451-455, 2011.

120. **Requena B, Zabala M, and Padial P.** Sodium bicarbonate and sodium citrate: ergogenic aids? *Journal of Strength and Conditioning Research* 19: 213-224, 2005.

121. **Robbins MK, Gleeson K, and Zwillich CW.** Effect of oxygen breathing following submaximal and maximal exercise on recovery and performance. *Medicine and Science in Sports and Exercise* 24: 720-725, 1992.

122. **Robergs RA, Pascoe DD, Costill DL, Fink WJ, Chwalbinska-Moneta J, Davis JA, et al.** Effects of warm-up on muscle glycogenolysis during intense exercise. *Medicine and Science in Sports and Exercise* 23: 37-43, 1991.

123. **Rogers M, Bohlken R, and Beets M.** Effects of creatine, ginseng, and astragalus supplementation on strength, body composition, mood, and blood lipids during strength-training in older adults. *Journal of Sports Science and Medicine* 5: 60-69, 2006.

124. **Roy BD, Bosman MJ, and Tarnopolsky MA.** An acute oral dose of caffeine does not alter glucose kinetics during prolonged dynamic exercise in trained endurance athletes. *European Journal of Applied Physiology* 85: 280-286, 2001.

125. **Rozenek R, Fobel B, and Banks J.** Does hyperbaric oxygen exposure affect high-intensity, short-duration exercise performance? *Journal of Strength and Conditioning Research* 21: 1037-1041, 2007.

126. **Shao A and Hathcock JN.** Risk assessment for creatine monohydrate. *Regul Toxicol Pharmacol* 45: 242-251, 2006.

127. **Shrier I.** Special communications: letters to the editor-in-chief. *Medicine and Science in Sports and Exercise* 36: 1832-1833, 2004.

128. **Siegler JC, Marshall PWM, Bray J, and Towlson C.** Sodium bicarbonate supplementation and ingestions timing: does it matter? *Journal of Strength and Conditioning Research* 26: 1953-1958, 2012.

129. **Siegler JC, Midgley AW, Polman RCJ, and Lever R.** Effects of various sodium bicarbonate loading protocols on the time-dependent extracelluar buffering profile. *Journal of Strength and Conditioning Research* 24: 2551-2557, p. 576 2010.

130. **Simic L, Sarabon N, and Markovic G.** Does pre-exercise static stretching inhibit maximal muscular performance? A meta-analytical review. *Scandinavian Journal of Medicine and Science in Sports.* 23: 131-148, 2013.

131. **Smith-Ryan AE, Fukuda DH, Stout JR, and Kendall KL.** High-velocity intermittent running:

effects of beta-alanine supplementation. *Journal of Strength and Conditioning Research* 26: 2798-2805, 2012.

132. **Spriet LL.** Exercise and sport performance with low doses of caffeine. *Sport Medicine.* 44 (Suppl 2): S175-S184, 2014.

133. **Spriet LL.** Caffeine and performance. *International Journal of Sport Nutrition* 5 (Suppl): S84-99, 1995.

134. **Stellingwerff T, Glazier L, Watt MJ, LeBlanc PJ, Heigenhauser GJ, and Spriet LL.** Effects of hyperoxia on skeletal muscle carbohydrate metabolism during transient and steady-state exercise. *Journal of Applied Physiology: Respiratory, Environmental and Exercise Physiology* 98: 250-256, 2005.

135. **Tallis J, Duncan MJ, and James RS.** What can isolated skeletal muscle experiments tell us about the effects of caffeine on exercise performance. *British Journal of Pharmacology.* 172: 3703-3713, 2015.

136. **Tarnopolsky MA.** Effect of caffeine on the neuromuscular system: potential as an ergogenic aid. *Applied Physiology, Nutrition and Metabolism* 33: 1284-1289, 2008.

137. **Tarnopolsky MA, Atkinson SA, MacDougall JD, Sale DG, and Sutton JR.** Physiological responses to caffeine during endurance running in habitual caffeine users. *Medicine and Science in Sports and Exercise* 21: 418-424, 1989.

138. **Tesch P, Sjodin B, Thorstensson A, and Karlsson J.** Muscle fatigue and its relation to lactate accumulation and LDH activity in man. *Acta Physiologica Scandinavica* 103: 413-420, 1978.

139. **Thacker SB, Gilchrist J, Stroup DF, and Kimsey CD, Jr.** The impact of stretching on sports injury risk: a systematic review of the literature. *Medicine and Science in Sports and Exercise* 36: 371-378, 2004.

140. **Trexler ET, Smith-Ryan AE, Stout JR, Hoffman JR, Wilborn CD, Sale C, Kreider RB, Jäger R, Earnest CP, Bannock L, Campbell B, Kalman D, Ziegenfuss TN, and Antonio J.** International society of sports nutrition position stand: beta-alanine. *Journal of the International Society of Sports Nutrition.* 12: 30 DOI 10.1186, 2015.

141. **Trivedi B, and Danforth WH.** Effect of pH on the kinetics of frog muscle phosphofructokinase. *Journal of Biological Chemistry* 241: 4110-4112, 1966.

142. **United States Anti-Doping Agency.** Reasoned decision: United States Anti-Doping Agency vs. Lance Armstrong. http://d3epuodzu3wuis.cloudfront.net/ReasonedDecision.pdf, 2012.

143. **Van Handel P.** Caffeine. In *Ergogenic Aids in Sports,* edited by Williams M. Champaign, IL: Human Kinetics, 1983.

144. **Van Thuyne W, and Delbeke FT.** Distribution of caffeine levels in urine in different sports in relation to doping control before and after the removal of caffeine from the WADA doping list. *International Journal of Sports Medicine* 27: 745-750, 2006.

145. **VanThuyne P, VanEenoo P, and Delbeke F.** Nutritional supplements: prevalence of use and contamination with doping agents. *Nutrition Research Reviews* 19: 147-158, 2006.

146. **Volek J.** What we now know about creatine. *ACSM's Health & Fitness Journal* 3: 27-33, 1999.

147. **Voss S, Thevis M, and Schinkothe T.** Detection of homologous blood transfusion. *International Journal of Sports Medicine* 28: 633-637, 2007.

148. **Warren GL, Park ND, Maresca RD, Mckibans KI, and Millard-Stafford ML.** Effect of caffeine ingestion on muscular strength and endurance: a meta-analysis. *Medicine and Science in Sports and Exercise* 42: 1375-1387, 2010.

149. **Welch H.** Effects of hypoxia and hyperoxia on human performance. In *Exercise and Sports Sciences Reviews,* edited by Pandolf K. New York, NY: Macmillan, 1987, pp. 191-222.

150. **Welch HG, Bonde-Petersen F, Graham T, Klausen K, and Secher N.** Effects of hyperoxia on leg blood flow and metabolism during exercise. *Journal of Applied Physiology: Respiratory, Environmental and Exercise Physiology* 42: 385-390, 1977.

151. **Weldon SM and Hill RH.** The efficacy of stretching for prevention of exercise-related injury: a systematic review of the literature. *Manual Therapy* 8: 141-150, 2003.

152. **Wilcox A.** *Bicarbonate Loading.* Gatorade Sports Science Institute, Barrington, Il.

153. **Wilcox A.** *Caffeine and Endurance Performance.* Gatorade Sports Science Institute, 1990.

154. **Wilcox A.** Nutritional ergogenics and sport performance. In *The President's Council on Physical Fitness and Sports Research Digest,* edited by Corbin C, and Pangrazi B, Washington, D.C.: Department of Health and Human Services, 1998.

155. **Williams MH, Anderson DE, and Rawson ES.** *Nutrition for Health, Fitness & Sport.* New York, NY: McGraw-Hill, 2017.

156. **Williams MH, Wesseldine S, Somma T, and Schuster R.** The effect of induced erythrocythemia upon 5-mile treadmill run time. *Medicine and Science in Sports and Exercise* 13: 169-175, 1981.

157. **Wilmore J.** Oxygen. In *Ergogenic Aids and Muscular Performance,* edited by Morgan W. New York, NY: Academic Press, 1972, pp. 321-342.

158. **Wilson GD and Welch HG.** Effects of hyperoxic gas mixtures on exercise tolerance in man. *Medicine and Science in Sports* 7: 48-52, 1975.

159. **Wilson GD, and Welch HG.** Effects of varying concentrations of N_2/O_2 and He/O_2 on exercise tolerance in man. *Medicine and Science in Sports and Exercise* 12: 380-384, 1980.

160. **Wilson GJ, Wilson JM, and Manninen AH.** Effects of beta-hydroxy-beta-methylbutyrate (HMB) on exercise performance and body compostion across levels of age, sex, and training experience: a review. *Nutrition & Metabolism* 5: Article No. 1, 2008.

161. **Witvrouw E, Mahieu N, Danneels L, and McNair P.** Stretching and injury prevention: an obscure relationship. *Sports Medicine* 34: 443-449, 2004.

162. **World Anti-Doping Agency.** *The 2013 Prohibited List: International Standard.* Switzerland: World Anti-Doping Agency, 2012.

163. **Yang YT and McElligott MA.** Multiple actions of beta-adrenergic agonists on skeletal muscle and adipose tissue. *Biochemical Journal* 261: 1-10, 1989.

164. **Yeo SE, Jentjens RL, Wallis GA, and Jeukendrup AE.** Caffeine increases exogenous carbohydrate oxidation during exercise. *Journal of Applied Physiology: Respiratory, Environmental and Exercise Physiology* 99: 844-850, 2005.

165. **Zanchi NE, Gerlinger-Romero F, Guimaraes-Ferreira L, de Siqueira MA, Felitti V, Lira FS, et al.** HMB supplementation: clinical and athletic performance-related effects and mechanisms of action. *Amion Acids* 40: 1015-1025, 2011.

166. **Zeno SA, Purvis D, Crawford C, Lee C, Lisman P, and Deuster PA.** Warm-ups for military fitness testing: rapid evidence assessment of the literature. *Medicine and Science in Sports and Exercise* 45: 1369-1376, 2013.

167. **Zhang Y, Coca A, Casa DJ, Antonio J, Green JM, and Bishop PA.** Caffeine and diuresis during rest and exercise: a meta analysis. *Journal of Science and Medicine in Sport.* 18: 659-574, 2015.

Calculation of Oxygen Uptake and Carbon Dioxide Production

Calculation of Oxygen Consumption

Calculation of oxygen consumption is a relatively simple process that involves subtracting the amount of oxygen exhaled from the amount of oxygen inhaled:

(1) Oxygen consumption ($\dot{V}O_2$) =
[volume of O_2 inspired] – [volume of O_2 expired]

The volume of O_2 inspired (I) is computed by multiplying the volume of air inhaled per minute ($\dot{V}_I$) by the fraction (F) of air that is made up of oxygen. Room air is 20.93% O_2. Expressed as a fraction, 20.93% becomes .2093 and is symbolized as F_IO_2. When we exhale, the fraction of O_2 is lowered (i.e., O_2 diffuses from the lung to the blood) and the fraction of O_2 in the expired (E) gas is represented by F_EO_2. The volume of expired O_2 is the product of the volume of expired gas ($\dot{V}_E$) and F_EO_2. Equation (1) can now be symbolized as:

(2) $\dot{V}O_2 = (\dot{V}_I \cdot F_IO_2) - (\dot{V}_E \cdot F_EO_2)$

The exercise values for F_IO_2, F_EO_2, $\dot{V}_I$, and $\dot{V}_E$ for a subject are easily measured in most exercise physiology laboratories. In practice, F_IO_2 is not generally measured but is assumed to be a constant value of .2093 if the subject is breathing room air. F_EO_2 will be determined by a gas analyzer, and $\dot{V}_I$ and $\dot{V}_E$ can be measured by a number of different laboratory devices capable of measuring airflow. Note that it is not necessary to measure both $\dot{V}_I$ and $\dot{V}_E$. This is true because if $\dot{V}_I$ is measured, $\dot{V}_E$ can be calculated (and vice versa). The formula used to calculate $\dot{V}_E$ from the measurement of $\dot{V}_I$ is called the "Haldane transformation" and is based on the fact that nitrogen (N_2) is neither used nor produced in the body. Therefore, the volume of N_2 inhaled must equal the volume of N_2 exhaled:

(3) $[\dot{V}_I \cdot F_IN_2] = [\dot{V}_E F_EN_2]$

Therefore, $\dot{V}_I$ can be computed if $\dot{V}_E$, F_IO_2, and F_EO_2 are known. For example, to solve for $\dot{V}_I$:

(4) $\dot{V}_I = \dfrac{(\dot{V}_E \cdot F_EN_2)}{F_IN_2}$

Likewise, if $\dot{V}_I$ was measured, $\dot{V}_E$ can be computed as:

(5) $\dot{V}_E = \dfrac{(\dot{V}_I \cdot F_IN_2)}{F_EN_2}$

The values for F_IN_2 and F_EN_2 are obtained in the following manner. If the subject is breathing room air, F_IN_2 is considered to be a constant .7904. The final remaining piece to the puzzle is F_EN_2. Recall that the three principal gases in air are N_2, O_2, and CO_2 and the sum of their fractions must add up to 1.0 (i.e., $F_ECO_2 + F_EO_2 + F_EN_2 = 1.0$). Therefore, F_EN_2 can be computed by subtracting the sum of F_ECO_2 and F_EO_2 from 1 (i.e., $F_EN_2 = 1 - (F_ECO_2 + F_EO_2)$). Because the expired fractions of O_2 and CO_2 will be determined by gas analyzers, F_EN_2 can then be calculated.

Calculation of Carbon Dioxide Production

The volume of carbon dioxide produced ($\dot{V}CO_2$) can be calculated in a manner similar to $\dot{V}O_2$. That is, the volume of CO_2 produced is equal to:

(6) $\dot{V}CO_2 = $ [Volume of CO_2 expired]
– [Volume of CO_2 inspired]
or
(7) $\dot{V}CO_2 = (\dot{V}_E \cdot F_ECO_2) - (\dot{V}_I \cdot F_ICO_2)$

The steps in performing this calculation are the same as in the computation of $\dot{V}O_2$. That is, $\dot{V}_E$ and $\dot{V}_I$ must be measured (or calculated) and the fraction of expired carbon dioxide (F_ECO_2) must be determined by a gas analyzer. Similar to F_IO_2, the fraction of inspired carbon dioxide (F_ICO_2) is considered to be a constant value of .0003.

By convention, $\dot{V}O_2$ or $\dot{V}CO_2$ are expressed in liters · min^{-1} and standardized to a reference condition called "STPD." STPD is an acronym for "standard temperature pressure dry." In a similar manner, pulmonary ventilation is expressed in liters · min^{-1} and standardized to a reference standard called BTPS, an acronym for "body temperature pressure saturated." The purpose of these reference standards is to allow comparison of gas volumes measured in laboratories throughout the world, which may vary in ambient temperature and barometric pressures. Standardization of gas volumes to a specified temperature and pressure is necessary because gas volume is dependent upon both temperature and pressure. For instance, a given number of gas molecules will occupy a greater volume at a higher temperature and lower pressure than at a lower temperature and higher pressure. This means that a fixed number of gas molecules would change volume as a function of the ambient temperature and barometric pressure. This poses a serious problem to researchers trying to make comparisons of respiratory gas exchange, because temperature and pressures vary day by day and vary from one laboratory to another. By standardizing temperature and pressure conditions for gases, the scientist or technician knows that two equal volumes of gas contain the same number of molecules. For these reasons, respiratory gases must be corrected to a reference temperature and volume.

CORRECTION OF GAS VOLUMES TO REFERENCE CONDITIONS

Before we begin a discussion of "how to" calculate gas volume corrections, it is necessary to introduce two important gas laws. The first, called "Charles's Law," states that the relationship between temperature and gas volume is directly proportional. That is, the gas volume is directly related to temperature, so that increasing or decreasing the temperature of a gas (at a constant pressure) causes a proportional volume increase or decrease, respectively. This relationship is expressed mathematically in the following way:

$$(8) \quad \frac{T_1}{T_2} = \frac{V_1}{V_2}$$

The units for temperature in equation (8) are the Kelvin (K) or Absolute (A) scale, where $0°$ C = $273°$ K [i.e., $20°$ C = $(273° + 20°) = 293°$ K]. In using Charles's Law for gas temperature corrections, we rearrange equation (8) to solve for V_2:

$$(9) \quad V_2 = \frac{V_1 \cdot T_2}{T_1}$$

Let's leave Charles's Law for the moment and introduce a second gas law known as Boyle's Law. Boyle's Law states that at a constant temperature, the number of gas molecules in a given volume varies inversely with the pressure and is represented mathematically in the following equation:

$$(10) \quad P_1 V_1 = P_2 V_2$$

Again, rearranging equation (10) to solve for V_2:

$$(11) \quad V_2 = \frac{P_1 \cdot V_1}{P_2}$$

Pressure in equations (10) and (11) is expressed in mm Hg or Torr. Note that when respiratory gases are corrected for pressure differences, a correction is often made for water vapor, even though water vapor pressure is dependent only upon temperature (because respiratory gas is saturated with water vapor). When the gas volume is to be corrected to "0" water vapor pressure or "dried" as in STPD, the vapor pressure of water (PH_2O) at the ambient temperature is subtracted from the ambient or initial pressure (P_1) in Boyle's Law as follows:

$$(12) \quad V_2 = \frac{V_1(P_1 - PH_2O)}{P_2}$$

COMBINED CORRECTION FACTORS

We can now combine Charles's Law and Boyle's Law (complete with water vapor correction) into one equation for STPD and BTPS conditions. Let's consider the STPD correction first.

STPD Correction

Gas volumes measured in the laboratory under room conditions of temperature and pressure are expressed as "ambient temperature pressure and saturated" (ATPS). This means that the gas volume is not a standardized volume but rather a volume that is subject to the ambient conditions of temperature and pressure. As previously stated, because ATPS conditions may vary from laboratory to laboratory, there is a need to correct $\dot{V}O_2$ and $\dot{V}CO_2$ volumes to the reference volume, STPD. Correcting a volume to STPD requires the standardization of temperature to $0°$ C ($273°$ K), pressure to 760 mm Hg (sea level), and a correction for vapor pressure. For simplicity we will divide the gas correction procedure into two parts: (1) temperature and (2) pressure correction.

Step 1: Temperature Correction Let's consider the temperature correction first. For this correction, we use equation (9) (Charles's Law):

$$V_2 = \frac{V_1 \cdot T_2}{T_1}$$

where:

- V_2 = volume corrected to standard temperature (V_{ST})
- V_1 = ATPS volume (V_{ATPS})
- T_1 = absolute temperature in ambient surroundings ($273° K + T_a° C$)

  where: T_a = ambient temperature
- T_2 = absolute standard temperature ($273° K$)

Therefore, correcting an ATPS gas volume to V_{ST} is performed using the following equation:

$$(13)\ V_{ST} = V_{ATPS} \left[\frac{273°}{(273° + T_a)} \right]$$

Step 2: Barometric Pressure and Water Vapor Pressure Correction To correct for barometric pressure and vapor pressure, we use equation (12), where:

- V_1 = volume ATPS
- V_2 = volume corrected to standard pressure and dry (V_{SPD})
- P_1 = ambient barometric pressure in mm Hg
- P_2 = standard barometric pressure (760 mm Hg)
- PH_2O = partial pressure of water vapor at ambient temperature (see Table A.1 for a list of vapor pressures at various ambient temperatures)

Therefore, when correcting V_{SPD} from ATPS volumes, the following equation is used:

$$(14)\ V_{SPD} = V_{ATPS} \left[\frac{P_1 - PH_2O}{760 \text{ mm Hg}} \right]$$

At this point we are ready to combine both the temperature correction factor equation (13) and the pressure and vapor pressure correction factor equation (14) into one equation and compute one single STPD correction factor. Combining equations (13) and (14) we arrive at:

$$(15)\ V_{STPD} = V_{ATPS} \left[\frac{273°}{(273° + T_a)} \right] \left[\frac{(P_1 - PH_2O)}{760 \text{ mm Hg}} \right]$$

Let's consider a sample problem to illustrate correction of ATPS volumes to STPD volumes.

Given:

- V_{ATPS} = 90.0 liters
- Laboratory temperature = 21° C
- Ambient barometric pressure = 742 mm Hg
- H_2O vapor pressure at 21° C (from Table A.1) = 18.7 mm Hg

TABLE A.1 Water Vapor Pressure as a Function of Ambient Temperature

Temperature (°C)	Saturation Water Vapor Pressure (PH$_2$O), mm Hg
18	15.5
19	16.5
20	17.5
21	18.7
22	19.8
23	21.1
24	22.4
25	23.8
26	25.2
27	26.7

Using the above sample conditions and equation (15), the STPD correction would be as follows:

$$V_{STPD} = 90 \left[\frac{273°}{(273° + 21°)} \right] \left[\frac{742 - 18.7}{760} \right]$$

$$= 79.5 \text{ liters STPD}$$

It is important to point out that if inspired gas volumes are measured and the relative humidity of the inspired gas is not 100%, then equation (15) must be modified by multiplying the relative humidity (RH) of the inspired gas (expressed as a fraction) by the partial pressure of water vapor at ambient temperature (e.g., if RH = 80%, then use $.8 \times PH_2O$).

BTPS Correction

As previously mentioned, all ventilatory volumes are corrected to BTPS conditions. This correction procedure is similar to the STPD correction procedure with two exceptions: (1) Standard temperature is 310°K instead of 273°K (e.g., 310° = 273°K + 37°C [normal core temperature]). This correction is necessary because body temperature is usually greater than ambient temperature and results in an increase in gas volume. (2) The partial pressure of vapor pressure at body temperature is subtracted from P_1 in equation (14). This correction is necessary because the partial pressure of water vapor at body temperature is generally greater than PH_2O at ambient conditions (i.e., at 37° the PH_2O = 47 mm Hg).

Therefore, correcting from ATPS to BTPS would involve the following equation:

$$(16)\ V_{BTPS} = V_{ATPS} \left[\frac{310°}{273° + T_a} \right] \left[\frac{P_1 - PH_2O}{P_1 - 47} \right]$$

Let's consider a sample calculation of converting V_{ATPS} to V_{BTPS} using the following conditions:

- Laboratory temperature = 20° C
- Ambient barometric pressure = 752 mm Hg
- PH_2O at 20° C = 17.5 mm Hg
- V_{ATPS} = 60 liters

Therefore:

$$V_{BTPS} = 60 \left[\frac{310°}{273° + 20°} \right] \left[\frac{752 - 17.5}{752 - 47} \right]$$

$$= 65.4 \text{ liters BTPS}$$

Problems

1. Calculate $\dot{V}O_2$ and $\dot{V}CO_2$ given:

   $\dot{V}_E$ (ATPS) = 100 liters · min^{-1}
   F_EO_2 = .1768
   F_ECO_2 = .0351
   Assume F_IO_2 = .2093 and F_ICO_2 = .0003
   Ambient temperature = 21° C
   Barometric pressure = 749 mm Hg

2. Calculate the respiratory exchange ratio (R) from $\dot{V}O_2$ and $\dot{V}CO_2$ values computed in question 1.

3. Calculate V_{BTPS} and V_{STPD} given:

   V_{ATPS} = 45.3 liters
   Laboratory temperature = 19° C
   Ambient barometric temperature = 746 mm Hg
   Body temperature = 37° C

Answers

1. $\dot{V}O_2$ = 2.73ℓ · min^{-1}
   $\dot{V}CO_2$ = 3.54ℓ · min^{-1}
2. R = 1.15
3. V_{BTPS} = 50.19 liters
4. V_{STPD} = 40.65 liters

Dietary Reference Intakes: Estimated Energy Requirements

Estimated Energy Requirements (EER) for Men and Women 30 Years of Age[a]
Food and Nutrition Board, Institute of Medicine, National Academies

Height (m [in])	PAL[b]	Weight for BMI[c] of 18.5 kg/m² (kg [lb])	Weight for BMI of 24.99 kg/m² (kg [lb])	EER, Men[d] (kcal/day) BMI of 18.5 kg/m²	BMI of 24.99 kg/m²	EER, Women[d] (kcal/day) BMI of 18.5 kg/m²	BMI of 24.99 kg/m²
1.50 (59)	Sedentary	41.6 (92)	56.2 (124)	1,848	2,080	1,625	1,762
	Low Active			2,009	2,267	1,803	1,956
	Active			2,215	2,506	2,025	2,198
	Very Active			2,554	2,898	2,291	2,489
1.65 (65)	Sedentary	50.4 (111)	68.0 (150)	2,068	2,349	1,816	1,982
	Low Active			2,254	2,566	2,016	2,202
	Active			2,490	2,842	2,267	2,477
	Very Active			2,880	3,296	2,567	2,807
1.80 (71)	Sedentary	59.9 (132)	81.0 (178)	2,301	2,635	2,015	2,211
	Low Active			2,513	2,884	2,239	2,459
	Active			2,782	3,200	2,519	2,769
	Very Active			3,225	3,720	2,855	3,141

[a]For each year below 30, add 7 kcal/day for women and 10 kcal/day for men. For each year above 30, subtract 7 kcal/day for women and 10 kcal/day for men.
[b]PAL = physical activity level.
[c]BMI = body mass index.
[d]Derived from the following regression equations based on doubly labeled water data:

Adult man: $EER = 662 - 9.53 \times age\ (yr) + PA \times (15.91 \times wt\ [kg] + 539.6 \times ht\ [ml])$
Adult woman: $EER = 354 - 6.91 \times age\ (yr) + PA \times (9.36 \times wt\ [kg] + 726 \times ht\ [ml])$

where PA refers to coefficient for PAL.

PAL = total energy expenditure ÷ basal energy expenditure

PA = 1.0 if PAL ≥ 1.0 < 1.4 (sedentary)
PA = 1.12 if PAL ≥ 1.4 < 1.6 (low active)
PA = 1.27 if PAL ≥ 1.6 < 1.9 (active)
PA = 1.45 if PAL ≥ 1.9 < 2.5 (very active)

SOURCE: *Dietary Reference Intakes for Energy, Carbohydrate, Fiber, Fat, Fatty Acids, Cholesterol, Protein, and Amino Acids* (2002).

Dietary Reference Intakes: Vitamins

Dietary Reference Intakes (DRIs): Recommended Intakes for Individuals, Vitamins Food and Nutrition Board, Institute of Medicine, National Academies						
Life Stage Group	Vit A (µg/d)[a]	Vit C (mg/d)	Vit D (µg/d)[b,c]	Vit E (mg/d)[d]	Vit K (µg/d)	Thiamin (mg/d)
Infants						
0–6 mo	400*	40*	5*	4*	2.0*	0.2*
7–12 mo	500*	50*	5*	5*	2.5*	0.3*
Children						
1–3 yr	300	15	5*	6	30*	0.5
4–8 yr	400	25	5*	7	55*	0.6
Males						
9–13 yr	600	45	5*	11	60*	0.9
14–18 yr	900	75	5*	15	75*	1.2
19–30 yr	900	90	5*	15	120*	1.2
31–50 yr	900	90	5*	15	120*	1.2
51–70 yr	900	90	10*	15	120*	1.2
>70 yr	900	90	15*	15	120*	1.2
Females						
9–13 yr	600	45	5*	11	60*	0.9
14–18 yr	700	65	5*	15	75*	1.0
19–30 yr	700	75	5*	15	90*	1.1
31–50 yr	700	75	5*	15	90*	1.1
51–70 yr	700	75	10*	15	90*	1.1
>70 yr	700	75	15*	15	90*	1.1
Pregnancy						
14–18 yr	750	80	5*	15	75*	1.4
19–30 yr	770	85	5*	15	90*	1.4
31–50 yr	770	85	5*	15	90*	1.4
Lactation						
14–18 yr	1,200	115	5*	19	75*	1.4
19–30 yr	1,300	120	5*	19	90*	1.4
31–50 yr	1,300	120	5*	19	90*	1.4

NOTE: This table (taken from the DRI reports, see www.nap.edu) presents Recommended Dietary Allowances (RDAs) in **bold** type and Adequate Intakes (AIs) in ordinary type followed by an asterisk (*). RDAs and AIs may both be used as goals for individual intake. RDAs are set to meet the needs of almost all (97%–98%) individuals in a group. For healthy breastfed infants, the AI is the mean intake. The AI for other life stage and gender groups is believed to cover needs of all individuals in the group, but lack of data or uncertainty in the data prevent from being able to specify with confidence the percentage of individuals covered by this intake.

[a]As retinol activity equivalents (RAEs). 1 RAE = 1 µg retinol, 12 µg β-carotene, 24 µg α-carotene, or 24 µg β-cryptoxanthin. The RAE for dietary provitamin A carotenoids is twofold greater than retinol equivalents (RE), whereas the RAE for preformed vitamin A is the same as RE.

[b]As cholecalciferol. 1 g cholecalciferol = 40 IU vitamin D.

[c]In the absence of adequate exposure to sunlight.

[d]As α-tocopherol. α-Tocopherol includes RRR-α-tocopherol, the only form of α-tocopherol that occurs naturally in foods, and the 2R-stereoisomeric forms of α-tocopherol (RRR-, RSR-, RRS-, and RSS-α-tocopherol) that occur in fortified foods and supplements. It does not include the 2S-stereoisomeric forms of α-tocopherol (SRR-, SSR-, SRS-, and SSS-α-tocopherol), also found in fortified foods and supplements.

Riboflavin (mg/d)	Niacin (mg/d)^e	Vit B$_6$ (mg/d)	Folate (μg/d)^f	Vit B$_{12}$ (μg/d)	Pantothenic Acid (mg/d)	Biotin (μg/d)	Choline (mg/d)^g
0.3*	2*	0.1*	65*	0.4*	1.7*	5*	125*
0.4*	4*	0.3*	80*	0.5*	1.8*	6*	150*
0.5	6	0.5	150	0.9	2*	8*	200*
0.6	8	0.6	200	1.2	3*	12*	250*
0.9	12	1.0	300	1.8	4*	20*	375*
1.3	16	1.3	400	2.4	5*	25*	550*
1.3	16	1.3	400	2.4	5*	30*	550*
1.3	16	1.3	400	2.4	5*	30*	550*
1.3	16	1.7	400	2.4^i	5*	30*	550*
1.3	16	1.7	400	2.4^i	5*	30*	550*
0.9	12	1.0	300	1.8	4*	20*	375*
1.0	14	1.2	400^i	2.4	5*	25*	400*
1.1	14	1.3	400^i	2.4	5*	30*	425*
1.1	14	1.3	400^i	2.4	5*	30*	425*
1.1	14	1.5	400	2.4^h	5*	30*	425*
1.1	14	1.5	400	2.4^h	5*	30*	425*
1.4	18	1.9	600^j	2.6	6*	30*	450*
1.4	18	1.9	600^j	2.6	6*	30*	450*
1.4	18	1.9	600^j	2.6	6*	30*	450*
1.6	17	2.0	500	2.8	7*	35*	550*
1.6	17	2.0	500	2.8	7*	35*	550*
1.6	17	2.0	500	2.8	7*	35*	550*

^{e}As niacin equivalents (NE). 1 mg of niacin = 60 mg of tryptophan; 0–6 months = preformed niacin (not NE).

^{f}As dietary folate equivalents (DFE). 1 DFE = 1 μg food folate = 0.6 μg of folic acid from fortified food or as a supplement consumed with food = 0.5 μg of a supplement taken on an empty stomach.

^{g}Although AIs have been set for choline, there are few data to assess whether a dietary supply of choline is needed at all stages of the life cycle, and it may be that the choline requirement can be met by endogenous synthesis at some of these stages.

^{h}Because 10% to 30% of older people may malabsorb food-bound B$_{12}$, it is advisable for those older than 50 years to meet their RDA mainly by consuming foods fortified with B$_{12}$ or a supplement containing B$_{12}$.

^{i}In view of evidence linking folate intake with neural tube defects in the fetus, it is recommended that all women capable of becoming pregnant consume 400 μg from supplements or fortified foods in addition to intake of food folate from a varied diet.

^{j}It is assumed that women will continue consuming 400 μg from supplements or fortified food until their pregnancy is confirmed and they enter prenatal care, which ordinarily occurs after the end of the periconceptional period—the critical time for formation of the neural tube.

Dietary Reference Intakes: Minerals and Elements

Dietary Reference Intakes (DRIs): Recommended Intakes for Individuals, Elements Food and Nutrition Board, Institute of Medicine, National Academies

Life Stage Group	Calcium (mg/d)	Chromium (µg/d)	Copper (µg/d)	Fluoride (mg/d)	Iodine (µg/d)	Iron (mg/d)	Magnesium (mg/d)
Infants							
0–6 mo	210*	0.2*	200*	0.01*	110*	0.27*	30*
7–12 mo	270*	5.5*	220*	0.5*	130*	**11**	75*
Children							
1–3 yr	500*	11*	**340**	0.7*	**90**	**7**	**80**
4–8 yr	800*	15*	**440**	1*	**90**	**10**	**130**
Males							
9–13 yr	1,300*	25*	**700**	2*	**120**	**8**	**240**
14–18 yr	1,300*	35*	**890**	3*	**150**	**11**	**410**
19–30 yr	1,000*	35*	**900**	4*	**150**	**8**	**400**
31–50 yr	1,000*	35*	**900**	4*	**150**	**8**	**420**
51–70 yr	1,200*	30*	**900**	4*	**150**	**8**	**420**
>70 yr	1,200*	30*	**900**	4*	**150**	**8**	**420**
Females							
9–13 yr	1,300*	21*	**700**	2*	**120**	**8**	**240**
14–18 yr	1,300*	24*	**890**	3*	**150**	**15**	**360**
19–30 yr	1,000*	25*	**900**	3*	**150**	**18**	**310**
31–50 yr	1,000*	25*	**900**	3*	**150**	**18**	**320**
51–70 yr	1,200*	20*	**900**	3*	**150**	**8**	**320**
>70 yr	1,200*	20*	**900**	3*	**150**	**8**	**320**
Pregnancy							
14–18 yr	1,300*	29*	**1,000**	3*	**220**	**27**	**400**
19–30 yr	1,000*	30*	**1,000**	3*	**220**	**27**	**350**
31–50 yr	1,000*	30*	**1,000**	3*	**220**	**27**	**360**
Lactation							
14–18 yr	1,300*	44*	**1,300**	3*	**290**	**10**	**360**
19–30 yr	1,000*	45*	**1,300**	3*	**290**	**9**	**310**
31–50 yr	1,000*	45*	**1,300**	3*	**290**	**9**	**320**

NOTE: This table presents Recommended Dietary Allowances (RDAs) in **bold** type and Adequate Intakes (AIs) in ordinary type followed by an asterisk (*). RDAs and AIs may both be used as goals for individual intake. RDAs are set to meet the needs of almost all (97%–98%) individuals in a group. For healthy breastfed infants, the AI is the mean intake. The AI for other life stage and gender groups is believed to cover needs of all individuals in the group, but lack of data or uncertainty in the data prevent from being able to specify with confidence the percentage of individuals covered by this intake.

SOURCES: *Dietary Reference Intakes for Calcium, Phosphorous, Magnesium, Vitamin D, and Fluoride* (1997); *Dietary Reference Intakes for Thiamin, Riboflavin, Niacin, Vitamin B6, Folate, Vitamin B 1 2, Pantothenic Acid, Biotin, and Choline* (1998); *Dietary Reference Intakes for Vitamin C, Vitamin E, Selenium, and Carotenoids* (2000); *Dietary Reference Intakes for Vitamin A, Vitamin K, Arsenic, Boron, Chromium, Copper, Iodine, Iron, Manganese, Molybdenum, Nickel, Silicon, Vanadium, and Zinc* (2001); and *Dietary Reference Intakes for Water, Potassium, Sodium, Chloride, and Sulfate* (2004). These reports may be accessed via http://www.nap.edu.

Manganese (mg/d)	Molybdenum (µg/d)	Phosphorus (mg/d)	Selenium (µg/d)	Zinc (mg/d)	Potassium (g/d)	Sodium (g/d)	Chloride (g/d)
0.003*	2*	100*	15*	2*	0.4*	0.12*	0.18*
0.6*	3*	275*	20*	3	0.7*	0.37*	0.57*
1.2*	17	460	20	3	3.0*	1.0*	1.5*
1.5*	22	500	30	5	3.8*	1.2*	1.9*
1.9*	34	1,250	40	8	4.5*	1.5*	2.3*
2.2*	43	1,250	55	11	4.7*	1.5*	2.3*
2.3*	45	700	55	11	4.7*	1.5*	2.3*
2.3	45	700	55	11	4.7*	1.5*	2.3*
2.3*	45	700	55	11	4.7*	1.3*	2.0*
2.3*	45	700	55	11	4.7*	1.2*	1.8*
1.6*	34	1,250	40	8	4.5*	1.5*	2.3*
1.6*	43	1,250	55	9	4.7*	1.5*	2.3*
1.8*	45	700	55	8	4.7*	1.5*	2.3*
1.8*	45	700	55	8	4.7*	1.5*	2.3*
1.8*	45	700	55	8	4.7*	1.3*	2.0*
1.8*	45	700	55	8	4.7*	1.2*	1.8*
2.0*	50	1,250	60	12	4.7*	1.5*	2.3*
2.0*	50	700	60	11	4.7*	1.5*	2.3*
2.0*	50	700	60	11	4.7*	1.5*	2.3*
2.6*	50	1,250	70	13	5.1*	1.5*	2.3*
2.6*	50	700	70	12	5.1*	1.5*	2.3*
2.6*	50	700	70	12	5.1*	1.5*	2.3*

Percent Fat Estimate for Men: Sum of Triceps, Chest, and Subscapula Skinfolds

Sum of Skinfolds (mm)	Age to Last Lear								
	Under 22	23–27	28–32	33–37	38–42	43–47	48–52	53–57	Over 57
8–10	1.5	2.0	2.5	3.1	3.6	4.1	4.6	5.1	5.6
11–13	3.0	3.5	4.0	4.5	5.1	5.6	6.1	6.6	7.1
14–16	4.5	5.0	5.5	6.0	6.5	7.0	7.6	8.1	8.6
17–19	5.9	6.4	6.9	7.4	8.0	8.5	9.0	9.5	10.0
20–22	7.3	7.8	8.3	8.8	9.4	9.9	10.4	10.9	11.4
23–25	8.6	9.2	9.7	10.2	10.7	11.2	11.8	12.3	12.8
26–28	10.0	10.5	11.0	11.5	12.1	12.6	13.1	13.6	14.2
29–31	11.2	11.8	12.3	12.8	13.4	13.9	14.4	14.9	15.5
32–34	12.5	13.0	13.5	14.1	14.6	15.1	15.7	16.2	16.7
35–37	13.7	14.2	14.8	15.3	15.8	16.4	16.9	17.4	18.0
38–40	14.9	15.4	15.9	16.5	17.0	17.6	18.1	18.6	19.2
41–43	16.0	16.6	17.1	17.6	18.2	18.7	19.3	19.8	20.3
44–46	17.1	17.7	18.2	18.7	19.3	19.8	20.4	20.9	21.5
47–49	18.2	18.7	19.3	19.8	20.4	20.9	21.4	22.0	22.5
50–52	19.2	19.7	20.3	20.8	21.4	21.9	22.5	23.0	23.6
53–55	20.2	20.7	21.3	21.8	22.4	22.9	23.5	24.0	24.6
56–58	21.1	21.7	22.2	22.8	23.3	23.9	24.4	25.0	25.5
59–61	22.0	22.6	23.1	23.7	24.2	24.8	25.3	25.9	26.5
62–64	22.9	23.4	24.0	24.5	25.1	25.7	26.2	26.8	27.3
65–67	23.7	24.3	24.8	25.4	25.9	26.5	27.1	27.6	28.2
68–70	24.5	25.0	25.6	26.2	26.7	27.3	27.8	28.4	29.0
71–73	25.2	25.8	26.3	26.9	27.5	28.0	28.6	29.1	29.7
74–76	25.9	26.5	27.0	27.6	28.2	28.7	29.3	29.9	30.4
77–79	26.6	27.1	27.7	28.2	28.8	29.4	29.9	30.5	31.1
80–82	27.2	27.7	28.3	28.9	29.4	30.0	30.6	31.1	31.7
83–85	27.7	28.3	28.8	29.4	30.0	30.5	31.1	31.7	32.3
86–88	28.2	28.8	29.4	29.9	30.5	31.1	31.6	32.2	32.8
89–91	28.7	29.3	29.8	30.4	31.0	31.5	32.1	32.7	33.3
92–94	29.1	29.7	30.3	30.8	31.4	32.0	32.6	33.1	33.4
95–97	29.5	30.1	30.6	31.2	31.8	32.4	32.9	33.5	34.1
98–100	29.8	30.4	31.0	31.6	32.1	32.7	33.3	33.9	34.4
101–103	30.1	30.7	31.3	31.8	32.4	33.0	33.6	34.1	34.7
104–106	30.4	30.9	31.5	32.1	32.7	33.2	33.8	34.4	35.0
107–109	30.6	31.1	31.7	32.3	32.9	33.4	34.0	34.6	35.2
110–112	30.7	31.3	31.9	32.4	33.0	33.6	34.2	34.7	35.3
113–115	30.8	31.4	32.0	32.5	33.1	33.7	34.3	34.9	35.4
116–118	30.9	31.5	32.0	32.6	33.2	33.8	34.3	34.9	35.5

Jackson, A. S., and Pollock, M. L., "Practical Assessment of Body Composition," *Physician and Sportsmedicine* 13(5): 85. Minneapolis, MN: McGraw-Hill Healthcare Group, 1985.

Percent Fat Estimate for Women: Sum of Triceps, Abdomen, and Suprailium Skinfolds

Sum of Skinfolds (mm)	Age to Last Year								
	18–22	23–27	28–32	33–37	38–42	43–47	48–52	53–57	Over 57
8–12	8.8	9.0	9.2	9.4	9.5	9.7	9.9	10.1	10.3
13–17	10.8	10.9	11.1	11.3	11.5	11.7	11.8	12.0	12.2
18–22	12.6	12.8	13.0	13.2	13.4	13.5	13.7	13.9	14.1
23–27	14.5	14.6	14.8	15.0	15.2	15.4	15.6	15.7	15.9
28–32	16.2	16.4	16.6	16.8	17.0	17.1	17.3	17.5	17.7
33–37	17.9	18.1	18.3	18.5	18.7	18.9	19.0	19.2	19.4
38–42	19.6	19.8	20.0	20.2	20.3	20.5	20.7	20.9	21.1
43–47	21.2	21.4	21.6	21.8	21.9	22.1	22.3	22.5	22.7
48–52	22.8	22.9	23.1	23.3	23.5	23.7	23.8	24.0	24.2
53–57	24.2	24.4	24.6	24.8	25.0	25.2	25.3	25.5	25.7
58–62	25.7	25.9	26.0	26.2	26.4	26.6	26.8	27.0	27.1
63–67	27.1	27.2	27.4	27.6	27.8	28.0	28.2	28.3	28.5
68–72	28.4	28.6	28.7	28.9	29.1	29.3	29.5	29.7	29.8
73–77	29.6	29.8	30.0	30.2	30.4	30.6	30.7	30.9	31.1
78–82	30.9	31.0	31.2	31.4	31.6	31.8	31.9	32.1	32.3
83–87	32.0	32.2	32.4	32.6	32.7	32.9	33.1	33.3	33.5
88–92	33.1	33.3	33.5	33.7	33.8	34.0	34.2	34.4	34.6
93–97	34.1	34.3	34.5	34.7	34.9	35.1	35.2	35.4	35.6
98–102	35.1	35.3	35.5	35.7	35.9	36.0	36.2	36.4	36.6
103–107	36.1	36.2	36.4	36.6	36.8	37.0	37.2	37.3	37.5
108–112	36.9	37.1	37.3	37.5	37.7	37.9	38.0	38.2	38.4
113–117	37.8	37.9	38.1	38.3	39.2	39.4	39.6	39.8	39.2
118–122	38.5	38.7	38.9	39.1	39.4	39.6	39.8	40.0	40.0
123–127	39.2	39.4	39.6	39.8	40.0	40.1	40.3	40.5	40.7
128–132	39.9	40.1	40.2	40.4	40.6	40.8	41.0	41.2	41.3
133–137	40.5	40.7	40.8	41.0	41.2	41.4	41.6	41.7	41.9
138–142	41.0	41.2	41.4	41.6	41.7	41.9	42.1	42.3	42.5
143–147	41.5	41.7	41.9	42.0	42.2	42.4	42.6	42.8	43.0
148–152	41.9	42.1	42.3	42.4	42.6	42.8	43.0	43.2	43.4
153–157	42.3	42.5	42.6	42.8	43.0	43.2	43.4	43.6	43.7
158–162	42.6	42.8	43.0	43.1	43.3	43.5	43.7	43.9	44.1
163–167	42.9	43.0	43.2	43.4	43.6	43.8	44.0	44.1	44.3
168–172	43.1	43.2	43.4	43.6	43.8	44.0	44.2	44.3	44.5
173–177	43.2	43.4	43.6	43.8	43.9	44.1	44.3	44.5	44.7
178–182	43.3	43.5	43.7	43.8	44.0	44.2	44.4	44.6	44.8

Jackson, A. S., and Pollock, M. L., "Practical Assessment of Body Composition," *Physician and Sportsmedicine* 13(5): 85. Minneapolis, MN: McGraw-Hill Healthcare Group, 1985.

Glossary

absolute $\dot{V}O_2$ the amount of oxygen consumed over a given time period; expressed as liters · min^{-1}.

acclimation the change that occurs in response to repeated environmental stresses and results in the improved function of an existing homeostatic system. In general, acclimation is commonly used to refer to a rapid physiological adaptation that occurs within days to a few weeks.

acclimatization a gradual, long-term adaptation of an organism (e.g., humans) to a change in the environment (e.g., heat exposure). Acclimatization results in the improved function of an existing homeostatic system. Although acclimatization and acclimation are similar terms, acclimatization is often used to describe a gradual physiological adaptation that occurs within months to years of exposure to the environmental stress.

Acetyl-CoA a two carbon molecule formed from pyruvate produced by glycolysis or from the oxidation of fatty acids or amino acids. Acetyl-CoA can the citric acid cycle and undergoes oxidation resulting in the release of electrons into the electron transport chain.

acidosis an abnormal increase in blood hydrogen ion concentration (i.e., arterial pH below 7.35).

acids compounds capable of giving up hydrogen ions into solution.

acromegaly a condition caused by hypersecretion of growth hormone from the pituitary gland; characterized by enlargement of the extremities, such as the jaw, nose, and fingers.

actin a structural protein of muscle that works with myosin in permitting muscular contraction.

action potential the all-or-none electrical event in the neuron or muscle cell in which the polarity of the cell membrane is rapidly reversed and then reestablished.

activation energy energy required to initiate a chemical reaction. The term *activation energy* is sometimes referred to as the *energy of activation*.

adaptation the term adaptation refers to a change in the structure and function of a cell or organ system that results in an improved ability to maintain homeostasis during stressful conditions.

adenosine diphosphate (ADP) a molecule that combines with inorganic phosphate to form ATP.

adenosine triphosphate (ATP) the high-energy phosphate compound synthesized and used by cells to release energy for cellular work.

adenylate cyclase enzyme found in cell membranes that catalyzes the conversion of ATP to cyclic AMP.

adequate intake (AI) recommendations for nutrient intake when insufficient information is available to set an RDA standard.

adiponectin is a protein hormone that modulates a number of metabolic processes, including glucose regulation and fatty acid oxidation.

adrenal cortex the outer portion of the adrenal gland. Synthesizes and secretes corticosteroid hormones, such as cortisol, aldosterone, and androgens.

adrenaline *see* epinephrine.

adrenocorticotrophic hormone (ACTH) a hormone secreted by the anterior pituitary gland that stimulates the adrenal cortex.

aerobic in the presence of oxygen.

afferent fibers nerve fibers (sensory fibers) that carry neural information back to the central nervous system.

afferent neuron sensory neuron carrying information toward the central nervous system.

Air Quality Index (AQI) a measure of the quality of the air for five major air pollutants regulated by the Clean Air Act: ground-level ozone, particulate matter, carbon monoxide, sulfur dioxide, and nitrogen dioxide.

aldosterone a corticosteroid hormone involved in the regulation of electrolyte balance.

alkalosis an abnormal increase in blood concentration of OH$^-$ ions, resulting in a rise in arterial pH above 7.45.

alpha receptors a subtype of adrenergic receptors located on cell membranes of selected tissues.

alveolar ventilation ($\dot{V}_A$) the volume of gas that reaches the alveolar region of the lung.

alveoli microscopic air sacs located in the lung where gas exchange occurs between respiratory gases and the blood.

amenorrhea the absence of menses.

AMPK (5'adenosine monophosphate activated protein kinase) an important signaling molecule that is activated during exercise due to changes in muscle fiber phosphate/energy levels. AMPK regulates numerous energy produc-

ing pathways in muscle by stimulating glucose uptake and fatty acid oxidation during exercise and is also linked to the control of muscle gene expression by activating transcription factors associated with fatty acid oxidation and mitochondrial biogenesis.

anabolic steroid a prescription drug that has anabolic, or growth-stimulating, characteristics similar to that of the male androgen testosterone.

anaerobic without oxygen.

anaerobic threshold a commonly used term meant to describe the level of oxygen consumption at which there is a rapid and systematic increase in blood lactate concentration. Also termed the *lactate threshold.*

anatomical dead space the total volume of the lung (i.e., conducting airways) that does not participate in gas exchange.

androgenic steroid a compound that has the qualities of an androgen; associated with masculine characteristics.

androgens male sex hormones. Synthesized in the testes and in limited amounts in the adrenal cortex. Steroids that have masculinizing effects.

angina pectoris chest pain due to a lack of blood flow (ischemia) to the myocardium.

angiotensin I and II these compounds are polypeptides formed from the cleavage of a protein (angiotensinogen) by the action of the enzyme renin produced by the kidneys, and converting enzyme in the lung, respectively.

anorexia nervosa an eating disorder characterized by rapid weight loss due to failure to consume adequate amounts of nutrients.

anterior pituitary the anterior portion of the pituitary gland that secretes follicle-stimulating hormone, luteinizing hormone, adrenocorticotrophic hormone, thyroid-stimulating hormone, growth hormone, and prolactin.

antidiuretic hormone (ADH) hormone secreted by the posterior pituitary gland that promotes water retention by the kidney.

aortic bodies receptors located in the arch of the aorta that are capable of detecting changes in arterial PO$_2$.

apophyses sites of muscle-tendon insertion in bones.

arrhythmia abnormal electrical activity in the heart (e.g., a premature ventricular contraction).

arteries large vessels that carry arterialized blood away from the heart.

arterioles a small branch of an artery that communicates with a capillary network.

articular cartilage cartilage that covers the ends of bones in a synovial joint.

atherosclerosis a pathological condition in which fatty substances collect in the layer (intima) of arteries.

atmospheric pressure downward force exerted in the earth's surface due to the weight of the air above that point.

ATPase enzyme capable of breaking down ATP to ADP + P$_i$ + energy.

ATP-PC system term used to describe the metabolic pathway involving muscle stores of ATP and the use of phosphocreatine to re-phosphorylate ADP. This pathway is used at the onset of exercise and during short-term, high-intensity work.

atrioventricular node (AV node) a specialized mass of muscle tissue located in the interventricular septum of the heart; functions in the transmission of cardiac impulses from the atria to the ventricles.

autocrine signaling signaling that occurs when a cell produces and releases a chemical messenger into the extracellular fluid that acts upon the cell producing the signal. The autocrine agent refers to the chemical messenger that is released by the cell.

autologous transfusion blood transfusion whereby the individual receives his or her own blood.

autonomic nervous system portion of the nervous system that controls the actions of visceral organs.

autoregulation mechanism by which an organ regulates blood flow to match the metabolic rate.

axon a nerve fiber that conducts a nerve impulse away from the neuron cell body.

basal metabolic rate (BMR) metabolic rate measured in supine position following a 12-hour fast and 8 hours of sleep.

bases compounds that ionize in water to release hydroxyl ions (OH$^-$) or other ions that are capable of combining with hydrogen ions.

B-cells cells in the pancreas that secrete insulin into the blood to increase the uptake of glucose and amino acids by tissues.

beta oxidation breakdown of free fatty acids to form acetyl-CoA.

beta-receptor agonist (β-agonist) a molecule that is capable of binding to and activating a beta receptor.

beta receptors adrenergic receptors located on cell membranes. Combine mainly with epinephrine and, to some degree, with norepinephrine.

bioenergetics the chemical processes involved with the production of cellular ATP.

biological control systems a control system capable of maintaining homeostasis within a cell or organ system in a living creature.

blood boosting a term that applies to the increase of the blood's hemoglobin concentration by the infusion of additional red blood cells. Medically termed *induced erythrocythemia*.

blood doping *see* blood boosting.

blood packing *see* blood boosting.

Bohr effect the right shift of the oxyhemoglobin dissociation curve due to a decrease of blood pH. Results in a decreased affinity for oxygen.

bradycardia a resting heart rate less than 60 beats per minute.

brain stem portion of the brain that includes midbrain, pons, and medulla.

buffer a compound that resists pH change.

bulimia an eating disorder characterized by eating and forced regurgitation.

bulk flow mass movement of molecules from an area of high pressure to an area of lower pressure.

calcitonin hormone released from the thyroid gland that plays a minor role in calcium metabolism.

calciuneurin a phosphatase activated by increases in cytosolic calcium; it participates in several adaptive responses in muscle, including fiber growth/regeneration and the fast-to-slow fiber type transition that occurs as a result of exercise training.

calmodulin-dependent kinase (CaMK) is activated during exercise in an intensity-related manner. This important kinase exerts influence on exercise-induced muscle adaptation by contributing to the activation of PCG-1α. The primary upstream signal to activate CaMK is increased cytosolic calcium levels.

capillaries microscopic blood vessels that connect arterioles and venules. Portion of vascular system where blood/tissue gas exchange occurs.

cardiac accelerator nerves part of the sympathetic nervous system that stimulates the SA node to increase heart rate.

cardiac output the amount of blood pumped by the heart per unit of time; equal to product of heart rate and stroke volume.

cardiovascular control center the area of the medulla that regulates the cardiovascular system.

carotid bodies chemoreceptors located in the internal carotid artery; respond to changes in arterial PO$_2$, PCO$_2$, and pH.

catecholamines organic compounds, including epinephrine, norepinephrine, and dopamine.

cell body the soma, or major portion of the body of a nerve cell. Contains the nucleus.

cell membrane the lipid-bilayer envelope that encloses cells. Called the *sarcolemma* in muscle cells.

cell signaling a system of communication that governs cellular activities and coordinates cell actions. Cell signaling can occur via numerous signaling pathways, including direct contact of cells.

cellular respiration process of oxygen consumption and carbon dioxide production in cells (i.e., bioenergetics).

central command the control of the cardiovascular or pulmonary system by cortical impulses.

central fatigue factors located prior to the neuromuscular junction that impair the force-generating capacity of muscle.

central nervous system (CNS) portion of the nervous system that consists of the brain and spinal cord.

cerebellum portion of the brain that is concerned with fine coordination of skeletal muscles during movement.

cerebrum superior aspect of the brain that occupies the upper cranial cavity. Contains the motor cortex.

chemiosmotic hypothesis the mechanism to explain the aerobic formation of ATP in mitochondria.

cholesterol a 27-carbon lipid that can be synthesized in cells or consumed in the diet. Cholesterol serves as a precursor of steroid hormones and plays a role in the development of atherosclerosis.

Citric acid cycle (also known as the Krebs cycle or tricarboxylic acid cycle) is a key metabolic pathway located in the mitochondria. Specifically, the citric acid cycle is a series of chemical reactions used to harness usable energy through the oxidation of acetyl-CoA derived from carbohydrates, fats, and proteins. The oxidation of acetyl-CoA ultimately results in the production of carbon dioxide and chemical energy in the form of adenosine triphosphate (ATP).

clo   unit that describes the insulation quality of clothing.

complement system   part of the innate immune system; it forms a second line of defense against infection. The more than 20 proteins that make up the complement system are present in high concentrations in the blood and tissues. When the body is exposed to a foreign agent (e.g. bacterium), the complement system is activated to attack the invader.

concentric action   occurs when a muscle is activated and shortens.

conduction   transfer of heat from warmer to cooler objects that are in contact with each other. This term may also be used in association with the conveyance of neural impulses.

conduction disturbances   refers to a slowing or blockage of the wave of depolarization in the heart, e.g., first-degree AV block, or bundle branch block.

conductivity   capacity for conduction.

convection   the transmission of heat from one object to another through the circulation of heated molecules.

Cori cycle   the cycle of lactate-to-glucose between the muscle and liver.

coronary artery bypass graft surgery (CABGS)   the replacement of a blocked coronary artery with another vessel to permit blood flow to the myocardium.

cortisol   a glucocorticoid secreted by the adrenal cortex upon stimulation by ACTH.

coupled reactions   the linking of energy-liberating chemical reactions to "drive" energy-requiring reactions.

critical power   a specific submaximal power output that can be maintained without fatigue.

cromolyn sodium   a drug used to stabilize the membranes of mast cells and prevent an asthma attack.

cycle ergometer   a stationary exercise cycle that allows accurate measurement of work output.

cyclic AMP   a substance produced from ATP through the action of adenylate cyclase that alters several chemical processes in the cell.

cytokines   hormone messengers that regulate the immune system by facilitating communication with other cells within the immune system.

cytoplasm   the contents of the cell surrounding the nucleus. Called *sarcoplasm* in muscle cells.

Daily Value   a standard used in nutritional labeling.

deficiency   a shortcoming of some essential nutrient.

degenerative diseases   diseases not due to infection that result in a progressive decline in some bodily function.

delayed-onset muscle soreness (DOMS)   muscle soreness that occurs 12 to 24 hours after an exercise bout.

dendrites   portion of the nerve fiber that transmits action potentials toward a nerve cell body.

deoxyhemoglobin   hemoglobin not in combination with oxygen.

diabetes mellitus   a condition characterized by high blood glucose levels due to inadequate insulin. People with type 1 diabetes are insulin dependent, whereas people with type 2 diabetes are resistant to insulin.

diabetic coma   unconscious state induced by a lack of insulin.

diacylglycerol   a molecule derived from a membrane-bound phospholipid, phosphatidylinositol, that activates protein kinase C and alters cellular activity.

diaphragm   the major respiratory muscle responsible for inspiration. Domeshaped–separates the thoracic cavity from the abdominal cavity.

diastole   period of filling of the heart between contractions (i.e., resting phase of the heart).

diastolic blood pressure   arterial blood pressure during diastole.

Dietary Guidelines for Americans   general statements related to food selection that are consistent with achieving and maintaining good health.

Dietary Reference Intakes (DRIs)   the framework for nutrient recommendations being made as a part of the revision of the 1989 RDA.

diffusion   random movement of molecules from an area of high concentration to an area of low concentration.

direct calorimetry   assessment of the body's metabolic rate by direct measurement of the amount of heat produced.

dose   the amount of drug or exercise prescribed to have a certain effect (or response).

double-blind research design   an experimental design in which the subjects and the principal investigator are not aware of the experimental treatment order.

double product   the product of heart rate and systolic blood pressure; estimate of work of the heart.

dynamic   refers to an isotonic muscle action.

dynamic stretching   stretching that involves controlled movement.

dynamometer   device used to measure force production (e.g., used in the measurement of muscular strength).

dysmenorrhea   painful menstruation.

dyspnea   shortness of breath or labored breathing. May be due to various types of lung or heart diseases.

eccentric action   occurs when a muscle is activated and force is produced but the muscle lengthens.

ectomorphy   category of somatotype that is rated for linearity of body form.

effect (response)   change in variable (e.g., $\dot{V}O_2$ max) due to a dose of exercise (e.g., 3 days per week, 40 min/day at 70% $\dot{V}O_2$ max).

effector   organ or body part that responds to stimulation by an efferent neuron (e.g., skeletal muscle in a withdrawal reflex).

efferent fibers   nerve fibers (motor fibers) that carry neural information from the central nervous system to the periphery.

efferent neuron   conducts impulses from the CNS to the effector organ (e.g., motor neuron).

ejection fraction   the proportion of end-diastolic volume that is ejected during a ventricular contraction.

electrocardiogram (ECG or EKG)   a recording of the electrical changes that occur in the myocardium during the cardiac cycle.

electron transport chain   a series of cytochromes in the mitochondria that are responsible for oxidative phosphorylation.

element   a single chemical substance composed of only one type of atom (e.g., calcium or potassium).

endergonic reactions   energy-requiring reactions.

endocrine gland   a gland that produces and secretes its products directly into the blood or interstitial fluid (ductless glands).

endocrine signaling   occurs when cells release chemical signals (hormones) into the blood, which are carried in the blood to all tissues in the body. However, only the cells with a receptor to which the hormone can bind will respond.

endocrine system   the endocrine system releases hormones (endocrine signals) into the blood to circulate to tissues to bring about a change in the tissue's activity.

endomorphy   the somatotype category that is rated for roundness (fatness).

endomysium the inner layer of connective tissue surrounding a muscle fiber.

endorphin a neuropeptide produced by the pituitary gland that has pain-suppressing activity.

end-plate potential (EPP) depolarization of a membrane region by a sodium influx.

energy of activation energy required to initiate a chemical reaction.

enzymes proteins that lower the energy of activation and, therefore, catalyze chemical reactions. Enzymes regulate the rate of most metabolic pathways.

epidemiology the study of the distribution and determinants of health-related states or events in specified populations, and the application of this study to the control of health problems.

epilepsy a neurological disorder manifested by muscular seizures.

epimysium the outer layer of connective tissue surrounding muscle.

epinephrine (E) a hormone synthesized by the adrenal medulla; also called *adrenaline*.

epiphyseal plate (growth plate) cartilaginous layer between the head and shaft of a long bone where growth takes place.

EPOC an acronym for "excess post-exercise oxygen consumption"; often referred to as the *oxygen debt*.

EPSP excitatory post synaptic potential. A graded depolarization of a post synaptic membrane by a neurotransmitter.

ergogenic aid a substance, appliance, or procedure (e.g., blood doping) that improves performance.

ergometer instrument for measuring work.

ergometry measurement of work output.

erythrocythemia an increase in the number of erythrocytes in the blood.

erythropoietin (EPO) hormone that stimulates red blood cell production.

Estimated Energy Requirement (EER) the average dietary energy intake that is predicted to maintain energy balance in a healthy adult of a defined age, gender, weight, height, and level of physical activity, consistent with good health.

estrogens female sex hormones, including estradiol and estrone. Produced primarily in the ovary and also produced in the adrenal cortex.

evaporation the change of water from a liquid form to a vapor form. Results in the removal of heat.

exercise a subclass of physical activity.

exercise immunology the study of exercise, psychological, and environmental influences on immune function.

exergonic reactions chemical reactions that release energy.

extensors muscles that extend a limb–that is, increase the angle at a joint.

FAD flavin adenine dinucleotide. Serves as an electron carrier in bioenergetics.

fasciculi a small bundle of muscle fibers.

fast-twitch fibers one of several types of muscle fibers found in skeletal muscle; also called type II fibers; characterized as having low oxidative capacity but high glycolytic capacity.

female athlete triad a syndrome in which amenorrhea, eating disorders, and bone mineral loss are collectively present.

ferritin the iron-carrying molecule used as an index of whole-body iron status.

field test a test of physical performance performed in the field (outside the laboratory).

flexors muscle groups that cause flexion of limbs–that is, decrease the angle at a joint.

follicle-stimulating hormone (FSH) a hormone secreted by the anterior pituitary gland that stimulates the development of an ovarian follicle in the female and the production of sperm in the male.

food records the practice of keeping dietary food records for determining nutrient intake.

free fatty acid (FFA) a type of fat that combines with glycerol to form triglycerides. Is used as an energy source.

free radicals highly reactive molecules that contain an unpaired electron in their outer orbital.

G protein the link between the hormone-receptor interaction on the surface of the membrane and the subsequent events inside the cell.

gain refers to the amount of correction that a control system is capable of achieving.

General Adaptation Syndrome (GAS) a term defined by Selye in 1936 that describes the organism's response to chronic stress. In response to stress, the organism has a three-stage response: (1) alarm reaction; (2) stage of resistance; and (3) readjustment to the stress, or exhaustion.

glucagon a hormone produced by the pancreas that increases blood glucose and free fatty acid levels.

glucocorticoids any one of a group of hormones produced by the adrenal cortex that influences carbohydrate, fat, and protein metabolism.

gluconeogenesis the synthesis of glucose from amino acids, lactate, glycerol, and other short carbon-chain molecules.

glucose a simple sugar that is transported via the blood and metabolized by tissues.

glucose polymer a complex sugar molecule that contains multiple simple sugar molecules linked together.

glycogen a glucose polymer synthesized in cells as a means of storing carbohydrate.

glycogenolysis the breakdown of glycogen into glucose.

glycolysis a metabolic pathway in the cytoplasm of the cell that results in the degradation of glucose into pyruvate or lactate.

Golgi tendon organ (GTOs) a tension receptor located in series with skeletal muscle.

graded exercise test *see* incremental exercise test.

gross efficiency a simple measure of exercise efficiency defined as the ratio of work performed to energy expended, expressed as a percent.

growth hormone (GH) hormone synthesized and secreted by the anterior pituitary that stimulates growth of the skeleton and soft tissues during the growing years. It is also involved in the mobilization of the body's energy stores.

HDL cholesterol cholesterol that is transported in the blood via high-density proteins; related to low risk of heart disease.

heart rate variability heart rate variability refers to the variation in the time between heartbeats measured as the R-R time interval using an EKG tracing.

heat cramps painful muscle cramps in the abdomen, legs, or arms following strenuous activity in the heat; use direct pressure on cramps, stretch muscles, and gentle ice massage.

heat exhaustion symptoms include heavy sweating, rapid pulse, dizziness, and nausea; it is linked to dehydration and can develop into heatstroke. Move to cool or shaded area, place in supine position with legs raised, and provide fluids and cooling.

heat shock proteins an important family of stress proteins that are produced in cells in response to cellular stresses. Following synthesis, heat shock protein can protect cells against disturbances in homeostasis.

heatstroke (also called exertional heatstroke) a life-threatening heat illness in which body temperature is extremely elevated (104°F or 40°C); possibility of central nervous system disturbances and organ failure. Rapid whole-body cooling measures should be initiated immediately; treat as medical emergency.

heat syncope sudden dizziness or fainting during or after exercising in the heat related to a drop in blood pressure; may be accompanied by feelings of excessive thirst, fatigue, headache, nausea, and vomiting. Move to cool area and provide fluids.

hemoglobin a heme-containing protein in red blood cells that is responsible for transporting oxygen to tissues. Hemoglobin also serves as a weak buffer within red blood cells.

high-density lipoproteins (HDLs) proteins used to transport cholesterol in blood; high levels appear to offer some protection from atherosclerosis.

homeostasis the maintenance of a constant internal environment.

homeotherms animals that maintain a fairly constant internal temperature.

homologous transfusion a blood transfusion using blood of the same type but from another donor.

hormone a chemical substance that is synthesized and released by an endocrine gland and transported to a target organ via the blood.

hydrogen ion (H⁺) a free hydrogen ion in solution that results in a decrease in pH of the solution.

Hydrostatic weighing see underwater weighing

hyperbaric chamber chamber where the absolute pressure is increased above atmospheric pressure.

hyperoxia oxygen concentration in an inspired gas that exceeds 21%.

hyperthermia elevated body temperature due to heat loss not keeping up with heat load from exercise and the environment; linked to heat illnesses.

hypertrophy an increase in cell size.

hypothalamic somatostatin hypothalamic hormone that inhibits growth hormone secretion.

hypothalamus brain structure that integrates many physiological functions to maintain homeostasis; site of secretion of hormones released by the posterior pituitary; also releases hormones that control anterior pituitary secretions.

hypothermia decreased body temperature due to heat loss being greater than heat production; defined clinically as body temperature below 35°C.

hypoxia a relative lack of oxygen (e.g., at altitude).

IGF-1/Akt/mTOR signaling pathway a pathway that plays an important role in the regulation of muscle growth (i.e., protein synthesis) resulting from resistance training. Contractile activity (i.e., muscle stretch) stimulates the secretion of IGF-1 from the active muscle fibers, which acts as an autocrine/paracrine signaling molecule, binding to its membrane receptor and initiating a cascade of molecular events to promote muscle protein synthesis. Binding of IGF-1 to its receptor on the muscle membrane activates the important signaling kinase, Akt. Active Akt then activates another downstream kinase called *mammalian target of rapamycin* (mTOR), which then promotes protein synthesis by improving translational efficiency.

immunity refers to all the mechanisms used in the body to protect against environmental agents that are foreign to the body. Immunity is achieved by a precise coordination of the innate and acquired immune system.

immunotherapy procedure in which the body is exposed to specific substances to elicit an immune response in order to offer better protection upon subsequent exposure.

incremental exercise test an exercise test involving a progressive increase in work rate over time. Often, graded exercise tests are used to determine the subject's $\dot{V}O_2$ max or lactate threshold. (Also called *graded exercise test*.)

Incretins: Incretins are a group of hormones secreted by endocrine cells in the GI tract when food is being ingested; they anticipate and augment the insulin response due to the rising blood glucose or amino acid levels.

indirect calorimetry estimation of heat or energy production on the basis of oxygen consumption, carbon dioxide production, and nitrogen excretion.

induced erythrocythemia causing an elevation of the red blood cell (hemoglobin) concentration by infusing blood; also called *blood doping* or *blood boosting*.

infectious diseases diseases due to the presence of pathogenic micro-

organisms in the body (e.g., viruses, bacteria, fungi, and protozoa).

inflammation part of the complex biological response to harmful stimuli such as bacteria entering the body through a wound in the skin, damaged cells, or other irritants. Clinical signs of local inflammation are redness, swelling, heat, and pain around the injured tissue.

inorganic relating to substances that do not contain carbon (C).

inorganic phosphate (P$_i$) a stimulator of cellular metabolism; split off, along with ADP, from ATP when energy is released; used with ADP to form ATP in the electron transport chain.

inositol triphosphate (IP$_3$) a molecule derived from a membrane-bound phospholipid, phosphatidylinositol, that causes calcium release from intracellular stores and alters cellular activity.

insulin hormone released from the beta cells of the islets of Langerhans in response to elevated blood glucose and amino acid concentrations; increases tissue uptake of both.

insulin-like growth factors groups of growth-stimulating peptides released from the liver and other tissues in response to growth hormone.

insulin shock condition brought on by too much insulin, which causes an immediate hypoglycemia; symptoms include tremors, dizziness, and possibly convulsions.

integrating center the portion of a biological control system that processes the information from the receptors and issues an appropriate response relative to its set point.

intercalated discs portion of cardiac muscle cell where one cell connects to the next.

intermediate fibers muscle fiber type that generates high force at a moderately fast speed of contraction, but has a relatively large number of mitochondria (type IIa).

intracrine signaling a hormone that acts inside a cell. Steroid hormones act through intracellular (mostly nuclear) receptors and, thus, are considered to be intracrines. In contrast, peptide or protein hormones, in general, act as endocrines, autocrines, or paracrines by binding to their receptors present on the cell surface.

ion a single atom or small molecule containing a net positive or negative charge due to an excess of either protons or electrons, respectively (e.g., Na⁺, Cl⁻).

IPSP inhibitory post-synaptic potential that moves the post-synaptic membrane farther from threshold.

irritability a trait of certain tissues that enables them to respond to stimuli (e.g., nerve and muscle).

isocitrate dehydrogenase rate-limiting enzyme in the Krebs cycle that is inhibited by ATP and stimulated by ADP and P_i.

isokinetic action in which the rate of movement is constantly maintained through a specific range of motion even though maximal force is exerted.

isometric action action in which the muscle develops tension, but does not shorten; also called a *static contraction*. No movement occurs.

isotonic contraction in which a muscle shortens against a constant load or tension, resulting in movement.

juxtracrine signaling a type of cell signaling that occurs between two adjacent cells that are in direct contact via a junction across the cell membrane that connects the cytoplasm of the two cells.

ketosis acidosis of the blood caused by the production of ketone bodies (e.g., acetoacetic acid) when fatty acid mobilization is increased, as in uncontrolled diabetes.

kilocalorie (kcal) a measure of energy expenditure equal to the heat needed to raise the temperature of 1 kg of water 1 degree Celsius; also equal to 1000 calories and sometimes written as calorie rather than kilocalorie.

kilogram-meter a unit of work in which 1 kg of force (1 kg mass accelerated at 1 G) is moved through a vertical distance of 1 meter; abbreviated as kg-m, kg · m, or kgm.

kinesthesia a perception of movement obtained from information about the position and rate of movement of the joints.

Krebs cycle (also known as the citric acid cycle or tricarboxylic acid cycle) is a key metabolic pathway located in the mitochondria. Specifically, the citric acid cycle is a series of chemical reactions used to harness usable energy through the oxidation of acetyl-CoA derived from carbohydrates, fats, and proteins. The oxidation of acetyl-CoA ultimately results in the production of carbon dioxide and chemical energy in the form of adenosine triphosphate (ATP).

lactate a three-carbon molecule that is a potential end-product of glucose metabolism.

lactate threshold a point during a graded exercise test when the blood lactate concentration increases abruptly.

lateral sac *see* terminal cisternae.

leptin hormone secreted by adipocytes. It influences appetite through a direct effect on the "feeding centers" in the hypothalamus, and acts on peripheral tissues to enhance insulin sensitivity.

LDL cholesterol form of low-density lipoprotein responsible for the transport of plasma cholesterol; high levels are indicative of a high risk of coronary heart disease.

leukocytes (also called white blood cells) a group of special cells designed to recognize and remove foreign invaders (e.g., bacteria) in the body.

lipase an enzyme responsible for the breakdown of triglycerides to free fatty acids and glycerol.

lipolysis the breakdown of triglycerides in adipose tissue to free fatty acids and glycerol for subsequent transport to tissues for metabolism.

lipoprotein protein involved in the transport of cholesterol and triglycerides in the plasma.

low-density lipoproteins (LDL) form of lipoprotein that transports a majority of the plasma cholesterol; *see* LDL cholesterol.

low-grade chronic inflammation characterized by a two- to three-fold increase in inflammatory cytokines (e.g., tumor necrosis factor alpha [TNF-α] and interleukin-6 [IL-6]) and c-reactive protein (CRP).

luteinizing hormone (LH) also called "interstitial cell stimulating hormone"; a surge of LH stimulates ovulation in the middle of the menstrual cycle; LH stimulates testosterone production in men.

macrophages phagocytes that engulf and kill invading bacteria. Macrophages are considered to be a portion of the innate immune system.

major minerals dietary minerals, including calcium, phosphorus, potassium, sulfur, sodium, chloride, and magnesium.

mast cell connective tissue cell that releases histamine and other chemicals in response to certain stimuli (e.g., injury).

maximal oxygen uptake ($\dot{V}O_2$ max) greatest rate of oxygen uptake by the body measured during severe dynamic exercise, usually on a cycle ergometer or a treadmill; dependent on maximal cardiac output and the maximal arteriovenous oxygen difference.

mesomorphy one component of a somatotype that characterizes the muscular form or lean body mass aspect of the human body.

MET (metabolic equivalent) an expression of the rate of energy expenditure at rest; equal to 3.5 ml · $kg^{-1} \cdot min^{-1}$, or 1 kcal · $kg^{-1} \cdot hr^{-1}$.

metabolism the total of all cellular reactions that occur in cells and includes chemical pathways that result in the synthesis of molecules (anabolic reactions) as well as the breakdown of molecules (catabolic reactions).

mineralocorticoids steroid hormones released from the adrenal cortex that are responsible for Na^+ and K^+ regulation (e.g., aldosterone).

mitochondrion the subcellular organelle responsible for the production of ATP with oxygen; contains the enzymes for the Krebs cycle, electron transport chain, and the fatty acid cycle.

mixed venous blood a mixture of venous blood from both the upper and lower extremities; complete mixing occurs in the right ventricle.

molecular biology branch of biochemistry involved with the study of gene structure and function.

motor cortex portion of the cerebral cortex containing large motor neurons whose axons descend to lower brain centers and spinal cord; associated with the voluntary control of movement.

motor neuron the somatic neuron that innervates skeletal muscle fibers (also called an *alpha motor neuron*).

motor unit a motor neuron and all the muscle fibers innervated by that single motor neuron; responds in an "all-or-none" manner to a stimulus.

muscle action term used to describe the muscle movement (e.g., shortening versus lengthening).

muscle spindle a muscle stretch receptor oriented parallel to skeletal muscle fibers; the capsule portion is surrounded by afferent fibers, and intrafusal muscle fibers can alter the length of the capsule during muscle contraction and relaxation.

muscular strength the maximal amount of force that can be generated by a muscle or muscle group.

myocardial infarction (MI) death of a portion of heart tissue that no longer conducts electrical activity nor provides force to move blood.

myocardial ischemia a condition in which the myocardium experiences an inadequate blood flow; sometimes accompanied by irregularities in the electrocardiogram (arrhythmias and ST-segment depression) and chest pain (angina pectoris).

myocardium cardiac muscle; provides the force of contraction to eject blood; muscle type with many mitochondria that is dependent on a constant supply of oxygen.

myofibrils   the portion of the muscle containing the thick and thin contractile filaments; a series of sarcomeres where the repeating pattern of the contractile proteins gives the striated appearance to skeletal muscle.

myoglobin   protein in muscle that can bind oxygen and release it at low PO_2 values; aids in diffusion of oxygen from capillary to mitochondria.

myosin   contractile protein in the thick filament of a myofibril that contains the cross-bridge that can bind actin and split ATP to cause tension development.

nicotinamide adenine dinucleotide (NAD)   coenzyme that transfers hydrogen and the energy associated with those hydrogens; in the Krebs cycle, NAD transfers energy from substrates to the electron transport chain.

natural killer cells   an important part of the innate immune system because they are versatile "killers" of foreign agents, including bacteria, viruses, cancer cells, and other unwanted invaders of the body.

negative feedback   describes the response from a control system that reduces the size of the stimulus, e.g., an elevated blood glucose concentration causes the secretion of insulin, which, in turn, lowers the blood glucose concentration.

net efficiency   the mathematical ratio of work output divided by the energy expended above rest.

neuroendocrinology   study of the role of the nervous and endocrine systems in the automatic regulation of the internal environment.

neuromuscular junction   synapse between axon terminal of a motor neuron and the motor end plate of a muscle's plasma membrane.

neuron   nerve cell; composed of a cell body with dendrites (projections) that bring information to the cell body, and axons that take information away from the cell body to influence neurons, glands, or muscles.

neutrophils   short-lived leukocytes that participate in phagocytosis of bacteria.

neurotransmitter   a chemical messenger used by neurons to communicate with each other. More specifically, a neurotransmitter is a chemical that transmits signals from a neuron to a target cell across a synapse.

NFκB   nuclear factor kappa B is a transcriptional activator that promotes the expression of several antioxidant enzymes that protect muscle fibers against free-radical mediated injury.

nitroglycerin   drug used to reduce chest pain (angina pectoris) due to lack of blood flow to the myocardium.

norepinephrine (NE)   a hormone and neurotransmitter released from postganglionic nerve endings and the adrenal medulla.

normocythemia   a normal red blood cell concentration.

normoxia   a normal PO_2.

nucleus   membrane-bound organelle containing most of the cell's DNA.

nutrient density   the degree to which foods contain selected nutrients, e.g., protein, relative to the number of kilocalories.

open-circuit spirometry   indirect calorimetry procedure in which either inspired or expired ventilation is measured and oxygen consumption and carbon dioxide production are calculated.

organic   describes substances that contain carbon.

osteoporosis   a decrease in bone density due to a loss of cortical bone; common in older women and implicated in fractures; estrogen, exercise, and Ca^{++} therapy are used to correct the condition.

overload   a principle of training describing the need to increase the load (intensity) of exercise to cause a further adaptation of a system.

overtraining   an accumulation of training stress that impairs an athlete's ability to perform training sessions and results in long-term decrements of performance.

oxidation   removal of electrons from an element of molecule.

oxidative phosphorylation   mitochondrial process in which inorganic phosphate (P_i) is coupled to ADP as energy is transferred along the electron transport chain in which oxygen is the final electron acceptor.

oxygen debt   the elevated post-exercise oxygen consumption (*see* EPOC); related to replacement of creatine phosphate, lactate resynthesis to glucose, and elevated body temperature, catecholamines, heart rate, breathing, etc.

oxygen deficit   refers to the lag in oxygen uptake at the beginning of exercise.

oxyhemoglobin   hemoglobin combined with oxygen; 1.34 ml of oxygen can combine with 1 g Hb.

p38   mitogen activated kinase p38 (p38) is an important signaling molecule that is activated in muscle fibers during endurance exercise. Once activated, p38 can contribute to mitochondrial biogenesis by activating PGC-1α.

pancreas   gland containing both exocrine and endocrine portions; exocrine secretions include enzymes and bicarbonate to digest food in the small intestine; endocrine secretions include insulin, glucagon, and somatostatin, which are released into the blood.

paracrine signaling   occurs when signals produced by cells act locally on nearby cells to bring about cellular responses.

parasympathetic nervous system   portion of the autonomic nervous system that primarily releases acetylcholine from its postganglionic nerve endings.

partial pressure   the fractional part of the barometric pressure due to the presence of a single gas, e.g., PO_2, PCO_2, and PN_2.

percent grade   a measure of the elevation of the treadmill; calculated as the sine of the angle.

percutaneous transluminal coronary angioplasty (PTCA)   a balloon-tipped catheter is inserted into a blocked coronary artery and plaque is pushed back to the artery wall to open the blood vessel.

perimysium   the connective tissue surrounding the fasciculus of skeletal muscle fibers.

peripheral fatigue   factors located after the neuromuscular junctions that impair the force-generating capacity of muscle (also called *muscular fatigue*).

peripheral nervous system (PNS)   portion of the nervous system located outside the spinal cord and brain.

PGC-1α (peroxisome proliferator-activated receptor-gamma coactivator 1α (PGC-1α)   an important signaling molecule activated by endurance exercise and is considered the master regulator of mitochondrial biogenesis in cells.

pH   a measure of the acidity of a solution; calculated as the negative $\log_{10}$ of the $[H^+]$ in which 7 is neutral; values that are >7 are basic and <7 are acidic.

phagocytes   cells that eat (engulf) foreign agents, such as bacteria.

phosphocreatine   a compound found in skeletal muscle and used to resynthesize ATP from ADP.

phosphodiesterase   an enzyme that catalyzes the breakdown of cyclic AMP, moderating the effect of the hormonal stimulation of adenylate cyclase.

phosphofructokinase (PFK) rate-limiting enzyme in glycolysis that is responsive to ADP, P_i, and ATP levels in the cytoplasm of the cell.

phospholipase C membrane-bound enzyme that hydrolyzes phosphatidylinositol into inositol triphosphate and diacylglycerol that, in turn, bring about changes in intracellular activity.

physical activity (PA) characterizes all types of human movement; associated with living, work, play, and exercise.

physical fitness a broad term describing healthful levels of cardiovascular function, strength, and flexibility; fitness is specific to the activities performed.

pituitary gland a gland at the base of the hypothalamus of the brain with an anterior portion that produces and secretes numerous hormones that regulate other endocrine glands and a posterior portion that secretes hormones that are produced in the hypothalamus.

placebo an inert substance that is used in experimental studies, e.g., drug studies, to control for any subjective reaction to the substance being tested.

pleura a thin lining of cells that is attached to the inside of the chest wall and to the lung; the cells secrete a fluid that facilitates the movements of the lungs in the thoracic cavity.

postactivation potentiation (PAP) PAP refers to the increase in muscle force production that occurs following a series of nonfatiguing, submaximal muscle contractions.

posterior pituitary gland portion of the pituitary gland secreting oxytocin and antidiuretic hormone (vasopressin) that are produced in the hypothalamus.

power a rate of work; work per unit time; $P = W/t$.

power test a test measuring the quantity of work accomplished in a time period; anaerobic power tests include the Margaria stair climb test and the Wingate test; aerobic power tests include the 1.5-mile run and cycle ergometer and treadmill tests in which power output and oxygen consumption are measured.

Preoptic-anterior hypothalamus (POAH) This small region of the brain serves as the body's thermostat and is responsible for the regulation of body temperature. In response to information from thermoreceptors, the POAH activates mechanisms that regulate heating or cooling of the body.

primary risk factor a sign (e.g., high blood pressure) or a behavior (e.g., cigarette smoking) that is directly related to the appearance of certain diseases independent of other risk factors.

progressive resistance exercise (PRE) a training program in which the muscles must work against a gradually increasing resistance; an implementation of the overload principle.

prolactin hormone secreted from the anterior pituitary that increases milk production from the breast.

proprioceptive neuromuscular facilitation (PNF) technique of preceding a static stretch with an isometric contraction.

proprioceptors receptors that provide information about the position and movement of the body; includes muscle and joint receptors as well as the receptors in the semicircular canals of the inner ear.

protein kinase C part of second messenger system that is activated by diacylglycerol and results in the activation of proteins in the cell.

provitamin a precursor of a vitamin.

pulmonary circuit the portion of the cardiovascular system involved in the circulation of blood from the right ventricle to the lungs and back to the left atrium.

pulmonary respiration term that refers to ventilation (breathing) of the lung.

Quebec 10-second test a maximal effort 10-second cycle test designed to assess ultra short-term anaerobic power during cycling.

radiation process of energy exchange from the surface of one object to the surface of another that is dependent on a temperature gradient but does not require contact between the objects; an example is the transfer of heat from the sun to the earth.

receptor in the nervous system, a receptor is a specialized portion of an afferent neuron (or a special cell attached to an afferent neuron) that is sensitive to a form of energy in the environment; *receptor* is also a term that applies to unique proteins on the surface of cells that can bind specific hormones or neurotransmitters.

reciprocal inhibition when extensor muscles (agonists) are contracted, there is a reflex inhibition of the motor neurons to the flexor muscles (antagonists), and vice versa.

Recommended Dietary Allowances (RDAs) standards of nutrition associated with good health for the majority of people. Standards exist for protein, vitamins, and minerals for children and adults.

reduction gain of electrons.

relative $\dot{V}O_2$ oxygen uptake (consumption) expressed per unit body weight (e.g., ml $\cdot$ kg^{-1} $\cdot$ min^{-1}).

releasing hormone hypothalamic hormones released from neurons into the anterior pituitary that control the release of hormones from that gland.

renin enzyme secreted by special cells in the kidney that converts angiotensinogen to angiotensin I.

repetition the number of times an exercise is repeated within a single exercise "set."

residual volume (RV) volume of air in the lungs following a maximal expiration.

respiration external respiration is the exchange of oxygen and carbon dioxide between the lungs and the environment; internal respiration describes the use of oxygen by the cell (mitochondria).

respiratory compensation the buffering of excess H^+ in the blood by plasma bicarbonate (HCO^-_3), and the associated elevation in ventilation to exhale the resulting CO_2.

respiratory exchange ratio (R) the ratio of CO_2 production to O_2 consumption; indicative of substrate utilization during steady-state exercise in which a value of 1.0 represents 100% carbohydrate metabolism and 0.7 represents 100% fat metabolism.

resting membrane potential the voltage difference measured across a membrane that is related to the concentration of ions on each side of the membrane and the permeability of the membrane to those ions.

resting metabolic rate (RMR) metabolic rate measured in the supine position following a period of fasting (4-12 hours) and rest (4-8 hours).

rest interval the time period between bouts in an interval training program.

reversibility a principle of training that describes the temporary nature of a training effect; adaptations to training are lost when the training stops.

sarcolemma the cell (plasma) membrane surrounding a muscle fiber.

sarcomeres the repeating contractile unit in a myofibril bounded by Z lines.

sarcopenia the loss of muscle mass associated with aging. Sarcopenia occurs primarily due to muscle atrophy, but can also occur due to a loss of muscle fibers.

sarcoplasmic reticulum a membranous structure that surrounds the myofibrils of muscle cells; location of the terminal cisternae or lateral sacs that store the Ca^{++} needed for muscle contraction.

satellite cells undifferentiated cell found adjacent to skeletal muscle fibers. These cells can fuse with existing muscle fibers and contribute to muscle growth (hypertrophy). It may also be possible that these fibers can differentiate and form a new muscle fiber following muscle injury.

Schwann cell the cell that surrounds peripheral nerve fibers, forming the myelin sheath.

second messenger a molecule (cyclic AMP) or ion (Ca^{++}) that increases in a cell as a result of an interaction between a "first messenger" (e.g., hormone or neurotransmitter) and a receptor that alters cellular activity.

secondary risk factor a characteristic (age, gender, race) or behavior that increases the risk of coronary heart disease when primary risk factors are present.

sensor a receptor in the body capable of detecting change in a variable.

set a basic unit of a workout containing the number of times (repetitions) a specific exercise is done (e.g., do three sets of five repetitions with 100 pounds).

sex steroids a group of hormones, androgens and estrogens, secreted from the adrenal cortex and the gonads.

sham reinfusion an experimental treatment at the end of a blood doping experiment in which a needle is placed in a vein, but the subject does not receive a reinfusion of blood.

sham withdrawal an experimental treatment at the beginning of a blood doping experiment in which a needle is placed in a vein, but blood is not withdrawn.

sinoatrial node (SA node) specialized tissue located in the right atrium of the heart that generates the electrical impulse to initiate the heartbeat. In a normal, healthy heart, the SA node is the heart's pacemaker.

System International (SI) units system used to provide international standardization of units of measure in science.

size principle the progressive recruitment of motor units beginning with the smallest motor neurons and progressing to larger and larger motor neurons.

sliding filament model a theory of muscle contraction describing the sliding of the thin filaments (actin) past the thick filaments (myosin).

slow-twitch fibers muscle fiber type that contracts slowly and develops relatively low tension, but displays great endurance to repeated stimulation; contains many mitochondria, capillaries, and myoglobin.

somatostatin hormone produced in the hypothalamus that inhibits growth hormone release from the anterior pituitary gland; secreted from cells in the islet of Langerhans and causes a decrease in intestinal activity.

somatotype body-type (form) classification method used to characterize the degree to which an individual's frame is linear (ectomorphic), muscular (mesomorphic), and round (endomorphic); Sheldon's scale rates each component on 1-7 scale.

spatial summation the additive effect of numerous simultaneous inputs to different sites on a neuron to produce a change in the membrane potential.

Specific heat the term *specific heat* refers to the amount of heat energy required to raise 1 kg of body tissue by 1°C.

specificity a principle of training indicating that the adaptation of a tissue is dependent on the type of training undertaken; for example, muscles hypertrophy with heavy resistance training, but show an increase in mitochondria number with endurance training.

spirometry measurement of various lung volumes.

static stretching stretching procedure in which a muscle is stretched and held in the stretched position for 10 to 30 seconds; in contrast to dynamic stretching, which involves motion.

steady state describes the tendency of a control system to achieve a balance between an environmental demand and the response of a physiological system to meet that demand to allow the tissue (body) to function over time.

steroids a class of lipids, derived from cholesterol, that includes the hormones testosterone, estrogen, cortisol, and aldosterone.

stress proteins the term *stress protein* refers to a family of proteins that are manufactured in cells in response to a variety of stresses (e.g.,

high temperature). One of the most important families of stress proteins are called heat shock proteins.

stroke volume the amount of blood pumped by the ventricles in a single beat.

strong acids an acid that completely ionizes when dissolved in water to generate H^+ and its anion.

strong bases a base (alkaline substance) that completely ionizes when dissolved in water to generate OH^- and its cation.

summation repeated stimulation of a muscle that leads to an increase in tension compared to a single twitch.

supercompensation an increase in the muscle glycogen content above normal levels following an exercise-induced muscle glycogen depletion and an increase in carbohydrate intake.

sympathetic nervous system portion of the autonomic nervous system that releases norepinephrine from its postganglionic nerve endings; epinephrine is released from the adrenal medulla.

sympathomimetic substance that mimics the effects of epinephrine or norepinephrine, which are secreted from the sympathetic nervous systems.

synapses junctions between nerve cells (neurons) where the electrical activity of one neuron influences the electrical activity of the other neuron.

systole portion of the cardiac cycle in which the ventricles are contracting.

systolic blood pressure the highest arterial pressure measured during a cardiac cycle.

tapering the process athletes use to reduce their training load for several days prior to competition.

target heart rate (THR) range the range of heart rates describing the optimum intensity of exercise consistent with making gains in maximal aerobic power; equal to 70% to 85% HR max.

T-cells a family of immune cells produced in the bone marrow. There are three main types of T-cells: (1) killer T-cells (also called cytotoxic T-cells; (2) helper T-cells; and (3) regulatory T-cells.

temporal summation a change in the membrane potential produced by the addition of two or more inputs occurring at different times (i.e., inputs are added together to produce a potential change that is greater than that caused by a single input).

terminal cisternae   portion of the sarcoplasmic reticulum near the transverse tubule containing the Ca^{++} that is released upon depolarization of the muscle; also called *lateral sac.*

testosterone   the steroid hormone produced in the testes; involved in growth and development of reproductive tissues, sperm, and secondary sex characteristics.

tetanus   highest tension developed by a muscle in response to a high frequency of stimulation.

theophylline   a drug used as a smooth muscle relaxant in the treatment of asthma.

thermogenesis   the generation of heat as a result of metabolic reactions.

thyroid gland   endocrine gland located in the neck that secretes triiodothyronine (T_3) and thyroxine (T_4), which increase the metabolic rate.

thyroid-stimulating hormone (TSH)   hormone released from the anterior pituitary gland; stimulates the thyroid gland to increase its secretion of thyroxine and triiodothyronine.

thyroxine   hormone secreted from the thyroid gland containing four iodine atoms (T_4); stimulates the metabolic rate and facilitates the actions of other hormones.

tidal volume   volume of air inhaled or exhaled in a single breath.

Tolerable Upper Intake Level (UL)   the highest average daily nutrient intake level that is likely to pose no risk of adverse health effects to almost all individuals in the general population. As intake increases above the UL, the potential risk of adverse effects may increase.

tonus   low level of muscle activity at rest.

total lung capacity (TLC)   the total volume of air the lung can contain; equal to the sum of the vital capacity and the residual volume.

toxicity   a condition resulting from a chronic ingestion of vitamins, especially fat-soluble vitamins, in quantities well above that needed for health.

trace elements   dietary minerals, including iron, zinc, copper, iodine, manganese, selenium, chromium, molybdenum, cobalt, arsenic, nickel, fluoride, and vanadium.

transferrin   plasma protein that binds iron and is representative of the whole-body iron store.

transverse tubule   an extension, invagination, of the muscle membrane that conducts the action potential into the muscle to depolarize the terminal cisternae, which contain the Ca^{++} needed for muscle contraction.

triiodothyronine   hormone secreted from the thyroid gland containing three iodine atoms (T_3); stimulates the metabolic rate and facilitates the actions of other hormones.

tropomyosin   protein covering the actin-binding sites that prevent the myosin cross-bridge from touching actin.

troponin   protein associated with actin and tropomyosin that binds Ca^{++} and initiates the movement of tropomyosin on actin to allow the myosin cross-bridge to touch actin and initiate contraction.

twenty-four-hour recall   a technique of recording the type and amount of food (nutrients) consumed during a twenty-four-hour period.

twitch   the tension-generating response following the application of a single stimulus to muscle.

type I fibers   fibers that contain large numbers of oxidative enzymes and are highly fatigue resistant.

type IIa fibers   fibers that contain biochemical and fatigue characteristics that are between type IIb and type I fibers.

type IIx fibers   fibers that have a relatively small number of mitochondria, a limited capacity for aerobic metabolism, and are less resistant to fatigue than slow fibers.

underwater weighing   (also known as hydrostatic weighing) procedure to estimate body volume by the loss of weight in water; result is used to calculate body density and, from that, body fatness.

vagus nerve   a major parasympathetic nerve.

variable-resistance exercise   strength training in which the resistance varies throughout the range of motion.

veins   the blood vessels that accept blood from the venules and bring it back to the heart.

ventilation   the movement of air into or out of the lungs (e.g., pulmonary or alveolar ventilation); external respiration.

ventilatory threshold (Tvent)   the "breakpoint" at which pulmonary ventilation and carbon dioxide output begin to increase exponentially during an incremental exercise test.

venules   small blood vessels carrying capillary blood to veins.

vestibular apparatus   sensory organ consisting of three semicircular canals that provides needed information about body position to maintain balance.

vital capacity (VC)   the volume of air that can be moved into or out of the lungs in one breath; equal to the sum of the inspiratory and expiratory reserve volumes and the tidal volume.

WBGT   wet-bulb globe temperature. This is a heat stress index that incorporates the dry-bulb, wet-bulb, and black-globe temperatures.

web of causation   an epidemiologic model showing the complex interaction of risk factors associated with the development of chronic degenerative diseases.

whole-body density   a measure of the weight-to-volume ratio of the entire body; high values are associated with low body fatness.

wind chill index   describes the impact of wind on the decrease in air temperature experienced by an individual on exposed skin.

Wingate test   anaerobic power test to evaluate maximal rate at which glycolysis can deliver ATP.

work   the product of a force and the distance through which that force moves ($W = F \times D$).

work interval   in interval training, the duration of the work phase of each work-to-rest interval.

Index

American Heart Association (AHA)
dietary and physical activity recommendations, 421t
physical inactivity, 8b
public health physical activity guidelines, 368
registry of VO$_2$ max values, 371
American Journal of Physiology, 11t
American Physiological Society (APS), 11
amino acids, 49, 58, 86, 532-534, 576t
AMP kinase, 496
AMP/ATP ratio, 307
amphetamines, 583
AMPK, 308
amylase, 47t
anabolic window (protein synthesis), 535b
anaerobic ATP production, 51-54
anaerobic exercise training, 314-315
anaerobic glycolysis, 418
anaerobic metabolism, 51, 450
anaerobic performance and ergogenic aids, 581-582
anaerobic power, 469-473
anaerobic threshold, 77
anaerobic training, 489, 490b
anaerobic/aerobic energy production, 68b
anatomical dead space, 231
Andean altitude residents, 553
androgens, 107, 108b
androstenedione (andro), 576t
anemia, 416
anerobic/aerobic ATP production, 64
angina pectoris, 218, 348, 352, 397
angiogenesis, 308
angioplasty, 336
angiotensin I, 104
angiotensin II, 104
angiotensin-converting enzyme (ACE) inhibitors, 397
angiotensinogen, 104
anorexia nervosa, 428, 509, 510f
anterior cruciate injury (ACL), 109, 513
anterior pituitary gland, 99
antibodies, 132, 133
antidiuretic hormone (ADH), 100-101
antigens, 132
anti-inflammatory cytokines, 112b, 135
anti-vivisectionists, 102b
antioxidant supplementation, 447b, 496
antioxidants, 304, 576t
aorta, 195f
aortic baroreceptors, 206f
aortic bodies, 246, 246f
aortic semilunar valve, 195, 195f
"Application of critical power in sport" (Vanhatalo et al.), 467, 476
Applied Body Composition Assessment (Heyward and Wagner), 423, 424, 436

APS (American Physiological Society), 11
AQI (air quality index), 568, 586f
Archimedes' principle, 424
arginine, 576t
arm crank ergometer, 19f, 76
arrhythmia, 270, 352, 398
arterial blood pressure, 199-202
blood pressure measurement, 200b
blood pressure regulation, 202
factors to consider, 201-202
graded exercise test (GXT), 352
hypertension, 201
mean arterial pressure, 201
resting conditions, 32f
systolic/diastolic blood pressure, 199
arterial hemoglobin content, 452
arterial-mixed venous oxygen content, 214
arterial oxygen content (CaO2), 452
arteries, 194
arteriole dilation, 209
arterioles, 194, 211
arteriovenous O$_2$ difference, 299
articular cartilage, 514
ascorbic acid, 415t
Asmussen, Erling, 4, 4f, 5
asthma, 392-395
attack, 392
buddy system, 395
diagnosis and causes, 392
EIA, 392-395
incidence/prevalence, 393
mechanism of attack, 393, 393f
prevention/relief, 392
screening (children), 394b
asthmatics, 517
Astrand and Rodahl protocol, 357t
Astrand and Ryhming nomogram, 360
astronauts, 448, 454b
atherosclerosis
heart disease, and, 203b
inflammation, 336
plumbing issue, 336
proinflammatory cytokines, 105b
treatment, 336
web of causation, 332f
athlete as machine, 456
athletic amenorrhea, 508-509
athletic performance
assessment. *See* laboratory assessment of performance
dehydration, 282b
distance running, 453b
factors to consider, 443f, 460f
fatigue. *See* fatigue/muscle fatigue
growth hormone (GH), 100b
intermediate-length performances, 452-453, 453f
long-term performances, 453-456
moderate-length performances, 452, 452f
muscle fiber, 183

pulmonary system, 250, 251b
short-term performances, 450-451, 451f
steroids, 108b
ultra-endurance events, 454b
ultra short-term performances, 450, 450f
Atkins diet, 431, 431f
atmospheric pressure, 549
ATP. *See* adenosine triphosphate (ATP)
ATPase, 50, 181, 182, 188
ATP-phosphocreatine (ATP-PC) system, 51, 63, 75, 314, 450, 469, 472, 481, 482t, 489, 490b
ATPS (ambient temperature pressure and saturated), A-2
atria, 195f
atrial fibrillation, 352
atrioventricular (AV) bundle, 202f
atrioventricular (AV) node, 202, 202f, 206f
atrioventricular (AV) valves, 195, 195f
August & Marie Krogh, 4, 14
August Krogh Institute, 4
Australian Institute of Sport, 575
autocrine signaling, 37, 36f
autologous transfusion, 579
autonomic motor division (PNS), 141
autonomic nervous system, 161-162
autoregulation, 216
AV bundle, 202f
AV node, 202, 202f, 206f
AV valves, 195, 195f
Aviation, Space and Environmental Medicine, 11t
axon, 142, 143f

B

Baldwin, K., 9
Balke, Bruno, 358b
Bannister, Roger, 486b
barometric pressure, 234
barometric pressure and water vapor pressure correction, A-3
Bar-Or, Oded, 516b
baroreceptors, 202, 206f, 220
basal metabolic rate (BMR), 432-433
base, 257
baseline effect, 400b
basophils, 130t
BAT (brown adipose tissue), 433
B-cell, 130t, 132-133
Beamon, Bob, 550b
Bean, Bruce, 179
behavioral risk factors, 331-332, 331f
bench step, 18, 19f
Bergström, Jonas, 527b
Bernard, Claude, 32b
beta-adrenergic blocking drugs, 113, 207b
β_2-agonists, 392, 585b
beta(β)-alanine, 263b, 576t
beta-blockers, 207b
beta oxidation, 58, 58b
beta receptors, 103, 103t

β_1 receptors, 103t
β_2 receptors, 103t
β_3 receptors, 103t
beta-receptor agonists, 392
beta (β) subunits, 97, 98f
BIA (bioelectrical impedance analysis), 425
bicarbonate, 240, 260
bicarbonate buffer system, 262, 581-582
bicarbonate ions, 257
bicuspid valve, 195, 195f
bicycle, 586-587. *See also* cycling
racing positions, 588f
Bigland-Ritchie, Brenda, 451b
binge eating, 428, 509
bioelectrical impedance analysis (BIA), 425
bioenergetics
aerobic ATP production, 54-61, 576t
anaerobic ATP production, 51-54
control of ATP-PC system, 63
control of citric acid cycle, 64
control of electron transport chain, 64
control of glycolysis, 63
defined, 41
biographical sketches. *See* important people in science
biological control system, 33, 33f
biological energy transformation, 43-48
cellular chemical reactions, 43-44
coupled reactions, 43-44
enzymes, 45-48
oxidation-reduction reactions, 44
biology, fields of, 42b
biotin, A-7
black globe temperature (T_g), 560
blood
components, 210
bicarbonate, 265
boosting, 579
buffer systems, 265, 266b
buffers, 581-582
cells, 129
doping, 579-581
lactate concentration, 79
packing, 579
physical characteristics, 210
potassium levels, 246-247
pressure. *See* arterial blood pressure
pressure measurement, 200b
pressure regulation, 202
proteins, 261-262
vessel graft, 398
vessel vasodilation, 216
viscosity, 210
blood flow
high-intensity exercise/hot environment, 283
local blood flow during exercise, 215
low-intensity exercise, 236
oxygen demands during exercise, 194
pressure/resistance, and, 211

metabolism, 41. *See also* exercise metabolism
meter (m), 17*t*
meters per second (m·s⁻¹), 17*t*
metric system, 17, 17*t*
Metropolitan Life Insurance height and weight tables, 423
Mexico City Olympic Games, 550, 550*b*, 550*t*, 551*t*
Meyerhof, Otto F., 3, 3*f*
MI (myocardial infarction), 397
micro-, 17*t*
midbrain, 156*f*, 157
Midcourse Report, 8*b*
mild hypothermia, 561, 566
military fitness testing, 589-590
milk, 404*b*
milli-, 17*t*
Milo of Crotona, 491
mineralocorticoids, 103
minerals
 calcium, 414, 416
 DRIs, A-8, A-9
 iron, 416, 540-541
 major, 414, 417*t*
 sodium, 416
 trace elements, 414, 417*t*
mitochondria, 41*f*
 afferent nerve fibers, 312
 BAT, 433
 capillary density, 313
 endurance training, 300, 302*f*
 exercise intensity, 301
 fatty acid beta-oxidation, 303
 intermyofibrillar, 301
 p38, 307
 powerhouse of the cell, 41-42
 pyruvate formation, 304
 subsarcolemma, 301
 VO₂ max, 299, 299*f*
mitochondrial biogenesis, 301*b*, 305, 308, 309, 323, 324*f*
mitochondrial turnover, 301*b*
mitogen-activated kinase p38 (p38), 293
mitophagy, 301*b*
mixed diet, 85*t*
mixed venous blood, 194, 236
"Models to explain fatigue during prolonged endurance cycling" (Abbiss/Laursen), 455-456
moderate hypothermia, 561, 566
moderate-intensity exercise, 370, 372*b*
moderate-length performances, 452-453, 452*f*
Modified Canadian Aerobic Fitness Test (mCAFT), 351
molecular biology, 41, 42*b*
molybdenum, 417*t*, A-9
Monark friction-braked cycle, 20-21, 359
monocytes, 130*t*
monosaccharides, 48
Montoye, H., 9
Morococha, Peru, 553
Morris, Jeremy N., 335*b*
Morrow, J. R., Jr., 7, 14
motor cortex, 157
motor-driven treadmill, 19*f*
motor functions, 159
motor neuron, 153-154, 171

motor unit, 153*f*, 153, 154*b*, 170
motor unit recruitment, 154, 154*b*
Mount Everest, 554-557, 566*b*
mountain climbing (Mount Everest), 554-557, 566*b*
movement. *See* nervous system
movement speed and efficiency, 27
MPS (muscle protein synthesis), 535*b*
mRNA (messenger RNA), 38*b*, 305, 319
MS (multiple sclerosis), 144*b*
MSH (melanocyte-stimulating hormone), 99
mTOR, 308, 319
multiple sclerosis (MS), 144*b*
"multiplying effect," 9
muscle
 actions, 184-185
 antioxidant activity, 318
 antioxidant capacity, 304
 cell, 41*f*. *See also* muscle fiber
 chemoreceptors, 153, 220
 contractile protein synthesis, 323
 contraction, 171-176
 cramps, 177-179
 cytokines, 112*b*
 endocrine gland, as, 112*b*
 excitation, 173, 170*b*, 175*f*
 fatigue, 157*b*. *See* fatigue/ muscle fatigue
 force-velocity relationship, 187-189
 hyperplasia, 317
 hypertrophy, 317
 in vivo (fatigue), 445*t*
 mechanoreceptors, 220
 oxidative capacity, 317
 power-velocity relationship, 189
 proprioceptors, 150-152
 protein synthesis (MPS), 535*b*
 pump, 208
 relaxation, 174-176, 174*b*
 skeletal. *See* skeletal muscle
 soreness, 497-499, 498*b*
 spindle, 150-151, 221
 strength. *See* muscular strength
 triglycerides, 86
Muscle Electrolytes, 527*b*
muscle fiber, 41*f*, 42*b*, 180-184
 biochemical properties, 180-181
 contractile properties, 181
 endurance training, 300-301
 energy efficiency, and, 26-27, 181
 exercise intensity, 448*f*
 fast fibers. *See* fast fibers
 fast-to-slow fiber type shift, 300
 immunohistochemical staining, 180*b*
 influence on intracellular buffer capacity, 261
 performance, and, 183-184
 slow fibers. *See* slow fibers
muscle glycogen, 84, 85*t*, 85, 113, 323, 529. *See also* glycogen

depletion, 281
 supercompensation, 527
muscle-glycogen utilization, 111-113
muscle protein synthesis, 318-319
Muscle soreness and delayed onset muscle soreness, 504
muscles of expiration, 230*f*
muscles of inspiration, 230*f*
muscles of respiration, 229*f*, 230*f*
muscular dystrophy, 188*b*
muscular endurance, 315-316
muscular strength, 315, 473-476. *See also* resistance training
 defined, 473
 free weight testing, 474
 isokinetic testing, 474-475
 isometric testing, 473-474
 variable resistance testing, 475-476
myocardial infarction (MI), 397
myocardial ischemia, 203*b*, 218, 352
myocardium, 195*f*, 196, 197*f*
myofibril, 168*f*, 169*f*
myofibrillar proteins, 317
myofilaments, 169*f*
myoglobin, 240
myoglobin-oxygen dissociation curve, 240, 240*f*
myokines, 112*b*
myonuclear domain, 169
myonuclei, 321
myosin, 168*f*, 169, 197, 317
 cross-bridges, 172*f*, 173, 447*b*
 isoforms, 181
myotatic reflex, 150
MyPlate, 422

N

N (Newton), 17*t*
N · m, 17*t*
N-acetyl-cysteine, 447*b*
N-balance, 532
N-balance studies, 532, 533
NAD+, 44, 44*f*, 53
NADH, 44, 44*f*, 54*b*, 59
Nagle, Francis J., 358*b*
nano-, 17*t*
nasal cavity, 226*f*
National Exercise and Heart Disease protocol, 356, 357*t*
National Strength and Conditioning Association, 12
National Weight Control Registry (NWCR), 435*b*
natural killer cells, 130, 130*t*, 134
Nautilus equipment, 491, 492-494, 493*t*
NE. *See* norepinephrine (NE)
needle biopsy technique, 527*b*
negative feedback, 34
negative N-balance, 532
nerve fiber, 142
nervous system, 140-163
 action potential, 145, 147*f*
 all-or-none law, 145
 anatomical divisions, 141, 141*f*
 autonomic nervous system, 161-162

brain, 156-159
 central fatigue, 444-445
 CNS/PNS, 141, 141*f*
 EPSPs, 148
 equilibrium, 155-156
 fatigue, 443-444
 functions, 141
 IPSP, 149
 irritability/conductivity, 142
 joint proprioceptors, 150
 motor functions, 159-160
 motor neuron, 153-155
 MS, 144*b*
 muscle chemoreceptors, 153
 muscle proprioceptors, 150-152
 neuron, 142, 143*f*
 opening/closing of "gates," 144-145, 145*f*
 reflexes, 149-152
 resting membrane potential, 143-145, 143*f*
 size principle, 154, 154*b*
 sodium/potassium pump, 145, 146*f*
 somatic motor function, 153-155
 spatial summation, 149
 spinal tuning, 159
 synapse, 145-146, 148*f*
 synaptic transmission, 143*f*, 145-149
 temporal summation, 149
 vestibular apparatus, 155-156
 voluntary movement, 160, 161*f*
net efficiency, 25, 26
neural input, 245, 247
neural theory (repeated bout effect), 498*b*
neuroendocrinology
 blood hormone concentration, 94-95
 defined, 93
 hormone-receptor interaction, 95-98
 mechanisms of hormone action, 95-98
neurohypophysis, 99
neuromuscular cleft, 170
neuromuscular junction, 170-171, 170*f*, 446
neuron, 142, 143*f*
neuron depolarization and repolarization, 145, 147*f*
neurotransmitter, 146
neutrophils, 130, 130*t*
Newton (N), 17*t*
Newton-meter (N · m), 17*t*
NFκB (nuclear factor kappa B), 307, 309
niacin, 415*t*, A-7
nicotinamide adenine dinucleotide (NAD⁺), 44, 53
Nielsen, Marius, 4, 4*f*, 5
Nieman, David, 133, 136*b*
Nissl substance, 143*f*
nitric oxide, 575
nitrogen(N)-balance studies, 532, 533
nitroglycerin, 397
Nixon, Richard, 7
NMR (nuclear magnetic resonance), 424